ANESTHESIA AND UNCOMMON PEDIATRIC DISEASES

SECOND EDITION

ANESTHESIA AND UNCOMMON PEDIATRIC DISEASES

SECOND EDITION

JORDAN KATZ, M.D.
Professor, Department of Anesthesiology
School of Medicine
University of California, San Diego
San Diego, California

DAVID J. STEWARD, M.B., F.R.C.P.C.
Director of Anesthesiology
Children's Hospital of Los Angeles
Professor of Anesthesiology
University of Southern California
Los Angeles, California

W.B. SAUNDERS COMPANY
A Division of Harcourt Brace & Company
Philadelphia London Toronto Montreal Sydney Tokyo

W.B. SAUNDERS COMPANY
A Division of
Harcourt Brace & Company

The Curtis Center
Independence Square West
Philadelphia, Pennsylvania 19106

Library of Congress Cataloging-in-Publication Data

Anesthesia and uncommon pediatric diseases / [edited by] Jordan Katz, David J. Steward.—2nd ed.

p. cm.

Includes bibliographical references.

ISBN 0–7216–6681–7

1. Anesthesia—Complications. 2. Rare diseases.
I. Katz, Jordan. II. Steward, David J.
[DNLM: 1. Anesthesia. 2. Pathology. WO 235 A579]

RD87.3.R35A5 1993

617.9′6—dc20

DNLM/DLC 92-48754

Anesthesia and Uncommon Pediatric Diseases, 2nd Edition ISBN 0–7216–6681–7

Printed in the United States of America.

Last digit is the print number: 9 8 7 6 5 4 3 2 1

To Ruby

Eamus quo ducit fortuna

Jordan

This book is dedicated to all children unfortunate enough to have an unusual disease. We hope that by reference to it the anesthesiologist gains a better insight into the child's disease and will thus be able to afford the most appropriate care.

JORDAN KATZ
DAVID STEWARD

CONTRIBUTORS

BERNARD M. BRAUDE, M.B., B.Ch., F.R.C.P.C., D.A.(S.A.), F.F.A.(S.A.)
Lecturer, Department of Anaesthesia, University of Toronto Faculty of Medicine; Staff Anaesthetist, Department of Anaesthesia, The Hospital for Sick Children, Toronto, Ontario, Canada
Immune Disorders

FREDERICK A. BURROWS, M.D., F.R.C.P.C.
Associate Professor, Department of Anaesthesia, University of Toronto Faculty of Medicine; Staff Anaesthetist, Department of Anaesthesia, The Hospital for Sick Children, Toronto, Ontario, Canada
Immune Disorders

D. RYAN COOK, M.D.
Professor of Anesthesiology, University of Pittsburgh School of Medicine; Chief of Anesthesiology, Children's Hospital of Pittsburgh, Pittsburgh, Pennsylvania
Pharmacology of Pediatric Anesthesia

G. MARK CRAMOLINI, M.D., F.A.A.P.
Assistant Clinical Professor of Pediatrics and Anesthesiology, University of California, San Francisco, School of Medicine, San Francisco; Attending Anesthesiologist and Pediatric Intensivist, Valley Children's Hospital, Fresno, California
Diseases of the Renal System

R. E. CREIGHTON, M.D., F.R.C.P.C.
Associate Professor, Department of Anaesthesia, University of Toronto Faculty of Medicine; Staff Anaesthetist, Department of Anaesthesia, The Hospital for Sick Children, Toronto, Ontario, Canada
Central Nervous System Diseases

PETER G. DUNCAN, M.D., F.R.C.P.C.
Professor and Chairman, Department of Anaesthesia, University of Saskatchewan College of Medicine; Active Staff, Royal University Hospital, Saskatoon, Saskatchewan, Canada
Neuromuscular Diseases

NANCY KNUTSEN FRANCE, M.D.
Associate Professor and Chief of Pediatric Anesthesia, Medical College of Wisconsin; Director of Pediatric Anesthesia, Children's Hospital of Wisconsin, Milwaukee, Wisconsin
Ophthalmological Diseases

MILTON GOLD, M.D., F.R.C.I.(C.)
Assistant Professor, Division of Allergy and Immunology, University of Toronto Faculty of Medicine, Toronto, Ontario, Canada
Immune Disorders

NISHAN G. GOUDSOUZIAN, M.D., M.S.
Associate Professor of Anaesthesia, Harvard Medical School; Anesthetist,

Massachusetts General Hospital, Boston, Massachusetts
Anatomy and Physiology in Relation to Pediatric Anesthesia

WILLIAM R. HAIN, M.B., B.S., F.F.A.R.C.S.
Late Clinical Teacher, University of Nottingham; Consultant Paediatric Anaesthetist, City Hospital and University Hospital, Nottingham, England
Diseases of Blood

INGRID B. HOLLINGER, M.D.
Professor of Anesthesiology, Associate Professor of Pediatrics, Albert Einstein College of Medicine; Clinical Director, Department of Anesthesiology, Montefiore Medical Center, New York, New York
Diseases of the Cardiovascular System

HELEN M. HOLTBY, M.B., B.S. (LOND.), F.R.C.P.C.
Assistant Professor, Department of Anaesthesia, University of Toronto Faculty of Medicine; Staff Anaesthetist, The Hospital for Sick Children, Toronto, Ontario, Canada
Orthopedic Diseases

SUSAN E. F. JONES, M.B., B.S., F.R.C.ANAES.
Consultant Anaesthetist, The Children's Hospital, Birmingham, England
Diseases of Blood

JORDAN KATZ, M.D.
Professor, Department of Anesthesiology, School of Medicine, University of California, San Diego, San Diego, California

THOMAS P. KEON, M.D.
Associate Professor of Anesthesia, University of Pennsylvania School of Medicine; Senior Anesthesiologist, The Children's Hospital of Philadelphia, Philadelphia, Pennsylvania
Diseases of the Endocrine System

JERROLD LERMAN, M.D., B.A.SC., F.R.C.P.C.
Associate Professor of Anaesthesia, University of Toronto Faculty of Medicine; Anaesthetist-in-Chief, The Hospital for Sick Children, Toronto, Ontario, Canada
Allergic Diseases

M. E. MCLEOD, M.D., F.R.C.P.C.
Assistant Professor, Department of Anaesthesia, University of Toronto Faculty of Medicine; Staff Anaesthetist, The Hospital for Sick Children, Toronto, Ontario, Canada
Central Nervous System Diseases

JAMES D. MORRISON, M.D., F.F.A.R.C.S.
Assistant Professor of Anaesthesia, Dalhousie University Faculty of Medicine; Chief of Anaesthesia, The Izaak Walton Killam Hospital for Children, Halifax, Nova Scotia, Canada
Otolaryngological Diseases

JOHN E. S. RELTON, M.B., F.F.A.R.C.S.(ENG.), F.R.C.P.C.
Associate Professor, Department of Anaesthesia, University of Toronto Faculty of Medicine; Staff Anaesthetist, The Hospital for Sick Children, Toronto, Ontario, Canada
Orthopedic Diseases

MICHAEL F. SMITH, M.D., F.R.C.P.C.
Clinical Assistant Professor, University of British Columbia; Attending Anaesthesiologist, British Columbia's Children's Hospital, Vancouver, British Columbia, Canada
Skin and Connective Tissue Diseases

LINDA C. STEHLING, M.D.
Former Professor of Anesthesiology and Pediatrics, State University of New York Health Science Center at Syracuse, Syracuse, New York; Director of Medical Affairs, Blood Systems, Inc., Scottsdale, Arizona
Genetic Metabolic Diseases

DAVID J. STEWARD, M.B., F.R.C.P.C.

Director of Anesthesiology, Children's Hospital of Los Angeles; Professor of Anesthesiology, University of Southern California, Los Angeles, California
Infectious Diseases; Diseases of the Gastrointestinal System

JOSEPHINE J. TEMPLETON, M.D.

Assistant Professor of Anesthesia, University of Pennsylvania School of Medicine; Senior Anesthesiologist, The Children's Hospital of Philadelphia, Philadelphia, Pennsylvania
Diseases of the Endocrine System

I. DAVID TODRES, M.D.

Associate Professor of Anesthesia (Pediatrics), Harvard Medical School; Director, Neonatal and Intensive Care Units; Anesthetist, Department of Anesthesia; Pediatrician, Children's Service, Massachusetts General Hospital, Boston, Massachusetts
Diseases of the Respiratory System

C. F. WARD, M.D.

Anesthesia Service Medical Group, Green Hospital of Scripps Clinic, University of California, San Diego, San Diego, California
Pediatric Head and Neck Syndromes

DAVID A. ZIDEMAN, Q.H.P.(C.), B.Sc.(Hon.), M.B., B.S., F.R.C. Anaesth.

Hon. Senior Lecturer, Royal Postgraduate Medical School, University of London; Consultant Anaesthetist, Department of Anaesthetics, Hammersmith Hospital, London, England
Infectious Diseases

PREFACE TO THE FIRST EDITION

There is a bewildering array of diseases of infancy and childhood, some relatively common but still challenging, some truly uncommon. Associated with many of these are surgically correctable malformations, either congenital or acquired, which will require repair under general anesthesia. In addition, unrelated surgical conditions may present in these children. The anesthesiologist, in the broader role as an acute care physician, may be asked to participate in the general management of some of these children. Hence, it is essential to understand the underlying pathophysiology of the disease process.

We, therefore, have attempted to assemble more than simply a book of anesthesia-related facts. We have designed this volume to provide a detailed summary of background knowledge related to each disease. We have added to this, where it is available, specific information that will be of additional direct importance to the anesthesiologist. Unfortunately, many diseases that are discussed in this book have not been the subjects of detailed anesthesia-oriented reviews, and there is little or no reported experience with these diseases in the anesthesia literature. In such instances it was necessary to extrapolate from the available knowledge of the disease process what might be the important anesthetic implications. This approach hopefully will enable the reader to meet the challenge of collaborating with specialists in other disciplines in providing optimal total care in and outside the operating room.

It is obvious that a book of this scope required the diligent effort of many dedicated physicians. We hope that the resultant text meets all of their expectations.

JORDAN KATZ
DAVID STEWARD

PREFACE TO THE SECOND EDITION

The critical acceptance of the first edition convinced us that an expanded text covering the ever-enlarging array of uncommon pediatric disorders was appropriate.

In this second edition we have encouraged our authors to update their contributions to include new diseases and to incorporate knowledge that has been gleaned from the more recently reported experience of our pediatric anesthesiologist colleagues around the world.

We believe that the resulting book is as complete a compendium on this subject matter as can be found. As such we trust that it will act as an essential reference guide, not only for the pediatric specialist, but for all anesthesiologists who become involved in the care of infants and children.

JORDAN KATZ
DAVID STEWARD

CONTENTS

CHAPTER

1 Anatomy and Physiology in Relation to Pediatric Anesthesia

NISHAN G. GOUDSOUZIAN, M.D.

Of primary importance for the clinical anesthesiologist is the realization that the newborn infant is not simply a small adult. The infant is unique both in distinctive anatomical and physiological features and in the variable rates of development. In relation to an adult, for instance, the neonate weighs about one twentieth, has a surface area of one eighth, and is slightly less than one third in length. With growth, weight increases markedly, doubling within the first 4 months, tripling in 1 year, and quadrupling in 2 years (Table 1–1). During these 2 years, height increases 1.5 times and surface area 2.5 times.

Infants are born with an excess of body water, most of which they lose in the first 2 to 3 days of life. The initial resultant weight loss (about 5 to 10 percent of total body weight) is usually regained in 10 to 14 days. During the first 3 months of life, an average baby gains 30 grams a day (120 grams a week), thereafter slowing to a gain of about 70 grams each week.

Table 1–1. APPROXIMATE VALUES FOR HEIGHT, WEIGHT, AND SURFACE AREA OF CHILDREN AND ADULTS

Age	Height (cm)	Weight (kg)	Surface Area (m^2)
Newborn	50	3.2	0.2
3 mo	60	5.7	0.3
1 yr	70	10	0.45
3 yr	84	15	0.6
7 yr	120	25	0.8
10 yr	140	32	1
12 yr	150	40	1.2
15 yr	165	53	1.5
Adult	170	70	1.7

The anatomical difference between the infant and the adult is nowhere more dramatic than in the head. At birth, the head accounts for 20 percent of the total body surface area (and even more in the premature baby), whereas in adulthood the head accounts for only 9 percent or so. This feature reflects the relatively large size of the infant brain, which also results in the relatively large size of the occiput in relation to the face. Postnatal skull growth is quite rapid during the first 2 years, when the brain increases in weight from 350 grams to about 800 grams. The brain reaches 90 percent of adult size (1400 g) by the fifth year and 95 percent by the tenth year.[1] As expected, the circumference of the skull increases similarly, expanding from 33 to 35 cm in the neonate to 47 cm at the second year and 53 cm in the adult.

The large head of the infant necessitates special clinical consideration. Because the head, which often has only a minimal amount of hair, is a source of heat loss, it must be covered to protect against hypothermia[2]; this is especially important in managing the hydrocephalic infant, whose head is shaved and is likely to be cleaned repeatedly with surgical preparation solutions. Bathing the head carefully, by contrast, can help cool a feverish infant. Since the head is usually accessible to the anesthesiologist, such maneuvers can be easily accomplished in the operating room.

CARDIOVASCULAR SYSTEM

One of the major transitions during delivery is the change from a fetal circulatory pattern (Fig. 1–1) to an adult pattern. At birth, the newborn infant's lungs must assume the function of gas exchange, which in the fetal stages was performed by the placenta.

FETAL CIRCULATION

In the fetus, blood enters the systemic arterial circulation from both ventricles because of the free communication between the left and right sides of the heart. This occurs via the foramen ovale, which connects both atria, and via the ductus arteriosus, which connects the aortic arch with the pulmonary trunk. About 45 percent of the combined output reaches the umbilical placental circulation. The unsaturated blood passes through the two umbilical arteries to reach the placenta, where it is oxygenated and then returns to the fetus via a single umbilical vein. The umbilical venous blood has an oxygen tension of 30 to 35 mm Hg (80 percent saturation), which is lower than that of the mother's mixed venous blood but is the highest present in the fetus.[3]

About half of the umbilical venous blood flow with this relatively high oxygen tension enters the inferior vena cava directly via the ductus venosus; the other half is distributed in the hepatic microcirculation, where it is mixed with blood draining from the gastrointestinal tract via the portal vein.[4]

The blood from the inferior vena cava as it reaches the heart is preferentially directed through the foramen ovale into the left atrium. The left atrium pumps this blood into the left

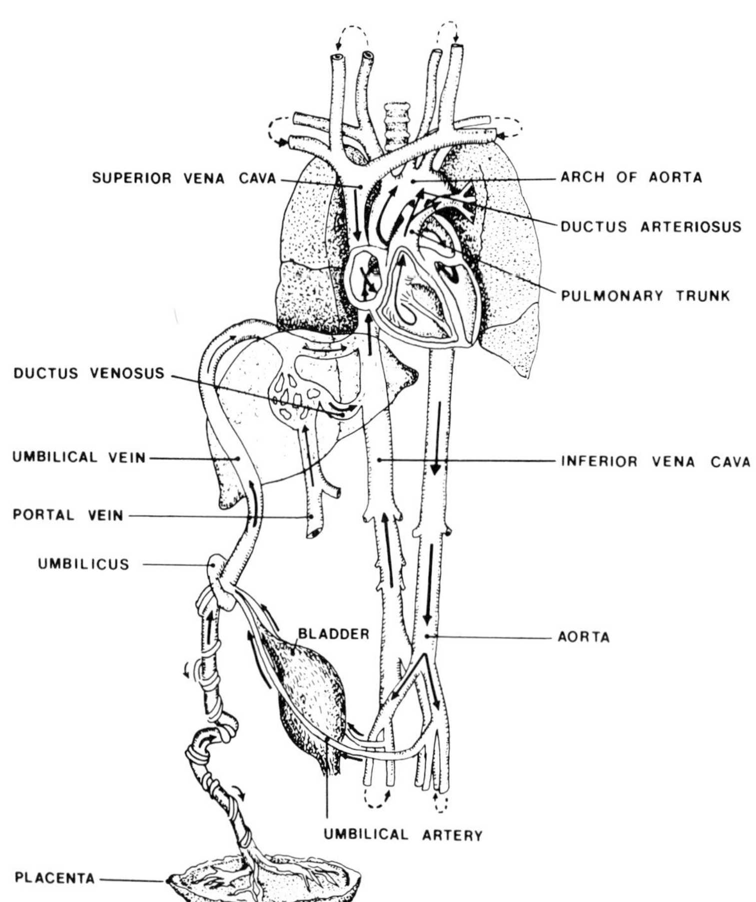

FIGURE 1–1. The fetal circulation. (From Goudsouzian N, Karamanian A: Physiology for the Anesthesiologist. 2nd ed. Norwalk, Conn., Appleton-Century-Crofts, 1984, p 110. Reproduced with permission of Appleton-Century-Crofts, Publishing Division of Prentice-Hall, Englewood Cliffs, N.J.)

ventricle, from which it is pumped into the ascending aorta and is distributed to branches principally supplying the head. Blood returning to the heart via the superior vena cava is directed mainly via the tricuspid valve into the right ventricle and pumped toward the lungs. The presence of high pulmonary resistance within the deflated fetal lungs assures that most of this blood will be diverted into the descending aorta via the ductus arteriosus. The ductus joins the aorta distal to the innominate and left carotid arteries. Thus much of the blood with the lowest saturation pumped by the right ventricle is directed peripherally and to the umbilical arteries to be oxygenated in the placenta. The ultimate result is that the blood with the highest saturation reaches the developing brain of the fetus, whereas the lower part of the body receives less oxygenated blood, much of which will pass to the placenta.

CIRCULATORY CHANGES AT BIRTH

With the delivery of the fetus, the sporadic ventilatory muscle activity present antenatally becomes continuous. These initial postnatal respiratory efforts create a markedly negative intrathoracic pressure (40 to 60 cm H_2O), which leads to the expansion of the lung and a dramatic decrease (four- to tenfold) in pulmonary vascular resistance. This causes a marked increase in pulmonary blood flow; consequently, oxygenation improves. This vasodilatation is reversible, however: hypoxia or acidosis or both can induce severe pulmonary vasoconstriction in infants. The capacity of the pulmonary vasculature in the neonate to respond to such stimuli is due to the presence of a thick layer of smooth muscle in the pulmonary vessels, extending more peripherally than later in life.[5]

The pulmonary vasculature of the newborn infant is also responsive to such chemical mediators as acetylcholine, histamine, bradykinin, beta-adrenergic catecholamines, and prostaglandins (PGE_1, PGE_2), all of which are known vasodilators.[6] Leukotrienes also seem to have important regulatory effects on the pulmonary circulation of the neonate.

Most of the decrease in pulmonary vascular resistance (80 percent) occurs shortly after birth, with a more gradual decline continuing for the next 8 weeks.[7] This later decrease in vascular resistance is due to gradual thinning of the muscular layer of the pulmonary vessels. In general, infants delivered by cesarean section have higher pulmonary vascular resistance at birth than do infants born by the vaginal route. In such infants a decrease to the normal range generally occurs within 3 hours of birth.[8]

Closure of the Foramen Ovale. This opening, covered by a flap-valve, is located in the central area of the atrial septum. It remains open during gestation because right atrial pressure exceeds that of the left, and the force of the jet of blood streaming from the inferior vena cava is strong. Upon delivery, the drop in pulmonary vascular resistance and the consequent increase in pulmonary blood flow direct more blood to the left atrium. This is further increased by the temporary left-to-right shunt through the ductus arteriosus. As left atrial pressure becomes higher than that in the right atrium, the flap-valve over the foramen ovale closes, restricting flow between the atria. It is important to note that this closure is in fact functional and can be reversed in the presence of any marked increase in right atrial pressure, such as might occur during coughing, severe crying, or the Valsalva maneuver, when pulmonary vascular resistance increases. Probe patency of the foramen ovale can be demonstrated until the age of 5 years in most children and also in some adults. The foramen ovale can thus be a potential avenue for paradoxical emboli, or it can be advantageous for catheterization of the left side of the heart without an arteriotomy.[9]

Closure of the Ductus Arteriosus. With interruption of the placental circulation, the systemic arterial pressure increases as pulmonary arterial pressure diminishes. This leads to a reversal of the shunt at the ductus, which fills with oxygenated blood from the aorta. Initially the flow at the ductus is bidirectional, but at 15 hours of age the shunt becomes entirely left to right. Prompt closure of the ductus arteriosus is more reliable in the full-term than in the preterm infant and depends mainly on the arterial oxygenation. Functional closure, which is due principally to contraction of the muscles in the wall of the ductus, usually occurs in the first 2 days of life. The contraction of the ductal smooth muscles leads to a thickening of its walls and intimal invagination. This functional closure is reversible by hypoxia or acidosis. Permanent anatomical closure takes another 2 to 3 weeks and results primarily from destruction of endothelium, proliferation of subintimal layers, and eventual fibrosis (creating the remnant known as the ligamentum arteriosum).

Several factors are involved in the closure of the ductus arteriosus. Of prime importance is oxygen, the effect of which is dose dependent; it probably acts by increasing the rate of oxidative phosphorylation within the ductal muscle cells.[10, 11] The ability of the fibers to constrict also depends on gestational age, with a greater effect being seen in full-term than in preterm infants. Furthermore, substances such as norepinephrine, epinephrine, acetylcholine, and bradykinin all potentially trigger an initial smooth muscle contraction that leads to functional ductal closure.

Prostaglandins are also involved. PGE_2 helps maintain patency of the ductus during gestation. During the last trimester, however, the sensitivity of the ductus to PGE_2 decreases and the sensitivity to oxygen increases. Premature infants have been shown to retain a degree of sensitivity to prostaglandins, an observation that has occasioned the use of PGE_1 in cyanotic congenital heart disease to keep the ductus open and of the prostaglandin inhibitor indomethacin to help closure of the ductus.[12, 13] The ductus venosus is usually the last structure to close, taking several more weeks. This pathway provides a shunt past the liver and might be a factor affecting the hepatic metabolism of drugs in the neonate.

Persistent Fetal Circulation. In this situation, the pulmonary hypertension present in the fetus persists in the postnatal stage; such an occurrence can be idiopathic but is more frequently due to respiratory disease, such as meconium aspiration. In these patients, hypoxia induces a further increase in the pulmonary hypertension, which in turn causes a rise in right ventricular and right atrial pressures; under these circumstances, blood will use the path of least resistance, traveling right to left at the atria and at the ductus arteriosus, with a dramatic decrease in peripheral arterial oxygen tension.[14] The first line of therapy for this potentially fatal condition is optimal oxygenation; affected infants also will benefit from hyperventilation, sedation, and paralysis. Tolazoline may be required to induce pulmonary vasodilatation, and in severe and persistent cases extracorporeal membrane oxygenation might be needed.[15]

A clinical implication of the anatomy of the ductus arteriosus is that in the immediate neonatal period, especially in cases of persistent fetal circulation, arterial blood sampling is more meaningful if it is performed from the right radial artery or the temporal arteries where the values in the blood reaching the brain and the coronary arteries are reflected. Sampling from the left radial artery may be misleading because of the close proximity of the left subclavian artery to the ductus, whereas sampling from the lower limbs might be completely misleading if the ductus is open. Similarly, pulse oximeter probes should be placed on the right upper limb or head region.

FUNCTIONAL BEHAVIOR OF THE MYOCARDIUM

Throughout the fetal and early neonatal stages, the myocardial tissues contain a large number of nuclei and mitochondria and an extensive endoplasmic reticulum to support rapid cell growth and protein synthesis. Since these tissues are not contractile, the neonatal myocardium is less compliant (stiffer) and probably less efficient than the adult myocardium. With diminished ventricular compliance, small changes in end-diastolic volume cause marked changes in end-diastolic pressure. Diminished compliance makes the Frank-Starling mechanism less effective in infants in increasing the stroke volume in response to increases of the preload; hence, in infants the stroke volume is relatively fixed. Consequently the only effective way to increase their cardiac output is to increase heart rate.

In contrast to adult cardiac muscle, which predominantly depends on oxygen for its metabolism, the fetal myocardium is capable of anaerobic glycolytic metabolism, probably because exogenous glucose can be metabolized during anaerobic conditions. This may be due to the presence of high concentrations of glycogen coupled with high hexokinase activity. This circumstance allows the fetal and newborn myocardium to be more resistant to the damaging effects of hypoxia, provided that oxygenation and perfusion are re-established within a reasonable interval.

With the infant's growth, the cardiac myofibers increase in numbers until all are formed, after which only their diameter and mass increase. The contractile elements become well organized and, during the first 3 months of extrauterine life, the left ventricle gradually becomes the dominant chamber owing to progressive ventricular remodeling.

INNERVATION OF THE HEART

The sympathetic innervation of the fetal and neonatal myocardium is relatively sparse. In fact, the fetal myocardium in animals has been shown to have a diminished store of catecholamines and an increased sensitivity to exogenous norepinephrine. The sympathetic system prob-

Table 1–2. CIRCULATORY VARIABLES IN INFANTS AND CHILDREN

Age	Heart Rate (beats/min)	Systolic Blood Pressure (mm Hg)	Diastolic Blood Pressure (mm Hg)	Cardiac Index (L/min/m^2)	Oxygen Consumption (ml/kg/min)
Preterm	150 ± 20	50 ± 3	30 ± 3		8 ± 1.4
Term	122 ± 18	80 ± 8	60 ± 8	2.5 ± 0.6	6 ± 1.0
6 mo	130 ± 20	100 ± 29	66 ± 10	2.0 ± 0.5	5 ± 0.9
1 yr	120 ± 20	105 ± 30	69 ± 25	2.5 ± 0.6	5.2 ± 0.1
2 yr	110 ± 25	105 ± 25	68 ± 25	3.1 ± 0.7	6.4 ± 1.2
5 yr	100 ± 10	109 ± 14	69 ± 9	3.7 ± 0.9	6.0 ± 1.1
12 yr	80 ± 17	120 ± 16	77 ± 9	4.3 ± 1.1	3.3 ± 0.6
Young adult	75 ± 5	122 ± 30	75 ± 20	3.7 ± 0.3	3.4 ± 0.6

Data adapted from Crone,[18] Kaplan and Graves,[30] and Task Force on Blood Pressure Control in Children.[118]

ably does not mature until 4 to 6 months of age.[16, 17] At birth, beta-receptor sensitivity (such as to isoproterenol) is well established, but the catecholamine degradation system is immature.

In contrast to the sympathetic supply, the parasympathetic supply to the myocardium is completely developed at birth, and the heart is sensitive to vagal stimulation.[18–20] This relative imbalance between cholinergic tone and sympathetic innervation predisposes the fetal and neonatal heart to bradycardia, as evidenced by the bradycardic response of the infant to hypoxia.[21, 22] A similar response is seen in infants upon the administration of a single dose of succinylcholine.[23, 24] In adults, such bradycardia occurs after a second dose but only very rarely after an initial dose.

As in adults, the neonate's heart rate varies with circumstances; it adapts to the metabolic needs of the body. There is wide variation in the normal range of the heart rate: it is substantially lower during sleep than during wakefulness and is higher during normal crying.[25] The resting heart rate normally decreases during the first month of life.

The anatomical and autonomic characteristics of the neonatal myocardium put a neonate at a disadvantage relative to an adult. Passive myocardial compliance, which is evaluated by measuring myocardial fiber tension along the length tension curve (Frank-Starling), is lower in the perinatal period than in later life. Similarly, active myocardial tension, which is a good indicator of contractility, is also lower in small infants. In older children, mild elevations in preload are associated with increased stroke volume: however, due to poor ventricular compliance, in neonates this effect is minimal and cardiac output is more dependent on heart rate. Therefore the infant's cardiac output can be increased by raising the heart rate, but little can be gained by changing the end-diastolic pressure. It has been demonstrated in fetal and newborn lambs that ventricular output is linearly related to heart rate over a wide range of up to more than 200 beats per minute.[20, 26] In the newborn infant, unbalanced cholinergic tone also predisposes to negative inotropy. Consequently, the neonate is more prone to develop congestive heart failure.[27] Further distinguishing the neonate is the fact that digoxin does not increase contractility as effectively as it does in older children and adults. The infant's myocardium performs in lower Frank-Starling curves of lesser slopes and cannot readily increase contractility by shifting to another curve.[28]

The vasomotor reflex arcs are functional in the newborn infant as in adults.[29] Stretching the baroreceptors of the carotid sinus by increasing its intramural pressure leads to an increase in the afferent firings via the glossopharyngeal nerve to the vasomotor center in the medulla; this leads to parasymapathetic stimulation and sympathetic inhibition.

Cardiovascular parameters are of course much different for the infant than for the adult. The infant's heart rate is higher, decreasing to adult levels at about age 5 years (Table 1–2). Cardiac output is also higher in infants, especially when calculated according to body weight, and it parallels oxygen consumption. Because fetal and newborn myocardium is less compliant than that of an adult, heart rate becomes the most important determinant of cardiac output. A more constant reading is obtained by relating cardiac output to surface area (cardiac index) because of the infant's high ratio of surface area to body weight. Blood pressure is lower in infants.[30] Coupled with a high cardiac output, this implies that the infant's systemic vascular resistance is lower, a factor that correlates well with oxygen consumption. This reflects the simple concept that cardiac output in normal situations is governed mostly by the requirement of the body tissue, whereas the control mechanisms and the intrinsic properties of the myocardium help in adjusting the system to perform at the most optimal levels.[31]

Oxygen Consumption. The full-term human infant's oxygen consumption at birth is about 4.6 ml/kg/min and within a week increases to 7 to 8 ml/kg/min, because of increased muscle activity and growth. It gradually decreases to reach adult values of 3.3 ml/kg/min after puberty. Oxygen consumption depends markedly on temperature; there is generally a 10 to 13 percent increase in oxygen consumption for each degree rise in core temperature.[15]

Neonatal Response to Stress. Early observations showed that newborn animals are better suited to survive hypoxia than are older animals.[32] For example, mature animals die after breathing 100 percent nitrogen for 3 minutes, whereas newborn animals survive for 7 minutes, and some species survive for about 50 minutes. Some factors that seem to contribute to the newborn's greater capacity to survive are the presence of increased carbohydrate stores and improved mobilization of glycogen, as well as the neonatal ability to generate anaerobic energy from glycolysis. In the fetus and newborn animal, hypoxia leads to the preferential redistribution of blood to vital organs such as the heart, brain, and adrenal gland, especially if it is accompanied by acidosis.[33]

RESPIRATORY SYSTEM

UPPER AIRWAY

The upper airway of the newborn infant, besides being smaller, is also anatomically different from that of adults. The tongue is relatively large and occupies most of the cavity of the mouth and oropharynx. Because the oral cavity is compromised by the absence of teeth, airway obstruction can easily occur. The airway usually can be cleared by holding the mouth in an open position while lifting the jaw; alternatively, an oropharyngeal airway can be inserted. The clinician must also remember that infants in the first few weeks of life (except when crying) are virtually *obligate nasal breathers* because the epiglottis, positioned high in the pharynx, almost meets the soft palate, making oral ventilation difficult. If the nasal airway of a neonate is occluded, the infant may not rapidly and effectively convert to oral ventilation. Consequently, it is extremely important to ensure that the nasal passages of the infant are clear during and after anesthesia. Nasal obstruction, if it does occur, usually can be relieved by causing the infant to cry.

In the infant, the larynx is located at a high position. The body of the hyoid bone is situated approximately at the level of the disc between the second and third cervical vertebrae, whereas in the adult it is at about the level of the fourth cervical vertebra.[34] The high position of the epiglottis and larynx allows the infant to breathe and swallow simultaneously.

The technique of endotracheal intubation in the neonate differs from that in the adult because of the baby's anatomical features.[35] The relatively large head obviates the need for its support by a pillow or a blanket. The angle of the jaw is approximately 140 degrees, whereas in the adult it is about 120 degrees. The epiglottis is more U-shaped, usually resembling the Greek letter omega (Ω), and it protrudes over the larynx at a 45-degree angle. Because the larynx of the infant is high and has an anterior inclination, the straight laryngoscope blade is most useful. The view can be markedly improved by external pressure on the larynx pushing it backward.

With the growth of the child the larynx descends. Most of this descent occurs in the first year, but the adult position is not reached until the fourth year. The change in position is essential for the development of speech and means that the child can no longer breathe and drink simultaneously.[1] The vocal cords of the neonate are slanted so that the anterior commissure is more caudal than the posterior commissure.

The narrowest area of an adult's airway is between the vocal cords, but that of the infant is in the cricoid region of the larynx.[35] Because the cricoid is a circular, cartilaginous structure and consequently not expansile, an endotracheal tube may pass easily through an infant's vocal cords but be tight at the cricoid area. The limiting factor here becomes the cricoid ring. The mucosa covering the cricoid ring is frequently the site of trauma, with resulting edema causing stridor after use of an oversized endotracheal tube.[36]

The diameter of the trachea in the newborn infant is 4 to 5 mm. Airflow resistance is directly related to the length and inversely related to the fourth power of the diameter of the tube. Consequently, 1 mm of edema in the trachea of the newborn baby will reduce its cross-sectional area by about 75 percent and will increase the resistance to airflow sixteenfold. The same degree of edema in an adult would decrease the cross-sectional area by only 44 percent and increase the flow resistance only threefold.[37]

The alignment of the trachea in the infant is directed caudally and posteriorly, whereas in the adult it is directly caudally. Consequently, cricoid pressure is more effective in facilitating passage of the endotracheal tube in an infant. This is especially important during nasotracheal intubation when the tube tends to get caught anteriorly in the subglottic region. The tonsils and the adenoids are very small in the neonate. They grow markedly during childhood, reaching their largest size at 4 to 7 years of age, and then recede gradually.

In the newborn infant the distance between the bifurcation of the trachea and the vocal cords is 4 to 5 cm. Thus an endotracheal tube must be very carefully positioned and fixed. Because of the large size of the infant's head, the tip of the tube can move about 2 cm during flexion or extension of the head. Therefore the anesthesiologist must check the position of the endotracheal tube every time the baby's head is moved.

In general, the right main bronchus is less angled than the left; hence, this is the one most frequently entered during endobronchial intubation, and the place where aspirated foreign bodies tend to lodge.

The compliant nature of the major airways of the infant further distinguishes them from those in adults. The diameter of infant airways changes more easily when exposed to distending or compressive forces, a factor that becomes important when there is any moderate-to-severe airway obstruction. For example, if there is obstruction to inspiration at the level of the larynx (e.g., subglottic edema), vigorous efforts at inspiration result in a very low intraluminal pressure in the extrathoracic trachea, which will tend to collapse and thus compound the obstruction. Conversely, if there is obstruction to expiration within the lower airways (e.g., asthma), the high intrathoracic pressures that are generated tend to compress intrathoracic airways further and prolong expiration. The higher airflows and changes in intrathoracic pressures brought on by crying can easily aggravate any such obstruction. For this reason it is very important to keep a child with airway obstruction as calm and quiet as possible.

The compliancy of the airways also may influence the clinical signs that can be elicited. With obstruction at the level of the larynx, stridor will occur mainly on inspiration. With obstruction of the airway at the level of the trachea (e.g., foreign body, vascular ring) stridor may be heard during both inspiration and expiration; by contrast, during lower airway obstruction (as in bronchiolitis or asthma), most of the dynamic collapse occurs during expiration, thus producing the characteristic expiratory wheezing.

The configuration of the thoracic cage differs in the infant and adult. The infant's ribs are more horizontal and do not rise as much as an adult's during inspiration. The diaphragm is therefore more important in ventilation, and the consequences of abdominal distention are worse. With growth, the thoracic wall changes. As the child learns to stand up, gravity pulls on the abdominal contents, thus encouraging the chest wall to lengthen; now the chest cavity can be expanded by raising the ribs into a more horizontal position.

The infant's thoracic cage is more cartilaginous, and hence more compliant (in fact it is five times as compliant as that of an adult); it is softer and more distensible. If compliance decreases or an obstruction is present in the airway, lung volumes will not be as well maintained as in adults.[38] Nor can the infant generate as much inspiratory pressure in the presence of obstruction, for the chest wall will move in a paradoxical fashion.

The diaphragmatic and intercostal muscles of infants are more liable to fatigue than are those of the adult, a fact attributable to a difference in muscle fiber type. In the adult diaphragm, 60 percent of the fibers are type I (a slow-twitch, high-oxidative, fatigue-resistant type) whereas in the newborn infant type II muscles (fast-twitch, low-oxidative, less energy-efficient) predominate (75 percent vs. 25 percent for type I); this difference is even more pronounced in premature infants. The same pattern is seen in the intercostal muscles.[39] Thus the preterm infant is prone to respiratory muscle fatigue and may be unable to cope when suffering from conditions that result in reduced lung compliance (e.g., respiratory distress syndrome).

THE LUNG

The newborn lung is not a miniature of the adult lung. Each of its components has a different pattern of growth. At the fetal stage, the pattern of the bronchial tree is fully developed by the 16th week of gestation. Alveoli develop later; they increase in number until the age of 8 years[40] and in size until the full development of the chest wall. Growth of the blood vessels is also variable. The preacinar vessels (arteries and veins) develop concomitantly with the airways, whereas the intra-acinar vessels develop with the alveoli. At about 26 to 28 weeks of gestation, proliferation of the capillary network surrounding the terminal airspaces enables pulmonary gas exchange.[41] Occasionally these morphological changes occur earlier, as evidenced by the fact that some infants have been known to survive after only 24 to 25 weeks of gestation. The number of alveoli increases from around 12 to 70 million at birth to 300 million by 8 years of age, at an average rate of a new alveolus every 8 seconds. After the age of 8 years, alveoli continue to grow in size but not in number.[42]

The lining of the respiratory saccules and the alveoli is derived from two types of cells: type I pneumocytes produce the lining and supporting cells of the alveoli and contribute to the blood gas interface; type II pneumocytes are more glandular and contain osmiophilic cytoplasmic inclusion granules. Pulmonary surfactant is synthesized in these granular pneumocytes (type II) and stored in the lamellar bodies. It is released by fusion of the lamellar body membrane with the cell wall (exocytosis).

The lung surfactant is a complex, multicomponent system containing various surface-active molecules, including phospholipids like phosphatidylcholine and phosphoglycerol with broad fatty acid distribution. It is similar, but not identical, to dipalmitoyl phosphatidylcholine[43]—85 percent of it is lipid in nature (mostly phospholipids), and 10 to 15 percent is protein unique to the lung.[44] The surfactant is so oriented that its hydrophilic choline group is in the aqueous phase and its hydrophobic palmitic side chains are above the air liquid interface. This arrangement reduces the surface tension at the air-tissue interface in the alveoli, thus preventing the alveoli from collapsing during expiration.[45]

Surfactant appears at approximately 20 weeks of gestational age. Its production increases slowly and then accelerates at about 30 to 34 weeks. Production can be hastened by the administration of glucocorticoids during pregnancy, and it increases during such compromised situations as prolonged rupture of the membranes (probably also glucocorticoid-mediated).[46] Whether glucocorticoids have a specific effect on normal surfactant development is speculative. In animals, thyroxine accelerates its production. Beta-adrenergic and cholinergic stimulation can release surfactant, whereas pure oxygen accelerates its breakdown. Instillation of artificial surfactant, either bovine or synthetic, into the lungs of premature infants helps improve lung function and helps relieve the clinical symptoms of respiratory distress symptom.[47, 48] In addition, essential phospholipids present in the surfactant-associated proteins (A, B, and C) enhance the rate of surface film formation[49]; this may be a factor that helps determine the beneficial effect of surfactant in full-term neonates with respiratory failure due to pneumonia or meconium aspiration.

ONSET OF RESPIRATION

In the human embryo, breathing movement can be detected as early as the 11th week of gestation. Such movement is irregular until the 20th week, after which it becomes more patterned; by 36 weeks it is entirely regular at a rate of 30 to 70 breaths per minute.[50] This intrauterine activity shows a circadian rhythm that is more accentuated in the evening than in the morning. Fetal breathing may decrease or even stop with alterations of fetal environment, such as those caused by bimanual examination, surgical procedures, and hypoglycemia. Hypoxemia, which in the postnatal stage stimulates respiration, serves to abolish respiratory movements in the fetus. Maternal alcohol ingestion or cigarette smoking will depress fetal breathing.[51] The significance or the value of fetal breathing is not clear; it has been suggested that the characteristic movements are sort of "prenatal practice" preparing the lung for its function after birth.[51] A corollary to this theory notes that bilateral phrenic nerve sections in animals lead to hypoplasia of the lung.[52]

At birth, under the combined influence of both physical stimuli, such as temperature and tactility, and a chemoreceptor response (hypoxemia, acidosis), respiratory movements usually become strong and continuous and are finally secured by the clamping of the cord. Initial inspiratory pressures of about 70 cm of water act against the viscosity of the fluids in the airways and the elastic recoil of the lungs and chest wall to establish the resting lung volumes. In the presence of adequate pulmonary surfactant, air is retained in the lungs after each successive gasp and creates sufficient surface for gas exchange in the next few minutes. As the alveoli expand, lower intrathoracic pressures are required to maintain air movement.

RESPIRATORY FUNCTION

When related to body weight, the respiratory parameters of the newborn infant, including tidal volume (VT), dead space (VD), VD/VT, vital capacity, functional residual capacity

(FRC), and specific compliance, are rather similar to those in the adult[38] (Table 1–3). Because of the infant's higher metabolic rate, more marked differences are seen in respiratory frequency and hence in alveolar ventilation. This high level of alveolar ventilation, when related to the functional residual capacity, makes the latter a less effective buffer between inspired gases and pulmonary circulation. This has important implications for the anesthesiologist; any interruption of ventilation will lead very rapidly to hypoxemia, and the fraction of anesthetic gases in the alveolus will equilibrate with the inspired fraction more rapidly than occurs in adults.

Lung compliance depends on the amount of elastic tissue present in the lungs and varies with age. At birth, the few elastic fibers present in the walls of terminal air sacs extend as far as the alveolar opening. With time, the elastic tissue increases as the alveoli grow in size. At the age of 18 years, elastic tissue is fully developed, and from there on it gradually deteriorates. Consequently, lung compliance is relatively low in the very young and the very old, with a peak in late adolescence.[53]

Since the infant's chest wall is soft and the ribs are cartilaginous and horizontal, the chest wall is more compliant and does not contribute significantly to respiratory motion; hence the negative intrapleural pressure is generated by diaphragmatic and abdominal muscles. The compliance of the chest wall and the lung lowers the resting lung volume, making the functional residual capacity more difficult to establish and maintain.

The functional residual capacity (FRC) is determined by the balance between the outward stretch of the thorax and the inward recoil of the lung; in a standing adult it is approximately equal to half the total lung capacity. These two opposing forces create a mean negative intrapleural pressure of 5 cm of H_2O in older children and adults. In small infants, by contrast, the relative lack of elastic recoil in the thorax and rib cage allows for only a slightly negative, almost atmospheric, pressure. The loss of muscle tone during anesthesia, therefore, causes a more profound reduction in FRC in the infant and may result in airway closure.[54]

The closing volume is the lung volume at which terminal airways begin to close off. It is

Table 1–3. RESPIRATORY VARIABLES IN INFANTS AND CHILDREN

	Neonate	1 Yr	8 Yr	Adult
Weight (kg)	3	10	25	70
Height (cm)	48	75	130	170
Respiratory frequency (breaths/min)	35	25	18	12
Tidal volume (v_T)				
ml	20	78	180	500
ml/kg	6.7	8	7	7
Dead space V_D				
ml	7	21	70	150
ml/kg	2	2	2.8	2
V_D/V_T	0.35	0.3	0.3	0.3
Alveolar ventilation				
ml/min	400	1200	2200	4000
ml/min/kg	130	120	80	60
Vital capacity				
ml	110	450	1800	4000
ml/kg	37	45	70	60
Functional residual capacity				
ml	80	250	1100	2400
ml/kg	28	25	44	35
Specific compliance C_L/FRC				
ml/cm H_2O/ml	0.04		0.06	0.05
Resting alveolar ventilation				
ml/min	400	1200	2200	3800
ml/kg/min	130	120	90	53
Hematocrit g/100 ml	55	35	40	42
PaO_2 (mm Hg)	60–90	90	95	95

Data adapted from Crone,[18] Kaplan and Graves,[30] Motoyama,[71] and Goudsouzian and Karamanian.[31]

much higher in neonates and infants than in adults because of the near absence of elastic tissue in the very young, a circumstance that would predispose to atelectasis in the terminal alveoli of the bases of the lungs at the end of each breath.[53] Healthy infants overcome this tendency through constant activity and reach total lung volume through crying. By contrast, in a sedated or anesthetized infant with shallow breathing or in an infant with residual muscle paralysis, airway closure can be exaggerated. An increase in positive end-expiratory pressure (PEEP) to 5 cm reverses this airway closure and increases FRC.

Ventilation/Perfusion Relationships. In the normal lung of a standing adult, V/Q ratios change from base to apex because the effect of gravity favors blood flow to the dependent parts of the lung. In infants and children, the distribution of pulmonary blood flow is more uniform because the pulmonary arterial pressure is relatively high and the effect of gravity is less. In the presence of general anesthesia, both FRC and diaphragmatic movements are reduced, so airway closure tends to be exaggerated and the dependent parts of the lung are poorly ventilated. Hypoxic pulmonary vasoconstriction, which diverts blood flow from areas of the lung that are underventilated, is abolished during anesthesia, thus increasing the hypoxic tendency.[54, 55]

RESPIRATORY RATE

In general, the rate and depth of respiration are regulated to expend the least amount of energy. At rates of 35 to 40 breaths per minute in a newborn infant or 12 to 16 breaths per minute in an adult, the work of the respiratory muscles to overcome elastic and resistive forces is at a minimum. At these rates, both the infant and the adult expend about 1 percent of their metabolic energy in ventilation.

In adults, respiration is stimulated by hypoxia and depressed by hyperoxia. In the neonate, however, the initial hyperventilation in the presence of hypoxia can be followed by a sustained decrease in ventilation.[44] This response, which tends to disappear in a few weeks in term infants, is more apparent in the premature, and can be aggravated by a cool environment.

Periodic breathing, which can be observed in the normal newborn infant and frequently occurs during REM sleep, is common in the preterm infant. It is usually manifested as rapid ventilation followed by a period of apnea of less than 10 seconds, during which the arterial oxygen tension remains in the normal range. Its incidence decreases significantly as the infant reaches 41 weeks of conceptual age,[56] and it is not seen in healthy infants after 6 weeks of age. However, periodic breathing is seen occasionally in infants who have survived an apneic episode related to sudden infant death syndrome.[57]

Administration of oxygen abolishes periodic breathing in preterm infants. Low concentrations of oxygen, on the other hand, increase the incidence of periodic breathing and lengthen the duration of apneic spells.

In premature infants, apneic spells longer than 20 seconds can be observed and are frequently associated with arterial desaturation and bradycardia. Such apneic episodes increase in frequency during stressful situations such as respiratory infections or the postanesthetic and postsurgical states.[58–60]

Two main types of apnea can occur in a premature infant: *central* and *obstructive*. Central apnea originates in the central nervous system, and breathing stops without any respiratory efforts. Obstructive apnea, by contrast, is due to upper airway obstruction, and respiratory efforts continue, with paradoxical movements of the thorax and abdomen. This latter type may be due to excessive relaxation of the genioglossus muscle during sleep, or obstruction elsewhere in the upper respiratory passages. Treatment with caffeine and theophylline has been effective in reducing apneic spells of both types in preterm infants[61, 62]; such drugs (xanthine) seem to act both by stimulating the central nervous system and by preventing fatigue in the respiratory muscles.[63]

Arterial P_{CO_2} is lower in both premature and term infants than it is in adults. It is interesting that term infants tend to respond to CO_2 like adults and so show an increase in the tidal volume, whereas premature infants show an increase in the respiratory rate and only a small increase in tidal volume.[44]

OXYGEN TRANSPORT

The blood volume of a healthy newborn baby is 70 to 90 ml/kg (depending on whether the cord is clamped early or late), and the hemoglobin content of the blood is high (19 g/dl), consisting mostly of fetal hemoglobin. The Hb concentration rises slightly in the first few days of life because of the decrease in the extracellular fluid volume; thereafter it declines to the

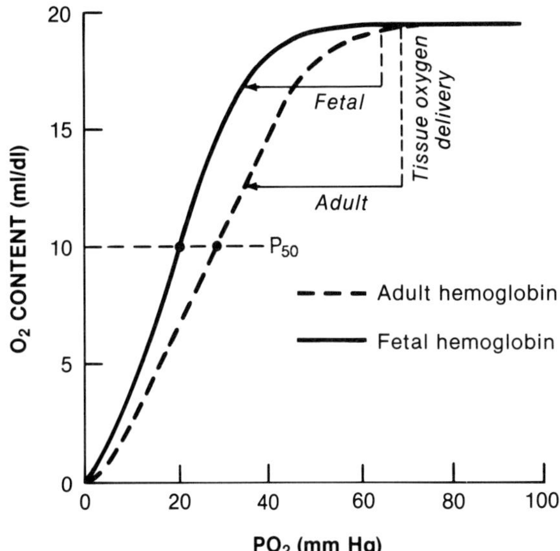

FIGURE 1–2. Oxygen dissociation curves of fetal and adult hemoglobin. Note that as O_2 tension decreases from arterial (95 mm Hg) to mixed venous (35 mm Hg) blood, approximately twice as much O_2 is released at the tissues from adult hemoglobin than from fetal hemoglobin.

level commonly referred to as the physiological anemia of infancy.

Fetal hemoglobin (Hb F) has a greater affinity for oxygen than does adult hemoglobin. In Hb F, one histidine molecule of the beta chain is replaced by serine, thus preventing 2,3-DPG from sliding easily between the beta chains. Hence, oxygen is more strongly attracted to the hemoglobin molecule than is 2,3-DPG.[64] By nature, fetal hemoglobin is able to load more oxygen from the mother at the placenta. In the fetal stage, the umbilical venous blood has an oxygen tension of 32 to 35 mm Hg, which is similar to that of maternal mixed venous blood. The presence of fetal hemoglobin, though, creates an oxygen saturation of about 80 percent in the fetal umbilical vein, up from 65 percent in maternal blood. Because the bridge between the arterial and tissue oxygen tensions crosses the steep part of the curve, fetal hemoglobin readily unloads sufficient oxygen to the tissues despite its relatively low saturation. However, because it does not give up the oxygen easily at the tissues, cyanosis occurs at lower Po_2 than in the adult. The P-50 (the partial pressure at which 50 percent of the hemoglobin is saturated with oxygen) is about 27 mm Hg in the normal adult, whereas in the neonate it is 20 mm Hg (Fig. 1–2).

After birth, the total hemoglobin level decreases rapidly as the proportion of fetal hemoglobin diminishes; indeed, it can drop below 10 g/dl at 2 to 3 months (Fig. 1–3), creating the so-called physiological anemia of infancy characteristic of this period.[65] Concurrently, though, the P-50 rapidly increases as the fetal hemoglobin is replaced by hemoglobin A, which has a high concentration of 2,3-DPG and so insures efficient oxygen off-loading at the tissues; the gradual decrease in oxygen-carrying capacity in the first few months of life is thus well tolerated by a normal, healthy infant.

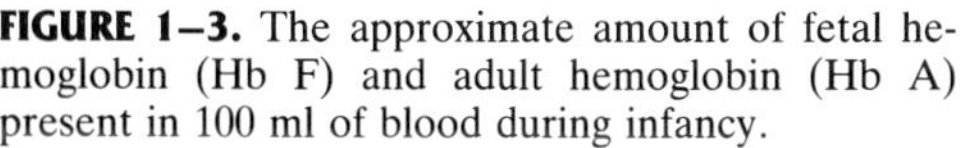
FIGURE 1–3. The approximate amount of fetal hemoglobin (Hb F) and adult hemoglobin (Hb A) present in 100 ml of blood during infancy.

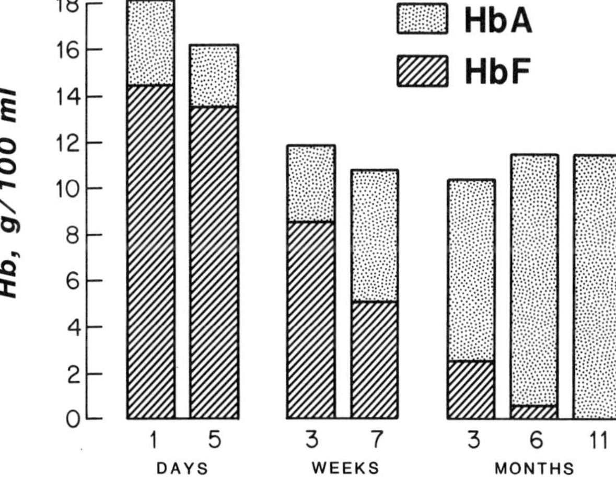

The early increase in P-50 brings it to a level in excess even of that in adults, which generally persists during the first decade of life.[66] A precise correlation does not exist between decreases in oxygen affinity in neonatal blood and the progressive decline in the concentration of fetal hemoglobin; the process seems to be due to an interplay between the levels of hemoglobin A and red blood cell 2,3-DPG.[67] In premature infants and those with respiratory distress syndrome, 2,3-DPG levels are lower than in term infants, a circumstance predisposing to an unfavorable outcome.[65]

The regulation of *erythropoiesis* in the newborn infant is a complicated process. In the fetus, anemia or hypoxia induces increased erythropoietin activity. In general, a gradual rise in plasma erythropoietin occurs coincident with a decline in hemoglobin below 11 g/dl.[67, 68] In the normal situation, the reticulocyte count and the hemoglobin concentration fall after the first day of life, and plasma erythropoietin is not detectable thereafter for 2 to 3 months. In situations of decreased oxygen supply to the tissues, such as severe anemia or congenital heart disease, increased plasma erythropoietin is seen, indicating that its production is probably modulated by tissue oxygen tension or oxygen requirements.[69]

There is no consensus in the literature about the lowest tolerable hemoglobin concentration for an infant; the old 10/30 rule of hemoglobin 10 g/dl, hematocrit 30 percent is no longer in vogue.[70] Obviously, the lowest limit will depend on such other factors as the duration of anemia, the acuity of blood loss, the intravascular volume, and, more important, the impact of other conditions that might interfere with oxygen transport. Clinical experience, however, has shown that children older than 3 months will tolerate hemoglobin levels as low as 8.2 g/dl (hematocrit 25 percent). With respect to younger infants, opinion is mixed; in this population, there is generally a high probability of associated conditions, and under such circumstances, a higher level than that recommended for children would probably be more acceptable.[71] Traditionally, in premature infants, the decision to transfuse has depended on such additional factors as tachypnea, tachycardia, poor weight gain, apnea, bradycardia, pallor, lethargy, decreased activity, or poor feeding. None of these symptoms, however, is predictably associated with symptoms classically attributed to anemia.[72] Therefore, the transfusion based on "nonphysiological anemia of prematurity" is decided on a case by case basis, and no decision is ever predicated on a single blood hematocrit measurement.

RENAL FUNCTION

In the fetus, the placenta is the main excretory organ. Although anephric infants survive intrauterine life, fetal malformation may occur owing to oligohydramnios caused by the absence of fetal urine. The formation of the glomeruli is not complete until the 34th week of gestation, most of the growth occurring in the third trimester.[73] Between 34 and 36 weeks, when the fetus weighs about 2000 grams, the glomeruli mature considerably. In infants born at less than 34 weeks of gestational age, glomerular function is markedly depressed and develops more slowly in the postnatal stage, whereas in infants born after this critical period, glomerular and tubular function increases at the same rate as in a term infant.[74]

The healthy term infant has a complete complement of nephrons at birth, but the glomeruli are smaller than their adult counterparts. However, their filtration surface related to body weight is similar. The tubules are not fully grown at birth and may not pass into the medulla.

The *glomerular filtration rate* at birth is about 30 percent of the adult value of 125 ml/min/1.73 m^2. It increases rapidly during the first 2 weeks of age but then is relatively slow to approach the adult level by the end of the first year.[75] The rate of increase is practically the same for premature infants born after 34 weeks' gestation and full-term infants, although the initial level is lower in the premature baby.[76]

Several factors contribute to the increase in glomerular function normally seen with development: an increase in cardiac output, changes of renovascular resistance, altered regional blood flow, and changes in the glomeruli. Maturation of glomerular function is complete at 5 to 6 months of age.

In general, maturation of *tubular function* lags behind that of the glomeruli. Reasons for decreased tubular function in the premature infant include low blood flow to peritubular regions, immaturity of the energy-supplying process, the small number of the tubular working cells, and the size of the tubules themselves. Peak renal capacity is reached at 2 to 3 years of age, after which it decreases at a rate of 2.5 percent per year.[77]

Tubular function and permeability are not fully mature in the term neonate and even less so in the premature infant. The neonate's kidney can excrete dilute urine up to 50 mOsm/L, but, owing in part to the lack of urea-forming solids in the diet, it can rarely concentrate to more than 700 mOsm/L (adults, 1200 mOsm/L). A second major reason for the reduced concentration of urine in the neonate is the hypotonicity of the renal medulla.[74] However, the kidney of the newborn infant does show some response to antidiuretic hormone. The inability to concentrate urine may result in plasma hyperosmolarity, especially when the child is dehydrated from diarrhea or high environmental temperature. This may occur when small infants are kept under radiant heat lamps for a prolonged period.

The diluting capacity generally becomes mature by 3 to 5 weeks' postnatal age. The ability to handle a water load is reduced, and the newborn infant may be unable to increase water excretion to compensate for excessive water intake.

Because of the anabolic state of the newborn baby and the small muscle mass relative to body weight, the normal value for creatinine is lower in infants than in adults (0.4 mg/dl vs. 1 mg/dl). The renal threshold for bicarbonate is also lower in the neonate (20 mmol/L vs. the adult 25 mmol/L). With a normal value of plasma bicarbonate at 20 mmol/L, the infant has a lower plasma pH of about 7.34.

In the intrauterine stage, the fetus excretes a large volume of hypotonic urine of low sodium content. Following birth (and lasting generally for a few hours to days), the infant enters a phase of relative oliguria, during which period the urine formed is hypertonic to plasma with an increased concentration of urea, potassium, and phosphate. This phase of relative oliguria is followed by a diuretic phase during which the extracellular space undergoes contraction; sodium from the extracellular space is the principal electrolyte lost at this point.[78] It is interesting to note that the onset of the diuretic phase is frequently related to the onset of improved respiratory function, and continuing diuresis then accompanies continuing respiratory improvement. The trigger to diuresis and extracelluar fluid contraction may be the release of a natriuretic agent brought about by a decrease in pulmonary vascular resistance and increased left atrial filling.[79]

THE LIVER AND METABOLISM

Glucose from the mother is the main metabolic energy source in the fetus. It is transferred through the placenta from the maternal circulation by the mechanism of facilitated diffusion and stored as fat and glycogen. The fetal plasma glucose level averages 70 to 80 percent of the maternal level throughout pregnancy, but storage occurs mostly in the last trimester. At a gestational age of 28 weeks, the fetus has practically no fat stored. At 34 weeks, 7 to 8 percent of fetal body weight is fat and 9 grams of glycogen are stored; at term, 16 percent of the body is fat, with 34 grams of stored glycogen.

In the first few hours following delivery, glucose is the infant's main energy source. During this period, hepatic and muscle glycogen stores are rapidly depleted. Fat then becomes the principal energy source. As it is metabolized, the respiratory quotient falls to 0.7. Ketone bodies and probably lactate are also utilized by the brain.

In the first 4 hours of extrauterine life, depletion of liver glycogen leads to a rapid drop in plasma glucose levels. The lower limit of normal is 30 mg/dl in the term infant but is as low as 20 mg/dl in the premature infant. Although at this level infants usually do not show any neurological signs or symptoms, they may develop pallor, sweating, or tachycardia. A blood glucose level below 20 mg/dl usually precipitates neurological signs such as apnea or convulsion. These blood glucose levels are simply guidelines for the careful clinical management of the affected infant. No specific value can be considered hypoglycemic; a more realistic approach recognizes that falling blood glucose levels can induce neurological dysfunction and that these may vary from one circumstance to another.[78, 79a]

Since glucose stores are limited at birth, it is imperative that the newborn infant not be kept for a long period without enteral or parenteral nutrition. This is especially true for premature infants, in whom the tendency to hypoglycemia may persist for weeks; babies who are small for their gestational age are also at risk. In the latter, hypoglycemia is most likely to occur during the first 12 hours of life and results from a high metabolic rate coupled with depleted glycogen stores. Carbohydrate stores in the vital organs (heart, liver, skeletal muscles) are often only 10 percent of the amount expected normally. By contrast, post-term infants do not differ from their term counterparts in their ability to regulate temperature or glucose during the first 24 hours.[80]

Hyperglycemia is also a concern in the premature baby, especially in the very low birth weight infant (less than 1000 grams), who has a long period of intravenous alimentation with 10 percent glucose. Here, the high rate of insensible water loss, the depressed insulin secretion in response to glucose, and the stress situation that makes the peripheral tissues less responsive to insulin all contribute to hyperglycemia.[81] This is an important risk factor in these vulnerable infants, since it may induce intraventricular hemorrhage and result in an osmotic diuresis that may cause dehydration, hyponatremia, and other electrolyte disorders.

The liver is of primary importance in neonatal metabolism and is relatively large compared with that of the adult. In utero, it performs several important functions essential for fetal survival.[82] Starting as early as 10 to 12 weeks after conception, it maintains glucose regulation, protein and lipid synthesis, and drug metabolism. Its excretory products (such as lipid-soluble unconjugated substances like bilirubin) traverse the placenta and are detoxified and excreted by the maternal liver.

In the neonate, the liver volume represents 4 percent of the total body weight, whereas in an adult it is 2 percent of body weight. The enzyme concentration and activity, however, are lower in the neonatal liver.[71, 82, 84]

Most of the metabolic biotransformation of drugs in the liver is affected through two major pathways. Phase I, or degradative reactions, include the oxidation, reduction, and hydrolysis reaction; most of the phase I reactions occur in the microsomal fraction of the liver under the influence of the cytochrome p450 enzyme system. Phase II, or synthetic reactions, occur mostly by conjugation. The enzyme systems responsible for phase II develop later than those responsible for phase I reactions; in consequence, neonates, and especially preterm infants, are less effective in conjugating bilirubin, chloramphenicol, sulfonamides, acetaminophen, and meprobamate.[85, 86] Glucuronide conjugation does not reach adult values until 3 years of age.[87] Increased hepatic metabolic activity usually manifests at about 3 months of age, reaches a peak at 2 to 3 years, by which time the enzymes are fully mature, and then starts declining, reaching adult values after puberty.

Renin, angiotensin, aldosterone, cortisol, and thyroxine levels are high in the newborn infant and decrease in the first few weeks of life.

TEMPERATURE REGULATION

Although neonates have an active central temperature regulatory mechanism, it is limited by certain anatomical and physiological factors and so succeeds in maintaining a constant body temperature only within a narrow range of environmental conditions. Oxygen consumption in the infant is at its minimum when the environmental temperature is within 3 to 5 percent (1 to 2°C) of body temperature (an abdominal skin temperature of 36°C).[88] This is known as the neutral thermal state, and a deviation in either direction will increase oxygen consumption. Whereas an adult can sustain body temperature in an environment as cold as 0°C, a full-term infant starts developing hypothermia at an ambient temperature of about 22°C. It is estimated that a term neonate in an incubator would gain thermal control over an ambient temperature range of 26 to 36°C and would feel comfortable within the thermoneutral range of 32.5 to 34°C.[88, 88a]

Premature infants are even more vulnerable, requiring higher environmental temperatures to maintain normothermia.[89] In the very premature infant, a cause for concern is the thinness of the skin which is only 2 to 3 cells thick, and the lack of keratin, which allows for a marked increase in evaporative water loss, even to a point in extreme situations well in excess of the infant's total rate of heat production; in the clinical situation, an infant at risk must always be adequately covered and nursed in the presence of high temperature and humidity.[89a]

The important mechanisms for heat production are metabolic activity, shivering, and nonshivering thermogenesis. Newborn babies usually do not shiver. Heat is produced instead by nonshivering thermogenesis. Exposure to cold leads to increased production of norepinephrine, which in turn increases the metabolic activity of brown fat.[90] Brown fat is highly specialized tissue with a great number of mitochondrial cytochromes; it is these that provide the brown color. The cells have several small vacuoles of fat and are richly endowed with sympathetic nerve endings. They are mainly located in the nape and between the scapulae but are found as well in the mediastinal and perirenal regions.

Once released, norepinephrine acts on the alpha- and beta-adrenergic receptors on the brown adipocytes. This stimulates the release of lipase,[91] which in turn splits triglycerides into glycerol and fatty acids, thus increasing heat production. The increase in brown fat metabolism raises the proportion of cardiac output diverted through the brown fat, which in turn facilitates the direct warming of blood. The increased level of norepinephrine causes peripheral vasoconstriction and mottling of skin.

The ability to generate heat ultimately depends on body mass, whereas heat loss to the environment is mainly a factor of surface area. Neonates, who have a ratio of surface area to mass about three times higher than that of adults, thus have difficulty thermoregulating in a cold environment.[92] One benefit of the large surface area is the ease with which the infant can be warmed by using a warming blanket in the operating room.[93]

A major source of heat loss in an infant is the respiratory system. A 3-kg infant with a minute ventilation of 500 ml spends 3.5 cal/min to raise the temperature of inspired gases. To saturate the gases with water vapor takes an additional 12 cal/min. The total of 15 cal/min (900 cal/h), or approximately 1 kcal/h, represents about 10 to 20 percent of the total oxygen consumption of an infant.[94]

In the spontaneously breathing child, the temperature of the inspired gases at the pharynx reaches 23°C with a relative humidity of 86 percent. Full saturation is achieved in the distal bronchi. In the anesthetized patient, an open breathing system delivers gases that are practically devoid of humidity; with a semiclosed system, relative humidity can be increased to 80 percent at 20°C (water content, 14 mg/L). The introduction of a heated humidifier into this system can ensure a water content of 30 mg/L at 30°C.[95] Such humidification is similar to that occurring normally at the pharynx and minimizes the calories lost through the respiratory system during the critical intraoperative period.

The sweating mechanism, although present in the neonate, is less effective than that of adults, possibly because of the immaturity of the cholinergic receptors in the sweat glands. In the intrauterine period, the active sweat mechanisms develop late in gestation; in fact, babies born 3 weeks before term sweat very little, and those born 8 weeks prematurely hardly sweat at all.[96, 97] Full-term infants display structurally well-developed sweat glands, but these do not function appropriately.[98] Sweating during the first days of life is actually confined mostly to the head.

DEVELOPMENT OF MYONEURAL JUNCTIONS

During development, several organizational changes occur in the myoneural junctions. In the early stages, polyneuronal innervation is a characteristic feature, and some axons innervate a very large number of muscle fibers. However, near full-term, these large motor units rapidly decrease in size as the superfluous nerve terminals are eliminated, probably by withdrawal.

As motor activity increases after birth, muscle stimulation is mediated to a great extent by acetylcholine, which induces the release of enzymes into the synaptic clefts. These enzymes tend to digest the nerve terminal; the ability of the terminal to survive ultimately will depend on the supply of reparative material that is received from the cell body. As the weaker terminals are withdrawn, the neuron is able to divert more reparative material to its surviving terminal, thus maintaining it.[99, 100]

Another maturational change is in the distribution of receptors in the muscle itself. In the normal adult, the postsynaptic receptors for the cholinergic transmitter are primarily located at the crests of the junctional folds as part of the integral membrane protein. These receptors can be delineated at the binding sites at an approximate concentration of 10,000 per μm^2. The deeper region of the junctional cleft and the remainder of the muscle membrane are practically devoid of receptors.[101, 102]

Normally, almost all the cholinergic receptors are localized around the nerve endings. These are known as junctional receptors. However, there are also a very small number of extrajunctional receptors on the muscle membrane. In abnormal states, the number of these extrajunctional receptors increases; denervation, for example, produces a fivefold to thirtyfold increase. Extrajunctional receptors spread over the muscle membrane are more loosely attached and have a rapid turnover rate, their half-life being on the order of 17 to 22 hours (vs. 1 to 2 weeks for junctional receptors). Characteristically, extrajunctional receptors are resistant to curare; up to three times the usual dose is required to prevent acetylcholine from opening these channels.[101]

Clinically, resistance to nondepolarizing muscle relaxants can be found in the affected side of a hemiplegic patient, during prolonged immobilization, or after a severe burn.[103–106] Extrapolating from animal studies, one can presume, then, that resistance to muscle relaxants is due to the development of extrajunctional receptors.

The presence of extrajunctional receptors is not unique to denervation or immobilization. They are also found in embryonic muscle fiber, though whether these are identical with the extrajunctional receptors of denervation is a matter of debate. In animal preparations, acetylcholine sensitivity is found all along the muscle of embryonal tissues. Further, the turnover rate of receptors here is quite rapid and in fact rather similar to that of the extrajunctional receptors common to other conditions (half-life of approximately 24 hours).[106–109] Within a few days of established innervation, however, the turnover rate increases to that of adult junctional receptors.[108] These developmental changes can vary from one animal to another and even in the same animals from one group of muscles to another.[109]

For obvious reasons, detailed studies of the myoneural junctions cannot be performed in human neonates. Indirect studies indicate immaturity of the junctions; for example, train-of-four values are lower in neonates than in older infants and children.[110, 111] Also, tetanus is poorly sustained.[112, 113]

Studies demonstrate that the same level of neuromuscular blockade seen in older children with a given plasma concentration of a relaxant can be achieved in infants with a similar or lesser concentration.[114, 115] However, an interesting feature of relaxant studies in infants is the marked variation in response: some infants are quite sensitive to nondepolarizers, whereas others are quite resistant.[114, 116] Animal data seem to indicate that the presence of immature myoneural junctions might predispose to sensitivity while a large number of extrajunctional receptors might result in resistance.[117] Within a short interval, probably in less than a month, this variation diminishes, and the myoneural junction of the infant behaves almost like that of the adult. The wide variation in the response of the infant to relaxant drugs suggests that it is wise to use a neuromuscular blockade monitor to judge the dose required for each patient.

REFERENCES

1. Crelin ES: Functional Anatomy of the Newborn. New Haven, Yale University Press, 1973, pp 1–40.
2. Goudsouzian NG: Anatomical differences between the child and the adult and their clinical sequelae. *In* Ramez-Salem M (ed): Pediatric Anesthesia: Current Practice. New York, Academic Press, 1981, pp 1–3.
3. Rudolph AM: Distribution and regulation of blood flow in the fetal and neonatal lamb. Circ Res *57*:811, 1985.
4. Rudolph AM: Hepatic and ductus venosus blood flows during fetal life. Hepatology *3*:254, 1983.
5. Perelman R, Engle MJ, Farrell P: Perspectives in fetal lung development. Lung *159*:53, 1981.
6. Cassin C, Winikow I, Tod M, et al: Effects of prostacyclin on the fetal pulmonary circulation. Pediatr Pharmacol *1*:197, 1991.
7. Rudolph AM: The changes in the circulation after birth: Their importance in congenital heart disease. Circulation *41*:343, 1970.
8. Jacobstein MD, Hirschfeld SS, Flinn C, et al: Neonatal circulatory changes following elective cesarean section. Pediatrics *69*:374, 1982.
9. Lynch JJ, Schuchard GH, Gross CM, et al: Prevalence of right-to-left atrial shunting in a healthy population: Detection by Valsalva maneuver contrast echocardiography. Am J Cardiol *53*:1478, 1984.
10. Heymann MA, Rudolph AM: Ductus arteriosus dilation by prostaglandin E_1 in infants with pulmonary atresia. Pediatrics *59*:325, 1977.
11. Heymann MA: Patent ductus arteriosus. *In* Adams FH, Emmanouilides GC (eds): Heart Disease in Infants, Children and Adolescents. Baltimore, Williams & Wilkins, 1983, pp 158–171.
12. Elliot RB, Starling MB, Neutze JM: Medical manipulation of the ductus arteriosus. Lancet *1*:140, 1975.
13. Lewis AB, Freed MD, Heymann MA, et al: Side effects of therapy with prostaglandin E_1 in infants with critical congenital heart disease. Circulation *64*:893, 1981.
14. Adams FH: Fetal and neonatal circulation. *In* Adams FH, Emmanouilides GC (eds): Heart Disease in Infants, Children and Adolescents. Baltimore, Williams & Wilkins, 1983, pp 11–17.
15. Schieber RA: Cardiovascular physiology in infants and children. *In* Motoyama EK, Davis PJ (eds): Anesthesia for Infants and Children. 5th edition. St. Louis, CV Mosby, 1990, pp 77–104.
16. Legato MJ: Ultrastructural changes during normal growth in the dog and rat ventricular myofiber. *In* Lieberman M, Sano T (eds): Developmental and Physiological Correlates of Cardiac Muscles. New York, Raven Press, 1976, pp 249–274.
17. Friedman WF: The intrinsic physiologic properties of the developing heart. Prog Cardiovasc Dis 15:87, 1972.
18. Crone RK: Pediatric critical care: Supporting the developing organ systems. *In* Shoemaker WC, Thompson WL, Holbrook PR (eds): Society of Critical Care Medicine: Textbook of Critical Care. Philadelphia, WB Saunders, 1984.
19. Spotnitz WD, Spotnitz HM, Truccone NJ, et al: Relation of ultrastructure and function. Sarcomere dimensions, pressure-volume curves and geometry of the intact left ventricle of the immature canine heart. Circ Res *44*:679, 1979.
20. Gootman PM: Perinatal neural regulation of cardiovascular function. *In* Gootman N, Gootman PM (eds): Perinatal Cardiovascular Function. New York, Marcel Dekker, 1983, p 287.
21. Mott JC: The ability of young mammals to withstand total oxygen lack. Br Med Bull *17*:145, 1961.
22. Enhoring G, Westin B: Experimental studies of the human fetus in prolonged asphyxia. Acta Physiol Scand *31*:359, 1954.
23. Craythorne NW, Turndorf H, Dripps RD: Changes in pulse rate and rhythm associated with the use of succinylcholine in anesthetized children. Anesthesiology *21*:465, 1960.
24. Goudsouzian NG: Turbe del ritmo cardiaco durante intubazione tracheale nei bambini. Acta Anesth Ital *32*:293, 1981.
25. Montague TJ, Taylor PG, Stockton R, et al: The spectrum of cardiac rate and rhythm in normal newborns. Pediatr Cardiol *2*:33, 1982.
26. Rudolph AM, Heymann MA: Cardiac output in the fetal lamb: The effects of spontaneous and induced changes of heart rate on the right and left ventricular output. Am J Obstet Gynecol *124*:183, 1976.
27. Rudolph AM, Heymann MA: Fetal and neonatal circulation and respiration. Annu Rev Physiol *36*:187, 1974.

28. Berman W Jr, Yabek SM, Dillon T, et al: Effects of digoxin in infants with a congested circulatory state due to ventricular septal defect. N Engl J Med *308*:363, 1983.
29. Gootman PM: Neural regulation of cardiovascular function in the perinatal period. *In* Gootman N, Gootman PM (eds): Perinatal Cardiovascular Function. New York, Marcel Dekker, 1983, p 265.
30. Kaplan RF, Graves SA: Anatomic and physiologic differences of neonates, infants and children. Semin Anesth *3*:1, 1984.
31. Goudsouzian N, Karamanian A: Physiology for the Anesthesiologist. Norwalk, Conn., Appleton-Century-Crofts, 1984, pp 242–254.
32. Cross KW, Flynn DM, Hill JR: Oxygen consumption in normal newborn infants during moderate hypoxia in warm and cool environments. Pediatrics *37*:565, 1966.
33. Rudolph AM, Heymann MA, Teramo KAW, et al: Studies on the circulation of the previable human fetus. Pediatr Res *5*:452, 1971.
34. Ardran GM, Kemp FH: The mechanism of changes in form of the cervical airway in infancy. Med Radiolog Photog *44*:26, 1968.
35. Eckenhoff JE: Some anatomic considerations of the infant larynx influencing endotracheal anesthesia. Anesthesiology *12*:401, 1951.
36. Koka BV, Jeon IS, Andre JM, et al: Postintubation croup in children. Anesth Analg *56*:501, 1977.
37. Coté CJ, Eavey R, Todres ID: Providing for the needs of the pediatric larynx. Wellcome Trends in Anesthesiology, Dec. 1983, p 2.
38. Motoyama EK: Pulmonary mechanics during early postnatal years. Pediatr Res *11*:220, 1977.
39. Keens TG, Bryan AC, Levison H, et al: Developmental patterns of muscle fiber types in human ventilatory muscles. J Appl Physiol *44*:909, 1978.
40. Reid L: The lung: Its growth and remodeling in health and diseases. Am J Roentgenol *129*:777, 1977.
41. Milner AD, Greenough A: Adaptation of the respiratory system. Br Med Bull *44*:909, 1988.
42. Langston C, Kida K, Reed M, Thurlbeck WM: Human lung growth in late gestation and in the neonate. Am Rev Resp Dis *129*:607, 1984.
43. Notter RH, Shapiro DL: Lung surfactant in an era of replacement therapy. Pediatrics *68*:781, 1981.
44. Roberton NRC: Perinatal physiology. *In* Godfrey S, Baum JD (eds): Clinical Paediatric Physiology. Oxford, Blackwell Scientific Publications, 1979, pp 134–192.
45. Rooney SA: The surfactant system and lung phospholipid biochemistry. Am Rev Resp Dis *131*:439, 1985.
46. Collaborative Group on Antenatal Steroid Therapy: Effect of antenatal doxamethasone on the prevention of respiratory distress syndrome. National Heart, Lung and Blood Institute, Bethesda, Md. Am J Obstet Gynecol *141*:276, 1981.
47. Avery ME, Merrit TA: Surfactant replacement therapy (editorial). N Engl J Med *324*:910, 1991.
48. Fujiwara T, Konishi M, Chida S, et al: Surfactant replacement therapy with a single postventilatory dose of a reconstituted bovine surfactant in preterm neonates with respiratory distress syndrome. Pediatrics *86*:753, 1990.
49. Takahashi A, Fujiwara T: Proteolipid in bovine lung surfactant: Its role in surfactant function. Biochem Biophys Res Commun *135*:527, 1986.
50. Jansen AH, Chernick V: Development of respiratory control. Physiol Rev *63*:437, 1983.
51. Dawes GS: Breathing before birth in animals and man. N Engl J Med *290*:557, 1974.
52. Alcorn D, Adamson TM, Maloney JE, et al: Morphological effects of chronic bilateral phrenectomy or vagotomy in the fetal lamb lung. J Anat *130*:683, 1980.
53. Mansell A, Bryan C, Levison H: Airway closure in children. J Appl Physiol *33*:711, 1972.
54. Motoyama EK, Glazener CH: Hypoxemia after general anesthesia in children. Anesth Analg *65*:267, 1986.
55. Mathers JM, Benumof JL, Wahrenbrock EA: General anesthetics and regional hypoxic pulmonary vasoconstriction. Anesthesiology *46*:111, 1977.
56. Glotzbach SF, Baldwin RB, Lederer NE, et al: Periodic breathing in preterm infants. Incidence and characteristics. Pediatrics *84*:785, 1989.
57. Finer NN, Barrington KJ, Peters KL: The relationship between periodic breathing and apneic spells in premature infants. Am Rev Resp Dis *137*:265S, 1988.
58. Liu LMP, Coté CJ, Goudsouzian NG, et al: Life-threatening apnea in infants recovering from anesthesia. Anesthesiology *59*:506, 1983.
59. Welborn LG, Ramirez N, Oh TH, et al: Postanesthetic apnea and periodic breathing in infants. Anesthesiology 65:658, 1986.
60. Welborn LG, Rice LJ, Hannalah RS, et al: Postoperative apnea in former preterm infants: Prospective comparison of spinal and general anesthesia. Anesthesiology *72*:838, 1990.
61. Kuzemko JA, Paala J: Apnoeic attacks in the newborn treated with aminophylline. Arch Dis Chil *48*:404, 1973.
62. Welborn LG, Desoto H, Hannalah RS, et al: The use of caffeine in the control of postanesthetic apnea in former premature infants. Anesthesiology *68*:796, 1988.
63. Aubier M, DeTroyer A, Sampson M, et al: Aminophylline improves diaphragmatic contractility. N Engl J Med *305*:249, 1981.
64. Perutz MF: Hemoglobin structure and respiratory transport. Sci Am *239*:92, 1978.
65. Stockman JA, Garcia JF, Oski FA: The anemia of prematurity. Factors governing the erythropoietin response. N Engl J Med *296*:647, 1977.
66. Oski FA: The unique fetal red cell and its function. Pediatrics *51*:494, 1973.
67. Stockman JA III: Anemia of prematurity. Current concepts in the issue of when to transfuse. Pediatr Clin North Am *33*:111, 1986.
68. Gairdner D, Marks J, Roscoe JD: Blood formation in infancy. I. The normal bone marrow. Arch Dis Child *27*:128, 1952.
69. Bard H, Prosmanne J: Elevated levels of fetal hemoglobin synthesis in infants with bronchopulmonary dysplasia. Pediatrics *86*:193, 1990.
70. Consensus Conference: Perioperative red blood cell transfusion. JAMA *260*:2700, 1988.
71. Motoyama EK: Respiratory physiology in infants and children. *In* Motoyama EK, Davis PJ (eds): Anesthesia for Infants and Children. St. Louis, CV Mosby, 1990, pp 11–76.
72. Keyes WG, Donohue PK, Spivak JL, et al: Assessing the need for transfusion of premature infants and role of hematocrit; clinical signs and erythropoietin level. Pediatrics *84*:412, 1989.
73. Arant BS Jr: Developmental patterns of renal functional maturation compared in the human neonate. J Pediatr *92*:705, 1978.
74. Aperia A, Broberger O, Elinder G, et al: Postnatal development of renal function in preterm and full-term infants. Acta Pediatr Scand *70*:183, 1981.
75. Fawer CL, Torrado A, Guignard JP: Maturation of renal function in full-term and premature neonates. Helv Paediatr Acta *34*:11, 1979.

76. Oh W: Renal function and clinical disorders in the neonate. Clin Perinatol *8*:213, 1981.
77. Rane A, Wilson JT: Clinical pharmacokinetics in infants and children. Clin Pharmacokinet *1*:2, 1976.
78. Modi N: Development of renal function. Br Med J *44*:935, 1989.
79. Kojima T, Hirata Y, Fukada Y, et al: Plasma atrial natriuretic peptide and spontaneous diuresis in sick neonates. Arch Dis Child *62*:667, 1987.
79a. Cornblath M, Schwartz R, Aynsley-Green A, et al: Hypoglycemia in infancy: The need for a rational definition. Pediatrics *85*:834, 1990.
80. Dweck H, Brans Y, Sumner J, Cassady G: Glucose intolerance in infants of very low birth weight. Biol Neonate *30*:261, 1976.
81. Goldman SL, Hirata T: Attenuated response to insulin in very low birth weight infants. Pediatr Res *14*:50, 1980.
82. De La Iglesia FA, Sturgess JM, McGuire EJ, et al: Quantitative microscopic evaluation of endoplasmic reticulum in developing human liver. Am J Pathol *82*:61, 1976.
83. Morselli PL: Clinical pharmacokinetics in neonates. Clin Pharmacokinet *1*:81, 1976.
84. Currin MR: Pharmacology of the neonate. S Afr Med J *56*:101, 1979.
85. Weiss CF, Glazko AJ, Weston JK: Chloramphenicol in the newborn infant: A physiological explanation of its toxicity when given in excessive doses. N Engl J Med *262*:787, 1960.
86. Yu WL, Aldrich RA: The glucuronide transferase system in the newborn infant. Pediatr Clin North Am *7*:381, 1960.
87. Dutton GJ: Developmental aspects of drug conjugation with special reference to glucuronidation. Annu Rev Pharmacol Toxicol *18*:17, 1978.
88. Adamsons K, Towell ME: Thermal homeostasis in the fetus and newborn. Anesthesiology *26*:531, 1965.
88a. Hull D: Thermal control in very immature infants. Br Med Bull *44*:971, 1988.
89. Heiser MS, Downes JJ: Temperature regulation in the pediatric patient. Semin Anesth *2*:37, 1980.
89a. Okken A, Jonxis JHP, Rispens P, Zijlstra WG: Insensible water loss and metabolic rate in low birthweight newborn infants. Pediatr Res *13*:1072, 1979.
90. Schiff DS, Stern L, Leduc J: Chemical thermogenesis in newborn infants. Catecholamine excretion and the plasma nonesterified fatty acid response to cold exposure. Pediatrics *37*:577, 1966.
91. Himms-Hagen J: Cellular thermogenesis. Annu Rev Physiol *38*:315, 1976.
92. Mitchell D, Laburn HP: Pathophysiology of temperature regulation. Physiologist *28*:507, 1985.
93. Goudsouzian NG, Morris RH, Ryan JF: The effects of a warming blanket on the maintenance of body temperature in anesthetized infants and children. Anesthesiology *39*:351, 1973.
94. Goudsouzian NG: Temperature regulation in the operating room. *In* Ramez-Salem M (ed): Pediatric Anesthesia: Current Practice. New York, Academic Press, 1981, pp 31–33.
95. Weeks DB, Broman KE: A method of quantitating humidity in the anesthesia circuit by temperature control: Semiclosed circle. Anesth Analg *49*:292, 1970.
96. Robertshaw D: Man in the extreme environments; Problems of the newborn and elderly. *In* Cena K, Clark JA (eds): Bioengineering, Thermal Physiology and Comfort. Amsterdam, Elsevier 1981, pp 169–179.
97. Harpin VA, Rutter N: Sweating in preterm babies. J Paediatr *100*:614, 1982.
98. Risenfeld T, Hammarlund K, Sedin G: The effect of warm environment on respiratory water loss in fullterm newborn infants on their first day after birth. Acta Paediatr Scand *79*:893, 1990.
99. Brown MC, Jansen JKS, van Essen D: Polyneuronal innervation of skeletal muscles in newborn rats and its elimination during maturation. J Physiol *261*:387, 1976.
100. O'Brien RAD, Östberg AJC, Vebova G: The reorganization of neuromuscular junctions during development in rats. *In* Hoffman JF, Giebisch GH (eds): Membranes in Growth and Development. New York, Alan R. Liss, 1982, pp 247–257.
101. Fambrough DM: Control of acetylcholine receptors in skeletal muscle. Physiol Rev *59*:165, 1979.
102. Peper K, Bradley RJ, Dreyer F: The acetylcholine receptor at the neuromuscular junction. Physiol Rev *62*:1271, 1982.
103. Graham DH: Monitoring neuromuscular block may be unreliable in patients with upper-motor-neuron lesions. Anesthesiology *52*:74, 1980.
104. Moorthy SS, Hilgenberg JC: Resistance to nondepolarizing muscle relaxants in paretic upper extremities of patients with residual hemiplegia. Anesth Analg *59*:624, 1980.
105. Martyn JAJ, Szyfelbein SK, Ali HH, et al: Increased D-tubocurarine requirement following major thermal injury. Anesthesiology *52*:352, 1980.
106. Bennett MR: Development of neuromuscular synapses. Physiol Rev *63*:915, 1983.
107. Reiness CG, Weinberg CB: Metabolic stabilization of acetylcholine receptors at newly formed neuromuscular junctions in rat. Develop Biol *84*:247, 1981.
108. Linden DC, Fambrough DM: Biosynthesis and degradation of acetylcholine receptors in rat skeletal muscles. Effects of electrical stimulation. Neuroscience *4*:517, 1979.
109. Nag AC, Cheng M: Differentiation of fibre types in an extraocular muscle of the rat. J Embryol Exp Morph *71*:171, 1982.
110. Goudsouzian NG: Maturation of neuromuscular transmission in the infant. Br J Anaesth *52*:205, 1980.
111. Goudsouzian NG, Crone RK, Todres ID: Recovery from pancuronium blockade in the neonatal intensive care unit. Br J Anaesth *53*:1303, 1981.
112. Koenigsberger MR, Patten B, Lovelace RE: Studies of neuromuscular function in the newborn. I. A comparison of myoneural function in the full-term and the premature infant. Neuropaediatrie *4*:350, 1973.
113. Crumrine RS, Yodlowski EH: Assessment of neuromuscular function in infants. Anesthesiology *54*:29, 1981.
114. Fisher DM, O'Keeffe C, Stanski DR, et al: Pharmacokinetics and dynamics of D-tubocurarine in infants, children and adults. Anesthesiology *57*:203, 1982.
115. Matteo RS, Lieberman IG, Salanitre E, et al: Distribution, elimination and action of D-tubocurarine concentration in neonates, infants, children and adults. Anesthesiology *63*:798, 1984.
116. Goudsouzian NG, Donlon JV, Savarese JJ, et al: Reevaluation of dosage and duration of action of D-tubocurarine in the pediatric age group. Anesthesiology *43*:416, 1975.
117. Goudsouzian NG, Standaert FG: The infant and the myoneural junction. Anesth Analg *65*:1208, 1986.
118. Task Force on Blood Pressure Control in Children. Report of the second Task Force on blood pressure control in children. Pediatrics *79*:1, 1987.

CHAPTER

2 Pharmacology of Pediatric Anesthesia

D. RYAN COOK, M.D.

The young infant, especially during the neonatal period, differs from the adult in quantitative responses to many anesthetic drugs and adjuncts. During the first several months of life there is rapid physical growth and rapid change and maturation in the factors involved in the uptake, distribution, redistribution, metabolism, and excretion of drugs.[1–6] Important differences in these processes between the infant and adult have been identified to explain the young infant's altered response to many drugs. In addition, variations in penetration of the blood brain barrier and in receptor sensitivity have been observed in infants for some anesthetics and adjuncts. This chapter discusses the factors that influence the infant's handling of drugs in general and gives examples of pharmacological differences for certain anesthetic drugs and adjuncts, along with their probable explanations.

DRUG ABSORPTION

Most anesthetic drugs (other than inhalation anesthetics) are given parenterally. The intravenous route is the most direct, bypassing the absorption barriers. Drugs in aqueous solution injected intramuscularly are often absorbed fairly rapidly; subcutaneously injected drugs are usually more slowly absorbed. Absorption from intramuscular and subcutaneous sites depends mainly on tissue perfusion, and, if perfusion is adequate, this absorption is similar in children and adults. The vasomotor instability in the newborn period theoretically might delay absorption from peripheral sites, although in practice the therapeutic effectiveness of drugs given via these routes suggests that this is not an important factor.[7]

On rare occasions, anesthesiologists give either oral or rectal medication (sedative-hypnotics) to infants, usually for neurodiagnostic procedures. Such drugs are given in solution, not as tablets or capsules, so that disintegration and dissolution are irrelevant. They are absorbed across the gut by passive diffusion, which depends upon the physicochemical properties of the drug and the surface area of the gut available for diffusion.[8, 9] Since most drugs are weak acids or weak bases, the un-ionized fraction that is available for diffusion will vary with the pH of the fluid in the gut (e.g., the pH of gastric fluid varies between 1.5 and 6.0, whereas the intestinal fluid is considerably more alkaline).

In adults, the total absorptional area of the small intestine is probably 200 m^2 compared with 1 m^2 for the stomach. Because of this larger surface area, acidic drugs are absorbed more rapidly from the alkaline small intestine than from the acidic stomach in spite of their being highly un-ionized in the intestine. In large part, therefore, the rate of gastric emptying is a controlling factor in drug absorption from the gut (i.e., slower gastric emptying delays a drug's access to the small intestine and vice versa). Gastric emptying may be slowed by food, drugs, or surgical conditions. Once a drug is in the small intestine, up to 4 to 10 hours are available for absorption; however, most drugs reach peak concentrations by 30 to 40 minutes. Thus, changes in intestinal transit time have little effect on drug absorption. Likewise, very few drugs are absorbed rapidly enough for blood flow to be a rate-limiting factor, although ethanol may be an exception. Methyldopa, levodopa, and 5-fluorouracil are the few drugs actively transported across cell membranes against a concentration gradient. Ethanol is probably the only drug that, in part, crosses the gut by filtration through pores.

There are no functional differences among the older infant, child, and adult that should affect gastrointestinal absorption. The rate, but not extent, of absorption of many drugs may be increased by using liquid preparations. In the newborn period and after the first day of life, gastric contents are less acidic, and the gastric emptying time and intestinal transit time are considerably slower than at any other age.[10] Consequently, drugs such as penicillin G and ampicillin, which are partially inactivated by a low pH, have greater overall absorption when swallowed. The slow gastric emptying time reduces the absorption of some drugs, whereas others may achieve greater absorption because of prolonged contact with the bowel wall during the longer transit period through the intestine.

DRUG DISTRIBUTION

The distribution process regulates the amount of drug reaching specific body compartments or tissues and hence the concentration of the drug at the receptor site. Distribution is influenced mainly by the degree of protein binding and red cell binding, tissue volumes, tissue solubility coefficients, and blood flow to various tissues. Extracellular inert binding to plasma proteins depends on the amount of binding protein available and the drug affinity constant for proteins; these factors are directly or indirectly modified by pathophysiological conditions and by other drugs and compounds.[11–18]

In blood, drugs may bind to albumin and several other serum proteins. The degree to which this occurs is usually measured as the percentage of total nondialyzable drug in the blood—i.e., that bound to large molecules. Binding to nonreceptor proteins also takes place outside the vascular compartment and may account for a significant fraction of the total drug in the body. The volume of distribution of a drug is directly proportional to the fraction of free drug in the plasma. Drug molecules bound to inert binding sites are not available for diffusion or interaction with receptors, but they are, however, in equilibrium with free drug. Thus alterations in the concentration of free drug will result in changes in the amount (but not the percentage) bound. Nonreceptor protein binding sites are not very specific; many weak acids with different pharmacological effects bind to the same or closely related plasma protein sites. Therefore, different drugs may compete for the same binding sites. This can have important consequences when a high percentage of a potent drug (A) is bound; the binding sites must be loaded to achieve a therapeutic concentration of free drug in the plasma. Addition of a second drug (B) which competes for the same inert binding site (but not the receptor site) may result in a marked increase in the concentration of free drug A and thereby precipitate toxicity.

A quantitative and qualitative reduction in plasma protein binding occurs in the newborn period.[19–21] At this stage, infants, particularly preterm infants, have lower plasma albumin concentrations than at other ages (30 to 40 g/L), and the albumin is qualitatively different and has a lower affinity for drugs. Further modification of plasma protein binding is likely to occur at this age as a result of the higher free fatty acid and bilirubin concentrations and the lower blood pH. Concentrations of α_1-acid glycoproteins that bind many basic drugs are lower in the neonate than in the adult. Decreased protein binding, therefore, may contribute to the larger apparent volume of distribution for many drugs, such as ketamine, for example.[22]

In the neonate, differences in the size of the body fluid compartments, relatively smaller muscle mass and fat stores, and presumably greater blood flow per unit of organ weight influence the distribution of drugs to their active site and secondary redistribution. Metabolism and excretion may take place during redistribution. Total body water, extracellular fluid, and blood volume of the neonate are larger on a weight basis than those of an adult (Table 2–1).[23] The initial larger volume for distribution of a parenterally administered drug may explain, in part, why neonates appear to require larger amounts of some drugs on a weight basis to produce a given effect. Differences in fat stores and muscle mass at different ages are shown in Table 2–1.[24] Table 2–2 gives developmental estimates of tissue volumes and tissue blood flow derived from physiological studies and from autopsy of normal tissue at the Children's Hospital of Pittsburgh.[24–27] A high proportion of the cardiac output is distributed to the vessel-rich organs, particularly to the brain. Smaller muscle mass and fat stores provide less uptake to inactive sites and tend to keep plasma concentration higher. The smaller amount of fat tissue in neonates provides a relatively small reservoir for fat-soluble drugs.

Table 2–2. AGE-RELATED ESTIMATES OF TISSUE VOLUME AND BLOOD FLOW

	Gas and Tissue Volumes (ml/kg)		**Tissue Blood Flows** (% CO)	
	Adult	***Infant***	***Adult***	***Infant***
Tidal volume	7	7		
Functional residual capacity	40	25		
Volume	70	90		
Brain	21	90	14.3	34
Heart	4	4.5	4.3	3
Splanchnic	57	70	28.6	25
Kidney	6	10	25.7	18
Muscle	425	180	11.4	10
Fat	150	100	5.7	5
Poorly perfused tissue	270	270	10.0	5

Data from Widdowson,[24] Smith and Nelson,[25] Guignard et al,[26] and Altman and Dittmer.[27]

BLOOD-BRAIN BARRIER

The blood-brain barrier, a lipid membrane interface between the endothelial cells of the brain vasculature and the extracellular fluid of the brain, may be "immature" at birth.[28–35] The intercellular clefts of brain are closed; these are tight junctions. The transport of drugs into and out of brain depends on principles identical to those determining the movement of substances across other biological membranes. The rate of penetration of un-ionized drugs into brain increases with the degree of lipid solubility. Active transport mechanisms or specific carrier systems allow rapid exchange of certain biologically active compounds and of certain inorganic and organic anions either into or from the brain. Some polar metabolites are cleared from the brain by diffusion into cerebral spinal fluid (i.e., sink action).

Table 2–1. BODY COMPOSITION DURING GROWTH

Body Compartment	**Premature** (1.5 kg)	**Full-Term** (3.5 kg)	**Adult** (70 kg)
Total body water (% body weight)	83	73	60
Extracellular fluid (% body weight)	62	44	20
Blood volume (ml/kg)	60	85–105	70
Intracellular water (% body weight)	25	33	40
Muscle mass (% body weight)	15	20	50
Fat (% body weight)	3	12	18

Data from Friss-Hansen[23] and Widdowson.[24]

Oldendorf has measured the blood-brain barrier permeability during a single capillary pass for a number of drugs relative to a highly diffusible tracer like water or butanol.[36–38] The uptake of the drug is expressed as a percentage of the uptake of the highly diffusible tracer, the brain uptake index (BUI). Drugs with an oil-water partition coefficient below 0.01 hardly penetrate the cerebral capillaries during a single pass, whereas those with a partition coefficient above 0.1 are likely to have 50 percent or more penetration. Drugs having a partition coefficient greater than about 0.03 will undergo substantially complete clearance during a single brain passage (Fig. 2–1). For example, in adults, morphine, with a limited lipid solubility, has rather limited brain uptake, whereas heroin, with a high lipid solubility, has high brain uptake. If the lipid solubility of a compound is very high, rapid diffusion across the barrier leads to rapid equilibration between blood and brain. The rate of entry is then determined by blood flow. Since in the infant the brain receives a large proportion of cardiac output, it is not surprising that the brain concentration of many drugs is higher in the infant than in the adult. Regional differences in brain perfusion will also affect the uptake of compounds into brain.

BIOTRANSFORMATION AND EXCRETION

Renal excretion plays a pivotal role in terminating the biologic activity of a few drugs that have small molecular sizes or have polar characteristics at physiological pH. Most drugs do

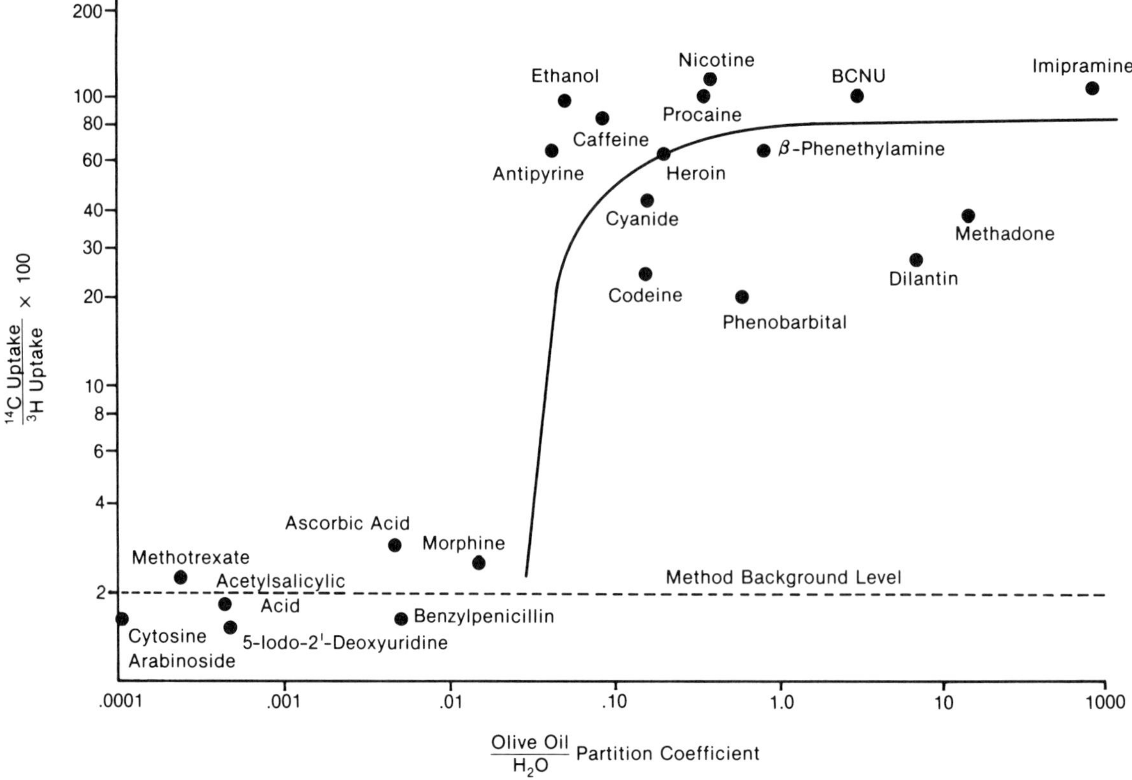

FIGURE 2–1. Percentage clearance of various drugs during a single brain circulatory passage vs. olive oil–water partition coefficients.

not possess such physicochemical properties. Pharmacologically active organic molecules tend to be highly lipophilic and remain un-ionized or only partially ionized at physiological pH. They are often strongly bound to plasma proteins. Such substances are not readily filtered at the glomerulus. The lipophilic nature of renal tubular membranes also facilitates the reabsorption of hydrophobic compounds following their glomerular filtration. Consequently, most drugs would have a prolonged duration of action if their termination depended solely on renal excretion.

An alternative process that may lead to the termination or alteration of biological activity is metabolism. In general, lipophilic drugs are transformed to more polar and hence more readily excretable products. Most metabolic biotransformations occur at some point between absorption of the drug into the general circulation and its renal elimination. A few transformations occur in the intestinal lumen or intestinal wall. In general, all these reactions can be assigned to two major categories called phase I and phase II reactions.

PHASE I REACTIONS

Phase I reactions usually convert the parent drug to a more polar metabolite by introducing or unmasking a functional group (—OH, —NH_2, —SH). Often these metabolites are inactive, although in some instances activity is only modified. Metabolic products are often less active than the parent drug and may even be inactive. However, some biotransformation products have enhanced activity or toxic properties, including mutagenicity, teratogenicity, and carcinogenicity.

If phase I metabolites are sufficiently polar, they may be readily excreted. However, many phase I products are not eliminated rapidly and undergo a subsequent reaction in which an endogenous substrate such as glucuronic acid, sulfuric acid, acetic acid, or an amino acid combines with the newly established functional group to form a highly polar conjugate. Such conjugations or synthetic reactions are the hallmarks of phase II metabolism. A great variety of drugs undergo these sequential biotransformation reactions, although in some instances the parent drug may already have a functional group that may form a conjugate directly.

Although at all ages every tissue has some ability to metabolize drugs, the liver is the principal organ of drug metabolism. The overall rate of metabolism probably depends on both the size of the liver and the metabolizing ability of the appropriate microsomal enzyme system. Liver volume relative to body weight decreases from birth to adulthood, the relative volume in the first year of life being twice that at 14 years. Other sites of considerable metabolic activity include the gastrointestinal tract, lungs, skin, and kidney. After oral administration, many drugs (e.g., isoproterenol, meperidine, pentazocine, and morphine) are absorbed intact from the small intestine and transported first via the portal system to the liver, where they undergo extensive metabolism. This process has been called a first-pass effect. Some orally administered drugs (e.g., clonazepam and chlorpromazine) are more extensively metabolized in the intestine than in the liver. Thus, intestinal metabolism may contribute to the overall first-pass effect. First-pass effects may so greatly limit the bioavailability of orally administered drugs that alternative routes of administration must be used to achieve therapeutically effective blood levels. The lower gut harbors intestinal microorganisms that are capable of many biotransformation reactions. In addition, drugs may be metabolized by gastric acid (penicillin), by digestive enzymes (polypeptides such as insulin), or by enzymes in the wall of the intestine (catecholamines).

Although drug biotransformation in vivo can occur by spontaneous, noncatalyzed chemical reactions, the great majority are catalyzed by specific cellular enzymes. Many drug-metabolizing enzymes are located in the lipophilic membranes of the endoplasmic reticulum of the liver and other tissues. When these lamellar membranes are isolated by homogenization and fractionation of the cell, they reform into vesicles called microsomes. Microsomes retain most of the morphological and functional characteristics of the intact membranes, including the rough and smooth surface features of the rough (ribosome-studded) and smooth (no ribosomes) endoplasmic reticulum. Whereas the rough microsomes tend to be dedicated to protein synthesis, the smooth microsomes are relatively rich in enzymes responsible for oxidative drug metabolism. In particular, they contain the important class of enzymes known as the mixed-function oxidases.

Microsomal drug oxidations require cytochrome P-450, cytochrome P-450 reductase, NADPH, and molecular oxygen. The relative abundance of cytochrome P-450, compared with that of the reductase in the liver, contributes to making cytochrome P-450 heme reduction the rate-limiting step in hepatic drug oxidations. The potent oxidizing properties of this activated oxygen permit oxidation of a large number of substrates. Substrate specificity is very low for this enzyme complex. High solubility in lipids is the only common feature of the wide variety of structurally unrelated drugs and chemicals that serve as substrates in this system.

PHASE II REACTIONS

Parent drugs or their phase I metabolites that contain suitable chemical groups often undergo coupling or conjugation reactions with an endogenous substance to yield drug conjugates. In general, conjugates are polar molecules that are readily excreted and often inactive. Certain conjugation reactions (*O*-sulfation of *N*-hydroxyacetylaminofluorene and *N*-acetylation of isoniazid) may lead to the formation of reactive species responsible for the hepatotoxicity of the drug. Conjugate formation involves high-energy intermediates and specific transfer enzymes. Such enzymes (transferases) may be located in microsomes or in the cytosol. They catalyze the coupling of an activated endogenous substance (such as the uridine 5′-diphosphate [UDP] derivative of glucuronic acid) with a drug or of an activated drug with an endogenous substrate. Because the endogenous substrates originate in the diet, nutrition plays a critical role in the regulation of drug conjugations.

The hepatic enzyme systems responsible for the metabolism of drugs are incompletely developed or absent in the neonate. Rats and ferrets develop the cytochrome P-450 system in liver microsomes to adult levels by age 10 to 20 days. Of phase I biotransformation processes, the ability to oxidize drugs is most deficient in neonates; the ability to reduce substrates is much less so; whereas the ability to hydrolyze substrates is as effective as that in adults. The activity of oxidative and reductive enzymes increases to adult levels within the first few days of life. Phase II processes—conjugation with sulfate, acetate, glucuronic acid, or amino acids—are severely limited at birth.[39, 40] Neonatal hepatic tissues, for example, are unable to synthesize glucuronides because of low tissue levels of uridine diphospate, glucuronic acid, and UDP-transferase, the latter of which catalyzes transfer of glucuronic acid to foreign molecules.[41] Conjugation reactions with acetate occur by 1 month of age, with glucuronide by 2 months, and with amino acids by 3 months. Some of these metabolized drugs are recirculated and excreted in the urine; other metabolites or unmetabolized drugs are excreted in the bile.

ENZYME INDUCTION AND INHIBITION

An interesting feature of some of these chemically dissimilar drug substrates is their ability, on repeated administration, to "induce" cytochrome P-450 by enhancing the rate of its synthesis or reducing its rate of degradation. Induction accelerates metabolism and usually results in a decrease in the pharmacological action of the inducer and also of coadministered drugs. However, in the case of drugs metabolically transformed to reactive intermediates, enzyme induction may exacerbate drug-mediated tissue toxicity. Various substrates appear to induce forms of cytochrome P-450 that have different molecular weights and exhibit different substrate specificities and immunochemical and spectral characteristics. In infants, the enzyme activity of the cytochrome P-450 systems can be increased by known enzyme inducers, such as benzopyrene or phenobarbital. Thus, the low enzyme activity for various substrates reflects lack of stimulation rather than inability of the enzyme system to be stimulated.[42] The age from birth is important for maturation of these enzyme systems, not the duration of gestation. Premature infants and mature-born infants developed the ability to metabolize drugs to the same degree at the same time period after birth.

Other drug substrates may inhibit cytochrome P-450 enzyme activity. Proadifen (SK&F 525-A) and cimetidine bind avidly to the cytochrome molecule and thereby competitively inhibit the metabolism of potential substrates.[43, 44] Some substrates irreversibly inhibit cytochrome P-450 via covalent interaction of a metabolically generated reactive intermediate that may react with either the apoprotein or the heme moiety of the cytochrome (e.g., ethinyl estradiol, norethindrone, and spironolactone; fluroxene, secobarbital, and allobarbital; carbon disulfide; and proplythiouracil).[44]

EXCRETION

The ultimate route of elimination of most drugs or their metabolites is by way of the kidney. Since many drugs are simply filtered by the kidney, the glomerular filtration rate (GFR) influences drug excretion and action. Inulin and thiosulfate clearances, which reflect GFR, are lower in neonates and young children than in adults. Volume clearance, when related to surface area, approaches adult values at about 3 months of age. If, on the other hand, clearance is related to weight, adult values are reached in about 10 days to 2 weeks. The time-clearance method resolves the question of which basis to select. The elimination half-life for thiosulfate is about three times slower in neonates than in older children or adults; by 3 weeks of age these differences disappear. The maturation of glomerular function may be related to changes in the permeability of the glomerular membrane or to conversion of nonfunctional glomeruli to functional participants in the process of filtration. Proximal tubular secretion assumes adult values in the first 4 to 5 months of age.[39] The glucuronide and sulfate metabolities of drugs may be secreted through the proximal tubules by an acid pump mechanism.

INHALATION ANESTHETICS

AGE-RELATED DIFFERENCES IN UPTAKE AND DISTRIBUTION

The uptake of nitrous oxide, cyclopropane, and halothane is more rapid in infants and small children than in adults.[45–50] Salanitre and Rackow[47] compared the uptake of nitrous oxide among infants 0 to 6 months of age, 15-year-old children, and two groups of adults. An FE/FI ratio of 1.0 occurred in infants in about 25 minutes, in children in about 30 minutes, and in adults in about 60 minutes. Steward and Creighton likewise noted more rapid washout of nitrous oxide in infants than in adults.[48] These age-related differences in anesthetic uptake are more striking with halothane, which has a fivefold higher blood solubility than does nitrous oxide. Salanitre and Rackow[46] showed that the uptake of halothane was more rapid in children 15 years of age than in adults. However, the uptake of halothane was determined concurrently with that of nitrous oxide. The rapid uptake of nitrous oxide may have influenced the early uptake of halothane because of the so called "second gas effect." More recently, Brandom, Brandom, and Cook measured the uptake of halothane in infants.[50] FE/FI for halothane in these infants increased more rapidly than has been described in adults (Fig. 2–2).

Major differences between adults and infants in blood-gas solubility coefficients, body composition, alveolar ventilation, and the distribution of cardiac output explain the concomitant differences in their rates of uptake of anesthetic. Tidal volume on a weight basis (7 ml/kg) is relatively constant throughout life. However, the infant has a relatively high alveolar ventilation, particularly in relation to functional reserve capacity (FRC). The alveolar ventilation to FRC ratio is about 5:1 in infants, contrasted with 1.4:1 in adults. The lung time constant is estimated to be 0.19 minute in infants and 0.73 minute in adults, for a gas with limited blood solubility (helium and nitrous oxide). Thus, lung washin or lung washout of inhalation anesthetics is relatively more rapid in infants than in adults. In infants, controlled ventilation that increased alveolar ventilation would further increase this ratio; in adults it would appear difficult to utilize tidal breaths approaching FRC in magnitude.

The blood-gas solubility coefficients for halothane have been shown to vary with age.[51, 52] Halothane is less soluble in blood taken from the fetal circulation of the placenta than it is in blood taken from adults. The influence of hematocrit, hemoglobin type, and plasma protein fractions on anesthetic solubility has not been well defined. The blood-gas solubility coefficient of nitrous oxide varied about 3 percent as hematocrit increased from 30 percent to 52 percent. If all other things were equal, the high cardiac output of the infant (on a weight basis about twice that of the adult) would retard the uptake of inhalation anesthetics. However, this effect is minimized by other factors. More important, a larger percentage of the infant's cardiac output is distributed to the vessel-rich tissue group. Compared with the adult, the infant has increased brain mass and limited muscle mass and fat; significant differences in tissue blood flow correspond to these differences in tissue compartments.

We constructed an 11-compartment model incorporating age-dependent differences in respiratory variables, lung and tissue volumes, and (tissue regional) blood flow to illustrate these differences.[50] Such a model allows one to predict FE/FI ratios over time and, more importantly, tissue anesthetic concentrations for any given anesthetic. Tissue solubility coefficients for adults were used in this model and may have introduced minor errors. For example, brain water content decreases with increasing age;

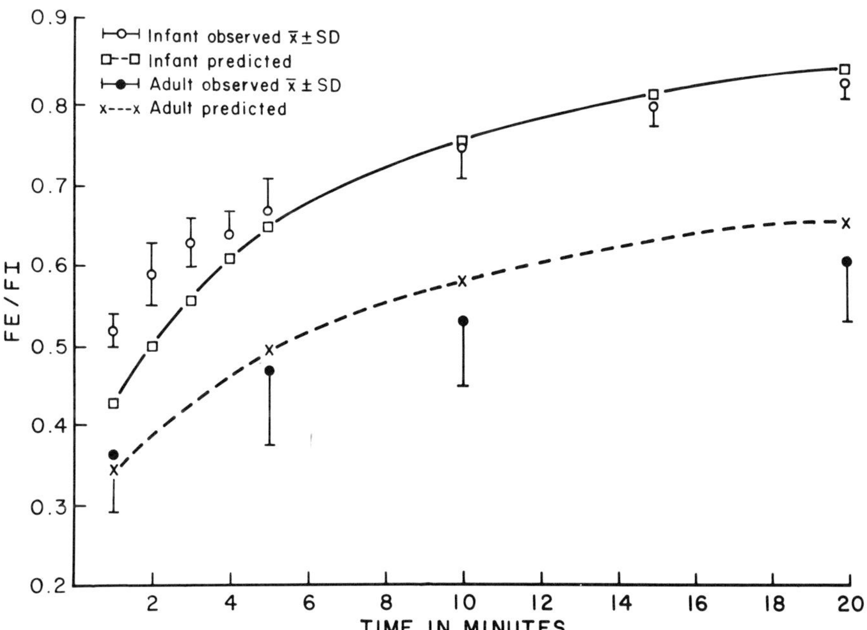

FIGURE 2–2. Predicted versus observed FE/FI for halothane in infants and adults.

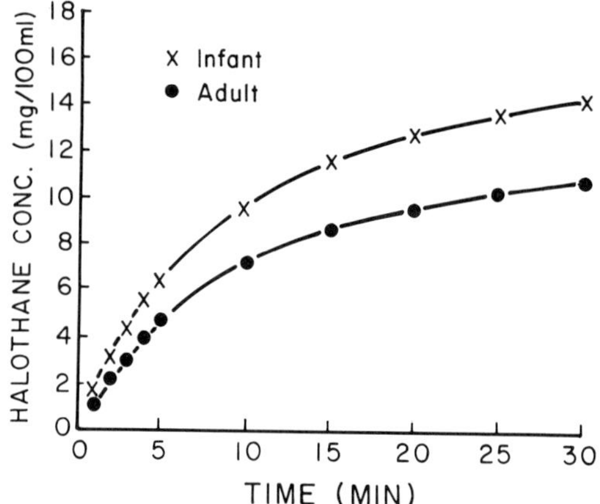

FIGURE 2–3. Predicted concentration of halothane in the brain. The values in Figure 2–4 were derived from our computerized model of anesthetic uptake and distribution. The model infant weighed 4 kg; the model adult weighed 70 kg. In both cases, normal ventilation and a constant inspired fraction of 0.5 percent halothane were employed. Tissue levels are given in mg/100 ml of tissue.

this may influence the brain tissue solubility coefficient.[53] Our model predicts that the concentration of halothane in tissues will increase more rapidly in infants (e.g., the brain and heart) (Figs. 2–3 and 2–4) than in adults, given the same inspired concentration of halothane. The reduced muscle mass of the infant compared with the adult, and the concurrent reduction of the proportion of cardiac output perfusing muscle, tends to concentrate the cardiac output in infants toward the more highly perfused vessel-rich organs such as the brain and heart.

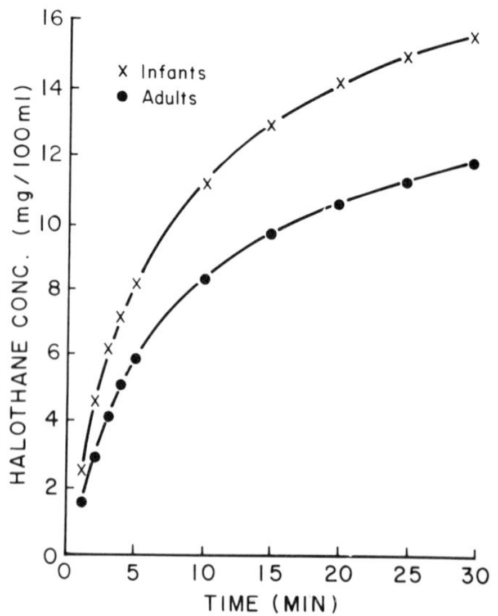

FIGURE 2–4. Predicted concentration of halothane in the heart. See Figure 2–3 for legend.

Early in an anesthetic induction the infant has a higher tissue concentration of anesthetic than the adult; at some relatively infinite time, both will have the same tissue concentrations, if one assumes the partition coefficients to be the same in infants and adults. Another way to state this difference is in terms of tissue time constants, $\dot{V}/Q$ (blood-tissue solubility coefficient times volume divided by tissue blood flow). Given the same concentration of anesthetic in arterial blood, the anesthetic concentration will increase more rapidly in a tissue with a shorter time constant. We derived tissue time constants for infants and adults using the anatomical and physiological assumptions of our model (Table 2–3). Time constants of infant tissues are less than the corresponding time constants in the adult. Although the volume of some vessel-rich tissues (brain) relative to total body weight is greater in the infant than in the adult, these tissues have so much more blood flow in the infant that their time constants are smaller than those in adults.

INFLUENCE OF INTRACARDIAC SHUNTS ON UPTAKE

Intracardiac shunts can alter the uptake of inhalation anesthetics.[54, 55] Their influence is more pronounced with relatively insoluble agents. A right-to-left shunt slows the uptake of anesthetic as the anesthetic tension or concentration in the arterial blood increases more slowly. Induction of anesthesia is prolonged. Using overpressure to achieve a more rapid induction in infants with significant right-to-left shunts from congenital heart disease can be hazardous. If significant cardiovascular depression occurs from a relative anesthetic overdose, it is equally difficult to decrease the anesthetic concentration. The influence of a left-to-right shunt on anesthetic uptake depends on the size of the shunt and on whether a right-to-left shunt exists. A large (greater than 78 percent) left-to-right shunt increases the rate of anesthetic trans-

Table 2–3. TIME CONSTANTS (MINUTES)

	Adult	Infant
Brain	3.4	2.2
Heart	2.3	1.4
Splanchnic	5.0	2.5
Kidney	0.35	0.30
Muscle	49.0	8.4
Fat	2000.0	540.0

Tissue time constants = $\lambda\ \dot{V}/Q$. (See text.)

fer from the lungs to the arterial blood; smaller shunts (less than 50 percent) have a neglible effect on uptake. A left-to-right shunt may speed induction when it coexists with a large right-to-left shunt. Increases in pulmonary vascular resistance or decreases in systemic vascular resistance occasionally can reverse left-to-right shunts.

ANESTHETIC REQUIREMENTS

The anesthetic requirements for various inhalation anesthetics (cyclopropane, halothane, and enflurane) generally are related inversely to age.[56-60] Anesthetic requirements are usually quantified by the alveolar concentration of anesthetic at which 50 percent of the patients move (or do not move) in response to a surgical stimulus (minimum alveolar concentration, MAC). Alternatively, one can estimate MAC for an individual patient as an intermediate concentration between a concentration associated with movement and a concentration associated with no movement. The MAC, or median effective dose (ED_{50}), for halothane in infants and children has been determined by several groups of investigators.

In the first months of life, the relation between age and MAC is somewhat complex. During the first week of life the response of the neonate to pain is attenuated even in the awake state. During the first few months of life, both the sensitivity to pain and the behavioral response to pain rapidly mature. Gregory and associates noted that the MAC for halothane is lower in the fetal lamb than in the newborn lamb; in addition, the MAC for halothane increased over the first 12 hours of life in the newborn lambs.[60] The increase in MAC in the newborn lambs was associated with a decrease in serum progesterone. At pharmacological doses, progesterone is an anesthetic in the rat. No causal relationship exists.[61] Increased metabolic rate and oxygen consumption after birth may also contribute to the increase in anesthetic requirements. Increased plasma peptide concentrations have been documented in neonates during the immediate postnatal period; in the first month of life these concentrations decrease to adult concentrations.[62] In adults, peptides do not cross the blood-brain barrier. In neonates, one could postulate increased permeability of the blood-brain barrier to these peptides, although cerebrospinal fluid concentrations have not been documented. However, Gregory and colleagues could not reverse the early "analgesia" in newborn lambs with naloxone.[60]

Equally as perplexing as the progressive increase in MAC through the first month or so of life is the gradual and progressive decrease after 6 months. Is this related to changes in oxygen consumption, is it related to differences in anesthetic solubilities, or is it a conundrum of definition?

MAC is an indirect measurement of the anesthetic partial pressure at the anesthetic sites of action. At equilibrium, the partial pressure of anesthetic is equal in all tissue compartments of the body. However, the tissue concentration (mg/100 g tissue) of anesthetic will vary with the solubility of the anesthetic in that tissue. Miller and associates have suggested that a certain anesthetic molar concentration at the sites of action is necessary to produce anesthesia.[63] The molar concentration of anesthesia at the site of action is the product of the anesthetic partial pressure and the anesthetic solubility at the site. Measuring of anesthetic concentration in the brain allows one to estimate the molar concentration required in the brain to produce anesthesia. Cook and colleagues noted that the ED_{50} for halothane was higher in 15-day-old rats than in 30- or 60-day-old rats.[53] In contrast, the concentration of halothane in the brain under anesthesia was lower in the 15-day-old rats than in the older rats. This difference in brain concentration for halothane as a function of age is most likely due to the difference in water content in the younger rats. When corrected for differences in water content, the estimated halothane concentrations in brain dry weight appear comparable in the three age groups of rats. This suggests that nearly equal concentrations of halothane in the nonaqueous phase of the brain are achieved at the end-point of anesthesia in different-aged animals. A higher partial pressure of anesthetic (ED_{50}, or MAC) may be necessary in the younger animal to compensate for the high water content of the developing brain.

Age-related differences in blood gas solubility coefficients also may influence the brain anesthetic concentration and hence contribute to age-related differences in MAC. B.W. Brandom examined this issue using our model of anesthetic distribution (unpublished data). She altered the blood gas solubility coefficient of halothane while holding all other physiological variables constant, to assess the effect of this change on brain anesthetic concentrations. With a blood-gas solubility coefficient of 2.3, the FE/FI ratio was 0.813 after 45 minutes of exposure to 0.5 percent halothane; the corresponding estimate of brain halothane concentration was 15.6 mg/dl. With a solubility coefficient of 1.9, that measured in neonatal cord blood, the FE/FI ratio was 0.843 after 45 minutes; the corresponding brain halothane concentration was 13.2 mg/dl. The decrease in blood-gas solubility coefficient caused a more rapid increase in FE/FI and a slower increase in tissue anesthetic concentration. FE/FI was 3 percent higher with the less soluble anesthetic, but the associated brain concentration was 17 percent lower. These data suggest that changes in blood gas solubility may contribute to age-dependent differences in the movement of anesthetic through the body to the brain, and hence to age-dependent differences in anesthetic requirements.

CARDIOVASCULAR EFFECTS OF INHALATION ANESTHETICS

The incidence of bradycardia, hypotension, and cardiac arrest during induction of anesthesia is higher in infants and small children than in adults.[58, 64–66] This has been attributed to an increased sensitivity of the cardiovascular system to potent agents. Rao and associates noted that halothane, isoflurane, and enflurane depress the force of contraction in isolated neonatal rat atria significantly more than in adult atria.[67] This may be related to the decreased contractile element in the neonatal myocardium. However, the greater incidence of untoward effects can be attributed partly to differences in uptake and to the use of higher than necessary inspired concentrations of potent agents. The myocardial and brain concentration of anesthetic at equal inspired concentrations may be higher early in anesthetic induction in the infant than in the adult. These higher tissue concentrations may produce what appears to be augmented cardiovascular effect.

To define clearly the issue of age-related cardiovascular sensitivity, it is necessary to measure simultaneously the determinants of cardiac output in anesthetized patients (or animals), at known end-tidal concentrations of anesthetic and at known MAC multiples. In addition, it is necessary to define the sensitivity of cardiovascular "protective" reflexes (baroreceptor reflex) at MAC multiples of the anesthetic. Direct measurement of cardiac output, contractility, preload, and afterload involves invasive techniques. Few patient studies have been done, but the results of several key animal studies are available.

The hemodynamic effects of halothane have been determined in the developing piglet.[68] MAC for halothane in piglets (aged 1 to 11 days) was 0.87 percent (range: 0.73 to 0.99 percent). Cardiac index, mean arterial pressure, heart rate, and all contractility indexes (LV peak dP/dT, SF, and VCF) decreased relative to concentration after 0.5 percent and 1 percent halothane (Table 2–4). When heart rate was kept constant with atrial pacing, $dP/dT/DP_{40}$ (diastolic pressure of 40), cardiac index, and mean arterial pressure remained severely depressed at the two concentrations of halothane. Estimates of preload, stroke volume index, and total peripheral vascular index did not change significantly. Thus, the major adverse hemodynamic effect of halothane was its negative inotropic action, not negative chronotropic or loading activity. This effect occurred at a concentration less than MAC. These cardiovascular changes were not age-related.

In piglets studied by Bailie and associates, profound bradycardia and hypotension were associated with an unexplained increase in peripheral resistance.[69] The change in cardiovascular response to halothane with age in the piglet is similar to that in newborn infants and children. In our study, the degree of change of each variable with the administration of 1 percent halothane did not correlate with age over the first 2.5 weeks of life. However, the pattern of cardiovascular response to halothane in pigs appears to change with increasing age beyond this period. At equal end-tidal halothane concentrations supplemented by 60 to 70 percent nitrous oxide, 3-month-old pigs (21 to 28 kg) studied by Merin and colleagues had a depression of cardiac index comparable to that observed in our younger animals.[70] However, mean aortic pressure was considerably lower in the older animal study than in ours and was accompanied by peripheral vasodilation and marked reduction in dP/dT. Our newborn piglets had less profound reductions in CI, MAP, and dP/dT and no important change in peripheral resistance. We note that bradycardia occurred regularly only in the newborn piglets. These differences in heart rate (HR) among pigs of different ages under halothane anesthesia were probably due to the more highly developed baroreceptor responses of the older animals.[71] Recently, Lerman and associates found that at equipotent concentrations of halothane, the incidence of hypotension and bradycardia was equal in neonates and infants.[59] These data agree with our findings that the maximal degrees of change in MAP and HR did not correlate significantly with age.

Table 2–4. HEMODYNAMIC VALUES FOR END-TIDAL HALOTHANE IN PIGLETS

Variable	Control	0.5%	1%	0.5%	0%
MAP (mm Hg)	96.2 (21.2)	81.0 (17.4)	63.5 (20.3)	78.8 (18.0)	88.5 (15.5)
CI (L/min/kg)	0.288 (0.098)	0.237 (0.054)	0.205 (0.056)	0.264 (0.073)	0.293 (0.086)
dP/dT (mm Hg/sec)	3640 (860)	2480 (800)	1560 (600)	2260 (720)	3500 (920)
SF	0.45 (0.11)	0.30 (0.15)	0.21 (0.10)	0.21 (0.11)	0.35 (0.09)
VCF (circ/sec)	3.40 (1.35)	2.32 (0.73)	1.51 (0.86)	1.76 (0.64)	2.93 (0.93)
LVEDP (mm Hg)	4.1 (3.5)	4.9 (3.2)	6.6 (4.4)	5.0 (4.3)	4.4 (3.6)
LVIDd (cm)	1.49 (0.36)	1.46 (0.32)	1.63 (0.37)	1.63 (0.31)	1.45 (0.44)
HR (beats/min)	215 (41)	185 (40)	156 (33)	186 (51)	229 (54)
SVI (ml/beat/kg)	1.39 (0.54)	1.13 (0.61)	1.24 (0.51)	1.32 (0.78)	1.39 (0.64)
TPRI (mm Hg/L/min/kg)	0.364 (0.133)	0.357 (0.097)	0.323 (0.094)	0.317 (0.114)	0.328 (0.112)

Values are means ± 1 standard deviation.
MAP = mean aortic pressure; CI = cardiac index; dP/dT = maximum first derivative of left ventricular (LV) pressure with respect to time; SF = LV shortening fraction; VCF = mean rate of LV circumferential fiber shortening; LVEDP = LV end-diastolic pressure; LVIDd = LV internal diastolic dimension; HR = heart rate; SVI = stroke volume index; TPRI = total peripheral resistance index.
Variables were obtained at end-tidal halothane values ascending to 1 percent and then returning to 0 percent.

In a similar study by my group, the MAC for isoflurane in piglets was determined to be 1.20 percent ± 0.4 percent (unpublished data). At 0.5 MAC, isoflurane caused a large, significant reduction in MAP, total peripheral resistance index (TPRI), and dP/dT/DP_{40} (Table 2–5). At 1 MAC, MAP and dP/dT/DP_{40} decreased further, and TPRI and SF remained depressed. At 1.3 MAC, these four variables remained low. Preload (LVEDP) and SVI did not change significantly during the study period. CI and HR were significantly less than baseline only at 1.3 MAC, although bradycardia did not occur in all animals. We used atrial pacing at baseline HR in 5 piglets who developed bradycardia at 1.3 MAC, to determine the influence of HR on the other variables. CI then remained within 2 percent of baseline, while MAP and TPRI each decreased 49 percent and dP/dT/DP40 decreased 45 percent from baseline values. The large decrease in MAP at 1 MAC isoflurane was offset by a similar decrease in afterload, leaving CI unchanged. During pacing, dP/dT/DP40 is a particularly reliable indicator of LV contractility, since it is independent of changes in HR, preload, and afterload. The large reduction in afterload also may have partly offset the effect of reduced contractility on CI. However, the reduced MAP should have caused tachycardia via the baroreceptor response. The lack of tachycardia signifies either an immature baroreflex or a drug-induced attenuation of baroreceptor responsiveness.

Isoflurane had fewer adverse cardiovascular effects than 1.3 MAC halothane in the same animal model. Although the drugs similarly reduced dP/dT and HR at 1.3 MAC, isoflurane reduced TPRI three times as much and MAP 1.5 times as much as did halothane; the resulting reduction in CI with isoflurane was thus only half that with halothane. At 0.5 MAC, isoflurane increased CI, whereas halothane reduced it. During newborn anesthesia, isoflurane may permit greater hemodynamic stability than halothane. The alarming reduction in MAP caused by isoflurane may reflect only a decrease in peripheral resistance in the face of normal cardiac output.

Desflurane, a new, potent inhalational anesthetic agent, is currently undergoing clinical trials. Desflurane has a blood gas solubility of 0.46, an oil gas coefficient of 18.7, and a boiling point of about 20°C. Consequently, it requires a pressurized, heated vaporizer for delivery of anesthetic gases. In healthy adults, the minimal alveolar concentration is between 6 and 7. On exposure to soda lime, desflurane is markedly stable and undergoes negligible metabolism or degradation.[72] In children, Taylor and Lerman[73] have noted age-related changes in MAC that are similar to those of the other potent inhalational agents. Studies in pediatric patients are

Table 2–5. HEMODYNAMIC VALUES FOR ISOFLURANE

	Baseline	0.5 MAC	1 MAC	1.3 MAC
CI (L/min/kg)	0.263 (0.039)	0.293 (0.051) + 11%	0.251 (0.039) − 5%	0.225 (0.042) − 14%
MAP (mm Hg)	120 (23)	92 (20) − 23%	76 (16) − 37%	66 (15) − 45%
HR (beats/min)	194 (43)	187 (41) −4%	164 (22) − 15%	157 (24) − 19%
dP/dT (mm Hg/sec)	3457 (843)	2360 (577) − 33%	1827 (328) − 48%	1573 (433) − 56%
dP/dT/DP40 (mm Hg/sec)	2560 (519)	2040 (448) −20%	1733 (327) −32%	1480 (319) −42%
SF (%)	40 (10)	35 (8) −13%	32 (9) −20%	28 (7) −30%
TPRI (mm Hg/L/min/kg)	.444 (.137)	.314 (.77) −29%	.303 (.79) −32%	.298 (.73) −33%
SVI (ml/beat/kg)	1.5 (0.5)	1.7 (0.4) −13%	1.7 (0.4) −13%	1.6 (0.3) −7%
LVEDP (mm Hg)	4.0 (3.4)	2.9 (2.8)	4.7 (1.7)	4.5 (1.8)

Abbreviations as in Table 2–4.

limited. Although hemodynamic stability appears maintained with desflurane, coughing and laryngospasm upon induction of anesthesia are major problems. Clinical experience suggests that these side effects will significantly delay the onset of anesthesia regardless of the low solubility of the gas.

Little information is available on the cardiovascular effects of desflurane in humans. In swine, the cardiovascular effects of desflurane appear similar to the effects of isoflurane.[74] In humans, desflurane appears to decrease mean arterial blood pressure and vascular resistance more than isoflurane. At concentrations of less than 1.5 MAC, desflurane maintained cardiac output by increasing heart rate.[75] In chronically instrumented dogs with multivessel coronary artery obstruction, desflurane does not appear to redistribute coronary blood flow away from collateral-dependent myocardium.[76]

Effects of Anesthetics on Baroreceptor Reflexes

Baroreceptor reflexes modulate changes in blood pressure by altering heart rate, myocardial contractility, and systemic vascular resistance. In the unanesthetized infant, particularly the premature infant, these protective reflexes may be limited. Anesthetic agents may further blunt these reflexes. To evaluate baroresponses, Gregory examined the relationship among changes in heart rate and blood pressure in premature infants anesthetized with halothane for ligation of a patent ductus arteriosus.[77] After the ductus was ligated and systemic blood flow increased, the arterial pressure had increased 38 percent (to about control values) without a change in heart rate. These data suggest that potent anesthetics abolish baroreceptor activity in premature infants.

In subsequent studies, the effect of halothane and nitrous oxide on the baroresponse in adult and baby rabbits was evaluated.[78, 79] In these studies, the baroreceptor response was tested by increasing the systolic pressure 20 percent to 30 percent with phenylephrine. When the baroreflexes are functioning, this increase in systolic pressure decreases heart rate (Fig. 2–5). The slope of the heart rate vs. systolic pressure curve, a reflection of baroreflex sensitivity, was decreased in adults and babies with halothane in a concentration-, or dose-, dependent manner (Table 2–6). More importantly, the sensitivity of the reflex was lower in the awake baby rabbits than in the awake adults, as it was at equal MAC multiples of halothane. Halothane (1.0 MAC) effectively abolished the baroresponse in baby rabbits. In the newborn rabbit, nitrous oxide also diminishes baroreceptor activity in a concentration-dependent manner, to the same degree as does halothane (at equal MAC multiples).

The reasons why anesthesia depresses the baroreceptor reflexes more in baby rabbits are unknown. Most likely they are related to developmental differences in the autonomic nervous system. Baroresponses may be mediated in part by acute changes in plasma catecholamines. Young animals have significant amounts of norepinephrine in their adrenergic terminals, but the nerves fail to arborize and incompletely penetrate the myocardium. In addition, the vascular response to vasopressors is also less in the neonate than in the adult. The baroresponse included a reduction in sympathetic outflow. Since the neonate's sympathetic nervous system is inadequately developed, an increase in systolic pressure may not permit the heart rate to decrease as much. The parasympathetic nervous system is very active in the neonate.

The lack of responsiveness of the baroreflexes places the infant at considerable disadvantage

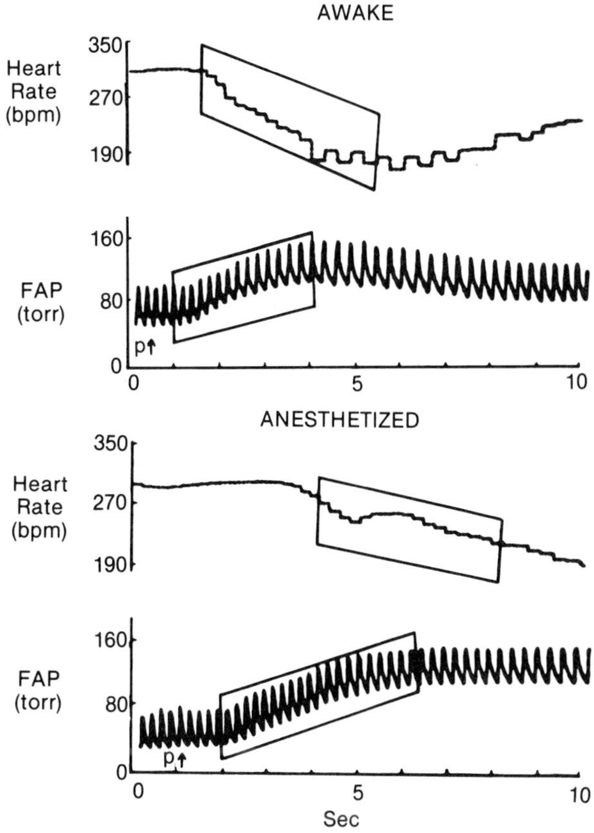

FIGURE 2–5. Relationship between heart rate and arterial pressure (FAP) in a baby rabbit. P ↑ indicates the point at which phenylephrine was injected. With the rabbit awake, the heart rate began to decrease within three beats after the initial rise in arterial pressure. During anesthesia the decrease in heart rate occurred later (after nine beats). The time from the onset of the rise in pressure to the onset of the decrease in heart rate is defined as the lag time.

during anesthesia with potent inhalation anesthetics. For reasons previously discussed, the incidence of hypotension and bradycardia is high in this age group.

Margin of Safety

The separation between MAC and the lethal concentration of a potent inhalation anesthetic defines the safety margin or therapeutic ratio. Wolfson and associates determined the therapeutic ratio (TR) of the potent anesthetic in adult rats:

$$TR = \frac{\text{mean anesthetic heart concentration at cardiovascular failure}}{\text{mean anesthetic heart concentration at anesthesia}}$$

In their study, isoflurane had a higher therapeutic ratio than did halothane.[80, 81] Kissen and colleagues confirmed this and in addition noted

Table 2–6. RELATIONSHIP BETWEEN HALOTHANE AND BARORECEPTOR RESPONSE

	Slope of Heart Rate vs. Systolic Pressure (MS/mm Hg)		Log Time (S)	
	Baby	***Adult***	***Baby***	***Adult***
Awake	1.94 ± 0.27	2.90 ± 0.41	0.67 ± 0.25	0.75 ± 0.67
0.5 MAC	0.40 ± 0.21*	1.33 ± 0.28*	1.11 ± 0.26*†	1.19 ± 0.61*
1.0 MAC	0.23 ± 0.08*	1.05 ± 0.35*	1.75 ± 0.51*	1.50 ± 0.63*†
1.5 MAC	0.07 ± 0.08*†	0.60 ± 0.20*†	2.44 ± 0.44*†	1.87 ± 0.30*†

Values are means ± 1 standard deviation.
*Significantly different from values obtained when animals were awake ($p<0.001$).
†Significantly different from values obtained at 0.5 MAC halothane ($p<0.005$)

that the standard safety margin, the percentage by which the ED_{95} has to be increased before LD_{50} is reached, is also higher with isoflurane than with halothane.[82]

Cook and colleagues noted that the therapeutic ratio for halothane was decreased about 50 percent in young rats compared with older rats.[53] This study suggests that at higher anesthetic concentrations myocardial contractility and protective cardiovascular reflexes are not preserved in the infant. Recently, we determined that isoflurane and halothane have similar therapeutic ratios in the newborn piglet (2.5:1) (unpublished data).

BIOTRANSFORMATION OF INHALATION ANESTHETICS

Significant biotransformation of inhalation anesthetics occurs in the liver. The metabolites may be toxic to tissue. Carbon tetrachloride and chloroform are hepatotoxic in adult animals; however, they are not hepatotoxins in animals less than 1 to 2 weeks of age. In the newborn rat, the metabolism of halothane takes several weeks to reach adult levels. Serum bromine levels following halothane exposure are reported to be lower in infants and young children than in adults.[83] Free fluoride concentration, a nephrotoxic metabolite of methoxyflurane, is lower in infants and children.[84] Nephrotoxicity from free fluoride has, likewise, been reported after enflurane anesthesia in obese patients. This is unlikely in infants because of their limited fat deposits. Also, biotransformation of isoflurane is unlikely. Differences in the relative rates of metabolism of inhalation anesthetics in infants and adults have not been studied, nor has any determination been made of differences in intermediate metabolites.

INTRAVENOUS DRUGS

SEDATIVE-HYPNOTICS

A variety of sedative-hypnotic drugs appear to have increased toxic effects in the neonate.[85] The mechanism of this increased sensitivity has been elucidated for some of the barbiturates and benzodiazepines.

DIAZEPAM

Diazepam is a widely used sedative-hypnotic and anti-convulsant agent. Infants born of mothers who have had diazepam for sedation during labor have shown lethargy and impaired thermoregulation for several days. The probable reasons for this prolongation of effect are several. Brain levels of diazepam and *N*-demethyldiazepam, a metabolite, have been noted to be higher in newborn rats and guinea pigs for up to 180 minutes after subcutaneous administration. This higher brain concentration probably explains why diazepam also gives greater protection against metrazol convulsions in newborn rats and guinea pigs than in adult animals.[86]

The plasma half-life of diazepam varies with maturity. The ability of the liver to metabolize diazepam is reduced in neonates as compared with adults. A demethylated derivative of diazepam, *N*-demethyldiazepam, could not be measured in plasma in premature infants until 4 hours after injection, although its plasma concentration was still rising at 48 hours. In contrast, *N*-demethyldiazepam was measured in the plasma of older children by 1 hour and had peaked by 24 hours. In adults, 71 percent of diazepam or its metabolites was excreted in the urine and about 10 percent in the feces. Urinary excretion of diazepam has not been quantified in infants and children. Older children were shown to excrete a considerable amount of hydroxylated metabolites in urine; term infants, a limited amount; and premature infants, none. All three groups had trace amounts of diazepam and *N*-demethyldiazepam in the urine.[87]

The plasma half-life of diazepam and the nature of the diazepam metabolites formed vary with maturity.[87] The premature infant and the mature infant at term eliminate diazepam at a slower rate than do older infants, children, and adults. Also, in premature infants a demethylated derivative of diazepam, *N*-demethyldiazepam, could not be measured in plasma until 4 hours after injection; its plasma concentration was still rising at 48 hours. In contrast, *N*-demethyldiazepam was measured in the plasma of older infants and children by 1 hour and had peaked by 24 hours. In the premature infant, hydroxylated metabolites of diazepam did not form; in term infants they formed in limited amounts. In adults, 71 percent of diazepam or its metabolites was excreted in the urine and about 10 percent in the feces. No quantification of urinary excretion has been performed in infants or children.

MIDAZOLAM

Midazolam is a new, water-soluble, short-acting benzodiazepine.[87] Cardiovascular stability, transient mild respiratory depression, minimal venous irritation, antegrade amnesia, and short duration of action are all useful anesthetic properties of midazolam.[88-95] Anesthesia induction times following midazolam are comparable to those of diazepam. Midazolam is metabolized in the liver; less than 1 percent is excreted unchanged in the urine. The terminal elimination phase ranges from 1 to 4 hours.[96] Protein binding is extensive, with a free fraction of 3 to 6 percent. Following oral administration, midazolam has an intermediate rate of absorption (0.5 to 1.5 hours) and a bioavailability of 30 to 50 percent. In healthy patients there is no significant difference in hemodynamic effects between induction doses of 0.25 mg/kg of midazolam and 4 mg/kg of thiopental.[97] Midazolam can cause transient respiratory depression and apnea in some individuals and can also inhibit the ventilatory response to carbon dioxide.[93]

In children, midazolam has been used as an effective preanesthetic medication. In a double-blind study, Rita and associates have shown that intramuscular midazolam (0.8 mg/kg) was a better drug for preanesthetic sedation than morphine (0.15 mg/kg).[98] More recently, Feld and colleagues demonstrated in a randomized, double-blind, placebo-controlled study that orally administered midazolam (0.5 to 0.75 mg/kg) is an effective preanesthetic medication.[99] Another means of administering midazolam is transmucosally.

Following rectal administration, Saint-Maurice and associates reported that 0.35 mg/kg of midazolam produced a noticeable effect by 10 minutes but required 20 to 30 minutes for more reliable sedation.[100] Wilton and colleagues have shown that 0.2 mg/kg of intranasal midazolam can provide anxiolysis and sedation in preschool-aged children.[101]

Plasma concentrations following 0.1 mg/kg intravenous and intranasal administration of midazolam have been reported by Walbergh and group.[102] Intranasal midazolam achieved peak concentrations of 72.2 ng/ml ± 27.3 (mean ± SD) 10 minutes following administration. These peak plasma concentrations were 57 percent of that observed in the intravenous group after 10 minutes. In pediatric patients of similar age and weight undergoing closed or open cardiac surgical procedures, the pharmacokinetic profile of midazolam was determined following a single intravenous dose (in the group undergoing open heart procedures, midazolam was administered after cardiopulmonary bypass). There was no significant difference between these two groups with respect to half-life (2.8 ± 0.89 hr vs. 3.3 ± 0.53), clearance (719 ± 400 ml/kg/hr vs. 512 ± 108), or volume of distribution at steady state (1.89 ± 0.243 L/kg vs. 1.85 ± .283).[103] However, the half-life observed in the children with cardiac disease was longer than the values reported in healthy children (1.42 ± 0.49 hr) undergoing elective surgery with a variable anesthetic background.[104]

Barbiturates

On a milligram per kilogram basis, barbiturates are more lethal to neonatal than to more mature animals.[105-107] The sleeping times of newborn animals are markedly prolonged at sublethal doses given on an equal milligram per kilogram basis.[107] Greater penetration of the blood-brain barrier by barbiturates has been found in neonates as opposed to older animals.[108] We have recently determined the brain uptake index (BUI) at 15 seconds for pentobarbital in developing rats (Table 2–7). BUI was higher in the younger rats and exceeded 100 percent. These data suggest that capillary transit time is less than 15 seconds in younger rats. High brain blood flow rather than differential permeability probably explains these observations for pentobarbital, which is highly lipid soluble. In addition, the brain levels of hexobarbital on arousal or following death from respiratory failure are lower in neonates than in adults. This suggests that the barbiturates are more potent in the neonatal brain.

Neonates have a decreased ability to metabolize barbiturates.[109] The longer-acting barbiturates, which are in part excreted unmetabolized in the urine, would be expected to have prolonged or elevated blood levels.[110, 111] Glucuronic acid conjugation of barbiturates develops rapidly and increases thirtyfold during the first 3 weeks of life.[40] For the ultrashort-acting barbiturates, redistribution is as important as metabolism in the liver in lowering the brain concentration.[112] Blood concentrations of thiopentone

Table 2–7. AGE-RELATED CHANGES IN BRAIN UPTAKE OF MORPHINE AND PENTOBARBITAL

Age (Days)	Brain Uptake Index (%)		Brain Water Content (%)
	Morphine	*Pentobarbital*	
7	36.2 ± 3.5	213.3 ± 20.6	87.9 ± 0.05
15	17.2 ± 3.2	78.0 ± 1.5	84.1 ± 0.1
30	7.4 ± 0.8	61.2 ± 5.0	79.6 ± 0.1
60	5.6 ± 1.3	44.0 ± 3.0	78.0 ± 0.1

Mean ± standard error.

decrease about as rapidly in neonates as in their mothers.[113] The use of these ultrashort-acting barbiturates for induction of anesthesia is, therefore, not a pharmacological problem, although the lack of a suitable intravenous route is often a practical deterrent.

PROPOFOL

Propofol, a rapidly acting hypnotic agent with no analgesic properties, is now being reconstituted in 10 percent intralipid to avoid anaphylactoid hypersensitivity reactions.[114] Its rapid redistribution and metabolism make for a short duration of action and allow for repeat injections or continuous infusions without any accumulation of drug.[115, 116] Induction time is dependent on dose and speed of injection.[117] Propofol compares favorably with althesin in smoothness of induction and lack of excitatory side effects.[118] Continuous infusion regimens both with and without use of nitrous oxide have been developed.[119–121] Following 2 mg/kg induction doses, Al-Khudhairi and colleagues noted a 19 percent increase in heart rate, a 23 percent decrease in mean arterial pressure, a 19 percent decrease in systemic vascular resistance, and a 26 percent decrease in stroke volume, with no change in the cardiac output.[122] Propofol causes minimal respiratory depression following induction doses.

Little information on propofol in children is available. Hannallah and associates noted in children that the ED_{50} and ED_{95} for loss of eyelash reflex were 1.3 and 2.0 mg/kg, and the ED_{50} and ED_{95} for acceptance of a face mask were 1.5 and 2.3 mg/kg.[123] In this study, blood pressure decreased by 20 percent in 48 percent of the children who received 1 to 3 percent halothane following the propofol infusion. In a study comparing bolus and continuous infusion of propofol to thiopental bolus followed by halothane maintenance, Borgeat and colleagues noted that children receiving propofol had significantly shorter times to extubation, shorter times to discharge, and fewer side effects (nausea, vomiting, and agitation were less than those in the thiopental/halothane-anesthetized children).[124] Following the bolus of propofol, arterial pressure decreased 14 percent, similar to the decline following thiopental. Similar hemodynamic results have been demonstrated by Valtonen et al.[125]

The pharmacokinetics of propofol in children have also been characterized by Valtonen and group.[125] The final elimination phase, the volumes of distribution, and the clearance volumes were similar to values obtained in adults. As with adult studies, the clearance values of propofol observed in children surpass hepatic blood flow. Therefore, extrahepatic sites of metabolism probably are involved with propofol metabolism and elimination.

KETAMINE

Ketamine is a nonbarbiturate cyclohexamine derivative that produces dissociation of the cortex from the limbic system; it may also act on the brain stem. There is frequently electroencephalographic seizure activity, particularly in the limbic system and cortex, without clinical manifestations. This may be the mechanism of its action. On a microgram per kilogram basis, the amount of ketamine required to prevent gross movements is four times greater in infants under 6 months than in 6-year-olds.[126] Acute studies show little metabolism of ketamine by the newborn infant.[127]

Waterman and Livingston noted that after ketamine the sleeping times of rats decreased with increasing age; the onset time of sleep was significantly shorter in younger rats than in older ones.[128] The demethylated metabolite of ketamine was present at recovery from anesthesia in 1-week-old rats; the oxidated metabolite was not present until 2 to 4 weeks of age. A dramatic decrease in sleeping time after ketamine was associated with the appearance of the oxidated metabolite.

Recently we determined the pharmacokinetics of ketamine in different-aged patients (Table 2–8). In infants less than 3 months of age, the volume of distribution was similar to that in older infants, but the elimination half-life was prolonged. Hence, clearance was reduced in the younger infants. Reduced metabolism and renal excretion in the young infant are the likely causes.

In the "anesthetic" state associated with ketamine, respiration and blood pressure are

Table 2–8. PHARMACOKINETICS OF KETAMINE AS A FUNCTION OF AGE

Age	β	AUC (μg/kg/min)	Cl (ml/min/kg)	Vd (L/kg)	t½ β min
< 3 months	0.004	153.8	12.9	3.46	184.7
4–12 months	0.012	58.7	35.0	3.03	65.1
4 years	0.023	83.6	25.1	1.18	31.6
Adults	0.315	99.0	20.0	0.75	107.3

AUC = area under the curve; Cl = clearance, Vd = volume of distribution.

usually well maintained. However, use of ketamine in infants, particularly at the high doses required for lack of movement, has been associated with respiratory depression and apnea.[129] Generalized extensor spasm with opisthotonos also has been seen in infants.[130] Intracranial pressure may increase in infants with hydrocephalus.[131] In addition, acute increases in pulmonary artery pressure occasionally have been seen in an infant with congenital heart disease when ketamine was used as an anesthetic for cardiac catheterization.[132] Recent studies suggest that pulmonary vascular resistance is not changed by ketamine in infants with either normal or elevated pulmonary vascular resistance as long as the airway and ventilation are maintained.[133, 134]

Morphine and Meperidine

Meperidine (0.5 to 1 mg/kg) and morphine (0.05 to 0.1 mg/kg) are used to reinforce nitrous oxide–oxygen anesthesia in the neonate. Such low doses attenuate the cardiovascular responses to surgical stress. In the past, high-dose meperidine and morphine anesthesia was given with oxygen-air to critically ill infants, particularly those requiring palliative heart surgery. The cardiovascular effects of these narcotics seemed minimal.

Narcotics are more toxic to newborn animals than to older animals.[84] In neonates, morphine depresses respiration more than meperidine does, at a ratio of 1:10; in adults, 10 mg of morphine produces respiratory depression equal to that from 100 mg of meperidine.[135] The blood-brain barrier is more permeable to morphine and dihydromorphinone in newborn animals than in older animals. Brain concentration of morphine several hours after injection was two to four times greater in brains of younger rats despite equal blood concentration. This finding may be related to greater perfusion or greater permeability or both in the newborn infant. We recently determined the brain uptake index (BUI) for morphine in developing rats (Table 2–7). The BUI was higher in younger rats than in older rats. Such developmentally increased permeability is not seen with meperidine.[136] This is not surprising since the lipid solubility of meperidine is quite high.

Morphine is inactivated by *N*-demethylation and glucuronide conjugation; the inactive forms are largely excreted in the urine. In spite of the inefficient metabolism of morphine, there is little difference in the plasma half-life of morphine between newborn and older animals.[137] Meperidine in inactive forms is also largely excreted. De-esterification and *N*-demethylation occur mainly in the liver. In adults, the rate of transformation ranges from 10 to 20 percent per hour.[41] In newborn animals the plasma half-life of meperidine is about twice that of the adult. Neonates excrete 25 to 40 percent of a dose of meperidine in about 48 hours, almost exclusively in the demethylated form.[137]

Fentanyl

Fentanyl (3 to 5 μg/kg) is used to reinforce nitrous oxide–oxygen anesthesia in the neonate; high-dose fentanyl (25 to 50 gmg/kg) is popular as the primary anesthetic in infants undergoing cardiac anesthesia. Bradycardia and chest wall rigidity are potential features of high-dose fentanyl anesthesia. For these reasons it is common to administer muscle relaxants with wanted cardiovascular side effects (i.e., pancuronium or gallamine) to ameliorate the effects of fentanyl. The cardiovascular effects of fentanyl at doses of 30 to 75 μg/kg (with pancuronium) are minimal.[138] Modest decreases in mean arterial pressure and systemic vascular resistance index were noted by Hickey and group.[139] Other indexes of cardiac function were unchanged. Schieber and associates documented that the cardiovascular effects of fentanyl (without relaxant) are concentration dependent;[140] a similar relationship between decreases in systolic blood pressure and concentration was noted by Koren and colleagues.[141] Respiratory depression is likely concentration related.

The dose of fentanyl needed to guarantee satisfactory anesthesia for infants is unknown. The dose of fentanyl needed to guarantee adequate anesthesia depends on the type and duration of surgery. Yaster has noted that in neonates undergoing several types of surgery, fentanyl in initial doses of 10 to 12.5 μg/kg provided adequate anesthesia (as defined by changes in heart rate and blood pressure) for 75 minutes.[142] Ellis and Steward have reported that in children undergoing hypothermic cardiopulmonary bypass and limited exogenous dextrose infusions who were anesthetized with greater than 50 μg/kg of fentanyl had blood glucose concentrations that were less than 200 mg/dl.[143] Age-related differences in the kinetics and sensitivity to fentanyl and changes in kinetics associated with profound pathophysiological conditions make generalizations difficult.[144–147] In neonates, the volume of distribution is longer, the elimination half-life longer, and the clearance comparable or faster compared with pharmacokinetic parameters in adults. In premature infants undergoing patent ductus arteriosus ligation, Collins and colleagues have noted the elimination half-life of fentanyl to be markedly prolonged, ranging in time from 6 to 32 hours.[148] In addition to age-related pharmacokinetic changes, the disease process may influence fentanyl pharmacology. Koehntop and colleagues, in a study of neonates undergoing various types of surgery, noted that in neonates with increased intra-abdominal pressure fentanyl half-life was markedly prolonged.[149] In a study of children undergoing repair of congenital heart disease, changes in fentanyl volume of distribution depended on the severity of the hemodynamic disturbance, whereas changes in drug clearance were a function of patient age.[150]

In addition to intravenous routes of administration, fentanyl can also be administered transmucosally. In healthy pediatric patients, oral transmucosal fentanyl citrate (OTFC) in doses of 15 to 20 μg/kg has been shown to be a safe and efficacious means of delivering preanesthetic medication.[99, 151, 152] However, in patients with congenital heart disease, Goldstein Dresner and associates noted that when compared with a standard oral premedication of atropine, demerol, and diazepam, higher doses of OTFC (20 to 25 μg/kg) resulted in similar emotional status scores at the time of parental separation and anesthetic induction, but OTFC was associated with significantly more side effects, namely, preoperative emesis and pruritus.[153]

SUFENTANIL

Sufentanil, a new potent synthetic opioid, is an N-4 substituted derivative of fentanyl. It is a highly lipophilic compound that is distributed rapidly and extensively to all tissues. Sufentanil is approximately five to ten times more potent than fentanyl and has an extremely high margin of safety. The median lethal to median effective dose (LD_{50}:ED_{50}) is about 10:1.[154] Dogs have survived intravenous doses of 5 mg/kg without respiratory assistance. Infusions of 40 μg/kg in mechanically ventilated animals given atropine produced few hemodynamic changes.[155] Little is known about the effects of sufentanil on human cerebral metabolism, cerebral blood flow, and intracranial pressure. The major pathways for sufentanil metabolism involve *O*-demethylation and *N*-dealkylation; minimal amounts are excreted unchanged in urine.

Pharmacokinetic and pharmacodynamic studies of sufentanil have been conducted in infants, children, and adults. In adults, compared with fentanyl, sufentanil's smaller volume of distribution (2.48 L/kg) and high clearance rate (11.3 ml/kg/min) contribute to its short terminal elimination half-life (149 min). Meuldermans and coworkers demonstrated that sufentanil is more protein bound (92 percent) than fentanyl (84 percent) and that pH affects protein binding.[156] Decreasing pH from 7.4 to 7.0 increased protein binding by 28 percent; conversely, increasing pH from 7.4 to 7.8 decreased protein binding by 28 percent. The shorter elimination half-life of sufentanil should allow for a shorter duration of action. Clinical studies by deLang and Howie and colleagues,[157, 158] using recovery times or time to extubation, have not demonstrated significant clinical differences between sufentanil and fentanil, whereas studies by Smith and coworkers[159] support shorter periods of postoperative ventilation in patients treated with sufentanil.

Clinical studies assessing the hemodynamic and endocrine stress response of sufentanil have been conducted in patients undergoing cardiopulmonary bypass. In patients maintained on high-dose beta-adrenergic blocking agents and with good left ventricular function, sufentanil produced no significant hemodynamic changes.[157, 160, 161] Bovill and colleagues, comparing comparable doses of fentanyl and sufentanil, found that the incidence of hypertension necessitating vasodilator therapy was less in the patients anesthetized with sufentanil.[162] If hypertension did occur, supplemental doses of sufentanil were more effective in blood pressure control than equipotent doses of fentanyl.[157] However, in a double-blind study Rosow and group found the drugs to be comparable with regard to hemodynamic stability.[163] The neuroendocrine response in patients undergoing cardiothoracic surgery has been evaluated following sufentanil infusions[161, 164] and is variable. Sufentanil appears to block some of the stress responses to cardiac surgery. Stress-induced increases in antidiuretic hormone (ADH) and growth hormone (GH) appear to be blocked before, during, and after cardiopulmonary bypass, while the catecholamines (norepinephrine, epinephrine and dopamine) show a large surge during the bypass and postbypass periods.

The pharmacodynamic and pharmacokinetic effects of sufentanil in children are relatively unknown. Hickey and Hansen compared the hemodynamic responses of 5 and 10 μg/kg of sufentanil to 50 to 75 μg/kg of fentanyl in patients with complex congenital heart disease.[165] Although heart rate and blood pressure changed slightly, they noted marked improvement in the patient's oxygenation with both fentanyl and sufentanil. They concluded that both sufentanil and fentanyl were safe anesthetics in high doses and that both agents favorably decreased pulmonary vascular resistance and thereby increased pulmonary blood flow and systemic oxygenation in patients with cyanotic heart disease.[165] Henderson and colleagues examined both the pharmacodynamics and pharmacokinetics of high-dose sufentanil (15 μg/kg) and oxygen in infants and children undergoing cardiac surgery.[166] Sufentanil provided marked hemodynamic stability after an infusion and during the stress periods of incision and sternotomy. The hemodynamic responses to sufentanil were similar to those noted by Hickey and Hansen.[165] The pharmacokinetic data best fit a two-compartment model. In infants younger than 10 months and children older than 10 months who were not surface cooled, elimination half-lives were similar, as were clearance values. However, the volume of distribution was significantly smaller in the infants compared with the older children. In infants younger than 10 months who were surface cooled, elimination half-life was longer and the volume of distribution larger, but the clearance rate was similar compared with age- and weight-matched infants.

As with fentanyl, transmucosal administration of sufentanil has also been reported. Henderson and others have reported that in doses of 1.5 to 3.0 μg/kg, nasal sufentanil is an effective preanesthetic medication. However, in doses greater than 3.0 μg/kg, truncal rigidity with decreased ventilatory compliance occurs, thereby decreasing the usefulness of the drug.[166] Helmers and associates studied the pharmacodynamics and plasma decay curves of intravenous and nasal sufentanil.[167] In this study, the onset of sedation was rapid in both groups but more so with the intravenous group. After 20 minutes, the degree of sedation was similar in both groups. After 30 minutes, the plasma concentrations were identical regardless of the route of administration.

ALFENTANIL

Alfentanil, a new, potent ultrashort-acting analogue of fentanyl, is rapidly distributed to brain and central organs and then rapidly redistributed to more remote sites. It is about one fourth as potent as fentanyl and has one third the duration of action. It is a safe drug; the $LD_{50}:ED_{50}$ ratio is 1080.[168] Alfentanil's ultrashort duration of action, relative hemodynamic stability, and lack of cardiac depressant effect provide great flexibility in anesthetic management. The drug's decreased volume of distribution results in a significantly shorter elimination half-life. Its low lipid solubility allows less penetration of the blood-brain barrier. Thus, brain tissue concentration is markedly less than that of the plasma. The duration of narcotic effect appears to be governed by redistribution and elimination. These two mechanisms are influenced by dosage and method of infusion (bolus injection or constant infusion). The redistribution principle operates in small, single-dose infusions, whereas elimination determines the effect of a large single bolus, multiple small bolus infusions, or continuous infusions. Alfentanil is metabolized in the liver by oxidative *N*-dealkylation and *O*-demethylation. The pharmacologically inactive metabolites are excreted in the urine.[169]

Protein-binding has a significant influence on the pharmacokinetics of alfentanil. Protein binding is independent of alfentanil concentrations and is independent of changes in blood pH. Alfentanil is 88 to 95 percent protein bound in the plasma. The plasma protein most responsible for binding of alfentanil is alpha-1 acid glycoprotein. Changes in the binding and in the pharmacokinetics of alfentanil occur during and after cardiopulmonary bypass.[170] These changes have been associated with altered concentrations of alpha-1 acid glycoprotein. The pharmacokinetics of alfentanil have been studied in both pediatric and adult patients. In children, renal failure and cholestatic liver disease do not appear to affect alfentanil's pharmacokinetics.[171] Large interpatient variability with respect to alfentanil pharmacokinetics occurs in both children and adults. Little information is available on the developmental pharmacology of alfentanil. In children, the half-life of alfentanil appears faster than in adults. In the study by Meistelman and group comparing children with adults, the shorter half-life in children was influenced by the smaller volume of distribution;[172] in the study by Roure and colleagues, volumes of distribution were similar, but children had smaller clearance values than did adult patients.[173]

In studies of alfentanil in premature infants, Davis and associates demonstrated that newly born premature infants in the first 3 days of life had larger volumes of distribution, longer elimination half-lives, and smaller clearance rates compared with older children.[174] Killian and associates noted that there was no correlation of gestational age to the pharmacokinetic parameters of alfentanil.[175]

The pharmacodynamics of alfentanil have been extensively investigated in adults but not in infants and children.[176–178] McDonnell and coworkers have shown the ED_{50} and ED_{90} of unconsciousness to be III μg/kg and 164 μg/kg, respectively, in the unpremedicated healthy patient.[176] Nauta and colleagues found that the ED_{50} and ED_{90} could be reduced to 40 and 50 μg/kg in the patient premedicated with atropine and lorazepam.[177] Premedication also affects the drug's onset time. In patients premedicated with lorazepam, alfentanil has an onset time of 75 seconds, whereas in unpremedicated patients the onset time is 135 seconds.[177] In addition to a rapid onset time, recovery time from alfentanil infusions is rapid. Rapid recovery from alfentanil is felt to be a function of the drug's redistribution and elimination mechanics as well as its ability to dissociate from its opioid receptors in the central nervous system.[179]

As with other narcotics, alfentanil produces a shift to the right in the ventilatory response curve. Though this shift is dose dependent, the ventilatory depressant effects are dissipated by 30 to 50 minutes following the dose.[180, 181]

The cardiovascular effects of alfentanil have been assessed during both low- and high-dose infusions. In low-dose infusions (1.6 μg/kg and 6.4 μg/kg) administered at slow rates to healthy volunteers, no hemodynamic changes occurred.[180] In patients undergoing minor surgical procedures, Kay and Stephenson demonstrated the hemodynamic stability of low-dose alfentanil.[181] At higher doses of 150 μg/kg, heart rate, mean arterial pressure (MAP) and systemic vascular resistance (SVR) were noted to decrease. Pulmonary capillary wedge pressure, pulmonary vascular resistance, right atrial pressure, and pulmonary artery pressure increased slightly.[182] In other studies following induction with high-dose alfentanil, small, transient decreases in mean arterial pressure and systolic pressure occurred. These changes were not associated with changes in cardiac output or venous pressures. However, with the surgical stimulus of sternotomy, both arterial and central venous pressures increased.

The neuroendocrine stress response has been studied by Stanley[183] and deLange[184] and their coworkers. The ability of high-dose alfentanil to blunt the stress response is incomplete. In Stanley's study, high-dose alfentanil was found to blunt the stress response of growth hormone (GH), antidiuretic hormone (ADH), and cortisol before, during, and after bypass. In deLange's study, catecholamines (epinephrine and norepinephrine) were measured following high-dose alfentanil infusion. Plasma norepinephrine and epinephrine concentrations were unaltered until the bypass period. With the onset of bypass there was a marked elevation in their concentrations.

LOCAL ANESTHETICS

The rates of plasma decay for lidocaine and mepivacaine are similar in adults and newborn infants. However, the plasma levels of lidocaine and mepivacaine in the neonate that produce cardiovascular and respiratory depression are about one half those in adults.[137] The convulsive dose for infants on a milligram per kilogram basis of either ester-type (benzocaine) or amide-type (lidocaine) local anesthetics is not known. The rate of metabolism of the ester-type local anesthetics is decreased in the infant because pseudocholinesterase levels are low.[185] The neonate metabolizes lidocaine;[186] the rates of metabolism of the amide-type local anesthetics in the neonate are not known.[187, 188]

ATROPINE

Strong cholinergic stimulation, such as from cyclopropane, halothane, methoxyflurane, and succinylcholine, can produce profound bradycardia and reduce cardiac output in infants. The primary purpose of atropine in pediatric anesthesia is to protect against cholinergic challenge; its secondary purpose is to inhibit the production of secretions.

If atropine is given intravenously in incremental doses, more atropine is needed in children less than 2 years of age on a weight basis to accelerate the heart rate; however, acceleration uniformly occurs with 14.3 μg/kg.[189] A dose of 30 μg/kg appears to be vagolytic in infants, children, and adults. This dose provides adequate protection against a cholinergic challenge. In all age groups, 5 to 10 μg/kg of atropine will minimally decrease salivation.[190]

MUSCLE RELAXANTS

Throughout infancy, the neuromuscular junction matures physically and biochemically, the contractile properties of skeletal muscle change, the amount of muscle in proportion to body weight increases, and the neuromuscular junction is variably sensitive to relaxants. In addition, the apparent volume of distribution of relaxants, their redistribution and excretion (clearance), and possibly their rate of metabolism change. These factors influence the dose-response relationship of relaxants and the duration of neuromuscular blockade. It is not surprising, therefore, that the infant's or child's response to relaxants is different from that of the adult.[191]

STRUCTURAL AND FUNCTIONAL DEVELOPMENT OF THE NEUROMUSCULAR SYSTEM

The structural and functional development of the neuromuscular system is incomplete at birth.[192–196] The conduction velocity of motor nerves increases throughout gestation as nerve fibers myelinate. The myotubules connect to mature muscle fibers in the latter part of intrauterine life and in the first several weeks after birth. Some slow-contracting muscle (intrinsic muscles of the hand) is progressively converted to fast-contracting muscle, with a concomitant change in the force-velocity relationship. Both the diaphragm and intercostal muscles in infants increase the percentage of slow muscle fibers in the first months of life. Synaptic transmission is relatively slow at birth, but more importantly, the rate at which acetylcholine is released during repetitive nerve stimulation is limited in the infant. This margin of safety for neurotransmission is reduced in infants compared with adults.

Unanesthetized newborn infants appear to have less neuromuscular reserve during tetanic stimulation than do adults. In neonates there is no fade of twitch height with repetitive stimulation at rates of 1 to 2 Hz; at 20 Hz, however, there is significant fade. Premature infants may show post-tetanic exhaustion for 15 to 20 minutes.[197] Goudsouzian noted slower contraction times of the thumb following slow and rapid rates of stimulation in term infants (1 to 10 days of age, anesthetized with halothane) than in older children.[198] The percent of fading at 20, 50, or 100 Hz did not differ between the infants and the older children; however, the tetanic stimulus was applied for only 5 seconds. The train-of-four ratio (the ratio of the amplitude of the fourth evoked response to the amplitude of the first response in the same train), the degree of post-tetanic facilitation, and the tetanus twitch ratio increase with age. Crumrine and Yodlowski noted a decrease in the amplitude of the frequency sweep electromyogram (FS-EMG) at frequencies of 50 to 100 Hz in infants less than 12 weeks of age (Fig. 2–6).[199] The frequency sweep-EMG is a recording of the action potential from an electrical stimulus rate that increases exponentially from 1 pulse per second to 100 Hz over a stimulation period of 10 seconds. The exponential increase in frequency allows assessment of neuromuscular transmission at tetanic rates without inducing fatigue. In older infants and children, Crumrine and Yodlowski found that there was little or no decrement in the FS-EMG at the higher frequencies of stimulation. Similarly, the FS-EMG response of full-term infants less than 12 weeks old was depressed after administration of 70 percent nitrous oxide, whereas that of the older patients did not change.

AGE-RELATED DIFFERENCES IN SENSITIVITY OF THE CHOLINERGIC RECEPTOR TO RELAXANTS

The sensitivity of the postjunctional cholinergic receptor to acetylcholine may vary with age. When allowance is made for differences in the volume of distribution and for type and concentration of anesthesia, infants appear relatively resistant to succinylcholine and relatively sensitive to nondepolarizing relaxants.

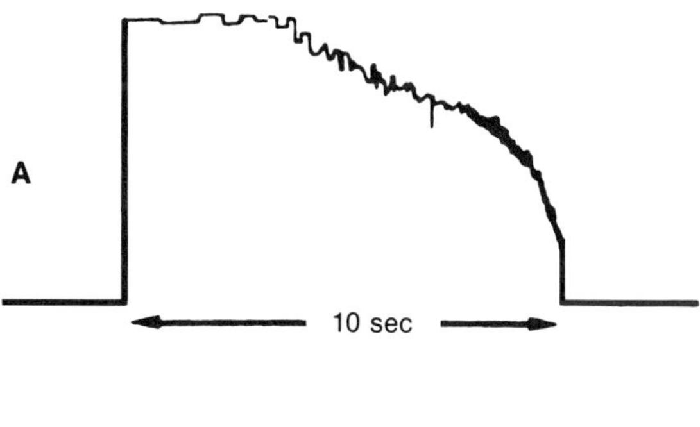

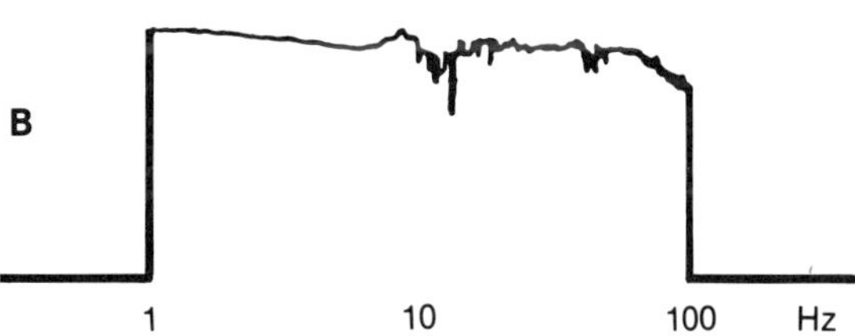

FIGURE 2–6. Tracings of the frequency sweep electromyogram (FS-EMG) responses from the tibialis anterior muscles of a 1-day-old infant (*A*) and a 4-month-old infant (*B*) premedicated with methohexital.

Depolarizing Muscle Relaxants

On a weight basis, more succinylcholine is needed in infants than in older children or adults to produce apnea, to depress respiration, or to depress neuromuscular transmission. Cook and Fischer noted that in infants succinylcholine (1 mg/kg) produced neuroblockade about equal to that produced by 0.5 mg/kg in children ages 6 to 8 years.[200] At these equipotent doses, there is no statistically significant difference between the times to recover to 50 percent (T50) and 90 percent (T90) of neuromuscular transmission in the two groups. Complete neuromuscular blockade develops in children given 1.0 mg/kg of succinylcholine. The ED_{95} of succinylcholine (the estimated dose of relaxant required to give 95 percent neuromuscular blockade) in infants is 2.2 mg/kg (Fig. 2–7).[200, 201]

Goudsouzian and Liu needed threefold higher infusion rates of succinylcholine (mg/kg/hr) to maintain 90 percent twitch depression in young infants than in older infants or children.[202] Phase II block occurred after a slightly larger dose of succinylcholine in infants than in the other age groups. Differences in cholinesterase activity, receptor sensitivity, or volume of distribution may explain these age-related differences in succinylcholine requirements.

The infant has about one half the pseudocholinesterase activity of the older child or adult.

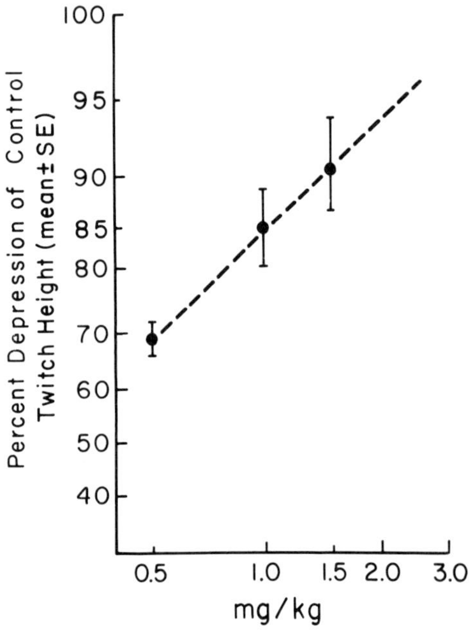

FIGURE 2–7. Mean dose-response curve (log-probit) for succinylcholine (mg/kg) for infants. Data calculated from Cook and Fischer.[200, 201]

Thus it is unlikely that augmented cholinesterase activity is responsible for the infant's resistance to succinylcholine. When succinylcholine was given in equal doses on a surface area basis (40 mg/m²), Walts and Dillon found no difference between infants and adults in the times to recover to 10, 50, or 90 percent neuromuscular transmission; this dose of succinylcholine produced complete neuromuscular blockade in all patients.[203] Cook and Fischer noted a linear relationship between the log dose on a milligram per square meter basis and the maximum intensity of neuromuscular blockade for infants, children, and adults.[200] They also saw a linear relationship between the logarithm of the dose on a milligram per square meter basis and to either 50 or 90 percent recovery time for infants and children as a combined group. Because of its relatively small molecular size, succinylcholine is rapidly distributed throughout the extracellular fluid. The blood volume and extracellular fluid (ECF) volume of the infant are significantly greater than the child's or adult's on a weight basis. Therefore, on a weight basis (mg/kg), twice as much succinylcholine is needed in the infant as in adults to produce 50 percent neuromuscular blockade. Since ECF and surface area bear a nearly constant relationship throughout life (6 to 8 L/m²), it is not surprising that there is a good correlation between succinylcholine dose (in mg/m²) and response throughout life. The data of Goudsouzian and Liu suggest that relative resistance to succinylcholine persists in some infants even when the dose is transformed to mg/m²/min.[202] These data suggest that the acetylcholine receptor matures with age.

Nondepolarizing Muscle Relaxants

Long-Acting Relaxants. On the basis of clinical criteria, it has been suggested that the neonate is sensitive to D-tubocurarine (dtc). However, electromyographic studies demonstrate no increased sensitivity of hand muscles to dtc in infants compared with adults. In infants, respiratory depression parallels the neuromuscular blockade noted in the hands; in adults, neuromuscular blockade of the hand occurs before respiratory depression.[204] This important observation suggests that the respiratory muscles of the infant may be more sensitive to dtc than those of the adult, or that the infant has less respiratory reserve than the adult. Both may be true.

In adults, Donlon and coworkers have determined cumulative dose-response curves and noted recovery times for dtc, gallamine, pancuronium, and metocurine during nitrous oxide–oxygen-narcotic anesthesia.[205] At equipotent doses of these relaxants, the recovery time from 95 percent block to 50 percent block averaged 45 minutes. Similar studies by other investigators have been performed in children during halothane and balanced anesthesia.[206–210] The ED_{95} for these relaxants during balanced anesthesia in children tended to be higher than that in adults, and the recovery times tended to be shorter. The dose requirements (ED_{95}) for pancuronium, metocurine, D-tubocurarine, and gallamine are reduced by halothane anesthesia in children as they are in adults. During halothane–nitrous oxide anesthesia, there was little difference in the ED_{95} on a weight basis for the longer-acting muscle relaxants in infants and children (Table 2–9).

The dose of D-tubocurarine on a surface-area basis that would be needed to produce 95 percent twitch depression in infants, in children, and in adults during halothane anesthesia has been estimated.[211] In this estimate, compensation is needed for the wide variation in extracellular fluid volume that exists in infants, children, and adults. The extracellular fluid volume mirrors the volume of distribution for the nondepolarizing muscle relaxants. Also, the comparison is between like anesthetics—halothane with halothane. The adult and child require about 7 to 8 mg/m^2 of D-tubocurarine; the 6- to 9-month-old infant, 5 to 6 mg/m^2; but the neonate, only about 4 mg/m^2. This suggests that the neonate, and to a lesser degree the infant, is quite sensitive to D-tubocurarine if compensation is made for the wide variation in volumes of distribution.

Fisher and coworkers documented the sensitivity to D-tubocurarine of infants as compared with older patients during equipotent nitrous oxide–halothane anesthesia.[212] Since the MAC of halothane is higher in infants than in adults, infants received higher end-tidal concentrations of halothane. The volume of distribution for D-tubocurarine is quite high in the newborn infant compared with the older child or adult, but plasma clearance of D-tubocurarine does not differ with age (Table 2–10). The volume of distribution for D-tubocurarine appears relatively constant on a liter per square meter basis. More importantly, the plasma concentration associated with 50 percent neuromuscular block (Cpss) was age-related; Cpss in neonates was about one third that noted for adults. The largest variability in elimination half-life and volumes of distribution was seen in the data for the neonates. Likewise, Goudsouzian and associates noted wide variations in the ED_{95} for D-tubocurarine in neonates during halothane

Table 2–9. COMPARISON OF AGE-RELATED DOSE REQUIREMENTS OF NONDEPOLARIZING RELAXANTS AND RECOVERY TIMES

Age	ED_{95} (mg/kg)*	Recovery Times T_5–T_{25} (min)†
D-Tubocurarine		
1–7 yr	0.32	28.3
2–12 mo	0.29	17.8
11–60 d	0.34	22.4
1–10 d	0.34	32.7
Metocurine		
1–7 yr	0.18	49.7
10 d–1 yr	0.22	36.7
0–9 d	0.19	25.7
Pancuronium		
5 wk–7 yr	0.05	23.6
2–10 yr	0.06	—
Gallamine		
2–10 yr	1.90	—

*ED_{95} = Estimated dose of relaxant required to produce 95 percent neuromuscular blockade.
†T_5–T_{25} = Time for neuromuscular transmisson to recover from 5 percent to 25 percent.

Table 2–10. PHARMACOKINETIC AND PHARMACODYNAMIC VALUES OF D-TUBOCURARINE

Patient Group	N	t½ β (min)	Vl (L/kg)	Vdss (L/kg)	Cl (mg/kg/min)	Cpss50 (μg/ml)
Neonates	7	174 ± 60	0.19 ± 0.13	0.74 ± 0.33	3.7 ± 2.1	0.18 ± 0.09
Infants	7	130 ± 54	0.16 ± 0.07	0.52 ± 0.22	3.3 ± 0.4	0.27 ± 0.06
Children	9	90 ± 23	0.14 ± 0.05	0.41 ± 0.12	4.0 ± 1.1	0.42 ± 0.14
Adults	8	89 ± 18	0.11 ± 0.02	0.30 ± 0.10	3.0 ± 0.8	0.53 ± 0.14
Significance ($p<0.05$)		*	NS	†	NS	‡

Values are means ± 1 standard deviation.
NS = not significant.
*t½ β: Neonates > children and adults.
†Vdss: Neonates > infants, children, and adults.
‡CPss50: Neonates and infants < children and adults.

anesthesia.[209] Some infants were paralyzed with 0.18 mg/kg and others required 0.6 mg/kg; the mean ED_{95} was similar to that in older children. This suggests that the neonate's response to nondepolarizing relaxants is quite unpredictable and that the clinician should titrate the dose of relaxant to produce the desired effect. The recovery times from all relaxants is dose-related: if the infant were overdosed by a factor of two, recovery time would be quite prolonged.

Pipecuronium and doxacurium, new long-acting relaxants without cardiovascular effects, have recently been introduced into clinical practice. Both have a duration of action in adults and children similar to that of pancuronium, but unlike pancuronium, they appear to be devoid of cardiovascular effects.[213–215] Renal failure can prolong the effect of these relaxants.[216, 217] Children require higher doses of each relaxant than do adults to achieve the same degree of neuromuscular blockade during equivalent anesthetic backgrounds. At equipotent doses of pipecuronium and doxacurium, the time to recovery of neuromuscular transmission to 25 percent (T_{25}) is shorter in children than in adults. Infants appear to be more sensitive to the neuromuscular blocking effects of pipecuronium. However, the clinical duration of action (T_{25}) of pipecuronium following cumulative dosing is about 20 minutes in infants and 30 minutes in children. Spontaneous recovery indexes are not prolonged in the younger patients.

Intermediate-Acting Relaxants. Atracurium, a muscle relaxant of intermediate duration, is metabolized by nonspecific esters and spontaneously decomposes by Hofmann degradation. Both processes are sensitive to pH and temperature. Under physiological conditions the breakdown of atracurium is mainly by ester hydrolysis; Hofmann elimination plays a minor role. Deficient or abnormal pseudocholinesterases have little or no effect on atracurium degradation.[218, 219]

We and others have studied the effects of both age and potent inhalation agents on dose-response relationships of atracurium in infants, children, and adolescents.[220–224] On a weight basis (μg/kg), the ED_{95} for atracurium was similar in infants (1 to 6 months of age) and adolescents, whereas children had a higher dose requirement (Table 2–11). On a surface area basis (μg/m²), the Ed_{95} for atracurium was similar in children and adolescents; the ED_{95} (μg/m²) for atracurium in infants was much lower (Fig. 2–8).

At equipotent doses (1 times ED_{95}), the duration of effect (time from injection to 95 percent recovery) was 23 minutes in infants and 29 minutes in children and adolescents, compared with 44 minutes in adults. The time from injection to T_{25} (25 percent neuromuscular transmission) was 10 minutes in infants, 15 minutes in children and adolescents, and 16 minutes in adults. At T_{25}, supplemental doses are needed to maintain relaxation for surgery. At higher multiples of the ED_{95}, the duration of effect will be longer, but the times from T_5 to T_{25} will be the same. The shorter duration of effect in the infant may represent a difference in pharmacokinetics.

The pharmacokinetics of atracurium differ between infants and children or infants and adults. We have determined the kinetics of atracurium in infants and children; comparable data exist for adults.[225] The kinetic variables are shown in Table 2–12. The more striking differences are between infants and children. The volume of distribution is larger and the elimi-

Table 2–11. MEAN ED_{50} and ED_{95} VALUES FOR ATRACURIUM IN ANESTHETIZED CHILDREN

Anesthetic	ED_{50} μg/kg	ED_{95} μg/kg	ED_{50} μg/m²	ED_{95} μg/m₂
Thiopental-fentanyl	170	350	3900	8200
Halothane	130	260	3300	6600
Isoflurane	120	280	3000	8600

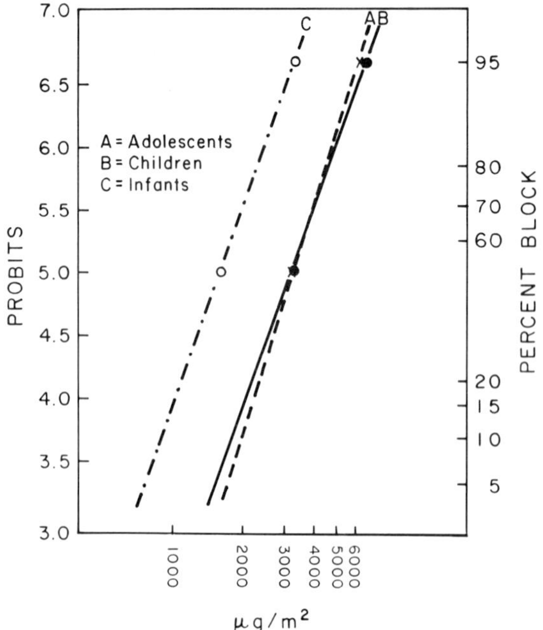

FIGURE 2–8. Mean dose-response curves for atracurium (μg/m²) for adolescents (A), children (B), and infants (C).

Table 2–12. AGE-RELATED PHARMACOKINETICS OF ATRACURIUM

Parameter	Children	Infants
t½ α	2.1 ± 0.56	104 ± 0.34*
t½ β	19.1 ± 4.5	13.6 ± 1.4*
V_1 (ml/kg)	52.6 ± 5.66	50.55 ± 6.3
Vd (ml/kg)	139.0 ± 23.48	176.6 ± 22.2*
Cl (ml/kg/min)	5.1 ± 0.56	9.0 ± 1.65*

*$p < 0.05$.

nation half-life is shorter in infants than in children or adults. For both reasons, clearance in infants is more rapid. Although there is little difference in the kinetics of atracurium among children aged 2 to 10 years, there are age-related differences in the volume of distribution, elimination half-life, and clearance. The volume of distribution is higher in the younger patients, and elimination half-life is shorter; clearance is little different.

In children, "light" isoflurane anesthesia (1 percent end-tidal) reduces the atracurium required by about 30 percent from that needed with thiopental-narcotic anesthesia. There was no statistically significant difference in the isoflurane or halothane dose response curve (Fig. 2–9). For clinical purposes, both potent agents should be viewed as potentiating atracurium to the same degree.[222]

We have recently used a continuous infusion of dilute atracurium (200 μg/ml) following a bolus to maintain neuromuscular blockade at 95 ± 5 percent (Fig. 2–10).[222] To maintain this degree of steady-state block, an infusion rate of 4 to 5 μg/kg/min was required during halothane or isoflurane anesthesia, and 8 to 10 μg/kg/min were required with thiopental-narcotic anesthesia following an initial bolus (Table 2–13). No accumulation was seen with prolonged infusion; recovery of neuromuscular transmission was prompt. The recovery of neuromuscular transmission from the same degree of blockade was similar with all three anesthetics. From these infusion data, one can estimate the removal of atracurium. At steady state, the infusion rate

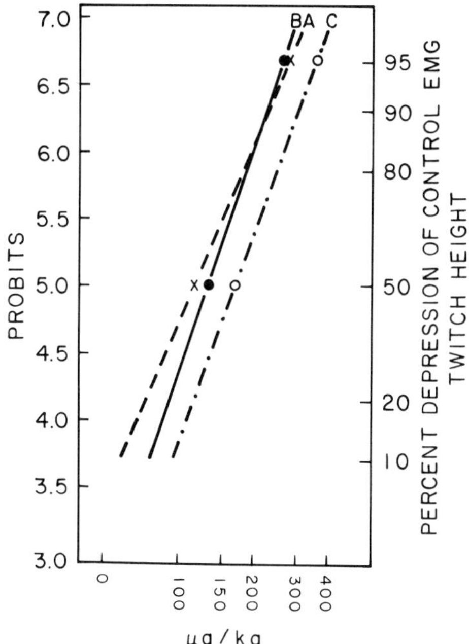

FIGURE 2–9. Mean dose-response curves for atracurium (μg/kg) during halothane (A), isoflurane (B), or nitrous oxide–narcotic (C).

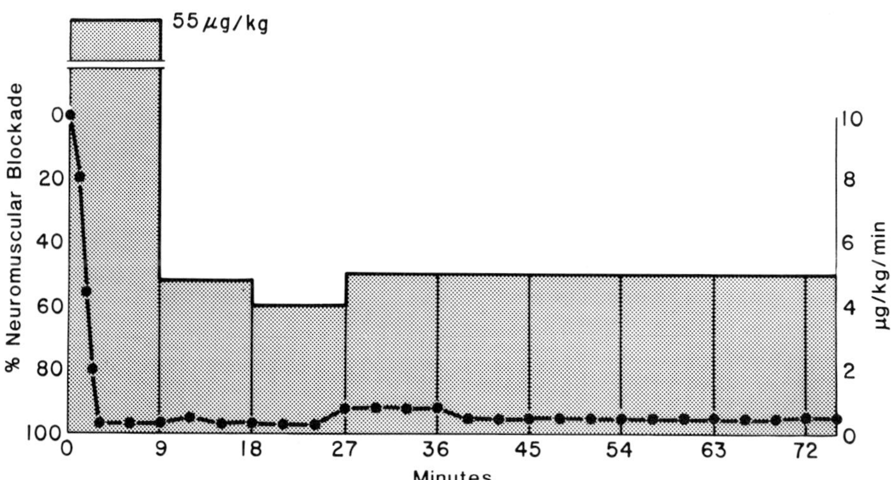

FIGURE 2–10. Evolution of atracurium requirements calculated for a 9-minute period (shaded area) to maintain neuromuscular blockade (solid dots) in a typical patient. The first 9-minute period represents in large part the bolus injection.

Table 2–13. ATRACURIUM INFUSION REQUIREMENTS FOR SURGICAL RELAXATION DURING ANESTHESIA INDUCED BY VARIOUS DRUGS IN CHILDREN

Anesthetic	Infusion Rate* (μg/kg/min)	Infusion Rate* (μg/m²/min)
Thiopental-fentanyl	9.3 ± 0.8 (6.6–13.6)	226 ± 15 (171–309)
Halothane	†6.8 ± 0.5 (4.8–9.3)	†175 ± 19 (104–274)
Isoflurane	†5.9 ± 0.7 (4.4–9.3)	†147 ± 16 (94–217)

*Mean ± SE (range).
†Different from thiopental-fentanyl $p < 0.05$.

(Iss) equals the removal rate (Rss) of atracurium. Removal is directly related to the clearance and steady-state plasma concentration associated with 95 percent neuromuscular blockade. Hence:

$$\text{Iss} = \text{Rss} = \text{clearance} \times \text{CPss95}$$

From this relationship one can estimate CPss95 from clearance and the steady-state infusion rate. In children, during the potent anesthetics, CPss95 is about 1 μg/ml; during balanced anesthesia, it is about 2 μg/ml. Comparable studies are in progress in infants. Atracurium infusion requirements in children during nitrous oxide–narcotic anesthesia can be compared with those noted in several age-groups of adults during similar anesthesia. D'Hollander and associates noted that in patients 16 to 85 years old the steady-state atracurium infusion rate averaged 14.4 mg/m²/hr; this corresponds to 240 μg/m²/min.[226] This value is similar to the 226 μg/m²/min we noted.

Vecuronium. Vecuronium, a steroidal relaxant related to pancuronium, is taken up largely by the liver, then excreted unchanged via the hepatobiliary system (40 percent to 50 percent) or, alternatively, excreted through the kidneys (4 percent to 14 percent). Limited biotransformation of vecuronium to the 3-hydroxy-, 17-hydroxy-, and 3,17-dihydroxy-metabolites occurs. Only 3-hydroxy-vecuronium is known to have neuromuscular blocking effects.[227] These routes of elimination may be affected by physiological changes at the extremes of life.[228, 229]

The ED_{95} for vecuronium is somewhat higher in children than in infants and adults (Table 2–14).[228, 230] At equipotent doses (2 times ED_{95}) of vecuronium, the duration of effect (time from injection to 90 percent recovery) was longest for infants (73 minutes), compared with that for children (35 minutes) and adults (53 minutes). Thus, vecuronium does not have intermediate duration in infants. Vecuronium is potentiated by potent inhalation anesthetics but not in a dose-dependent manner.[231, 232]

Table 2–14. AGE-RELATED POTENCY AND TIME COURSE FOR VECURONIUM

	Potency			Time Course (70 μg/kg)	
	ED₅₀ (μg/kg)	***ED₉₅*** (μg/kg)	***ED₉₅ Multiple***	***Onset Time*** (min)	***Duration*** (min)
Infants	16.5	27.7	2.5	1.5 ± 0.6	73 ± 27
Children	19.0	45.5	1.5	2.4 ± 1.4	35 ± 6
Adults	15.0	33.8	2	2.9 ± 0.2	53 ± 21

Fisher and associates determined the pharmacodynamics and pharmacokinetics of vecuronium in infants and children (Table 2–15).[233] The volume of distribution and mean residence time were greater in infants than in children. Clearance was similar in the two groups; the CPss50 was lower in infants than in children. The combination of a large volume of distribution in infants and fixed clearance results in a longer mean residence time. After a single dose of relaxant, recovery of neuromuscular transmission depends on both distribution and elimination. The combination of a longer mean residence time and a lower sensitivity for vecuronium explains the prolongation of neuromuscular blockade in infants.

ORG-9426. ORG-9426, an intermediate steroidal derivative of vecuronium, is less potent than vecuronium but has a shorter onset time of neuromuscular blockade and a similar duration of action. It has minimal cardiovascular effects. The ED_{95} of ORG-9426 in adults receiving balanced anesthesia is 300 μg/kg.[234] At 2 times ED_{95}, the onset time of complete neuromuscular blockade is about 1.5 minutes. At these doses the clinical duration (i.e., time to T_{25}) was 40 minutes, which is comparable to that of vecuronium at equal multiples of the ED_{95}. Cardiovascular changes were minimal. S. K. Woelfel and colleagues (unpublished data)

Table 2–15. PHARMACOKINETICS AND PHARMACODYNAMICS OF VECURONIUM

	ED₉₅ (μg/kg)	t½ β (min)	Cl (ml/kg/min)	Vdss (ml/kg)	CPss50 (ng/ml)
Infants	27.7	64.7 ±30.2	5.6 ±1	357 ±70	57.3 ±17.7
Children	45.5	41.0 ±15.1	5.9 ±2.4	204 ±116	109.8 ±28.1
Adults	33.8	70.7 ±20.4	5.2 ±0.7	269 ±42	93.7 ±33.5

determined the ED_{50} and ED_{95} of ORG-9426 in children during halothane anesthesia to be 179 μg/kg^{-1} and 303 μg/kg^{-1}, respectively. The initial recovery index (T_{10} to T_{25}) after an ED_{95} dose (given in incremental doses) was 3.2 minutes. Thus, the duration of neuromuscular blockade is somewhat shorter in children than in adults.

Short-Acting Relaxants. Mivacurium, a short-acting relaxant, is metabolized by plasma cholinesterase. When administered in doses less than two times the ED_{95} to adults, mivacurium appears to be devoid of cardiovascular effects; larger doses may be associated with a transient decrease in blood pressure from histamine release. Compared with adults, children require significantly more mivacurium (microgram per kilogram) during comparable anesthetic backgrounds. When referenced to body surface area (microgram per square meter), however, the dosage requirements are not significantly different. This suggests that age-related dosage requirements for mivacurium may be associated with age-related differences in volume of distribution. At equal potent doses, the onset time of mivacurium is faster in children than in adults; the clinical duration is likewise shorter in children. We observed cutaneous flushing in three children given high doses of mivacurium and a transient 32 percent decrease in mean arterial pressure in one of these patients. Flushing was not always associated with hypotension. Pseudocholinesterase activity influences the clearance and hence infusion roles in children. Mivacurium can be administered by infusion for several hours with no evidence of cumulation and with rapid spontaneous or pharmacologically induced return of neuromuscular function after termination of the infusion. The mivacurium infusion rates are higher in children than in adults.[235]

REVERSAL OF NEUROMUSCULAR BLOCK

Fisher and colleagues examined the doses of neostigmine and edrophonium required in infants, children, and adults to reverse a 90 percent block from a continuous D-tubocurarine infusion.[236, 237] In infants and children, 15.0 μg/kg of neostigmine produced a 50 percent antagonism of the D-tubocurarine block; in adults, 23 μg/kg was required. It was claimed that the duration of antagonism was equal in all three groups, although the elimination half-life was clearly shorter for infants. A larger dose than that recommended apparently would give a higher sustained blood concentration. Whether this is of pharmacological benefit in the absence of a continuous infusion of relaxant is doubtful. The dissociation between the elimination half-life and the duration of antagonism may result from the carbamylation of cholinesterase by neostigmine. In infants, 145 μg/kg of edrophonium produced a 50 percent antagonism of the D-tubocurarine block; in children, 233 μg/kg was required; and in adults, 128 μg/kg. The volume of distribution of edrophonium was similar in all age groups. The elimination half-life of edrophonium was shorter in infants than in children or adults; hence, clearance was more rapid in infants. Since the molecular interaction between edrophonium and cholinesterase is readily reversible, Fisher and associates suggest that the shorter elimination half-life for edrophonium might limit the value of edrophonium in pediatric patients. This is doubtful.

Meakin and associates compared the rate of recovery from pancuronium-induced neuromuscular blockade with several doses of neostigmine (0.036 or 0.07 mg/kg) or edrophonium (0.7 or 1.43 mg/kg) in infants and children.[238] In the first 5 minutes, recovery of neuromuscular transmission was more rapid after edrophonium than neostigmine in all age groups; the speed of recovery was faster in infants and children than in adults. By 10 minutes there was no difference in neuromuscular transmission achieved in infants and children with either reversal agent (at either dose); adults had lower neuromuscular transmission at the lower dose (0.036 mg/kg) of neostigmine. Thus, if speed of initial recovery is a critical issue, then edrophonium is better than neostigmine, and a high dose of neostigmine is better than a low dose. At 30 minutes after injection of either reversal agent (at any dose), there was no differences between neuromuscular transmission between age groups.

REFERENCES

1. Sereni F: Developmental pharmacology. Annu Rev Pharmacol *8*:453–470, 1968.
2. Jusko WJ: Pharmacokinetic principles in pediatric pharmacology. Pediatr Clin North Am *19*:81–100, 1972.
3. Brown TCK: Pediatric pharmacology. Anaesth Intensive Care *1*:473–479, 1973.
4. Cook DR: Neonatal anesthetic pharmacology: A review. Anesth Analg *53*:544–548, 1974.
5. Yaffe SJ, Juchau JR: Perinatal pharmacology. Annu Rev Pharmacol *14*:219–238, 1974.
6. Cook DR: Pediatric anesthesia: Pharmacological considerations. Drugs *12*:212–221, 1976.

7. Rylance G: Clinical pharmacology: Drugs in children. Br Med J *282*:50–51, 1981.
8. Orme M: Drug absorption in the gut. Br J Anaesth *56*:59–67, 1984.
9. DeBoer AG, DeLeede LGJ, Breimer DD: Drug absorption by sublingual and rectal routes. Br J Anaesth *56*:69–82, 1984.
10. Huang NN, High RH: Comparison of serum levels following the administration of oral and parenteral preparations of penicillin to infants and children of various age groups. J Pediatr *42*:567–568, 1958.
11. Borga G, Piafsky KM, Nilsen OG: Plasma protein binding of basic drugs. I. Selective displacement from alpha-1 acid glycoprotein by *tris*-butoxyethyl phosphate. Clin Pharmacol Ther *22*:539–544, 1977.
12. Brem RF, Giardina EGV, Bigger JT: Time course of alpha-1 acid glycoprotein and its relationship to imipramine plasma protein binding. Clin Pharmacol Ther *31*:206, 1982.
13. Edwards DJ, Lalka D, Cerra G, Slaughter RL: Alpha-1 acid glycoprotein concentration and protein binding in trauma. Clin Pharmacol Ther *31*:62–67, 1982.
14. Grossman SH, Davis D, Kitchell BB, Shand D, Routledge PA: Diazepam and lidocaine plasma protein binding in renal disease. Clin Pharmacol Ther *31*:350–357, 1982.
15. Kornguth ML, Hutchins LG, Eichelman BS: Binding of psychotropic drugs to isolated alpha-1 acid glycoprotein. Biochem Pharmacol *30*:2435–2441, 1981.
16. Piafsky KM: Disease-induced changes in the plasma binding of basic drugs. Clin Pharmacokinet *5*:246–262, 1980.
17. Piafsky KM, Borga O, Odar-Cederlog I, Johansson C, Sjoqvist F: Increased plasma protein binding of propranolol and chlorpromazine mediated by disease-induced elevations of plasma acid glycoprotein. N Engl J Med *299*:1435–1439, 1978.
18. Pike E, Skuterud B, Kierugg P, Fredstad D, Abdel Sayed SM, Lunde PKM: Binding and displacement of basic, acidic and neutral drugs in normal and orosomucoid-deficient plasma. Clin Pharmacokinet *6*:367–374, 1981.
19. Nation RL: Meperidine binding in maternal and fetal plasma. Clin Pharmacol Ther *29*:472–479, 1981.
20. Pruitt AW, Dayton PG: A comparison of the binding of drugs to adult and cord plasma. Eur J Clin Pharmacol *4*:59, 1971.
21. Wood J, Wood AJJ: Changes in plasma drug binding and alpha-1 acid glycoprotein in mother and newborn infant. Clin Pharmacol Ther *29*:522–526, 1981.
22. Dayton PG, Stiller RL, Cook DR, Perel JM: The binding of ketamine to plasma proteins: Emphasis on human plasma. Eur J Clin Pharmacol *24*:825–831, 1983.
23. Friss-Hansen B: Body composition during growth. Pediatrics *47*:264–274, 1971.
24. Widdowson EM: Changes in body proportions and composite during growth. *In* Davis JA, Dobbing J (eds): Scientific Foundations of Pediatrics. Philadelphia, WB Saunders, 1974, pp 153–163.
25. Smith CA, Nelson NM: The Physiology of the Newborn Infant. 4th edition. Springfield, Ill, Charles C Thomas, 1976, pp 179, 181, 188, 209.
26. Guignard JP, Torrado A, Cunha OD, Gautier E: Glomerular filtration rate in the first three weeks of life. J Pediatr *87*:268–272, 1975.
27. Altman PL, Dittmer DS: Respiration and Circulation Handbook. (Revised edition.) Bethesda, Md, Federation of American Society of Experimental Biologists, 1971, pp 426–427.
28. Oldendorf WH: The blood-brain barrier. *In* Bito LZ, Davson H, Fenstermacher JD, (eds): The Ocular and Cerebrospinal Fluids. New York, Academic Press, 1977, pp 177–190.
29. Behnsen G: Farbstoffversuche mit trypanblan an der schranke zwischen blut und zentralnervensystem der wachsenden maus. Munch Med Wschr *73*:1143–1147, 1926.
30. Behnsen G: Uber die farbstoffspeicherung im zentralnervensystem der weissen maus in verschiedenen alterszugstanden. Z Zellforsch *4*:515–572, 1927.
31. Barlow CF, Domek NS, Goldberg MA, Roth LJ: Extracellular brain space measured by ^{35}S-sulphate. Arch Neurol *5*:102–110, 1961.
32. Davson H: Physiology of the Cerebral Spinal Fluid. London, Churchill, 1967.
33. Ferguson RK, Woodbury DM: Penetration of ^{14}C-inulin and ^{14}C-sucrose into brain, cerebrospinal fluid, and skeletal muscle in developing rats. Exp Brain Res *7*:181–194, 1969.
34. Evans CAN, Reynolds JM, Reynolds ML, Saunders NR, Segal MB: The development of a blood-brain barrier mechanism in foetal sheep. J Physiol *238*:371–386, 1974.
35. Evans CAN, Reynolds JM, Reynolds ML, Saunders NR: The effect of hypercapnia on a blood-brain barrier mechanism in foetal and newborn sheep. J Physiol *255*:701–714, 1976.
36. Oldendorf WH: Measurement of brain uptake of radio-labeled substances using a tritiated water internal standard. Brain Res *24*:372–376, 1970.
37. Oldendorf WH, Braun LD: [^{3}H]-Tryptamine and ^{3}H water as diffusible internal standard for measuring brain extraction of radio-labelled substances following carotid injection. Brain Res *113*:219–224, 1976.
38. Oldendorf WH, Hyman S, Braun L, Oldendorf SZ: Blood-brain barrier: Penetration of morphine, codeine, heroin and methadone after carotid injection. Science *178*:984–986, 1972.
39. Gladtke E, Heimann G: The rate of development of elimination functions in kidney and liver of young infants. *In* Morselli PC, Garattini S, Sereni F (eds): Basic and Therapeutic Aspects of Perinatal Pharmacology. New York, Raven Press, 1975, pp 377–392.
40. Brown AK, Zwelzin WW, Burnett HH: Studies on the neonatal development of the glucuronide conjugating system. J Clin Invest *37*:332–337, 1958.
41. Greene NM: The metabolism of drugs employed in anesthesia. Anesthesiology *29*:127–137, 1968.
42. Yaffe SJ: Neonatal pharmacology. Pediatr Clin North Am *13*:527–532, 1966.
43. Somogyi A, Gugler R: Drug interactions with cimetidine. Clin Pharmacokinet *7*:23–41, 1982.
44. Katzung GB: Basic and Clinical Pharmacology. Los Altos, Cal, Lange Medical Publications, 1984.
45. Eger EI II: Anesthesia Uptake and Action. Baltimore, Williams and Wilkins, 1974.
46. Salanitre E, Rackow H: The pulmonary exchange of nitrous oxide and halothane in infants and children. Anesthesiology *30*:388–394, 1969.
47. Rackow H, Salanitre E: The pulmonary equilibration of cyclopropane in infants and children. Br J Anaesth *46*:35–42, 1974.
48. Steward DJ, Creighton RE: The uptake and excretion of nitrous oxide in the newborn. Can Anaesth Soc J *25*:215–217, 1978.
49. Eger EI, II, Bahlman SH, Munson ES: The effect of age on the rate of increase of alveolar anesthetic concentration. Anesthesiology *35*:365–372, 1971.
50. Brandom BW, Brandom RB, Cook DR: Uptake and

distribution of halothane in infants: In vivo measurements and computer simulations. Anesth Analg *62*:404–410, 1983.
51. Gibbs CP, Munson ES, Tham MK: Anesthetic solubility coefficients for maternal and fetal blood. Anesthesiology *43*:100–103, 1975.
52. Lerman J, Gregory GA, Willis MM, Eger EI, II: Age and solubility of volatile anesthetics in blood. Anesthesiology *61*:139–143, 1984.
53. Cook DR, Brandom BW, Shiu G, Wolfson BW: The inspired median effective dose, brain concentration at anesthesia, and cardiovascular index for halothane in young rats. Anesth Analg *60*:182–185, 1981.
54. Stoelting RK, Longnecker DE: Effect of right-to-left shunt on rate of increase in arterial anesthetic concentration. Anesthesiology *36*:352–356, 1972.
55. Tanner G, Angers D, Barash PG, Mulla A, Miller P, Rothstein P: Does a left- to-right shunt speed the induction of inhalational anesthesia in congenital heart disease? Anesthesiology *57*:A427, 1982.
56. Deming MV: Agents and techniques for induction of anesthesia in infants and young children. Anesth Analg *31*:113–117, 1952.
57. Gregory GA, Eger EI, II, Munson ES: The relationship between age and halothane requirements in man. Anesthesiology *30*:488–491, 1969.
58. Nicodemus HF, Nassiri-Rahimi C, Bachman L: Median effective dose (ED_{50}) of halothane in adults and children. Anesthesiology *31*:344–348, 1969.
59. Lerman J, Robinson S, Willis MM, Gregory G: Anesthetic requirements for halothane in young children 0–1 month and 1–6 months of age. Anesthesiology *59*:421–424, 1983.
60. Gregory GA, Wade JG, Beihl DR, Ong BY, Sitar DS: Fetal anesthetic requirement (MAC) for halothane. Anesth Analg *62*:9–14, 1983.
61. Moss IR, Conner H, Yee WFH, Iorio P, Scarpelli EM: Human β-endorphin in the neonatal period. J Pediatr *101*:443–446, 1982.
62. Bayon A, Shoemaker WJ, Bloom FE, Mauss A, Gullemin R: Perinatal development of the endorphin- and enkephalin-containing systems in rat brain. Brain Res *179*:93, 1979.
63. Miller KM, Paton WDM, Smith EB, Smith RA: Physiochemical approaches to the mode of action of general anesthetics. Anesthesiology *36*:339–351, 1972.
64. Rackow H, Salanitre E, Green LT: Frequency of cardiac arrest associated with anesthesia in infants and children. Pediatrics *28*:697–704, 1961.
65. Friesen RH, Lichtor JL: Cardiovascular depression during halothane anesthesia in infants: A study of three induction techniques. Anesth Analg *61*:42–45, 1982.
66. Friesen RH, Lichtor JL: Cardiovascular effects of inhalation induction with isoflurane in infants. Anesth Analg *62*:411–414, 1983.
67. Rao CC, Bayer M, Krishna G, Paradise RR: Effects of halothane, isoflurane and enflurane on the isometric contraction of the neonatal isolated rat atria. Anesthesiology *61*:A424, 1984.
68. Boudreaux JP, Schieber RA, Cook DR: Hemodynamic effects of halothane in the newborn piglet. Anesth Analg *63*:731–737, 1984.
69. Bailie MD, Alward CT, Sawyer DC, Hook JB: Effect of anesthesia on cardiovascular and renal function in the newborn piglet. J Pharmacol Exp Ther *208*:298–302, 1979.
70. Merin RG, Verdouw PD, deJong JW: Dose-dependent depression of cardiac function and metabolism by halothane in swine (*Sus scrofa*). Anesthesiology *46*:417–423, 1977.
71. Gootman PM, Gootman N, Buckley BJ: Maturation of central autonomic control of the circulation. Fed Proc *42*:1648–1655, 1983.
72. Eger EI: Stability of I-653 in soda lime. Anesth Analg *66*:983–985, 1987.
73. Taylor RH, Lerman J: Minimum alveolar concentration of desflurane and hemodynamic responses in neonates, infants, and children. Anesthesiology *75*:975–979, 1991.
74. Weiskopf RB, Holmes MA, Eger EI II, et al: Cardiovascular effects of I-653 in swine. Anesthesiology *69*:303–309, 1988.
75. Weiskopf RB, Cahalan MK, Yasuda N, et al: Cardiovascular actions of desflurane (I-653) in humans. Anesth Analg *70*:S426, 1990.
76. Hartman JC, Pagel PS, Kampine JP, et al: Influence of desflurane on regional distribution of coronary blood flow in chronically instrumented canine model of multivessel coronary artery obstruction. Anesth Analg *72*:289–299, 1991.
77. Gregory GA: The baroresponses of preterm infants during halothane anesthesia. Can Anaesth Soc J *29*:105–107, 1982.
78. Duncan P, Gregory GA, Wade JA: The effects of nitrous oxide on the baroreceptor response of newborn and adult rabbits. Can Anesth Soc J *28*:339–341, 1981.
79. Wear R, Robinson S, Gregory GA: The effect of halothane on the baroresponse of adult and baby rabbits. Anesthesiology *56*:188–191, 1982.
80. Wolfson B, Kielar CM, Lake C, Hetrick WD, Siker ES: Anesthetic index—a new approach. Anesthesiology *38*:583–586, 1973.
81. Wolfson B, Hetrick WD, Lake C, Siker ES: Anesthetic indices—further data. Anesthesiology *48*:187–190, 1978.
82. Kissen I, Morgan PL, Smith LR: Comparison of isoflurane and halothane safety margins in rats. Anesthesiology *58*:556–561, 1983.
83. Resurreccion MA, Casthely P, Pimental C, Cottrell JE, Velcek F: Serum bromide post halothane in infants and young children. Anesthesiology *55*:A327, 1981.
84. Stoelting RK, Peterson C: Methoxyflurane anesthesia in pediatric patients: Evaluation of anesthetic metabolism and renal function. Anesthesiology *42*:26–29, 1975.
85. Goldenthal EI: A compilation of LD_{50} values in newborn and adult animals. Toxicol Appl Pharmacol *18*:185–207, 1971.
86. Marcucci F, Mussini E, Airoldi L, Guaitani A, Garattini S: Diazepam metabolism and anticonvulsant activity in newborn animals. Biochem Pharmacol *22*:3051–3059, 1973.
87. Morselli PL, Mandelli M, Tognoni G, Principi N, Pardi G, Sereni F: Drug interactions in the human fetus and in the newborn infant. *In* Morselli PL, Cohen SN (eds): Drug Interactions. New York, Drug Interactions, 1974, pp 320–333.
88. Smith M, Eadie M, Brophy T: The pharmacokinetics of midazolam in man. Eur J Clin Pharmacol *19*:271–278, 1981.
89. Fragen R, Gahl F, Caldwell N: A water soluble benzodiazepine RO21-3981, for induction of anesthesia. Anesthesiology *49*:41–43, 1978.
90. Nilsson A, Lee P, Revenas B: Midazolam as induction agent prior to inhalational anesthesia: A comparison with thiopentone. Acta Anaesth Scand *28*:249–251, 1984.

91. Gamble J, Kawar P, Dundee J, Moore J, Briggs L: Evaluation of midazolam as an intravenous induction agent. Anaesthesia *36*:868–873, 1981.
92. Berggren L, Eriksson I: Midazolam for induction of anesthesia in outpatients: A comparison with thiopentone. Acta Anaesth Scand *25*:492–496, 1981.
93. Brown C, Sarnquist F, Canup C, Pedley T: Clinical electroencephalographic and pharmacokinetic studies of a water-soluble benzodiazepine, midazolam maleate. Anesthesiology *50*:467–470, 1979.
94. Massaut J, D'Hollander A, Barvais L, Dubois-Primo J: Haemodynamic effects of midazolam in the anaesthetized patients with coronary artery disease. Acta Anaesth Scand *27*:299–302, 1983.
95. Reeves J, Samuelson P, Lewis S: Midazolam maleate induction in patients with ischemic heart disease: Haemodynamic observation. Can Anaesth Soc J *26*:402–407, 1979.
96. Greenblatt D, Arendt R, Abernethy D, Giles H, Sellers E, Shader R: In vitro quantitation of benzodiazepine lipophilicity; Relation to in vivo distribution. Br J Anaesth *55*:985–989, 1983.
97. Lebowitz P, Cote E, Daniels A, Ramsey F, Martyn J, Teplick R, Davison K: Comparative cardiovascular effects of midazolam and thiopental in healthy patients. Anesth Analg *61*:771–775, 1982.
98. Rita L, Seleny FL, Goodarzi M: Intramuscular midazolam for pediatric preanesthetic sedation: A double-blind controlled study with morphine. Anesthesiology *63*:528–531, 1985.
99. Feld LH, Champeau MW, van Steennis CA, Scott JC: Preanesthetic medication in children: A comparison of oral transmucosal fentanyl citrate versus placebo. Anesthesiology *71*:374–377, 1989.
100. Saint-Maurice C, Meistelman C, Rey E, Esteve C, DeLauture D, Olive G: The pharmacokinetics of rectal midazolam for premedication in children. Anesthesiology *65*:536–538, 1986.
101. Wilton NCT, Leigh J, Rosen DR, Pandit UA: Preanesthetic sedation of preschool children using intranasal midazolam. Anesthesiology *69*:972–975, 1988.
102. Walbergh EJ, Wills RJ, Eckhert J: Plasma concentrations of midazolam in children following intranasal administration. Anesthesiology *74*:233–235, 1991.
103. Mathews HML, Carson IW, Lyons SM, Orr IA, Collier PS, Howard PJ, Dundee JW: A pharmacokinetic study of midazolam in paediatric patients undergoing cardiac surgery. Br J Anaesth *61*:302–307, 1988.
104. Salonen M, Kanto J, Iisalo E, Himberg JJ: Midazolam as an induction agent in children: A pharmacokinetic and clinical study. Anesth Analg *66*:625–628, 1987.
105. Carmichael EB: The median lethal dose (LD_{50}) of pentothal sodium for both young and old guinea pigs and rats. Anesthesiology *8*:589–593, 1947.
106. Carmichael EB: The median lethal dose of Nembutal (pentobarbital sodium) for young and old rats. J Pharmacol Exp Ther *62*:284–286, 1938.
107. Weatherall JA: Anaesthesia in newborn animals. Br J Pharmacol *15*:454–459, 1960.
108. Domek NS, Barlow CF, Roth LJ: An octogenetic study of phenobarbital C-14 in cat brain. J Pharmacol Exp Ther *130*:285–290, 1960.
109. Mirkin BL: Perinatal pharmacology. Anesthesiology *43*:156–169, 1975.
110. Boreus LO, Jalling B, Kallberg N: Clinical pharmacology of phenobarbital in the neonatal period. *In* Morselli PL, Garattini S, Sereni F: Basic and Therapeutic Aspects of Perinatal Pharmacology. New York, Raven Press, 1975, pp 331–340.
111. Knauer B, Draffen GA, Williams FM: Elimination kinetics of amobarbital in mothers and their newborn infants. Clin Pharmacol Ther *14*:442–447, 1973.
112. Sorbo S, Hudson RJ, Loomis JC: The pharmacokinetics of thiopental in pediatric surgical patients. Anesthesiology *61*:666–670, 1984.
113. Kosaka Y, Takahashi T, Mark LC: Intravenous thiobarbiturate anesthesia for cesarean section. Anesthesiology *31*:489–506, 1969.
114. Briggs L, Clarke R, Watkins J: An adverse reaction to the administration of disoprofol (diprivam). Anaesthesia *37*:1099–1101, 1982.
115. Kay B, Rolly G: ICI 35868; A new intravenous induction agent. Acta Anaesth Belg *28*:303–316, 1977.
116. Adam H, Briggs L, Bahar M, Douglas E, Dundee J: The pharmacokinetic evaluation of ICI 35868 in man. Single induction dose with different rates of infusion. Br J Anaesth *55*:97–103, 1983.
117. Kay B, Stephenson D: Alfentanil (R39209); Initial clinical experience with a new narcotic analgesic. Anaesthesia *35*:1197–1201, 1980.
118. Rogers K, Dewar K, McCubbin T, Spence A: Preliminary experience with ICI 35,868 as an I.V. induction agent: Comparison with althesin. Br J Anaesth *35*:807–810, 1980.
119. Fragen R, Hanssen H, Denissen P, Booij L, Crul J: Disoprofol (ICI 35868) for total intravenous anaesthesia. Acta Anaesth Scand *27*:113–116, 1983.
120. Prys-Roberts C, Davies J, Calverley R, Goodman N: Haemodynamic effects of infusions of di-isopropyl phenol (ICI 35,868) during nitrous oxide anaesthesia in man. Br J Anaesth *55*:105–111, 1983.
121. O'Callaghan A, Normandale J, Grundy E, Lumley J, Morgan M: Continuous intravenous infusion of disoprol (ICI 35,868, diprivan); Comparison with althesin to cover surgery under local analgesia. Anaesthesia *37*:295–300, 1982.
122. Al-Khudhairi D, Gordon G, Morgan M, Whitman J: Acute cardiovascular changes following disoprofol. Anaesthesia *37*:1007–1010, 1982.
123. Hannallah RS, Baker SB, Casey W, et al: Propofol: Effective dose and induction characteristics in unpremedicated children. Anesthesiology *74*:217–219, 1991.
124. Borgeat A, Popovic V, Meier D, Schwander D: Comparison of propofol and thiopental/halothane for short-duration ENT surgical procedures in children. Anesth Analg *71*:511–515, 1990.
125. Valtonen M, Iisalo E, Kanto J, Rosenberg P: Propofol as an induction agent in children: Pain on injection and pharmacokinetics. Acta Anaesthesiol Scand *33*:152–155, 1989.
126. Lockhart CH, Nelson WL: The relationship of ketamine requirements to age in pediatric patients. Anesthesiology *40*:507–508, 1974.
127. Chang T, Glazko T: Biotransformation and distribution of ketamine. Int Anesth Clin *12*:157–177, 1974.
128. Waterman AE, Livingston A: Effects of age and sex on ketamine anesthesia in the rat. Br J Anaesth *50*:885–889, 1978.
129. Eng M, Bonica JJ, Akamatsu TJ, Berges PU, Ureland K: Respiratory depression in newborn monkeys at cesarean section following ketamine administration. Br J Anaesth *47*:917–920, 1975.
130. Radney PA, Badola RP: Generalized extensor spasm in infants following ketamine anesthesia. Anesthesiology *39*:459–460, 1973.
131. Lockhart CH, Jenkins JJ: Ketamine-induced apnea in patients with increased intracranial pressure. Anesthesiology *37*:92–93, 1972.

132. Gasser S, Cohen M, Aygen M: The effect of ketamine on pulmonary artery pressure. Anaesthesia *29*:141–146, 1974.
133. Morray JP, Lynn AM, Stamm SJ, Herndon P, Kawabori I, Stevenson JG: Hemodynamic effects of ketamine in children with congenital heart disease. Anesth Analg *63*:895–899.
134. Hickey PR, Hansen DD, Cramolini GM: Pulmonary and systemic hemodynamic responses to ketamine in infants with normal and elevated pulmonary vascular resistance. Anesthesiology *61*:A438, 1984.
135. Way WL, Costley EC, Way EL: Respiratory sensitivity of the newborn infant to meperidine and morphine. Clin Pharmacol Ther *6*:454–459, 1965.
136. Kupferberg HJ, Way EL: Pharmacologic basis for the increased sensitivity of the newborn rat to morphine. J Pharmacol Exp Ther *141*:105–109, 1963.
137. Mirkin BL: Developmental pharmacology. Ann Rev Pharmacol *10*:255–272, 1970.
138. Hickey PR, Hansen DD: Fentanyl- and sufentanil-oxygen-pancuronium anesthesia for cardiac surgery in infants. Anesth Analg *63*:117–124, 1984.
139. Hickey PR, Hansen DD, Wessell D: Responses to high dose fentanyl in infants: Pulmonary and systemic hemodynamics. Anesthesiology *61*:A445, 1984.
140. Schieber RA, Stiller RL, Cook DR: Cardiovascular and pharmacodynamic effects of high-dose fentanyl in newborn piglets. Anesthesiology *63*:166–171, 1985.
141. Koren G, Crean P, Goresky G, Klein J, MacLeod SM: Fentanyl anesthesia for cardiac surgery in children: a) Fentanyl-oxygen vs. fentanyl-N_2O; b) Relationship between drug concentrations and pharmacodynamics. Anesthesiology *61*:A444, 1984.
142. Yaster M: The dose response of fentanyl in neonatal anesthesia. Anesthesiology *66*:433–435, 1987.
143. Ellis DJ, Steward DJ: Fentanyl dosage is associated with reduced blood glucose in pediatric patients after hypothermic cardiopulmonary bypass. Anesthesiology *72*:812–815, 1990.
144. Koehntop DE, Rodman JH, Brundage DM, Hegland MG, Buckley JJ: Pharmacokinetics of fentanyl in neonates. Anesth Analg *65*:227–232, 1986.
145. Singleton MA, Rosen JI, Fisher DM: Pharmacokinetics of fentanyl for infants and adults. Anesthesiology *61*:A440, 1984.
146. Johnson KL, Erickson JP, Holley FO, Scott JC: Fentanyl pharmacokinetics in the pediatric population. Anesthesiology *61*:A441, 1984.
147. Collins G, Koren G, Crean P, Klein J, Ray WL, MacLeod SM: The correlation between fentanyl pharmacokinetics and pharmacodynamics in preterm infants during PDA ligation. Anesthesiology *61*:A442, 1984.
148. Collins G, Koren G, Crean P, et al: Fentanyl pharmacokinetics and hemodynamic effects in preterm infants; Ligation of patent ductus arteriosus. Anesth Analg *64*:1078, 1985.
149. Koehntop DE, Rodman JH, Brundage DM, et al: Pharmacokinetics of fentanyl in neonates. Anesth Analg *65*:227, 1986.
150. Koren G, Goresky G, Crean P, Klein J, MacLeod SM: Unexpected alterations in fentanyl pharmacokinetics in children undergoing cardiac surgery: Age related or disease related? Dev Pharmacol Ther *9*:183–191, 1986.
151. Nelson PS, Streisand JB, Mulder SM, Pace NL, Stanley TH: Comparison of oral transmucosal fentanyl citrate and an oral solution of meperidine, diazepam, and atropine for premedication in children. Anesthesiology *70*:616–621, 1989.
152. Streisand JB, Stanley TH, Hague B, van Vreeswijk H, Ho GH, Pace NL: Oral transmucosal fentanyl citrate premedication in children. Anesth Analg *69*:28–34, 1989.
153. Goldstein-Dresner MC, Davis PJ, Kretchman E, Siewers RD, Certo N, Cook DR: Double-blind comparison of oral transmucosal fentanyl citrate with meperidine, diazepam, and atropine as preanesthetic medication in children with congenital heart disease. Anesthesiology *74*:28–33, 1991.
154. Niemegers C, Schellenkens K, VanBever W, Janssen P: Sufentanil, a very potent and extremely safe intravenous morphine-like compound in mice, rats and dogs. Arzheim Forsch *26*:1551, 1976.
155. Reddy P, Liu W, Port D, Gillmore S, Stanley T: Comparison of haemodynamic effects of anaesthetic doses of alphaprodine and sufentanil in the dog. Can Anaesth Soc J *27*:345–356, 1980.
156. Meuldermans W, Hurkmans R, Heykants J: Plasma protein binding and distribution of fentanyl, sufentanil, alfentanil and lofentanil in blood. Arch Int Pharmacodyn Ther *25*:4–19, 1982.
157. deLange S, Boscoe M, Stanley T, Pace N: Comparison of sufentanil-oxygen and fentanyl-oxygen for coronary artery surgery. Anesthesiology *56*:112–118, 1982.
158. Howie M, Rietz J, Reilley T, Harrington K, Smith D, Dasta J: Does sufentanil's shorter half-life have any clinical significance? Anesthesiology *59*:A146, 1983.
159. Sanford TJ, Smith NT, Dec-Silver H, Harrison WK: A comparison of morphine, fentanyl and sufentanil anesthesia for open-heart surgery; Induction, emergence, and extubation. Anesth Analg *65*:259–266, 1986.
160. Sebel P, Bovill J: Cardiovascular effects of sufentanil anesthesia. Anesth Analg *61*:115–119, 1982.
161. deLange S, Boscoe M, Stanley T, DeBruijn N, Philbin D, Coggins C: Antidiuretic and growth hormone response during coronary artery surgery with sufentanil-oxygen and alfentanil-oxygen anesthesia in man. Anesth Analg *61*:434–438, 1982.
162. Bovill J, Sebel P, Blackburn C, Heykants J: The pharmacokinetics of alfentanil (R39209): A new opiate analgesic. Anesthesiology *57*:439–443, 1982.
163. Rosow C, Philbin D, Moss J, Keegan C, Schneider R: Sufentanil vs. fentanyl. I. Suppression of hemodynamic responses. Anesthesiology *59*:A323, 1983.
164. Bovill J, Sebel P, Fiolet J, Touber J, Kok K, Philbin D: The influence of sufentanil on endocrine and metabolic responses to cardiac surgery. Anesth Analg *62*:391–397, 1983.
165. Hickey P, Hansen D: Fentanyl and sufentanil-oxygen-pancuronium anesthesia for cardiac surgery in infants. Anesth Analg *63*:117–124, 1984.
166. Henderson JM, Brodsky DA, Fisher DM, et al: Preinduction of anesthesia in pediatric patients with nasally administered sufentanil. Anesthesiology *68*:671–675, 1988.
167. Helmers JH, Noorduin H, Van Peer A, Van Leeuwen L, Zuurmond WWA: Comparison of intravenous and intranasal sufentanil absorption and sedation. Can J Anaesth *36*:5; 494–497, 1989.
168. DeCastro J, Van De Weter A, Wouter L, Xhouneux R, Reneman R, Kay B: Comparative study of cardiovascular, neurological and metabolic side-effects of 8 narcotics in dogs. Acta Anaesth Belg *30*:5–99, 1979.
169. Camu F, Gepts E, Rucquoi M, Heykants J: Pharmacokinetics of alfentanil (R39709) in man. Anesth Analg *61*:657–661, 1982.
170. Hug C: Alfentanil: Pharmacology and Uses in Anaesthesia. Aukland, New Zealand, Adis Press, 1984.

171. Davis PJ, Stiller RL, Cook DR, et al: Effects of cholestatic hepatic disease and chronic renal failure on alfentanil pharmacokinetics in children. Anesth Analg *68*:579–583, 1989.
172. Meistelman C, Saint-Maurice C, Lepaul M, et al: A comparison of alfentanil pharmacokinetics in children and adults. Anesthesiology *66*:13, 1987.
173. Roure P, Jean N, Leclerc A-C, et al: Pharmacokinetics of alfentanil in children undergoing surgery. Br J Anaesth *59*:1437, 1987.
174. Davis PJ, Killian A, Stiller RL, et al: Pharmacokinetics of alfentanil in newborn premature infants and older children. Dev Pharmacol Ther *13*:21–27, 1989.
175. Killian A, Davis PJ, Stiller RL, Cicco R, Cook DR, Guthrie RD: Influence of gestational age on pharmacokinetics of alfentanil in neonates. Dev Pharmacol Ther *15*:82–85, 1990.
176. McDonnell T, Bartkowski R, Williams J: ED_{50} of alfentanil for induction of anesthesia in unpremedicated young adults. Anesthesiology *60*:136–140, 1984.
177. Nauta J, Delange S, Koopman D, Spierdijk J, Stanley T: Anesthetic induction with alfentanil; A new, short-acting narcotic analgesic. Anesth Analg *61*:267–272, 1982.
178. deLange S, Boscoe M, Stanley T, Pace N: Comparison of sufentanil-oxygen and fentanyl-oxygen for coronary artery surgery. Anesthesiology *56*:112–118, 1982.
179. Leysen J, Commern W, Niemegers C: Sufentanil—a superior ligand for u-opiate receptors: Binding properties and regional distribution in rat brain and spinal cord. Eur J Pharmacol *87*:209–225, 1983.
180. Kay B, Pleuvry B: Human volunteer studies of alfentanil (R39209), a new short-acting narcotic analgesic. Anaesthesia *35*:952–956, 1980.
181. Kay B, Stephenson D: Alfentanil (R39209): Initial clinical experiences with a new narcotic analgesic. Anaesthesia *35*:1197–1201, 1980.
182. Kramer M, Kling D, Walter P, Bormann B, Hempelmann G: Alfentanil, a new short-acting opioid: Haemodynamic and respiratory aspects. Anesthetist *32*:265–271, 1983.
183. Stanley T, Pace N, Liu W, Gillmor S, Willard K: Alfentanil-N_2O vs. fentanyl-N_2O balanced anesthesia: Comparison of plasma hormonal changes, early postoperative respiratory function and speed of postoperative recovery. Anesth Analg *62*:285, 1983.
184. deLange S, Boscoe M, Stanley T, DeBruijn N, Berman L, Robertson D: Catecholamine and cortisol response to sufentanil-oxygen and alfentanil-oxygen anaesthesia during coronary artery surgery. Can Anaesth Soc J *30*:248–254, 1983.
185. Ecobichon DJ, Stephen DS: Perinatal development of human blood esterases. Clin Pharmacol Exp Ther *14*:44–46, 1973.
186. Blankenbaker WL, DiFazio CA, Berry FA Jr: Lidocaine and its metabolites in the newborn. Anesthesiology *42*:325–330, 1975.
187. Moore RG, Thomas J, Triggs DB, et al: The pharmacokinetics and metabolism of anilide anesthetics in neonates. Eur J Clin Pharmacol *14*:203, 1978.
188. Morgan D, McQuillan D, Thomas J: Pharmacokinetics and metabolism of the anilide local anesthetics in neonates. Eur J Clin Pharmacol *13*:365, 1981.
189. Dauchot P, Gravenstein JS: Effects of atropine on the electrocardiogram in different age groups. Clin Pharmacol Exp Ther *12*:274–280, 1971.
190. Gaviotaki A, Smith RM: Use of atropine in pediatric anesthesia. Int Anesthesiol Clin *1*:1:97–114, 1962.
191. Cook DR: Clinical use of muscle relaxants in infants and children. Anesth Analg *60*:335–343, 1981.
192. Anggard L, Ottoson D: Observations on the functional development of the neuromuscular apparatus in fetal sheep. Exp Neurol *7*:294–304, 1963.
193. Close R: Dynamic properties of fast and slow skeletal muscles of the rat during development. J Physiol *173*:74–95, 1964.
194. Close R: Force-velocity properties of mouse muscles. Nature *206*:718–719, 1965.
195. Close R: Effects of cross-union of motor nerves to fast and slow skeletal muscles. Nature *206*:831–832, 1965.
196. Buller AJ: Developmental physiology of the neuromuscular system. Br Med Bull *22*:45–48, 1966.
197. Koenigsberger MR, Patten B, Lovelace RE: Studies of neuromuscular function in the newborn—a comparison of myoneural function in the full-term and premature infant. Neuropaediatrie *4*:350–361, 1973.
198. Goudsouzian NG: Maturation of neuromuscular transmission in the infant. Br J Anaesth *52*:205–213, 1980.
199. Crumrine RS, Yodlowski EH: Assessment of neuromuscular function in infants. Anesthesiology *54*:29–32, 1981.
200. Cook DR, Fischer CG: Neuromuscular blocking effects of succinylcholine in infants and children. Anesthesiology *42*:662–665, 1975.
201. Cook DR, Fischer CG: Characteristics of succinylcholine neuromuscular blockade in infants. Anesth Analg *57*:63–66, 1978.
202. Goudsouzian NG, Liu LMP: The neuromuscular response of infants to a continuous infusion of succinylcholine. Anesthesiology *60*:97–101, 1984.
203. Walts LF, Dillon JB: The response of newborns to succinylcholine and D-tubocurarine. Anesthesiology *31*:35–38, 1969.
204. Churchill-Davidson HC, Wise RP: The response of the newborn infant to muscle relaxants. Can Anaesth Soc J *11*:1–5, 1964.
205. Donlon JV, Ali HH, Savarese JJ: A new approach to the study of four nondepolarizing relaxants in man. Anesth Analg *53*:924–39, 1974.
206. Goudsouzian NG, Liu LMP, Cote CJ: Comparison of equipotent doses of nondepolarizing muscle relaxants in children. Anesth Analg *60*:862–866, 1981.
207. Goudsouzian NG, Liu LMP, Savarese JJ: Metocurarine in infants and children: Neuromuscular and clinical effects. Anesthesiology *49*:266–269, 1978.
208. Goudsouzian NG, Ryan JF, Savarese JJ: The neuromuscular effects of pancuronium in infants and children. Anesthesiology *41*:95–98, 1974.
209. Goudsouzian NG, Donlon JV, Savarese JJ, Ryan JF: Re-evaluation of dosage and duration of action of D-tubocurarine in the pediatric age group. Anesthesiology *43*:416–425, 1975.
210. Goudsouzian NG, Martyn JJA, Liu LMP: The dose response effect of long-acting non-depolarizing neuromuscular blocking agents in children. Can Anaesth Soc J *3*:246–250, 1984.
211. Cook DR: Sensitivity of the newborn to tubocurarine. Br J Anaesth *53*:320, 1981.
212. Fisher DM, O'Keefe C, Stanski DR, Cronnelly R, Miller RD, Gregory GA: Pharmacokinetics and pharmacodynamics of D-tubocurarine in infants, children, and adults. Anesthesiology *57*:203–208, 1982.
213. Pittet JF, Tassonyi E, Morel DR, et al: Neuromuscular effect of pipecuronium bromide in infants and children during nitrous oxide–alfentanil anesthesia. Anesthesiology *72*:432–435, 1990.
214. Sarner JB, Brandom BW, Cook DR, et al: Clinical pharmacology of doxacurium chloride (BW A938U) in children. Anesth Analg *67*:303–306, 1988.

215. Sarner JB, Brandom BW, Dong ML, et al: Clinical pharmacology of pipecuronium in infants and children during halothane anesthesia. Anesth Analg *71*:362–366, 1990.
216. Cook DR, Freeman JA, Lai AA, et al: Pharmacokinetics and pharmacodynamics of doxacurium in normal patients and those with hepatic or renal failure. Anesth Analg *72*:145–150, 1991.
217. Caldwell JE, Canfell PC, Castagnoli KP, et al: The influence of renal failure on the pharmacokinetics and duration of action of pipecuronium bromide in patients anesthetized with halothane and nitrous oxide. Anesthesiology *70*:7–12, 1989.
218. Stiller RL, Cook DR, Chakravorti S: In vitro degradation of atracurium in human plasma. Br J Anaesth *57*:1085–1088, 1985.
219. Stiller RL, Brandom BW, Cook DR: Determinations of atracurium by high-performance liquid chromatography. Anesth Analg *64*:58–62, 1985.
220. Brandom BW, Woelfel SK, Cook DR, Fehr BL, Rudd GD: Clinical pharmacology of atracurium in infants. Anesth Analg *63*:309–312, 1984.
221. Brandom BW, Rudd GD, Cook DR: Clinical pharmacology of atracurium in pediatric patients. Br J Anaesth *55*:117s–121s, 1983.
222. Brandom BW, Cook DR, Woelfel SK, Lineberry CG, Fehr BL, Rudd GD: Atracurium infusion in children during fentanyl, halothane, and isoflurane anesthesia. Anesth Analg *64*:471–476, 1985.
223. Goudsouzian NG, Liu L, Cote CJ, Gionfriddo M, Rudd GD: Safety and efficacy of atracurium in adolescents and children anesthetized with halothane. Anesthesiology *39*:459–462, 1983.
224. Goudsouzian NG, Liu LMP, Gionfriddo M, Rudd GD: Neuromuscular effects of atracurium in infants and children. Anesthesiology *62*:75–79, 1985.
225. Brandom BW, Cook DR, Stiller RL, Woelfel S, Chakravorti S, Lai A: Pharmacokinetics of atracurium in infants and children. Br J Anaesth *58*:1210–1213, 1986.
226. D'Hollander AA, Luyckx C, Barvais L, DeVille A: Clinical evaluation of atracurium besylate requirement for a stable muscle relaxation during surgery: Lack of age-related effects. Anesthesiology *59*:237–240, 1983.
227. Durant NN: Norcuron, a new, nondepolarizing neuromuscular blocking agent. Semin Anesth *1*:47–56, 1982.
228. Fisher DM, Miller RD: Neuromuscular effects of vecuronium (ORG NC45) in infants and children during N_2O, halothane anesthesia. Anesthesiology *58*:519–523, 1983.
229. d'Hollander AA, Massaux F, Nevelsteen M, Agoston S: Age-dependent dose-response relationship of ORG NC45 in anaesthetized patients. Br J Anaesth *54*:653–657, 1982.
230. Goudsouzian NG, Martyn J, Liu LMP, et al: Safety and efficacy of vecuronium in adolescents and children. Anesth Analg *62*:1083, 1983.
231. Rupp SM, Miller RD, Gencarelli PJ: Vecuronium-induced neuromuscular blockade during enflurane, halothane, and isoflurane in humans. Anesthesiology *60*:102–105, 1984.
232. Miller RD, Rupp SM, Fisher DM, Cronnelly R, Fahey MR, Sohn YJ: Clinical pharmacology of vecuronium and atracurium. Anesthesiology *61*:444–453, 1984.
233. Fisher DM: Pharmacodynamics of vecuronium in infants and children. Clin Pharm Exp Ther *37*:402–406, 1985.
234. Foldes FF, Nagashima H, Nguyen HD, et al: The neuromuscular effects of ORG9426 in patients receiving balanced anesthesia. Anesthesiology *75*:191–196, 1991.
235. Brandom BW, Sarner JB, Woelfel SK, et al: Mivacurium infusion requirements in pediatric surgical patients during nitrous oxide–halothane and during nitrous oxide–narcotic anesthesia. Anesth Analg *71*:16–22, 1990.
236. Fisher DM, Cronnelly R, Miller RD, Sharma M: The neuromuscular pharmacology of neostigmine in infants and children. Anesthesiology *59*:220–225, 1983.
237. Fisher DM, Cronnelly R, Sharma M, Miller RD: Clinical pharmacology of edrophonium in infants. Anesthesiology *61*:428–433, 1984.
238. Meakin G, Sweet PT, Bevan JC, Bevan DR: Neostigmine and edrophonium as antagonists of pancuronium in infants and children. Anesthesiology *59*:316–321, 1983.

CHAPTER

3 Infectious Diseases

DAVID A. ZIDEMAN, M.B., and DAVID J. STEWARD, M.B.

Infections are common during infancy and childhood. The anesthesiologist may encounter infants and children who require surgical treatment related to infectious disease, or more often this disease may be present in a child who requires surgery for an unrelated lesion. In the latter case, the risks of anesthesia in the presence of the infectious disease must be balanced against the urgency of the surgical procedure. Some of these judgments will be very difficult, and in all patients the anesthesia technique must be modified to accommodate any special aspects of the infectious disease.

Some childhood infectious diseases are extremely contagious, and anesthesiologists must be familiar with the mode of transmission if they are to take adequate precautions to prevent the spread of infection to other patients and hospital staff. Many of the conditions to be discussed are now quite rare, and because of the rarity many physicians are less familiar with the special care that is required.

FEVER

Fever is defined as elevation of the body temperature above the normal. When it is associated with infection, this elevation of body temperature is a part of the patient's response to that infection. Indeed, there is some evidence to suggest that fever may assist the body in combating the infective agent.[1] Certainly, during an infection the patient's thermoregulatory responses tend to maintain the elevated core temperature.

Low birth weight infants may not develop a fever in response to sepsis and, in fact, may become hypothermic. This lack of a febrile reaction might contribute to increased mortality from infection in newborn infants.[2]

The mechanism of production of fever is as follows: Infecting agents stimulate the production of pyrogen by leukocytes, macrophages, and other cells. This pyrogen, which is a polypeptide, acts upon the hypothalamus, either directly or via a prostaglandin, catecholamine, and cyclic adenosine monophosphate (cAMP) pathway. The result is a hypothalamic-induced increase in heat production centered principally in skeletal muscle in older children and adults. Young infants may become febrile as a result of nonshivering thermogenesis.[3]

The rise in body temperature during a fever is associated with an increased metabolic rate for oxygen. In adults, this increase approximates

13 percent for each degree centigrade above normal body temperature.[4] The energy cost of fever in infants and small children will be higher as a result of greater heat loss from a relatively larger body surface area.[2]

The clinical manifestations of fever include chills, headache, rigors, and tachycardia. Sweating may occur as the fever resolves. Delirium and coma may occur during high fever, and convulsions may occur in children (see later). Fluid losses via the skin and respiratory tract are increased and may result in dehydration, particularly if fluid intake is reduced owing to anorexia or vomiting.

Therapy to reduce fever can be justified if this benefits the general comfort of the child, improves the outcome of the illness, or reduces the incidence of febrile convulsions. Favorable response of a fever to antipyretic therapy does not indicate that the illness is trivial,[5] but this may induce a false sense of security in parents and physicians and mask the early signs of serious illness. There is little evidence that reduction of fever improves the outcome of childhood infections. Antipyretic drugs may cause toxicity; however, they may be indicated when there is an urgent indication to lower the body temperature (for example, febrile convulsions or preexisting heart disease).

The treatment of fever generally should be directed at the underlying infective process. Active measures to reduce the body temperature of a febrile, infected patient may cause harm; if the child is placed in a cool environment, heat losses will increase, but may be matched by increased thermogenesis unless the hypothalamic setpoint is lowered. This increased thermogenesis will be accompanied by a further increase in the metabolic demand for oxygen.

FEBRILE CONVULSIONS

About 4 percent of children aged 6 months to 6 years will have a febrile convulsion.[6] These are generally benign. A simple febrile convulsion is characterized by a brief, generalized (nonfocal) seizure during a fever without evidence of serious intracranial disease. There is prompt recovery to a normal state of consciousness, and no other signs of neurological or metabolic disease. There may be a family history or past history of febrile convulsions. It is most important that other causes of seizures be sought and excluded before accepting a diagnosis of seizure due to fever. Antecedent brain injury is often present in patients with febrile convulsions.

Treatment is directed at the cause of the fever but must also ensure rapid termination of the seizure. Prompt reduction of the fever with antipyretics and tepid sponging is advised. Intravenous diazepam, 0.3 mg/kg, administered at a rate of 1 mg/min, may be given until the seizure stops.[6] Appropriate steps should be taken to preserve the airway and minimize the risk of aspiration.

There is controversy about the danger of neurological or intellectual sequelae of a febrile convulsion. Children who have repeated febrile convulsions may be placed on long-term anticonvulsant therapy, though this too is controversial.

ANESTHESIA FOR PATIENTS WITH FEVER

Patients with increased body temperature will have an increased metabolic rate for oxygen and carbon dioxide. The increase is directly related to the extent of pyrexia. Hence, special consideration should be given to ensuring a high concentration of inspired oxygen and an increased level of alveolar ventilation. Any interruption of oxygenation is very poorly tolerated by pyrexial patients; should hypoxia proceed to cardiac arrest, the neurological result may be very much worse than in normothermic patients. A perfect continuous airway and very adequate oxygenation and ventilation must be absolutely assured.

Some other considerations also apply for the patient with pyrexia. Atropine should not be given as a premedicant as it will prevent sweating and hence may lead to further preoperative pyrexia. If necessary, atropine can be given once anesthesia is induced, as temperature management is more readily accomplished during anesthesia. The patient should be placed on a cooling blanket and ice packs used if required to restore normothermia. Volatile anesthetic agents such as halothane and isoflurane may be useful to produce vasodilation of skin vessels and so increase heat loss from pyrexial patients. Neuromuscular blocking drugs should be given to prevent shivering, especially if active cooling measures are taken.

SEPTICEMIA

Septicemia (sepsis) implies a severe and overwhelming infection[7] with a bacteremia. The diagnosis is based on findings of fever, shock, debility, and possible disseminated intravascular coagulation in a patient who is susceptible to, or has a likely source of, infection.

Sepsis in pediatric patients is most commonly seen in the neonate, but fulminating sepsis may also occur in older children, especially with meningococcal, pneumococcal, staphylococcal, or streptococcal infections.

NEONATAL SEPSIS

This may affect 1 to 8 per 1000 live births.[8] Despite advances in antibiotic therapy, the mortality remains as high as 25 percent.

Several factors predispose the newborn infant to sepsis. Both cellular and humoral responses to infection are limited, especially in the preterm infant.[9] Leukocytes have impaired chemotaxis, phagocytosis, and bactericidal action. Immunoglobulin deficiency is also present, especially in the preterm infant, as transplacental transfer of globulins varies with the length of gestation.

This vulnerability to infection, when associated with conditions that tend to introduce microorganisms into the infant's environment, may result in severe sepsis. Antenatal factors, such as prolonged rupture of the membranes and maternal colonization with group B streptococcus, increase the risk of sepsis, as does perinatal asphyxia.[10] The risk of infection is high in the neonatal nursery.[11] Endotracheal intubation, venous infusions, and invasive monitoring lines all provide routes for infection. Preterm infants who undergo surgical procedures have a higher incidence of sepsis than others. Failure to observe strict hand washing prior to handling of infants is a leading cause of infection.

The organisms most commonly involved in neonatal sepsis have been gram-positive group B streptococci and the gram-negative *Escherichia coli*.[12] In the past 10 years, however, the coagulase-negative staphylococci have emerged as a very frequent cause of infection (see later).

The clinical picture of neonatal sepsis is varied, and the early signs are frequently missed. Classic signs of sepsis are lethargy, pyrexia or temperature instability, abdominal distention, jaundice, respiratory distress, and apnea. In addition, changes in activity, feeding, and muscle tone may be noted. Later, cardiovascular changes result in hypotension; mottling of the skin and a bleeding tendency may become apparent.

The diagnosis of sepsis is confirmed by blood, urine, and cerebrospinal fluid (CSF) culture, which may also identify the organism involved and its antibiotic sensitivities. Unfortunately, there is a high false-negative rate for blood culture in the septic neonate.[10] Other laboratory tests may assist in diagnosis. Abnormal leukocyte counts and the presence of neutrophil vacuolization or toxic granulation is a good indication of sepsis. C-reactive protein levels are increased within 24 hours in most infants with sepsis. Thrombocytopenia is often present. Gram stains of blood smears may sometimes reveal the presence of bacteria. The diagnosis is therefore not always easily confirmed, and the use of a series of biochemical tests as a "sepsis screen" may be useful.[13]

The treatment of neonatal sepsis must begin early (before culture results are available). Antibiotic therapy should be based on the likely organism involved. Various regimens have been used as initial therapy before the causative organism is identified. These are selected on the basis of the likely organism involved in the particular infant, with the knowledge of patterns of infection within the particular neonatal nursery. The reader is referred to texts of neonatal medicine for specific recommendations.[12, 14]

In addition to antibiotic therapy, the neonate with sepsis requires aggressive further treatment. The infant should be carefully maintained in a neutral thermal environment, electrolyte and acid-base disturbances corrected, and oxygenation ensured. The infant should be carefully monitored to detect apnea. Oral feedings should be discontinued and a gastric tube inserted to prevent gastric dilatation. Blood component therapy may be required to correct coagulopathy and anemia; platelet infusions or exchange transfusions or both may reduce the mortality rate, especially in beta-streptococcal sepsis.[15] The seriously ill neonate with sepsis may require therapy with inotropic drugs.

The anesthesiologist may be involved in the surgical care of the infant with sepsis. It is important that the preoperative cardiorespiratory, metabolic, acid-base and electrolyte, and hematological status be accurately evaluated. Meticulous care during transport and intraoperatively must be directed at maintaining all therapy and avoiding further physiological stress. Cold stress, hypoglycemia, and fluid overload must be prevented. Asepsis must be ensured in all anesthesia-related procedures (for example, venipuncture, endotracheal intubation).

SEPSIS IN OLDER INFANTS AND CHILDREN

Sepsis after the neonatal period is most commonly due to meningococcal, pneumococcal, staphylococcal, or streptococcal infections.

Meningococcal Sepsis

The meningococcus, *Neisseria meningitidis*, is a gram-negative diplococcus that is frequently found in the nasopharynx, where it may cause a mild pharyngitis or result in no symptoms. From such carriers the disease is spread and may be manifested as meningococcal meningitis, meningococcal bacteremia, or sepsis.

Meningococcal sepsis is a fulminating disease characterized by high fever and a petechial or purpuric rash. The rash may become widespread (purpura fulminans) with mucous membrane involvement. In some cases the rash may not be present and this may delay diagnosis.[16] Meningitis may or may not be present. Arthritis is common and may be the presenting feature. Vomiting and diarrhea may occur. Pneumonia may be present on initial presentation.

The disease may proceed extremely rapidly, with circulatory failure and death within a few hours. Myocarditis may complicate meningococcal sepsis, and disseminated intravascular coagulation (DIC) may occur. This DIC may lead to vascular insufficiency caused by both direct vessel occlusion and release of vasoconstrictor substances, with eventual gangrene. Severe meningococcal sepsis in children may be complicated by adrenal insufficiency[17] due to bilateral adrenal hemorrhage (the Waterhouse-Friderichsen syndrome).

Prompt diagnosis of meningococcal sepsis is important so that early antibiotic therapy can be initiated and also to ensure that contacts can be given prophylactic therapy to prevent spread of the disease.

The first objective in treatment of meningococcal sepsis is to restore the circulating blood volume. Appropriate hemodynamic monitoring must be established to achieve this. An arterial line, central venous pressure line, and urinary catheter should be inserted. Plasma or 5 percent albumin, together with appropriate multiple electrolyte solutions, should be infused to achieve an optimal filling pressure. If blood pressure remains low, inotropic drugs are required. A low urine output with adequate fluid intake and a normal blood pressure indicates the onset of renal failure.

The use of corticosteroids has been controversial, but many authorities had advised their use in the absence of any firm evidence of their lack of efficacy.[18] Recently there is increasing evidence that early therapy with dexamethasone may reduce meningeal inflammation and improve the outcome.[19]

The choice of antibiotics for serious meningococcal infections has previously been ampicillin with chloramphenicol. The new generation cephalosporins are now being used more frequently, and ceftriaxone appears to be emerging as the drug of choice.[20] Continuous lumbar epidural blockade with 0.125 percent bupivacaine has been used to alleviate pain and improve perfusion in a patient with severe vascular compromise of the lower extremities secondary to meningococcal purpura fulminans.[21] This patient had normal coagulation indices at the time this therapy was instituted.

Pneumococcal Sepsis

This disease is characteristically seen in patients with a nonfunctioning or absent spleen.[22, 23] The pneumococcus is especially dangerous to such children as it is an encapsulated bacterium; splenic function is thought to aid phagocytosis of such organisms by production of opsonins.[24] A critical illness with widespread purpura and DIC may occur. The peripheral blood smear may demonstrate the bacteria on Gram staining. The risk of sepsis is highest in infants under 2 years of age and in recently splenectomized children.

Prophylactic antibiotics are recommended for asplenic patients, but their value in preventing sepsis is unproved. A conservative approach to splenic trauma is recommended.[25] A pneumococcal vaccine is available and is advised for children over 2 years of age with impaired splenic function.

Staphylococcal Sepsis

Acute staphylococcal sepsis may occur without a previous focus of infection[26] but usually can be related to a focal infection. Osteomyelitis, arthritis, and wound infections are common primary foci. Staphylococcal infections may appear as a complication of vascular cannulation, hence the anesthesiologist must always strive for optimal asepsis. Toxic shock syndrome resulting from staphylococcal involvement in a bacterial tracheitis complicating respiratory syncytial virus infection has been described.[27]

The patient with staphylococcal sepsis appears very ill and toxic. Skin rashes similar to those of meningococcal sepsis may occur. Hematuria, jaundice, seizures, and cardiac murmurs may occur as the disease progresses.[28] Disseminated intravascular coagulation is common.

The treatment of staphylococcal sepsis depends upon active fluid replacement and aggressive antibiotic therapy. Nafcillin and cefazolin are recommended drugs.

In the neonatal intensive care unit, coagulase-negative staphylococci, and particularly *Staphylococcus epidermidis*, have become the most common pathogens. Sepsis due to these organisms is associated with significant mortality and morbidity and often results in prolonged hospitalization.[28] The signs of sepsis due to coagulase-negative staphylococci are similar to those already outlined, but focal lesions may also be present. In such cases there will be persistent bacteremia, and infected lesions may be found in the heart, central nervous system, bowel, or lungs. These lesions may be associated with indwelling catheters, shunts, endotracheal tubes, or chest drains.

Patients with infections due to coagulase-negative staphylococci are generally treated with vancomycin. The prevention of nosocomial infection by these organisms is a matter of some importance for the anesthesiologist. Strict adherence to hand-washing routines can minimize spread between patients. The use of a careful surgical technique for central venous catheter insertion and management is essential. Catheter insertion sites should be inspected every 72 hours, and peripheral intravenous cannulae should be removed after 72 hours if possible.[29]

It is possible that the material of some intravenous cannulae may encourage the growth of coagulase-positive staphylococci, hence it is also possible that particular cannulae will be found to be preferable for use in the neonate at risk.

STREPTOCOCCAL SEPSIS

Streptococcal sepsis may complicate cellulitis, chickenpox, or wound infections. Occasionally sepsis occurs without an obvious focal infection.

SEPTIC SHOCK

Shock is a frequent manifestation of acute sepsis and is associated with a high mortality.[30] In fact, there has probably been an increase in the incidence of septic shock in children over the past decade. This is due to the increasing complexity of surgical procedures, widespread antibiotic use, prolongation of life of patients with defective immunity, and the use of invasive techniques that provide portals for infection.[30]

The common pathogens are gram-negative organisms: *E. coli* and *N. meningitidis* were frequently implicated, but recently a variety of other organisms, including *Haemophilus influenzae* type B and *Streptococcus pneumoniae* have been shown to be commonly associated with pediatric septic shock.[31] Less commonly, *S. aureus* and other gram-positive organisms may be involved. The initial disturbances of septic shock are mediated by endotoxins and result in changes in the microcirculation. Later, the cardiovascular effects of secondary products (complement, kallikrein, and so forth) and other vasoactive agents become superimposed. In addition, there is failure of oxygen extraction at the cellular level, activation of compensatory mechanisms, and the effect of underlying host disease factors.[32]

The end result is an unpredictable pattern of circulatory insufficiency with inadequate tissue oxygenation. Three stages of the circulatory response to sepsis are generally recognized: hyperdynamic compensated, hyperdynamic uncompensated, and cardiogenic.[33] The early stages are characterized by tachycardia, tachypnea, bounding pulses, and normotension or hypertension, with a decreased systemic vascular resistance and a high cardiac index. Later the tachycardia persists but is accompanied by hypotension, reduced cardiac index, and increased systemic vascular resistance. Hypoxemia is present throughout and in the last stages is accompanied by acidosis (respiratory and metabolic) and oliguria. A coagulopathy appears as the disease progresses. Multiple organ failure is the final outcome unless the process can be reversed.

The diagnosis of septic shock is based on the finding of persisting hypotension (<2 standard deviations [SDs] of mean normal for age), plus clinical evidence of sepsis, fever or hypothermia, tachycardia, and dyspnea, combined with signs of inadequate tissue perfusion (disordered mentation, oliguria, hypoxemia, or metabolic acidosis).[32]

The treatment of septic shock aims to preserve the central nervous system, the myocardium, and renal function.[33] Intensive cardiovascular monitoring is essential to guide fluid therapy and drug administration. Cardiorespiratory support measures may be required from the outset. The important therapeutic steps are:[34]

1. Appropriate cardiorespiratory support, which is directed at ensuring the best possible oxygenation and an adequate alveolar ventilation.
2. Intravenous fluid therapy to maintain the central venous pressure above 10 mm Hg and the hematocrit at 35 to 40 percent. Rapid

early fluid resuscitation using volumes in excess of 40 ml/kg in the first hour has been demonstrated to improve survival in pediatric septic shock.[35] This volume was made up of approximately 60 percent crystalloid (Ringer's lactate or normal saline) and 40 percent colloid (5 percent albumin or other blood products); such therapy was not associated with an increased incidence of cardiogenic pulmonary edema or adult respiratory distress syndrome.[35]
3. Aggressive intravenous antibiotic therapy.
4. Correction of acid-base and electrolyte disturbances, hypoglycemia, and hypocalcemia.
5. Dopamine infusion to reverse hypotension and oliguria when the central venous pressure is above 10 μg/kg/min may be required, depending upon response.
6. Corticosteroids: methylprednisolone, 30 to 60 mg/kg intravenously every 4 hours, until hypotension is corrected.
7. Appropriate surgical treatment of localized infections or other lesions.

Anesthesia for the Patient with Septic Shock

It may be necessary to anesthetize the patient in shock to drain localized infections or to resect infected or infarcted tissues. Although it is important that optimal therapy for the shock state be in progress, surgical treatment should not be delayed unduly. The physical status of the patient may continue to deteriorate because of infected tissues. Hypovolemia and acidosis should be corrected and fever reduced prior to operation; hypoxia should be reversed as much as possible; and hypoventilation, if present, should be treated by controlled ventilation. Corticosteroid therapy should be augmented and inotropic therapy used to the maximum.

Anesthesia techniques for the patient in septic shock should be selected to spare the cardiovascular system. Ketamine may be useful to induce anesthesia. Fentanyl and oxygen with neuromuscular blocking drugs are recommended for maintenance of anesthesia.[36]

PERINATAL INFECTIONS

Several serious perinatal infections may cause death or lasting damage to a child. The anesthesiologist should have some knowledge of the mode of transmission and the effects of these important diseases.

CYTOMEGALOVIRUS

Cytomegalovirus (CMV) is a DNA virus of similar structure to the herpes virus. CMV is the most frequently recognized congenital infection and is a common cause of later mental retardation. In adults, the infection is usually symptomless and innocuous. The virus is frequently found in cervical secretions and breast milk of the mother, but only some infants will acquire the infection and develop symptoms.

Cytomegalovirus is carried, probably in the leukocyte, in asymptomatic hosts and may be transmitted by blood transfusion. Transfusion-acquired CMV disease may occur in infants with serious sequelae. Blood transfused to infants should be screened for CMV.[37] The infant with CMV may infect the mother, and this may result in fetal CMV infection during subsequent pregnancies.[36]

The clinical manifestations of CMV disease depend upon the time of infection and the immune status of the infant: transplacental immunity may modify the disease. Intrauterine infection of the fetus may result in severe congenital deformity; microcephaly with mental retardation is common.[38] Intracranial periventricular calcification may be present. Other features of congenital CMV infection are hepatosplenomegaly, jaundice, thrombocytopenia, and eye disease (optic atrophy, chorioretinitis, coloboma, and cataracts).

Postnatal infection may result in pneumonia, hepatosplenomegaly, lymphadenopathy, and atypical lymphocytosis.

No specific treatment for congenital CMV has been shown to be effective. Antiviral agents have little effect on the course of the disease.

CONGENITAL RUBELLA

In older children and adults, rubella is a mild infectious disease with an incubation period of 10 to 21 days. The systemic signs are very mild and are often missed. They include fever, sore throat, and lymphadenopathy in the sternomastoid and occipital regions. The maculopapular rash usually develops in the face and spreads to the trunk and limbs. Occasional complications include arthritis and encephalitis, which are rare. Thrombocytopenic purpura may occur with rubella.[40] The rubella syndrome that follows intrauterine infection is the most serious complication of the disease.[41]

Rubella Syndrome

Maternal rubella may cause severe fetal defects, especially if infection occurs during early gestation (less than 12 weeks). The classic rubella syndrome results in a low birth weight child with congenital heart disease (patent ductus arteriosus, pulmonary stenosis), eye defects (cataracts, glaucoma, and microphthalmia), and microcephaly. Deafness is also a common feature. In 1964, a severe epidemic of rubella in the United States resulted in other features of the syndrome being recognized. These include hepatosplenomegaly with jaundice, thrombocytopenic purpura, encephalitis, and myocarditis.[41]

A "late onset" rubella syndrome is also recognized. Affected infants show minimal signs at birth but after 3 to 6 months develop multisystem disease.[42] Pneumonia, skin rash, diarrhea, and hypogammaglobulinemia circulating immune complexes may be present.[43] Infants with rubella syndrome may develop hypotonia and convulsions later. Diabetes mellitus has also occurred during childhood in patients with rubella syndrome.

Anesthetic Implications. The child with rubella syndrome may present for surgery of the various component defects of the syndrome, for complications thereof, or for any other surgical disease of childhood.

Special attention must be directed to the cardiovascular status, but other defects also demand consideration. Microcephaly may lead to difficulty with airway management and intubation, as may the presence of cleft palate and dental deformities. Anemia and thrombocytopenia may be present and require correction prior to anesthesia and surgery. The small size of the patient is frequently compounded by a generalized muscular weakness, and the response to and recovery from neuromuscular blocking drugs should be carefully assessed.

Finally, it must be recognized that the rubella virus persists in some body fluids of the child for prolonged periods; thus, the possibility of cross-infection must be considered and suitable isolation precautions taken.

HERPES SIMPLEX INFECTION

Herpes simplex virus (HSV) has a DNA structure very similar to that of CMV. In the adult, infection characteristically produces cutaneous lesions about the mouth (type 1 virus, or HSV-1) or in the genital region (type 2 virus, or HSV-2). Oral lesions due to HSV-1 may be spread to other skin areas by direct contact, and digital infections are common in anesthesiologists.[44] HSV-2 infection is sexually transmitted.

The fetus may become infected in utero, but more commonly the neonate acquires the infection from the mother during birth. The extent of the disease in the infected neonate depends upon the baby's immune status.[45] Neonatal herpes may also be acquired from other infants and hospital personnel.[46]

Neonatal herpes infection usually becomes apparent in the first month of life and may range from isolated skin lesions to widespread infection. The skin lesions typically are groups of vesicles. The disseminated infection presents with fever, pneumonia, hepatomegaly and jaundice, and coagulopathy.[47] Mortality is high in disseminated herpes, and many survivors have neurological or ocular damage or both.

Treatment is with antiviral drugs such as acyclovir, but the long-term outcome is as yet uncertain. Prevention of maternal herpes and avoidance of nosocomial spread of the disease in the newborn infant are therefore of vital importance. Cesarean section had been recommended for mothers with active genital herpes, but this is now controversial as further observations suggest that there is a low incidence of neonatal disease in infants delivered vaginally.[48] Infants with suspected infection should be carefully isolated. The anesthesiologist who has a suspected active herpes infection should not become involved in the care of the neonate (or the immunosuppressed patient).[49] A gown and gloves should be worn by all personnel when handling infected infants.

Herpes simplex encephalitis is an uncommon disease, with 25 to 30 percent of cases involving children. The presenting signs of fever and altered mental status progress to include focal neurological deficits, seizures, and increasing coma. The CSF characteristically contains erythrocytes and may contain an HSV antigen. Brain biopsy may be required to confirm the diagnosis. Patients with advanced disease require respiratory support and measures to control intracranial pressure. Antiviral therapy with acyclovir should be initiated as soon as possible to optimize the outcome.[50]

NEONATAL HEPATITIS

Acute hepatitis in the mother may result in premature birth and neonatal infection. Maternal hepatitis type A may also increase the risk of abortion.[51] The neonate may also become infected after delivery: hepatitis A infection usually results in a mild disease. Hepatitis B in neonates is more serious as it may proceed to chronic active hepatitis and even hepatoma later.[52]

Infected infants should be isolated. Those with type A hepatitis, which is spread by fecal contamination, should be in a single room with careful disposal of items that may be contaminated, such as used linens. Gowning, gloving, and meticulous hand washing by attendant staff are recommended. Hepatitis type B is spread primarily by blood and secretions. (For a full discussion of isolation requirements in hepatitis, see page 66.) Active and passive immunization is recommended for treatment of infants exposed to hepatitis B.[53]

CONGENITAL TOXOPLASMOSIS

Toxoplasma gondii is a protozoan parasite of mammals and birds. The intermediate stage oocyst forms only in the cat intestine. Human infection results from contact with infected material from household pets, or from ingestion of the organism in undercooked meats. Infection is often almost asymptomatic in adults but may cause severe damage to the developing fetus.

Congenital toxoplasmosis may manifest with obstructive hydrocephalus, encephalitis, and scattered intracranial calcification.[54] These neurological signs may not appear until 2 to 3 months of age. Hepatosplenomegaly and anemia may be present. Chorioretinitis may develop later and cause blindness.

Infected infants are treated with pyrimethamine, sulfadiazine, and folinic acid for 3 weeks, and this regimen is repeated twice during the first year of life. This therapy is not thought to eliminate the organism completely, but it may halt progression of the disease. No isolation techniques are suggested for affected infants.

CONGENITAL SYPHILIS

Syphilis is caused by the spiral bacterium *Treponema pallidum*. It is becoming more common in adults in the United States, and therefore an increase in congenital syphilis might be expected.

Intrauterine infection with syphilis may cause widespread damage to the fetus but only rarely causes abortion. Most affected infants appear normal at birth, and the classic features of the disease develop over the first months and years of life. Some infants may be small and premature, and some may show lymphadenopathy, hepatosplenomegaly, and jaundice at birth. A nasal discharge, sometimes blood-stained, may be present and may contain *T. pallidum* in high concentration. A maculopapular rash may develop over 2 to 3 weeks and may ulcerate, in which case the infectious organism is usually present in high concentration.

The clinical manifestations of congenital syphilis that appear in the first 2 years of life include bone lesions (panosteitis), central nervous system disease (meningitis, hydrocephalus, convulsions), iritis, and skin rashes.[55] Mucous patches may develop on the palate. Hepatosplenomegaly and a mild anemia are common. The later manifestations are bony abnormalities (deformed maxilla, frontal bossing); abnormal short, narrow, wide-spaced teeth (Hutchinson's teeth); interstitial keratitis, which may lead to blindness; nerve deafness; and chronic skin lesions.

The diagnosis of congenital syphilis is usually made on the serological testing of the mother and clinical signs in the infant. Serological testing of the infant is complicated by the fact that maternal antibody is passively acquired via the placenta. Isolation of the pathogen from lesions on the infant confirms the diagnosis. Treatment of the infant is with penicillin; a single dose of benzathine penicillin G, 50,000 IU intramuscularly, or, if neurosyphilis cannot be excluded, aqueous penicillin G, 50,000 IU intramuscularly per day for 10 days.

Lesions should become noninfectious after 48 hours of antibiotic therapy. The anesthesiologist who must handle an infant with active congenital syphilis (an ulcerating rash or nasal discharge) is advised to wear gloves.

CANDIDA

Widespread systemic fungal infection is a disease that has been seen in the neonatal intensive care unit with increasing frequency over the past decade.

Candida is an important neonatal pathogen. The organism very commonly occurs in the oral cavity (acute pseudomembranous candidiasis, or "thrush") and around the perineum, causing a skin rash. In otherwise healthy neonates, infection in these sites can be effectively treated with nystatin preparations and does not represent a risk factor for the development of disseminated candidiasis. However the sick infant, especially the preterm, who has an immature immune response and may be treated with broad-spectrum antibiotics and intravenous alimentation, is at high risk for the development of systemic fungal infection.

Candida albicans is the commonest fungal infecting agent, but *C. tropicalis*, *C. parapsilosis*, and others such as cryptococcus are sometimes implicated.

Congenital candidiasis is a rare disease that may be associated with ascending infection following prolonged rupture of the membranes. It is usually characterized by an extensive maculopapular or vesicular skin rash, from which the organism may be recovered. The rash usually responds well to treatment with local antifungal agents. In some patients there may also be pulmonary involvement, with associated pneumonia; in such cases, the prognosis is less certain, and early diagnosis with aggressive antifungal therapy is essential.

In the newborn infant, systemic candidiasis is a serious disease that may occur as catheter-associated sepsis affecting a central intravenous line or as disseminated candidiasis.[56] In catheter-related sepsis, the fungus can be isolated from the central line or blood, but the disease is controlled on removal of the line and institution of antifungal therapy. In infants with disseminated candidiasis, however, *Candida* persists following catheter removal or is apparent in other normally sterile systemic sites.

Risk factors for the development of systemic candidiasis include prematurity, low birth weight, the use of broad-spectrum antibiotics, prolonged venous cannulation, total parenteral nutrition, and prolonged endotracheal intubation. The immature immune system of the infant, especially the preterm, is an important predisposing cause of infection.[57] The mechanism of infection in systemic candidiasis has been suggested to be as follows: The use of broad-spectrum antibiotics favors the overgrowth of *Candida* in the bowel or on the skin; then, in the absence of a competent immune system, penetration of the organism into deep tissues, lymphatics, and blood vessels occurs, and systemic spread follows. Intestinal diseases such as necrotizing enterocolitis may facilitate the spread of infection from the bowel. The presence of intravascular catheters or endotracheal tubes provides an additional portal of entry. The use of corticosteroids or theophylline may further suppress the immune response and predispose the neonate to infection.[57]

The clinical manifestations of neonatal infection are varied. A positive blood culture may be the only finding in catheter-related sepsis. However, in disseminated infection there may be involvement of the meninges, the kidneys, the lungs, the endocardium, the peritoneum, the eye, and the joints. Proliferation of the fungus in these varied anatomical sites may result in hydrocephalus, urinary obstruction, or an intracardiac fungal mass and may cause extensive tissue damage. The diagnosis can be confirmed by blood culture in a large percentage of neonates, but this should be supplemented by culture of CSF, urine, and endotracheal secretions. Lung biopsy may be required in the diagnosis of pneumonia.

The treatment of systemic candidiasis is by removal of infected catheters and the use of antifungal drugs. Disseminated candidiasis may require long periods of therapy, and, unfortunately, the drugs used have serious toxic side effects. Amphotericin B, which is widely used, may cause hepatotoxicity, nephrotoxicity, and bone marrow depression. These problems are compounded by the drug's pharmacokinetic parameters, which show wide variation in small infants. Intracardiac or intrarenal fungal masses will require surgical removal.[58]

In older children, systemic *Candida* infection usually occurs in those patients with impaired immunity and in association with prolonged antibiotic therapy. Patients having bone marrow or liver transplantation are particularly vulnerable.

The anesthesiologist has a role to play in the prevention of this disease and must recognize the risk of colonization from intravenous and intra-arterial lines, and from the equipment connected to these devices (transducers, and so on). Great care must be taken to ensure that all this equipment is properly sterilized, and that appropriate aseptic precautions are taken during cannulations.

RESPIRATORY INFECTIONS OF THE NEONATE

Pneumonia in the neonate may result from transplacental infection, intrauterine infection, infection during birth, or postnatal infection.[59] The newborn infant is especially vulnerable to infections of the lungs, since mucociliary clearance mechanisms are incompletely developed and IgA is relatively deficient in respiratory secretions.[60]

Congenital or intrauterine pneumonia is seen at autopsy of infants who die at or shortly after birth. Though there is a marked inflammatory reaction in the lungs, bacteria often are not seen and cultures may be negative. It is therefore not clear whether the changes seen are due to infection or hypoxia.[61] Indeed, it has been suggested that amniotic fluid may protect the fetus and newborn infant, as cases of bacterial pneumonia are rare.[60]

Pneumonia acquired during or after birth is similar to that seen in older patients. There are vascular congestion, hemorrhage, and areas of cellular infiltration and necrosis.[62] Bacteria are commonly present. The infecting agents are most usually *Streptococcus pneumoniae, Streptococcus pyogenes, Staphylococcus aureus, H. influenzae*, and the viruses.

Though some infants may be critically ill, the clinical manifestations of pneumonia in a neonate may be nonspecific: pallor, poor feeding, tachypnea, and tachycardia. Physical examination of the chest is unreliable as a means to diagnose the condition with certainty, and chest radiographs are essential.

Symptoms in an infant who has a history of early rupture of the membranes or premature delivery, especially if the amniotic fluid appeared infected, should prompt a radiological investigation of the chest. Bacteriological diagnosis may be obtained by culture of tracheal aspirate, but this should be obtained at direct laryngoscopy to avoid contamination by upper respiratory tract flora. Blood or CSF, or, if present, pleural fluid culture may also indicate the pathogen. Lung puncture may be necessary to provide an immediate diagnosis in the critically ill neonate.[63]

The management of infants with pneumonia must include immediate optimal antibiotic therapy, which should be modified as soon as cultures are completed. Initial therapy with penicillin, ampicillin, or, if staphylococcal infection is likely, a penicillinase-resistant penicillin, together with an aminoglycoside, is presently recommended.[60] Other measures should include appropriate oxygen therapy and respiratory care; maintenance of fluid, electrolyte, and acid-base status; and drainage of effusions if present.

RESPIRATORY SYNCYTIAL VIRUS INFECTIONS

Respiratory syncytial virus (RSV) is a cause of respiratory infection in all age groups, but in infants and young children it is the leading cause of bronchiolitis and pneumonia. The organism is a paramyxovirus that can be isolated from the nasophayngeal secretions of affected patients. In small infants, the signs of the disease may be minimal, but those with underlying cardiopulmonary disease or immune deficiency may develop a very severe illness. RSV occurs in epidemics, usually in winter and spring, and may rapidly spread among hospital personnel and patients, particularly in the Intensive Care Unit and Neonatal ICU. Transmission is by direct contact or droplet, and the virus may survive for long periods on the hands and on equipment. Previously healthy infants with RSV should be isolated but may recover with only supportive care.

Infants at risk of severe disease require isolation and aggressive therapy. Treatment of RSV is with ribavirin, which inhibits viral protein synthesis. It must be administered by small-particle aerosol, which will deposit the drug into the terminal airways. The administration of the drug is by nebulization into a hood, mask, or tent over a period of 12 to 18 hours per day for 3 to 7 days. Patients on mechanical ventilation may be given the drug in the ventilator circuit, but there is a concern that deposits of the drug in the ventilator components (particularly the expiratory valve) might lead to ventilator malfunction. Hence a one-way valve should be used in the inspiratory line before the nebulizer, and a filter should be placed in the expiratory line. The patient's ventilation, of course, should be carefully monitored throughout. There is also a concern that during treatment disseminated ribavirin particles may be inhaled by other persons. Ribavirin may have teratogenic effects in some species, though the risk to humans is unknown. The risk to health care workers is considered to be low, but it is recommended that pregnant women should not care for patients receiving ribavirin by tent or hood. Appropriate scavenging of excess aerosol is obviously desirable.

Prevention of the spread of RSV among patients, and especially high-risk groups, is obviously essential. Contact isolation is advised for infants and young children. Masks and eye-nose goggles are recommended to prevent droplet spread. Strict attention to hand washing is necessary.

INFECTIOUS DISEASES OF CHILDHOOD

MEASLES (RUBEOLA)

This is a very infectious viral disease spread by droplet infection. The incubation period is 7 to 12 days, but the child can infect others during the last few days of this time.

The clinical features of the disease include a high fever, severe cough, and conjunctivitis. After 3 to 4 days a rash appears, usually beginning on the face and neck and spreading to involve the whole body. An enanthem consisting of small white papules appears on the buccal mucosa 1 to 2 days before the typical maculopapular exanthem. The skin rash becomes confluent and lasts about 7 days.

The complications of measles can be severe. Respiratory infections are common, and pneumonitis is present in 20 percent of patients.[64] In some children this may progress to a severe pneumonia, and this may occur in those who have received killed measles vaccine.[65] Pleural effusions may appear with atypical measles infection. Pneumomediastinum, pneumothorax, and subcutaneous emphysema have occurred in association with measles.[66]

Laryngitis is a frequent complication of measles in some countries and is a leading cause of mortality in young, malnourished children. Upper airway obstruction is often accompanied by lung disease, so tracheotomy or endotracheal intubation may not be followed by immediate improvement.[67] Myocarditis has been described in association with measles and may be diagnosed by electrocardiographic changes.[68]

Abdominal complications of measles include diarrhea, which may lead to severe fluid disturbances, especially if malnutrition is present. Lymphoid hyperplasia may result in abdominal pain and rarely may precipitate appendicitis.

Hematological changes occur with measles and include a marked leukopenia. Thrombocytopenia is much less common but may result in severe episodes of bleeding.[69]

The most common neurological complication of measles is encephalitis.[70] This occurs within a few days of the onset of measles and has a clinical course of 1 to 2 weeks. The disease may be due to direct invasion by the virus or may be an allergic demyelinating disorder.[70] Symptoms include lethargy, irritability, tremors, and later convulsions and depressed consciousness. Meningeal signs are usually present. A later and rarer neurological complication is subacute sclerosing panencephalitis (SSPE). This is characterized by mental deterioration, myoclonic seizures, and eventual death and may follow several years after the initial measles infection. SSPE is thought to be due to persistent infection of the central nervous system by the measles virus and is usually seen in patients who had the initial infection in their first year of life.[71] There is no specific treatment.

Other neurological complications that may be associated with measles include the Guillain-Barré syndrome.[72] Muscle weakness and depressed tendon reflexes appear 1 to 2 weeks after the appearance of the measles rash and progress to the typical clinical picture of Guillain-Barré syndrome.

No specific isolation recommendations are made for children in the home, but those in the hospital should be isolated from the onset of the catarrhal stage until the third day of the rash, to reduce possible exposure to those children at high risk (for example, immunosuppressed patients).

VARICELLA (CHICKENPOX) AND HERPES ZOSTER

Varicella is a common, extremely contagious disease. It is usually a relatively benign disease, but serious complications may develop in the very young or in immunosuppressed patients. Because of the highly contagious nature of the disease and the potential for severe complications in some patients (such as those on immunosuppressive drugs or with leukemia), it is most important that children who may have varicella are not inadvertently admitted to the hospital. Thus pediatric surgical patients who develop an illness or rash should be carefully examined prior to admission.

The first sign of varicella is usually the appearance of a "dewdrop" rash, mainly on the trunk. The prodromal symptoms are mild. The rash rapidly progresses through macular to papular to vesicular stages. The vesicles then dry and crust.

In the immunosuppressed patient, varicella may rapidly progress to a hemorrhagic disseminated infection. Death from pneumonia or encephalitis may ensue.[73]

Herpes zoster is caused by the same virus and is more common in adults, but it can occur in children and even in infants.[74] There is usually a history of a previous attack of varicella. Herpes zoster presents with pain and a varicella-like rash along the course of a peripheral sensory nerve. The pain of herpes zoster is less in children than in older patients, and the rash heals more rapidly. Post-herpetic neuralgia is uncommon in children.

Varicella may be complicated by coagulopathy, which may be secondary to thrombocytopenia, factor V deficiency, low fibrinogen or prothrombin level, and an associated vasculitis. Another serious disease that has been associated with varicella is Reye's syndrome (see page 93); as many as 15 percent of patients with this syndrome may give a history of an associated varicella infection.

MUMPS (EPIDEMIC PAROTITIS)

This is a viral infection that is most common in school-age children, though it may occur in adults. The disease is characterized by fever, malaise, and swelling of the parotid glands. The disease tends to cause milder symptoms in the younger age groups. The etiological agent is myxovirus parotidis, which is found in the saliva of patients with the disease.

The parotid glands become painful and enlarge within 24 hours of the onset of symptoms. The disease is sometimes limited to one side but may involve both parotid glands and the submandibular and sublingual salivary glands.

The most common complication in older patients and adults is orchitis, which may occur in up to 35 percent of male adults with mumps. In female patients, oophoritis may occur, and if the right ovary is involved the symptoms may resemble appendicitis. Meningoencephalitis may occur with mumps, and the virus may be found in the CSF in 10 percent of all patients. Neurological involvement is usually followed by complete recovery.

Other complications include deafness, possibly due to endolymphatic labyrinthitis, myocarditis, and possibly endocardial fibroelastosis (EFE).[75] The latter association is based on the finding of positive mumps antigen skin testing in children with EFE.[75] It has been suggested that mumps virus might be implicated in the etiology of juvenile diabetes mellitus.[76]

ROSEOLA INFANTUM

This is a common infectious disease of infants. The disease results in a high fever (39.5 to 40°C) for a period of 3 to 4 days followed by a sudden fall to normal levels and the appearance of a measles-like rash. The patient usually does not appear as ill as the temperature would indicate, but convulsions may occur during the febrile period. No specific treatment is required, and recovery is complete.

INFECTIOUS MONONUCLEOSIS

This disease of children, adolescents, and young adults is caused by Epstein-Barr virus (EBV) infection. The illness is characterized by lassitude, fever, pharyngitis, lymphadenopathy, and hepatosplenomegaly and usually runs a benign course, though serious complications can develop. EBV infection may cause serious disease or death in immunosuppressed patients.

Complications of EBV infection that may concern the anesthesiologist include airway obstruction due to massively enlarged tonsils, splenic rupture, and Guillain-Barré syndrome. Patients with impending airway obstruction may benefit from steroid therapy, though tracheotomy is sometimes required. Rupture of the spleen is a rare (0.2 percent) complication but is extremely serious[77] and may occur up to 3 months after the development of the illness. Neurological complications of EBV infection may occur in 1 to 8 percent of cases and account for 50 percent of deaths from the disease. Guillain-Barré syndrome is seen in approximately 20 percent of those with nervous system involvement. The mortality rate with ascending polyneuritis is reported to be as high as 25 percent.[78]

Hepatic function may be impaired in patients with infectious mononucleosis, and jaundice may occur. Abnormal liver isoenzymes are found in the majority of patients.

DIPHTHERIA

This is an acute infectious disease caused by *Corynebacterium diphtheriae*, which is a club-shaped gram-positive rod. The organism invades the nose and throat, causing a nasopharyngitis, and also produces a powerful exotoxin that causes major myocardial and neurological damage.[79] Diphtheria is now a very rare disease in Western countries as a result of successful immunization programs. Sporadic cases do occur, however, and there is a continuing danger that recent immigrants might introduce the infection to unimmunized segments of the population. Because of airway, myocardial, and neurological involvements, the disease is of importance to anesthesiologists.

The incubation period of diphtheria is 2 to 5 days, and the onset is insidious, with a mild sore throat and pyrexia of 37.7 to 38.9°C. The pharynx is initially red, but within 24 hours whitish spots appear that coalesce to form a thin, adherent membrane. The membrane becomes thicker and darker in color, with distinct margins. Attempts to remove the membrane result in bleeding and formation of a new membrane. The process subsides after 5 to 6 days, the membrane loosens, and symptoms resolve.

However, cardiac and neurological damage may occur after even a mild infection.

In some patients, infection and membrane formation are limited to the nasopharynx. The symptoms then are those of a mucoid or sanguineous nasal discharge. Systemic effects may be minimal owing to the poor absorption of toxin via the nasal mucosa. At the other extreme, the most severe form of diphtheria demonstrates rapid spread of the infection. The membrane spreads to cover pharynx, buccal cavity, and nasopharynx. There is marked cervical lymphadenopathy and swelling of the tissues of the neck, resulting in a "bull-neck" appearance. Such patients develop severe systemic symptoms of high fever, vomiting and diarrhea, muscle weakness, and central nervous system depression. Death may occur from respiratory obstruction or myocardial failure.

Laryngeal diphtheria occurs in up to 25 percent of cases. Voice changes occur early, and the disease may progress rapidly to encroach on the airway. Sudden obstruction by a fragment of membrane is a constant potential threat. The patient must be kept under very close continuous observation by staff who are expert in emergency airway support.

Myocardial changes are due to a direct effect of the exotoxin and consist of cloudy swelling of muscle fibers that may proceed to complete degeneration.[79] Some degree of myocardial involvement is evident in up to 50 percent of patients with diphtheria. Early signs include tachycardia and a low pulse volume. Electrocardiographic changes include prolongation of the P-R interval, T-wave inversion, and later bundle branch block or complete heart block.[80] As the myocardial involvement progresses, evidence of congestive cardiac failure appears. Myocarditis is likely to be most severe in patients who show evidence of this complication during the first 10 days of a diphtheria infection. Occasionally myocardial fibrosis may follow as a permanent complication of diphtheria.[81]

The neurological complications of diphtheria affect the cranial nerves and their nuclei and the spinal cord. Paralysis of some form is common, and muscles of the palate are most frequently affected. Paralysis, however, may be widespread and may affect the muscles of ventilation, requiring ventilatory therapy.[82]

The diagnosis of diphtheria is confirmed by isolation and culture of the infecting agent. Cultures should be taken before antibiotics are given. Treatment is with antitoxin and must be commenced early, usually before the diagnosis is confirmed by culture. Antitoxin is given intravenously in one dose diluted in normal saline. Penicillin or erythromycin should be given in addition. Cardiac failure requires therapy with digitalis. Arrhythmias must be treated as appropriate, and cardiac pacing may be necessary for heart block. Severe diphtheria interferes with oral feeding, and intravenous therapy is required.

TETANUS

Tetanus is caused by infection of a wound with the spore-bearing, anaerobic, gram-positive organism *Clostridium tetani*, which produces a powerful neurotoxin. This toxin is formed by the organism in the wound and spreads to the central nervous system via the motor nerves or bloodstream. The neurotoxic effects produce a characteristic clinical picture. The disease is now rare in developed countries as a result of immunization programs, but sporadic cases still occur in unprotected children. In developing countries the disease is still very common and often presents in the neonate following infection of the umbilicus. Tetanus is still a major cause of death worldwide.[83]

The clinical signs usually develop 3 to 21 days after infection. In general, the shorter the incubation period, the more severe is the disease. Trismus is the common presenting sign in older children. This is a result of the neurotoxin affecting the facial nerve centers in the region of the fourth cerebral ventricle. Muscle rigidity spreads to affect all the facial muscles, producing a classic fixed facial expression—risus sardonicus. Generalized painful tonic and clonic spasms of skeletal muscle follow as the disease progresses. Initially, these spasms are intermittent and are triggered by sensory stimuli, including touch, noise, and bright light. Later the spasms become continuous. Muscle spasms occur as a result of the depressant effects of the neurotoxin on inhibitory internuncial neurons.

As the disease progresses, spasms become more severe and continuous and eventually result in opisthotonos, flexion and adduction of the arms, and extension of the legs and feet. Spasms of the ventilatory muscles or larynx may lead to respiratory failure and death.

The autonomic nervous system is also involved, and this may lead to alterations in heart rate, labile hypertension, disordered temperature control, and serious cardiac arrhythmias.[84]

Neonatal tetanus has a short incubation period and presents as inability to suck.[83] This is rapidly followed by generalized stiffness and convulsions. Spasms of the muscles of ventilation may lead to apnea. Aspiration pneumonia is common. The differential diagnosis of neonatal tetany includes intracranial injury, hypocalcemia, sepsis, and meningitis.

The treatment of tetanus includes antitoxin and antibiotic therapy; penicillin and tetracycline* are effective against *C. tetani*. The child should be nursed in a quiet area and all external stimuli avoided to decrease reflex spasms. Diazepam has been widely used to control spasms, but many patients will require neuromuscular blocking drugs and mechanical ventilation. Ileus is common, so patients will require intravenous alimentation. All general supportive and nursing care is essential during the period of weeks for which therapy may be required.

Cardiovascular instability secondary to autonomic involvement may require therapy with antihypertensives, and it has been suggested that D-tubocurarine is preferable to pancuronium for neuromuscular blockade in such patients.[85] It is also suggested that isoflurane may be the inhalation agent of choice for the patient with tetanus who requires general anesthesia.[86] Isoflurane can be administered to achieve good control of blood pressure, and arrhythmias may be less troublesome than with halothane.

BOTULISM

Botulism is a disease of the neuromuscular system caused by the exotoxin produced by the infecting agent *C. botulinum*. The disease usually follows the ingestion of the organisms, together with preformed toxin, in improperly preserved foods. In infants the disease is rare, but it may be caused by toxin formed in the patient's gastrointestinal tract following infection by the same organism.[87]

In older children and adults the disease results from ingestion of the toxin in uncooked foods—the toxin is destroyed by heat. The disease is characterized by muscle weakness, which results from the effect of the botulism toxin on neuromuscular transmission. The toxin has now been shown to interfere with acetylcholine release at the presynaptic motor nerve ending;[88] synthesized acetylcholine is blocked from release from its storage sites in the synaptic vesicles. The resulting progressive paralysis results in generalized weakness and ventilatory failure. Diplopia, dysarthria, dysphasia, dry mouth, and dilated pupils are constant early symptoms. Fever is usually absent.

In infants with botulism resulting from gastrointestinal colonization by *C. botulinum*, the onset of symptoms is more insidious. Constipation is a common early sign and may be present for 7 to 10 days prior to the onset of progressive muscle weakness, poor feeding, and lethargy.[87] Weakness of the respiratory muscles may lead to ventilatory failure. The diagnosis of infantile botulism is supported by the demonstration of the "staircase phenomenon" on electrical stimulation of a peripheral nerve.[88] Evoked muscle action potentials show a positive incremental response at stimulation frequencies above 10 Hz. This response may also be seen in antibiotic toxicity, the Eaton-Lambert syndrome, and snakebite by some species.

The pattern of muscle weakness in infant botulism is characteristic; diaphragmatic function tends to be preserved as peripheral weakness progresses, so that ventilatory failure occurs later in the disease. During recovery, diaphragmatic activity appears before there is much evidence of peripheral muscle strength.

Treatment of infantile botulism must include respiratory and nutritional support as indicated. Infants who lose the ability to cough, gag, or swallow should be considered for endotracheal intubation to protect the airway. In one series of infants, 77 percent of patients required intubation and 68 percent required mechanical ventilation.[89] The average period for which controlled ventilation is required is 3 to 4 weeks. The only recorded deaths have followed failure to maintain adequate artificial ventilation. Nasogastric feedings have been successfully used and will usually maintain weight and avoid the need for intravenous alimentation.[89] Penicillin is effective against the organism but may not clear the infection. Purgatives may be indicated to hasten excretion of toxin. The use of antitoxin has been successful only in some patients.[90]

VIRAL HEPATITIS

Viral hepatitis may occur in children in three different forms: hepatitis A, hepatitis B, and non-A/non-B hepatitis.

Hepatitis A infections are common in school-age children, often as a cyclical epidemic disease. The usual mode of transmission is by ingestion of the virus in contaminated food. Parenteral transmission is rare. The incubation

*Because of the risk of discoloration of permanent teeth, tetracyclines should not be used in children less than 8 years of age unless other drugs are contraindicated or would be ineffective.

period of the disease is 2 to 6 weeks, and the clinical course tends to be milder in children than in adults. Asymptomatic infection and anicteric disease are common in children.[91] Hepatitis A does not usually lead to chronic liver disease or a carrier state.

Hepatitis B virus causes a variety of responses in infected persons. Some maintain an asymptomatic carrier state with little or no liver damage. Others display varying degrees of liver dysfunction and may proceed to chronic active hepatitis. Hepatitis B is accompanied by a number of important extrahepatic manifestations that may concern the anesthesiologist. Glomerulonephritis, purpura, aplastic anemia, and polyarteritis may occur. Pleural effusion, pericarditis, and myocarditis have been described in children.[92]

A principal concern for the anesthesiologist caring for the child with hepatitis B infection is to avoid communicating the infection to other patients or to himself or herself. Transmission of hepatitis B is principally via parenteral inoculation, but the virus can be found in urine, saliva, and other body fluids. Disposable equipment should be used for infected patients and be safely disposed of. The anesthesiologist should be careful to avoid self-inoculation and should obtain appropriate prophylactic immunization against hepatitis B.[93]

Non-A/non-B hepatitis is a disease that is similar to hepatitis B in transmission and symptomatology, though it is usually not as severe.[91] It is most commonly transmitted during blood transfusion.

GASTROINTESTINAL INFECTIONS

Gastrointestinal infections are second only to respiratory tract infections as a cause of morbidity and mortality in children. The peak incidence of gastroenteritis is in the first year of life, and at this age, infants are particularly vulnerable to the dehydrating and debilitating effects of diarrhea and vomiting. As in respiratory infections the most common pathogens are viruses, such as rotavirus, Norwalk virus, and enteroviruses. Bacteria that are commonly involved are *Salmonella, Shigella, Campylobacter*, and *E. coli*.

Of particular concern to the anesthesiologist is the gastroenteritis that spreads in the infant wards of a hospital. Many infants who are admitted for surgery run the risk of such a hospital-acquired infection. The anesthesiologist must adhere strictly to the procedures for isolation of infected infants and contacts, so that she or he does not become a vector for the disease.

Rotavirus infection is a common cause of diarrhea in hospitalized infants, but adults also may become infected. In infants, the gastrointestinal symptoms of rotavirus infection are often accompanied by an upper respiratory infection.[94] Most infections are self-limiting, but the disease may be serious in immunodeficient patients and others who are debilitated. Complications of rotavirus infection include intussusception and encephalitis. The most important prophylactic measures to prevent the spread of rotavirus infection are those of meticulous hand washing and proper disposal of soiled diapers and other linens.

Salmonella infections are also common in the infant wards of hospitals, and infants under 3 months of age are particularly at risk.[95] Such infants commonly excrete *Salmonella* organisms from the bowel for several weeks after the symptoms of gastroenteritis have resolved.

TUBERCULOSIS

Tuberculosis is still a major cause of childhood disease worldwide. In developed nations, the disease is rarer and confined mainly to children in the lower socioeconomic groups. Because of the comparative rarity of the disease, there is a danger that tuberculosis will be missed as a diagnosis. The infective agent is *Mycobacterium tuberculosis* in most cases, though *M. bovis* is also pathogenic in humans. These bacteria are relatively resistant to drugs, can survive in a dried state for prolonged periods, and remain viable in tissues for prolonged periods but are destroyed by direct sunlight or ultraviolet light.

Most tuberculous infections are due to airborne spread of the bacillus,[96] and pulmonary infection follows inspiration of infected air. The most contagious patients are those with an intrapulmonary infected cavity and large numbers of organisms in the sputum. Children with pulmonary or extrapulmonary tuberculosis are usually not contagious and need not be isolated.[97]

Primary tuberculosis infection involves the lungs and appears several weeks after infection. Many children are asymptomatic and the infection is apparent only on tuberculin testing. Most infected children will show enlarged hilar lymph nodes that may cause segmental atelectasis. Some patients have pulmonary infiltrates and a pleural effusion. Most patients heal spontaneously without therapy, but if the disease is diagnosed, treatment may be ordered to prevent progression to other tissues or relapses. In a minority of patients the disease progresses to cavity formation in the lungs or extrapulmonary infections. The other tissues most commonly involved are the cervical lymph glands, bone, meninges, and kidneys.

The children who progress to chronic tuberculous infection commonly do so as a result of altered resistance to the disease. Factors that may predispose to chronic disease include young age, poor nutrition, other infections (for example, measles, pertussis), and surgical trauma.

The anesthesiologist may be involved with many aspects of the treatment of children with tuberculosis. The multiplicity of tissues that may be involved and require surgical intervention dictates that a great variety of critical problems may be present. Each child, therefore, must be fully assessed to determine the full effects of the disease. Contamination of anesthesia equipment is a possible hazard, so disposable items should be used whenever possible. Anesthetic and ventilator circuits should be protected by bacterial filters. All equipment that is not disposable should be treated by boiling for 3 minutes or being placed in an antiseptic solution (such as 0.1 percent chlorhexidene) for 1 hour. All other items that might have become infected and cannot be treated this way should be gas sterilized using ethylene oxide. Large items of equipment in the operating room should be washed with a chemical disinfectant (such as 70 percent alcohol).[98]

PARASITIC DISEASES

ROUNDWORMS (ASCARIASIS)

Ascaris lumbricoides is a large roundworm 20 to 45 cm in length and up to 6 mm in diameter. Ascariasis is common in the tropics and extends to the temperate climates. Infection usually occurs as a result of ingesting *Ascaris* eggs from soil that later hatch in the duodenum. The larvae migrate through the intestinal wall and pass via the lymphatics or venules into the liver and thence via the bloodstream to the lungs. In the lungs the larvae grow and later migrate via the glottis into the esophagus. They are then swallowed to infest the small intestine.

During the lung phase, large numbers of larvae may produce an atypical pneumonia (Löffler's syndrome). The larvae at this stage may also induce an allergic response characterized by bronchospasm, urticaria, and eosinophilia.

As the mature worms grow in the intestine, the most common symptom in children is colic. Occasionally a mass of worms may cause intestinal obstruction, intussusception, or ileus; perforation of the intestine has occurred.

The treatment of roundworm infestion is with piperazine citrate. This drug may cause further gastrointestinal disturbance and, rarely, visual effects and ataxia.

HOOKWORMS

The hookworm *Ancylostoma duodenale* is an intestinal parasite that is widespread in tropical and subtropical countries. *Necator americanus* is a similar species found in many countries of the Western hemisphere. Hookworm embryos develop into larvae in warm, moist soil and gain access to the body through the skin of feet or hands. The larvae migrate to the lungs, where they may cause hemorrhagic pneumonia. The larvae then pass via the glottis into the gastrointestinal tract, where they grow to maturity.

The most important symptoms of hookworm disease are those that result from chronic blood loss.[99] The resultant anemia is hypochromic and microcytic and may result eventually in cardiomegaly, congestive heart failure, and severe weakness.

Treatment of hookworm infections is with mebendazole, which may also cause diarrhea and abdominal pain. In addition, the anemia must be treated with oral or parenteral iron. Patients who require urgent surgery should have packed cell infusions to increase the hemoglobin level preoperatively.

TRICHINOSIS

The parasite *Trichinella spiralis*, which causes an intestinal and tissue infection, is ingested usually in uncooked pork or bear meat. The adult worm inhabits the intestine, causing abdominal pain and diarrhea. The larvae invade other tissues, particularly skeletal muscle, causing edema, myalgia, and eosinophilia. Eventually calcification of encysted larvae occurs. Occasionally the larvae enter cardiac muscle, causing myocarditis with chest pain, tachycardia, hypotension, and electrocardiographic changes. Steroid therapy is indicated for patients with myocardial involvement.

ECHINOCOCCOSIS AND HYDATID DISEASE

Echinococcus granulosus is a tapeworm that infests the intestine of the dog; humans and sheep are among the species that serve as intermediate hosts. If eggs are ingested by humans, the embryo hatches and penetrates the abdominal wall, enters lymphatic or venous channels, and is transported to one of several organs. Here it develops into the hydatid cyst. This cyst is fluid-filled and unilocular and is surrounded by an outer laminated layer and an inner germinal layer. The germinal layer produces protoscoleces, which may number up to 2 million and are capable of infecting the primary host if ingested.

The symptoms produced by the hydatid cyst vary according to the site. The structure most commonly affected is the liver (63 percent), followed by lung (25 percent), muscle (5 percent), bone (3 percent), and brain (1 percent). Hepatic cysts may be asymptomatic for years before presenting with abdominal pain and a palpable mass. Lung cysts are usually found on routine radiograph but may cause cough, chest pain, and hemoptysis. The diagnosis is made from the history of a slow-growing mass, an eosinophilia that is usual but not constant, and sometimes by intradermal testing (Casoni's test). The latter test is not reliable and has a high false-positive rate.[100] The definitive diagnosis is made after excision of the cyst.

The treatment of hydatid cyst is surgical excision of the intact cyst. Aspiration for diagnosis or treatment is contraindicated owing to the potential danger of leakage of fluid into body cavities. Rupture of the cyst, whether spontaneous or during attempted removal, may be followed by an anaphylactic reaction. In some cases intraoperative aspiration of the cyst and injection of 20 percent saline, or absolute alcohol, have been performed to prevent possible seeding of the contents.[101] If rupture and anaphylaxis occur during surgery, vasopressors such as epinephrine, a bronchodilator such as isoproterenol, and large doses of corticosteroid drugs are indicated.[102]

ANTIBIOTIC THERAPY AND ANESTHESIA

Many patients who present for general anesthesia are receiving antibiotic therapy, and in some instances it may be necessary to administer antibiotics during the course of an anesthetic. It is therefore necessary that the anesthesiologist have some knowledge of the potential side effects and possible interactions with anesthetic drugs of these antibiotics in general use. Table 3–1 summarizes the doses of antibiotics used for serious infections and lists their potential adverse reactions.

PENICILLINS

These drugs may cause hypersensitivity reactions. Penicillin is now one of the most common causes of anaphylaxis, with an incidence of 0.015 to 0.04 percent.[103] There is no evidence to suggest that patients with a history of atopy are at greater risk. Anaphylaxis develops within seconds of injection of the drug, with bronchospasm, hypotension, and an erythematous rash. Prompt therapy is essential for survival. Epinephrine administration, endotracheal intubation, and ventilation with oxygen must be immediately performed. Bronchodilators, corticosteroids, and antihistamines may help to reverse further the anaphylactic state. Despite therapy, the mortality rate may be as high as 10 percent; therefore, prevention of the state is highly desirable. Meticulous history-taking for evidence of antibiotic allergies is essential. Though penicillin is most commonly involved, anaphylaxis may also follow administration of ampicillin, streptomycin, vancomycin, and the sulfonamide drugs.[105]

Penicillin is also sometimes followed by less acute hypersensitivity reactions. Skin rashes, including urticaria and angioedema, may form immediately or appear a few days after the drug is given. More rarely, severe dermatological conditions, including Stevens-Johnson syndrome, exfoliative dermatitis, and epidermal necrolysis may occur. Serum sickness, characterized by fever, rash, arthritis, and lymphadenopathy, may develop, usually appearing after an interval of 4 to 12 days.

Penicillin therapy has been associated with central nervous system complications, particularly when the drug is given in large doses.[105] Grand mal seizures may occur,[106] and depression of consciousness and coma may develop.

Hemopoietic disease may result from penicillin therapy.[107] Hemolytic anemia, neutropenia, and thrombocytopenic purpura may occur. The semisynthetic penicillins are more often a cause of hematological disease than are the naturally occurring penicillins.

Renal diseases, including glomerulonephritis and interstitial nephritis, are rare complications,

Table 3–1. ANTIBIOTIC THERAPY IN PEDIATRIC PATIENTS

Drug	Route	Daily Dose (mg/kg/day in divided doses)*	Comments and Adverse Reactions
N.B. All antibiotics given intravenously should be infused slowly. Use caution in patients with renal failure, as excretion may be prolonged and toxic levels may occur.			
penicillin G	IV, IM	100,000–400,000 IU/kg in 4 doses (Infants: 25,000 q12h)	May cause hypersensitivity reactions. Leukopenia, myoclonic seizures (high doses)
Penicillinase-Resistant Penicillins			
methicillin (Staphcillin)	IV, IM	150–200 in 4–6 doses (Infants: 25 q6–12h)	Interstitial nephritis may occur with hematuria in up to 4% of patients. Hypersensitivity, leukopenia
oxacillin (Prostaphlin)	IV, IM	150–200 in 4–6 doses (Infants: 25 q6–12h)	Hypersensitivity and leukopenia
nafcillin (Unipen)	IV, IM	150–200 in 4–6 doses (Infants: 25 q6–12h)	As above
Broad-Spectrum Penicillins			
ampicillin (Ampicin)	IV, IM	200–300 in 4 doses (Infants: 25 q8–12h)	Hypersensitivity, leukopenia, eosinophilia. Thrombocytopenia and prolonged bleeding time. Rash in 10% of patients
azlocillin (Azlin)	IV, IM	200–300 in 4–6 doses	Hypersensitivity, rash, leukopenia
carbenicillin (Geopen)	IV, IM	400–600 in 4–6 doses	As above
mezlocillin, piperacillin, ticarcillin	IV, IM	200–300 in 4–6 doses	As above
Cephalosporins			
cefamandole (Mandol)	IV, IM	100–150 in 4–6 doses	Hypersensitivity
cefazolin (Kefzol, Ancef)	IV, IM	50–150 in 3–4 doses	As above
cefotaxime (Claforan)	IV, IM	150–200 in 3–4 doses	May cause thrombocytopenia. Hypersensitivity
cefoxitin (Mefoxin)	IV, IM	80–160 in 4–6 doses	Hypersensitivity
ceftazidime (Fortaz)	IV, IM	125–150 in 3 doses	Useful for *Pseudomonas* infection. Hypersensitivity
ceftizoxime (Cefizox)	IV, IM	150–200 in 3 doses	Hypersensitivity
ceftriaxone (Rocephin)	IV, IM	80–100 in 2 doses (Infants: 50 q24h)	May displace albumin-bound bilirubin. Hypersensitivity
cefuroxime (Zinacef)	IV, IM	175–240 in 3 doses	Hypersensitivity
cephalothin (Keflin)	IV, IM	100–150 in 4–6 doses	As above
cephapirin (Cefadyl)	IV, IM	40–80 in 4 doses	As above
moxalactam (Moxam)	IV, IM	150–200 in 4 doses	May displace albumin-bound bilirubin. May cause hypoprothrombinemia
Aminoglycosides			
amikacin (Amikin)	IV, IM	15–30 in 2 doses	Ototoxic and nephrotoxic. May cause neuromuscular blockade
gentamicin (Garamycin)	IV, IM	3–7.5 in 3 doses	Ototoxic and nephrotoxic. May cause neuromuscular blockade, especially with relaxants or calcium channel blockers
kanamycin (Kantrex)	IV, IM	15–30 in 2–3 doses	As above
netilmicin (Netromycin)	IV, IM	3–7.5 in 3 doses	As above
tobramycin (Nebcin)	IV, IM	3–7.5 in 3 doses	As above
Other			
chloramphenicol (Chloromycetin)	IV	50–100 in 4 doses (Infants: 25 q12–24h)	May cause dose-related reversible depression of the hemopoietic system or rarely idiosyncratic aplastic anemia; cimetidine increases this risk. May cause gray baby syndrome
clindamycin (Cleocin)	IV, IM	25–40 in 3–4 doses (Infants: 5 q6–12h)	May cause myocardial depression. Hypersensitivity. Rarely, hepatic failure
erythromycin	IV	15–50 in 4 doses	Must be given slowly over 1 hour. Rarely, hypersensitivity
vancomycin (Vancocin)	IV	40–60 in 4 doses (Infants: 10 q8–12h)	Must be given slowly over 1 hour. Hypotension and cardiac arrest with rapid infusion. Nephrotoxic and ototoxic

*Infants: Mg/kg at intervals.

particularly of methicillin therapy. This complication is more likely to occur in those with preexisting renal disease.

CEPHALOSPORINS

Allergic reactions to cephalosporins (cefamandole, cephaloridine, cefazolin, and so forth) may occur, and there is probably a cross-reactivity with penicillin. Thus patients known to be allergic to penicillin, especially if urticaria or anaphylaxis occurs, should not receive cephalosporins. Cephalosporins may also induce allergic reactions in patients who are not allergic to penicillin.

Hematological reactions to cephalosporins are uncommon, but coagulation disorders may rarely occur. Thrombocytopenia may follow therapy with cefotaxime and some other first and second generation cephalosporins. This thrombocytopenia usually occurs after a prolonged course of therapy and is rapidly corrected when treatment ceases. Hypoprothrombinemia may occur following moxalactam or cefoperazone therapy. This is particularly likely in a patient with impaired renal function. The effect is likely multifactorial but is partly due to eradication of vitamin K, producing intestinal flora. It may be corrected with intravenous vitamin K.[108] Cephaloridine administration in high dosage rarely may cause renal damage.[109]

Cephalosporins (especially ceftriaxone) may displace bilirubin from its binding sites on serum albumin, and this could be clinically significant in the jaundiced neonate.

AMINOGLYCOSIDES

Aminoglycosides may cause serious side effects, and therefore their use should be limited to infections for which they are essential therapy. Renal damage and ototoxicity are the most important complications and are usually related to high blood levels of the drug.

These drugs are also recognized as causes of neuromuscular blockade. This is thought to be due to inhibition of acetylcholine release at the prejunctional site. Patients with hypocalcemia, hypermagnesemia, botulism, or myasthenia gravis, and those given other neuromuscular blocking drugs, are particularly likely to develop skeletal muscle weakness.[110] It has been observed that therapeutic levels of gentamicin and tobramycin prolong the effect of vecuronium but not that of atracurium.[111] Hence it has been suggested that atracurium might be considered the relaxant of choice for patients taking these aminoglycosides. If abnormal weakness persists in patients on aminoglycoside therapy following surgery, artificial ventilation and all appropriate respiratory care should be continued until the condition resolves.[112] Attempts to reverse neuromuscular blocks caused by antibiotics with the use of pharmacological agents are not usually completely successful.

VANCOMYCIN

The most common side effect of this drug is ototoxicity, which is dose related. There are some other rarer, but important, complications. Severe hypotension and cardiac arrest have been reported following vancomycin administration during anesthesia.[113] These complications have usually followed inadvertent rapid administration and/or large doses but have also been reported during slow infusion of the drug. It is recommended that vancomycin be given to pediatric patients using a volumetric pump, and the infusion should be monitored carefully. If a preoperative infusion of vancomycin is not completed before anesthesia is to be induced, then the induction should be delayed.[113] Vancomycin also has been demonstrated to potentiate the neuromuscular blocking effects of vecuronium.[114]

The "red neck" syndrome is an anaphylactoid reaction associated with rapid intravenous infusion of the drug. It is a histamine-like reaction, with erythematous rash, bronchospasm, and hypotension, which may lead to death.[115] Slow administration of the drug will prevent this reaction.

Hypersensitivity reactions with aminoglycosides are rare, but fever and a skin rash may occur in a small percentage of patients.

CHLORAMPHENICOL

Very rarely, chloramphenicol may cause aplastic anemia. Much more commonly the drug results in a predictable degree of reversible bone marrow suppression. Thus blood studies should be performed at regular intervals.

The gray baby syndrome affects preterm and term neonates who are treated with large doses of chloramphenicol (more than 100 mg/kg/day) for several days. The condition is characterized by rapid onset of abdominal distention, cyanosis, tachycardia, hypotonia, and eventual cardiovascular collapse.[116] This condition is thought to be due to the inadequacy of neonatal liver function to metabolize the drug and the inability of the neonate's kidneys to excrete unconjugated drug.

Hypersensitivity reactions to chloramphenicol are extremely rare.

ERYTHROMYCIN

Erythromycin is widely regarded as one of the safest antibiotics. Gastrointestinal reactions, including pseudomembranous enterocolitis, may occur, and cholestatic hepatitis may develop in children over 12 years of age. Erythromycin has been demonstrated to delay the metabolism of some drugs, including alfentanil and theophylline.[117] Hence caution is recommended when administering alfentanil to patients receiving erythromycin. Theophylline toxicity may be precipitated by concurrent erythromycin therapy.[118]

Rapid intravenous infusion of erythromycin may result in very severe hypotension.

LINCOMYCIN AND CLINDAMYCIN

Lincomycin and clindamycin may cause myocardial depression, and cardiac arrest has been reported following a rapid infusion of lincomycin.[119] It is suggested that the principal effects of lincomycin may be on conduction mechanisms in the heart rather than contractility.

Hepatotoxicity is common with lincomycin, but hepatic failure rarely develops. Interactions of lincomycin with neuromuscular blocking drugs have occurred.

True anaphylaxis to lincomycin may occur but is rare. Severe skin rashes, including the Stevens-Johnson syndrome, have occurred.

BACITRACIN

Bacitracin may induce anaphylaxis, and there are case reports of such reactions during anesthesia as a result of wound irrigation with the drug.[120] In reported cases the anesthesiologist was not told that the drug had been used, bronchospasm was absent, and cutaneous manifestations were not obvious, thus leading to a delay in the diagnosis of anaphylaxis. Profound hypotension and tachycardia were the sole signs. Therefore, the anesthesiologist should be informed of the use of any antibiotics in irrigation solutions and should be alert for any subsequent effect.

In summary, all antibiotics are capable of producing severe side effects. The anesthesiologist must diligently seek a history of antibiotic drug allergy and must observe appropriate caution in the use of these drugs. Rapid intravenous injections must be avoided, as they are associated with the highest incidence of severe reactions.

REFERENCES

1. Kluger MJ, Ringler DH, Anver MR: Fever and survival. Science *188*:166, 1975.
2. Heim T: Homeothermy and its metabolic cost. *In* Davis JA, Dobbing J (Eds.): Scientific Foundations of Pediatrics. 2nd edition. London, Heinemann, 1981, p 118.
3. Mathsaniotis N, Pastelis V, Agathopoulos A, et al: Fever and biochemical thermogenesis. Pediatrics *47*:571, 1971.
4. Dubois EF: The Mechanism of Heat Loss and Temperature Regulation. Lance Memorial Lectures. Palo Alto, Cal, Stanford University Press, 1937.
5. Baker MD, Fossarelli PD, Carpenter RO: Childhood fever: Correlation of diagnosis with temperature response to acetaminophen. Pediatrics *80*:315, 1987.
6. Addy D: Febrile convulsions. *In* Ross E, Reynolds E (Eds.): Paediatric Perspectives on Epilepsy. Chichester, Wiley, 1985, pp 73–77.
7. Moffet HL: Pediatric Infectious Diseases. 2nd ed. Philadelphia, JB Lippincott, 1981, p 263.
8. Placzek MM, Whitelaw A: Early and late neonatal septicemia. Arch Dis Child *58*:728, 1983.
9. Miller E: Chemotactic function in the human neonate: Humoral and cellular aspects. Pediatr Res *5*:487, 1971.
10. Gerdes JS: Clinicopathological approach to the diagnosis of neonatal sepsis. Clin Perinatol *18*:361–381, 1991.
11. Keay AS, Simpson R: Prevention of infection in nurseries for the newborn. Postgrad Med J *53*:583, 1977.
12. Remington JS, Klein JO: Infectious Diseases of the Fetus and Newborn Infant. Philadelphia, WB Saunders, 1983.
13. Philip AGS, Hewitt JR: Early diagnosis of neonatal sepsis. Pediatrics *65*:1036, 1980.
14. Klaus MH, Fanaroff AA: Care of the High-Risk Neonate. Philadelphia, WB Saunders, 1979, p 275.
15. Sheoka A, Hall R, Hill H: Blood transfusion in group B streptococcal sepsis. Lancet *1*:636, 1978.
16. Wong VK, Hitchcock W, Mason WH: Meningococcal infections in children: A review of 100 cases. Pediatr Infect Dis J *8*:224–227, 1989.
17. Bosworth DC: Reversible adrenocortical insufficiency in fulminant meningococcemia. Arch Intern Med *139*:823, 1979.
18. Reichgott MJ, Melmon KL: Should corticosteroids be used in shock? Med Clin North Am *57*:1211, 1983.
19. Odio CM, Faingezicht I, Paris M, et al: The beneficial effects of early dexamethasone administration in infants and children with bacterial meningitis. N Engl J Med *324*:1526–1531, 1991.
20. Lebel MH, Hoyt MJ, McCracken GH: Comparative efficacy of ceftriaxone and cefuroxime for treatment of bacterial meningitis. J Pediatr *114*:1049–1054, 1989.

21. Anderson CTM, Berde CB, Sethna NF, Pribaz JJ: Meningococcal purpura fulminans: Treatment of vascular insufficiency in a 2 year old child with lumbar epidural sympathetic blockade. Anesthesiology *71*:463–464, 1989.
22. Coonrod JD, Leach RP: Antigenemia in fulminant pneumococcemia. Ann Intern Med *84*:561, 1976.
23. Dicerman JD: Splenectomy and sepsis: a warning. Pediatrics *63*:638, 1979.
24. Trigg ME: Immune function of the spleen. South Med J *72*:593, 1979.
25. Sherman NJ, Aach MJ: Conservative surgery for splenic injuries. Pediatrics *61*:267, 1978.
26. Hiebert JP, Nelson AJ, McCracken GH: Acute disseminated staphylococcal disease in childhood. Am J Dis Child *131*:181, 1977.
27. Jordan CN, Donaldson JD, Halperin S: Bacterial tracheitis associated with respiratory syncytial virus infection and toxic shock syndrome. Can Med Assoc J *142*:233–234, 1990.
28. Martin MA, Pfaller MA, Wenzel RP: Coagulase-negative staphylococcal bacteremia. Mortality and hospital stay. Ann Intern Med *110*:9, 1989.
29. Decker MD, Edwards KM: Central venous catheter infections. Pediatr Clin North Am *35*:579, 1988.
30. Heirro FR, Palomequee A, Calvo M, et al: Septic shock in pediatrics. Pediatrician *8*:93, 1979.
31. Jacobs RF, Sowell MK, Moss M, Fiser DH: Septic shock in children: bacterial etiologies and temporal relationships. Pediatr Infect Dis J *9*:196–200, 1990.
32. Perkin RM, Levin DL: Shock in the pediatric patient. Part I. J Pediatr *101*:163, 1982.
33. Marks MI:, Pediatric Infectious Diseases. New York, Springer-Verlag, 1985, pp 731–735.
34. Zimmerman JJ, Dietrich KA: Current perspectives on septic shock. Pediatr Clin North Am *34*:131–163, 1987.
35. Carcillo JA, Davis AL, Zaritsky A: Role of early fluid resuscitation in pediatric septic shock. JAMA *266*:1242–1245, 1991.
36. Stanley TH, Reddy P: Fentanyl oxygen in septic shock. Anesthesiology *51*:S100, 1979.
37. Adler SP, Chandrika T, Lawrence L, et al: Cytomegalovirus infections in neonates acquired by blood transfusions. Pediatr Infect Dis *2*:114, 1983.
38. Yeager AJ: Transmission of cytomegalovirus to mothers by infected infants: Another reason to prevent transfusion-acquired infections. Pediatr Infect Dis *2*:295, 1983.
39. Pass RF, Stagno S, Myers GJ, et al: Outcome of symptomatic congenital cytomegalovirus infection: results of long-term longitudinal follow-up. Pediatrics *66*:758, 1980.
40. Ozsoylu S, Kanra G, Savas G: Thrombocytopenic purpura related to rubella infection. Pediatrics *62*:567, 1978.
41. Korones SB, Ainger LE, Monif GRG: Congenital rubella syndrome: A study of 22 infants. Am J Dis Child *110*:434, 1965.
42. Mioller E, Cradock-Watson JE, Pollock TM: Consequences of confirmed maternal rubella at successive stages of pregnancy. Lancet *2*:781, 1982.
43. Tradieu M, Grospierre B, Durandy A, et al: Circulating immune complexes containing rubella antigens in late onset rubella syndrome J Pediatr *97*:370, 1980.
44. Louis DS, Silva J: Herpetic whitlow: herpetic infections of the digits. J Hand Surg *4*:90, 1979.
45. Yeager AS, Arvin AM, Urbani LJ, et al: Relationship of antibody to outcome in neonatal herpes simplex virus infections. Infect Immun *29*:532, 1980.
46. Light IJ: Postnatal acquisition of herpes simplex virus by the newborn infant: A review of the literature. Pediatrics *63*:480, 1971.
47. Miller DR, Hanshaw JB, O'Leary DS, et al: Fatal disseminated herpes simplex virus infection and hemorrhage in the neonate. J Pediatr *76*:409, 1970.
48. Prober CG, Sullender WM, Yasukawa LL, et al: Low risk of herpes simplex virus infections in neonates exposed at the time of vaginal delivery to mothers with recurrent genital herpes simplex virus infections. N Engl J Med *316*:240–244, 1987.
49. Adams G, Stover BH, Kennlyside RA, et al: Nosocomial herpetic infections in a pediatric intensive care unit. Am J Epidemiol *113*:126, 1981.
50. Kohl S: Herpes simplex virus encephalitis in children. Pediatr Clin North Am *35*:465–483, 1988.
51. Stevens CE, Krugman S, Szmuness W, et al: Viral hepatitis in pregnancy: problems for the clinician dealing with the infant. Pediatr Rev *2*:121, 1980.
52. Dupey JM, Giraud P, Dupey C, et al: Hepatitis B in children J Pediatr *92*:200, 1978.
53. Chin J: Prevention of chronic hepatitis B virus infection from mothers to infants in the United States. Pediatrics *72*:289, 1983.
54. Desmonts G, Couvrer J: Toxoplasmosis in pregnancy and its transmission to the fetus. Bull NY Acad Med *50*:146, 1974.
55. Fiumara NJ: Syphilis in newborn children. Clin Obstet Gynecol *18*:183, 1975.
56. Butler KM, Baker CJ: *Candida*: an increasingly important pathogen in the nursery. Pediatr Clin North Am *35*:543–563, 1988.
57. Baley JE: Neonatal candidiasis: the current challenge. Clin Perinatol *18*:263–280, 1991.
58. Foker JE, Bass JL, Thompson T, et al: Management of intracardiac fungal masses in premature infants. J Thorac Cardiovasc Surg *87*:244, 1984.
59. Klein JO: Bacterial infections of the respiratory tract. *In* Remington JS, Klein JO (Eds.): Infectious Diseases of the Fetus and Newborn Infant. Philadelphia, WB Saunders, 1983, p 744.
60. Marks MI: Pediatric Infectious Diseases for the Practitioner. New York, Springer-Verlag, 1985, p 179.
61. Barter RA: Congenital pneumonia. Lancet *1*:165, 1962.
62. Berstein J, Wang J: The pathology of neonatal pneumonia. Am J Dis Child *101*:350, 1961.
63. Klein JO: Diagnostic lung puncture in the pneumonias of infants and children. Pediatrics *44*:486, 1969.
64. Kohn JL, Koiransky H: Successive roentgenograms of the chest of children during measles. Am J Dis Child *28*:258, 1929.
65. Gokiert JC, Beamish WE: Altered reactivity to measles virus in previously vaccinated children. Can Med Assoc J *103*:724, 1970.
66. Bloch A, Vardy P: Pneumonediastinum and subcutaneous emphysema in measles. Clin Pediatr *7*:7, 1968.
67. O'Donovan C: Measles in Kenyan children. East Afr Med J *48*:5226, 1971.
68. Ross LJ: Electrocardiographic findings in measles. Am J Dis Child *83*:282, 1952.
69. Hudson JB, Weinstein L, Chang T: Thrombocytopenic purpura in measles. J Pediatr *48*:48, 1956.
70. Kipps A, Dick G, Moodie JW: Measles and the central nervous system. Lancet *2*:1406, 1983.
71. Modlin JF, Halsey NA, Eddins DL, et al: Epidemiology of subacute panencephalitis. J Pediatr *94*:231, 1979.
72. Lidin-Janson G, Stannegard O: Two cases of Guillain-Barré syndrome and encephalitis after measles. Br Med J *2*:572, 1972.

73. Feldman S, Hughes WT, Daniel CB: Varicella in children with cancer: Seventy seven cases. Pediatrics *56*:388, 1975.
74. Winkleman RK, Perry HO: Herpes zoster in children. JAMA *171*:876, 1959.
75. Noren GR, Adams P, Anderson RC: Positive skin reactivity to mumps virus antigen in endocardial fibroelastosis. J Pediatr *62*:604, 1963.
76. Sultz HA, Hart BA, Zielezny M: Is mumps virus an etiologic factor in juvenile diabetes mellitus? J Pediatr *86*:654, 1975.
77. Rutkow IM: Rupture of the spleen in infectious mononucleosis. Arch Surg *113*:718, 1978.
78. Grose C, Feorino PM: Epstein-Barr virus and Guillain-Barré syndrome. Lancet *2*:1285, 1972.
79. Hodes HL: Diphtheria. Pediatr Clin North Am *26*:445, 1979.
80. Nihoyannopoulos J, Agoroyannis S: Disorders of cardiac rhythm in diphtheria: fascicular blocks and their prognostic value. Proc Assoc Pediatr Cardiol *8*:61, 1972.
81. Sayers EG: Diphtheritic myocarditis with permanent heart damage. Ann Intern Med *48*:146, 1958.
82. Bowler DP: Post-diphtheritic polyneuritis with respiratory paralysis. Med J Aust *47*:733, 1960.
83. Stoll BJ: Tetanus. Pediatr Clin North Am *26*:415, 1979.
84. Hollow VM, Clark GN: Autonomic manifestations of tetanus. Anaesth Intens Care *3*:142, 1975.
85. De Michele JF, Da Silva AMT: Cardiovascular findings in a patient with severe tetanus. Crit Care Med *11*:828, 1983.
86. Haselby KA: Infectious diseases. *In* Stoelting RK, Dierdorf SF (Eds.): Anesthesia and Co-existing Disease. New York, Churchill-Livingstone, 1983.
87. Polin RA, Brown LW: Infant botulism. Pediatr Clin North Am *26*:345, 1979.
88. Kao I, Drachman DB, Price DL: Botulinum toxin: Mechanism of presynaptic blockade. Science *193*:1256, 1976.
89. Schreiner MS, Field E, Ruddy R: Infant botulism: A review of 12 years' experience at the Children's Hospital of Philadelphia. Pediatrics *87*:159–165, 1991.
90. Arnon SS, Midura TF, Clay AS, et al: Infant botulism: Epidemiological, clinical and laboratory aspects. JAMA *237*:1946, 1977.
91. Seto DSY: Viral hepatitis. Pediatr Clin North Am *26*:305, 1979.
92. Adler R, Takahashi M, Wright HT: Acute pericarditis associated with hepatitis B infection. Pediatrics *61*:716, 1978.
93. du Moulin GC, Hedley-White J: Hospital-associated viral infection and the anesthesiologist. Anesthesiology *59*:51, 1983.
94. Steinhoff MC: Rotavirus: The first five years. J Pediatr *96*:611, 1980.
95. Nelson SJ, Granoff D: *Salmonella* gastroenteritis in the first three months of life: A review of management and complications. Clin Pediatr *21*:709, 1982.
96. Riley RL, Mills CC, O'Grady F, et al: Infectiousness of air from a tuberculosis ward. Am Rev Resp Dis *85*:511, 1962.
97. David SD, Rosenzweig DY: Tuberculosis: diseases due to *Mycobacterium tuberculosis* and atypical mycobacteria. *In* Wedgewood RJ, David SD, Ray DF, et al (Eds.): Infections in Children. Philadelphia, JB Lippincott, 1982, p 978.
98. The experts opine. Surv Anesth *22*:587, 1978.
99. Roche M, Layusse M: The nature and causes of hookworm anemia. Am J Trop Med Hyg *15*:1031, 1966.
100. Kagan IG, Osiman JJ, Varela JC, et al: Evaluation of intradermal and serologic tests for the diagnosis of hydatid disease. Am J Trop Med Hyg *15*:172, 1966.
101. Lewis JW, Koss N, Kerstein MD: A review of echinococcal disease. Ann Surg *181*:390, 1975.
102. Jakubowski MS, Barnard DE: Anaphylactic shock during operation for hydatid disease. Anaesthesiology *34*:197, 1971.
103. Idsoe E, Guthe T, Wilcox RR, et al: Nature and extent of penicillin side-reactions, with particular reference to fatalities from anaphylactic shock. Bull WHO *38*:159, 1968.
104. Martin MJ, Wellman WE: Clinically useful antimicrobial agents. Postgrad Med J *33*:327, 1963.
105. Weinstein L, Lerner PI, Chew WH: Clinical and bacteriological studies of the effect of massive doses of penicillin G on infections caused by gram-negative bacilli. N Engl J Med *271*:525, 1964.
106. Smith H, Lerner PI, Weinstein L: Neurotoxicity and massive intravenous therapy with penicillin. Arch Intern Med *120*:47, 1967.
107. Wilkowske CJ: The penicillins. Mayo Clin Proc *52*:616, 1977.
108. Weinstein AJ: The new cephalosporins and penicillins. Compr Ther 8:26, 1982.
109. Fleming PC, Jaffe D: The nephrotoxic effect of cephaloridine. Postgrad Med J (Suppl) 43:89, 1967.
110. Pittinger C, Adamson R: Antibiotic blockage of neuromuscular function. Annu Rev Pharmacol *12*:169, 1972.
111. Dupuis JY, Martin R, Tetrault JP: Atracurium and vecuronium interaction with gentamicin and tobramycin. Can J Anaesth *36*:407–411, 1989.
112. Harwood TN, Moorthy SS: Prolonged vecuronium-induced neuromuscular blockade in children. Anesth Analg *68*:534–536, 1989.
113. Best CJ, Ewart M, Sumner E: Perioperative complications following the use of vancomycin in children: A report of two cases. Br J Anaesth *67*:576–577, 1989.
114. Huang KC, Heise A, Schrader AK, Tsueda K: Vancomycin enhances the neuromuscular blockade of vecuronium. Anesth Analg *71*:194–196, 1990.
115. Newfield P, Roizen MF: Hazards of rapid administration of vancomycin. Ann Intern Med *91*:581, 1979.
116. Weiss CF, Glazko AJ, Weston JK: Chloramphenicol in the newborn infant. A physiologic explanation of its toxicity when given in excessive doses. N Engl J Med *262*:787, 1960.
117. Bartkowski RR, Mcdonnell TE: Prolonged alfentanil effect following erythromycin administration. Anesthesiology *73*:556–568, 1990.
118. Cummins LH, Kozak PP, Gillman SA: Erythromycin's effect on theophylline blood levels. Pediatrics *59*:144, 1977.
119. Daubeck JL, Daugherty MJ, Petty C: Lincomycin-induced cardiac arrest: A case report. Anesth Analg *53*:563, 1974.
120. Sprung J, Schedewie HK, Kampine J: Intraoperative anaphylactic shock after bacitracin irrigation. Anesth Analg *71*:430–433, 1990.

CHAPTER

4 Central Nervous System Diseases

M. E. McLEOD, M.D. and R. E. CREIGHTON, M.D.

Anesthesia for neurosurgery in the infant and child differs from adult practice in many ways. Many procedures are for congenital anomalies of the central nervous system or for resection of brain tumors, which represent a significant proportion of childhood neoplasms. In contrast, carotid artery disease is rare.

The open fontanelle in the infant and the higher metabolic rate of infancy and childhood also influence anesthetic management. In the infant, the open fontanelle not only increases cranial compliance but also provides a means to assess the intracranial pressure noninvasively. While palpation of the fontanelle will aid in clinical assessment of the degree of intracranial hypertension, the application of a transducer to the fontanelle can provide an accurate, noninvasive estimate of actual intracranial pressure (ICP).[1] In the older child, as in the adult, the skull must be considered as a rigid and essentially closed container in which the pressure depends on the total volume of brain substance, interstitial fluid, cerebrospinal fluid (CSF), and blood. The familiar pressure-volume curve of intracranial compliance shows that with initial volume changes in one compartment, compensation is possible, and only a small change in pressure results (Fig. 4–1).[2] This is achieved by displacement of CSF into the relatively distensible spinal dural sac, as well as by changes in the volume of the intracranial vascular bed.[3] Once the limit of compensation is reached, a small change in intracranial volume will result in a more dramatic change in intracranial pressure. Since manipulations of CSF volume are possible only if access to the ventricular system is available, the control of ICP by the anesthesiologist usually depends on alterations in cerebral blood volume or the volume of intracellular and interstitial fluid.

Through modifications of the nitrous oxide method, cerebral blood flow (CBF) has been measured in small children, and it is evident that both CBF and cerebral metabolic rate

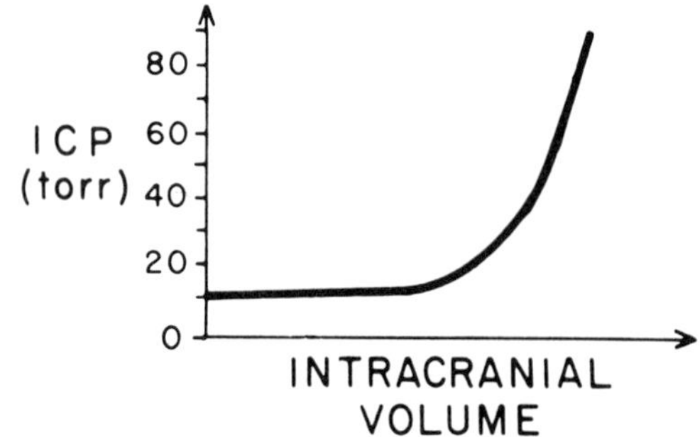

FIGURE 4–1. Idealized intracranial volume-pressure relationship. (From Shapiro HM: Intracranial hypertension: Therapeutic and anesthetic considerations. Anesthesiology *43*:445, 1975.)

($CMRO_2$) are significantly higher in children, whereas cerebrovascular resistance is lower.[4] Noninvasive measurement of cerebral blood flow velocity can be made either transcranially or via the fontanelle, using pulsed Doppler techniques, and the resistance index calculated. This can be used to measure the effects of therapeutic interventions on CBF.[5]

Changes in cerebral blood flow, when associated with changes in cerebral blood volume, can produce rapid alterations in ICP. Normally, CBF is controlled by $Paco_2$, Pao_2, and mean arterial pressure (Fig. 4–2). In the normal adult, cerebral blood flow remains relatively constant between mean arterial pressures of 50 and 150 torr, provided changes are not abrupt.[2] This autoregulation, however, can be abolished by trauma, acidosis, and various drugs.[6] The exact limits of autoregulation in infants and children have not been defined. In the neonate with birth asphyxia or respiratory distress syndrome, it has been shown that autoregulation may be entirely absent, and as a result, the cerebral circulation becomes pressure-passive.[7] This can increase the risk of intraventricular hemorrhage if wide swings in arterial pressure occur.

Except at extremes, arterial oxygen tension has little influence on cerebral blood flow. When Pao_2 falls to a threshold level of 50 torr, however, cerebral blood flow increases rapidly.[8] In humans, the $Paco_2$ is the most important regulator of cerebrovascular resistance and cerebral blood flow. Indeed, a linear relationship exists: over the range of 15 to 76 torr, for each torr change in $Paco_2$ the cerebral blood volume changes 0.041 ml/100 gm of perfused tissue, and the CBF changes 1.8 ml/100 gm/min.[9] Thus, hyperventilation plays an important role in the management of the patient with raised ICP, and end-tidal CO_2 measurement is an important component of patient monitoring.

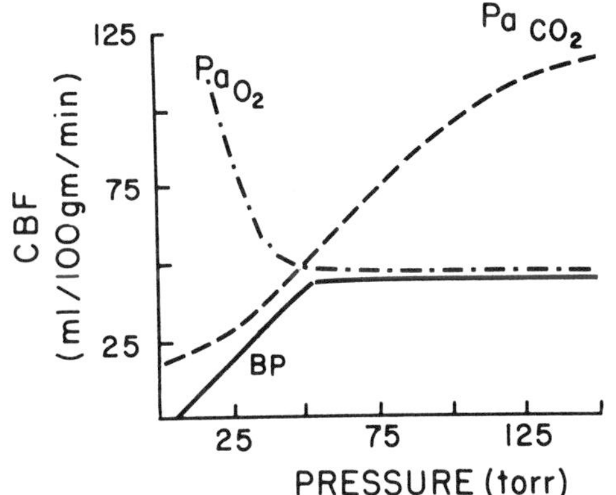

FIGURE 4–2. Changes in cerebral blood flow secondary to $Paco_2$ (---), Pao_2 (•—•—), and blood pressure (——). (From Shapiro HM: Intracranial hypertension: Therapeutic and anesthetic considerations. Anesthesiology *43*:445, 1975.)

Reductions in ICP also can be achieved by reducing the cerebral interstitial volume with diuretics. Osmotic agents, in particular mannitol, have proved to be effective in lowering ICP.[10] This is achieved by an increase in plasma osmolality and withdrawal of fluid from the intracellular and interstitial spaces. This action may result in transient increases in cerebral blood volume and ICP prior to the onset of diuresis.[11] To avoid this initial elevation in ICP, nonosmotic diuretics have been used to reduce cerebral blood volume. Furosemide, in doses of 1 mg/kg, will reduce ICP in the clinical situation without producing significant changes in serum osmolality or electrolytes.[11, 12] It provides a reasonable alternative to mannitol for the patient undergoing craniotomy. The precise mechanism by which furosemide lowers ICP is unclear, but it is thought to be due to effects on brain sodium levels and water transport.[13] The use of mannitol and furosemide together may be even more effective than either agent alone. Pollay and colleagues have shown that a combination of mannitol, 1 gm/kg, and furosemide, 0.7 mg/kg, results in a greater and more prolonged drop in ICP than that achieved with single drug therapy.[14]

The use of steroids in neurosurgery has long been a subject of controversy. Although steroid pretreatment has been shown to reduce cerebral edema and glucocorticoids have been shown to reduce CSF production,[15, 16] the efficacy of steroids in reducing edema in patients with cerebral trauma or encephalopathy remains unconfirmed.

When the operation is elective and dexamethasone therapy precedes the surgical treatment of tumors or vascular lesions, experimental evidence suggests that steroids should be of value.[15] The head-injured patient who is treated after the insult is less likely to derive the same benefit.

ANESTHETIC DRUGS

INTRAVENOUS AGENTS

The drugs used in anesthetic practice may increase, decrease, or have no effect on intracranial pressure. This factor determines their usefulness in the neurosurgical patient.

One of the most hazardous periods for the patient with elevated ICP coincides with induction of anesthesia and the establishment of the airway. The effectiveness of barbiturates in reducing intracranial pressure has long been recognized.[17] The dose-dependent decreases in both cerebral blood flow and metabolism make thiopentone an ideal induction agent for the patient with raised ICP.

Ketamine should not be used as an induction agent in neurosurgery. In dogs, an 80 percent increase in CBF and a 16 percent increase in $CMRO_2$ occur after ketamine injection, and these values remain above control for 30 minutes.[18] In hydrocephalic children, ketamine has been shown to produce two- to threefold increases in CSF pressure when given either intramuscularly or intravenously.[19]

Propofol, which can be used both as an induction and maintenance agent, is reported to decrease both cerebral blood flow and metabolism.[20] In baboons, Van Hemelrijck and colleagues have demonstrated that autoregulation is preserved during propofol anesthesia.[21] Falls in mean arterial pressure after rapid bolus doses, however, may result in falls in cerebral perfusion pressure; thus Pinaud and associates, in a study of brain-injured patients, have recommended reducing propofol doses for both induction and maintenance in patients at risk.[22]

In spite of induction of anesthesia with thiopentone, laryngoscopy and intubation may produce significant changes in mean arterial pressure and in ICP in patients with space-occupying lesions. The use of lidocaine, 1.5 mg/kg intravenously at induction, attenuates the blood pressure response and protects against increases in ICP.[23, 24] This technique has advantages over lidocaine aerosol in that blood levels are achieved prior to laryngoscopy, and accurate doses can be given to small children. Lidocaine, like thiopentone, is also effective in lowering ICP when acute elevations occur intraoperatively.[25]

Narcotics are useful for the maintenance of anesthesia in pediatric neurosurgical patients, although they are rarely used for premedication because of the danger of respiratory depression. Intravenous morphine has been shown to have little effect on cerebral blood flow, and autoregulation remains intact.[26] The high-dose fentanyl technique has also been used successfully in neuroanesthesia, but the need for postoperative naloxone infusion makes it impractical for the average patient.[27] Fentanyl in combination with droperidol results in small decreases in ICP,[28] making both neuroleptanesthesia and neuroleptanalgesia useful techniques. In contrast to the ICP stability typical of fentanyl, alfentanil has been shown to produce an increase in CSF pressure in patients with brain tumors.[29] Although sufentanil does not appear to increase CBF when given in small doses to healthy volunteers,[30] the increases in CBF seen in anesthetized animals[31] suggest that it, too, may be less appropriate for neuroanesthesia than fentanyl.

In addition to its beneficial effects in controlling seizures, diazepam produces decreases in both cerebral blood flow and oxygen consumption.[32] Midazolam maleate, like diazepam, decreases cerebral blood flow and metabolism,[33] and because of its short duration of action may prove to be of great benefit in neuroanesthesia.

The neuromuscular blocking drugs have little effect on the cerebral circulation. Pancuronium and atracurium in the presence of halothane have been shown to have no effect on CBF, ICP, or $CMRO_2$, although at sub–minimal alveolar concentrations (MAC) of halothane, the electroencephalographic arousal effects of atracurium's metabolite, laudanosine, can be observed.[34] Suxamethonium, on the other hand, produces an initial fall in ICP followed by a rise above baseline levels.[35]

INHALATION AGENTS

Nitrous oxide is thought to have minimal effect on cerebral blood flow, although some investigators have reported increases in both cerebral blood flow and metabolism in dogs.[36] Studies in rats suggest that there is a disproportionate increase in CBF compared with cerebral metabolism.[37] The electroencephalogram (EEG) shows progressive loss of alpha rhythm as the concentration is increased above 30 percent.[38]

Volatile anesthetics are known to be cerebral vasodilators and must be used with caution in the patient with raised ICP. Therefore, the induction of anesthesia with inhalation agents is not recommended for patients with significantly elevated ICP. Because it produces epileptiform activity on the EEG, enflurane generally should be avoided in neurosurgical patients.[38] In the experimental animal, enflurane also causes an increase in CSF production,[39] in contrast to halothane, which decreases the output of CSF.[40] Although both halothane and enflurane abolish autoregulation at 1.0 MAC, the cerebral vasculature remains responsive to changes in Pa_{CO_2}.[41] It has been shown that the prior establishment of hypocapnia minimizes the increase in ICP associated with halothane[42] and that cerebral blood flow begins to return toward control values after 30 minutes of halothane anesthesia.[43] Isoflurane, which is commonly used in neuroanesthesia, also increases CBF at levels of greater than 1.1 MAC, but the increase is less than occurs with halothane,[44] and the ICP returns to control levels more rapidly after the establishment of hypocapnia.[45] At 1.0 MAC, isoflurane autoregulation appears to be preserved, but at higher concentrations, as with the other agents, the cerebral vasculature becomes pressure-passive.[46] At higher inspired concentrations, a decrease in $CMRO_2$ is also seen, which may provide some measure of protection against ischemic insult.[47] In addition, its relatively rapid elimination permits early postoperative neurological assessment.

In animal studies, sevoflurane appears to be similar to isoflurane in its effects on the cerebral circulation. Cerebral metabolism is reduced, and no increase in CBF is seen at concentrations of up to 1.0 MAC.[48] Desflurane also reduces $CMRO_2$ in a similar fashion, but it is a more potent cerebral vasodilator.[49]

POSITIONING

Patient positioning is important in neuroanesthesia because of the effects on the airway, circulation, and intracranial pressure. In some centers, the sitting position is commonly used for procedures in the posterior fossa. The major disadvantages of this position are the increased risk of air embolism and the potential for cardiovascular instability. Ernst and coworkers found decreases in CBF and spinal cord blood flow when the sitting position was used in the presence of elevated ICP.[50] A widely varying incidence of air embolism has been reported in patients undergoing surgery in the sitting position, which probably is similar in children and adults.[51] Cucchiara and Bowers found the frequency of air embolism in children detected by Doppler to be 33 percent.[51] In this study, the incidence of hypotension associated with air embolism was 69 percent in contrast to an incidence of only 36 percent in a group of adults. The precordial Doppler has been shown to be more sensitive than pulmonary artery pressure, end-tidal carbon dioxide concentrations, and end-tidal nitrogen in detecting even small volumes of entrained air. However, the noise produced by electrocautery may render it less informative, and small changes in Doppler position or in the patient's systemic blood pressure may alter the sounds.[52] The high incidence of hypotension associated with air embolism in children necessitates an immediate response by the anesthesiologist when air embolus is suspected. Nitrous oxide, if in use, must be discontinued, the surgeon must flood the operative site with saline, and the head must be lowered. Attempts to aspirate air from a right atrial catheter are reported to be less successful in children.[51]

The prone position provides an alternative to the sitting position for posterior fossa operations and is also commonly used for operations on the back and cervical spinal cord. Care must be taken to secure the airway and support the anesthetic circuit so that accidental extubation or disconnection cannot occur. A nasotracheal tube is more easily secured than an oral tracheal tube in this position since the fixative tape is less likely to be loosened by secretions. Depending on the size of the child, either a U-shaped bolster or a Hall-Relton frame can be used to ensure free excursion of the diaphragm without obstruction of abdominal venous return. If a horseshoe headrest is used, careful padding and positioning of the face are required to avoid pressure on the eyes.

When patients are operated on in the supine position, a 15- to 30-degree anti-Trendelenburg tilt is often used since this amount of elevation does decrease ICP,[53] although it may increase the risk of air embolism. If the head is to be turned to either side to an excessive degree, the lateral decubitus position is preferable, as this avoids obstruction of the jugular venous system by keeping the head in a neutral position.

Regardless of the position chosen when the patient is placed on the operating table, the chest must be carefully auscultated after final positioning to ensure that turning the head or flexing the neck has not resulted in either kinking of the endotracheal tube or endobronchial intubation. Use of an armored endotracheal tube will decrease the risk of tube kinking but will result in an airway of smaller diameter because of the wall thickness of armored tubes.

CRANIOSYNOSTOSIS

Craniosynostosis results from premature fusion of cranial sutures. It may involve single, bilateral, or multiple sutures and may be part of a syndrome involving other anomalies. The bones of the calvarium arise from widely separated centers of ossification that spread centrifugally toward each other. The separation of adjacent bones is a result of expansion of underlying cranial contents and is compensated for by the addition of new bone at the sutural edges. Premature fusion will result in inhibition of the normal direction of growth of the neurocranial capsule.[54] The incidence of craniosynostosis is approximately 1 in 2000.[55] Premature fusion of the sagittal suture is the most common lesion, and boys are more often affected than girls.[56] Other cranial sutures and multiple sutures are affected in fewer than half the cases (Table 4–1).[57] There may be a family history in as many as 39 percent of cases of synostosis.[58] Some cases, such as Crouzon's syndrome, which consists of craniosynostosis, maxillary hypoplasia, and shallow orbits with proptosis, and Apert's syndrome, in which craniosynostosis is associated with syndactyly, can be inherited as autosomal-dominant conditions.[59]

Operation for craniosynostosis is usually carried out in infancy. It may be necessary at a very early age if multiple suture involvement produces constriction of the brain. Additionally, in early correction the bone is more malleable, and the rapidly growing brain will assist in remodeling of the cranial contours.[58] Up to 20 percent of patients will also have hydrocephalus that will require operation in early infancy. Hydrocephalus is seen more commonly in those patients with craniofacial syndromes than in those with isolated suture involvement.[60, 61]

Anesthetic Considerations

The surgical correction of these defects ranges from simple strip craniectomy in the case of single suture synostosis to major craniofacial reconstructions required for patients with complex syndromes. In the infant presenting for sagittal craniectomy, the most common of these procedures, the major anesthetic concerns are positioning (usually prone) and the potential for rapid blood loss.

When a cranial vault reshaping is the planned procedure, it is important to evaluate the child for ease of airway management and any associated anomalies. Preservation of CNS homeostasis, blood and fluid replacement, and temperature maintenance are the major intraoperative concerns. Brain relaxation may be necessary in vault reconstructions and can be achieved by hyperventilation and diuresis. Although these procedures are done in the supine position, there is still a risk of venous air embolism.[62] Blood loss may be considerable owing to the extent of the surgery and the vascularity of the structures. As losses are extremely difficult to measure accurately during these procedures, monitoring of central venous and intra-arterial pressures is important, as is measurement of urine output. The use of controlled hypotension to decrease blood loss should be restricted to primarily facial procedures. In intracranial operations, the risk of cerebral ischemia may be increased if deliberate hypotension is combined with brain retraction, which may by itself lead to focal ischemia.[63]

At the end of the procedure, patients must be wide awake so that neurological function, especially vision, can be assessed. Any patient with a difficult airway who has had a facial component to the operation should be left intubated until any risk of airway obstruction caused by postoperative swelling has passed.

Table 4–1. INCIDENCE OF CONGENITAL SYNOSTOSES

Suture	Percent
Sagittal	56
Single coronal	11
Bilateral coronal	11
Metopic	7
Lambdoid	1
Three or more	14

Reproduced by permission from Harwood-Nash DC, Fitz CR: Neuroradiology in Infants and Children. Volume 1. St. Louis, CV Mosby, 1976, p 76.

NEURAL TUBE DEFECTS

Although the neural tube defects of anencephaly, spina bifida, and encephalocele are among the most widely studied of birth defects, the precise etiology of these malformations is unknown. Most investigators have concluded that both genetic and environmental factors play a role.[64]

ENCEPHALOCELE

Encephalocele, also known as cranium bifidum, is a herniation of cerebral tissue and meninges through a defect in the skull that may occur anywhere in the midline, from the foramen magnum to the nasal cavity.[56] The incidence of encephalocele is between 1 and 3 per 10,000 live births.[65]

Anterior encephalocele commonly presents as a mass in the nasopharynx (Fig. 4–3). Although small lesions may go unnoticed for years, patients with larger masses may present with continous nasal discharge or recurrent meningitis. In the case of basal encephalocele, there may

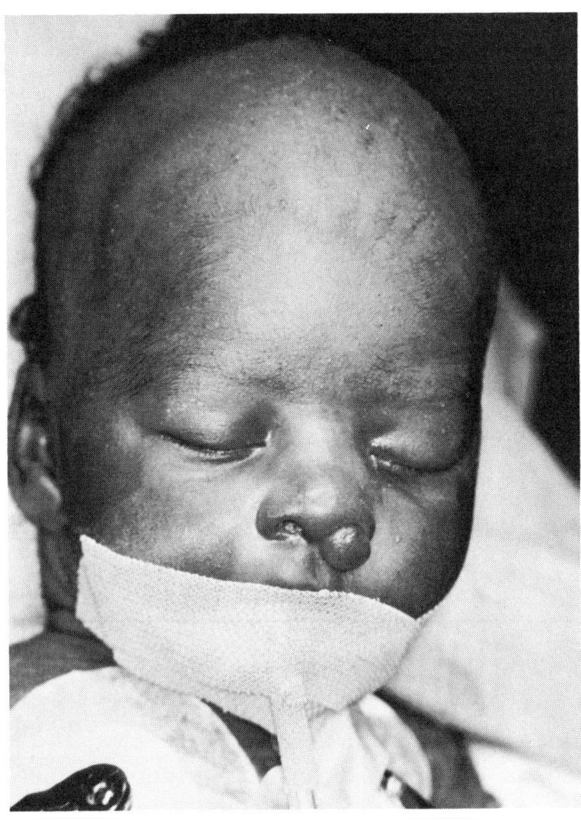

FIGURE 4–3. Infant with nasopharyngeal encephalocele.

be associated feeding difficulties or airway obstruction. The size of the defect and the contents of the sac (potentially hypothalamus and pituitary) may preclude resection. Operative mortality for treatment of basal encephalocele has been reported to be as high as 50 percent.[66]

More commonly encountered in the neonatal period is the posterior encephalocele. These occipital lesions account for 66 to 89 percent of encephaloceles and represent 8 to 15 percent of congenital dysraphic syndromes.[67] In addition to the obvious occipital abnormality, Karch and Urich demonstrated anomalies throughout the neuraxis in these infants. Hydrocephalus, epilepsy, paraplegia, spasticity, and blindness have been reported in survivors.[65] The Klippel-Feil deformity and cleft lip and palate are also frequently associated with encephalocele.[68] In addition, defects in thermoregulation have been demonstrated in infants with central nervous system abnormalities.[69]

Anesthetic Considerations

In the patient with a large anterior encephalocele and facial clefts, intubation may prove to be difficult, and appropriate precautions should be taken. Securing the airway may also pose some problems in the infant with a large occipital encephalocele, as the patient's head may be difficult to position for intubation (Fig. 4–4). If difficulty with intubation is not anticipated, a smooth intravenous induction is preferable to awake intubation in the older infant. Spontaneous ventilation has been used in the past as a monitor of brain stem integrity. However, in the neonate there is a significant risk of depression by anesthetic agents, and controlled ventilation is advisable. Changes in heart rate and rhythm will serve to warn of brain stem compromise. There is a danger that brain stem centers will be within the occipital encephalocele, but with magnetic resonance imaging a preoperative assessment of the encephalocele contents can be made.[67] In a large Nigerian series of occipital encephaloceles, operative mortality was 6 percent, and all infants who died had brain substance within the sac.[70]

MYELOMENINGOCELE

The commonly used term *spina bifida* merely refers to a failure of fusion of the vertebral arches. In 5 to 10 percent of cases, it occurs as spina bifida occulta, in which skin and soft tissues cover the defect, usually at L5.[71] The alternative form is spina bifida aperta, in which the defect communicates with the outside either as a meningocele (sac covered by meninges but containing no neural elements), or as a myelomeningocele in which the sac contains nerve roots and often part of the spinal cord. The roots below the level of the lesion do not function, resulting in muscle paralysis and a neurogenic bowel and bladder. The incidence of myelomeningocele is estimated at 0.2 to 4 per 1000 live births, and it is more common in caucasians and girls.[72] Maternal screening for alpha-fetoprotein, high-resolution ultrasonography, and amniocentesis now permit early diagnosis as well as assessment of the level of the lesion. Ventriculomegaly, if present, in utero, can also be detected.[73]

The majority of these children, between 65 and 85 percent, will have associated hydrocephalus. Stein and Schut found that 80 percent of 156 children with myelomeningocele developed hydrocephalus, although only in 15.3 percent was it evident at birth. Aqueductal stenosis was the cause of the hydrocephalus in 73.4 percent of patients.[74]

The urgency for operation in these patients is

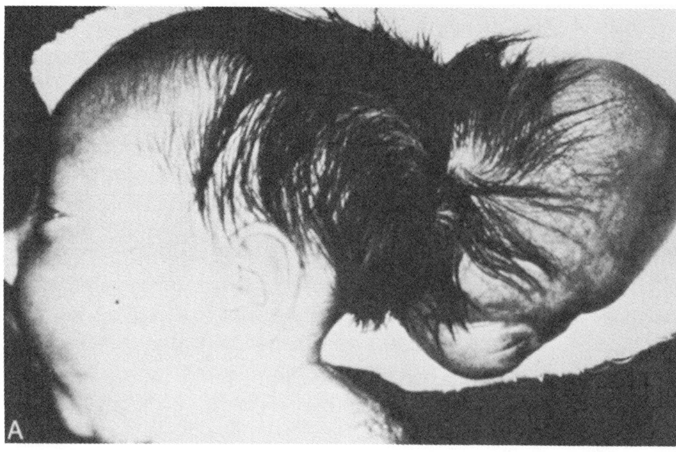

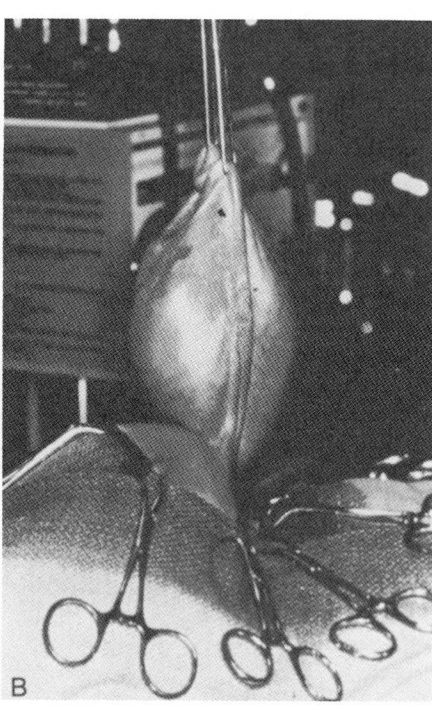

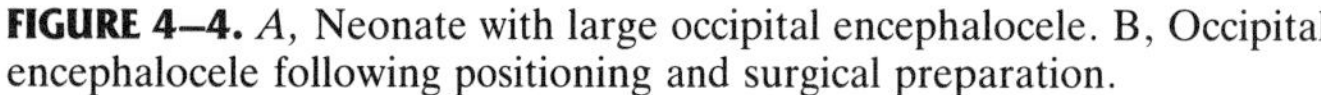

FIGURE 4–4. *A,* Neonate with large occipital encephalocele. B, Occipital encephalocele following positioning and surgical preparation.

a result of the potential for infection of the central nervous system, particularly if the sac has ruptured. Closure within the first 24 to 48 hours of life is preferred. Operation for closure of the meningocele is usually the first of many trips to the operating room for these patients. In infants with overt hydrocephalus at birth, a ventriculoperitoneal shunt is sometimes inserted as part of the initial procedure, but more commonly the hydrocephalus becomes symptomatic later and a second operation is required.

Skeletal anomalies are also frequently associated with myelomeningocele. Club foot and congenital dislocation of the hip are the most common.[75] Scoliosis also occurs frequently, but only a small percentage is congenital and associated with additional vertebral anomalies. In the majority of myelomeningocele patients, scoliosis is acquired and is due to abnormal neuromuscular control. The severity is therefore related to age and level of the myelomeningocele.[76] Those patients with thoracic lesions may develop progressive kyphoscoliosis with eventual cardiorespiratory compromise and may require spinal instrumentation and fusion. Complications resulting from a neurogenic bladder may also lead to multiple urologic procedures.[77]

Anesthetic Considerations

The problems of anesthetizing these patients for closure of the myelomeningocele include those of any neonatal procedure. In addition, there are the problems of positioning, the potentially large blood and fluid losses from the operative site, and heat loss. To minimize the risk of trauma to the sac, the infants are best intubated on the side. Because this is an unusual position for securing the airway, awake intubation is prudent. The patient may be placed supine if a sufficiently large cushioned ring is available to protect the sac.

Actual blood and fluid losses are difficult to measure but may be considerable if extensive undermining of the skin is required to facilitate closure of the defect. In very large lesions, either myocutaneous flaps or staged procedures with the insertion of tissue expanders may be necessary to obtain closure.[78] Changes in vital signs, especially systolic blood pressure, will closely parallel blood volume changes in the neonate. Although blood transfusion is usually unnecessary because of the high hemoglobin in the neonate, colloid solutions such as albumin may be of benefit.

Close monitoring is necessary in the postoperative period, since associated hydrocephalus and Arnold-Chiari malformation may cause significant hypoventilation or apnea. Ward and coworkers reported that infants with myelomeningocele, even without a history of apnea, showed abnormal ventilatory patterns during sleep.[79]

These children may remain at risk for respiratory complications following anesthesia as they grow older and return to the operating room for other procedures. A significantly lower hypercapnic ventilatory response has been demonstrated in adolescents with myelomeningocele compared with controls, which may result in hypoventilation in the perioperative period.[80] There is also an increased risk of endobronchial intubation in this group of patients: Wells and co-workers found that 36 percent of 87 patients with myelomeningocele had short tracheas.[81]

HYDROCEPHALUS

Hydrocephalus is a condition in which there is a disproportionately large volume of cerebrospinal fluid relative to other cranial contents. It may arise because of a congenital abnormality, or it may be secondary to obstruction caused by neoplasm, infection, or trauma. In noncommunicating hydrocephalus, the CSF is excluded from the subarachnoid space by the obstruction of flow in any part of the ventricular system—in particular, the cerebral aqueduct (aqueduct stenosis), the interventricular foramen, or the foramina of Luschka and Magendie. In communicating hydrocephalus, CSF flows unimpeded to the spinal subarachnoid space but is either excluded from the cerebral subarachnoid space or cannot be absorbed into the cerebral venous sinuses via the arachnoid villi.

A large portion of the CSF is formed by the choroid plexuses, and it has been shown that this is not dependent on hydrostatic pressure.[82] CSF continues to be produced in spite of increasing intracranial pressure, and the ventricles gradually dilate, between the plexus and the obstruction. As the process continues, the ventricles enlarge in conjunction with cortical thinning. In the infant, in whom the sutures have not yet fused, the head gradually increases in circumference.

Neonatal hydrocephalus is associated with a variety of congenital anomalies, including myelomeningocele, aqueduct stenosis, arachnoid cyst, porencephaly, and intracranial tumor. The Arnold-Chiari syndrome, in which there are multiple posterior fossa abnormalities, and the Dandy-Walker syndrome, in which the fourth ventricle is isolated, are much less common.[56] Hydrocephalus may also develop following hemorrhage or infection. More than 65 percent of preterm infants with severe intraventricular hemorrhage will develop progressive ventricular dilatation.[83]

Hydrocephalus is not invariably a progressive disorder, but signs of increased intracranial pressure or rapid increase in head circumference are indications for surgical intervention. Vomiting, behavior change (including irritability in the infant), drowsiness, and headache are the commonest symptoms, and increasing head circumference, tense anterior fontanelle, widening of sutures, and scalp vein distention are the commonest clinical signs. On occasion, children with raised ICP will have no clinical signs. In a review by Kirkpatrick and co-workers, half the infants with hydrocephalus had no symptoms, and one fourth of patients who had CSF shunts in place and elevated ICP by direct measurement had no clinical signs.[84]

Operation for hydrocephalus involves correction of the precipitating cause, if possible, and/or a CSF shunting procedure.

Ventriculoperitoneal shunt is the operation most commonly performed in noncommunicating hydrocephalus. Either the pleural space or the right atrium can be used in cases in which adhesive peritonitis makes the peritoneal route unusable. Ventriculoatrial shunts are inserted using electrocardiographic control to ensure placement within the atrium.[85] This shunting technique, while very effective, is less commonly employed than previously because of the risk of thrombus formation, multiple microemboli from the catheter tip, and superior vena cava obstruction.[86, 87] In communicating hydrocephalus, a lumboperitoneal shunt is often used.

With present therapy, infants with hydrocephalus at birth have approximately an 85 percent chance of survival and a 72 percent probability of normal or borderline intellectual function.[88]

Anesthetic Considerations

As a general rule, preoperative sedation should not be used, as narcotics or sedatives may depress ventilation, resulting in further increases in ICP. Lidocaine should be added to the induction sequence if there are signs of significant elevation of ICP, and the patient should be hyperventilated following induction of anesthesia.

These patients may be positioned in the supine postion with the head turned and the neck extended, in the lateral decubitus position, or even face-down with the body rotated (fourth ventricle–peritoneal shunt or cyst-peritoneal shunt in Dandy-Walker syndrome). Appropriate precautions should be taken to protect the face and airway and to maintain ventilation, depending on the position. Occasionally, the rapid decrease in ICP caused by shunt insertion may result in cardiac dysrhythmias.[89]

ARNOLD-CHIARI MALFORMATION AND SYRINGOMYELIA

The Arnold-Chiari (Chiari II) malformation is the most common anomaly involving the cerebellum. It is present in most children with myelomeningocele but is frequently asymptomatic. The malformation consists of an elongation of the cerebellar vermis and herniation of the caudal vermis and choroid plexus through the foramen magnum, with kinking of the medulla and upper cervical cord.[90]

In approximately 20 percent of patients with myelomeningocele, the Arnold-Chiari malformation will become symptomatic, and more than half of those who do require treatment will be seen before the age of 3 months.[91, 92] The usual signs and symptoms are swallowing difficulty, apneic episodes, stridor, aspiration, arm weakness, and opisthotonos. Swallowing difficulties are manifested by feeding problems and pooling of oral secretions. In these infants, the gag reflex may be diminished or absent. In Sieben and associates' series, all patients with symptomatic Arnold-Chiari malformations showed multiple cranial nerve involvement.[92] Mortality is increased in those infants who progress to vocal cord paralysis, arm weakness, or cardiorespiratory arrest within 2 weeks of initial presentation.

Anesthetic Considerations

Since recurrent aspiration is one of the presenting features of this condition and is unlikely to cease without intervention, respiratory function may be less than optimal at the time of surgery. Occasionally a patient will require intubation and ventilation preoperatively.

Surgical therapy involves posterior fossa decompression with upper cervical laminectomy and opening of the dura to decompress the herniated cerebellar tongue. This procedure is performed with the infant prone and the neck in flexion. Particular care must be taken with positioning of the nasotracheal tube, as the extremely flexed posture may result in endobronchial intubation in these patients who may have short tracheas.[81] Controlled ventilation is essential as these children are prone to apneic episodes. Changes in heart rate and rhythm will warn of further brain stem compromise.

In those infants with vocal cord paresis and depressed gag reflex, it may be necessary to leave an endotracheal tube in place postoperatively as recovery of function may not be immediate. Some will eventually require tracheotomy, and some will also need a gastrostomy to decrease the risk of aspiration. Although stridor is frequently improved in the postoperative period, all patients require close monitoring for the first few days after surgery. Ventilatory abnormalities, as shown by abnormal hypoxic and hypercapneic arousal responses, may persist after surgery.[93]

Syringomyelia

In older children and adults, the Arnold-Chiari malformation is commonly associated with syringomyelia. These patients typically present with upper extremity weakness with or without sensory abnormalities. The diagnosis is made when a thickened cord is seen on CT scan in conjunction with an Arnold-Chiari malformation or adhesions around the foramen magnum. Occasionally, a delayed scan will actually show contrast entering the syrinx from the fourth ventricle.[94]

Surgical therapy of this condition consists of either plugging the obex or draining the hydromyelia, in addition to decompressive laminectomy. Problems of positioning for posterior fossa or upper cervical surgery apply to these patients. It is also important to assess them preoperatively for bulbar symptoms, as these may have implications for postoperative airway management.

CEREBROVASCULAR ABNORMALITIES

ARTERIOVENOUS MALFORMATION

Cerebral arteriovenous malformations (AVMs) are congenital lesions arising from an abnormality of development of the primitive arteriolar-capillary network normally interposed between the arteries and veins of the brain.[95] Signs and symptoms may not arise until later childhood or early adult life: only about 18 percent of AVMs that become symptomatic do so before the age of 15 years.[96] Intracranial hemorrhage is the commonest form of presentation, occurring in about 70 percent of children.[97, 98] Seizure disorder is also a frequent sign at the time of diagnosis of the AVM.

The risk of rebleeding after the initial event is significant. Graf and colleagues, in their review, estimated the risk of recurrent hemorrhage at 2 percent per year after the first year, in which the rate was 6 percent.[99] In So's series, the risk of rebleeding within 5 years was 25 percent.[97]

Treatment of these lesions, if accessible, is frequently surgical. Intravascular embolization techniques permit the treatment of lesions that have multiple feeders or are nonresectable by virtue of their location or size (Fig. 4–5).

Anesthetic Considerations

The anesthetic management of children with cerebral AVMs is determined by the preoperative state. Of the patients seen with hemorrhage, some will be unconscious and require immediate resuscitative therapy prior to transfer to the operating room for evacuation of clot, and others will have only signs of subarachnoid bleeding and can be scheduled for operation after a period of stabilization. The first group requires airway support and should be considered to have an expanding space-occupying lesion in the form of intracerebral clot. The sympathetic stimulation associated with intubation may result in a recurrence of bleeding from the lesion. These patients therefore require adequate sedation and complete paralysis prior to airway manipu-

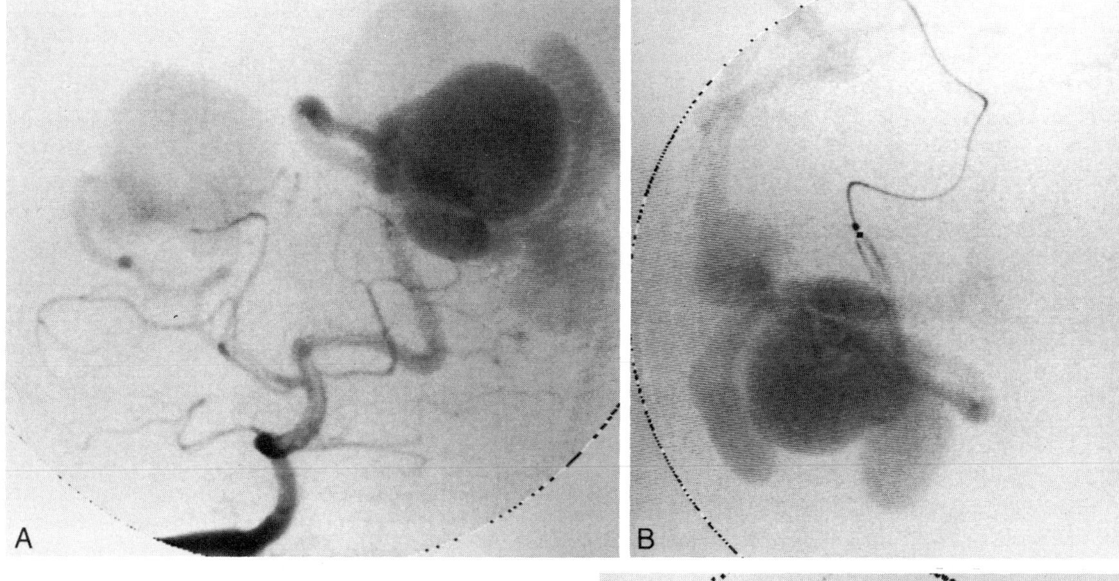

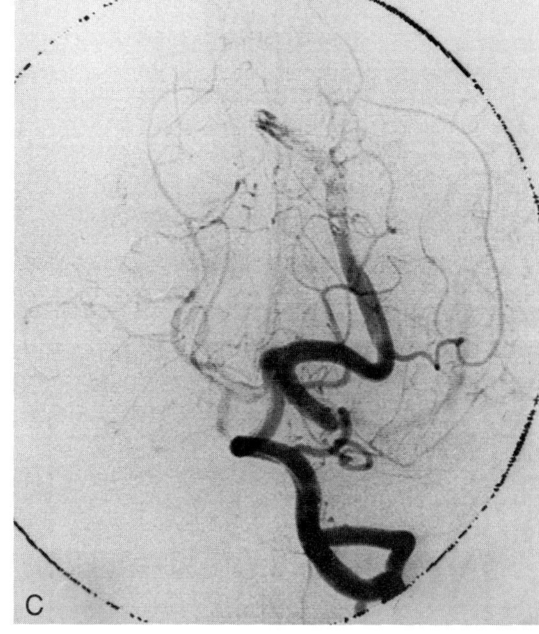

FIGURE 4–5. Angiograms of a 10-year-old child with bilateral occipital A-V fistula. *A*, Pre-embolization, showing fistulae from right and left posterior cerebral arteries (PCA). *B*, Pre-embolization, with microcatheter in feeding branch of left PCA. *C*, Immediately postembolization of left PCA and 1 week postembolization of right PCA. (Courtesy of Dr. P. Burrows.)

lation. The usual precautions for elevated ICP and the potentially full stomach should be taken. Hyperventilation should be instituted as soon as the endotracheal tube is in place.

Children scheduled for elective operation of an AVM should be sedated preoperatively with the aim of achieving as smooth an induction as possible. A combination of fentanyl citrate and droperidol is useful in this situation. As with the urgent group of patients, they must be deeply anesthetized and completely paralyzed prior to airway manipulation.

In some cases, induced hypotension will be of benefit in the surgical management of the AVM, particularly if the lesion is deep-seated and difficult to approach. The safe level and duration of controlled hypotension in children has not been defined, although their normally lower blood pressures and the absence of cerebrovascular disease lead one to expect that children tolerate pressures at least as low as those tolerated by adults. The ideal method of inducing hypotension is yet to be found. A variety of methods, including oligemia, ganglionic blockade, deep inhalational anesthesia, and direct vasodilatation, have been employed. Isoflurane has been used as a hypotensive agent in aneurysm operations in adults and appears to be effective and easy to control.[100] Rebound hypertension does not occur, increases in cerebral blood flow are minimal provided hypocapnia is maintained, and cerebral metabolism is reduced.[47, 100]

General anesthesia is usually required for embolization in children, although a neuroleptic technique has been recommended for adults as this permits neurological assessment during the procedure.[101] Embolization may be a lengthy procedure, especially if the lesion is a large AVM with multiple feeding vessels. End-tidal monitoring of CO_2 is essential, as hyperventilation may constrict vessels around the AVM and limit access of catheters. Normocarbia should therefore be maintained. Fluids must be carefully managed, as the contrast initially expands circulating volume and then causes an osmotic diuresis during long procedures. Hypotensive techniques occasionally may be required to allow the bucrylate glue to occlude feeders without passing too rapidly into the venous system.[101] In high-flow lesions associated with cardiac failure, however, hypotensive techniques may result in myocardial ischemia by decreasing the already low diastolic pressure.

ANEURYSM

Ruptured intracranial aneurysm occurs less commonly in children than in adults, the incidence of rupture being about 3 percent in those under the age of 20 years and 1 percent in those under the age of 15 years.[102] Many children with intracranial aneurysms will have had significant signs and symptoms, such as syncopal episodes, focal headache, or neurological deficit, prior to the event that precipitates hospital admission.[103] Cerebral aneurysms are more common in males, and lesions in children may occur in different locations than do those in the adult population.[104] As with arteriovenous malformations, most children will present with an acute hemorrhage, and subsequent morbidity and mortality are related to the neurological signs at the time of initial presentation. Perioperative mortality is 22 percent overall, but only 8 percent in those patients who present with good preservation of neurological function (Botterell grades I and II).[104, 105]

Anesthetic considerations in these patients are similar to those for children with arteriovenous malformations. Hypotensive techniques usually will be required, but the duration of hypotension will be shorter.

ANEURYSM OF THE VEIN OF GALEN

An uncommon vascular lesion in infants and children is aneurysm or arteriovenous malformation of the great cerebral vein of Galen. The age at which these patients present is related to the size of the lesion, and patients can be divided into four groups by clinical presentation. Neonates have the poorest prognosis and present with cranial bruit and severe congestive heart failure. Many die of cardiovascular complications before surgical therapy or embolization can be undertaken, and others die in the early postoperative period.[106] Subendocardial damage due to pressure and volume overload of the neonatal heart, combined with impaired myocardial perfusion, contributes to the high mortality.[107] The second group of patients presents later in infancy, with craniomegaly and a cranial bruit, and some will have mild congestive heart failure. Slightly older children, the third group, will also have an enlarged head at the time of presentation and may have a bruit, but heart failure is unusual.[106] In the fourth and rarest group, patients come to medical attention in late childhood or early adult life with headache and exercise syncope and are found to have a calcified rim in the pineal region.[108] The latter three groups can be managed as for other AVMs.

The neonatal group presents the greatest anesthetic challenge because of their compromised myocardial function and the greater risk of catastrophic bleeding due to the size of the lesion. Cardiopulmonary bypass and deep hypothermia have been used successfully in older infants,[109] but in the neonate this technique has not proved to be of benefit.[110] Controlled hypotension has also been recommended and has been used effectively in the older infant.[111] In spite of the advantage of the hypotension in decreasing the resistance to left ventricular outflow once the low resistance runoff has been occluded, this approach is unwise in the neonate. The myocardium is already at risk because of the excessive workload and the low diastolic perfusion pressure; any further decrease in myocardial perfusion due to induced hypotension may result in ischemia and cardiac arrest.

A more recent approach to treatment of this lesion in the neonate is closed embolization. Staged partial occlusion avoids one of the problems that may occur with complete surgical obliteration of a large AVM—that of sudden volume overload and severe heart failure.[112] In the neonate with high-output cardiac failure, one must pay particularly close attention to the volumes of flush solution and contrast used during catheter manipulation, as congestive failure can be significantly worsened by volume overload prior to actual embolization. Because these procedures tend to be lengthy, problems of temperature homeostasis are also encountered.

MOYAMOYA DISEASE

Moyamoya disease is a spontaneous, progressive occlusion of the internal carotid arteries of unknown etiology. Moyamoya means puff of smoke in Japanese, referring to the angiographic appearance of the haze of collateral vessels that develop at the base of the brain. Originally thought to be specific to Japan, this condition has now been reported in numerous ethnic groups.[113] There appear to be two peaks in onset, one in childhood and one in the third and fourth decades, and it is more common in females. The condition typically presents with one of four clinical patterns: hemorrhage, infarction, transient ischemic attacks (TIA), or epilepsy. Children under 10 years of age tend to present with TIA or epilepsy.[114] The disease is of particular interest to anesthetists as severe neurological sequelae may follow induced hypocapnia.

Studies by Taki and colleagues suggest that the actual reduction in CBF in moyamoya is small because peripheral resistance vessels are maximally dilated to maintain flow, and as a result transit time is increased.[115] Kuwabara and group have also demonstrated increased oxygen extraction in these tissues in children with moyamoya.[116] The response to an increase in CO_2 is therefore limited, and a decrease in $Pa{CO_2}$ may result in inadequate flow reaching these vessels from surrounding normal tissue.

The surgical treatment of moyamoya consists of one of three forms of revascularization: anastomosis of the superficial temporal artery to the middle cerebral artery; encephalomyosynangiosis (EMS), which is the apposition of a temporal muscle flap to the cortical surface to develop superficial collaterals; and encephaloduroarteriosynangiosis (EDAS), in which the superficial temporal artery with a plug of galea aponeurotica is applied to the dura. The latter method seems to be most effective in children.[113]

Anesthetic Considerations

Considerations are the same for the diagnostic angiogram and the subsequent revascularization. Although autoregulation appears to be maintained, vessels in the affected area are maximally dilated and transit time is prolonged, so that falls in blood pressure may result in ischemia. An anesthetic that is primarily a narcotic-relaxant with a low concentration of a volatile agent is therefore the anesthetic technique of choice. Hypocapnia may result in ischemia, owing to vasoconstriction of normal anastomotic or moyamoya vessels; therefore, normocapnia should be maintained throughout the procedure.

CNS TUMORS

Tumors of the central nervous system are the second most common malignancy of childhood, with an incidence reported to range between 1.3 and 5 percent.[117] The peak incidence of brain tumors in children occurs between 5 and 8 years of age, with only 3 percent occurring before the age of 1 year.[118] In the first year of life, supratentorial tumors are more common than infratentorial lesions, but the overall incidence throughout childhood is approximately equal.[117]

Astrocytoma, choroid plexus papilloma, and teratoma are the most commonly reported neoplasms of the CNS in children under 1 year of age, whereas in older children astrocytoma, medulloblastoma, and ependymoma are most frequently seen. Choroid plexus papilloma and teratoma are very uncommon after the first 12 months of life.[119]

Hydrocephalus is a common finding at the time of presentation, as about half of all brain tumors in children are located near the midline.[120] In infants, the most common signs of tumors are a full fontanelle, rapidly increasing head size, vomiting, abducens palsy, lethargy, and irritability.[117] In the older child, headache and vomiting signal the increase in intracranial pressure and are often the presenting symptoms of tumor, followed in frequency by unsteadiness of gait and impaired consciousness.[56] Although the majority of patients with brain tumor undergo craniotomy, in deep-seated lesions in which open biopsy may risk significant neurological deficit, stereotactic biopsy may be performed. A positive diagnosis can be made in approximately 90 percent of cases using this technique.[121, 122] A neuroleptic anesthetic is frequently used in adults for stereotactic biopsy, but in children general anesthesia is required.

Anesthetic Considerations

For stereotactic biopsy, the procedure is usually started in the radiology department with application of the stereotactic frame and subsequent CT scan. The patient is then transferred to the operating room where the biopsy is performed. It is important to secure the airway from the outset, as once the frame is positioned, access to the airway will be limited severely. The metal components of the circuit must be removed for the scan, and a transport stretcher equipped with anesthetic gases, resuscitation equipment, portable suction, and monitoring devices must be available. The anesthetic management of these patients should be as for any patient with a space-occupying lesion.

SUPRATENTORIAL TUMORS

Children undergoing operation for supratentorial lesions may or may not have raised ICP. Even if intracranial pressure is not elevated, heavy narcotic premedication is best avoided in these children, since the space-occupying lesion may put them at the limits of intracranial compensation. A smooth intravenous induction with thiopentone and a muscle relaxant allows placement of an oral armored tube or RAE tube and the rapid institution of hyperventilation to a Pa_{CO_2} of less than 30 mm Hg. If signs of increased ICP are present, intravenous lidocaine and fentanyl should be added to the induction sequence. If a nondepolarizing relaxant is used, a second small dose of thiopentone just prior to airway instrumentation may be of benefit.

These patients frequently receive dexamethasone preoperatively to reduce edema around the tumor. A repeat dose should be given prior to any manipulation of the brain. In many cases a diuretic will be required to reduce brain bulk. An intra-arterial catheter and a central venous line are useful if considerable blood loss is anticipated, or if the procedure is expected to be prolonged. Maintenance of anesthesia with a nitrous-narcotic-relaxant technique with a low dose of inhalation agent will provide a good surgical field.

The patient usually will be placed in the supine or lateral position with the head elevated 10 to 15 degrees. In positioning the head, care must be taken that venous return is not obstructed.

INFRATENTORIAL TUMORS

Operation for infratentorial neoplasm poses some additional problems to the anesthesiologist. Many of these patients will present with hydrocephalus, as the lesions are frequently midline. In order to improve the patient's fluid and nutritional status and reduce congestion of the operative site, it is sometimes advisable to insert a ventriculoperitoneal shunt prior to the definitive surgery.[123]

For the excision of the tumor, these patients will be placed in either the prone or the sitting position. (The advantages of the prone position have already been discussed.) The use of a nasal tube in prone patients allows secure fixation without the risk of tape being loosened by oral secretions. As with supratentorial tumors, a smooth intravenous induction is the method of choice, and controlled ventilation is commenced immediately. Anesthesia can be maintained with any of the commonly used techniques.

Air embolism and cardiac dysrhythmias are the intraoperative complications encountered most frequently in posterior fossa surgery. The use of the prone position decreases the risk of air embolism, and monitors such as a precordial Doppler and end-tidal carbon dioxide measurement assist in early diagnosis. Arrhythmia is often a result of tumor manipulation and may indicate proximity to brain stem centers.[124] It is therefore essential to communicate with the surgeon regarding any significant changes in vital signs. In some cases brain stem reflexes may be impaired by the surgery, and this should be assessed prior to extubation.

SUPRASELLAR TUMORS

These tumors are considered separately because of the associated endocrine abnormalities. This group of lesions includes craniopharyngioma, optic chiasm glioma, and germ cell tumors and represents 15 percent of brain tumors in children.[125] The most common sign in these patients at the time of presentation is decreasing visual acuity or a visual field defect. Sixty percent of patients with craniopharyngiomas have evidence of optic atrophy at the time of diagnosis, and approximately 65 percent have papilledema.[126] With germ cell tumors, symptoms of diabetes insipidus appear early, whereas this is uncommon in craniopharyngioma. About 30 percent of both groups have stunting of growth or delayed puberty.[125] Thomsett and associates found that 24 percent of patients had decreased levels of ACTH preoperatively, and 72 percent had decreased levels of growth hormone.[127] It is therefore essential to have a complete endocrine assessment preoperatively and to treat the patient with steroids if necessary.

There are two major approaches to surgical resection of suprasellar tumors: the trans-sphenoidal approach and the frontal craniotomy. The former is rarely used in small children. The anesthetic considerations are similar to those for any other supratentorial lesion once the endocrine status has been established and corrected if necessary. Cardiac arrhythmias, particularly bradycardia, are common during dissection around the optic nerves. This bradycardia can be reversed with a small dose of intravenous atropine.

In the postoperative period, these patients require close monitoring of fluid and electrolyte balance in addition to continued steroid treatment. Grant and Lyen found that 46 of 58 children undergoing resection of a craniopharyngioma had postoperative diabetes insipidus, and 23 of 35 had ACTH deficiency.[128] It is important that pitressin therapy be started early, as attempts to replace urinary water losses may lead to hyperglycemic coma.[129]

SPINAL TUMORS

Spinal tumors account for only a small proportion of CNS tumors occurring in childhood. Spinal tumors overall occur in a ratio of about one to every seven brain tumors and the commonest presenting features include extremity weakness, pain, and spinal deformity.[130] Primary intramedullary tumors have an incidence of approximately one in a million, and astrocytoma is the most common intramedullary tumor in children.[131] Extramedullary tumors include neuroblastoma, neurofibroma, meningioma, and metastases.

ANESTHETIC CONSIDERATIONS

The major anesthetic consideration in these patients is positioning for surgery. Proper positioning on a Hall-Relton frame or U-shaped bolster will provide support while not limiting diaphragmatic excursion. In the case of upper thoracic or cervical lesions, it will not be possible to turn the head to the side, so a nasal tube is more appropriate. Care must be taken to avoid pressure on the eyes in the face-down position.

If significant neurological deficit has been present for some time, succinylcholine should be avoided in these patients because of the risk of hyperkalemia.

NEUROBLASTOMA

Neuroblastoma is one of the most common soft tissue malignant tumors of childhood. Arising from postganglionic adrenergic cells of the sympathetic nervous system, neuroblastoma and ganglioneuroblastoma occur with an incidence of 9 to 10 per million children per year.[132] The adrenal glands and the cervical, thoracic, and abdominal sympathetic ganglia are the most frequent primary locations. Metastases are present at the time of initial presentation in two thirds of patients.[133] Prognosis is related to age, site of tumor, and stage of the disease at the time of diagnosis.[134] Survival decreases with increasing age at first diagnosis. Nonadrenal locations of the primary tumor have a better prognosis.[132]

Neuroblastoma sometimes occurs as a "dumbbell," with a primary in the mediastinum or retroperitoneum and extension into the spinal canal. The two components are joined via the intervertebral foramen. Compression of the spinal cord by tumor often results in neurological abnormalities in these patients.[135] Surgery is carried out in two stages. Laminectomy and excision of the spinal portion usually precede resection of the mediastinal component, since manipulation of the extraspinal tumor could result in edema or hemorrhage in the intraspinal component.[135]

Increased excretion of catechol metabolites is detectable in most of these patients.[132, 133] Hypertension generally is not considered to be a problem, but as many as 19 percent of patients with neurogenic tumors may have hypertension at some stage of the disease process.[136] Arrhythmias are very rare.

Coagulation abnormalities are common in children with metastatic neuroblastoma, and disseminated intravascular coagulation has been reported.[137, 138]

Anesthetic Considerations

Potential problems in these patients depend on the size and location of the tumor, the stage of the disease, and the extent of the planned surgical excision. In addition, patients with more advanced stages of neuroblastoma may receive preoperative chemotherapy. The possible side effects of these agents must also be considered (see also page 655).

When radical excision of a large tumor is planned, blood loss can be massive since these tumors may encroach on large blood vessels. Kiely reported blood replacement of up to three times the child's blood volume in long procedures.[139] Appropriate monitors include intraarterial and central venous pressure lines in addition to the usual monitors. Blood-warming devices should also be used. As the possibility for intraoperative hypertension with tumor manipulation exists, antihypertensive agents should be available in the operating room. In patients with advanced disease, preoperative coagulation studies are essential.

NEUROFIBROMATOSIS

Neurofibromatosis, or von Recklinghausen's disease, is a disorder of neural crest derivation with proliferation of nerve fibers and Schwann's cells, affecting skin, bone, soft tissues, and the central nervous system.[140] It occurs with a frequency of about 1 in 3000 live births,[141] and a positive family history following an autosomal-dominant inheritance pattern is obtained in approximately 50 percent of cases.[140] Physical signs of this condition may be present at birth and tend to increase with age. Diagnosis is usually made before puberty. Malignant change does occur in neurofibromatosis, but neurofibrosarcoma is more often found outside the pediatric age group.[142]

Although café au lait spots are the commonest clinical manifestation of this condition, multisystem involvement is typical. The central nervous system is involved in many cases, with clinical manifestations varying from mental retardation or seizure disorder to signs of a space-occupying lesion in the cranium or spinal cord.[143] Optic glioma and hypothalamic glial tumors are the most common intracranial tumors in children with neurofibromatosis.[141]

Scoliosis is the commonest skeletal abnormality and may be either the idiopathic type or a much more angulated dysplastic curve.[140] Giant plexiform neurofibromas may occur in the head and neck and result in ptosis, hemifacial gigantism, and visual problems if the lesion is in or around the orbit.[144] Attempts to excise these tumors may involve major craniofacial reconstructions.

The incidence of vascular anomalies has been reported to be as high as 9 percent.[143] Although hypertension may be more common with advancing age as the neurofibromatous change produces extensive small vessel disease, renal artery stenosis does occur in children with neurofibromatosis.[145] In addition, hypertension may be present as a result of another tumor of neural crest origin. Pheochromocytoma occurs with increased frequency in patients with neurofibromatosis.[146]

Anesthetic Considerations

In patients with neurofibromatosis and intracranial space-occupying lesions, the usual precautions should be taken. When a neurofibroma involves the head and neck, careful assessment of the airway with respect to potential intubation difficulty is mandatory. There is also a risk of cervical instability. Tumor infiltration or abnormalities of spinal ligaments will occasionally result in atlantoaxial dislocation.[147] Major vessel anomaly and pheochromocytoma should be ruled out preoperatively in the patient with neurofibromatosis who is hypertensive at the time of presentation. Increased sensitivity to pancuronium has also been reported.[148]

TEMPORAL LOBE EPILEPSY

The incidence of epilepsy in the general population is about six per thousand, and approximately one third of patients suffer from seizures of temporal lobe origin.[149] Temporal lobe epilepsy may present as psychomotor seizures or complex partial seizures. The latter form usually begins with an aura and is most often followed by a fixation of movements or by automatic, semipurposeful movements such as mastication, swallowing, or repetitive gestures. This form of epilepsy is refractory to medical therapy in 30 to 60 percent of cases.[150] In Meyer and associates' series, the age of onset of complex partial seizures in children was 7.5 years.[149] The uncontrolled seizures combined with high doses of anticonvulsants can have a significant effect on the psychosocial development of the child. When medical management fails, surgical resection of an area of cortex or a portion of the temporal lobe may be the treatment of choice. In approximately one third of cases considered for operation, investigation may reveal a mass lesion such as a tumor or vascular malformation.[151]

When there is no identifiable mass lesion, laterality of seizure activity must be established to plan surgical therapy. Electroencephalography (EEG) is the mainstay of diagnosis, as clinical signs are often unreliable. Cable telemetry, which provides a computer record of the EEG immediately before and during seizure activity, has been shown to be of value in determining the laterality of the lesion.[152] Depth EEG electrodes, put in place with the patient under anesthesia, have also been used to demonstrate a predominant focus when the surface EEG is inconclusive.[153]

When the dominant hemisphere is involved, the laterality of language function and independent memory capability of the contralateral temporal lobe are assessed using the Wada test. The Wada test consists of the intracarotid injection of amobarbital to inactivate the anterior two thirds of one hemisphere, followed by the assessment of language and independent memory function in the opposite hemisphere.[154, 155] While this may not be possible in the very young child, the child 8 or more years of age should be able to cooperate for this investigation. Since arterial catheterization is required, sedation and supervision by an anesthesiologist are usually necessary. Once the Wada test has been performed, general anesthesia is induced for completion of the arteriogram.

Resection of the seizure focus appears to be an effective treatment, as half to two thirds of patients will be seizure-free and only 10 to 12 percent will show no improvement postoperatively.[149, 150]

ANESTHETIC CONSIDERATIONS

It is important that sedation for the Wada test be minimal, as the amobarbital itself will have a sedating effect and may limit cooperation for injection of the second side. Small doses of fentanyl and droperidol or nitrous oxide and oxygen by mask, combined with local anesthesia, are usually sufficient for insertion of the femoral arterial catheter by the radiologist. The nitrous oxide is discontinued prior to arterial injection. It is important that the amobarbital solution be warmed prior to injection so that a shivering response is not induced following passage through the hypothalamus. Once language, memory, and EEG have been assessed, the patient can be given a general anesthetic for arteriography.

To minimize the risk of neurological damage during resection, craniotomy for temporal lobectomy is frequently performed under a neuroleptic technique when the patient is old enough to cooperate. It is important to develop rapport with the child preoperatively so that verbal responses will be obtained when required during cortical mapping and after resection. Diazepam and barbiturates should be avoided as premedicants, because these drugs may suppress epileptogenic foci, and resection will be based on cortical EEG recording intraoperatively.

These patients will require all the usual monitors. In addition, an intra-arterial catheter will eliminate the need for disturbing the patient with frequent inflations of a blood pressure cuff, and a urinary catheter will help the patient remain comfortable during the procedure.

Sedation is achieved by giving incremental doses of fentanyl and droperidol intravenously so that the patient is comfortable yet responsive to questions and maintains a $Pa{CO_2}$ of less than 50 mm Hg. End-tidal CO_2 can be measured by taping the sampling catheter below an external naris. A mixture of 0.5 percent lidocaine and 0.375 percent bupivicaine with epinephrine 1:200,000 is used for local infiltration of the pin sites of the head rest and the incision line. An oxygen mask is placed over the face prior to draping, and further sedation is added as required.

In patients too young to cooperate or for those in whom the speech area is not at risk, a general anesthetic technique can be employed. A continuous infusion technique of 0.1 percent methohexital in combination with nondepolarizing relaxant, morphine, and droperidol has been used effectively in epilepsy surgery.[156] If nitrous oxide is used, it should be discontinued prior to cortical recording because of its potential effects on the EEG.[157] Somatosensory evoked potentials may also be of use in predicting potential neurological deficits when general anesthesia is used.[156]

Anticonvulsants should be continued intravenously in the postoperative period as seizures are common in the first 7 to 10 days after surgery and are not necessarily predictive of final outcome. An elevated temperature is common in these patients postoperatively, presumably owing to the irritant effect of breakdown products of blood in the CNS.

CEREBRAL INFECTION

BRAIN ABSCESS

The overall incidence of cerebral abscess in childhood has decreased in recent years with the advent of antibiotics that achieve significant concentrations in the CSF. In spite of this, mortality remains at 6 to 30 percent.[158] The presenting signs and symptoms include fever, vomiting, headache, and focal neurological deficits. Brain abscess most commonly occurs in infants and children in association with meningitis, otitis, cyanotic congenital heart disease, sinusitis, shunt infection, and trauma.[159] In neonates, brain abscess occurs primarily as a result of meningitis or septicemia, and seizures and signs of sepsis are the most common presenting signs.[160]

A wide variety of both gram-positive and gram-negative organisms may be isolated from the abscess, depending on the site of the original infection. In neonates, *Citrobacter* and *Proteus* species are common.[159, 160] In the immunocompromised child, yeast or fungal infections may occur.[158, 159]

Tetralogy of Fallot is the congenital heart lesion in which cerebral abscess is seen most frequently.[161] The incidence appears to be decreasing, however, either as a result of earlier total correction of cyanotic lesions or better prophylactic antiobiotic coverage during periods of high risk.[158] Drainage of the lesion in conjunction with appropriate antibiotic therapy is the treatment of choice. Depending on the location of the abscess and the condition of the patient, the abscess can be drained either by craniotomy and excision or aspiration, with the assistance of CT scan and a stereotactic frame. In Johnson and associates' series of intracranial abscesses associated with sinusitis, no patient was successfully treated with antibiotics alone.[162]

SUBDURAL EMPYEMA

Subdural empyema accounts for 13 to 20 percent of intracranial bacterial infections and represents 5 percent of space-occupying lesions involving the subdural space.[163] Both subdural and epidural abscesses are frequently due to infection of contiguous structures: sinusitis, otitis, and mastoiditis.[162–164] Fever and headache are the most common symptoms. Many cases can be treated with burr hole drainage; others, particularly if they are multiloculated, will require formal craniotomy to evacuate the abscess cavity adequately.

ANESTHETIC CONSIDERATIONS

In both brain abscess and subdural or epidural empyema, one is faced with a septic patient with a space-occupying lesion. Induction and anesthetic maintenance are therefore as for any patient with raised ICP. In addition, febrile patients may require higher minute ventilation to maintain an acceptable Pa_{CO_2} because of the increased metabolic rate. Preoperative atropine should be avoided as it will affect sweating and therefore temperature regulation. An intravenous dose can be given at induction.

There may also be anesthetic considerations relating to the underlying condition: the immunosuppressed patient or the patient with cyanotic congenital heart disease. Patients with cyanotic heart disease are at risk of increased morbidity from even a small air embolism due to the right-to-left shunt. Nitrous oxide is therefore best avoided in these children. Dehydration with mannitol or furosemide is also inadvisable if the hematocrit is high.

HEAD INJURY

Head injury is common in infants and children and is a major cause of morbidity and mortality. Although young children appear to have a greater capacity than adults to recover from severe head injuries even after a protracted period of coma, mortality is greater in patients under the age of 5 years than in the 5- to 19-year age group.[165] Head injury encompasses a wide group of pediatric patients. The head-injured child may present with a simple depressed skull fracture and no other injuries or may arrive in the emergency department unconscious with multiple associated injuries. Primary brain injury has occurred at the time of the initial event. The aim of the anesthetic management of the child with severe cerebral trauma is to prevent secondary physiological brain injury caused by hypoxemia, hypercapnia, intracranial hypertension, or systemic hypotension. Oxygen therapy should be started immediately, as more than 30 percent of patients with head injury have a PaO_2 of less than 60 mm Hg, which is associated with poor outcome.[166] Control of the airway is therefore an essential step in limiting secondary head injury and frequently must be carried out prior to radiographic examination of the cervical spine. The presence of a coexisting cervical spine injury must be assumed, and precautions taken, during intubation. In fact, a negative radiograph will *not* guarantee an intact spinal cord in the unconscious child, since the anatomy of the developing spine permits transient subluxation without bone injury.[167] In the hemodynamically stable pediatric patient, a rapid-sequence induction including thiopentone and lidocaine will provide some measure of cerebral protection during laryngoscopy and intubation.

The head and neck should be stabilized in the neutral position during intubation by the application of axial traction. Although it has been suggested that this may result in excessive distraction or subluxation,[168] there is significantly less cervical spine movement during intubation when in-line traction is applied.[169]

In performing the initial resuscitation, it is essential to make some estimate of the severity of the head injury. The use of the Glasgow Coma Scale (GCS) (Table 4–2), which evaluates a series of responses, permits meaningful sequential assessment of patients with severe head injuries.[170]

Following stabilization in the emergency room, investigation of the injuries can proceed.

Table 4–2. GLASGOW COMA SCALE

	Observation	Score
Eye opening	spontaneous	4
	to speech	3
	to pain	2
	nil	1
Best motor response	obeys	6
	localizes	5
	withdraws	4
	abnormal flexion	3
	extends	2
	nil	1
Verbal response	oriented	5
	confused conversation	4
	inappropriate words	3
	incomprehensible sounds	2
	nil	1

Total score: 3–15 points.

From Jennet B, Teasdale G: Aspects of coma after severe head injury. Lancet *1*:878, 1977.

The majority of children will not require surgical treatment of the head injury. Comparisons of reported series of severe head injuries in children show that only 22 to 58 percent of patients with severe cerebral injuries will have mass lesions.[171, 172] Diffuse cerebral swelling is the most common initial finding with computed tomography (CT) in children, occurring in 20 to 34 percent;[172, 173] it is most frequently associated with a Glasgow score of less than 8.[173] This severe cerebral swelling is associated with a marked increase in cerebral blood volume.[173] Poor outcome has been associated with both high and reduced cerebral blood flow postinjury and may be a result of uncoupling of flow and metabolism.[174] Jaggi and colleagues have shown that a decrease in cerebral metabolic rate is more reliably predictive of unfavorable outcome than is CBF.[175]

Continuous recording of ICP in these comatose patients in the intensive care unit permits early identification of those with significant elevations in pressure and allows early intervention. Once the airway is controlled, therapy to reduce ICP can be instituted. Hyperventilation remains one of the simplest and most effective methods of lowering ICP. High-dose steroids have been found to have no effect on the outcome in severely injured patients who are comatose at the time of admission.[176] Although thiopentone is useful in acutely lowering ICP, the use of high-dose barbiturates in severely head-injured patients remains controversial. Pittman and group found that in the presence of pentobarbital, children with severe head injuries survived prolonged periods of low cerebral perfusion pressure,[177] but a controlled trial by Ward and co-workers demonstrated no benefit from barbiturate coma in patients over 12 years of age and a significant incidence of side effects from this treatment.[178]

The head-injured child with a mass lesion or with associated injuries requiring surgical therapy will present in the operating room following resuscitation. Extradural hematoma accounts for just over 3 percent of head trauma in children and is often an isolated injury, although there may be an associated intradural component.[179] Subdural hematoma is of particular interest to the anesthesiologist. Because of raised ICP, these patients may be normotensive at the time of surgery. In the infant or small child, it is possible for a large subdural hematoma to contain up to 27 percent of the normal circulating blood volume.[180] There is therefore a significant risk of hypotension when the ICP is suddenly lowered by the aspiration of the clot.

Uchida and coworkers found that 41 percent of all children became hypotensive with drainage of the hematoma, and 88 percent had a fall in blood pressure if the subdural collection contained more than 8 percent of the estimated blood volume.[180] Careful monitoring of volume is crucial, particularly if there are associated injuries and ongoing occult losses.

In spite of aggressive therapy of intracranial pressure and other injuries, the mortality after severe head injury remains close to 30 percent.[172, 181] Children with isolated head trauma appear to do better than those with multiple injuries,[182] and head injuries occurring in the first year of life have a poorer outcome.[183]

CERVICAL SPINE INJURY

Injury to the spinal column in children is relatively uncommon and accounts for only 0.65 to 9.5 percent of all spinal cord injuries.[184] However, a disproportionate number of these injuries involve the upper cervical spine. Hadley and colleagues found that in the 0- to 9-year age group, 72 percent of spinal injuries involved the cervical spine, and half of these occurred between the occiput and C-2.[185] In children, the cause of cervical spine trauma is most commonly a fall or a motor vehicle accident, and there is a significant incidence of spinal cord injury without radiological evidence.[167] In two large series of pediatric spinal trauma cases, almost half of the children were neurologically intact at the time of admission, whereas 17 to 19 percent had complete spinal cord lesions.[184, 185]

The anatomical differences that may account for the pattern of injury seen in children are the relatively large head and underdeveloped paraspinous musculature, the increased mobility due to laxity of ligaments, the orientation of the facets, and the shape of the incompletely ossified vertebrae.[185]

In addition, several subgroups of pediatric patients are at increased risk of cervical spine injury. The Klippel-Feil syndrome, which is characterized by congenital fusion of vertebrae, is also associated with spinal stenosis, scoliosis, and anomalies of the occipitoatlantal junction, which predispose these children to neurologic injury, although they frequently do not present until the second or third decade.[186] Subluxation of C1 on C2 has been reported in Hurler's syndrome as a result of failure of development of the dens.[187] Patients with Down's syndrome are also reported to have an increased incidence of atlantoaxial instability, but the actual risk of spinal cord injury due to this ligamentous laxity is unknown.[188] Deformities of the vertebral column are also common in neurofibromatosis, and atlantoaxial dislocation has been shown to occur in these patients.[147] Cervical instability may also be found in patients with athetoid cerebral palsy. This occurs mainly at the C3-4 and C4-5 levels.[189]

The majority of children with cervical spine injuries can be treated nonoperatively in a halo-vest or other form of external immobilization. Indications for early surgery include spinal cord compression in the face of an incomplete neurological injury, nonreducible or very unstable fractures, and significant subluxation without fracture.[185] Posterior fusion is the most common form of treatment in those requiring surgical stabilization. However, the transoral approach to the upper cervical spine may be necessary for decompression in some cases of subluxation.

Anesthetic Considerations

Controlling the airway is the most important anesthetic consideration. The objective is to intubate the patient without jeopardizing the intact spinal cord or causing further harm to an already damaged cord. When intubation is urgent in the acutely injured patient, a rapid sequence induction and intubation with manual in-line traction will minimize the effects of laryngoscopy and achieve airway control rapidly to prevent secondary hypoxemic damage. Fluid resuscitation may also be necessary because of spinal shock or other associated injuries.

In the elective situation, awake fiberoptic intubation is the ideal method and is possible in the older child with topical anesthesia and sedation. Patients can then be positioned for operation and reassessed neurologically prior to induction of general anesthesia. In young children, when cooperation cannot be expected, intubation with manual in-line traction following an inhalation induction can be performed. If the child is already stabilized in a halo-vest, an angled laryngoscope handle is helpful.

In the presence of a chronic spinal cord injury, succinylcholine should be avoided and consideration given to the autonomic instability that is common in lesions above T6.[190]

The transoral approach to the cervical spine allows access to the arch of C1, the odontoid process, and the bodies of C2 and C3 as well as the granulation tissue that forms anteriorly as a result of the instability.[191] When the transoral approach is used, tracheostomy may be performed prior to surgery.[192] However, it is possible to intubate orally with a RAE tube, which will sit under the mouth gag and allow adequate surgical access. This does add the problem of the shared airway, as the mouth gag may compress the endotracheal tube. It is important to release the gag at regular intervals to prevent edema of the tongue. These procedures are usually performed by a combined surgical team of otolaryngologists and neurosurgeons. In some cases, division of the soft palate will be required to gain access to superior structures. This has implications for postoperative management, because swelling of intraoral structures may make postoperative airway support necessary. Anterior fusion may be performed at the same operation, but more commonly posterior fusion is carried out, either at the time or in a subsequent procedure.

CEREBRAL PALSY

Cerebral palsy is a term used to describe a variety of disabilities, usually motor dysfunction or a movement disorder. These problems are a result of developmental problems or perinatal injury of the central nervous system. The incidence is approximately 7 per 1000 live births.[193] Hemiplegia, spastic diplegia, and quadriplegia are the most common manifestations. Swallowing disorders, manifested by poor sucking, nasopharyngeal regurgitation, coughing, and gagging during feeding frequently are seen in patients with severe cerebral palsy.[194] The most common etiological factor is prematurity.[195]

Patients with cerebral palsy may require multiple surgical procedures. Orthopedic operations to improve function in extremities are common, and some patients will require correction of progressive spinal deformity. In children with cerebral palsy and scoliosis, the degree of pulmonary compromise may be difficult to assess, since children may be unable to cooperate for pulmonary function testing. In addition, severe contractures may make both venous access and positioning for surgery difficult.

Spasticity is sometimes disabling in these children and may require surgical as well as medical treatment. Motor point injection with dilute phenol solutions is sometimes used for temporary relief of symptoms. The use of phenol is associated with cardiac dysrhythmias, and this may be a factor during halothane anesthesia.[196] Long-term improvement in spasticity can be obtained by selective posterior rhizotomy. This technique involves stimulation of the dorsal roots intraoperatively, with observation of muscle response. Those rootlets in which stimulation is followed by widespread dissemination of the response are severed, leaving intact those with less spread. Ketamine has proved to be an effective anesthetic for this procedure, providing analgesia while maintaining muscle tone.[197] Otherwise, a technique including nitrous oxide and isoflurane (0.5 to 1 percent) with small doses of fentanyl (2 μg/kg) and controlled ventilation is very satisfactory. Neuromuscular blocking drugs should be avoided. The patients most likely to benefit from this procedure are those with pure spasticity without contracture and mainly lower limb involvement.[198]

In patients with swallowing difficulties, drooling may be a significant disability. Surgical therapy for this problem consists of salivary gland excision, duct relocation or ligation, or neurectomy of parasympathetic secretomotor fibers.[199] Duct relocation is one of the most effective of these procedures, as it maintains salivary gland function while improving drooling.[200] A nasotracheal tube is required for this procedure, and throat packing is advisable in the early stages of the dissection to minimize the risk of aspiration of blood and secretions. When duct relocation is performed, close postoperative observation is essential because of the possible airway compromise by excessive swelling in the floor of the mouth. In addition, swallowing may prove difficult in the early postoperative period, and patients will require intravenous hydration and assistance with secretions.

REYE'S SYNDROME

Reye's syndrome, first described in 1963, is a disease of unknown etiology that occurs in children, usually following a viral illness.[201] The syndrome is characterized by encephalopathy and fatty degeneration of the viscera, particularly the liver. Although described following an upper respiratory infection, it has also been associated with other viral infections, particularly varicella and influenza A and B infections.[202] An association between Reye's syndrome and the use of salicylates to treat the initial viral infection was postulated. Indeed, since the use of salicylates in children has declined in North America, the incidence of Reye's syndrome has fallen dramatically.[203]

In the recovery phase of a viral illness, the child develops vomiting and subsequent alteration of consciousness. The clinical criteria for diagnosis include the typical history of an antecedent viral infection, neurological disturbance, elevation of liver enzymes, increased ammonia levels, and the exclusion of other disease processes and specific toxins.[201] Early diagnosis and therapy are considered essential if the disease is to be successfully treated. Diagnosis can also be made by liver biopsy if the history is atypical. Liver biopsy shows a distinctive pattern, with 20 to 30 percent triglyceride infiltration and evidence of mitochondrial injury.[204]

As a means of assessing the severity of the disease and to follow its progression, Lovejoy has described staging in Reye's syndrome (Table 4–3). Mortality rates of 22 to 54 percent are reported, and the mortality is higher in children under the age of 6 years[202] and in those whose therapy is started at later stages of the disease.[205–208]

The management of Reye's syndrome is determined by the stage of the disease. Patients in stage 1 require intravenous fluids, electrolytes, glucose, and close metabolic and neurological monitoring. Hypoglycemia must be prevented by glucose infusions and regular, frequent (2 to 4 hourly) blood glucose determinations. Children treated thus have an excellent prognosis.[209] Children with stage 2 or more advanced disease require treatment in an intensive care unit. Death in Reye's syndrome is usually related to intracranial hypertension, and treatment of the advanced disease is directed toward control of the intracranial pressure. The brain lesion appears to be a result of acute cytotoxic injury with astrocyte swelling, myelin bleb formation, and mitochondrial abnormality.[204]

In order to control ICP, intubation and ventilation are recommended, though there is some controversy as to the stage at which this should be instituted. There may be some advantage to commencing this early in stage 2 when patients are combative and hyperventilating.[208] Continuous monitoring of ICP is useful in determining the need for further therapeutic intervention.[210] In addition to fluid restriction, mannitol, and dexamethasone to reduce cerebral edema, pentobarbital and hypothermia have been used to control ICP. The latter therapy has been associated with increased pulmonary complications. Exchange transfusion and dialysis have been used in an attempt to moderate the metabolic disturbance, particularly the high blood ammonia level. Liver transplantation has been suggested for advanced cases.

The treatment of the advanced cases is very complex, and it is uncertain which modalities will have a clear benefit. Early recognition of the condition remains the most important factor in the treatment of Reye's syndrome.

Table 4–3. STAGING IN REYE'S SYNDROME

Stage I	Vomiting, lethargy, extensor plantar response, liver dysfunction
Stage II	Disorientation, combativeness, semicoma, hyperventilation, progressive liver dysfunction
Stage III	Coma, hyperventilation, decortication, continued liver dysfunction
Stage IV	Deepening coma, decerebration, continued liver function abnormalities
Stage V	Coma, medullary dysfunction, respiratory arrest, possible improvement in liver function abnormalities

From Lovejoy FJ, Bresnan MJ, Lombroso CT, et al: Anticerebral oedema therapy in Reye's syndrome. Arch Dis Child *50*:933, 1975.

REFERENCES

1. Hill A, Volpe JJ: Measurement of intracranial pressure using the Ladd intracranial pressure monitor. J Pediatr *98*:974, 1981.
2. Shapiro HM: Intracranial hypertension: Therapeutic and anesthetic considerations. Anesthesiology *43*:445, 1975.
3. Lofgren J, Zwetnow NN: Cranial and spinal components of the cerebrospinal pressure-volume curve. Acta Neurol Scand *49*:575, 1973.
4. Kennedy C, Sokoloff L: An adaptation of the nitrous oxide method to the study of the cerebral circulation in children: Normal values for cerebral blood flow and cerebral metabolic rate in childhood. J Clin Invest *36*:1130, 1957.
5. Chadduck WM, Seibert JJ: Intracranial duplex Doppler: Practical uses in pediatric neurology and neurosurgery. J Child Neurol *4*:S77, 1989.
6. Lassen NA, Christensen MS: Physiology of cerebral blood flow. Br J Anaesth *48*:719, 1976.
7. Lou HC, Lassen NA, Friis-Hansen B: Impaired autoregulation of cerebral blood flow in the distressed newborn infant. J Pediatr *94*:118, 1979.
8. Lassen NA: Control of cerebral circulation in health and disease. Circ Res *34*:749, 1974.
9. Grubb RL Jr, Raichle ME, Eichling JO, et al: The effects of changes in Pa_{CO_2} on cerebral blood volume, blood flow, and vascular mean transit time. Stroke *5*:630, 1974.
10. Harbaugh RD, James HE, Marshall LF, et al: Acute therapeutic modalities for experimental vasogenic cerebral edema. Neurosurgery *5*:656, 1979.
11. Cottrell JE, Robustelli AS, Post K, et al: Furosemide- and mannitol-induced changes in intracranial pressure and serum osmolality and electrolytes. Anesthesiology *47*:28, 1977.
12. Samson D, Beyer CW Jr: Furosemide in the intraoperative reduction of intracranial pressure in the patient with subarachnoid hemorrhage. Neurosurgery *10*:167, 1982.
13. Buhrley LE, Reed DJ: The effect of furosemide on sodium-22 uptake into cerebrospinal fluid and brain. Exp Brain Res *14*:503, 1972.

14. Pollay M, Fullenwider C, Roberts A, et al: Effect of mannitol and furosemide on blood-brain osmotic gradient and intracranial pressure. J Neurosurg *59*:845, 1983.
15. Eisenberg HM, Barlow CF, Lorenzo AV: Effect of dexamethasone on altered brain vascular permeability. Arch Neurol *23*:18, 1970.
16. Weiss MH, Nulsen FE: The effect of glucocorticoids on CSF flow in dogs. J Neurosurg *32*:452, 1970.
17. Shapiro HM, Galindo A, Wyte SR, et al: Rapid intraoperative reduction of intracranial pressure with thiopentone. Br J Anaesth *45*:1057, 1973.
18. Dawson B, Michenfelder JD, Theye RA: Effects of ketamine on canine cerebral blood flow and metabolism: Modification by prior administration of thiopental. Anesth Analg *50*:443, 1971.
19. Crumrine RS, Nulson FE, Weiss MH: Alterations in ventricular fluid pressure during ketamine anesthesia in hydrocephalic children. Anesthesiology *42*:758, 1975.
20. Vandesteene A, Trempont V, Engelman E, et al: Effect of propofol on cerebral blood flow and metabolism in man. Anaesthesia *43*(Suppl):42, 1988.
21. Van Hemelrijck J, Fitch W, Mattheussen M, et al: Effect of propofol on cerebral circulation and autoregulation in the baboon. Anesth Analg *71*:49, 1990.
22. Pinaud M, Lelausque J-N, Chettanneau A, et al: Effects of propofol on cerebral hemodynamics and metabolism in patients with brain trauma. Anesthesiology *73*:404, 1990.
23. Bedford RF, Winn HR, Tyson G, et al: Lidocaine prevents increased ICP after endotracheal intubation. *In* Shulman K, et al (eds): Intracranial Pressure. 4th edition. New York, Springer-Verlag, 1980.
24. Abou-madi MN, Keszler H, Yacoub JM: Cardiovascular reactions to laryngoscopy and tracheal intubation following small and large intravenous doses of lidocaine. Can Anaesth Soc J *24*:12, 1977.
25. Bedford RF, Persing JA, Peberskin L, et al: Lidocaine or thiopental for rapid control of intracranial hypertension. Anesth Analg *59*:435, 1980.
26. Jobes DR, Kennell E, Bitner R, et al: Effects of morphine-nitrous oxide anesthesia on cerebral autoregulation. Anesthesiology *42*:30, 1975.
27. Shupak RC, Harp JR, Stevenson-Smith W, et al: High-dose fentanyl for neuroanesthesia. Anesthesiology *58*:579, 1983.
28. Fitch W, Barker J, Jennett WB, et al: The influence of neuroleptanalgesic drugs on cerebrospinal fluid pressure. Br J Anaesth *41*:800, 1969.
29. Jung R, Shah N, Reinsel R, et al: Cerebrospinal fluid pressure in patients with brain tumors: Impact of fentanyl versus alfentanil during nitrous oxide–oxygen anesthesia. Anesth Analg *71*:419, 1990.
30. Mayer N, Weinstabl C, Podreka I, Spiss CK: Sufentanil does not increase cerebral blood flow in healthy human volunteers. Anesthesiology *73*:241, 1990.
31. Milde LN, Milde JH, Gallagher WJ: Effects of sufentanil on cerebral circulation and metabolism in dogs. Anesth Analg *70*:138, 1990.
32. Cotev S, Shalit MN: Effects of diazepam on cerebral blood flow and oxygen uptake after head injury. Anesthesiology *43*:117, 1975.
33. Hoffman WE, Miletich DJ, Albrecht RA: The effects of midazolam on cerebral blood flow and oxygen consumption and its interaction with nitrous oxide. Anesth Analg *65*:729, 1986.
34. Lanier WL, Milde JH, Michenfelder JD: The cerebral effects of pancuronium and atracurium in halothane-anesthetized dogs. Anesthesiology *63*:589, 1985.
35. Ducey JP, Deppe SA, Foley KT: A comparison of the effects of suxamethonium, atracurium and vecuronium on intracranial haemodynamics in swine. Anaesth Intens Care *17*:448, 1989.
36. Theye RA, Michenfelder JD: The effect of nitrous oxide on canine cerebral metabolism. Anesthesiology *29*:1119, 1968.
37. Baughman VL, Hoffman WE, Miletich DJ, Albrecht RF: Cerebrovascular and cerebral metabolic effects of N_2O in unrestrained rats. Anesthesiology *73*:269, 1990.
38. Clarke DL, Rosner BS: Neurophysiologic effects of general anesthetics. Anesthesiology *38*:564, 1973.
39. Artru AA, Nugent M, Michenfelder JD: Enflurane causes a prolonged and reversible increase in the rate of CSF production in the dog. Anesthesiology *57*:255, 1982.
40. Artru AA: Effects of halothane and fentanyl on the rate of CSF production in dogs. Anesth Analg *62*:581, 1983.
41. Miletich DJ, Ivankovich AD, Albrecht RF, et al: Absence of autoregulation of cerebral blood flow during halothane and enflurane anesthesia. Anesth Analg *55*:100, 1976.
42. Adams RW, Gronert GA, Sundt TM, et al: Halothane, hypocapnia, and cerebrospinal fluid pressure in neurosurgery. Anesthesiology *37*:510, 1972.
43. Albrecht RF, Miletich DJ, Madala LR: Normalization of cerebral blood flow during prolonged halothane anesthesia. Anesthesiology *58*:26, 1983.
44. Eger EI II: Isoflurane: A review. Anesthesiology *55*:559, 1981.
45. Adams RW, Cucchiara RF, Gronert GA, et al: Isoflurane and cerebrospinal fluid pressure in neurosurgical patients. Anesthesiology *54*:97, 1981.
46. McPherson RW, Traystman RJ: Effects of isoflurane on cerebral autoregulation in dogs. Anesthesiology *69*:493, 1988.
47. Newberg LA, Michenfelder JD: Cerebral protection by isoflurane during hypoxemia or ischemia. Anesthesiology *59*:29, 1983.
48. Scheller MS, Tateishi A, Drummond JC, Zornow MH: The effects of sevoflurane on cerebral blood flow; Cerebral metabolic rate for oxygen, intracranial pressure, and the electroencephalogram are similar to those of isoflurane in the rabbit. Anesthesiology *68*:548, 1988.
49. Lutz LJ, Milde JH, Milde LN: The cerebral, functional, metabolic and hemodynamic effects of desflurane in dogs. Anesthesiology *73*:125, 1990.
50. Ernst PS, Albin MS, Bunegin L: Intracranial and spinal cord hemodynamics in the sitting position in dogs in the presence and absence of increased intracranial pressure. Anesth Analg *70*:147, 1990.
51. Cucchiara RF, Bowers B: Air embolism in children undergoing suboccipital craniotomy. Anesthesiology *57*:338, 1982.
52. Matjasko J, Petrozza P, Mackenzie CF: Sensitivity of end-tidal nitrogen in venous air embolism detection in dogs. Anesthesiology *63*:418, 1985.
53. Durward QJ, Amacher AL, Del Maestro RF, et al: Cerebral and cardiovascular responses to changes in head position in patients with intracranial hypertension. J Neurosurg *59*:938, 1983.
54. Moss ML: Functional anatomy of cranial synostosis. Child's Brain *1*:22, 1975.
55. Hockley AD, Wake MJ, Goldin H: Surgical management of craniosynostosis. Br J Neurosurg *2*:307, 1988.
56. Till K: Paediatric Neurosurgery. Oxford, Blackwell Scientific, 1975.
57. Harwood-Nash DC, Fitz DR: Neuroradiology in In-

fants and Children. Volume 1. St. Louis, CV Mosby, 1976.
58. Marchac D, Renier D: Treatment of craniosynostosis in infancy. Clin Plast Surg *14*:61, 1987.
59. Cohen MM Jr: An etiologic and nosologic overview of craniosynostosis syndromes. Birth Defects *11*:137, 1975.
60. Golabi M, Edwards MSB, Ousterhout DK: Craniosynostosis and hydrocephalus. Neurosurgery *21*:63, 1987.
61. Collman H, Sorensen N, Kraub J, Muhling J: Hydrocephalus in craniosynostosis. Child's Nerv Syst *4*:279, 1988.
62. Harris MM, Strafford MA, Rowe RW, et al: Venous air embolism and cardiac arrest during craniectomy in a supine infant. Anesthesiology *65*:547, 1986.
63. Rosenørn J, Diemer NH: Reduction of regional cerebral blood flow during brain retraction pressure in the rat. J Neurosurg *56*:826, 1982.
64. Sever LE: An epidemiologic study of neural tube defects in Los Angeles County. II. Etiologic factors in an area with low prevalence at birth. Teratology *25*:323, 1982.
65. Karch SB, Urich H: Occipital encephalocele: A morphologic study. J Neurol Sci *15*:89, 1972.
66. Modesti LM, Glasauer FE, Terplan KL: Sphenoethmoidal encephalocele. Child's Brain *3*:140, 1977.
67. Chapman PH, Swearingen B, Caviness VS: Subtorcular occipital encephaloceles. J Neurosurg *71*:375, 1989.
68. Hendrick EB: Neurosurgery of congenital malformations. *In* Thompson RA, Green JR (eds): Pediatric Neurology and Neurosurgery. New York, Spectrum Publications, 1978.
69. Cross KW, Hey EN, Kennaird DL, et al: Lack of temperature control in infants with abnormalities of the central nervous system. Arch Dis Child *46*:437, 1971.
70. Shokunbi T, Adeloye A, Olumide A: Occipital encephaloceles in 57 Nigerian children: A retrospective analysis. Child's Nerv Syst *6*:99, 1990.
71. Bahnson DH: Myelomeningocele and its problems. Pediatr Ann *11*:528, 1982.
72. O'Brien MS, McLanahan CS: Review of the neurosurgical management of myelomeningocele at a regional pediatric medical center. *In* Concepts in Pediatric Neurosurgery I:202, 1981.
73. Hogge WA, Dungan JS, Brooks MP, et al: Diagnosis and management of prenatally detected myelomeningocele: A preliminary report. Am J Obstet Gynecol *163*:1061, 1990.
74. Stein SC, Schut L: Hydrocephalus in myelomeningocele. Child's Brain *5*:413, 1979.
75. Brown SF: Congenital malformations associated with myelomeningocele. J Iowa Med Soc *LXV*:101, 1975.
76. Samuelsson L, Eklof O: Scoliosis in myelomeningocele. Acta Orthop Scand *59*:122, 1988.
77. McLorie GA, Perez-Marero R, Csima A, Churchill BM: Determinants of hydronephrosis and renal injury in patients with myelomeningocele. J Urol *140*:1289, 1988.
78. Teichgraeber JF, Riley WB, Parks DH: Primary skin closure in large myelomeningoceles. Pediatr Neurosci *15*:18, 1989.
79. Davidson Ward SL, Jacobs RA, Gates EP, et al: Abnormal ventilatory patterns during sleep in infants with myelomeningocele. J Pediatr *109*:631, 1986.
80. Swaminathan S, Paton JY, et al: Abnormal control of ventilation in adolescents with myelodysplasia. J Pediatr *115*:898, 1989.
81. Wells TR, Jacobs RA, et al: Incidence of short trachea in patients with myelomeningocele. Pediatr Neurol *6*:109, 1990.
82. Bering EA Jr, Sato O: Hydrocephalus: Changes in formation and absorption of cerebrospinal fluid within the cerebral ventricles. J Neurosurg *20*:1050, 1963.
83. Volpe JJ: Current concepts in neonatal medicine: Neonatal intraventricular hemorrhage. N Engl J Med *304*:886, 1981.
84. Kirkpatrick M, Engelman H, Minns RA: Symptoms and signs of progressive hydrocephalus. Arch Dis Child *64*:124, 1989.
85. Creighton RE: Paediatric neuroanaesthesia. *In* Steward DJ (ed): Some Aspects of Paediatric Anaesthesia. Amsterdam, Elsevier/North Holland, 1982.
86. Nugent GR, Lucas R, Judy M, et al: Thrombo-embolic complications of ventriculo-atrial shunts. Angiocardiographic and pathologic correlations. J Neurosurg *24*:34, 1966.
87. Hammon WM: Evaluation and use of the ventriculoperitoneal shunt in hydrocephalus. J Neurosurg *34*:792, 1971.
88. McCullough DC, Balzer-Martin LA: Current prognosis in overt neonatal hydrocephalus. J Neurosurg *57*:378, 1982.
89. Alfery DD, Shapiro HM, Gagnon RL: Cardiac arrest following rapid drainage of cerebrospinal fluid in a patient with hydrocephalus. Anesthesiology *52*:443, 1980.
90. Ellsworth CA, Shaw C-M, Sumi SM: Central nervous system developmental abnormalities. *In* Thompson RA, Green JR (eds): Pediatric Neurology and Neurosurgery. New York, Spectrum, 1978.
91. Park TS, Hoffman HJ, Hendrick EB, et al: Experience with surgical decompression of the Arnold-Chiari malformation in young infants with myelomeningocele. Neurosurgery *13*:147, 1983.
92. Sieben RL, Hamida MB, Shulman K: Multiple cranial nerve deficits associated with the Arnold-Chiari malformation. Neurology *21*:673, 1971.
93. Davidson Ward SL, Nickerson BG, van der Hal A, et al: Absent hypoxic and hypercapneic arousal responses in children with myelomeningocele and apnea. Pediatrics *78*:44, 1986.
94. Cahan LD, Bentson JR: Considerations in the diagnosis and treatment of syringomyelia and the Chiari malformation. J Neurosurg *57*:24, 1982.
95. Drake CG: Cerebral arteriovenous malformations: Considerations for and experience with surgical treatment in 166 cases. *In* Carmel PW (ed): Clinical Neurosurgery. Baltimore, Williams and Wilkins, 1979.
96. Mori K, Murata T, Hashimoto N, et al: Clinical analysis of arteriovenous malformations in children. Child's Brain *6*:13, 1980.
97. So SC: Cerebral arteriovenous malformations in children. Child's Brain *4*:242, 1978.
98. McLeod ME, Creighton RE, Humphreys RP: Anaesthesia for cerebral arteriovenous malformation in children. Can Anaesth Soc J *29*:299, 1982.
99. Graf CJ, Perrett GE, Torner JC: Bleeding from arteriovenous malformations as part of their natural history. J Neurosurg *58*:331, 1983.
100. Lam AM, Gelb AW: Cardiovascular effects of isoflurane-induced hypotension for cerebral aneurysm surgery. Anesth Analg *62*:742, 1983.
101. O'Mahony BJ, Bolsin SNC: Anaesthesia for closed embolization of cerebral arteriovenous malformations. Anaesth Intens Care *16*:318, 1988.
102. Østergaard JR, Voldby B: Intracranial arterial aneurysms in children and adolescents. J Neurosurg *58*:832, 1983.
103. Storrs BB, Humphreys RP, Hendrick EB, et al: Intracranial aneurysms in the pediatric age-group. Child's Brain *9*:358, 1982.

104. Amacher AL, Drake CG: The results of operating upon cerebral aneurysms and angiomas in children and adolescents. Child's Brain *5*:151, 1979.
105. Botterell EH, Lougheed WM, Scott JW, et al: Hypothermia and interruption of carotid or carotid and vertebral circulation in the surgical management of intracranial aneurysms. J Neurosurg *13*:1, 1956.
106. Amacher AL, Shillito J Jr: The syndromes and surgical treatment of aneurysms of the great vein of Galen. J Neurosurg *39*:89, 1973.
107. Jedeikin R, Rowe RD, Freedom RM, et al: Cerebral arteriovenous malformation in neonates. The role of myocardial ischemia. J Cardiol *4*:29, 1983.
108. Russell W, Newton TH: Aneurysm of the vein of Galen. Am J Roentgenol *92*:756, 1964.
109. Hood JB, Wallace CT, Mahaffey JE: Anesthetic management of an intracranial arteriovenous malformation in infancy. Anesth Analg *56*:236, 1977.
110. Hoffman HJ, Chuang S, Hendrick EB, et al: Aneurysms of the vein of Galen. J Neurosurg *57*:316, 1982.
111. Takehara Y, Araki S, Motomasu K, et al: Anesthesia for Galen aneurysm. Jpn J Anesthesiol *28*:737, 1979.
112. Godersky JC, Menezes AH: Intracranial arteriovenous anomalies of infancy: Modern concepts. Pediatr Neurosci *13*:242, 1987.
113. Olds MV, Griebel RW, Hoffman HJ: The surgical treatment of childhood moyamoya disease. J Neurosurg *66*:675, 1987.
114. Maki Y, Enomoto T: Moyamoya disease. Child's Nerv Syst *4*:204, 1988.
115. Taki W, Yonekawa Y, Kobayashi A, et al: Cerebral circulation and oxygen metabolism in moyamoya disease of ischemic type in children. Child's Nerv Syst *4*:259, 1988.
116. Kuwabara Y, Ichiya Y, Otsuka M, et al: Cerebral hemodynamic change in the child and adult with moyamoya disease. Stroke *21*:272, 1990.
117. Raimondi AJ, Tomita T: Brain tumors during the first year of life. Child's Brain *10*:193, 1983.
118. Ellams ID, Neuhauser G, Agnoli AL: Congenital intracranial neoplasms. Child's Nerv Syst *2*, 1986.
119. Schreiber D, Janisch W, Gerlach H: CNS tumours in infancy, childhood and adolescence. *In* Voth D, Gutjahr P, Langmaid C (eds): Tumours of the Central Nervous System in Infancy and Childhood. Berlin, Springer-Verlag, 1982.
120. Jacobi G: Clinical presentation of space-occupying lesions of the central nervous system. *In* Voth D, Gutjahr P, Langmaid C (eds): Tumours of the Central Nervous System in Infancy and Childhood. Berlin, Springer-Verlag, 1982.
121. Godano U, Frank F, Fabrizi AP, Ricci RF: Stereotactic surgery in the management of deep intracranial lesions in infants and adolescents. Child's Nerv Syst *3*:85, 1987.
122. Pattisapu JV, Walker ML, Heilbrun MP: Stereotactic surgery in children. Pediatr Neurosci *15*:62, 1989.
123. Park TS, Hoffman HJ, Hendrick EB, et al: Medulloblastoma: Clinical presentation and management. J Neurosurg *58*:543, 1983.
124. Meridy HW, Creighton RE, Humphreys RP: Complications during neurosurgery in the prone position in children. Can Anaesth Soc J *21*:445, 1974.
125. Sung DI: Suprasellar tumours in children. Cancer *50*:1420, 1982.
126. McLone DG, Raimondi AJ, Naidich TP: Craniopharyngiomas. Child's Brain *9*:188, 1982.
127. Thomsett MJ, Conte FA, Kaplan SL, et al: Endocrine and neurologic outcome in childhood craniopharyngioma: Review of effect of treatment in 42 patients. J Pediatr *97*:728, 1980.
128. Grant DB, Lyen K: Hypopituitarism after surgery for craniopharyngioma. Child's Brain *9*:201, 1982.
129. Friedenberg GR, Kosnik EJ, Sotos JF: Hyperglycemic coma after suprasellar surgery. N Engl J Med *303*:863, 1981.
130. Peacock WJ, Lazareff JA: Spinal tumors of childhood. S Afr Med J *70*:668, 1986.
131. Hardison HH, Packer RJ, Rorke LB, et al: Outcome of children with primary intramedullary spinal cord tumors. Child's Nerv Syst *3*:89, 1987.
132. Wagner HP, Kaser H: The role of surgery, radio- and chemotherapy in the treatment of neuroblastoma and ganglioneuroblastoma. Prog Pediatr Surg *16*:1, 1983.
133. Evans AE, D'Angio GJ, Koop CE: Diagnosis and treatment of neuroblastoma. Pediatr Clin North Am *23*:161, 1976.
134. Coldman AJ, Fryer CJH, Elwood JM, et al: Neuroblastoma: Influence of age at diagnosis, stage, tumor site, and sex on prognosis. Cancer *46*:1896, 1980.
135. King D, Goodman J, Hawk T, et al: Dumbbell neuroblastomas in children. Arch Surg *110*:888, 1975.
136. Weinblatt ME, Heisel MA, Siegel SE: Hypertension in children with neurogenic tumors. Pediatrics *71*:947, 1983.
137. Thompson EN, Bosley A: Disseminated intravascular coagulation in association with congenital neuroblastoma. Postgrad Med J *55*:814, 1979.
138. Scott JP, Morgan E: Coagulopathy of disseminated neuroblastoma. J Pediatr *103*:219, 1983.
139. Kiely EM: Surgery for neuroblastoma. *In* Spitz L, et al (eds): Progress in Pediatric Surgery. Volume 22. Berlin, Springer-Verlag, 1989.
140. Crawford AH: Neurofibromatosis in childhood. Acta Orthop Scand (Suppl) *218*:1, 1986.
141. Gray J, Swaiman KF: Brain tumors in children with neurofibromatosis: Computed tomography and magnetic resonance imaging. Pediatr Neurol *3*:335, 1987.
142. Dales RL, McEver VW III, Quispe G, Davies RS: Update on biologic behavior and surgical implications of neurofibromatosis and neurofibrosarcoma. Surg Gynecol Obstet *156*:636, 1983.
143. Fienman NL, Yakovac WC: Neurofibromatosis in childhood. Pediatrics *76*:339, 1970.
144. Jackson IT, Laws ER, Martin RD: The surgical management of orbital neurofibromatosis. Plast Reconstr Surg *71*:751, 1983.
145. Daniels SR, Loggie JMH, McEnery PT, Towbin RB: Clinical spectrum of intrinsic renovascular hypertension in children. Pediatrics *80*:698, 1987.
146. Griffiths DFR, Williams GT, Williams ED: Multiple endocrine neoplasia associated with von Recklinghausen's disease. Br Med J *287*:1341, 1983.
147. Isu T, Miyasaka K, Abe H, et al: Atlantoaxial dislocation associated with neurofibromatosis. J Neurosurg *58*:451, 1983.
148. Nagao H, Yamashita M, Shinozaki Y, et al: Hypersensitivity to pancuronium in a patient with von Recklinghausen's disease. Br J Anaesth *55*:253, 1983.
149. Meyer FB, Marsh WR, Laws ER, et al: Temporal lobectomy in children with epilepsy. J Neurosurg *64*:371, 1986.
150. Cahan LD, Engel J Jr: Surgery for epilepsy: A review. Acta Neurol Scand *73*:551, 1986.
151. Drake J, Hoffman HJ, Kobayashi J, et al: Surgical management of children with temporal lobe epilepsy and mass lesions. Neurosurgery *21*:792, 1987.
152. Olivier A: Surgical management of complex partial seizures. *In* Nistico G, et al (eds): Epilepsy: An Update on Research and Therapy. New York, Alan R Liss, 1983.

153. King DW, Flanigin HF, Gallagher BB, et al: Temporal lobectomy for partial complex seizures: Evaluation, results, and 1-year follow-up. Neurology *36*:334, 1986.
154. Fisher RS, Uematsu S: Surgical therapy of complex partial epilepsy. Johns Hopkins Med J *151*:332, 1982.
155. Blume WT, Grabow JD, Darley FL, et al: Intracarotid amobarbital test of language and memory before temporal lobectomy for seizure control. Neurology *23*:812, 1973.
156. Ford EW, Morrell F, Whisler WW: Methohexital anesthesia in the surgical treatment of uncontrollable epilepsy. Anesth Analg *61*:997, 1982.
157. Rasmussen T: Cortical resection in the treatment of focal epilepsy. Adv Neurol *8*:197, 1975.
158. Moss SD, McLone DG, Arditi M, Yogev R: Pediatric cerebral abscess. Pediatr Neurosci *14*:291, 1988.
159. Sáez-Llorens XJ, Umaña MA, Odio CM, et al: Brain abscess in infants and children. Pediatr Infect Dis J *8*:449, 1989.
160. Renier D, Flandin C, Hirsch E, Hirsch J-F: Brain abscesses in neonates: A study of thirty cases. J Neurosurg *69*:877, 1988.
161. Kagawa M, Takeshita M, Yato S, Kitamura K: Brain abscess in congenital cyanotic heart disease. J Neurosurg *58*:913, 1983.
162. Johnson DL, Markle BM, Wiedermann BL, Hanahan L: Treatment of intracranial abscesses associated with sinusitis in children and adolescents. J Pediatr *113*:15, 1988.
163. Pattisapu JV, Parent AD: Subdural empyemas in children. Pediatr Neurosci *13*:251, 1987.
164. Smith HP, Hendrick EB: Subdural empyema and epidural abscess in children. J Neurosurg *58*:392, 1983.
165. Jennet B, Teasdale G: Aspects of coma after severe head injury. Lancet *1*:878, 1971.
166. Lewelt W, Jenkins LW, Miller JD: Effects of experimental fluid-percussion injury of the brain on cerebrovascular reactivity to hypoxia and hypercapnia. J Neurosurg *56*:332, 1982.
167. Pang D, Wilberger JE: Spinal cord injury without radiographic abnormalities in children. J Neurosurg *57*:114, 1982.
168. Bivins HG, Ford S, Bezmalinovic Z, et al: The effect of axial traction during orotracheal intubation of the trauma victim with an unstable cervical spine. Ann Emerg Med *17*:25, 1988.
169. Majernick TG, Bieniek R, Houston JB, Hughes HG: Cervical spine movement during orotracheal intubation. Ann Emerg Med *15*:417, 1986.
170. Jennet B, Teasdale G: Management of Head Injuries. Philadelphia, FA Davis, 1981.
171. Bruce DA, Schut L, Bruno LA, et al: Outcome following severe head injuries in children. J Neurosurg *48*:689, 1978.
172. Humphreys RP, Jaimovich R, Hendrick EB, Hoffman HJ: Severe head injuries in children. *In* Concepts in Pediatric Neurosurgery. Volume 4. Basel, Karger, 1983.
173. Bruce DA, Alavi A, Bilaniuk L, et al: Diffuse cerebral swelling following head injuries in children: The syndrome of "malignant brain edema." J Neurosurg *54*:170, 1981.
174. Obrist WD, Genneralli TA, Segawa H, et al: Relation of cerebral blood flow to neurological status and outcome in head-injured patients. J Neurosurg *51*:292, 1979.
175. Jaggi JL, Obrist WD, Gennarelli TA, Langfitt TW: Relationship of early cerebral blood flow and metabolism to outcome in acute head injury. J Neurosurg *72*:176, 1990.
176. Braakman R, Schouten HJA, Dishoeck MB, Minderhoud JM: Megadose steroids in severe head injury. J Neurosurg *58*:326, 1983.
177. Pittman T, Bucholz R, Williams D: Efficacy of barbiturates in the treatment of resistant intracranial hypertension in severely head-injured children. Pediatr Neurosci *15*:13, 1989.
178. Ward JD, Becker DP, Miller JD, et al: Failure of prophylactic barbiturate coma in the treatment of severe head injury. J Neurosurg *62*:383, 1985.
179. Dhellemmes P, Lejeune J-P, Christiaens J-L, Combelles G: Traumatic extradural hematomas in infancy and childhood. J Neurosurg *62*:861, 1985.
180. Uchida M, Yamaoka H, Imanishi Y: Hypotension during surgery for subdural hematoma and effusion in infants. Crit Care Med *10*:5, 1982.
181. Mahoney WJ, D'Souza BJ, Haller JA, et al: Long-term outcome of children with severe head trauma and prolonged coma. Pediatrics *71*:756, 1983.
182. Walker ML, Storrs BB, Mayer T: Factors affecting outcome in the pediatric patient with multiple trauma. Child's Brain *11*:387, 1984.
183. Raimondi AJ, Hirschauer J: Head injury in the infant and toddler; Coma scoring and outcome scale. Child's Brain *11*:12, 1984.
184. Ruge JR, Sinson GP, McLone DG, Cerullo LJ: Pediatric spinal injury: The very young. J Neurosurg *68*:25, 1988.
185. Hadley MN, Zabramski JM, Browner CM, et al: Pediatric spinal trauma. Review of 122 cases of spinal cord and vertebral column injuries. J Neurosurg *68*:18, 1988.
186. Nagib MG, Maxwell RE, Chou SN: Identification and management of high-risk patients with Klippel-Feil syndrome. J Neurosurg *61*:523, 1984.
187. Brill CB, Rose JS, Godmilow L, et al: Spastic quadriparesis due to C1-C2 subluxation in Hurler syndrome. J Pediatr *92*:441, 1978.
188. Davidson RG: Atlantoaxial instability in individuals with Down syndrome: A fresh look at the evidence. Pediatrics *81*:857, 1988.
189. Ebara S, Harada T, Yamazaki Y, et al: Unstable cervical spine in athetoid cerebral palsy. Spine *14*:1154, 1989.
190. Schonwald G, Fish KJ, Perkash I: Cardiovascular complications during anesthesia in chronic spinal cord injured patients. Anesthesiology *55*:550, 1981.
191. Harris JP, Godin MS, Krekorian TD, Alksne JF: The transoropalatal approach to the atlantoaxial-clival region: Considerations for the head and neck surgeon. Laryngoscope *99*:467, 1989.
192. Di Lorenzo N: Transoral approach to extradural lesions of the lower clivus and upper cervical spine: An experience of 19 cases. Neurosurgery *24*:37, 1989.
193. Eiben RM, Crocker AC: Cerebral palsy within the spectrum of developmental disabilities. *In* Thompson GH (ed): Comprehensive Management of Cerebral Palsy. New York, Grune and Stratton, 1982.
194. Alvarez N: Neurologic examination. *In* Thompson GH (ed): Comprehensive Management of Cerebral Palsy. New York, Grune and Stratton, 1982.
195. O'Reilly DE, Walentynowicz JE: Etiological factors in cerebral palsy: An historical review. Dev Med Child Neurol *23*:633, 1981.
196. Morrison JE Jr, Matthews D, Washington R, et al: Phenol motor point blocks in children: Plasma concentrations and cardiac dysrhythmias. Anesthesiology *75*:359, 1991.
197. Fasano VA, Broggi G, Barolat-Romana G, et al: Surgical treatment of spasticity in cerebral palsy. Child's Brain *4*:289, 1978.

198. Peacock WJ, Arens LJ, Berman B: Cerebral palsy spasticity. Selective posterior rhizotomy. Pediatr Neurosci *13*:61, 1987.
199. Crysdale WS: The drooling patient: Evaluation and current surgical options. Laryngoscope *90*:775, 1980.
200. Crysdale WS: Submandibular duct relocation for drooling. J Otolaryngol *11*:286, 1982.
201. Reye RDK, Morgan G, Baral J: Encephalopathy and fatty degeneration of the viscera. A disease entity in childhood. Lancet *2*:749, 1963.
202. Luscombe FA, Monto AS, Baublis JV: Mortality due to Reye's syndrome in Michigan: Distribution and longitudinal trends. J. Infect Dis *142*:363, 1980.
203. Hurwitz ES, Barret MJ, Bregman D, et al: Public health study of Reye's syndrome and medications: Report on the main study. JAMA *257*:1905, 1987.
204. Partin JC, Partin JS, Schubert WK, et al: Brain ultrastructure in Reye's syndrome. J Neuropathol Exp Neurol *34*:425, 1975.
205. Lovejoy FH, Smith AL, Bresnan MJ, et al: Clinical staging in Reye's syndrome. Am J Dis Child *128*:36, 1974.
206. Huttenlocher RP: Reye's syndrome: Relation of outcome to therapy. Pediatr Pharm Ther *80*:845, 1972
207. Samaha FJ, Blau E, Berardinelli JL: Reye's syndrome: Clinical diagnosis and treatment with peritoneal dialysis. Pediatrics *53*:336, 1974.
208. Glascow JFT: Clinical features and prognosis of Reye's syndrome. Arch Dis Child *59*:230, 1984.
209. Heubi JE, Daugherty CC, Partin JS, Partin JC, et al: Grade 1 Reye's syndrome—Outcome and predictors of progression to deeper coma grades. N Engl J Med *311*:1539, 1984.
210. Shaywitz BA, Levethal JM, Kramer MS, et al: Prolonged continuous monitoring of intracranial pressure in Reye's syndrome. Pediatrics *59*:595, 1977.

CHAPTER

5 Diseases of the Respiratory System

I. DAVID TODRES, M.D.

This chapter reviews the clinical presentation and diagnosis of diseases of the respiratory system and details specific anesthetic implications for each condition. The basic principles of thoracic anesthesia that apply in every situation are summarized in Table 5–1. Selected disorders are discussed in more detail because of their important anesthetic implications.

LUNG GROWTH AND DEVELOPMENT

The respiratory system is frequently diseased at birth, and as it is essential for independent existence, such disease may lead to significant morbidity and mortality. An appreciation of normal lung development in utero provides an understanding of the pathological processes that may occur in the respiratory system following birth.

Normal lung growth is governed by three laws relating to the development of the conducting airways, alveoli, and pulmonary vessels. Disturbances of growth and the gestational age at which these disturbances occur may be appreciated from an understanding of these laws:[1–3]

Airways. The bronchial tree, including the terminal bronchioles, is fully developed by the 16th week of intrauterine life. Respiratory airways are formed between 16 weeks and birth and also in infancy.

Alveoli. Alveoli develop mainly after birth, increasing in number until the child is approximately 8 years of age. Alveolar size increases until growth of the chest cage is complete.

Blood Supply (Pulmonary Vessels). The arteries and veins (preacinar vessels) follow the development of the airways. The intra-acinar

Table 5–1. GENERAL PRINCIPLES OF THORACIC ANESTHESIA

Preoperative

Complete history, physical examination, chest roentgenograms, assessment of arterial blood gases, pulmonary function tests

Optimize medical condition of child, with attention to special problems of the neonate

Avoid respiratory depressant drugs

Anticipate possible major hemorrhage in surgery, and order adequate blood for transfusion

Psychological preparation: what patient can expect postoperatively in the form of pain relief, intubation, and mechanical ventilation

Emergency surgery: do not compromise efforts to optimize medical condition, but recognize priorities and modify plan accordingly

Work out plan for surgery with team approach: surgeon, anesthesiologist, pediatrician, appropriate consultants

Operative

Recognize effect on $\dot{V}/\dot{Q}$ ratios with thoracotomy and lung surgery leading to potential hypoxemia; therefore increase FIO_2 and monitor oxygen saturation and PaO_2

Ensure reliable and adequate venous access to permit urgent and rapid transfusions

Anesthetic agents will depend upon the underlying physical condition of the patient and postoperative needs (inhalational or N_2O plus relaxants); avoid N_2O when there is a potential for increase in size of a life-threatening air space, e.g., congenital lobar emphysema

Recheck proper tube position following positioning of patient

Secretions and blood easily obstruct the endotracheal tube and airways; keep airway clear at all times

Retractions of lung may obstruct airway, impair ventilation, and compress heart and great veins, reducing venous return and causing a decrease in cardiac output and blood pressure; therefore, monitor ventilation continuously

Operative *(Continued)*

Monitor blood loss closely

Perform intermittent re-expansion of collapsed lung to optimize oxygenation; this requires close coordination between surgeon and anesthesiologist

Mechanical ventilation must be optimal, maintaining the $PaCO_2$ in the normal range (end-tidal CO_2 monitoring, blood gases); manual ventilation at times helpful in detecting changes in airway resistance and lung compliance

Intraoperative Monitoring

Precordial stethoscope to monitor heart and breath sounds

Esophageal stethoscope

Oscilloscope display of the ECG with audible signal

Blood pressure: Doppler probe, oscillometric, intra-arterial catheter

Oxygen saturation: pulse oximetry

Blood gases, pH: intra-arterial catheter

Temperature probe (esophageal when possible)

Central venous pressure in selected cases

Urine output via Foley catheter (should be at least 1 ml/kg/h)

Postoperative

Extubate when patient is alert, muscle relaxation has been adequately reversed as determined by clinical evaluation and blockade monitor, and patient is able to cough effectively

Postoperative pain relief with intercostal blocks, cryopexy, or appropriate narcotic dosages, including patient-controlled analgesic for older children

Monitor blood gases

Look for atelectasis or pneumothorax on chest roentgenograms

Monitor chest drains

Data from Bland JW Jr, Reedy JC, Williams WH: Pediatric and neonatal thoracic surgery. *In* Kaplan JA (ed): Thoracic Anesthesia. New York, Churchill Livingstone, 1983, pp 505–574; and Steward DJ: Manual of Pediatric Anesthesia. 2nd edition. New York, Churchill Livingstone, 1985, pp 181–203.

vessels follow the alveoli. Arterial smooth muscle development is completed only at adolescence.

EMBRYONIC AND FETAL DEVELOPMENT

By the fifth week of the embryonic period, the lobar bronchi to each lung have formed, and by the sixth week all subsegmental bronchi are present. Following the embryonic period, the fetal period consists of three stages of development:[4]

1. The glandular period (6 to 16 weeks) consists of the formation of the preacinar airways, which are blind-ending tubes lined by epithelium and lying within loose mesenchymal stroma. Cartilage differentiation in the trachea and main bronchi occurs.

2. The glandular period is followed by the canalicular stage (16 to 24 weeks), with increase in the caliber of the peripheral airways. At this

stage the pulmonary capillaries invade the mesenchyme and develop with the airways to form the beginnings of the blood-air interface, a potentially viable gas-exchanging surface. Toward the end of this stage, types I and II lining cells appear. Type II cells, or granular pneumocytes, have cytoplasmic lamellar bodies that appear at about 25 weeks and are associated with the production of surfactant.

3. The alveolar period, from 24 weeks to term (40 weeks), is a time of further differentiation into respiratory bronchioles, alveolar sacs, and primitive alveoli. Of the 27 generations of airways, the first 19 generations (two main bronchi, lobar bronchi, segmental bronchi, lobular bronchi) are nonrespiratory airways. These are followed by eight generations that form the respiratory bronchioles and alveolar ducts, which participate in gas exchange. Further growth of these structures is in part determined by a direct effect of growth hormone on the lung. During the alveolar period the amount of surfactant increases with the duration of gestation. Surfactant is critical in the prevention of respiratory distress syndrome (hyaline membrane disease). Glucocorticoids administered to the mother pass into the fetus and accelerate the production of surfactant as well as enhancing structural maturation of the lung.

The lung develops as a hollow, fluid-filled organ from the canalicular phase to term. Fluid is secreted into the airways and contributes to amniotic fluid. The presence of the lung fluid appears to be important for lung growth to occur.[5]

In the respiratory epithelium, specialized cells secrete the lung liquid and also produce hormones that may affect lung growth. Sympathetic stimulation appears to be a factor in terminating secretion of lung liquid at birth.[6]

Respiratory movements in the fetus are noted early in the second trimester and particularly involve the diaphragm. These movements are depressed by barbiturates, hypoxia, and hypoglycemia. Fetal respiratory movements appear to be important for normal lung growth.[7]

At birth the "alveoli" are primitive spaces or saccules that will eventually develop into well-formed alveoli. There are approximately 20 million "alveoli" at birth, and by 8 years of age there are approximately 300 million.[8] It should be appreciated that the lung of the premature infant not only is smaller than that of the full-term infant but has less than the normal number of respiratory units.[9]

Normal lung growth can be impaired postnatally by a number of insults, such as severe infections of the respiratory tract (adenovirus); prolonged oxygen therapy, which may result in reduced numbers of alveoli; and artificial ventilation, particularly in infants with bronchopulmonary dysplasia.[10, 11] Therapeutic irradiation in a child may affect the lung by affecting acinar development.[12]

The arteries and veins (preacinar vessels) follow the development of the airways, so that by the 16th week of gestation all preacinar vessels are present. In utero, the pulmonary artery trunk is exposed to systemic pressures and thus has relatively thick muscle within its wall. In more peripheral vessels also the muscle layer is relatively well developed, consistent with the high pulmonary vascular resistance in utero. This muscle layer thins out and eventually disappears at a level proximal to the terminal bronchioles. Thus, the arteries to the acinus are nonmuscular. However, in persistent pulmonary hypertension found in conditions such as meconium aspiration associated with severe hypoxemia, the alveolar wall arteries are all muscularized. This degree of muscularization represents the normal state in the adult.

ABNORMAL AIRWAY GROWTH

For abnormal airway growth—that is, reduction in bronchial airway generations—to have occurred, impairment of lung growth must have taken place before the 16th week of intrauterine life. Examples include congenital diaphragmatic hernia and renal agenesis. Should the pathological process follow the period of airway development, then alveolar multiplication receives the brunt of the insult, as seen, for example, in kyphoscoliosis.

COMPENSATORY GROWTH

Following resection of a portion of the lung, there is a compensatory increase in weight, volume, and alveolar size in the remaining lung.[13] If resection occurs during the period of alveolar multiplication, there is a more rapid multiplication of alveoli, but the total number of alveoli that develops is not greater than normal.[14, 15]

ASSOCIATION OF CONGENITAL LUNG ABNORMALITIES WITH OTHER ANOMALIES

Congenital abnormalities of the lung may be associated with other anomalies. This is especially important when medical and surgical treatment is undertaken for a specific pulmonary abnormality, since the associated anomaly may add significantly to the morbidity risks. Any infant or child who rapidly develops severe respiratory distress in a matter of hours following a mild respiratory illness should be evaluated immediately for an underlying pulmonary malformation.

PULMONARY AGENESIS AND PULMONARY APLASIA

Arrested lung bud development early in pregnancy will result in either pulmonary agenesis or pulmonary aplasia. Arrested development later in pregnancy will result in failure of alveolar differentiation, leading to pulmonary hypoplasia.

Unilateral pulmonary agenesis, that is, failure of the lung to develop, is compatible with normal life. The contralateral lung is larger owing to compensatory hypertrophy. Other anomalies involving particularly the cardiovascular, gastrointestinal, and genitourinary systems may be present in greater than 50 percent of cases and will significantly affect morbidity.

A small mainstem bronchial stump arising from a recognizable carina may exist with absence of lung tissue. When this occurs, it is referred to as pulmonary aplasia, which is more commonly seen than pulmonary agenesis.[16–18]

CLINICAL PRESENTATION

Recurrent pulmonary infections occur. These may be severe because the bronchial stump acts as a nidus for infection. Severe respiratory distress may occur because of a marked shift of mediastinal structures and inadequate respiratory reserve, but clinical examination may reveal few signs. In agenesis of the right lung the heart sounds may be best heard in the right chest.[19]

Chest roentgenograms show marked deviation of the mediastinal structures, and the normal lung may be seen herniating across the mediastinum to the opposite side.

Diagnosis may be confirmed by bronchoscopy, bronchography, and radionuclide perfusion scans. Associated cardiac anomalies may be present.

Right-sided agenesis has twice the mortality of left-sided agenesis, probably as a result of greater mediastinal shift with cardiac displacement.

TREATMENT

Surgical treatment is occasionally required because of repeated infections of the bronchial stump. Excision of the stump will relieve the symptoms.

ANESTHETIC IMPLICATIONS

Standard thoracotomy procedures are required. Accidental intubation of the bronchial stump in right lung agenesis may lead to life-threatening hypoxemia.

PULMONARY HYPOPLASIA

Pulmonary hypoplasia represents failure of the lung to develop to its normal size while containing essential anatomical elements for function. The condition is associated with a decrease in lung volume and weight. Pulmonary function is decreased to a degree commensurate with the degree of hypoplasia. A smaller than normal pulmonary artery may supply the hypoplastic lung and is best demonstrated with perfusion scans. Prolonged rupture of the membranes contributes to pulmonary hypoplasia.[20] Bilateral pulmonary hypoplasia occurs in approximately 1 in 1000 births.[21] Outcome depends on associated anomalies and is worse with those who have renal abnormalities.[22] A severe form of hypoplasia is seen in Potter's syndrome, which consists of bilateral pulmonary hypoplasia associated with renal agenesis or dysplasia. A history of oligohydramnios in the mother is characteristic. The oligohydramnios appears to be the result of lung hypoplasia rather than its cause.[23] Thus, pathologically it should be considered a form of primary hypoplasia. Pathologically, the lungs show reduced airway generations. The alveoli are small and fewer in number. When pulmonary hypoplasia of undetermined origin is found, a search for renal abnormalities should be made. Secondary hypoplasia occurs when the intrathoracic volume is reduced. This may be unilateral or bilateral. Causes may include congenital diaphragmatic hernia (the most common cause), thoracic or skeletal dystrophy, and large pleural effusions.

CLINICAL PRESENTATION

With unilateral pulmonary hypoplasia, either lung may be affected. Clinical symptoms will depend upon the degree of hypoplasia and associated anomalies. Children may present with

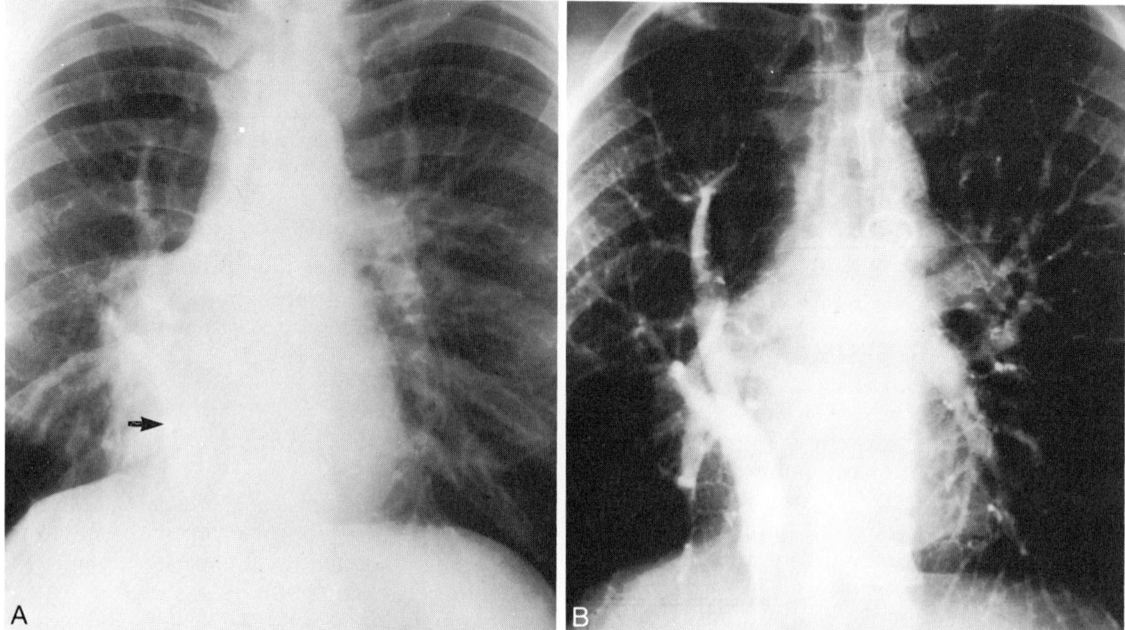

FIGURE 5–1. Scimitar syndrome. *A,* Anomalous pulmonary vein *(arrow)* with hypoplastic right lung. *B,* Angiogram defining the anomalous pulmonary vein. Note also the presence of right pulmonary artery hypoplasia. (Courtesy of Thomas Herman, M.D.)

recurrent pulmonary infections. In some cases the child is asymptomatic and the pathology is recognized as an incidental finding on a chest roentgenogram, which shows mediastinal and tracheal deviation to the affected side. The hemithorax is smaller, and the ribs appear "crowded" together. The lungs appear more radiodense, which can be confused with collapse-consolidation. Bilateral lung hypoplasia is also seen with other defects, especially cardiac. With secondary hypoplasia, the contralateral lung compression seen in congenital diaphragmatic hernia will further aggravate the respiratory distress because of the infant's inability to establish an adequate functional residual capacity (FRC).

ANESTHETIC IMPLICATIONS

The anesthesiologist should be particularly careful in the use of positive-pressure ventilation, since the hypoplastic lung tends to resist expansion. Excessive positive pressure may lead to bronchiolar rupture with interstitial emphysema and tension pneumothorax.

The treatment for the hypoplastic lung is basically conservative. However, if the lung should contain malformed bronchial tissue, recurring infections may necessitate resection.

SCIMITAR SYNDROME (DYSPLASTIC RIGHT LUNG)

The scimitar syndrome is a special form of pulmonary hypoplasia occurring mostly in females. It is a dysmorphic condition of the right lung that includes pulmonary hypoplasia.[24, 25] Its name derives from the radiological picture showing a curvilinear shadow of an anomalous pulmonary vein draining the right upper lobe lung into the right atrium or inferior vena cava (Fig. 5–1). Occasionally it drains into the portal or hepatic veins. The condition may be asymptomatic (detected on an incidental chest roentgenogram) or associated with recurrent pulmonary infections. It may be associated with serious congenital anomalies, especially of the heart (ventricular septal defect, patent ductus arteriosus, coarctation of the aorta, and tetralogy of Fallot). Vertebral anomalies are usually present.

PULMONARY HYPOPLASIA WITH HORSESHOE LUNG

In this condition, right and left lungs are joined behind the pericardial sac.[26] Embryologically, a delay or failure in the formation and fusion of the pleuropericardial and pleuroperitoneal folds occurs. Hypoplasia of the right lung contributes to the cardiac dextroversion. Surgical removal of the hypoplastic lung may be necessary because of recurrent pulmonary infections.

PULMONARY SEQUESTRATION

In this condition, embryonic and nonfunctioning lung tissue is sequestered from normal lung.[27–29] The abnormal lung receives its blood supply via systemic arteries. On rare occasions, high-output cardiac failure may occur because of a large arteriovenous malformation in the sequestration.[30–32] Abnormal embryological development of the lung gives rise to a supernumerary lung bud or buds. Two forms of sequestration occur:

1. Intralobar sequestration results when there is early incorporation of the abnormal lung bud within the normal lung and its visceral pleura.[33]
2. Extralobar sequestration results when the abnormal lung bud development occurs after the pleura has already formed; thus, the extralobar lung is separated from the normal lung but related to it.[34]

The sequestered lung tissue is embryonic, with multiple cysts and disorganized arrangement of airless alveoli, bronchi, and cartilage receiving its blood supply via a systemic artery. The affected lobe is frequently infected. Occasionally the sequestered lung tissue may communicate with the alimentary tract. Most commonly such a communication involves the esophagus, in which case it is known as a bronchopulmonary foregut malformation.[35] More commonly, the communication obliterates and disappears completely or remains as a fibrous stalk. The sequestered lung tissue receives its blood supply from a systemic artery, the aorta, or one of its branches.

INTRALOBAR SEQUESTRATION

Intralobar sequestration usually occurs in the lower lobes, mostly in the left posterior basal segment. It is rarely associated with other abnormalities. The sequestered lobe consists of multiple cysts of varying size filled with mucus, mucopurulent material, and air. Pathological changes due to infection are present. The arterial supply to the sequestered lobe is from an anomalous systemic artery from the descending thoracic aorta. In 10 to 15 percent of patients the arterial supply comes from below the diaphragm. Venous drainage is via the pulmonary veins. Patent communications with the gastrointestinal tract are rare.

CLINICAL PRESENTATION

In neonates and infants, the condition is frequently asymptomatic. Over half the cases are diagnosed after adolescence. The gender incidence is equal. The intralobar form usually presents with signs of pulmonary infection in the first two decades of life. A persistent fistula between the esophagus and respiratory system may lead to severe respiratory distress. Pulmonary infections are progressive and recurrent, with development of lung abscesses. The child presents with fever, cough, weight loss, and possibly hemoptysis.

A chest roentgenogram shows intralobar sequestration as a dense mass that may contain cysts, with fluid levels occurring usually in the posterior basal portion of the left lobe. An upper gastrointestinal series will exclude a communication between the sequestration and gastrointestinal tract. Perfusion scans will identify the aberrant systemic arterial supply and aid the surgeon in approaching the resection of the sequestered lobe.

EXTRALOBAR SEQUESTRATION

This consists of bronchial and alveolar structures often found behind the lung. The majority of extralobar sequestrations (90 percent) are found on the left at any level from the thoracic inlet to the upper part of the abdomen. Intra-abdominal pulmonary sequestration is extremely rare.[32] More than half the cases are diagnosed before the patient reaches 1 year of age. Extralobar sequestration occurs in males three times more commonly than in females. It is associated with diaphragmatic hernias or other congenital anomalies in approximately 50 percent of cases. These associated anomalies add considerably to the morbidity.[31] The arterial supply is from the aorta, and the venous drainage is via the azygos vein. Pathologically there is interstitial fibrosis with cystic spaces, destroyed lung tissue, and dilated bronchioles.

CLINICAL PRESENTATION

Extralobar sequestration is more commonly associated with congenital anomalies, most often congenital diaphragmatic hernia. Other associated anomalies include congenital heart disease and pulmonary arteriovenous malformations. Clinically, extralobar sequestration presents in infancy with recurrent infections and an area of infiltrate identifiable in the same location. Severe systemic arteriovenous shunting through aberrant vessels may cause cardiomegaly and high-output congestive heart failure.[30, 36]

On chest roentgenogram, extralobar sequestrations are usually identified as triangular densities in the posterior and medial left base. The diagnosis should be suspected when repeated clinical episodes of infection are associated with localization of roentgenographic findings to the same area. With abscess formation there may be fluid level. The sequestered lung may appear normal before changes of chronic infection set in. Ultrasonography is helpful in identifying the lesion.[37]

Treatment and Anesthetic Implications

The sequestered lung tissue is usually resected with excellent results. The extralobar sequestration is excised, and the intralobar sequestration is removed by lobectomy. Communication with the gastrointestinal tract, if present, is severed. The aberrant artery or arteries may bleed readily, necessitating close monitoring of blood loss and its replacement. The sequestered tissue may contain significant amounts of purulent material, making excision a slow and deliberate process. Antibiotics are given for infection. Mortality and morbidity are low, especially when operation is performed before repeated infections have occurred.

CYSTIC DISEASE OF THE LUNG

CONGENITAL PULMONARY CYSTS

Congenital pulmonary cysts have been classified as (1) bronchogenic type, (2) alveolar type, and (3) a combination of bronchogenic and alveolar. Note, however, that acquired cystic disease is much more common. Embryologically, congenital cystic disease is thought to arise as an anomalous development of the bronchopulmonary system at the stage of terminal bronchiolar or early alveolar development.[38, 39] The cyst arises on the basis of expiratory obstruction through bronchiolar narrowing. The most common form is a single peripheral air-filled cyst with a tracheobronchial communication. Cysts may be multiple. With infection it is difficult to distinguish histologically between a congenital cyst and an acquired cyst such as staphylococcal pneumatocele or a lung abscess. Cysts developing following an infection with staphylococci or *Klebsiella* are more common in children with an associated immune deficiency syndrome. The cyst is filled with air either directly or through the pores of Kohn. An increase in the size of the cyst leads to tension and distress in the neonate. Compression of normal lung occurs with shift of the mediastinum and a decrease in functioning lung tissue.

Clinical Presentation

The clinical findings depend upon the degree of distention of the cyst with air. Tension pneumothorax may develop and result in severe cardiopulmonary distress that demands emergency treatment. In late infancy and childhood, infection of the cyst usually occurs with symptoms of fever, cough, sputum, and possibly hemoptysis, with the cyst developing into a lung abscess.

The chest roentgenogram will show a large, distended cyst with mediastinal shift. There is compression atelectasis of the upper and lower lobes, and the roentgenographic picture may resemble lobar emphysema. Diaphragmatic hernia occasionally may resemble multiple lung cysts. A staphylococcal pneumatocele will undergo resolution with antibiotic treatment. Some cysts occur in sequestered lobes; therefore, careful evaluation of the blood supply to the lung is required. Blood flow in this case will be systemic and may make operation more difficult. Ventilation/perfusion scan and digital vascular imaging will help define the potential problem.

Treatment

Thoracotomy is indicated because of the potential for serious complications, namely, tension pneumothorax, abscess formation, bronchopleural fistula, and progressive and dangerous enlargement of the cyst. Elective lobectomy is therefore carried out. At times, however, emergency resection is required.[40] Note that aberrant systemic arteries may exist, especially with lower lobe cysts.

Anesthetic Implications

Excision of the cyst may be difficult because of recurrent infection and abscess formation, hence there may be significant blood loss.

CONGENITAL LOBAR EMPHYSEMA

This condition is characterized by overinflation and air trapping in the affected lobe, with compression atelectasis of the adjacent lung parenchyma and shift of the mediastinum. The left upper lobe is most often affected, followed by right middle and right upper lobes. Overinflation is greater in younger patients.

Males are affected twice as often as females. Bronchial obstruction may be due to congenital deficiency of bronchial cartilages, bronchial stenosis, or extrinsic vascular compression, usually by the pulmonary artery. It may be a manifestation of generalized lung disease resulting from loss of elastic recoil of the lungs. Rarely, it may be caused by intraluminal bronchial obstruction. Congenital heart disease is associated in 10 to 15 percent of cases.

Clinical Presentation

Progressive respiratory distress occurs in the newborn period or early infancy. The respiratory distress may be intermittent and is aggravated by feeding and crying. Tachypnea, retractions, wheezing, and cyanosis occur. Rapid deterioration may occur, requiring urgent operation. The emphysematous lobe displaces the mediastinum to the opposite side and causes compression atelectasis of the contralateral lung. The shift of the mediastinum causes increased intrathoracic pressure, impeding venous return and leading to decreased cardiac output. The emphysematous lobe does not participate in gas exchange; this, combined with atelectasis of the opposite lung, results in severe compromise of gas exchange. The infant may present with failure to gain weight and respiratory infections with cough, wheezing, and tachypnea. Associated congenital heart disease occurs in a significant number of children (10 to 15 percent).

The chest roentgenogram shows the emphysematous lobe, with atelectasis of the lower lobe. There is mediastinal shift with contralateral lung atelectasis. The emphysematous lobe appears to herniate across the mediastinum. Congenital lobar emphysema must be differentiated from postpneumonic pneumatocele, pulmonary cystic disease, and tension pneumothorax. Note that bronchovascular markings are present in congenital lobar emphysema, in contrast to a pneumothorax or lung cyst.

Treatment

Bronchoscopy is indicated if there is a possibility of intraluminal obstruction causing emphysema of a lobe. Otherwise, treatment consists of removal of the affected lobe. Surgical excision in the neonate may be urgent if the lobe is expanding rapidly.[41] The outcome after operation is good, with compensation for loss of lung parenchyma by expansion of the remaining lung.[42] In the older infant with few symptoms, nonsurgical treatment may be considered.[43]

Anesthetic Implications

An associated cardiac anomaly needs to be considered in the anesthetic and surgical management. During induction of anesthesia, vigorous positive pressure may further inflate the emphysematous lobe, with an increase in cardiopulmonary distress. Therefore, spontaneous ventilation is advised until the chest is open and the thorax decompressed. Nitrous oxide is avoided because of its potential for increasing the size of the emphysematous lobe.[44]

CONGENITAL CYSTIC ADENOMATOID MALFORMATION

This is a very rare condition. It may be associated with other congenital anomalies. It usually is unilateral and affects one or more lobes, usually the lower lobe. Differentiation from cystic disease of the lung is not always clear (Fig. 5–2). The condition has been classified into types I, II, and III based on gross and histological criteria.[45]

Clinical Presentation

Routine prenatal ultrasound examination has been helpful in detecting this lesion prior to birth.[46] The child presents either in acute respiratory distress in the newborn period or is seen late with recurrent pulmonary infections. Type I lesions have large cysts that may expand rapidly after birth, causing mediastinal shift and increasing respiratory distress. The cysts communicate with each other and with the bronchus. A lack of bronchial cartilage leads to bronchial collapse during expiration. Type II lesions consist of multiple small cysts resembling dilated terminal bronchioles. Type III lesions consist of a solid, airless mass of cystic bronchioles. Type III disease has a very poor prognosis.

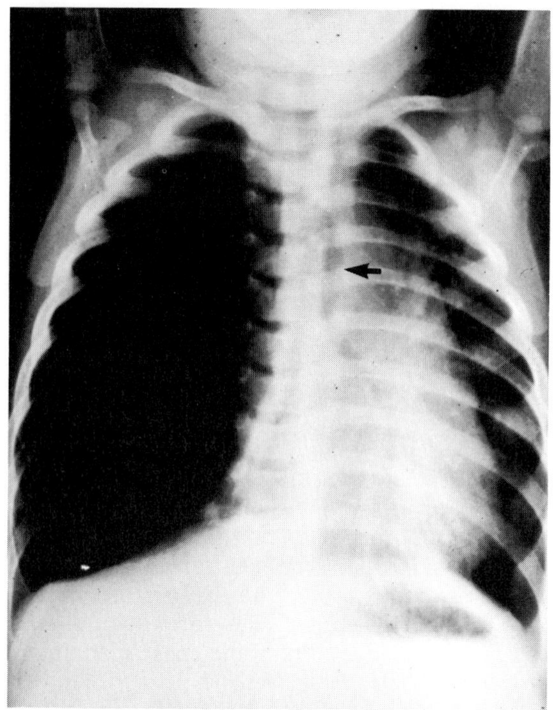

FIGURE 5–2. Chest roentgenogram showing cystic adenomatoid malformation of the right lung. Note the lower lobe inflation and the upper lobe herniating across the midline *(arrow)*. The radiological picture resembles that of congenital lobar emphysema. (Courtesy of David Kushner, M.D.)

The differential diagnosis on chest roentgenogram includes congenital and acquired cystic disease, lobar emphysema, and congenital diaphragmatic hernia. The position of the gastric bubble and a barium meal will help differentiate cystic adenomatoid malformation from congenital diaphragmatic hernia.

Treatment

In the neonate, operation may be urgent because of tension from enlarging cysts causing severe cardiopulmonary distress similar to that seen in obstructive emphysema. Lobectomy is performed. In older children, chronic infection, which is inevitable, should be treated, followed by thoracotomy and lobectomy. Prognosis following removal of the affected lung is good. The remaining lung compensates for the excised part.[47] Resection is recommended because of life-threatening respiratory distress, chronic infection,[48] or associated malignancy.[49]

BRONCHOGENIC CYST

Bronchogenic cysts may occur at any age but usually present in older children. They are unilocular cysts lined with respiratory epithelium and may have cartilage and bronchial glands in the wall. They usually do not communicate with the tracheobronchial tree.

Clinical Presentation

Bronchogenic cysts may be asymptomatic and are discovered on a routine chest roentgenogram. Otherwise, they may present with respiratory infections, cough, and possibly dysphagia. However, the cyst may cause severe respiratory distress through compression of a mainstem bronchus, in which case the cyst is commonly situated beneath the carina and compresses the left mainstem bronchus.[50] The cysts contain mucus and frequently become infected. Barium swallow, bronchography, and CT scanning help delineate the pathology.

CHYLOTHORAX

In this condition, a pleural chylous effusion forms. In the neonate, it is caused by a congenital abnormality or following traumatic rupture of the thoracic duct during the birth process.[51] It has been described as a complication of chest tube placement in the neonate.[52] The congenital abnormality may represent a failure of the proper fusion of mediastinal and pulmonary lymphatics and the production of multiple lymphatic fistulas. It is usually right-sided, but rarely may be bilateral.[53] Chylothorax may exist alone or be part of a generalized lymphangiectasia. The fluid fills the hemithorax and displaces the mediastinum.

Large fluid, protein, and fat losses occur through this effusion. The fluid aspirated is straw colored until milk is ingested, after which the fluid becomes milky in color. There is also a high concentration of lymphocytes in the fluid. Prolonged loss of fluid may lead to hypoproteinemia and fluid imbalance. Metabolic acidosis from loss of lymph has been described.[54]

In later childhood, chylothorax occurs from trauma or following surgical procedures, especially repair of patent ductus arteriosus, coarctation of the aorta, or the Blalock-Taussig shunt.[55] Chylothorax may be seen secondary to superior vena caval obstruction.[56] Occasionally, the chylous fluid enters the pericardial sac and causes chylopericardial tamponade, in which case it is important to assess the respiratory difficulty in terms of a cardiac versus a pulmonary basis.[57]

Clinical Presentation

Chylothorax is a rare cause of neonatal respiratory distress. The infant is tachypneic with chest retractions and is cyanotic. Examination of the chest shows dullness to percussion and diminished breath sounds on the affected side.

A chest roentgenogram shows opacification on the affected side, usually the right, with mediastinal shift and compression of the underlying lung.

Treatment

Thoracentesis or chest tube drainage will relieve the problem of respiratory distress.[58, 59] Drainage usually ceases in 1 to 2 weeks. In the meantime the infant should receive nutrition in the form of medium-chain triglycerides and, if necessary, total parenteral nutrition.[60] Prolonged drainage of chylous fluid leads to significant protein loss and depletion of lymphocytes. Operation is rarely necessary, but should it be required, thoracotomy is performed and ligation of the thoracic duct is carried out.[61, 62] In some cases identification of the thoracic duct is helped by feeding the patient neutral fats stained with dyes to outline lymphatic channels. The overall prognosis is very good.

ESOPHAGEAL ATRESIA AND TRACHEOESOPHAGEAL FISTULA

In the first month of the developing human embryo, the dorsal foregut (the forerunner of the esophagus) separates from the ventral trachea. This separation starts at the carina and extends in a cephalad direction. By the 26th day of gestation the trachea and esophagus have separated as two parallel tubes up to the level of the larynx. When this separation is incomplete, a tracheoesophageal fistula (TEF) arises. Esophageal atresia results when the lateral esophageal grooves continue distally in the process of separating the dorsal esophagus from the ventral trachea.

Tracheoesophageal fistula is one of the lesions found in the VATER syndrome, in which a disturbance in embryogenesis produces a well-recognized association of anomalies: *v*ertebral anomalies, *a*nal malformations, *t*racheo*e*sophageal fistula, *r*adial limb dysplasia, and *r*enal deformities.

The esophageal atresia and TEF malformations can be classified into five categories.

1. Esophageal atresia (7 percent). In this condition, the upper esophageal pouch ends blindly. The distal esophageal segment may be widely separated from the upper pouch, but there is no fistula.
2. Esophageal atresia with proximal TEF (2 percent).
3. Esophageal atresia with proximal and distal TEFs (1 percent).
4. Esophageal atresia with distal TEF (85 percent). This is the most common form. The distal esophageal segment is usually separated from the upper pouch by a distance of 1 to 2 cm and communicates with the airway just above the carina and posteriorly.
5. Tracheoesophageal fistula without atresia, "H-type" fistula (5 percent). The fistula is most often located at the thoracic inlet.

Clinical Presentation

There is an incidence of 1 in 3000 live births. Polyhydramnios is frequently present in the mother. Prematurity occurs in about one third of cases of esophageal atresia and TEF. Associated anomalies occurring in 50 percent of cases are presently the most significant cause of morbidity and mortality; particularly important are cardiac anomalies, which occur in 14 percent of cases.[63] Combined esophageal and duodenal atresia has been described.[64]

Pulmonary complications are a potentially serious consequence of esophageal atresia. The infants salivate excessively because of their inability to swallow. Choking, coughing, and regurgitation classically occur with the first feeding. Cyanosis and apnea may occur.

In esophageal atresia, the distended upper pouch compresses the cartilage of the tracheal wall, weakening its structure and causing tracheomalacia.[65, 66] The degree of tracheomalacia usually results in airway obstruction associated with a characteristic "barking" cough. The degree of obstruction may be severe enough to compromise the airway so much that a tracheostomy is required.

Aspiration into the tracheobronchial tree occurs from the fluid in the pharynx which cannot be swallowed because of the esophageal atresia. The distal TEF allows air to distend the stomach, especially with the infant crying. With gastric distention, diaphragmatic movements are markedly impeded. Reflux occurs readily, and gastric juice is aspirated into the lungs, producing pneumonitis.

The diagnosis is made by passing a catheter through the mouth or nose to the stomach. Obstruction is met at approximately 11 cm from the infant's nares. A roentgenogram will confirm the diagnosis with the tube held up in the upper pouch. The presence of air in the stomach and intestines is indicative of a distal TEF.

Isolated TEF without atresia is more difficult to diagnose and usually presents in older infants. Choking, coughing with feeding, and pneumonitis should suggest the diagnosis. Symptoms may be subtle, however. A contrast esophageal study usually shows the communication. If the study is negative, however, bronchoscopy is necessary to identify the fistula in the posterior tracheal wall. A significant number of cases have associated anomalies. They vary from minor to life-threatening. Cardiac and gastrointestinal anomalies occur most commonly. Cardiac anomalies are particularly significant in determining the outcome.

TREATMENT

Preoperative. Pulmonary complications preoperatively contribute to morbidity and mortality. These should be prevented until operation can be performed. The infant is kept NPO and positioned semi-upright to minimize regurgitation of gastric juice through the fistula. The proximal segment is suctioned continually through a Replogle tube to prevent aspiration of nasopharyngeal secretions. Atelectasis and pneumonitis tend to occur, particularly in the right upper lobe.

With severe hypoxemia and respiratory failure, endotracheal intubation and ventilation are required. Other aspects of newborn care must be optimized—namely, maintaining body temperature and treatment of hypoglycemia and other problems such as respiratory distress syndrome and hyperbilirubinemia. If the infant is critically ill, a gastrostomy is performed (sometimes using local anesthesia), and thoracotomy is postponed until respiratory function has improved. However, the respiratory status usually will not improve until the fistula is ligated. A careful search is made for associated anomalies, such as cardiac anomalies, anal atresia, and renal anomalies—that is, those anomalies associated with the VATER syndrome. The electrolyte status is assessed and corrected as necessary. A type and cross-match is performed for packed red blood cells. Broad-spectrum antibiotics are administered if pneumonitis is suspected.

Operative. Primary definitive repair is performed when the infant is more than 1800 grams in weight, without pneumonitis or other serious congenital anomalies. With very low birth weight or critically ill infants, the operative procedure is staged.[67] Gastrostomy for feeding and division of the distal tracheoesophageal fistula are performed. The proximal pouch is suctioned continuously to prevent pneumonitis. When the infant has gained weight and is physically stable, definitive repair—anastomosis of the upper and lower portions of the esophagus—is carried out.

Management of TEF in a premature infant with hyaline membrane disease has recently been re-evaluated. Traditionally, the surgical procedure to divide the fistula was often postponed to treat the medical condition, that is, the hyaline membrane disease, preferentially and proceed with operative repair when the infant has stabilized. This approach has its problems. Mechanical ventilation may lead to escape of air via the fistula into the stomach, leading to underventilation of the lungs.[68, 69] In addition, distention of the stomach may result in gastric perforation, pneumoperitoneum, and elevation of the diaphragm, producing potentially lethal hypoxemia. To avoid gastric distention and its potentially serious sequelae, a gastrostomy may be performed. However, this does not resolve the problem of preferential escape of air via the fistula. Retrograde positioning of a balloon catheter in the lower esophagus when the infant undergoes gastrostomy[69] or placement of a Fogarty balloon catheter in the fistula under bronchoscopic control has been advocated.[70] An approach that includes early thoracotomy (in the first 12 hours of life before the hyaline membrane disease has progressed to a more severe form) and division of the TEF has been very successful in infants of less than 34 weeks' gestation.[71]

Parenteral nutrition has contributed significantly to improving the outcome by optimizing the caloric intake and thus maintaining the infant in the best possible condition both pre- and postoperatively. With esophageal atresia without a fistula, bougienage stretching of the upper pouch is carried out over several weeks to prepare for a primary anastomosis.

ANESTHETIC IMPLICATIONS

A precordial stethoscope is placed in the left axilla to help detect intraoperative airway obstruction and to monitor the heart sounds. An arterial catheter to monitor pressure and blood gases is set up. The infant is premedicated with atropine, 0.02 mg/kg intravenously.

Tracheal intubation is carried out with the patient awake after the esophageal pouch has been suctioned. Topical analgesia with lidocaine gel to the tongue and palate may reduce the reaction of the infant to laryngoscopy and intubation. The endotracheal tube optimally should be positioned just distal to the fistula to avoid gaseous distention of the stomach. Gastric distention will impede ventilatory efforts and venous return and, if severe, may lead to cardiopulmonary arrest or gastric rupture.[72–74] The fistula, however, may be quite near or even at the level of the carina. In practice the tube is advanced into the right mainstem bronchus and then withdrawn to a position when bilateral breath sounds are heard. It can now be assumed that the tip of the tube is just above the carina.

Anesthesia is carried out with nitrous oxide, oxygen, and low concentrations of halothane or isoflurane, to avoid cardiovascular depression. Positive pressure should be avoided if possible until the chest is open. However, it may be necessary to employ positive pressure to prevent hypoxemia and hypercapnia, in which case it must be performed in a very gentle manner so as to avoid the danger of gastric distention. In performing a gastrostomy, the addition of local anesthesia is helpful because it eliminates the need to use high concentrations of volatile anesthetic agents. A nondepolarizing muscle relaxant is added for optimal operating conditions.

Hyperoxia in premature infants should be avoided because of the potential for retinopathy of prematurity and its possible sequela, retrolental fibroplasia. Serial blood gas analysis for PaO_2 and $PaCO_2$ is carried out. Pulse oximetry to monitor oxygen saturation and maintain this at 90 to 95 percent provides a continuous means to assure safe oxygenation. Suctioning of the endotracheal tube and airways is critical because of the likelihood of secretions and blood obstructing the airway. Airway obstruction may occur at any time from surgical manipulation of the trachea.

Maintaining the infant's body temperature at normal levels is critical, and a number of factors that help to do so are implemented: the use of a warming blanket, delivery of warmed, humidified gases, and keeping the operating room environment appropriately warmed. Warm intravenous fluids with dextrose are given at 4 ml/kg/h (check blood glucose levels to titrate accordingly), and an additional 6 to 8 ml/kg/h of lactated Ringer's solution is given for intraoperative evaporative and "third space" losses. Blood loss is measured in the suction bottle and by weighing sponges, and replacement is provided, if necessary, using warmed blood.

POSTOPERATIVE CARE AND COMPLICATIONS

Postoperative care is given in the intensive care unit, with special attention to the possible development of atelectasis and pneumonitis from retained secretions in the tracheobronchial tree. Careful suctioning should avoid introducing the catheter too far into the esophagus so as not to disturb the anastomosis. The infant may require tracheal intubation to help reexpand the lung and may need to remain intubated and ventilated. Careful positioning of the tube is required to avoid its impinging on the operative repair of the fistula.

The most important complications relevant to the operation include anastomotic leaks and strictures.[75, 76] Anastomotic leakage is an important cause of morbidity and mortality. In a series of 199 patients operated on for TEF, anastomotic leaks occurred in 17 percent. Major leakage occurred in 3.5 percent of patients.[77] The risk of anastomotic stricture increases markedly following anastomotic leakage. Should major anastomotic leakage occur, respiratory distress is noted, usually 2 to 4 days following the operation. Large amounts of saliva or mucus may be seen coming out of the chest drain. Surgical intervention is required to treat the problem. Minor leakage is usually treated successfully by nonoperative means. Total parenteral hyperalimentation is carried out while the anastomotic leak is allowed to heal. The anastomotic stricture problem may be compounded and aggravated by the presence of gastroesophageal reflux, in which case a fundoplication procedure may be necessary.[78] This usually results in marked decreases in symptoms and frequency of dilatation procedures.

Tracheomalacia occurs postoperatively in about 25 percent of cases. Symptoms vary from mild to severe. Characteristically, in the mild forms, there is a "barking" cough for months to years. In more severe cases the infant may suffer alarming blue or gray spells during feeding. This is due to the expanded proximal esophagus compressing the soft trachea against the aortic arch. The airway obstruction resulting from tracheomalacia may be resolved in some cases by fixing the aortic arch to the sternum and in this way preventing continued tracheal pressure.[79] All infants following repair of the esophageal atresia have some degree of dysphagia from disordered peristalsis.[80]

Overall survival rate is 82 percent, including all categories, with excellent results in those infants who have no associated life-threatening congenital anomalies. Supportive measures in addition to skilled anesthesia and surgery are crucial in affecting survival.[81] Follow-up lung function studies have shown a high incidence of lung damage and hypersensitive airways, which probably results from continuing subclinical aspiration of esophageal contents.[82]

H-TYPE TRACHEOESOPHAGEAL FISTULA

This condition, which has an incidence of 5 percent of all tracheoesophageal fistulas, is frequently missed. Although familiarly referred to as an H-type, the fistula is really closer to an N configuration, i.e., the fistula runs obliquely from the upper trachea (cephalad) to the esophagus (caudal). Associated anomalies of the airway and gastrointestinal system, as well as other organs, may occur.[83]

Clinical Presentation

Symptoms usually commence shortly after birth, but the diagnosis is often missed. H-type fistula should be suspected in an infant when symptoms after birth include (1) choking, coughing, and cyanosis caused by aspiration of feeds via the fistula into the lungs; (2) recurrent respiratory infections; and (3) improvement following gavage feeding.

Diagnosis is made on the basis of the clinical history and confirmed by radiological and endoscopic examination of the trachea and esophagus. Endoscopy is valuable in ruling out other anomalies of the airway and esophagus.

Treatment and Anesthetic Implications

Following diagnosis of the lesion, the infant's clinical status should be stabilized, such as treatment of pulmonary infections. During anesthesia, care should be taken to avoid gastric distention with positive-pressure ventilation. In addition, there are often abundant tracheal secretions, so appropriate suctioning of the airway is essential. The surgical approach is usually cervical. The fistula is usually located at the thoracic inlet. Operative division of the fistula may be associated with damage to the recurrent laryngeal nerves, necessitating close monitoring of the infant's airway for laryngeal palsy following extubation.

CONGENITAL LARYNGOTRACHEOESOPHAGEAL CLEFT

This rare anomaly has a high mortality rate. It has been classified according to extent. Type I cleft is limited to the larynx; type II is a partial cleft; type III is a complete cleft from the larynx to the carina; and type IV cleft extends beyond the carina into the mainstem bronchi.[84] The first successful management and repair of an infant with complete laryngoesophageal cleft was reported in 1984.[85]

Embryologically, at 28 days of gestation, bilateral indentations of the mesoderm begin to separate the foregut tube into the anterior trachea and posterior esophagus. The separation begins caudally and proceeds in a cephalad direction, reaching the larynx by 33 days. Interference with this advance will determine the extent of the defect.[86, 87]

Clinical Presentation

The clinical presentation will depend on the severity of the lesion and the presence of associated anomalies. Mild forms of cleft often escape detection in the first few weeks of life. The physician should suspect the diagnosis when seeing a patient with a history of a hoarse or muffled cry, excess mucus production, and cyanotic spells, with exacerbation of these symptoms during feeding. Episodes of coughing and apnea and atelectasis or pneumonitis may occur from recurrent aspiration of feedings. Severe defects are usually discovered soon after birth because of the severe respiratory distress in the infant.

The clinical picture should make one suspect the diagnosis, and further studies such as radiological studies, laryngoscopy, and bronchoscopy must be carried out to confirm it. A definitive diagnosis is made at the time of bronchoscopy.[88] Note that smaller clefts that involve the larynx and cricoid only are easily missed on laryngoscopy and bronchoscopy because the edges of the cleft are approximated. A chest roentgenogram may show areas of infiltrate, atelectasis, and overaeration. Contrast studies with barium will demonstrate overflow of contrast into the distal tracheobronchial tree.

Anesthetic Implications

Preoperative preparation includes antibiotics for aspiration pneumonia. Prior to definitive repair, gastrostomy is performed and tracheostomy may be necessary. Parenteral hyperalimentation is given via a central vein. A specially modified endotracheal tube is used. This tube has endobronchial bifurcations, which are placed in each mainstem bronchus to ensure ventilation of both lungs and thus avoid the danger of gastric inflation.

From the anesthetic point of view, stabilization of the airway is crucial.[89] Surgical technique is critical in preventing recurrences following repair.[90] The surgical procedure in the type III and type IV clefts involves both cervical and thoracic approaches and requires close teamwork between anesthesiologists and surgeons. Postoperatively, the anesthesiologist should be involved in caring for the infant's airway, which will involve keeping the infant paralyzed with nondepolarizing agents and ventilated to eliminate motion and high swings in intraluminal pressure. The postoperative care requires the highest standards in integrated teamwork, involving intensive care specialists, surgeons, anesthesiologists, and nursing staff.

TRACHEAL STENOSIS

Tracheal stenosis in infants and children may be congenital or acquired.

CONGENITAL TRACHEAL STENOSIS

This is a rare, life-threatening condition.[91] Pathologically, the luminal narrowing is due to the presence of complete tracheal rings. This lesion may occur alone or exist with other anomalies.[92] The presence of other significant anomalies is important in determining the outcome.[93, 94] An example is the condition of an aberrant left pulmonary artery or pulmonary artery sling, in which compression and narrowing of the posterior tracheal wall are due to an anomalous origin of the left pulmonary artery, from the right pulmonary artery near its origin. The anomalous left pulmonary artery passes behind the trachea to supply the left lung.[95, 96] Surgical correction of this defect still leaves the child with tracheal stenosis because of the underlying tracheal defect. With other vascular anomalies—for example, double aortic arch—compression of the trachea may also occur. Correction of the vascular anomaly will improve the airway problem greatly. Innominate artery compression of the trachea may be responsible for symptoms of tracheal stenosis. Surgical correction is a disputed subject.[96]

ACQUIRED TRACHEAL STENOSIS

Tracheal stenosis may be acquired in a number of different circumstances, for example: postintubation (endotracheal tube or tracheostomy), posttraumatic, thermal and chemical burns, or primary tumors.[97, 98] Of special concern to the anesthesiologist is the iatrogenic complication of tracheal stenosis following prolonged endotracheal intubation or tracheostomy. In neonates, stenosis is uncommon. However, in older children the problem is more frequently encountered. Pressure necrosis from the tube leads to the formation of granulation tissue, perichondritis, and finally scar formation with stricture. Symptoms of obstruction are delayed following the removal of the tube. Increasing respiratory distress from further stricture becomes life-threatening.

CLINICAL PRESENTATION

Upper respiratory infection may precipitate respiratory failure acutely because of mucus plugs and inflammatory reaction. Respiratory distress, stridor, and chest retractions increase with agitation and crying in the child, as a result of dynamic collapse of the airway associated with increased respiratory efforts. Airway obstruction is aggravated from inability to clear mucus. Depending on the site of the tracheal obstruction, wheezing may be heard and may be misdiagnosed as "allergic asthma." Thus, a thorough history is necessary, and a suspicion of this complication should exist if a history of recent intubation or tracheostomy is obtained, particularly if the patient's condition has been diagnosed as asthma, which has not responded well to standard therapeutic maneuvers. Physical examination will reveal diffuse inspiratory and expiratory wheezing that may resemble asthma.

Roentgenograms of the posteroanterior and lateral cervical neck and the chest define the location and extent of the tracheal pathology. Airway fluoroscopy demonstrates the dynamic movements of the airway with respirations and the degree of tracheomalacia present. Bronchography evaluation of the airway is potentially dangerous, because reactions to the agents may precipitate mucus plugging of a tight stenosis. In addition, any further restriction of the airway may be particularly dangerous in a radiological facility far removed from the controlled environment of the operating room and the presence of surgical and anesthesia personnel. Computed tomography (CT) is helpful in demonstrating the extent and severity of the lesion. Patients who require these studies and have an endotracheal tube in place are at potentially grave risk when extubated for radiological studies. An anesthesiologist should be in attendance in the radiology facility to reinsert the endotracheal tube if necessary. Barium swallow is carried out to determine the presence of a vascular ring, a condition that has a significantly high association with tracheal stenosis.

Bronchoscopy provides the definitive diagnosis. Bronchoscopy may be attended by bleeding and edema and may provoke increasing airway difficulty. This should be anticipated; the child should be carefully observed in the intensive care unit following the procedure. Inhalation of racemic epinephrine may alleviate some obstruction due to edema. In an emergency prior to intubation, if this is required, positive pressure with 100 percent oxygen, using a face mask with an adjustable "pop-off" valve, can deliver oxygen into the lungs by counteracting the dynamic airway collapse that occurs with increasing respiratory efforts.

Anesthetic Implications

The anesthesiologist must have a clear understanding of (1) the airway obstruction and its effect on the patient and (2) the general medical condition, especially the cardiopulmonary status, because of the possibility of associated anomalies.[99–103]

Preoperatively, the child should be in an intensive care unit, where airway compromise may be carefully monitored and treated should deterioration occur. The use of premedication will be dictated by the underlying condition of the patient. If significant airway obstruction is present, narcotics and sedatives should not be given, as they may cause central respiratory depression and respiratory failure.

Atropine may produce drying of secretions, which can lead to further airway obstruction. Atropine should be used only at the time of induction, and then its primary purpose is to prevent bradycardia from vagal stimuli. Blood gas analysis is not particularly helpful, as values may be normal despite significant airway obstruction.

Standard monitoring for a thoracotomy is employed, including esophageal stethoscope, ECG, blood pressure monitoring, and arterial cannulation. The right radial artery should not be used. During surgery the innominate artery, which is in close proximity to the trachea, is compressed, and thus the radial artery pulse is lost. Oxygenation can be measured with pulse oximetry, and carbon dioxide elimination with analysis of end-tidal gases. An assortment of airway equipment, including different sizes of endotracheal tubes, is essential to deal with unanticipated degrees of airway obstruction.

Induction of anesthesia is best carried out with spontaneous ventilation and assisted breaths, with nitrous oxide, oxygen, and increasing concentrations of halothane. Induction is prolonged because of the stenosis. Relaxants should be avoided, as it may be impossible to ventilate the patient with a face mask and positive pressure under these conditions. At an adequate depth of inhaled anesthesia, topical anesthesia with lidocaine (2 percent) provides optimal conditions for the bronchoscopy that usually precedes the surgical resection. The surgeon must be present to dilate the stenosis should increasing obstruction occur. If the obstruction is found to be critical on bronchoscopy, the surgeon may elect to dilate the obstruction so that ventilation may be more effective, thus preventing serious hypercapnia and the increased potential for cardiac arrhythmias during the surgical procedure.

An appropriate-sized endotracheal tube is passed to a point above the obstruction or through and beyond it. Tube position and patency are critical at all times. Anesthesia is maintained with nitrous oxide, oxygen, and halothane, and ventilation is controlled by hand. When the trachea is exposed and the resection procedure commences, a close understanding between the anesthesiologist and the surgeon is essential. Once the trachea is transected below the lesion, the lower trachea is intubated by the surgeon using a sterile armored tube. In the case of very low lesions, separate tubes may be passed into each main bronchus. Sterile connecting equipment is passed to the anesthesiologist for continuation of the anesthesia and controlled ventilation. This procedure must be well orchestrated to avoid the potential for hypoxemia.

The lesion is resected and the upper and lower ends are brought together, with removal of the distal armored tube when the posterior wall portion of the tracheal anastomosis is complete. The original endotracheal tube is then passed beyond the anastomosis into the distal trachea under direct vision. The position of the distal end of the tube is critical, because flexion of the neck to bring the ends of the anastomosis together may lead to accidental mainstem bronchial intubation. A technique using high-frequency jet ventilation for tracheal resection has also been described.[104]

At the conclusion of the procedure, the child is allowed to breathe spontaneously. Extubation at the conclusion is preferred, since the presence of a foreign body in the trachea may predispose to breakdown of the anastomosis. Extubation is attempted in the operating room with the patient under moderate-to-deep anesthesia, to avoid a marked increase in intraluminal pressures and tension on the sutures. However, reintubation may be necessary. The child is then transferred to the intensive care unit for postoperative care. Should the child have to remain intubated, endotracheal tube positioning is critical, because the infant's shortened trachea and flexed head may predispose to accidental mainstem intubation or extubation with minimal movement.

A variety of techniques have been utilized in selected cases before undertaking resection. These include dilatations, diathermic resection, cryosurgery, laser therapy, and steroid injections. These techniques may be helpful while granulation tissue is present or while the scar is still in the early stages. Once the scar tissue becomes hard and fibrous, resection appears to offer the best chance for success. Resection of tracheal stenosis is possible even in small infants.[98, 105–107] Conservative treatment is favored if it will tide the child over the difficulty to an age at which resection would be considered to be a safer undertaking. When possible, primary anastomosis is carried out. However, with extensive tracheal stenosis, new techniques, such as the interposition of cartilage grafts or pericardial patch, have been successfully carried out.[108, 109] More recently, balloon dilation of long-segment tracheal stenosis has been effective, avoiding the risks of tracheal anastomosis.[110]

LARYNGOMALACIA

This congenital abnormality is best referred to as a "flabby larynx."[111, 112] The fibrous and cartilaginous support of the supraglottic larynx is flaccid as a result of immaturity in development. Laryngomalacia is the most common cause of persistent stridor in the infant.[113]

Clinical Presentation

The stridor is present at birth or in the first few days or weeks following birth. It is classically an inspiratory stridor caused by an infolding of the supraglottic structures (epiglottic and aryepiglottic folds), leading to obstruction of the glottic opening. The inspiratory stridor may be intense, yet the child is not clinically ill. The infant's cry is normal. The stridor is markedly improved during sleep and with the infant in the prone position. The intensity of the stridor increases with increased negative pressure, as occurs with crying, and secondary to obstruction from upper respiratory infections. The condition resolves spontaneously within the first 2 to 3 years of life.

The history and clinical picture are very characteristic. However, further investigations should be performed to confirm the diagnosis, since many other conditions causing stridor may be much more serious. Fluoroscopy of the upper airway will demonstrate the supraglottic structures drawing in with inspiration. Laryngoscopy will confirm the diagnosis. Fiberoptic visualization at the bedside is less traumatic and provides a dynamic visualization free of the stress of direct laryngoscopy.

Anesthetic Implications

These infants are usually clinically well. The inspiratory stridor and airway obstruction clear as anesthesia is induced. Hence, diagnostic laryngoscopy should be performed when the infant is awake or recovering from anesthesia. The use of continuous positive airway pressure (CPAP) may help stabilize the airway. Very rarely, intubation or tracheostomy is required.

TRACHEOMALACIA

Tracheomalacia is a condition of abnormal flaccidity or "softening" of the tracheal wall, leading to tracheal collapse, especially during expiration.[111] Congenital tracheomalacia as a primary defect is very rare. The condition is found associated with tracheoesophageal fistula when there is a deficiency of tracheal cartilage or when extrinsic compression occurs with vascular anomalies (e.g., double aortic arch, aberrant left pulmonary artery) and mediastinal masses.[114–116] Acquired tracheomalacia may follow tracheostomy and prolonged tracheal intubation, especially with cuffed endotracheal tubes. With expiration and positive pressure within the chest, the tracheal wall collapses, and this leads to airway obstruction. In severe cases, total obstruction leads to apnea, requiring positive-pressure ventilation to "splint" open the airway and ventilate the child.

Clinical Presentation

The clinical history of previous intubation or tracheostomy may suggest the diagnosis in a child who has symptoms of airway obstruction that are particularly aggravated by crying and agitation. These children often present with persistent cough associated with retention of secretions and recurrent infections. Inability to cough up sputum leads to airway obstruction with wheezing.

Airway fluoroscopy defines the dynamic aspects of tracheomalacia, with constriction and dilatation of the tracheal wall related to phases of respiration. Barium swallow is performed to exclude extensive compression of the trachea (e.g., vascular ring). Bronchoscopy at light levels of anesthesia with spontaneous ventilation confirms the radiological findings and the level and extent of the tracheomalacia.

Treatment

The natural tendency for the trachea is to stiffen with age, and thus surgery is rarely indicated. Underlying causes for the secondary tracheomalacia should be identified and treated. These include division of vascular rings or correction of anomalous blood vessels compressing the trachea.[115] Very occasionally, innominate artery compression causes the obstruction, and aortopexy (stitching the aorta to the back of the sternum) relieves the symptoms. The vascular abnormalities causing tracheal compression are occasionally familial.[116] Occasionally, tracheostomy may be required until the trachea has firmed up and stabilized. Surgical treatment using an implanted splint has been successfully carried out.[117] Other methods of stabilizing the trachea include tracheopexy,[119] external airway splinting,[117, 120, 121] and wedge tracheoplasty.[122] Tracheomalacia may require long-term treatment with continuous positive airway pressure (CPAP).[123]

BRONCHOMALACIA

Severe bronchomalacia may result from compression of the mainstem bronchus by a bronchogenic cyst. Various methods have been employed to "splint" open the bronchus. A recent report describes suspension of the bronchial wall to the ligamentum arteriosum to stabilize the airway.[118] Airway splinting has been employed for both tracheomalacia and bronchomalacia.[117]

CONGENITAL DIAPHRAGMATIC HERNIA

Congenital diaphragmatic hernia (CDH) has an incidence of 1 per 2500 live births. The condition has been considered the result of the premature return of the midgut to the abdominal cavity during its embryonic development, before the diaphragm has completely formed. As a result, the abdominal viscera appear in the chest.[124] This usually includes the stomach, the small or large intestine, and occasionally the liver and spleen. There may be an associated malrotation of the gut.

The herniation occurs most often through the pleuroperitoneal sinus (foramen of Bochdalek) on the left. Pulmonary hypoplasia occurs on the affected side and in many cases in the opposite lung as well. Severe pulmonary hypoplasia is usually the cause of death in these infants.[125] However, occasionally and possibly if the herniation occurs later in the development of the lungs, there is more functional lung tissue and the outcome is more favorable. Approximately one in four neonates with CDH has associated congenital anomalies, the severity of which may significantly affect the infant's chances of survival. Much less commonly the herniation occurs through the substernal sinus (foramen of Morgagni); such hernias are not usually associated with severe pulmonary hypoplasia.

Clinical Presentation

The infant may be cyanotic and tachypneic with marked chest retractions immediately after birth. There is decreased chest movement on the affected side, with a shift of the cardiac impulse to the opposite side. The abdomen is scaphoid as a result of the bowel being displaced into the chest. Breath sounds are absent on the affected side. In some infants, respiratory distress may not be evident at birth but develops later; a later presentation is generally a good prognostic sign.

Roentgenographic studies are diagnostic, showing gas-filled loops of bowel in the chest, with a marked shift of the mediastinum to the opposite side and compression of the contralateral lung. This may be confused with congenital cystic lung disease (Fig. 5–3).

The infant is usually severely hypoxemic. Hypercapnia and acidemia may also be prominent.

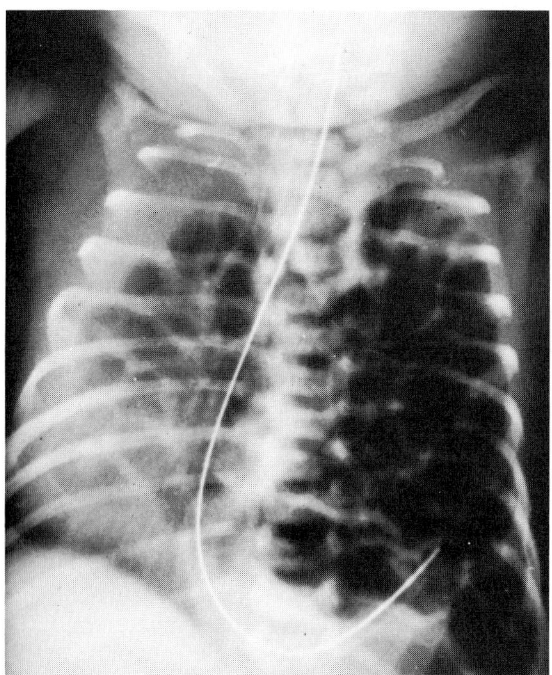

FIGURE 5–3. Congenital diaphragmatic hernia on the left with shift of the mediastinum to the right and atelectasis of the contralateral lung. Note presence of nasogastric tube in the chest.

Hypercapnia that is unresponsive to vigorous hyperventilation is associated with a mortality rate of 90 percent. Pathologically, these infants have bilateral pulmonary hypoplasia and severe preductal shunting. Those who respond well to hyperventilation with a reduction in $Pa\text{CO}_2$ have a more favorable outcome.[126] Further respiratory compromise may be the result of pneumothorax from the contralateral lung, which may occur pre-, intra-, or postoperatively and must be constantly suspected. This possibility should always be uppermost in the mind of the anesthesiologist. A decreased incidence of pneumothorax has been correlated with an improved survival with CDH.[127]

TREATMENT AND ANESTHETIC IMPLICATIONS

Congenital diaphragmatic hernia remains one of the most challenging problems for the surgeon and the anesthesiologist. In the severely distressed infant, the first priority in management consists of establishing an airway by awake oral intubation and instituting rapid, low-volume, controlled respirations to avoid high-peak inflation pressures. The patient should be sedated and paralyzed to minimize movement and intrathoracic pressure. The stomach should be decompressed through insertion of a nasogastric tube. A reliable intravenous line is secured. Monitoring includes electrocardiography, use of an esophageal stethoscope, a Doppler flow probe for blood pressure, and pulse oximetry and end-tidal carbon dioxide measurements for blood oxygen tension.

Traditionally, repair of CDH has been undertaken as a surgical emergency. Despite this aggressive approach, CDH is still associated with a high mortality in neonates who are significantly symptomatic within the first 12 hours following birth. A major factor in determining the outcome in these infants is the development of persistent pulmonary hypertension that is refractory to conventional medical management.[128] In addition, it has been noted that respiratory compliance frequently deteriorates immediately following repair.[129] A new approach to repair has been a strategy of delay during which the infant's condition is stabilized with conventional medical treatment or with extracorporeal membrane oxygenation (ECMO).[130, 131] This approach has led to an improved survival, but the mortality in one series despite this approach showed that almost half the patients still have fatal pulmonary hypoplasia or persistent pulmonary hypertension.[132] Others have described infants with CDH as responders or nonresponders. Preoperative stabilization is helpful in the responder group, in which responders were defined as those who had a preoperative postductal $P\text{O}_2$ at any time preoperatively of greater than 100 mm Hg.[133] One approach to determining the optimal time for operation has been to assess pulmonary artery pressure using Doppler echocardiographic monitoring and to carry out a period of preoperative stabilization until pulmonary artery pressure, i.e., pulmonary vascular resistance, decreased to acceptable levels.[134] Surgical repair of CDH has been associated with an increase in blood levels of thromboxane—a chemical mediator that causes active vasoconstriction of the smooth muscle cells of the pulmonary vascular tree.[135] In a recent series, 43 percent of patients were unsalvageable despite the addition of delayed operative management and preoperative ECMO.[136] However, ECMO may improve overall survival.[137]

Anesthetic agents should include a narcotic, such as fentanyl, to provide adequate analgesia and suppress autonomic responses, which may increase pulmonary vascular resistance. Nondepolarizing muscle relaxants are administered. Nitrous oxide is avoided because of its potential for increasing bowel distention. Initially, potent inhalational agents should be avoided because myocardial depression may occur and further potentiate any existing cardiovascular compromise. Once the chest is decompressed, inhalational agents may be used to supplement the anesthesia.

Surgical repair while the infant is on ECMO has been described. A principal concern is to ensure that the ECMO lines do not become kinked during the procedure.

Postoperative Care

Pulmonary artery hypertension is a major factor in the postoperative period. Relentless and progressive pulmonary hypertension with periods of improvement ("flip-flop") is frequently seen. Thus, efforts to reduce pulmonary artery hypertension caused by a hyperactive pulmonary vasculature is the keystone of postoperative care. During the period of increased pulmonary artery pressure, blood flow is rerouted away from the lungs through the ductus arteriosus and foramen ovale. This leads to progressive hypoxemia and acidemia. Unless this deterioration is rapidly checked, death ensues.

Factors that provoke pulmonary artery vasoconstriction, namely, hypoxemia, hypercapnia, acidemia, and hypothermia, must therefore be avoided.[138] Noxious stimuli such as pain and endotracheal tube suctioning may contribute to the development of pulmonary artery hypertension. Therefore, to minimize these effects, a prolonged "anesthetic state" is maintained with the use of infusions of narcotics, such as fentanyl, and muscle relaxants.[139] Hyperventilation to a pH of 7.5 to 7.6 is used to augment pulmonary vasodilation.[140]

Pharmacological vasodilator therapy remains controversial. Reports of early successes with vasodilators such as tolazoline, isoproterenol, PGE_1, and nitroglycerin have not always been followed with consistently good results. In addition to its alpha-adrenergic blocking effect, tolazoline inhibits platelet thromboxane synthesis.[141] Dopamine is frequently used for its inotropic effects and maintenance of systemic vascular resistance. Extracorporeal membrane oxygenation (ECMO) has been used with success in selected infants with severe ductal and foramen ovale shunting following repair of the diaphragmatic hernia[142, 143] or, as described earlier, as a means of stabilizing the critically ill infant prior to surgical repair of the diaphragmatic hernia. A follow-up of 20 patients with CDH showed that functional impairment from pulmonary hypoplasia was insignificant, as evidenced by the existence of a normal working capacity and maintenance of a normal alveolar gas exchange during exercise on a high work load.[144]

EVENTRATION OF THE DIAPHRAGM

In eventration of the diaphragm, an entire hemidiaphragm bulges into the chest. It may resemble a diaphragmatic hernia with a sac. In some cases the eventration maybe bilateral.[145, 146]

Clinical Presentation

The condition may be asymptomatic, or it may be associated with a history of respiratory infections and effort intolerance due to a reduced pulmonary functional reserve. Roentgenographic studies will show the elevated hemidiaphragm. It may resemble diaphragmatic paralysis. However, with paralysis there is paradoxical motion that is not seen with eventration. Ultrasound studies of the diaphragm are particularly hclpful in arriving at the diagnosis. A diagnostic pneumoperitoneum or radionucleotide scans of the liver and spleen may be necessary to establish the diagnosis.

Treatment

Operative repair consists of plication of the diaphragm through either a thoracic or an abdominal approach. No specific or unusual problems are related to anesthesia for this condition.

TRAUMATIC DIAPHRAGMATIC HERNIA

This condition is associated with severe trauma to the abdomen. Usually other associated injuries are present. In evaluating the patient with trauma, the physician focuses on the head, neck, chest, and abdomen and may readily overlook the partition between the chest and abdomen, the diaphragm. A major concern with traumatic rupture of the diaphragm is the danger of bowel strangulation.[147, 148]

A chest roentgenogram will be abnormal and may show bowel in the chest. In selected cases diagnostic studies include pneumoperitoneum, gastrointestinal barium study, and liver and spleen scans.

TREATMENT

Treatment usually will involve operative repair of the ruptured diaphragm as well as associated injuries.

ANESTHETIC IMPLICATIONS

The anesthetic technique used will depend, to a large extent, upon the associated injuries of other organ systems.

PNEUMONIA

Pneumonia in infancy and childhood is an important cause of morbidity, particularly in infants and young children.[149]

Neonatal pneumonia may be classified as early (within 48 hours of birth) or late onset (after 48 hours). The early-onset type is most commonly due to ascending infection from the maternal genital tract. Usually the infant is septicemic at birth. Late-onset pneumonia is usually nosocomial in origin.

Early-onset pneumonia is mostly due to group B streptocci infection. It may be difficult to distinguish from hyaline membrane disease. Early-onset pneumonia in neonates is associated with a high mortality, particularly in preterm infants. For this reason, it is reasonable practice to administer antibiotics intravenously to all preterm infants in respiratory distress for 48 to 72 hours pending the results of the blood cultures. A recent study indicates that there is a poor correlation between blood cultures and cultures from endotracheal tubes and nasopharyngeal aspirates.[150] Also, surveillance cultures are of limited value in predicting the etiology of neonatal sepsis.[151]

There may be a seasonal variation in the incidence of some pneumonias; for example, respiratory syncytial virus (RSV) causes winter epidemics of bronchiolitis and pneumonia. The peak incidence of pneumonia is between 6 months and 5 years of age. The age of the child is an important influence on susceptibility to specific organisms. In neonates, the organism is usually group B streptococcus or gram-negative bacteria (*Escherichia coli* and *Klebsiella pneumoniae*). Other less common causes include *Listeria monocytogenes,* cytomegalovirus (CMV), herpes simplex, and *Chlamydia trachomatis.*[152] *Chlamydia trachomatis* is a common cause of pneumonia in the first 3 months of life.[153] Between 1 month and 4 years of age, the most common cause of pneumonia is viral, with RSV being the most important pathogen. Other important causes are parainfluenza, influenza, and adenovirus. Bacterial causes are the pneumococcus and *Haemophilus influenzae* B. Over 4 years of age, the pneumococcus and *Mycoplasma pneumoniae* are the most frequent bacterial causes.

Clinical symptoms, such as fever, cough, and dyspnea, occur equally in viral or bacterial pneumonias, making differentiation difficult.[154] Wheezing tends to occur more often in viral infections. However, it is also common in mycoplasmal pneumonia.[155]

Chest roentgenograms are not always helpful in distinguishing viral from bacterial causes of pneumonia. However, the radiograph of staphylococcal pneumonia shows a characteristic pneumatocele (Fig. 5–4).[156] Sputum sampling is difficult to obtain from children. Often, the specimens obtained are contaminated by pharyngeal organisms. Blood cultures are positive in about 10 percent of children with bacterial pneumonia.[157]

For any child with recurrent pneumonia, one should consider the possibility of an underlying disorder such as cystic fibrosis, immunodeficiency condition, or congenital anomaly of the lung (sequestration).

PNEUMONIA IN A COMPROMISED HOST

Pneumocystis carinii is an important cause of pneumonia in children with immunodeficiency, in those suffering from malignant disease and receiving chemotherapy, and more recently in children with HIV infection. In these conditions, the organism may produce a life-threatening interstitial pneumonitis. The clinical examination of the chest is unrevealing. A chest roentgenogram shows widespread granular densities, which are initially perihilar.

Pneumonia may at times be part of a larger systemic illness involving other organ systems, for example, Goodpasture's disease or Wegener's granulomatosis. Goodpasture's disease is an autoimmune disease that affects adolescents and presents with pulmonary hemorrhages, followed by renal failure due to glomerulonephritis. Wegener's granulomatosis presents with upper and lower airway disease caused by necrotizing granulomas. Pulmonary destruction leads to respiratory failure. The kidneys are also involved, and renal failure develops.

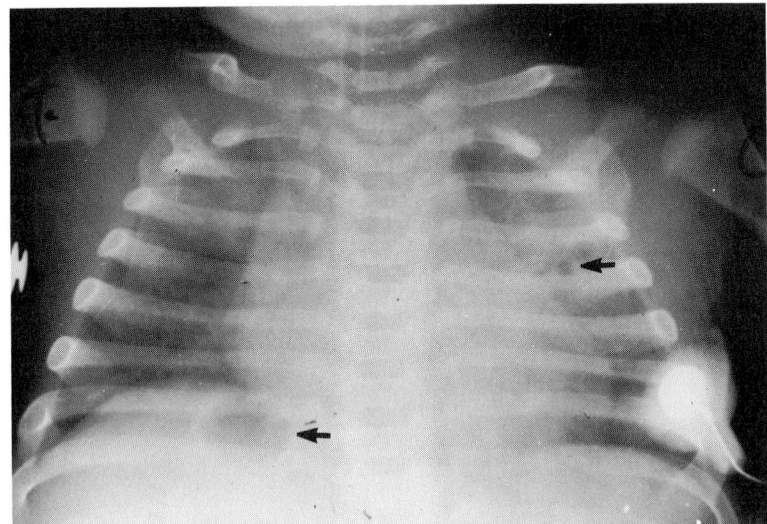

FIGURE 5–4. Radiograph of infant with staphylococcal pneumonia, showing presence of pneumatoceles *(arrows).*

ASPIRATION PNEUMONIA

Aspiration pneumonia may result from mechanical (e.g., foreign body), chemical, or bacterial causes. For a foreign body aspiration, bronchoscopy provides the diagnosis and is therapeutic. Inhalation of a foreign body such as a peanut results in an acute exudative response in the tracheobronchial tree within 24 hours. Chemical aspiration into the lung occurs during swallowing or vomiting, e.g., accidental ingestion of gasoline, furniture polish, or charcoal lighter fluid. Aspiration pneumonia in children commonly involves anaerobic bacteria, as is seen when there are central nervous system disorders and tracheoesophageal malformations.[157]

Open lung biopsy is commonly performed for the diagnosis of diffuse pulmonary lesions.[158, 159] One study showed that clinical diagnosis gave a correct diagnosis in 55 percent of patients, but lung biopsy and histological examination gave the final answer in all patients.[160] *Pneumocystis carinii* was found to be the causative organism in 67 percent of the immunosuppressed patients. Open lung biopsy is recommended as a procedure that should be performed earlier in the clinical course than is often the practice. The benefits of biopsy appear to outweigh the risks of its complications.

Thoracoscopic evaluation of intrathoracic lesions in children has been advocated as a safe and valuable procedure carried out under local or light general anesthesia.[161]

Anesthetic Implications for Open Lung Biopsy

General anesthesia is usually well tolerated. For this reason, the open lung biopsy is preferred to thoracoscopy, since it provides direct access for control of any bleeding or pulmonary air leaks. General anesthesia with controlled ventilation will optimize oxygenation and carbon dioxide elimination. Postoperatively, the potential for a tension pneumothorax exists.

PNEUMONIA ASSOCIATED WITH PLEURAL EFFUSION AND EMPYEMA

The presence of a pleural effusion is generally indicative of a bacterial pneumonia. The organism responsible is most commonly the pneumococcus or group A streptococcus. Other organisms implicated are *E. coli, Klebsiella, Pseudomonas,* and *M. tuberculosis.* Empyema may be a presenting sign of pneumonia due to *Haemophilus influenzae.* Staphylococcal pneumonia is frequently associated with empyema. Viral infections of the lung usually do not give rise to a pleural effusion. Chest roentgenograms will confirm the clinical findings. Ultrasound studies are helpful in assessing the extent of the effusion and identifying structures deep to the effusion, which may on radiograph obliterate an entire lung.

Empyema evolves in three stages: exudative, fibropurulent, and organizing. In the early part of its course, the exudative phase, the empyema may be drained by needle thoracentesis. Later in the course, more aggressive therapy to drain the pus is necessary. Drainage of pus is a critical part of the treatment, in addition to the administration of the appropriate antibiotics.

A study of the clinical course of empyema and long-term follow-up of empyema in 16 children showed the organisms responsible to be predominantly *Haemophilus influenzae, Staphylococcus aureus,* and *Streptococcus pneumoniae.* Chest tube drainage and antibiotic therapy were necessary in all patients. Three patients required an open thoracotomy because of an unsatisfactory clinical response. The long-term outcome was excellent.[162]

LUNG ABSCESS

This may be a primary event when it is due to *Staphylococcus* or *Klebsiella* organisms. It is secondary when it follows an event such as a foreign body aspiration. The condition is much less common today because of effective antibiotic therapy. Lung abscesses occur in children at any age but are rare in the neonate. Secondary abscesses occur more often in younger children.

The organisms responsible include bacteria, viruses, fungi, and protozoa. *Staphylococcus aureus* is the most common organism cultured. In the neonatal period, Group B streptococcus, *Klebsiella pneumoniae,* and *E. coli* are implicated.

Pathologically, a focus of inflammation is followed by central necrosis, with progressive fibrosis of the enclosing wall. Histologically, there is an accumulation of inflammatory cells, with suppurative destruction of the lung parenchyma, bronchi, and arteries with central cavitation. Bronchi may connect with the abscess cavities, leading to the presence of an air/fluid level on radiograph. Large abscesses may affect ventilation and perfusion, causing hypoxemia.

CLINICAL PRESENTATION

In older children, fever, malaise, and weight loss occur. There may be a history of cough, dyspnea, sputum production, and hemoptysis. The abscess may be invaded with anaerobic organisms, namely *Bacteroides* or microaerophilic streptococci. Chest physical signs may be minimal compared with the more overt signs in the adult, particularly following foreign body aspiration. Chest roentgenography may show solitary or multiple abscesses. An air-fluid level is often present. Computed tomography may be helpful in defining a cavity, if present, and distinguishing the abscess from an empyema.[163] Blood cultures may be positive in secondary lung abscesses. In children, determination of the organism is difficult because of the lack of sputum production.

TREATMENT

Antibiotics are essential in the therapy. In children with a primary abscess, antibiotic therapy alone causes resolution of the problem.[164] All secondary abscesses must be drained. Clinical resolution usually occurs in 2 weeks, but roentgenographic resolution may take months.

CYSTIC FIBROSIS

Cystic fibrosis is the most common cause of suppurative lung disease in children. Cystic fibrosis (CF) occurs in 1 in 2500 Caucasian live births. The disease is extremely rare in blacks and orientals. The disease is inherited as an autosomal recessive. The gene for cystic fibrosis has recently been identified.[165] It is the most common lethal genetic disorder. Survival rates are improving with advances in therapy;[166] up to 75 percent of affected individuals now reach adult life. There are newly recognized instances in which the condition has first been diagnosed in middle and later life.[167] Multiple organs are involved with obstructive lesions and disordered mucus and electrolyte secretion. The increase in the levels of sodium and chloride in sweat is a feature of the disease and is the basis for the diagnostic test for CF.[168] The pulmonary involvement leads to undue susceptibility to lower respiratory tract infection, with progressive deterioration of lung function. Obstruction of bile canaliculi leads to biliary cirrhosis and portal hypertension. Pancreatic insufficiency seriously affects the patient's nutritional status.

Of special concern to the anesthesiologist is the involvement of the respiratory system. The basic pathological change in the lungs is suppurative bronchitis and bronchiolitis, which eventually produces permanent damage in the airways. Complete obliteration of some smaller airways is common, and varying degrees of bronchiectasis occur. *Staphylococcus aureus* is the most common organism in younger children. In infants under 24 months of age, gram-negative organisms, especially *Pseudomonas aeruginosa,* are prevalent. *Pseudomonas cepacia* is an emerging problem in CF.[169] Fibrosis occurs in areas of chronic infection. Localized areas of pneumonia are common and may progress to abscess formation. Lung abscess associated with aspiration may occur.[170] Respiratory viral infections have been associated with pulmonary deterioration in patients with CF.[171] Hemoptysis is usually seen in the older CF patient with advanced lung disease. It occurs in about 60 percent of adolescents or adults.[172–174]

Increased airway resistance is associated with tracheobronchial collapse, rendering expectoration of purulent sputum ineffective. As a result of airways disease, patchy areas of collapse and hyperinflation occur in the lungs. Partial obstruction of small airways leads to maldistribution of ventilation and perfusion, resulting in hypoxemia.[175] Hypercapnia develops when the airway obstruction becomes widespread.[176] Pulmonary hypertension develops with extensive pulmonary disease, probably as a result of hypoxemia. Muscular hypertrophy of the small pulmonary arteries occurs, with muscle extending distally into the arterioles. Eventually the pulmonary hypertension becomes irreversible. Right heart failure is a frequent terminal event. Spontaneous pneumothorax, pneumomediastinum, and hemoptysis are complications of pulmonary involvement in adolescents.

Clinical Presentation

Cystic fibrosis may present in the newborn period as meconium ileus. The infant fails to pass meconium, and this is subsequently found to be thick and inspissated, leading to intestinal obstruction. The infant's abdomen is markedly distended, and bile-stained vomiting occurs. This occurs in 10 to 15 percent of newborn infants with cystic fibrosis. Intrauterine perforation may have occurred, leading to meconium peritonitis. A significant number of infants with meconium ileus have other anomalies, such as intestinal atresia.

Recurrent or persistent respiratory infections are the most common presentation beyond the newborn stage. Respiratory infections frequently take the form of a bronchiolitis.[177] Digestive tract manifestations of the disease are the result of exocrine pancreatic insufficiency. Maldigestion of fat and protein is the major manifestation of exocrine pancreatic insufficiency.[178] The clinical manifestations are failure to gain weight and chronic diarrhea, with bulky, foul, pale stools and abdominal distention. In a significant number of patients, hypoproteinemia leads to edema. Rectal prolapse occurs in 20 to 30 percent of cases and usually occurs during the second year of life.

As a result of defective bile salt absorption, cholelithiasis develops in at least 10 percent of patients. This may lead to cholecystitis or biliary colic with obstructive jaundice.

Hepatic involvement occurs in 20 to 50 percent of patients with CF. As the child grows, the liver becomes hard and nodular. Hepatic failure is rare; however, clotting factors are reduced. Biliary cirrhosis develops in a small number of older children and adolescents and may be complicated by portal hypertension with splenomegaly, hypersplenism, and bleeding esophageal varices.

Chronic sinusitis is invariably present in older patients with CF, and nasal polyps are prevalent.[179]

There are many emotional problems for patient and family that require understanding and support.

Anesthetic Implications

Increased airway resistance leads to gas trapping and an increase in functional reserve capacity (FRC). There is an imbalance of ventilation and perfusion ($\dot{V}/\dot{Q}$), leading to significant hypoxemia. The Pa_{CO_2} is usually normal; an elevation would be an indication of advanced lung disease. With pulmonary fibrosis giving rise to low $\dot{V}/\dot{Q}$ areas, induction of anesthesia and emergence are prolonged. It is important to appreciate that the patient may be responsive to a hypoxic respiratory drive, and thus with oxygen administration ventilatory assistance may be necessary.

Pulmonary vasoconstriction occurs because of underlying hypoxemia, especially when the Pa_{O_2} is less than 50 mm Hg, eventually leading to right heart hypertrophy. In addition, there may be evidence of left ventricular enlargement. Cor pulmonale and cardiac failure ultimately occur in the late stages of CF.[180]

Preoperative. Patients have excessive bronchial secretions, therefore their lung function should be brought to optimum prior to surgery with appropriate chest physiotherapy and postural drainage.[181, 182] In addition, lung function studies, e.g., peak expiratory flow rate, forced vital capacity (FVC), FEV_1, flow/volume curve, and oxygen saturation, are carried out if the child is of appropriate age. Narcotics are avoided because of their respiratory depressant effect. These patients may be on diuretic therapy, therefore a possible electrolyte imbalance should be checked. Bronchoscopy and lavage to improve ventilation and oxygenation may be necessary. Some patients respond well to steroid therapy.[183] Bacterial infections, such as *Staphylococcus aureus* and *Pseudomonas aeruginosa,* are common, as are fungal infections, e.g., *Aspergillus.* Patients frequently present with wheezing.

Selective bronchial arteriography and bronchial artery embolization may be necessary to control massive hemoptysis in children with CF.[184, 185] Thoracotomy and pleural stripping may be required to control recurrent pneumothorax.

Operative. Occasionally, pulmonary resection—mainly lobectomy—is required for complications of the cystic fibrosis, namely, bronchiectasis, abscess, and hemoptysis, and when there has been an inadequate response to conservative medical therapy.[186]

The anesthetic management for patients with cystic fibrosis depends upon the nature of the operative procedure.[187] Regional anesthesia is preferred whenever this is possible. The most common operation performed is nasal polypectomy. Ketamine should be avoided because of its association with increased bronchial secretions. For pulmonary resection when a lung abscess is present, endobronchial blockers are necessary. Nitrous oxide should be avoided when there is obstruction of bullae, pneumothorax, or intestinal obstruction.[188, 189] Anesthesia is effectively carried out with volatile anesthetic agents such as halothane or isoflurane or with a balanced technique (muscle relaxant and narcotic). The patient should be kept well hydrated, as dehydration leads to further inspissation of secretions.

A recent paper provides guidelines about the advisability of pulmonary resection in cystic fibrosis patients. Improvement was found with localized disease when FEV_1 and FVC were greater than the 30 percent expected. A FEV_1 or FVC of less than 30 percent was indicative of diffuse pulmonary disease, a condition that precluded the benefits of surgery.[190]

Postoperative. Chest physiotherapy is vital in this phase of care, as is adequate control of pain. For this purpose regional analgesia is ideal. Antibiotic needs must be carefully determined, and it should be appreciated that high doses may be needed because of an increase in renal clearance.[191] Significant deterioration in lung function may occur after general anesthesia in patients with cystic fibrosis.

BRONCHIECTASIS

Bronchiectasis consists of a permanent dilation of bronchi usually associated with inflammation. The condition is relatively uncommon and is associated with chronic and frequent repeated lung infections. The disease usually follows bronchitis or pneumonia during the first or second year of life. Severe adenovirus pneumonia is particularly likely to be followed by this complication. Bronchiectasis may also follow aspiration of a foreign body. In addition, recurrent pulmonary aspiration of gastric contents in a patient who has difficulty swallowing may contribute to the development of bronchiectasis. Conditions predisposing to the development of bronchiectasis include recurrent lower airway disease, cystic fibrosis, and immotile cilia syndrome.

Small airways become obstructed with secretions secondary to inflammation. The ciliated epithelium of the airway is destroyed, making it difficult to clear the airway of secretions. In addition, there is an increase in secretions from hypertrophied glands. As a result, atelectasis occurs distal to the obstruction. Abscess formation follows, with destruction and weakening of the bronchial wall.[192] This leads to dilatation of the airways from negative intrathoracic pressure and traction from surrounding fibrous tissue. Mechanical forces alone may not be adequate as an explanation for the pathological picture. The changes may affect one or both lungs. The bronchial arteries undergo hypertrophy of their walls. There is shunting of blood by bronchopulmonary anastomoses, with pulmonary hypertension.

Clinical Presentation

Bronchiectasis is characterized by chronic and frequent recurrent infections of the respiratory tract. Persistent cough and purulent sputum are classic symptoms, but bronchiectasis may still be present in the absence of sputum. Hemoptysis may also occur but is relatively uncommon. As the disease progresses, the child becomes progressively more dyspneic. Bronchiectasis occurs most commonly in the left lower lobe, lingula, and right middle lobe. However, most children have the disease more diffusely. There is clubbing of fingers. Failure to thrive occurs in the chronic case.

A chest roentgenogram may show characteristic findings, especially in advanced cases.[193] However, the diagnosis rests upon the demonstration of bronchiectasis by bronchography. CT scanning and ventilation/perfusion lung scans may aid in the diagnosis of bronchiectasis.

Bronchiectasis has been observed with certain syndromes, especially the unilateral hyperlucent lung (Swyer-James or Macleod's syndrome) that follows infections or foreign body aspiration.[194] Bronchiectasis is also a part of Kartagener's syndrome, which includes situs inversus and chronic sinusitis.[195] A disorder of the cilia with bronchiectasis and dextrocardia has been described.[196]

TREATMENT AND ANESTHETIC IMPLICATIONS

Treatment with appropriate antibiotics is essential. Mucus plugging of the airways is treated aggressively, with chest physiotherapy, postural drainage, and if necessary bronchoscopy. Bronchoscopy can be particularly helpful in obtaining appropriate sputum specimens for culture and sensitivity studies. Bronchography traditionally has been performed with the patient under general anesthesia.[197, 198] A technique using the blind passage of an endotracheal catheter in lightly sedated children may be successful and avoid general anesthesia. Fiberoptic bronchoscopy combined with selective bronchography appears to be an advance in diagnostic capabilities.[199]

General anesthesia in children requires endotracheal intubation. During anesthesia, the child is closely monitored for potential hypoxemia, both clinically and with the aid of a pulse oximeter for oxygen saturation. Wheezing following extubation may occur. Also, fever has been noted in one third of the patients.[200]

Pulmonary resection, that is, lobectomy, although relatively uncommon, may be necessary in selected cases.[201–203] Surgery is usually delayed if possible until the child is 6 to 12 years of age, to allow for resolution of the disease.

Anesthetic problems relate to the possible spread of purulent material to the healthy lung. For this reason, use of bronchial blockers and one-lung anesthesia (in the adolescent) is necessary. Bronchoscopic aspiration of affected lobes immediately prior to surgical resection may aid in decreasing the risk of contamination of the remaining lung tissue.

TUMORS OF THE LUNG

Primary lung tumors are very uncommon in infants and children. Metastatic tumors are seen more commonly.

BENIGN TUMORS

Plasma cell granuloma or myofibroblastic tumor is probably the most common benign tumor of the lung in childhood.[204] It is regarded by some to be a postinflammatory pseudotumor. The tumor is composed primarily of plasma cells; also present are histiocytes, small lymphocytes, and spindle cells. The child is usually asymptomatic. However, the tumor may obstruct a bronchus and produce respiratory distress. Chest roentgenography shows a solitary, circumscribed parenchymal lesion or coin lesion. Surgery is the treatment of choice, with a good prognosis.

MALIGNANT TUMORS

Primary malignant tumors are rare in childhood. They include fibrosarcoma, leiomyosarcoma, and rhabdomyosarcoma. Bronchial adenomas include bronchial carcinoid, cylindroma, and mucoepidermoid tumors, with bronchial carcinoid being the most common.[205, 206]

Primary carcinoma of the lung is very rare in childhood.

METASTATIC TUMORS

Metastases to the lung is a significant problem in childhood cancer. The metastases are usually very large. They may be either few or great in number. Metastases to the lung (nodular densities) are common in Wilm's tumor, osteosarcoma, Ewing's sarcoma, hepatoblastoma, and neuroblastoma.[207] The lungs may also be involved in leukemia, non-Hodgkin's lymphoma, and Hodgkin's disease, which tend to produce infiltrates or reticulonodular densities. Usually lung function is not compromised. However, if there are large numbers of metastases, pulmonary function may be affected. Bronchial infiltration of the tumor may cause bronchial stenosis.

TREATMENT

An aggressive approach to resecting the metastatic tumors is favored. This may involve multiple thoracotomies and resections.[208, 209] Results appear best with Wilm's tumor metastases. The aggressive surgical approach has led to a reduction in the need for radiotherapy with its potential for long-term sequelae. Pulmonary metastases secondary to hepatoblastoma and hepatocellular carcinoma have been successfully treated with aggressive excision, with survival despite the usually dismal prognosis.[210]

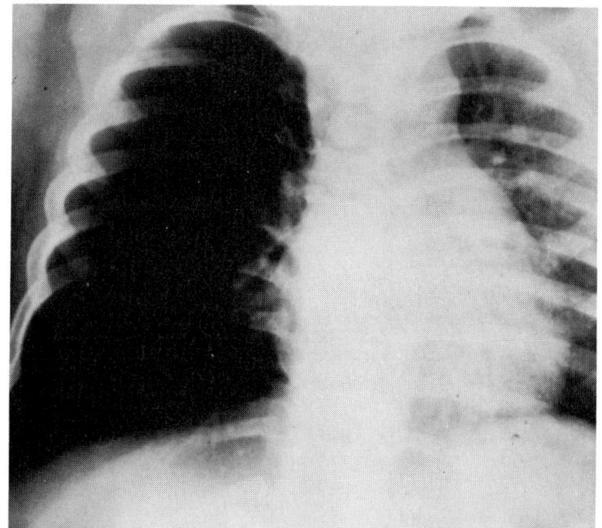

FIGURE 5–5. Foreign body in right main stem bronchus causing hyperaeration of the lung and shift of the mediastinum to the opposite side.

ANESTHETIC IMPLICATIONS

Biopsies of bronchial adenomas may lead to severe bleeding; the lesion, therefore, should be removed surgically. For tumors of the lung in children, the surgical procedure is relatively safe with a standard anesthetic approach to thoracotomy. The potential for postoperative pneumothorax should be monitored.

FOREIGN BODIES

Foreign body aspiration causes airway obstruction that may be life threatening. Frequently, the episode goes undetected, in which case it may result in severe lung damage. Children in the first 2 to 3 years of life are particularly prone to aspirate foreign objects. Sixty-five percent of food asphyxiation deaths occur in infants younger than 2 years of age.[211] Foreign body aspiration (of a balloon) has been reported even in a 3-month-old infant![212] Therefore, foreign body aspiration must be considered in all cases of sudden respiratory distress, regardless of age.

INTRABRONCHIAL FOREIGN BODIES

This is a common cause of respiratory illness in young children.[213–216] In two thirds of children, the diagnosis is made within the first few days. In a significant number, however, there is a considerable delay in making the diagnosis. Boys are involved more often than girls by a ratio of 2 to 1, with 80 percent of cases occurring in children under 4 years of age. The most common foreign bodies are peanuts, hot dogs, popcorn, grapes, and seeds. The most common site for the foreign body to lodge is in the right mainstem bronchus. Sharp foreign bodies such as pins impact in the larynx and produce symptoms of acute laryngeal edema. One should also suspect that a "foreign body aspiration" may be multiple foreign bodies.

CLINICAL PRESENTATION

The clinical picture is modified by the interval that has elapsed from the time of foreign body aspiration. With cases diagnosed within 24 hours, there is a history of a sudden episode of severe coughing and severe respiratory distress with cyanosis while the child is eating or playing with toys. Wheezing may be present. Suspicion of a foreign body aspiration should be aroused if a child without a history of wheezing suddenly begins to wheeze without obvious signs of respiratory infection. However, the classic triad of wheezing, coughing, and decreased breath sounds over the affected side is more common in the case diagnosed later. More often this diagnostic triad is incomplete.[217]

Chest roentgenography and fluoroscopy are useful diagnostic procedures. Note that the majority of aspirated foreign bodies are not radiopaque. One may see overinflation of the lung, which is partially obstructed (Fig. 5–5). As the air becomes absorbed, atelectasis develops (Fig. 5–6).

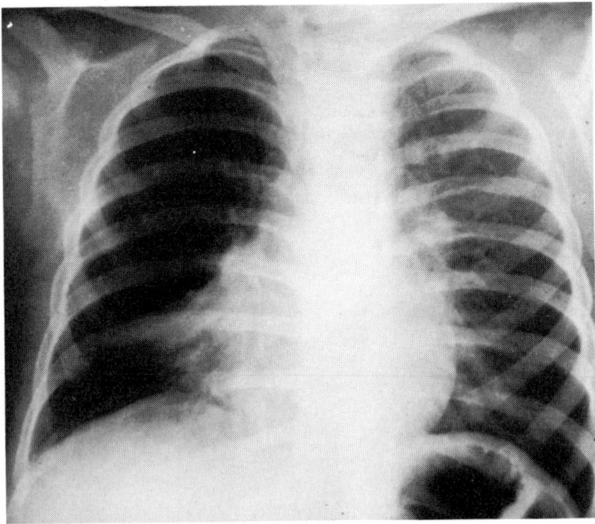

FIGURE 5–6. Foreign body in right main stem bronchus leading to right middle lobe collapse and right upper lobe overinflation.

If there has been delay in diagnosis, pneumonitis may be detected. Recurrent persistent localized pneumonitis that does not resolve with standard medical therapy should make one suspect an underlying foreign body. In one study, more than half the patients with aspirated foreign bodies were diagnosed many days after the event. *The anesthesiologist must appreciate that children who wheeze are not necessarily "asthmatic," and a foreign body aspiration may well be the underlying cause!*

Foreign bodies impacting on the esophagus, especially at sites of anatomical constriction, such as the postcricoid region and at the level of the aortic arch, may produce compression of the trachea and serious airway obstruction (Fig. 5–7).

Anesthetic Implications

The anesthesiologist should be familiar with emergency room measures to dislodge a foreign body that is producing a life-threatening crisis. Debate continues over the various maneuvers.[218] The Academy of Pediatrics and the American Heart Association recommend back blows followed by chest thrusts in those under 1 year of age. In infants, liver trauma is possible with abdominal thrusts, hence chest thrusts are preferred. Abdominal thrusts (Heimlich's maneuver) are advocated for children over 1 year of age.

Anesthesia and bronchoscopy for removal of the foreign body should be carried out by skilled personnel with appropriate equipment.[219] The Storz pediatric bronchoscope with the Hopkins' rod lens telescope provides excellent visualization of the foreign body and allows for the introduction of a forceps to remove it.[220, 221]

Preoperatively, narcotics and sedatives are avoided. The child is calmed to prevent dynamic

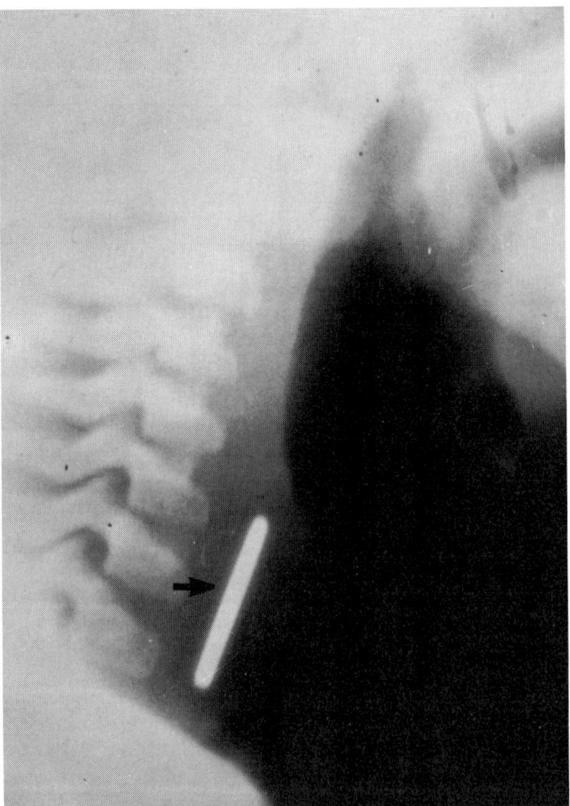

FIGURE 5–7. Coin in esophagus *(arrow)* impacting on trachea and causing airway obstruction.

collapse of the airway from agitation, which can cause further obstruction. Electrocardiographic monitoring and a precordial stethoscope are set up to monitor cardiac activity, and a pulse oximeter is placed to record continuous oxygen saturation.

Anesthesia is induced with halothane and oxygen with spontaneous respirations. Induction is slow because of airway obstruction and associated ventilation/perfusion imbalance. An intravenous line is placed when an analgesic level of anesthesia is achieved. Atropine is given intravenously to reduce the potential for bradycardia with laryngeal and tracheobronchial stimulation. During induction of anesthesia, ventilation is spontaneous unless it is apparent that hypoventilation, reflected in decreased movement of the chest or cardiac arrhythmias, is occurring. In this situation, ventilation must be assisted despite the theoretical risks of forcing the foreign body further down. Once the child is well anesthetized, the larynx and trachea may be sprayed with a local analgesic solution. The bronchoscope is then inserted, and ventilation continues via the bronchoscope connected to the anesthetic circuit; if necessary, ventilation can be controlled. Removal of the foreign body is usually accomplished with a forceps. On occasion, a Fogarty embolectomy balloon catheter is used to dislodge an impacted foreign body.[222] The catheter is pulled back, together with the bronchoscope, to the pharynx, from which the foreign body is removed. Very rarely, the foreign body, if deeply lodged in the bronchus, may have to be removed via a thoracotomy and bronchotomy.

In some situations following removal of the foreign body, the child may still have symptoms because of the presence of residual foreign material. Flexible fiberoptic bronchoscopy appears to be a useful technique in this situation to screen for possible residual foreign matter.[223]

Following a difficult removal of a foreign body, the child may have glottic and airway edema and require steroid therapy and racemic epinephrine inhalations. Early extraction through bronchoscopy will reduce local damage and distal parenchymal complications such as bronchiectasis and lung abscess. Extraction may be difficult with foreign bodies that crumble, such as peanuts; also, there may be an intense bronchial mucosa reaction (edema) to the peanut oil, making extraction difficult, thus necessitating bronchoscopy without delay when a peanut is the offending agent.

MEDIASTINUM

PNEUMOMEDIASTINUM

Pneumomediastinum is a collection of air in the mediastinum resulting from a pulmonary air leak. This most often follows trauma associated with the use of mechanical ventilation, or with severe asthmatic attacks. The air usually tracks to the superior mediastinum. Generally, the pneumomediastinum resolves spontaneously and does not produce significant pathophysiological effects. However, on rare occasions, large collections of air may produce circulatory tamponade, in which case urgent decompression is essential.

Pneumomediastinum may predispose to intracranial hypertension from interference with venous drainage from the head. Intracranial hypertension refractory to therapy until the pneumomediastinum was decompressed by the placement of a mediastinal tube has been reported.[224]

MEDIASTINAL MASSES

Masses may occur in the anterior, middle, or posterior mediastinum, and their diagnosis is related to their anatomical position. The anesthesiologist is particularly concerned with the effect of mediastinal masses on the airways, lungs, and cardiovascular system.

Anterior mediastinal masses commonly are lymphoma, teratoma, cystic hygroma, thymoma, pericardial cysts, and diaphragmatic hernia (through the foramen of Morgagni). Middle mediastinal masses are lymphoma and those found in tuberculous glands. Posterior mediastinal masses are neurogenic tumors, esophageal duplication cysts, and diaphragmatic hernia (through the foramen of Bochdalek).

Of importance to the anesthesiologist is the recognition that anesthesia in these patients is potentially hazardous and that thorough investigation and preparation are therefore mandatory.

Anterior Mediastinum. Most anterior mediastinal masses are lymphomatous in origin (Hodgkin's and non-Hodgkin's lymphoma). It is important to appreciate that cervical masses—for example, cystic hygroma—may have a deep extension into the mediastinum. Mediastinal masses may go unsuspected and be found on a routine chest roentgenogram.

Clinical signs and symptoms related to anterior mediastinal masses include cough (especially in the supine position), superior vena caval obstruction, stridor, wheezing, chest retractions, and cardiac compression producing tamponade.

Keon described a 9-year-old child undergoing a cervical node biopsy who sustained a cardiopulmonary arrest during induction of anesthesia and in whom efforts at resuscitation were unsuccessful. Autopsy revealed a massive malignant lymphoma in the anterior mediastinum that enveloped the heart with infiltration of the pericardium, producing a pericardial tamponade effect.[225]

Posterior Mediastinum. Posterior mediastinal masses—for example, an esophageal duplication cyst—may cause respiratory distress through encroachment on pulmonary reserve. In addition, compression of the esophagus leads to dysphagia and the possibility of reflux and aspiration on induction of anesthesia.

In some situations, symptoms are attributed to more benign conditions. An 8-year-old child was referred with severe dyspnea and wheezing unresponsive to treatment with antispasmodic medications. Investigation disclosed the child to have a large mediastinal mass (neurogenic tumor) obstructing the airway (Fig. 5–8).

Anesthetic Implications

Children with mediastinal masses are at significant risk during anesthesia because tracheal or bronchial obstruction may occur quite unexpectedly.[226–228] Also, compression of the great vessels of the heart may lead to a critical fall in cardiac output.[229–233] Some mediastinal tumors are particularly radiosensitive, e.g., lymphomas; therefore, it has generally been advised that radiotherapy treatment prior to any surgical procedure be carried out to lessen preoperative risks. However, irradiation of the tumor distorts the cellular picture and interferes with making a clear histological diagnosis. Hence, a practice of general anesthesia prior to irradiation of anterior mediastinal masses has been proposed even in the presence of respiratory or cardiovascular symptoms.[232]

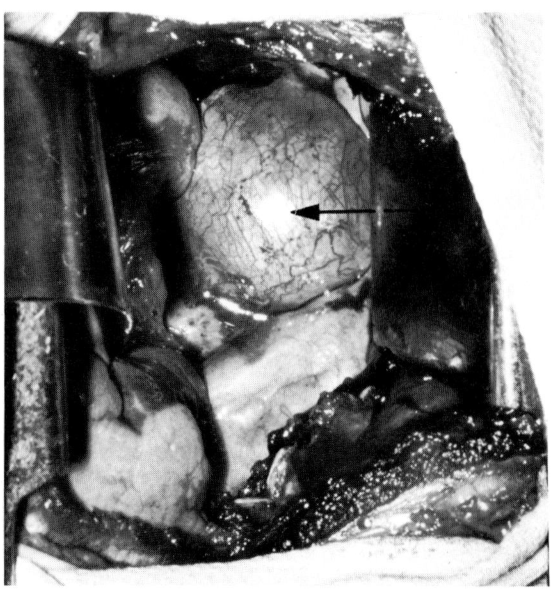

FIGURE 5–8. Neurogenic cyst exposed at thoracotomy. Airway compression gave rise to symptoms suggestive of "asthma." (Courtesy of Samuel Kim, M.D.)

Preoperative preparation of the child with a mediastinal mass focuses on (1) evaluation of the degree of airway obstruction, and (2) possible cardiovascular compromise. A history of orthopnea is ominous. In addition to clinical evaluation of airway patency and hemodynamic stability, other special studies are carried out. Roentgenography of the airway might include tomography and fluoroscopy. CT scans of the airway also provide better definition of any obstruction. Pulmonary flow volume loop studies, in both the upright and supine positions, provide sensitive indicators of obstructive lesions of the major airways. The peak flow rate may show a significant decrease even when the CT scan has revealed no airway obstruction.

In evaluating hemodynamic stability, the possibility of cardiac tamponade must be considered; thus, it is important to examine for pulsus paradoxus. Echocardiography is also performed with the patient in the upright and supine positions. Barium swallow examinations are performed in selected cases.

The position for induction of anesthesia must be one that produces the least cardiopulmonary compromise; this usually means having the child propped up. Drugs for resuscitation should be immediately available because of the high risks associated with induction of anesthesia. A rigid bronchoscope should be at hand. For this reason, too, the surgical team should be present at this time to assist in any crisis that may develop. Induction of anesthesia is best carried out under spontaneous ventilation, and assisted ventilation is performed should this become necessary. Muscle relaxants are best avoided at this time.

Local anesthesia for the biopsy procedure should be used in preference to general anesthesia if this is suitable in the particular patient. In rare situations, standby cardiopulmonary bypass equipment is necessary. Thoracotomy is usually necessary to make the specific diagnosis.

Excision of the entire mediastinal mass is undertaken if this is possible. Note that the extent of the pathology and its location may predispose to significant blood loss with excision.

If serious airway obstruction appears on induction of anesthesia or during maintenance, it is prudent to leave the child intubated in the pediatric ICU pending appropriate radiotherapy and chemotherapy. Following treatment, the airway obstruction will be relieved and the child should be safely extubated.

REFERENCES

1. Reid L: The lung: Its growth and remodeling in health and disease. AJR *129*:777, 1977.
2. Reid L: The pulmonary circulation: Remodeling in growth and disease. Am Rev Respir Dis *119*:531, 1979.
3. Reid L: Lung growth in health and disease. Br J Dis Chest *78*:113, 1984.
4. Hislop A, Reid L: Growth and development of the respiratory system—anatomical development. *In* Davies J, Dobbin J (eds): Scientific Foundations of Paediatrics. London, Heinemann, 1974, pp 214–253.
5. Alcorn D, Adamson TM, Lambert TF, et al: Effects of chronic tracheal ligation and drainage on the fetal lamb lung. J Anat *123*:649, 1977.
6. Brown MJ, Oliver RE, Ramsden CA, et al: Effects of adrenaline infusion and of spontaneous labor on lung liquid secretion and absorption in the fetal lamb. J Physiol *313*:13, 1981.
7. Boddy K, Davies GS: Fetal breathing. Br Med Bull *31*:3, 1975.
8. Thurlbeck WM: Postnatal growth of the lung. Am Rev Respir Dis *111*:803, 1975.
9. Hislop A, Reid L: Development of the acinus in the human lung. Thorax *29*:90, 1974.
10. Langston C, Kida K, Reed M, et al: Human lung growth in late gestation and in the neonate. Am Rev Respir Dis *129*:607, 1984.
11. Hislow A, Wigglesworth JS, Desai R: Alveolar development in the human fetus and infant. Early Hum Dev *13*:1, 1986.
12. Wohl MEB, Briscom MT, Traggis DG, et al: Effects of therapeutic irradiation delivered in early childhood upon subsequent lung function. Pediatrics *55*:507–516, 1975.
13. McBride J, Wohl ME, Streider DJ, et al: Lung growth and airway function after lobectomy for congenital lobar emphysema. J Clin Invest *66*:962, 1980.
14. Davies P, McBride J, Murray GF, et al: Structural changes in canine lung and pulmonary arteries after pneumonectomy. J Appl Physiol *53*:859, 1982.
15. Thurlbeck WM, Galaugher W, Mathers J: Adaptive response to pneumonectomy in puppies. Thorax *36*:424, 1981.
16. Sbokos CG, McMillan IKR: Agenesis of the lung. Br J Dis Chest *71*:183, 1977.
17. Borja AR, Ransdell HT, Villa S: Congenital developmental arrest of the lung. Ann Thorac Surg *10*:317, 1970.
18. McCormick TL, Kuhns LR: Tracheal compression by a normal aorta associated with right lung agenesis. Radiology *130*:659, 1979.
19. Maltz DL, Nadas AS: Agenesis of the lung: Presentation of eight new cases and review of the literature. Pediatrics *42*:175, 1968.
20. Nimrod C, Varela-Gittings G, Machin G, et al: The effect of very prolonged membrane rupture on fetal development. Am J Obstet Gynecol *148*:540, 1984.
21. Knox WF, Barzon AJ: Pulmonary hypoplasia in a regional perinatal unit. Early Hum Dev *14*:33, 1986.
22. Messinger AC, Fox HE, Higgin A, et al: Fetal breath movements are not a reliable indication of continued lung development in pregnancies complicated by oligohydramnios. Lancet *2*:1297, 1987.
23. Hislop A, Hey E, Reid L: The lungs in congenital bilateral renal agenesis and dysplasia. Arch Dis Child *54*:32, 1979.
24. Jue KL, Amplatz K, Adams P Jr, et al: Anomalies of great vessels associated with lung hypoplasia. The scimitar syndrome. Am J Dis Child *111*:35, 1966.
25. Partridge JB, Osborne JM, Slaughter RE: Scimitar etcetera. The dysmorphic right lung. Clin Radiol *39*:11, 1988.
26. Orzam F, Angelini P, Oglieth J, et al: Horseshoe lung: Report of two cases. Am Heart J *93*:501, 1977.
27. Buntain WC, Woolley MD, Mahour GH, et al: Pulmonary sequestration in children. A twenty-five year experience. Surgery *81*:413, 1977.
28. Khalik KG, Kilman JW: Pulmonary sequestration. J Thorac Cardiovasc Surg *70*:938, 1975.
29. Savic G, Birtel FJ, Tholen W, et al: Lung sequestration: Report of seven cases and review of 540 published cases. Thorax *34*:96, 1979.
30. Levine MM, Nudel DV, Gootman N, et al: Pulmonary sequestration causing congestive heart failure in infancy. A report of two cases and review of literature. Ann Thorac Surg *34*:581, 1982.
31. Luck SR, Reynolds M, Raffensperger JG: Congenital bronchopulmonary malformation. Curr Prob Surg *23*:250, 1986.
32. Black MD, Bass J, Martin DJ, et al: Intraabdominal pulmonary sequestration. J Pediatr Surg *26*:1381, 1991.
33. Heifhoff KG, Sane SM, Williams HJ, et al: Bronchopulmonary foregut malformations. A unifying etiological concept. Am J Roentgenol *126*:46, 1976.
34. Stocker JT, Kagan-Hallet K: Extralobar pulmonary sequestration. Analysis of 15 cases and review of 540 published cases. Am J Clin Pathol *72*:917, 1979.
35. Lewis JE, Murray RE: Pulmonary sequestration with bronchoesophageal fistula. J Pediatr Surg *3*:575, 1968.
36. Ransom JM, Norton JB, Williams GD: Pulmonary sequestration presenting as congestive failure. J Thorac Surg 7:68, 1969.
37. Mariona F, McAlpin G, Zador I, et al: Sonographic detection of fetal extrathoracic pulmonary sequestration. J Ultrasound Med *5*:283, 1986.
38. Bientain WL, Isaacs H, Payne VC, et al: Lobar emphysema, cystic adenomatoid malformation, pulmonary sequestration, and bronchogenic cysts in infancy and childhood: A clinical group. J Pediatr Surg *70*:260, 1975.
39. Demos NJ, Teresi A: Congenital lung malformation, a unified concept and a case report. J Thorac Cardiovasc Surg *70*:260, 1975.
40. Crawford TJ, Cahill JJ: The surgical treatment of pulmonary cystic disorders in infancy and childhood. J Pediatr Surg *6*:251, 1971.
41. Leape LL, Longine LA: Infantile lobar emphysema. Pediatrics *34*:246, 1964.
42. McBride JT, Wohl ME, Strieder DJ, et al: Lung growth and airway function after lobectomy in infancy for congenital lobar emphysema. J Clin Invest *66*:962, 1980.

43. Eigen H, Lemon RJ, Waring WW: Congenital lobar emphysema: Long-term evaluation of surgically and conservatively treated children. Am Rev Respir Dis *113*:823, 1976.
44. Cote CJ: Anesthetic management of congenital lobar emphysema. Anesthesiology *49*:296, 1974.
45. Stocker JT, Madewell JE, Drake RM: Congenital cystic adenomatoid malformation of the lung. Classification and morphologic spectrum. Hum Pathol *8*:155, 1977.
46. Adzick NS, Harrison MR, Glick PL, et al: Fetal cystic adenomatoid malformation: Prenatal diagnosis and natural history. J Pediatr Surg *20*:483, 1985.
47. Freckner B, Freyschuss U: Pulmonary function after lobectomy for congenital lobar emphysema and congenital cystic adenomatoid malformation: A follow-up study. Scand J Thorac Cardiovasc Surg *16*:293, 1982.
48. Neilson IR, Russo P, Laberge J-M, et al: Congenital adenomatoid malformation of the lung: Current management and prognosis. J Pediatr Surg *26*:975, 1991.
49. Wesley JR, Heidelberger KP, DiPietro MA, et al: Diagnosis and management of congenital cystic disease of the lungs in children. J Pediatr Surg *21*:202, 1986.
50. Eraklis AJ, Grisom NT, McGovern JB: Bronchogenic cysts of the mediastinum in infancy. N Engl J Med *281*:1150, 1969.
51. Bensoussan AL, Braun P, Guttman FM: Bilateral spontaneous chylothorax of the newborn. Arch Surg *110*:1243, 1975.
52. Kumar SP, Belik J: Chylothorax—a complication of chest-tube placement in a neonate. Crit Care Med *12*:411, 1984.
53. Van Aerde J, Campbell AN, Smyth JA, et al: Spontaneous chylothorax in newborns. Am J Dis Child *138*:961, 1984.
54. Siegler RL, Pearce MB: Metabolic acidosis from loss of thoracic lymph. J Pediatr *93*:465, 1978.
55. Hargus EP, Carson SC, McGrath RL, et al: Chylothorax and chylopericardial tamponade following Blalock-Taussig anastomosis. J Thorac Cardiovasc Surg *75*:642, 1978.
56. Seiber JJ, Golladay ES, Keller C: Chylothorax secondary to superior vena cava obstruction. Pediatr Radiol *12*:252, 1982.
57. Ducharme JC, Belanger R, Simard P, et al: Chylothorax, chylopericardium with multiple lymphangioma of bone. J Pediatr Surg *17*:365, 1982.
58. Brodman RF: Congenital chylothorax: Recommendations for treatment. NY State J Med *75*:553, 1975.
59. Stringel G, Mercer S, Bass J: Surgical management of persistent postoperative chylothorax in children. Can J Surg *27*:543, 1984.
60. Allen EM, von Heeckeren DN, Spector ML, et al: Management of nutritional and infectious complications of postoperative chylothorax in children. J Pediatr Surg *26*:1169, 1991.
61. Johnson DC, Cartmill TB: Low thoracic duct ligation for postoperative chylous effusions in infants and children. Aust NZ J Surg *47*:94, 1977.
62. Milson JW, Kron IL, Rheuban KS, et al: Chylothorax: An assessment of current surgical management. J Thorac Cardiovasc Surg *89*:221, 1985.
63. Greenwood RD, Rosenthal A: Cardiovascular malformations associated with tracheoesophageal fistula and esophageal atresia. Pediatrics *57*:87, 1976.
64. Spitz L, Ali N, Brereton RJ: Combined esophageal and duodenal atresia: Experience in 18 patients. J Pediatr Surg *16*:4, 1981.
65. Benjamin B, Cohen D, Glasson M: Tracheomalacia in association with congenital tracheoesophageal fistula. Surgery *79*:504, 1976.
66. Davies MRG, Cywes S: The flaccid trachea and tracheoesophageal congenital anomalies. J Pediatr Surg *13*:363, 1978.
67. Iko T, Sugito T, Nagaya M: Delayed primary anastomosis in poor-risk patients with esophageal atresia associated with tracheoesophageal fistula. J Pediatr Surg *19*:243, 1984.
68. Holmes SJK, Kiely EM, Spitz L: Tracheo-esophageal fistula and the respiratory distress syndrome. Pediatr Surg Int *2*:16, 1987.
69. Karl HW: Control of life-threatening air leak after gastrostomy in an infant with respiratory distress syndrome and tracheoesophageal fistula. Anesthesiology *62*:670, 1985.
70. Filston HC, Chitwood WR, Schkolne B, et al: The Fogarty balloon catheter as an aid to management of the infant with esophageal atresia and tracheoesophageal fistula complicated by severe RDS or pneumonia. J Pediatr Surg *17*:149, 1982.
71. Beasley SW, Myers NA, Auldist AW: Management of the premature infant with esophageal atresia and hyaline membrane disease. J Pediatr Surg *27*:23, 1992.
72. Calverley RK, Johnston AE: The anesthetic management of tracheoesophageal fistula: A review of 10 years' experience. Can Anaesth Soc J *19*:270, 1972.
73. Jones TB, Kirchner SG, Lee FA, et al: Stomach rupture associated with esophageal atresia, tracheoesophageal fistula and ventilatory assistance. Am J Radiol *134*:675, 1980.
74. Salem MR, Wong AY, Lin YH, et al: Prevention of gastric distension during anesthesia for newborns with tracheoesophageal fistulas. Anesthesiology *38*:82, 1973.
75. Filler RM, Rossello PJ, Lebowitz RL: Life-threatening anoxic spells caused by tracheal compression after repair of esophageal atresia: Correction by surgery. J Pediatr Surg *11*:739, 1976.
76. Kafrouni G, Baick CH, Woolley MM: Recurrent tracheoesophageal fistula: A diagnostic problem. Surgery *68*:889, 1970.
77. Chittmittrapap S, Spitz L, Kiely EM, et al: Anastomotic leakage following surgery for esophageal atresia. J Pediatr Surg *27*:29, 1992.
78. Pieretti R, Shandling B, Stephens CA: Resistant esophageal stenosis associated with reflux after repair of esophageal atresia: A therapeutic approach. J Pediatr Surg *9*:355, 1974.
79. Schwartz MZ, Filler RM: Tracheal compression as a cause of apnea following repair of tracheoesophageal fistula: Treatment by aortopexy. J Pediatr Surg *15*:842, 1980.
80. Duranceau A, Fisher SR, Flye MW, et al: Motor function of the esophagus after repair of esophageal atresia and tracheoesophageal fistula. Surgery *82*:116, 1977.
81. Koop CD, Schnaufer L, Broennle AM: Esophageal atresia and tracheoesophageal fistula. Supportive measures that affect survival. Pediatrics *54*:558, 1974.
82. Milligan DWA, Levison H: Lung function in children following repair of tracheoesophageal fistula. J Pediatr *95*:24, 1979.
83. Benjamin B, Pham T: Diagnosis of H-type tracheoesophageal fistula. J Pediatr Surg *26*:667, 1991.
84. Ryan DP, Muehvcke DD, Doody DP, et al: Laryngotracheoesophageal cleft (type IV): Management and repair of lesions beyond the carina. J Pediatr Surg *26*:962, 1991.
85. Donahoe PK, Gee PE: Complete laryngotracheoesophageal cleft: Management and repair. J Pediatr Surg *19*:143, 1984.

86. Felman AH, Talbert JL: Laryngotracheoesophageal cleft. Radiology *103*:641, 1972.
87. Donahoe PK, Hendren WH: The surgical management of laryngotracheoesophageal cleft with tracheoesophageal fistula and esophageal atresia. Surgery *73*:363, 1972.
88. Cotton RT, Schreiber JT: Management of laryngotracheoesophageal cleft. Ann Otol Rhinol Laryngol *90*:401, 1981.
89. Ruder CB, Glaser LC: Anesthetic management of laryngotracheoesophageal cleft. Anesthesiology *47*:65, 1977.
90. Hendren WH: Repair of laryngotracheoesophageal cleft using interposition of a strap muscle. J Pediatr Surg *11*:425, 1976.
91. Cotton RT: Pediatric laryngotracheal stenosis. J Pediatr Surg *19*:699, 1984.
92. Benjamin B, Pitkin J, Cohen D: Congenital tracheal stenosis. Ann Otol Rhinol Laryngol *90*:364, 1981.
93. Loeff DS, Filler RM, Vinograd I, et al: Congenital tracheal stenosis: A review of 22 patients from 1965–1987. J Pediatr Surg *23*:74, 1988.
94. Lobe TE, Hayden CK, Nicolas D, et al: Successful management of congenital tracheal stenosis in infancy. J Pediatr Surg *22*:1137, 1987.
95. Smith RJ, Smith MC, Glossop LP, et al: Congenital vascular anomalies causing tracheoesophageal compression. Arch Otolaryngol *110*:82, 1984.
96. Welz A, Reichert B, Weinhold C, et al: Innominate artery compression of the trachea in infancy and childhood: Is surgical therapy justified? Thorac Cardiovasc Surg *32*:85, 1984.
97. Berdon WE, Baker DH, Wung JT: Complete cartilage-ring tracheal stenosis associated with anomalous left pulmonary artery: The ring-sling complex. Radiology *152*:57, 1984.
98. Grillo HC, Zannini P: Management of obstructive tracheal disease in children. J Pediatr Surg *19*:414, 1984.
99. Clarkson WB, Davies JR: Anesthesia for cranial resection. Anesthesia *33*:815, 1978.
100. Ellis RH, Hinds CJ, Gadd LT: Management of anesthesia during tracheal resection. Anesthesia *31*:1076, 1976.
101. Geffin B, Bland J, Grillo HC: Anesthetic management of tracheal resection and reconstruction. Anesth Analg *48*:844, 1969.
102. Lee P, English ICW: Management of anesthesia during tracheal resection. Anesthesia *29*:305, 1974.
103. Wilson RS: Tracheostomy and tracheal reconstruction. *In* Kaplan JA (ed): Thoracic Anesthesia. New York, Churchill Livingstone, 1983, pp 426–445.
104. Neuman GG, Asher AS, Stern SB, et al: High-frequency jet ventilation for tracheal resection in a child. Anesth Analg *63*:1039, 1984.
105. Ein SH, Friedberg J, Williams WG, et al: Tracheoplasty—A new operation for complete congenital tracheal stenosis. J Pediatr Surg *17*:872, 1982.
106. Campbell DN, Lilly JR: Surgery for total congenital tracheal stenosis. J Pediatr Surg *21*:934, 1986.
107. Sorensen HR, Holsteen V: Resection of congenital stenosis of the trachea in an infant. Acta Paediatr Scand *73*:141, 1984.
108. Cohen RC, Filler RM, Konuma K, et al: The successful reconstruction of thoracic tracheal defects with free periosteal grafts. J Pediatr Surg *20*:852, 1985.
109. Idriss FS, DeLeon SY, Ilbawi MN, et al: Tracheoplasty with pericardial patch for extensive tracheal stenosis in infants and children. J Thorac Cardiovasc Surg *88*:527, 1984.
110. Bagwell CE, Talbert JL, Tepas JJ: Balloon dilatation of long-segment tracheal stenosis. J Pediatr Surg *26*:153, 1991.
111. Benjamin B: Endoscopy in congenital tracheal abnormalities. J Pediatr Surg *15*:164, 1980.
112. Holinger PH, Schild JA, Weprin L: Pediatric laryngology. Otolaryngol Clin North Am *3*:625, 1970.
113. Hollinger LD: Etiology of stridor in the neonate, infant and child. Ann Otol Rhinol Laryngol *89*:397, 1980.
114. Wailoo MP, Emery JL: The trachea in children with tracheoesophageal fistula. Histopathology *3*:329, 1979.
115. Roesler N, DeLeval M, Chrispin AR, et al: Surgical management of vascular ring. Ann Surg *197*:139, 1983.
116. Westby S, Dinwiddie R, Chrispin AR: Pulmonary artery sling in identical twins. Thorac Cardiovasc Surg *32*:182, 1984.
117. Filler RM, Buck JR, Bahoric A, et al: Treatment of segmental tracheomalacia and bronchomalacia by implantation of an airway splint. J Pediatr Surg *17*:597, 1982.
118. Koloske AM: Left mainstem bronchopexy for severe bronchomalacia. J Pediatr Surg *26*:260, 1991.
119. Conti VR, Lobe TE: Vascular string with tracheomalacia: Surgical management. Ann Thorac Surg *47*:310, 1989.
120. Blair GK, Cohen R, Filler RM: Treatment of tracheomalacia: Eight years' experience. J Pediatr Surg *21*:781, 1986.
121. Vinograd I, Filler RM, Bahoric A: Long-term functional results of prosthetic airway splinting in tracheomalacia and bronchomalacia. J Pediatr Surg *22*:38, 1987.
122. Hernandez-Cano AM, Lilly JR: Wedge tracheoplasty in infants. Surg Gynecol Obstet *165*:277, 1987.
123. Wiseman NE, Duncan PG, Cameron CB: Management of tracheobronchomalacia with continuous positive airway pressure. J Pediatr Surg *20*:489, 1985.
124. Reynolds M, Luck S, Lappen R: The "critical" neonate with diaphragmatic hernia: A 21 year perspective. J Pediatr Surg *19*:364, 1984.
125. Nguyen L, Guttman FM, De Chadarevian JP, et al: The mortality of congenital diaphragmatic hernia. Is total pulmonary mass inadequate, no matter what? Ann Surg *198*:666, 1983.
126. Bohn DJ, James I, Filler RM, et al: The relationship between $PaCO_2$ and ventilation parameters in predicting survival in congenital diaphragmatic hernia. J Pediatr Surg *19*:666, 1984.
127. Hansen F, James S, Burrington J, et al: The decreasing incidence of pneumothorax and improving survival of infants with congenital diaphragmatic hernia. J Pediatr Surg *19*:383, 1984.
128. Bartlett RH, Gazzaniga AB, Toomasian J, et al: Extracorporeal membrane oxygenation (ECMO) in neonatal respiratory failure: 100 cases. Ann Surg *204*:236, 1986.
129. Sakai H, Tamura M, Hosokawa Y, et al: Effect of surgical repair on respiratory mechanics in congenital diaphragmatic hernia. J Pediatr *111*:432, 1987.
130. Cartlidge PHT, Mann NP, Kapila L: Preoperative stabilization in congenital diaphragmatic hernia. Arch Dis Child *61*:1226, 1986.
131. Langer JC, Filler RM, Bohn DJ, et al: Timing of surgery for congenital diaphragmatic hernia. Is emergency surgery necessary? J Pediatr Surg *23*:731, 1988.
132. Breaux CW, Rouse TM, Cain WS, et al: Improvement in survival of patients with congenital diaphragmatic hernia, utilizing a strategy of delayed repair after medical and/or extracorporeal membrane oxygenation stabilization. J Pediatr Surg *26*:333, 1991.

133. Wilson JM, Lund DP, Lillehei CW, et al: Congenital diaphragmatic hernia: Predictors of severity in the ECMO era. J Pediatr Surg *26*:1028, 1991.
134. Haugen SE, Linker S, Eik-Nes S, et al: Congenital diaphragmatic hernia: Determination of the optimal time for operation by echocardiographic monitoring of the pulmonary arterial pressure. J Pediatr Surg *26*:560, 1991.
135. Boz AP, Tibboel D, Hazelrock FWJ, et al: Congenital diaphragmatic hernia: The impact of prostanoids on the perioperative period. Arch Dis Child *65*:994, 1990.
136. Wilson JM, Lund DP, Lillehei CW, et al: Delayed repair and preoperative ECMO does not improve survival in high-risk congenital diaphragmatic hernia. J Pediatr Surg *27*:368, 1992.
137. Stolar CJH, Snedecor SM, Bartlett RH: Extracorporeal membrane oxygenation and neonatal respiratory failure: Experience for its extracorporeal life support organization. J Pediatr Surg *26*:563, 1991.
138. Rudolph AM, Yuan S: Response of the pulmonary vasculature to hypoxia and H^+ ion concentration changes. J Clin Invest *45*:399, 1966.
139. Vacanti JP, Crone RK, Murphy JD, et al: The pulmonary hemodynamic response to perioperative anesthesia in the treatment of high-risk infants with congenital diaphragmatic hernia. J Pediatr Surg *19*:672, 1984.
140. Drummond WH, Gregory GA, Heymann MA, et al: The independent effects of hyperventilation, tolazoline, and dopamine on infants with persistent pulmonary hypertension. J Pediatr *98*:603, 1981.
141. Ford WD, James MJ, Walsh JA: Congenital diaphragmatic hernia: Association between pulmonary vascular resistance and plasma thromboxane concentrations. Arch Dis Child *59*:143, 1984.
142. Bartlett RH, Roloff DW, Cornell RD, et al: Extracorporeal circulation in neonatal respiratory failure: A prospective randomized study. Pediatrics *76*:479, 1985.
143. O'Rourke PP, Lillehei CW, Crone RK, et al: The effect of extracorporeal membrane oxygenation in the survival of neonates with high-risk congenital diaphragmatic hernia: 45 cases from a single institution. J Pediatr Surg *26*:147, 1991.
144. Freyschuss U, Lannergren K, Freckner B: Lung function after repair of congenital diaphragmatic hernia. Acta Paediatr Scand *73*:589, 1984.
145. Bishop HC, Koop CE: Acquired eventration of the diaphragm in infancy. Pediatrics *22*:1088, 1958.
146. Othersen HB, Lorenzo RL: Diaphragmatic paralysis and eventration: New approaches to diagnosis and operative correction. J Pediatr Surg *12*:309, 1977.
147. McElwee TB, Myers RT, Pennell TC: Diaphragmatic rupture from blunt trauma. Am Surg *50*:143, 1984.
148. Sharma LK, Kennedy RF, Heneghan WD: Rupture of the diaphragm resulting from blunt trauma in children. Can J Surg *20*:553, 1977.
149. Eichenwald HF: Pneumonia syndromes in children. Hosp Pract *2*:89, 1976.
150. Webber S, Wilkinson AR, Lindsell D, et al: Neonatal pneumonia. Arch Dis Child *65*:207, 1989.
151. Evans ME, Schaffner W, Federspiel CF: Sensitivity, specificity, and predictive value of body surface cultures on a neonatal intensive care unit. JAMA *259*:248, 1988.
152. Murphy TH, Henderson FW, Clyde WA, et al: Pneumonia: An eleven-year study in a pediatric practice. Am J Epidemiol *113*:12, 1981.
153. Rettig PJ: Infection due to *Chlamydia trachomatis* from infancy to adolescence. Pediatr Infect Dis *5*:449, 1986.
154. Turner RB, Lande AE, Chase P, et al: Pneumonia in pediatric outpatients: Causes and clinical manifestations. J Pediatr *111*:194, 1987.
155. Broughlan RA: Infections due to mycoplasma pneumonia in childhood. Pediatr Infect Dis *5*:71, 1986.
156. Chartrand SA, McCracken GH Jr: Staphylococcal pneumonia in infants and children. Pediatr Infect Dis *1*:19, 1982.
157. Brook I, Finegold SM: Bacteriology of aspiration pneumonia in children. Pediatrics *65*:1115, 1980.
158. Imoke E, Dudgeon DL, Colombani P, et al: Open lung biopsy in the immunocompromised pediatric patient. J Pediatr Surg *18*:816, 1983.
159. Prober CG, Whyte H, Smith CR: Open lung biopsy in immunocompromised children with pulmonary infiltrates. Am J Dis Child *138*:60, 1984.
160. Leijala M, Louhimo I, Lindfors EL: Open lung biopsy in children with diffuse pulmonary lesions. Acta Paediatr Scand *71*:717, 1982.
161. Janik JS, Nagaraj HS, Groff DB: Thoracoscopic evaluation of intrathoracic lesions in children. J Thorac Cardiovasc Surg *83*:408, 1982.
162. McLaughlin FJ, Goldmann DA, Rosenbaum DM, et al: Empyema in children: Clinical course and long-term follow up. Pediatrics *73*:587, 1984.
163. Stark DD, Federle MP, Goodman PC, et al: Differentiating lung abscess and empyema: Radiography and computed tomography. AJR *141*:163, 1983.
164. Asher MI, Spier S, Beland M, et al: Primary lung abscess in childhood. The long-term outcome of conservative management. Am J Dis Child *136*:491, 1982.
165. Kerem B, Rommens JM, Buchanan JA, et al: Identification of the cystic fibrosis gene: Genetic analysis. Science *245*:1073, 1989.
166. Wilmott RW, Tyson SL, Dinwiddie R, et al: Survival rates in cystic fibrosis. Arch Dis Child *58*:835, 1983.
167. Hunt B, Geddes DM: Newly diagnosed cystic fibrosis in middle and later life. Thorax *40*:23, 1985.
168. Gibson LE, Cooke RE: A test for the concentration of electrolytes in sweat in cystic fibrosis of the pancreas utilizing pilocarpine by iontophoresis. Pediatrics *23*:545, 1959.
169. Isles A, Maclusky I, Corey M, et al: *Pseudomonas cepacia* infection in cystic fibrosis: An emerging problem. J Pediatr *104*:206, 1984.
170. Lester LA, Egge A, Hubbard VS, et al: Aspiration and lung abscess in cystic fibrosis. Am Rev Respir Dis *127*:786, 1983.
171. Wang EEL, Prober CG, Manson B, et al: Association of respiratory viral infections with pulmonary deterioration in patients with cystic fibrosis. N Engl J Med *311*:165, 1984.
172. di Sant'Agnese PA, David PB: Cystic fibrosis in adults; 75 cases and a review of 232 cases in the literature. Am J Med *66*:121, 1979.
173. Schuster SR, Fellows KE: Management of major hemoptysis in patients with cystic fibrosis. J Pediatr Surg *12*:889, 1977.
174. Swersky RB, Chang JB, Wisoff BG, et al: Endobronchial balloon tamponade of hemoptysis in patients with cystic fibrosis. Ann Thorac Surg *27*:162, 1979.
175. Gurwitz D, Corey M, Francis PWJ, et al: Perspectives in cystic fibrosis. Pediatr Clin North Am *26*:603, 1979.
176. Corey M, Levison R, Crozier D: Five- to seven-year course of pulmonary function in cystic fibrosis. Am Rev Respir Dis *114*:1085, 1976.
177. Abman SH, Ogle HW, Butler-Simon N, et al: Role of respiratory syncytial virus in early hospitalization for

respiratory distress of young infants with cystic fibrosis. J Pediatr *113*:826, 1988.

178. Park RW, Grand RJ: Gastrointestinal manifestation of cystic fibrosis: A review. Gastroenterology *81*:1143, 1981.
179. Drake-Lee AB, Pitcher-Wilmott RW: The clinical and laboratory correlates of nasal polyps in cystic fibrosis. Int J Ped Otorhinolaryngol *4*:209, 1982.
180. Moss AJ: The cardiovascular system in cystic fibrosis. Pediatrics *70*:728, 1982.
181. Rossman CM, Waldes R, Sampson D, et al: Effect of chest physiotherapy on the removal of mucus in patients with cystic fibrosis. Am Rev Respir Dis *126*:131, 1982.
182. Slutton PP, Lopez-Vidriero M, Pavia D, et al: Effect of chest physiotherapy on the removal of mucus in patients with cystic fibrosis. Am Rev Respir Dis *127*:390, 1983.
183. Auerbach HS, Williams M, Kirkpatrick JA, et al: Alternate-day prednisolone reduces morbidity and improves pulmonary function in cystic fibrosis. Lancet *2*:686, 1985.
184. Fellows KE, Khaw KT, Schuster S, et al: Bronchial artery embolization in cystic fibrosis. Technique and long-term results. J Pediatr *95*:959, 1979.
185. Fellows KE, Stigol L, Shuster S, et al: Selective bronchial arteriography in patients with cystic fibrosis and massive hemoptysis. Radiology *114*:551, 1975.
186. Marmon L, Schidlow D, Palmer J, et al: Pulmonary resection for complications of cystic fibrosis. J Pediatr Surg *18*:811, 1983.
187. Lamberty JM, Rubin BK: The management of anesthesia for patients with cystic fibrosis. Anaesthesia *40*:448, 1985.
188. Eger EI, Saidman LJ: Hazards of nitrous oxide anesthesia in bowel obstruction and pneumothorax. Anesthesiology *26*:61, 1965.
189. Schuster SR, McLaughlin FJ, Mathews WJ Jr, et al: Management of pneumothorax in cystic fibrosis. J Pediatr Surg *18*:492, 1983.
190. Smith MB, Harden WD, Dressel DA, et al: Predicting outcome following pulmonary resection in cystic fibrosis patients. J Pediatr Surg *26*:655, 1991.
191. MacDonald NE, Anas NS, Peterson RG, et al: Renal clearance of gentamicin in cystic fibrosis. J Pediatr *103*:985, 1983.
192. Lewiston NJ: Bronchiectasis in childhood. Pediatr Clin North Am *31*:865, 1984.
193. Vandevivere J, Sphel M, Dab I, et al: Bronchiectasis in childhood. Comparison of chest roentgenograms, bronchoscopy and lung scintigraphy. Pediatr Radiol *9*:193, 1980.
194. Stokes D, Sigler A, Khouri NF, et al: Unilateral hyperlucent lung (Swyer-James syndrome) after severe *Mycoplasma pneumoniae* infections. Am Rev Respir Dis *117*:145, 1978.
195. Resouly A: Kartagener's syndrome: A case report and review of the literature. J Laryngol Otol *86*:1237, 1972.
196. Buchdahl RM, Reiser J, Ingram D, et al: Ciliary abnormalities in respiratory disease. Arch Dis Child *63*:238, 1988.
197. Levy M, Gick B, Springer C, et al: Bronchoscopy and bronchography in children. Am J Dis Child *173*:14, 1983.
198. Wilson JF, Peters GN, Fleshman JK: A technique for bronchography in children. Am Rev Respir Dis *105*:564, 1972.
199. Lundgren R, Hietala S, Adelroght E: Diagnosis of bronchial lesions by fiberoptic bronchoscopy combined with bronchography. Acta Radiol (Diagn) *23*:231, 1982.
200. Cameron EW, Holloway AM: Bronchography in children aged 3 years and under. Anesthetic techniques and results. S Afr Med J *54*:271, 1978.
201. Annest LS, Kratz JM, Crawford FA Jr: Current results of treatment of bronchiectasis. J Thorac Cardiovasc Surg *83*:546, 1982.
202. Campbell DN, Lilly JR: The changing spectrum of pulmonary operations in infants and children. J Thorac Cardiovasc Surg *83*:680, 1983.
203. Wilson JF, Decker AM: The surgical management of childhood bronchiectasis. Ann Surg *195*:354, 1982.
204. Hartman GE, Schochat SJ: Primary pulmonary neoplasms of childhood: A review. Ann Thorac Surg *35*:108, 1983.
205. Brandt B, Heintz SE, Rose EF, et al: Bronchial carcinoid tumors. Ann Thorac Surg *38*:63, 1984.
206. McCaughan BC, Martini N, Bains MS, et al: Bronchial carcinoids. Review of 124 cases. J Thorac Cardiovasc Surg *89*:8, 1985.
207. Price CHG, Zhuker K, Saezer-Kuntschik M, et al: Osteosarcoma in children. A study of 125 cases. J Bone Joint Surg *57*:341, 1975.
208. Beattie EJ: Surgical treatment of pulmonary metastases. Cancer *54*:2729, 1984.
209. Baldeyrou P, Lemoine G, Zucker GM, et al: Pulmonary metastases in children: The place of surgery. A study of 134 patients. J Pediatr Surg *19*:121, 1984.
210. Black CT, Luck SR, Musemeche CA, et al: Aggressive excision of pulmonary metastases is warranted in the management of childhood hepatic tumors. J Pediatr Surg *26*:1082, 1991.
211. Harris CS, Baker SP, Smith GA, et al: Childhood asphyxiation by food. JAMA *251*:2231, 1984.
212. Anas NG, Perkin MD: Aspiration of a balloon by a 3 month old. JAMA *250*:285, 1983.
213. Aytac A, Yardakl Y, Ikizler C, et al: Inhalation of foreign bodies in children: Report of 500 cases. J Thorac Cardiovasc Surg *74*:145, 1977.
214. Blazer S, Navelo Y, Friedman A: Foreign body in the airway. Am J Dis Child *134*:68, 1980.
215. Cotton E, Yasuda K: Foreign body aspiration. Pediatr Clin North Am *31*:937, 1984.
216. Majd NS, Mofenson HC, Greensher J: Lower airway foreign body aspiration in children. Clin Pediatr *16*:13, 1977.
217. Wiseman NE: The diagnosis of foreign body aspiration in childhood. J Pediatr Surg *19*:531, 1984.
218. Abman SH, Fan LL, Colton EK: Emergency treatment of foreign body obstruction of the upper airway in children. J Emerg Med *2*:7, 1984.
219. Hight EW, Phillipart AI, Hertzler JH: The treatment of retained foreign bodies in the pediatric airway. J Pediatr Surg *16*:694, 1981.
220. Black RE, Choi KJ, Sume WC, et al: Bronchoscopic removal of aspirated foreign bodies in children. Am J Surg *14*:77, 1984.
221. Cohen SR, Herbert WI, Lewis GB Jr, et al: Foreign bodies in the airway: Five-year retrospective study with special reference to management. Ann Otol Rhinol Laryngol *89*:437, 1980.
222. Hunsicker RC, Gartner WS: Fogarty catheter technique for removal of endobronchial foreign body. Arch Otolaryngol *103*:103, 1977.
223. Wood RE, Gauderer MW: Flexible fiberoptic bronchoscopy in the management of tracheobronchial foreign bodies in children: The value of a combined approach with open tube bronchoscopy. J Pediatr Surg *19*:693, 1984.

224. Tyler DC, Redding G, Hall D, et al: Increased intracranial pressure: An indication to decompress a tension pneumomediastinum. Crit Care Med *12*:467, 1984.
225. Keon TP: Death on induction of anesthesia for cervical node biopsy. Anesthesiology *55*:399, 1975.
226. Neuman G, Weingarten A, Abramowitz R, et al: The anesthetic management of patients with an anterior mediastinal mass. Anesthesiology *60*:144, 1984.
227. Maclive A, Watson C: Anesthesia and mediastinal masses. Anesthesia *39*:899, 1984.
228. Azizkham RG, Dudgeon DL, Buele, JR, et al: Life-threatening airway obstruction as a complication to the management of mediastinal masses in children. J Pediatr Surg *20*:816, 1985.
229. Ferrarri LR, Bedford RF: General anesthesia prior to treatment of anterior mediastinal masses in pediatric cancer patients. Anesthesiology *72*:991, 1990.
230. Bittar D: Respiratory obstruction associated with induction of general anesthesia in a patient with mediastinal Hodgkin's disease. Anesth Analg *54*:399, 1975.
231. Piro AH, Weiss DR, Hellman S: Mediastinal Hodgkin's disease: A possible danger for intubation anesthesia. Int J Radiat Oncol Phys *1*:415, 1976.
232. Todres ID, Reppert G, Hall D, et al: Management of critical airway obstruction in a child with a mediastinal tumor. Anesthesiology *45*:1000, 1976.
233. Neuman GG, Weingarten AE, Abramowitz RM, et al: The anesthetic management of the patient with an anterior mediastinal mass. Anesthesiology *60*:144, 1984.

CHAPTER

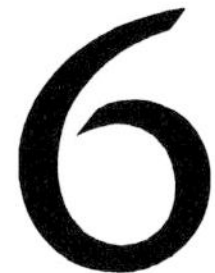

Diseases of the Cardiovascular System

INGRID B. HOLLINGER, M.D.

Safe anesthetic management of the infant or child with heart disease requires not only familiarity with anesthetic techniques and agents used in the pediatric age group but also a thorough understanding of the specific cardiac lesion, its pathophysiological consequences, and the possible effects of anesthetic techniques on these. In addition, the requirements of the proposed surgical therapy have to be considered.

This chapter reviews common and uncommon cardiac lesions, their current management, the results of therapy, and their implications for anesthetic management in noncardiac surgery.

In the appendices at the end of the chapter are outlined the current protocol for endocarditis prophylaxis, the pediatric dosages of commonly used cardiac medications, and a protocol for the reversal of chronic anticoagulation prior to elective or emergency surgery.

CONGENITAL CARDIAC LESIONS

Heart disease in infancy and childhood is due to congenital cardiac lesions in 90 percent of cases. These may be caused by deficiency of tissue leaving open communications between cardiac chambers, formation of excessive tissue causing obstruction at or near cardiac valves, persistence or development of anomalous connections between arteries or veins and cardiac chambers, or combinations of these problems. However, the most common congenital cardiac lesions, the floppy mitral valve and bicuspid aortic valve, are caused by improperly formed tissue that usually functions normally during infancy and childhood and generally does not lead to cardiac dysfunction until the later decades of life.

The incidence of congenital heart disease, with the exclusion of mitral valve prolapse and congenital bicuspid aortic valve, is approximately 6 to 8 per 1000 live births. This means that 24,500 children are born each year with congenital heart disease. In premature infants, the incidence of congenital heart disease is two to three times higher, even if persistent patency of the ductus arteriosus is excluded. Certain genetic syndromes and infectious or chemical teratogens can change the incidence of congenital heart disease. A listing of syndromes and teratogens and the commonly associated lesions is provided in Table 6–1.

Associated extracardiac defects may be present in children with congenital heart disease. Genitourinary tract anomalies are present in 4 to 15 percent of patients with congenital heart disease and should be sought at angiography. Approximately half of all infants with congenital heart disease require hospital admission for either medical or surgical therapy during the first year of life, the majority within the first 2 months. Approximately 30 percent become critically ill and either die from their disease or require surgical treatment. With advances in medical, surgical, and anesthetic management in recent years, early correction or palliation of the most severe anomalies is carried out within the first few weeks of life, and fewer children present now for noncardiac surgical therapy with their lesions uncorrected or nonpalliated.

Table 6–2 demonstrates the variability in the incidence of congenital cardiac lesions when grouped according to the time they are first diagnosed or first become symptomatic. Table 6–3 outlines the cardiac defects discussed in this chapter, their major physiologic consequences, and the special considerations for anesthetic management.

INTRACARDIAC DEFECTS PRODUCING PREDOMINANT LEFT-TO-RIGHT SHUNT

ATRIAL COMMUNICATIONS (Fig. 6–1)

PATENT FORAMEN OVALE

Functional closure of the foramen ovale occurs after birth, but anatomical closure is not complete until 2 to 3 months of age. Patency of the foramen ovale on probing persists in 34 to 50 percent of children and adolescents. In older patients, the patency rate is lower—20 percent over the age of 80 years. Because of the flaplike closure of this communication by the left-sided septum primum, shunting can occur only right-to-left after an increase in right atrial pressure. This is commonly associated with lesions causing increases in right ventricular pressure (e.g., pulmonic stenosis). However, if the foramen ovale is stretched by a distended left atrium, or if the flap valve is deficient, left-to-right shunting occurs through the opened communication. This latter situation is frequently observed in infants with a large patent ductus arteriosus or ventricular septal defect. Obstruction to left ventricular outflow, such as coarctation of the aorta or aortic stenosis, also may lead to large left-to-right shunts across a stretched foramen ovale,

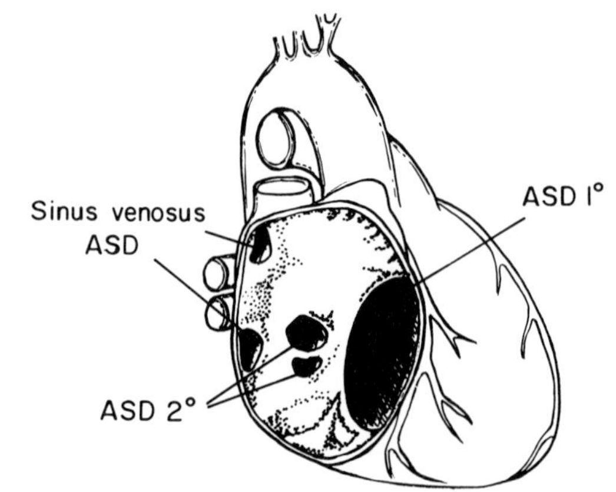

FIGURE 6–1. The atrial septum, showing several types of atrial septal defects as seen from the right atrium.

Table 6–1. SYNDROMES WITH CONGENITAL CARDIAC DEFECTS

	Incidence of Congenital Heart Disease (% of Patients)	*Cardiac Lesions in Order of Frequency (%)*
CHROMOSOMAL ABNORMALITIES		
Trisomy 21 (Down's)	40	ECD (32), VSD (29), ASD (11), TOF (8), PDA (7)
Trisomy 18	90	VSD (66), PDA (50), ASD (33), bicuspid PV (25), CoA (15), bicuspid AV (15)
Trisomy 13	80	PDA (63), VSD (43), ASD (40), abnormal valves (22), CoA (10)
$5p^-$ (Cri du chat)	25	VSD, PDA, ASD, PS
$4p^-$ (Wolf's)	50	VSD, ASD, PDA, PS
XO (Turner's)	10–30	CoA (50), AS, VSD, ASD
TERATOGENIC		
Alcohol	25–30	VSD, PDA, ASD
Amphetamines	5–10	VSD, PDA, ASD, TGA
Hydantoin	2–3	PS, AS, CoA, PDA
Trimethadione	15–30	TGA, TOF, hypoplastic LH
Thalidomide	5–10	TOF, VSD, ASD, truncus arteriosus
Rubella	35	Peripheral PS, PDA, VSD, ASD
Maternal diabetes	3–5	TGA, VSD, CoA
Maternal phenylketonuria	25–50	TOF, VSD, ASD
Maternal systemic lupus erythematosus	20–40	Congenital complete heart block

	Etiology	*Incidence of Congenital Heart Disease (% of Patients)*	*Characteristic Cardiac Defect*
GENETIC OR UNKNOWN ETIOLOGY			
Skeletal Defects Predominant			
Ellis–van Crefeld	R	50–60	Single atrium, ECD, PDA
Laurence-Moon-Biedl	R		TOF, VSD
Carpenter's	R		PDA, VSD
Holt-Oram	D	50	ASD, VSD, TOF, PS, PDA
Fanconi's	R		PDA, VSD
Thrombocytopenia, absent radius	R	10–15	ASD, TOF
Rubinstein-Taybi		15–20	CAV, ASD
VATER			Variable
Characteristic Facies			
Noonan's	D	50	PS (dysplastic PV), ASD
DiGeorge's	?	90–100	Interrupted aortic arch type B, aberrant right subclavian, right aortic arch, truncus arteriosus, TOF
Smith-Lemli-Opitz	R	15–20	VSD, PDA
Facial dysmorphism	D	10	PDA
de Lange's	?	20	VSD, PDA, ASD, TOF
Goldenhar's	?	50	TOF, VSD, PDA, CoA
Williams' elfin face	?	80	Supravalvular AS, peripheral AS, peripheral PS, interrupted arch
Asymmetric crying facies			Variable
Skin Lesions Prominent			
Forney's (deafness, freckles)	D		MI
Leopard (deafness, lentigines)	D		PS
Neurofibromatosis	D		PS, renal artery stenosis
Tuberous sclerosis	D		Rhabdomyoma
Situs Inversus			
Kartagener's (bronchiectasis)	R		Dextrocardia
Ivemark's asplenia or polysplenia	?		Complex cyanotic heart disease
Connective Tissue Disorders			
Marfan's	D	30–100	Dilation of proximal aorta (AI, aneurysm), MVP, cystic medial necrosis
Ehlers-Danlos	D	20–30	MVP, arterial rupture
Cutis laxa	R		Peripheral PS
Osteogenesis imperfecta	D, R		MVP, AI
Pseudoxanthoma elasticum	R		Coronary artery disease

Table continued on following page

Table 6–1. SYNDROMES WITH CONGENITAL CARDIAC DEFECTS *Continued*

	Etiology	*Characteristic Cardiac Defect*
GENETIC OR UNKNOWN ETIOLOGY		
Metabolic Disorders		
Glycogen storage disease II (Pompe's)	R	Massive cardiac enlargement due to glycogen deposition
Homocystinuria	R	Thrombosis of arteries
Mucopolysaccharidoses		
Type I, Hurler's	R	Pseudoatherosclerosis, AI, MI
Type II, Hunter's	X-linked	AI
Types IV, V, VI	R	Ai
Neuromuscular Disorders		
Friedreich's ataxia	R	Cardiomyopathy
Myotonic dystrophy	D	MVP, cardiomyopathy
Muscular dystrophy	X-linked	Cardiomyopathy
Arrhythmias		
Jervell and Lange-Nielsen (deafness)	R	Prolonged Q–T and R–T intervals, VF
Romano-Ward (no deafness)	D	Prolonged Q–T interval, VF
Refsum's (polyneuritis)	R	Arrhythmia, heart block
Familial periodic paralysis	D	Hypokalemia, SVT

Data from Noonan JA: Association of congenital heart disease with syndromes and their defects. Pediatr Clin North Am *25*:797, 1978; and Steinberg AG, et al: Progress in Medical Genetics. Volume V: Genetics of Cardiovascular Disease. Philadelphia, WB Saunders, 1983.

AI, Aortic insufficiency
AS, Aortic stenosis
ASD, Atrial septal defect
AV, Aortic valve
CAV, Canalis atrioventricularis
CoA, Coarctation of aorta
D, Dominant
ECD, Endocardial cushion defect
LH, Left heart
MI, Mitral insufficiency
MVP, Mitral valve prolapse
PDA, Patent ductus arteriosus
PS, Pulmonic stenosis
PV, Pulmonary valve
R, Recessive
SVT, Supraventricular tachycardia
TGA, Transposition of great arteries
TOF, Tetralogy of Fallot
VF, Ventricular fibrillation
VSD, Ventricular septal defect
?, Unknown

further aggravating pulmonary hyperperfusion or congestion or both.

Correction of the primary lesions generally will lead to a decrease in the size of the left atrium through reduction in right atrial pressure and disappearance of the left-to-right or right-to-left shunt across the foramen. If an intracardiac repair is performed, the foramen is generally closed surgically. Blood flow through a patent foramen ovale permits survival in certain congenital cardiac lesions, such as right ventricular obstruction, total anomalous pulmonary venous return, aortopulmonary transposition, and mitral atresia.

Isolated patency of the foramen ovale causes no clinical symptoms and cannot be diagnosed unless detected during cardiac catheterization; it may however be the route for paradoxical embolization.

Secundum Atrial Septal Defect (ASD)

Seventy-five percent of all atrial septal defects are of the secundum type, located at the fossa ovalis. This defect represents about 8 percent of all congenital heart disease. It is more common in females, with a male-to-female ratio of 1:2. Mitral valve prolapse is associated in 10 to 40 percent of patients. The magnitude and direction of the shunt are related to the relative inflow resistance of the right and left ventricles, since the atria are low-pressure systems and have a very small pressure difference. In infancy and early childhood, the right ventricle is relatively thicker and less compliant and offers more resistance to right atrial outflow. As pulmonary vascular resistance falls and the right ventricular wall becomes relatively thinner, right ventricular stroke volume and atrial shunt increase. This condition is usually not diagnosed before 2 or 3 years of age. Because of the difference in left and right atrial pressures, shunting is preferentially left-to-right, but a small right-to-left shunt of blood returning from the inferior vena cava is usually present. Immediately after a Valsalva maneuver, this venous blood flow is increased and may cause a drop in systemic arterial saturation. Pulmonary blood flow is usually markedly increased (often three to four times normal), but pulmonary artery pressure is normal

Table 6–2. INCIDENCE OF VARIOUS CONGENITAL CARDIAC LESIONS (% OF TOTAL)

In Normal Births*		All Congenital Heart Disease Seen in Infancy and Childhood†		Symptomatic in First Year of Life‡	
VSD	29.1	VSD	25	VSD	15.7
PS	8.1	PDA	12.5	D-TGA	9.9
PDA	7.7	PS	8.7	TOF	8.9
ASD secundum	7.4	TOF	7.9	CoA	7.5
CoA	6.5	CoA	6.6	Hypoplastic left heart	7.4
ECD	4.4	AS	6.3	PDA	6.1
TOF	3.5	ASD secundum	5.8	ECD	5.0
AS	3.5	D-TGA	4.5	Heterotaxia (dextrocardia, mesocardia, asplenia)	4.0
Hypoplastic left heart	3.5	ECD	3.1		
VSD + PS	2.4	Hypoplastic left heart	1.5	PS	3.3
Peripheral PS	2.4	Dextrocardia	1.5	Pulmonary atresia	3.1
D-TGA	2.5	Vascular ring	1.45	ASD secundum	2.9
EFE	2.2	PAPVR	1.4	TAPVR	2.6
Truncus arteriosus	2.0	TAPVR	1.3	Myocardial disease	2.6
Vascular ring	1.5	MI	1.15	Tricuspid atresia	2.6
Pulmonary atresia	1.5	Tricuspid atresia	1.14	Single ventricle	2.4
Tricuspid atresia	1.5	Single ventricle	1.0	AS	1.9
Anomalies of coronary arteries	1.5	EFE	1.0	DORV	1.5
DORV	1.1	Absent pulmonary valve	1.0	Truncus arteriosus	1.4
Single ventricle	0.9	AI	0.97	L-TGA	0.7
MI	0.7	Truncus arteriosus	0.74	Miscellaneous	10.4
EMF	0.7	L-TGA	0.58		
Miscellaneous	6.1	Pulmonary atresia	0.5		
		Ebstein's anomaly	0.5		
		Pulmonary atresia	0.5		
		Coronary anomalies	0.5		
		DORV	0.35		
		MS	0.3		
		Aortopulmonary window	0.24		
		Interrupted arch	0.175		
		Common atrium	0.17		
		Cor triatriatum	0.1		

*Data from Mitchell SC, et al: Congenital heart disease in 56,109 births. Circulation *63*:323, 1971.

†Data from Nadas AS, Fyler DC: Pediatric Cardiology. 3rd edition. Philadelphia, WB Saunders, 1972; and Keith JD, et al (eds): Heart Disease in Infancy and Childhood. 3rd edition. New York, Macmillan, 1978.

‡Data from Fyler DC, et al: Report of the New England Regional Infant Cardiac Program. Pediatrics *65*(Suppl):388, 1980.

VSD = ventricular septal defect; PS = pulmonic stenosis; PDA = patent ductus arteriosus; ASD = atrial septal defect; CoA = coarctation of aorta; ECD = endocardial cushion defect; TOF = tetralogy of Fallot; AS = aortic stenosis; TGA = transposition of great arteries; EFE = endocardial fibroelastosis; DORV = double outlet right ventricle; MI = mitral insufficiency; EMF = endomyocardial fibrosis; PAPVR = partial anomalous pulmonary venous return; TAPVR = total anomalous pulmonary venous return; AI = aortic insufficiency; MS = mitral stenosis; LH = left heart.

until adult life, and obstructive pulmonary vascular disease usually does not develop until the third or fourth decade of life. The main cause of deterioration of patients with secundum ASD in adult life is atrial arrhythmias, particularly atrial fibrillation and flutter.

Children with secundum ASD are usually asymptomatic. However, a small percentage of infants with secundum ASD is symptomatic, with failure to grow, recurrent lower respiratory tract infections, and congestive heart failure.

The attrition rate of unoperated ASD secundum after age 40 years is approximately 6 percent per year. With large shunts mild fatigue and dyspnea may be present. On auscultation, there is fixed splitting of the second heart sound. A systolic ejection murmur is heard maximally over the upper left sternal border. Echocardiography can distinguish secundum ASD from other lesions and eliminate the need for cardiac catheterization.

Treatment consists of elective surgical repair before school age. In recent years, transcatheter closure of atrial septal defects with a double-umbrella device has been performed in selected catheterization laboratories, eliminating the need for operation. These devices are at present still experimental. Between 7 and 20 percent of patients who have undergone surgical closure of a secundum ASD develop atrial arrhythmias; occasionally sick sinus syndrome may occur, requiring pacemaker implant years following the repair.

Sinus Venosus Defect. These defects account

Table 6–3. CARDIOVASCULAR DEFECTS IN INFANTS AND CHILDREN

Types of Lesions	*Special Considerations*
Intracardiac Defects ***A. Lesions producing dominant L-R shunt*** 1. Intra-atrial communications	
a. Patent foramen ovale b. Atrial septal defect c. Endocardial cushion defect i. Partial	Volume overload Paradoxical embolization Atrial arrhythmias
ii. Complete	Congestive heart failure Mitral regurgitation
2. Interventricular communications a. VSD, simple b. VSD, complicated (other associated cardiac lesions) c. Single ventricle d. Left ventricle to right atrium e. L-Transposition of the great vessels	Volume and pressure overload Pulmonary hypertension Shunt reversal with increased RV pressure Congestive heart failure Dependent shunting Delayed intravenous induction
f. Eisenmenger's syndrome	Fixed elevated pulmonary vascular resistance Reversed shunt
B. Lesions producing dominant R-L shunt with cyanosis	
1. Lesions with decreased pulmonary blood flow a. Tetralogy of Fallot b. Pulmonary atresia with VSD c. Double-outlet right ventricle with pulmonic stenosis d. Single ventricle with PS e. L-Transposition with VSD and PS	Dynamic RV outflow obstruction Low SVR increases R–L shunt Systemic embolization Polycythemia and thrombosis Reduced myocardial function postoperatively Tachyarrhythmias late postoperatively Rapid intravenous induction Delayed inhalation induction
2. Lesions with increased pulmonary blood flow a. D-Transposition of the great vessels b. Double-outlet right ventricle	Congestive heart failure Pulmonary hypertension Systemic embolization Atrial dysrhythmias
C. Obstructive lesions	
1. LV outflow—aortic stenosis a. Valvular b. Supravalvular c. Subvalvular d. Obstructive cardiomyopathy	Pressure overload—left ventricle High endocarditis risk Tachycardia causes ischemia Cardiac output fixed Peripheral vasodilation poorly tolerated Maintain preload and afterload Sudden death
2. RV outflow—pulmonic stenosis a. Valvular b. Infundibular c. Anomalous right ventricular bands d. Peripheral pulmonic stenosis e. Pulmonary atresia	Pressure overload—right ventricle Shunting across patent foramen ovale Syncope with stress in severe stenosis Myocardial fibrosis and limited cardiac reserve may persist postoperatively
3. LV inflow a. Mitral stenosis b. Parachute mitral valve (Shone's syndrome) c. Cor triatriatum d. Supravalvular ring e. Hypoplastic left heart syndrome	Increased left atrial pressure Pulmonary congestion Ventilatory abnormalities Tachycardia worsens symptoms Maintain preload and afterload
4. RV inflow a. Tricuspid atresia b. Tricuspid stenosis c. Ebstein's anomaly of tricuspid valve	R-L shunting Systemic embolization High endocarditis risk Maintain preload and afterload, sinus rhythm, and low pulmonary vascular resistance

Table 6–3. CARDIOVASCULAR DEFECTS IN INFANTS AND CHILDREN *Continued*

Types of Lesions	*Special Considerations*
D. Regurgitant lesions	
1. Aortic a. Aortic insufficiency b. Fenestration of aortic leaflets c. Aneurysm of sinus of Valsalva d. Aorto—left ventricular tunnel e. VSD with aortic insufficiency	Volume overload—left ventricle Regurgitation reduced by tachycardia and low peripheral vascular resistance Maintain myocardial contractility
2. Mitral a. Anomalous b. Cleft anterior or posterior leaflet c. Mitral valve prolapse d. Obstructive cardiomyopathy	Volume overload—left ventricle Regurgitation reduced by tachycardia and low peripheral vascular resistance Pulmonary congestion and ventilation abnormalities Monitor for arrhythmias with mitral valve prolapse
3. Pulmonic	
a. Pulmonary valve insufficiency	Usually well tolerated in the absence of pulmonary vascular disease
b. Absent pulmonary valve	Dilatation of pulmonary arteries leading to tracheal and bronchial compression Associated with VSD, may present as tetralogy of Fallot
4. Tricuspid a. Ebstein's anomaly b. Tricuspid insufficiency c. Uhl's anomaly	Volume overload—right ventricle R–L shunt at atrial level common Maintain right-sided filling pressures Tachycardia reduces regurgitation Maintain low pulmonary vascular resistance Intravenous induction prolonged
Malformations Involving the Great Vessels	
A. Arterial	
1. Systemic arteries	
a. Patent ductus arteriosus	Endocarditis risk preoperatively
b. Aortopulmonary window	Congestive failure, L–R shunting, and shunt reversal
c. Truncus arteriosus	Congestive failure, L–R shunting, shunt reversal, and RV–PA conduit postoperatively
d. Coarctation of aorta e. Interrupted aortic arch	Hypertension in upper extremity, may persist postoperatively
f. Vascular ring anomalies i. Double aortic arch ii. Aberrant right subclavian artery iii. Anomalous innominate artery iv. Right aortic arch v. Anomalous left carotid artery vi. Anomalous left pulmonary artery (vascular sling)	Tracheal or bronchial compression Esophageal compression Tracheomalacia may persist postoperatively
g. Congenital subclavian steal	Cerebral ischemia with exercise of affected arm Usually associated with coarctation or interrupted arch
2. Pulmonary arteries	
a. Anomalous origin of one pulmonary artery from the aorta	Severe pulmonary hypertension Development of obstructive pulmonary vascular disease
b. Congenital absence of one pulmonary artery	Associated pulmonary anomalies; recurrent infections; bronchiectasis; increased dead space
c. Congenital pulmonary arteriovenous fistula	Intrapulmonary R–L shunt; paradoxical embolization; polycythemia and systemic thrombosis
B. Venous	
1. Pulmonary veins	
a. Total anomalous pulmonary venous return i. Supracardiac ii. Cardiac iii. Infracardiac iv. Mixed	Pulmonary venous obstruction L–R shunt at atrial level Volume overload—right ventricle
b. Partial anomalous pulmonary venous return i. Superior vena cava ii. Right atrium iii. Inferior vena cava (scimitar syndrome)	Presentation similar to ASD Pulmonary infections common

Table continued on following page

Table 6–3. CARDIOVASCULAR DEFECTS IN INFANTS AND CHILDREN *Continued*

Types of Lesions	*Special Considerations*
***B. Venous** Continued* 2. Systemic veins a. Anomalous systemic venous return	
i. Persistent left superior vena cava to left atrium	Problems with cardiac catheterization
ii. Absence of inferior vena cava	Problems with cardiac catheterization and venous cannulation for bypass.
C. Anomalies of the Coronary Artery	
1. Aberrant left coronary artery (Bland-White-Garland syndrome)	Left ventricular ischemia and failure
2. Coronary arteriovenous fistula	L–R shunt through fistula; failure and ischemia rare
Cardiomyopathies: See Table 6–4.	
Tumors of the Heart A. Benign 1. Rhabdomyoma 2. Fibroma 3. Myxoma 4. Benign teratoma B. Malignant 1. Malignant teratoma 2. Rhabdomyosarcoma	 Obstruction to filling and blood flow Embolization of tumor fragments
Conduction Defects	
A. Congenital atrioventricular block B. Supraventricular tachycardia	Usually well tolerated past infancy May require temporary pacing for surgery
C. Wolff-Parkinson-White syndrome D. Lown-Ganong-Levine syndrome	Abnormal conduction pathway (Kent) Reentry tachycardia May be triggered by sympathetic stimulation Patients on digoxin
E. Prolonged Q–T interval	Imbalance of cardiac sympathetics Patients on beta-blockers Syncope due to ventricular fibrillation triggered by sympathetic stimulation Bradycardia may result in escape beats and ventricular fibrillation
Diseases of the Pericardium A. Pericardial defect B. Pericarditis C. Constrictive pericarditis D. Pericardial tumors	 Restriction to ventricular filling Pulsus paradoxus Fixed cardiac output Maintain heart rate, preload, afterload
Malpositions of the Heart A. Dextrocardia (asplenia syndrome) B. Ectopia cordis	 Associated congenital cardiac lesions common
Acquired Heart Disease	
A. Rheumatic heart disease	Valvular involvement usually mild in pediatric age group; penicillin prophylaxis and prevention of bacterial endocarditis
B. Kawasaki's syndrome	Coronary artery disease; aspirin therapy
C. Takayasu's disease	Hypertension

for about 5 to 10 percent of ASDs. They are located posterior to the fossa ovalis, with the vena cava frequently overriding the defect and the pulmonary veins from the entire right lung connected to either the right atrium or the superior vena cava.

Coronary Sinus ASD. The least common of all ASDs lies at the site of the anticipated coronary sinus ostium. It is usually associated with absence of the coronary sinus and a persistent left superior vena cava draining into the roof of the left atrium. It may be associated with a complete atrioventricular (AV) canal defect and the asplenia syndrome.

Clinical manifestations of both sinus venosus defect and coronary sinus ASD, when isolated, are similar to those of secundum ASD. Partial anomalous pulmonary venous return requires construction of a baffle to divert the anomalous pulmonary blood flow to the left atrium. The latter patients have a higher incidence of postoperative atrial dysrhythmias. Surgery is usually performed during childhood.

Endocardial Cushion Defect

Defects in the development and fusion of the endocardial cushions lead to incomplete septation of the primitive atrioventricular (AV) canal and various forms of atrial and/or ventricular communications, described as partial or complete endocardial cushion defect or AV canal. Endocardial cushion defects occur in 3 to 4 percent of children with congenital heart disease who are otherwise normal, but they are the predominant cardiac lesion (30 to 50 percent) in children with trisomy 21. At least 25 percent of children with endocardial cushion defect have Down's syndrome. Almost all patients with asplenia syndrome have some form of endocardial cushion defect. About half the patients with Ellis–van Crefeld syndrome have congenital heart disease, with the most frequent defect (40 percent) being single atrium, considered a form of endocardial cushion defect. Endocardial cushion defect is equally distributed between the sexes.

Partial AV canal is one fourth as frequent as secundum ASD and is characterized by nearly complete central fusion of the anterior and posterior cushions so that the mitral and tricuspid annuli are well formed (Fig. 6–2). The most common type is the ostium primum ASD with a cleft anterior mitral leaflet. The defect lies anterior and inferior to the fossa ovalis and is usually quite large. The lesion is frequently discovered during infancy because of the prominence of the cardiac murmur. Symptoms, including heart failure, may occur early, most commonly if the defect is associated with mitral insufficiency. Dyspnea, fatigue, and susceptibility to frequent respiratory infections may be present. Mitral insufficiency is rarely seen in infants but may become apparent by age 4 to 5 years.

Shunting in ostium primum defect occurs through two mechanisms; one similar to secundum defect depends on the difference in the inflow resistance of the right and left ventricle. With high pulmonary vascular resistance, there is minimal right-to-left shunt, whereas with low pulmonary vascular resistance there is left-to-right shunting proportional to the difference in pulmonary and systemic vascular resistances. This represents dependent shunting. Obligatory shunting occurs from a high-pressure to a low-pressure chamber, in this lesion from the left ventricle to the right atrium across the cleft mitral valve and ostium primum defect.

Pulmonary vascular disease rarely develops before adolescence. The electrocardiogram (ECG) typically shows left axis deviation, AV conduction abnormalities (usually first-degree block), and right ventricular conduction defect with or without hypertrophy. The heart is usually large on plain chest films, and there may be evidence of pulmonary hyperperfusion. Treatment consists of surgical repair of the defect with a patch of pericardium or prosthetic material and suture closure of the mitral cleft or mitral annuloplasty to provide mitral valve competence.

Mitral insufficiency may persist postoperatively and ultimately require mitral valve replacement. If no symptoms are present, repair is generally performed when the patient is between 5 and 7 years of age.

Anesthetic Considerations. Children with un-

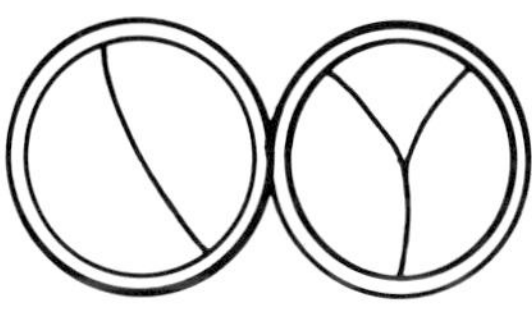

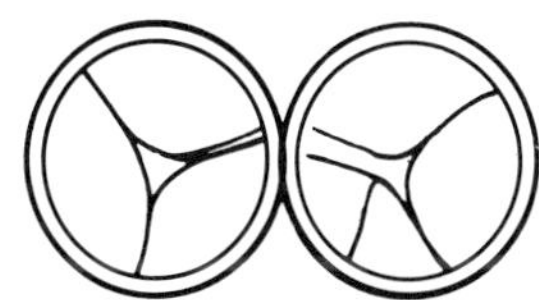

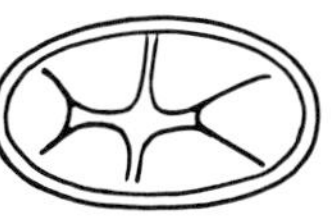

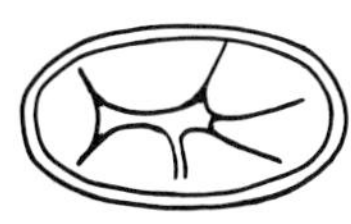

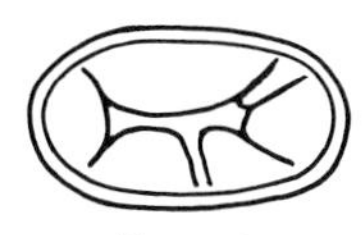

FIGURE 6–2. Schematic representation of partial and complete atrioventricular canal. Classification after Rastelli.

complicated ASD pose no unusual anesthetic risks. In noncardiac operation, the major concern has to be directed toward prevention of systemic air embolization, especially in coronary sinus ASD. Although the dominant direction of the shunt in ASD is from left to right atrium, reversal of the shunt direction can occur with sudden increases in right ventricular outflow resistance. This has been observed with embolization of air, as in neurosurgical procedures in the sitting position, and with marked increases in intrathoracic pressure during bronchoscopy with jet ventilation. Paradoxical embolization of air can occur through a persistent foramen ovale. Application of positive end-expiratory pressure (PEEP) under these circumstances may increase right-to-left shunting by increasing pulmonary vascular resistance. Hypoxia, hypercapnia, and acidosis all increase pulmonary vascular resistance and may lead to shunt reversal in ASD. Airway maintenance and prevention of hypoventilation during anesthesia are therefore particularly important. In small children and patients with Down's syndrome, endotracheal intubation should be considered for all but the most trivial procedures.

Endocarditis prophylaxis is necessary for patients with primum and sinus venosus defects pre- and postoperatively but not for patients with simple secundum defects pre- or postoperatively (if closed without prosthetic material).

Complete Endocardial Cushion Defect. Complete AV canal is associated with Down's syndrome in 69 percent of cases. The defect is characterized by a large combined atrial and ventricular septal defect and a single AV valve with five to six leaflets and commissures (see Figure 6–2). Angiography demonstrates the characteristic goose-neck deformity of the left ventricular outflow tract.

Symptoms invariably occur early in infancy owing to the large increase in pulmonary blood flow and pressure, which leads to pulmonary hypertension. Mitral regurgitation is present in at least 50 percent of patients. Congestive heart failure, pneumonia and failure to thrive are the common presenting features. Pulmonary vascular obstructive disease develops in two thirds of cases within the first year of life. With medical management, more than 50 percent of infants die within the first 12 months and 85 percent by the end of the second year of life. Left-to-right shunting occurs at the atrial and ventricular levels and becomes bidirectional or reversed, with progressive increase in pulmonary vascular resistance.

The treatment of choice at present is complete repair whenever unmanageable symptoms occur before 1 year of age. Pulmonary artery banding is ineffective in the presence of AV valve incompetence and carries over 30 percent mortality in complete AV canal. Late postoperative complications of complete AV canal repair in infancy include mitral valve insufficiency in 10 to 30 percent of patients and AV conduction disturbances, including complete heart block.

Anesthetic Considerations. Infants with uncorrected AV canal defects rarely undergo elective surgical procedures. Anesthetic management has to be directed toward maintenance of cardiac output in the presence of a failing myocardium. Patients are usually digitalized and on diuretic therapy. Congestive heart failure and electrolyte abnormalities should be controlled, and monitoring of intravascular volume and pressure should be established for major surgery. Anesthetic agents that are known to cause myocardial depression should be avoided.

Chronic pulmonary congestion may lead to airway closure and atelectasis. Large bronchi may be compressed by the pulmonary arteries or left atrium, small airway resistance is increased, compliance is decreased, and intrapulmonary right-to-left shunting occurs. Patients may be on the verge of respiratory failure. The airway should always be secured by endotracheal intubation and ventilation controlled to assure adequate gas exchange. In the presence of obstructive pulmonary vascular disease, pulmonary interstitial and alveolar edema may occur with fluid shifts because of the reduced pulmonary vascular bed.

Patients may require postoperative ventilation. Use of unnecessary high oxygen concentration may aggravate congestive heart failure by increasing left-to-right shunting because of a reduction in pulmonary vascular resistance. Hyperventilation, hypokalemia, and alkalosis may lead to ventricular arrhythmias in the digitalized patient. Serum potassium should be maintained above 4 mEq/L perioperatively. If cardiovascular deterioration occurs, use of intravenous inotropic agents (dopamine, dobutamine) should be considered. Patients require careful endocarditis prophylaxis.

Two thirds of patients who have undergone complete AV canal repair are in functional class I (NYHA classification). Anesthetic management is directed toward the general management of the patient with Down's syndrome and the prevention of bacterial endocarditis. If mitral regurgitation is present, maintenance of an adequate heart rate and low systemic vascular resistance is important. Myocardial depression can readily lead to congestive failure, especially when combined with operative fluid overload. Patients require very careful monitoring.

Common Atrium

Common atrium is characterized by virtually complete absence of the atrial septum. It is frequently combined with other cardiac anomalies, such as transposition, double-outlet right ventricle, univentricular heart, and anomalous pulmonary venous connection in association with asplenia or polysplenia syndrome. Nearly complete mixing of systemic and pulmonary blood occurs, but pulmonary blood flow exceeds systemic blood flow. Cyanosis may be constantly present or apparent only during exercise. Surgical repair is performed early in life to prevent development of pulmonary vascular disease. Endocarditis prophylaxis, prevention of systemic embolization, and shunt reversal are important considerations in anesthetic management.

INTERVENTRICULAR COMMUNICATIONS (Fig. 6–3)

Simple Ventricular Septal Defect

Isolated ventricular septal defect (VSD) is the most common congenital cardiac lesion causing symptoms in infants and children and is seen in 20 to 25 percent of all patients with congenital heart disease. It is slightly more common in females (56 percent) than in males (44 percent). Eighty percent of defects are located in the membranous portion of the ventricular septum beneath the crista interventricularis. Supracristal defects located beneath the pulmonic valve constitute approximately 5 to 7 percent of VSDs except in Japan or other Far Eastern countries, where they may constitute close to 30 percent. Defects may also be located in the muscular septum (frequently multiple) or beneath the septal leaflet of the tricuspid valve (AV canal type of defect).

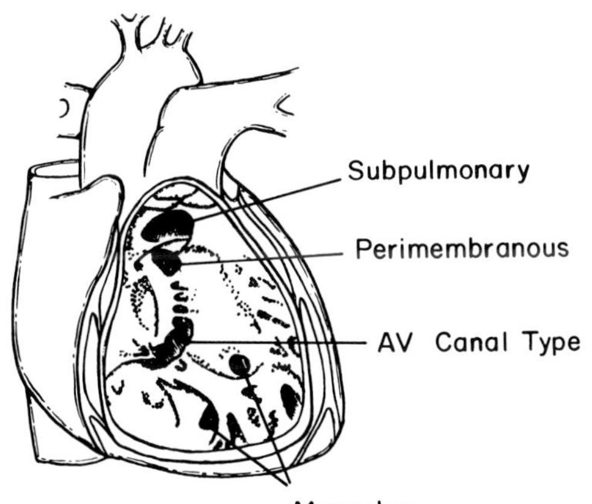

FIGURE 6–3. The ventricular septum, showing several types of ventricular septal defects as seen from the right ventricle.

The size of the defect largely determines the degree of pathophysiological derangement. With small-to-medium lesions, the size limits left-to-right shunting. With large defects (approximately the size of the aortic orifice), there is no restriction to flow, and shunting depends largely on differences between systemic vascular resistance and the resistance of the pulmonary vascular bed. Symptoms of left-to-right shunting usually develop between the second and third week of life with the normal decline in pulmonary vascular resistance. With very large defects and systemic pressures in the pulmonary arteries, the resistance of the pulmonary vascular bed declines more slowly, and congestive failure due to volume overload of the left ventricle may not occur until 2 to 3 months postnatally.

Spontaneous closure of the VSD is estimated to occur in 25 to 50 percent of small to moderate-sized defects, generally during the first year of life. Probably less than 5 percent of large VSDs undergo spontaneous closure. These infants are severely ill with congestive heart failure and pulmonary hypertension; if treated only medically, 25 percent die within the first 6 months. The high pulmonary artery pressures lead to progressive pulmonary vascular obstructive disease, particularly after the second year. Pulmonary artery banding has been performed in small infants in the past to protect the pulmonary vasculature, but the combined mortality of the initial procedure and the subsequent repair of the VSD with debanding approaches 25 percent. For this reason, primary surgical closure of the defect is presently recommended in the first year of life in infants with intractable congestive heart failure and failure to thrive, with a mortality quoted at 5 percent or less. All defects with significant pulmonary artery hypertension are generally closed before 24 months to prevent development of obstructive pulmonary vascular disease.

In moderate-sized defects with only mild elevation of pulmonary artery pressures, medical management is preferred during infancy; only if a large left-to-right shunt (greater than twice systemic blood flow) persists by 4 to 5 years of age is the defect then closed surgically. Operation is not recommended for small VSDs, but patients are followed at 2- to 3-year intervals to detect development of aortic regurgitation. All patients, even those with very small ventricular septal defects, require endocarditis prophylaxis.

Patients whose defects were closed during infancy show normal growth and development. Pulmonary artery pressures return to normal, as does left ventricular function. In patients operated upon during childhood, left ventricular function may remain mildly depressed and show abnormality with intense exercise, despite lack of clinical symptoms. Patients may have conduction defects after surgical closure, most commonly right bundle branch block or a combination of right bundle branch block with left anterior hemiblock. Complete heart block is fortunately rare.

Ventricular Septal Defect with Pulmonic Stenosis

Hypertrophy of the infundibulum of the right ventricle may occur in patients with large ventricular septal defects (particularly those with right aortic arch). This obstruction leads to progressive decrease in left-to-right shunting and protection of the pulmonary vascular bed from systemic pressures. If the muscle hypertrophy becomes severe enough, right-to-left shunting may eventually occur, initially only during exercise, and patients may have the same clinical features as those of tetralogy of Fallot.

Pulmonary stenosis rarely becomes prominent before 4 to 5 years of age. Treatment is surgical repair during childhood, with closure of the septal defect and resection of the infundibular muscle bands.

Ventricular Septal Defect with Aortic Insufficiency

Approximately 5 percent of patients with a VSD develop signs of aortic valve incompetence, which may become the predominant problem. It occurs more commonly in males. Supracristal or subpulmonary VSD is especially prone to this complication (25 percent). The right coronary cusp tends to herniate through the VSD in these patients and may cause some degree of right ventricular outflow obstruction. Aortic insufficiency in infracristal VSD is rare and usually is associated with anomalies of the aortic commissures (bicuspid aortic valve) and infundibular pulmonic stenosis. Mild aortic insufficiency may be treated by closure of the VSD alone. With more severe insufficiency, aortic valvuloplasty is performed at the time of VSD closure. The aortic regurgitation appears not to progress after repair. Surgical therapy is carried out as soon as prolapse of a cusp is noticed on angiography or if signs of aortic insufficiency occur.

Left Ventricular to Right Atrial Shunt

Communications between the left ventricle and right atrium constitute less than 1 percent of all congenital cardiac defects. There is a slight female preponderance. Approximately one third of the defects are located above the tricuspid valve, the remainder below in association with malformation of the septal leaflet. The shunt is always large because of the marked pressure difference between the left ventricle and right atrium during systole, which is present from birth. Volume overload of the right ventricle and enlargement of the pulmonary artery occur. The increased pulmonary venous return leads to volume overload of the left side, and heart failure may occur in the first months of life. There is always marked enlargement of the right atrium. The lesion may decrease in size, but spontaneous closure has not been observed.

There is a high incidence of endocarditis (6 percent of recorded cases) and atrial dysrhythmias (5 percent of recorded cases). Because of the large shunt and high endocarditis risk, surgical correction should be performed in early childhood. Long-term postoperative complications include complete heart block (4 percent) and atrial dysrhythmia (3 percent).

Single Ventricle

Connection of both atria, usually via two AV valves to a single ventricular chamber (or a large dominant ventricle with a diminutive second ventricular remnant), is a rare anomaly, accounting for approximately 1 to 1.5 percent of all congenital heart disease. There is a slight male preponderance. In nearly 75 percent of cases the single ventricle is a morphological left ventricle and the relationship of the great vessels is L-transposed. All patients with D-transposition have some degree of subaortic stenosis, while more than 50 percent of those with L-transposition tend to have subaortic and subpulmonary obstruction.

Half the patients are seen within the first month of life and close to 90 percent within the first 6 months. Without surgical intervention, three quarters of these infants die within this period. With various surgical interventions, approximately 75 percent of these patients survive at present.

Patients without obstruction to pulmonary blood flow are seen in early infancy with signs of a large left-to-right shunt, in congestive heart failure, with growth retardation and frequent respiratory infections. Despite nearly complete mixing of systemic and pulmonary venous blood in the systemic ventricle, cyanosis is not prominent in these children. In patients with obstruction to pulmonary outflow, cyanosis is present and heart failure rare. With pulmonary atresia, pulmonary blood flow may be ductus dependent.

The palliative procedure carried out during infancy consists of pulmonary artery banding in patients without pulmonary stenosis who have unremitting congestive heart failure. Development of secondary subaortic stenosis following this procedure may make a later septation operation impossible. In patients with pulmonary outflow obstruction, a systemic-to-pulmonary shunt is created. The mortality rate for banding ranges from 25 to 50 percent; for shunting, it is less than 20 percent. Long-term survival is poor with palliative operations because of development of progressive myocardial fibrosis, secondary subaortic obstruction, insufficient pulmonary blood flow, or development of elevated pulmonary vascular resistance.

Patients with favorable anatomy can undergo a septation procedure between 4 and 5 years of age. However, the majority of patients presently undergo a modified Fontan-type procedure (see Figure 6–14). Classically, it consists of connecting the right atrium to the pulmonary artery, closure of the right-sided inlet valve, and diversion of all ventricular output to the aorta. In recent years, creation of cavopulmonary shunts instead of systemic arterial-pulmonary shunts has become popular again. As a first stage for later complete Fontan's repair, a bidirectional cavopulmonary shunt is created connecting the superior vena cava to the pulmonary artery in an end-to-side anastomosis (see Figure 6–15). This allows for an increase in pulmonary blood flow without increasing ventricular work or pulmonary artery pressures and resistance. The completion of the Fontan repair is then carried out by baffling the inferior vena cava return to the pulmonary artery when the patient is 2 to 5 years old. In infants in the first year of life with refractory congestive heart failure and favorable anatomy, an initial septation procedure should be considered because of the poor results of septation following pulmonary artery banding. Mortality for "corrective" procedures ranges from 16 to 30 percent, with septation procedures carrying the highest mortality.

Long-term follow-up of patients after septation or the Fontan's operation indicates that septation is more likely to result in normal cardiac function. Only half of patients after the Fontan's operation were asymptomatic, and all patients were still on digitalis or diuretics, compared with only 10 percent of patients after septation. More than 50 percent of patients after Fontan's repair develop atrial arrhythmias.

L-TRANSPOSITION OF THE GREAT ARTERIES

Abnormal rotation of the bulboventricular loop results in ventricular inversion and transposition of the great arteries. The anatomical left ventricle receives the systemic venous return and ejects into the pulmonary artery, and the anatomical right ventricle receives the pulmonary venous return and ejects into the aorta (Fig. 6–4). If no additional anomalies exist, a hemodynamically normal heart is the result; hence the name corrected transposition.

This malfunction is rare, occurring in less than 1.5 percent of all congenital heart disease, with slight male preponderance. Only 1 percent of patients have physiologically normal hearts. Because of the ventricular inversion, the AV valves, the coronary arteries, and the conduction system are also inverted (Fig. 6–5). The left-sided tricuspid valve is frequently insuffi-

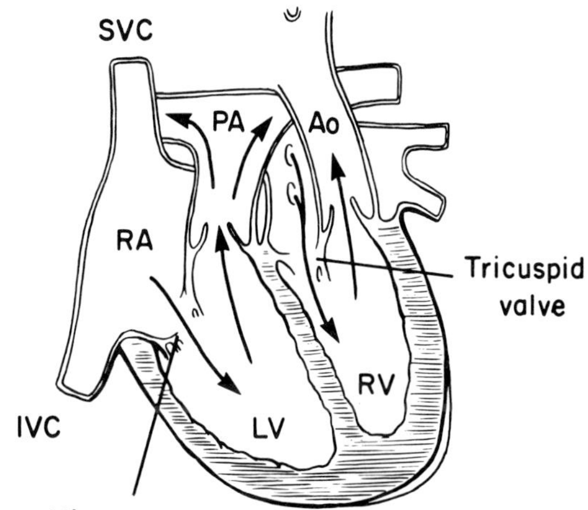

FIGURE 6–4. Circulation in corrected transposition. SVC = superior vena cava; IVC = inferior vena cava; RA = right atrium; PA = pulmonary artery; Ao = Aorta; RV = right ventricle; LV = left ventricle. (Redrawn from Kidd BSL: Transposition of the great arteries. *In* Keith JD, et al [eds]: Heart Disease in Infancy and Childhood. 3rd edition. New York, Macmillan, 1978.)

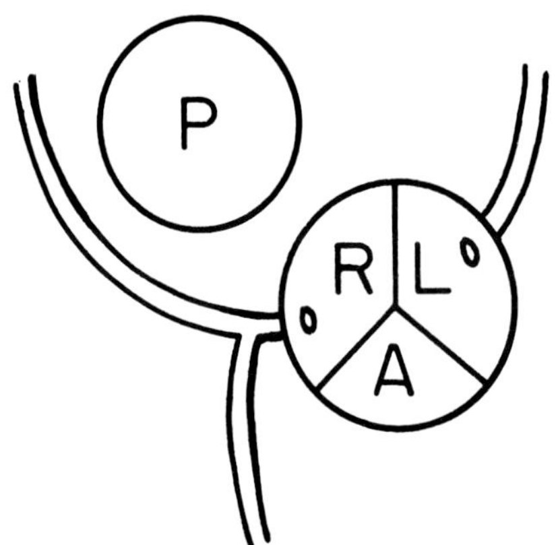

FIGURE 6–5. Coronary anatomy in corrected transposition. The right coronary artery gives off the anterior descending branch. The left coronary artery has only the circumflex distribution.

cient, often due to an Ebstein-type malformation. The left anterior descending coronary artery, originating on the right, traverses the pulmonary outflow tract. The bundle of His has a much longer course, which may explain the very high incidence of heart block, both spontaneously and following surgery. As many as 80 percent of patients have a large VSD or pulmonary outflow obstruction or both. Left-sided inflow or outflow lesions may be present in 10 to 15 percent of patients. Malposition of the heart (dextrocardia or mesocardia) is common.

The majority of patients are seen in the first month of life with signs of congestive failure in the presence of a large left-to-right shunt through the VSD, and with cyanosis and hypercyanotic spells with pulmonary outflow obstruction. Prognosis depends on the degree of hemodynamic abnormality. Patients with a large VSD and no pulmonary stenosis have a higher mortality (35 percent) during the first year of life than those with pulmonary outflow obstruction (20 percent).

Heart failure is initially treated with digitalis and diuretics, and if this is unsuccessful, banding of the pulmonary artery may be performed to relieve failure and protect the pulmonary vascular bed. Nearly 50 percent of children with pulmonary obstruction will require a systemic-to-pulmonary shunt for palliation of cyanosis. Total correction in corrected transposition is surgically difficult and carries a high mortality (40 percent). Because of the abnormal coronary arterial anatomy, a conduit repair is required for correction of severe pulmonic stenosis. Systemic AV valve insufficiency may require repair or replacement at the time of VSD closure. Conduction disturbance is present in 40 to 50 percent of patients postoperatively. Patients may develop sudden complete heart block after the age of 20 years.

Anesthetic Considerations. Uptake of inhalational anesthetic agents is only minimally influenced by a left-to-right shunt unless peripheral perfusion is poorly maintained. Under these circumstances, induction with an agent that has a low blood/gas solubility coefficient may be accelerated. Induction with intravenous agents, however, may be quite delayed, since a considerable portion of the drug will be recirculated through the lung. However, if the amount of drug injected is increased to achieve the desired effect more rapidly, side effects of overdose may appear after all drug finally reaches the brain and peripheral circulation.

Increases in peripheral vascular resistance tend to increase left-to-right shunting because of the obstruction to left ventricular outflow. Increases in pulmonary resistance tend to decrease the shunt. With marked obstruction to right ventricular outflow (for example, by embolization), however, reversal of the shunt and cyanosis can occur. In patients with a dynamic increase in pulmonary vascular resistance and a nonrestrictive VSD, administration of oxygen (a potent pulmonary vasodilator) may cause a very large increase in the left-to-right shunt owing to the reduction in pulmonary vascular resistance, resulting in congestive failure and peripheral collapse from insufficient systemic perfusion. Therefore, in patients with reactive pulmonary vascular resistance, oxygenation during anesthesia must be monitored carefully to avoid flooding the lung as a result of a marked reduction in pulmonary vascular resistance. Hypoxia may lead to shunt reversal through an increase in pulmonary vascular resistance.

Patients with small to moderate-sized VSDs most commonly may require anesthesia for elective surgery with the defect still open. If no signs of heart failure are present, they should not have any undue anesthetic risk. The main concern has to be directed toward prevention of endocarditis and air embolization.

In patients with large VSDs, heart failure should be optimally controlled prior to operation by the use of digitalis, diuretics, and if necessary a peripheral vasodilator (hydralazine). Because chronic pulmonary congestion leads to small airway disease, the airway should be secured by intubation, and oxygenation should be carefully monitored to avoid changes in pulmonary vascular resistance. Potent inhalational anesthetics are poorly tolerated by a failing myocardium and may cause severe hypotension. Narcotic-relaxant techniques are preferred for such patients coming for repair of their cardiac lesion or other extensive surgical procedures. Nitrous oxide increases pulmonary vascular resistance and may decrease the shunt. High-dose narcotics and ketamine appear to blunt the stress response in the pulmonary vascular bed. Ketamine, because of its indirect sympathomimetic effect, appears also to be well tolerated by patients with borderline myocardial reserve.

In patients with pulmonic obstruction, agents that cause a marked increase in inotropy (such as ketamine) should be avoided. Any increase in right ventricular outflow resistance may easily reverse the shunt. In patients with signs of aortic insufficiency, bradycardia and increases in peripheral vascular resistance may cause a significant increase in regurgitation. Mild tachycardia is desirable, as is mild reduction in left ventricular afterload. Isoflurane may be a useful agent under these circumstances. Patients who have undergone repair of their lesion during infancy should be normal postoperatively. They do, however, require endocarditis prophylaxis. Careful electrocardiographic monitoring is required in patients with postoperative conduction defects, although no instance of complete heart block occurring during anesthesia has been reported. Patients whose defects were closed later during childhood may not be able to respond to stress as well as normal controls do. Invasive hemodynamic monitoring to assess ventricular function and pulmonary artery pressures probably should be established early for an operation involving large and/or rapid fluid shifts. Patients may require mechanical ventilation postoperatively until fully recovered from anesthesia and operation, to minimize the work of breathing and optimize pulmonary vascular resistance.

Anesthetic management of patients with corrected transposition will be influenced by the pre-existing hemodynamic abnormality. The alteration in blood flow is similar either to that in patients with a large VSD without pulmonary obstruction or to that in patients with tetralogy of Fallot. All patients have to be carefully monitored for conduction disturbances. Endocarditis prophylaxis is indicated in all patients with associated defects. The hemodynamic effect in patients with a single ventricle who have undergone Fontan-type repair is physiologically similar to that in patients with "repaired" tricuspid atresia. Anesthetic considerations for these patients will be discussed later.

EISENMENGER'S COMPLEX AND SYNDROME

The development of a markedly elevated pulmonary vascular resistance with reversal of the left-to-shunt in the presence of a large VSD, first described by Victor Eisenmenger, has been termed the Eisenmenger complex. The designation of Eisenmenger's syndrome describes a pathophysiological entity in which pulmonary hypertension at systemic level because of a high pulmonary vascular resistance leads to a bidirectional or predominantly right-to-left shunt at the aortopulmonary, atrial, or ventricular level. Less than 10 percent of children with a large VSD develop this problem, but it is present in over 50 percent of adults with large aortopulmonary or ventricular communications. Because the underlying defect must allow for equalization of pressures between the ventricles, there is usually a history of congestive heart failure in infancy that improves as pulmonary vascular resistance increases. Obstructive pulmonary vascular disease may be present after the age of 2 years, and the presence of a fixed elevation in pulmonary vascular resistance renders the underlying defect inoperable. Children usually show few symptoms except for occasional dyspnea on exertion and fatigue. Cyanosis and failure are rare. Symptoms become increasingly prominent during the late twenties and early thirties of the patient. The average age at death, which frequently occurs suddenly, ranges between 33 and 36 years in various series.

Anesthetic Management. Perioperative dehydration should be avoided in patients who are cyanotic, since it may cause an increase in blood viscosity and result in thrombosis in the pulmonary and systemic vascular beds. Meticulous attention should be paid to intravenous lines to prevent embolization of air or clot to the systemic circulation. Since the pulmonary vascular resistance is fixed, shunting is largely determined by systemic vascular resistance. A fall in systemic vascular resistance will lead to increased cyanosis, owing to increased right-to-left shunting. High ventilation pressure may cause further reduction in pulmonary blood flow. Pulmonary function in these patients is abnormal, with reduction in total lung capacity, vital capacity, and compliance. Residual and closing volumes are increased.

Various reports of anesthetic management of patients with Eisenmenger's syndrome have been published. Recommendations include sedation to reduce preoperative anxiety and oxygen consumption, use of anesthetic agents with minimal effect on peripheral vascular resistance and myocardial contractility (narcotic or ketamine), prevention of hypoxia and hypoventilation intra- and postoperatively, and prevention of bradycardia by the use of anticholinergics. Regional anesthesia with attendant sympathetic blockade is relatively contraindicated in these patients. All patients require endocarditis prophylaxis.

INTRACARDIAC LESIONS PRODUCING PREDOMINANT RIGHT-TO-LEFT SHUNT WITH CYANOSIS

LESIONS WITH DECREASED PULMONARY BLOOD FLOW

TETRALOGY OF FALLOT

The combination of VSD, pulmonic valvular and/or infundibular stenosis, right ventricular hypertrophy, and straddling of the VSD by the aorta (malalignment defect) is known as tetralogy of Fallot. It is the most common cyanotic defect seen after the first year of life, contributing to 8 to 10 percent of all congenital cardiac lesions. Males are more often affected than females by a 3:2 ratio, and 25 to 30 percent of patients have a right-sided aortic arch.

The degree of pulmonic obstruction determines the onset and severity of cyanosis. With severe pulmonic stenosis, cyanosis appears with closure of the ductus arteriosus, and death occurs within the first 2 to 3 months, unless pulmonary blood flow is improved surgically. Many infants do not develop symptoms until 3 to 6 months of age and even then may not appear cyanotic at rest. However, episodes of severe cyanosis with hyperventilation and acidosis, known as hypercyanotic spells, may occur. They are caused by severe infundibular spasm, probably induced by changes in venous return and peripheral vascular resistance. Reduction in peripheral vascular tone leads to decreased pulmonary blood flow, since blood tends to be shunted to the systemic circulation. A fall in venous return further decreases pulmonary blood flow. Squatting may improve symptoms through an increase in venous return from the lower extremities and by increasing peripheral vascular resistance. Treatment consists of intravenous morphine, 0.1 to 0.2 mg/kg, or propranolol, 0.05 to 0.1 mg/kg.

In this context, it is important to remember that cyanosis is the clinical manifestation of reduced arterial oxygen saturation and clinically is generally recognized when 5 gm of reduced hemoglobin are present in arterial blood. With a hemoglobin concentration of 20 gm/dl and arterial saturation of 50 percent, 10 gm of reduced hemoglobin will be present in arterial blood with severe clinical cyanosis but adequate oxygen supply to the tissues, since 10 gm of hemoglobin will be fully saturated. With a hemoglobin concentration of 10 gm/dl and the same 50 percent arterial saturation, there will be 5 gm of reduced hemoglobin and only mild cyanosis; however, only 5 gm/dl of saturated hemoglobin will be available for oxygen supply, the equivalent of severe anemia.

In tetralogy of Fallot, both ventricles work at systemic pressure, but volume overload does not occur and congestive heart failure is rare. If pulmonary stenosis is moderate, the patient may be acyanotic and have signs of left-to-right shunt. With the progression of infundibular stenosis that occurs with time, cyanosis becomes apparent. Chronic hypoxemia leads to polycythemia and the development of collateral circulation to the lungs.

The mortality of untreated patients with tetralogy of Fallot approaches 50 percent by 5 years of age and 70 percent by the age of 10 years. Only 3 to 5 percent of patients survive to adulthood. Complications occurring early in patients with tetralogy of Fallot are cerebrovascular accidents, probably due to venous thrombosis from polycythemia, cerebral abscesses, and subacute bacterial endocarditis. In addition, an increasing number of patients with uncorrected tetralogy of Fallot develop aortic regurgitation. In infants and children with frequent spells, early corrective surgical therapy is presently advocated and results in low operative mortality (less than 10 percent). Infants with hypoplasia of the pulmonary arteries are not candidates for early correction. A systemic-to-pulmonary artery shunt is created to improve pulmonary blood flow and allow growth of the pulmonary vasculature.

The Blalock-Taussig operation is preferred if vessel size is adequate, or a Gore-tex graft may be inserted. Alternatively, the right ventricular outflow tract may be enlarged without closing the VSD. Pulmonary artery growth then appears to be more rapid with forward flow, and repair of the VSD may be possible sooner. The Potts' and Waterston-Cooley shunts have been associated with congestive failure and development of pulmonary vascular obstructive disease. Both significantly increase the risk of subsequent intracardiac repair.

Elective repair of tetralogy of Fallot is gen-

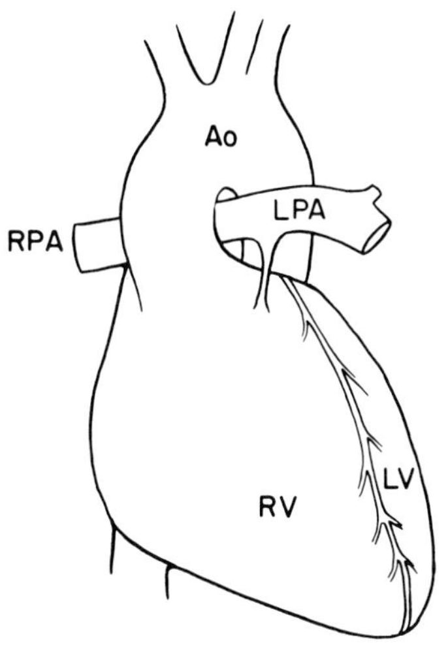

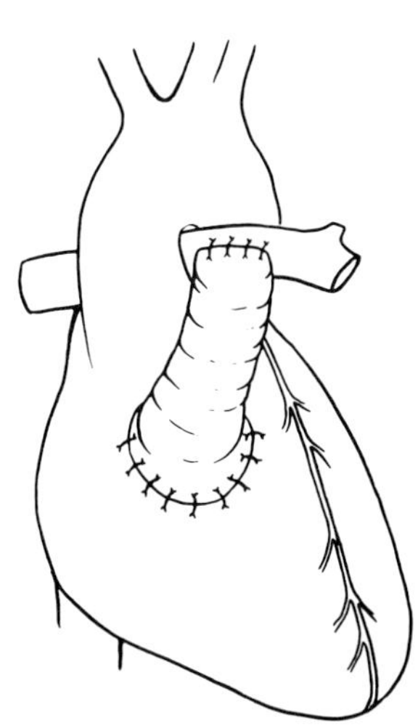

FIGURE 6–6. Pulmonary atresia before and after operation. Repair after Rastelli (conduit). Ao = Aorta; RPA = right pulmonary artery; LPA = left pulmonary artery; RV = right ventricle; LV = left ventricle.

erally carried out toward the end of the first year of life. The right ventricular obstruction has to be completely relieved, if necessary with a large patch crossing the pulmonary valve annulus and extending into the main pulmonary artery. The resulting pulmonary insufficiency appears to be well tolerated. Complications of reparative surgery include residual pulmonic stenosis (10 to 20 percent), residual VSD (5 percent), and, rarely, complete heart block. Right bundle branch block is commonly observed after right ventriculotomy. Between 8 and 11 percent of patients develop supraventricular tachycardia postoperatively. Twenty-three to forty-eight percent of patients develop premature ventricular contractions that occur with exercise. The majority of these patients have elevation of right ventricular pressure preoperatively. In one series, 30 percent of patients with premature ventricular contractions on a resting electrocardiogram died suddenly within 3 months to 8 years postoperatively. Approximately 7 percent of patients died within 15 years after intracardiac repair. However, these patients had late repairs and elevated right ventricular pressures postoperatively. In patients repaired before the age of 5 years, the risk of sudden death and ventricular arrhythmias appears to be less than 1 percent. Ventricular premature beats after intracardiac repair should be treated with propranolol or quinidine.

Left and right ventricular dysfunctions have been observed to persist after complete repair of tetralogy of Fallot even in the absence of residual hemodynamic defects. The response to maximal exercise is abnormal, with a reduction in maximal oxygen uptake and a reduced cardiac index. Repair before the age of 2 years appears to be associated with better preservation of myocardial function.

Pulmonary Atresia with Ventricular Septal Defect. Pulmonary atresia with VSD may be considered an extreme form of tetralogy of Fallot. The majority of infants born with this anomaly become cyanotic shortly after birth and may die within hours after the ductus arteriosus closes. They require a surgical shunt within the first few days of life or placement of a conduit between the right ventricle and main pulmonary artery with the VSD remaining open. The remainder of patients in this group have large and multiple aortopulmonary collaterals and may not exhibit cyanosis until childhood, when the collateral vessels may become inadequate or stenotic. With very large collateral vessels, obstructive pulmonary vascular disease may develop.

Definitive repair for these children consists of placement of a valved conduit between the right ventricle and pulmonary artery and closure of VSD (Fig. 6–6). Large collateral vessels are ligated surgically or embolized with coils in the catheterization laboratory. Reparative surgery is generally performed over the age of 1 year.

In patients with diminutive native pulmonary arteries, segments of collaterals to various parts of the lung may be anastomosed to the native pulmonary arteries or single shunt (unifocalization) in an attempt to create sufficient pulmonary arterial distribution to allow for later corrective surgery. Xenograft conduits, consisting of a Dacron conduit with either a porcine aortic or bovine pericardial valve, tend to degenerate early in young patients—generally within 5 years of implantation. Antibiotic sterilized or cryo-preserved aortic or pulmonary homografts are presently preferred in young patients and generally maintain excellent valve function for 15 to 20 years despite calcification of the walls, after which they tend to fail at a rate of 10 to 20 percent per year.

A number of anatomically different congenital cardiac lesions may present with clinical features similar to those of tetralogy of Fallot. These include double-outlet right ventricle with subaortic VSD and pulmonary stenosis, single ventricle with pulmonic stenosis, and truncus arteriosus. The physiological considerations important for anesthetic management are similar.

Anesthetic Management. The patient should arrive in the operating room well-sedated. However, excessive sedation should be avoided, since it may lead to hypoventilation and worsening cyanosis. Preoperative fluid restriction should be minimized and maintenance fluid given intravenously to prevent hemoconcentration and hypovolemia. Smooth induction is important to prevent increases in oxygen demand or hypercyanotic spells. The agents used should have minimal peripheral vasodilating effects. Mild myocardial depression (e.g., low-dose halothane) may relieve infundibular obstruction. If intravenous agents are used, they should be carefully titrated to prevent relative overdose. Intravenous barbiturate requirements may be reduced by half. The airway should be secured by intubation. Excessive airway pressures should be avoided. The adequacy of ventilation should be ascertained by arterial blood gas measurements, since end-tidal CO_2 measurements do not reflect arterial CO_2 tension in patients with severely reduced pulmonary blood flow. The arterial-to-end-tidal CO_2 gradient, in addition, can fluctuate during operation and anesthesia. Low-dose halothane or narcotic relaxant techniques may be used. Oxygenation is frequently improved under general anesthesia, probably by relaxation of the infundibular muscle, pulmonary vasodilation from higher oxygen concentrations, and reduced peripheral oxygen demands.

Monitoring blood pressure may become a problem in patients with previous shunting procedures that used the subclavian arteries. For major operation, intra-arterial and intravenous pressures should be measured directly. This will also allow blood sampling for blood gas and acid-base measurements. Because the major stress rests on the right ventricle in these patients, central venous pressures can be used to assess cardiac performance.

The presence of a right-to-left shunt prolongs induction with poorly soluble inhalational anesthetics. This may be offset by the presence of a surgically created systemic-to-pulmonary shunt. Intravenous induction is rapid, but conventional doses may produce undesirable side effects because of high systemic concentrations, since the drugs enter the systemic circulation without passage through the lung.

With a fixed obstruction to pulmonary outflow, right-to-left shunting is influenced by changes in peripheral vascular resistance. A decline in systemic vascular resistance may lead to increasing cyanosis, acidosis, and myocardial depression, creating a vicious circle. In patients with dynamic infundibular stenosis, severe infundibular spasm may be triggered intraoperatively by hyperventilation, hypovolemia, relative anemia, manipulation of intracardiac monitoring lines, and inotropic agents. Prompt treatment is essential. Intravenous morphine (0.1 to 0.2 mg/kg) or propranolol (0.05 to 0.1 mg/kg) should be used. Oxygen may have little effect in improving systemic oxygenation. Acidosis should be corrected and venous return improved by administration of fluids. If peripheral vasodilatation was a contributing factor, peripheral vascular resistance should be increased by a peripherally acting agent like phenylephrine (Neo-Synephrine) (5 to 10 μg/kg IV).

Maintenance of cardiac output is essential since the oxygen content of the blood is low. Bradycardia is very poorly tolerated for this reason. In patients with systemic-to-pulmonary shunts, adequate systemic blood pressure is necessary to maintain pulmonary perfusion.

All patients with right-to-left shunts are at an increased risk of systemic embolization of air or blood clots from intravenous lines. In patients with severe polycythemia, hemodilution to a hematocrit of 55 to 60 should be performed prior to elective operation. This will improve cardiac output, peripheral perfusion, and oxygen transport. It may also improve the coagulation defects commonly found in polycythemic patients. Hemodilution to normal levels may be very dangerous, however, as oxygen transport will then be seriously limited.

Endocarditis prophylaxis is essential for all surgical therapy associated with bacteremia. Patients with systemic pulmonary shunts are at particularly high risk.

Patients with cyanosis have a blunted response to hypoxia, which may persist after correction of the underlying lesion. In patients with reduced pulmonary blood flow, marked ventilation/perfusion inequalities exist. Positive-pressure ventilation may worsen this problem, leading to an increase in dead space ventilation and raised arterial P_{CO_2}.

Patients who have undergone correction present a lesser anesthetic problem. However, they may have some impairment of right and left ventricular function, and they have a tendency to develop arrhythmias. Ventricular extrasystoles should be treated, since they have been implicated in sudden death. Patients require endocarditis prophylaxis for their lifetime. The presence of residual defects should be determined prior to elective operation in postcorrection patients.

LESIONS WITH INCREASED PULMONARY BLOOD FLOW

D-TRANSPOSITION OF THE GREAT ARTERIES

In transposition of the great arteries, the aorta arises above the right ventricle and the pulmonary artery above the left ventricle (Fig. 6–7). The pulmonary and systemic circulations therefore run in parallel instead of in series, and systemic oxygenation depends on mixing between the circulations through anatomical communications.

It is a common malformation. The overall incidence is 5 percent of all congenital heart disease, but it is the most common lesion (17 percent) seen during the first week of life. Without treatment, 50 percent of afflicted babies die within the first 6 months, and 90 percent within the first year of life. There is a marked male preponderance (60 to 70 percent).

Blood shunted anatomically from left to right constitutes the effective systemic blood flow, and blood shunted right to left constitutes the effective pulmonary blood flow; the very large blood volume that is being recirculated constitutes physiological right or left shunting. Patients with transposition may be divided into subgroups depending on the presence of VSD and/or restriction to pulmonary blood flow. Transposition with an intact septum is the most common lesion (50 percent), followed by transposition with VSD (30 percent).

Patients present with hypoxemia, acidosis, and/or congestive heart failure in the newborn period or early infancy. If pulmonic stenosis is significant, signs of pulmonary underperfusion occur.

Patients with an intact septum usually are cyanotic within hours of birth as the ductus arteriosus closes and develop progressive acidosis and failure. They require immediate cardiac catheterization, at which time a balloon atrioseptostomy is carried out to allow mixing between the two circulations. The procedure permits survival until "corrective" operation can be performed. From 10 to 40 percent of infants

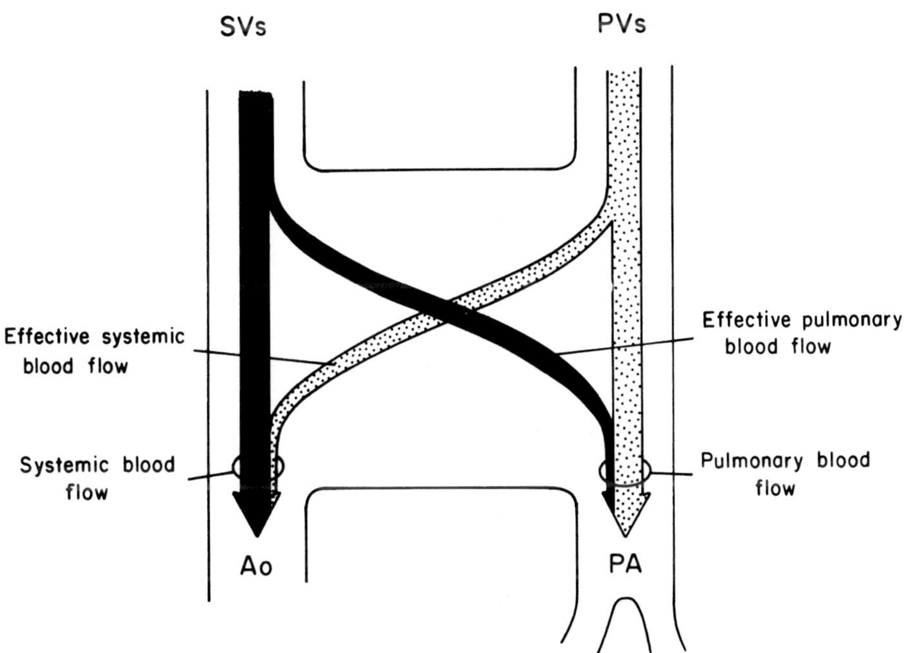

FIGURE 6–7. Transposition of the great vessels. Systemic and pulmonary blood flow in uncorrected transposition of the great vessels. SVs = Systemic veins; PVs = pulmonary veins; Ao = aorta; PA = pulmonary artery. (Redrawn after Kidd BSL: Transposition of the great arteries. *In* Keith JD, et al [eds]: Heart Disease in Infancy and Childhood. 3rd edition. New York, Macmillan, 1978.)

in whom only a balloon septostomy has been performed die within the first year. Patients with an intact septum and a large patent ductus arteriosus (PDA) may be less cyanotic, with reversal of flow through the ductus. The persistence of a large ductus is a lethal lesion in transposition, associated with a 90 percent mortality in the first 6 months with or without operation.

Infants with a large VSD will have adequate mixing despite the transposition and are usually only mildly cyanotic. However, they do develop severe congestive heart failure between 2 and 6 weeks of age that is often resistant to medical management, and they may require pulmonary artery banding or early correction for survival. Transposition is associated with the early development of pulmonary obstructive disease within the first year even in the absence of VSD or patent ductus arteriosus. The high pressures or flows in the pulmonary artery, combined with polycythemia, may be responsible for these changes. Most patients demonstrate preferential perfusion to the right lung. Patients with VSD and pulmonic stenosis may present later, as heart failure is rare and cyanosis mild. With severe pulmonary stenosis, a shunting procedure to improve pulmonary circulation may become necessary.

Although babies with transposition are commonly well developed at birth, they subsequently develop severe growth retardation.

At present, the trend in most surgical centers is toward early correction. The most commonly performed operations until 10 years ago were the Mustard and Senning procedures (Fig. 6–8). These were only physiological corrections, directing systemic venous return through the mitral valve into the left ventricle and pulmonary artery, and pulmonary venous return through the tricuspid valve into the right ventricle and aorta via placement of an intra-atrial baffle. An elective Mustard or Senning repair was commonly performed between 6 and 12 months to prevent pulmonary vascular disease. Mortality for this procedure ranges from 5 to 20 percent in patients in the first few weeks and months of life.

Anatomical correction by switching of the great arteries with coronary reimplantation, as advocated by Jatene for neonates with an intact septum (Fig. 6–9) has supplemented the atrial switching procedures. It is carried out within the first 2 weeks of life while pulmonary vascular resistance is still high. It is also used in patients with a large VSD to avoid the high combined mortality of a banding operation followed by

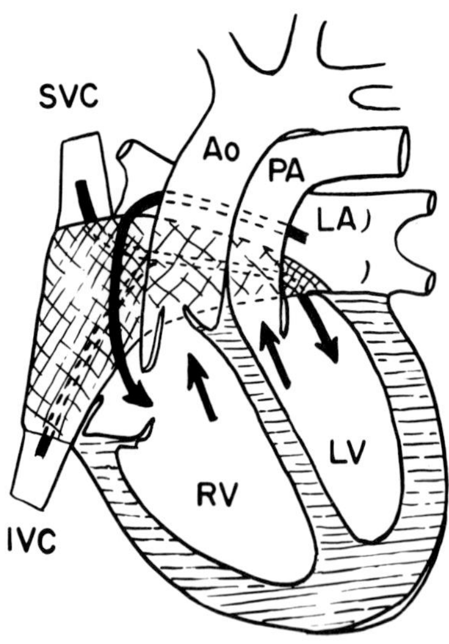

FIGURE 6–8. Transposition of the great vessels. Systemic and pulmonary blood flow after an atrial inversion procedure (Mustard or Senning). SVC = Superior vena cava; IVC = inferior vena cava; Ao = Aorta; PA = pulmonary artery; LA = left atrium; RV = right ventricle; LV = left ventricle.

late intra-atrial baffle repair. Since the left ventricle in these patients remains exposed to high pressures because of the large shunt across the VSD, the switching procedure can be delayed until the infant is 2 to 3 months old.

In the patient with left ventricular outflow obstruction, a Rastelli procedure is performed between 2 and 4 years of age. If inadequate blood flow is present in infancy, a systemic-to-pulmonary shunt is performed initially. In the Rastelli procedure, blood flow is diverted from the left ventricle via the VSD and a baffle to the aorta, and the pulmonary artery is divided and connected via prosthetic graft (usually homograft) to the right ventricle.

In patients with raised pulmonary vascular resistance, a palliative Mustard operation without closure of the VSD improves systemic oxygenation. Late complications after Mustard or Senning repair include systemic or pulmonary venous obstruction or both (22 percent), atrial dysrhythmia, including sick sinus syndrome (40 percent), tricuspid incompetence, and systemic (right) ventricular dysfunction, particularly with exercise. Obstruction of valved conduits occurs in up to 60 percent of patients within 10 years, depending on the material used. Patients who have undergone arterial switch appear to have a much better functional result. Left ventricular function appears to be normal, and the incidence of dysrhythmias is low. Approximately

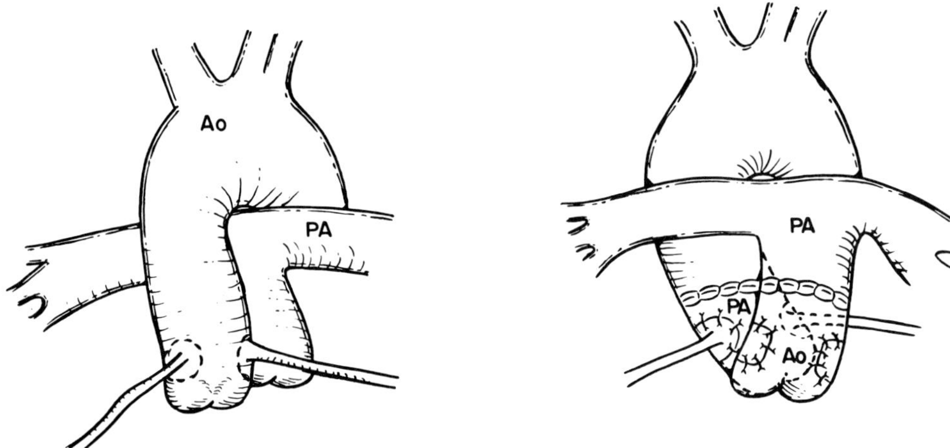

FIGURE 6–9. Repair of transposition of the great vessels, by arterial switch. *Left*, Before operation. *Right*, After operation. Ao = Aorta; PA = pulmonary artery. (Redrawn after Jatene AD, Iontes VF, Paulista PP: Anatomical correction of transposition of the great vessels. J Thorac Cardiovasc Surg *72*:364, 1976.)

15 percent of patients develop stenosis of the pulmonary artery at the site of the surgical anastomosis, with the need for reoperation in less than 5 percent of patients. Between 6 and 14 percent of patients exhibit mild aortic regurgitation. The fate of the reimplanted coronary arteries is at present not yet clear. A few patients have developed occlusion of one of the transplanted coronaries without changes in cardiac function because of development of collateral circulation from the remaining vessel. Whether these patients are at risk for development of premature coronary artery disease is not known.

Anesthetic Management. Other than patients with severe pulmonic obstruction who are awaiting Rastelli's procedure, it is rare that a patient with D-transposition will be encountered who requires cardiac surgical therapy prior to complete repair.

These patients are at a very high risk for systemic embolization. Patients with only balloon septostomy have a 10 to 20 percent incidence of cerebrovascular accidents, which are thought to be due to thrombosis. Perioperative dehydration increases the viscosity of the already hyperviscous polycythemic blood and may lead to thrombosis. The hematocrit should be kept below 60, if necessary by hemodilution. Endocarditis prophylaxis is mandatory.

Because of the low effective pulmonary blood flow, induction of anesthesia with inhalational agents is prolonged, and adverse side effects may linger after the anesthetic is discontinued. Intravenous agents must be used with caution; they have a rapid onset of action, since most of the venous return enters the aorta. Chronic congestive failure is often present, with congestion of the lung and low ventilatory volumes, which predispose the patient to atelectasis. Myocardial depression is poorly tolerated, and bradycardia is usually associated with acidosis. Because of the compromised cardiac and ventilatory function, postoperative mechanical ventilation may be advisable.

Anesthetic agents should have minimal cardiovascular side effects. Narcotic-relaxant techniques, particularly with fentanyl and/or ketamine, have been used with minimal side effects. Low concentrations (0.5 to 0.75 percent) of isoflurane may be used to supplement relaxant techniques. In patients with limited pulmonary blood flow, increases in pulmonary vascular resistance through coughing and struggling should be avoided. In the presence of a systemic-to-pulmonary shunt, maintenance of blood pressure is essential to allow pulmonary perfusion.

An ever-increasing number of children who have survived earlier reparative procedures may present for noncardiac operation in later years. Although they appear clinically normal without evidence of cyanosis or failure, they may not tolerate anesthesia and operation well. Atrial dysrhythmias are common after intra-atrial repairs and may become more frequent with time. The most serious of these is sick sinus syndrome, which may necessitate placement of a temporary pacemaker for surgical therapy if a permanent pacemaker is not already in place. There may be systemic venous obstruction at the baffle site, leading to signs of venous congestion. Significant baffle obstruction usually requires reoperation. Left-sided baffle obstruction (more common after the Senning procedure) may lead to pulmonary hypertension. Increases in peripheral vascular resistance will worsen the condition of the patient under these circumstances.

Insertion of pulmonary artery catheters in these patients is technically difficult because of the tortuous pathway of the venous blood flow, and this procedure may cause arrhythmias or baffle disruption. The right ventricle, carrying the systemic load, has limited reserve and may fail if stressed by rapid fluid shifts or use of myocardial depressing agents. Patients are still at risk for endocarditis, and patients with conduits are at a higher risk postoperatively than before. Arterial switching operations are relatively recent, and therefore little is known about the long-term effects of this procedure. Coronary artery disease may appear early in these patients, and the pulmonary valve in the systemic circulation may become incompetent. ECG monitoring for ischemia and an anesthetic technique that reduces myocardial oxygen demand are probably prudent choices despite the fact that these patients, until now, exhibit very little impairment of cardiac function or propensity for dysrhythmias.

Patients with late repairs of transposition with VSD may have progressive obstructive pulmonary vascular disease with impairment of the pulmonary ventricle.

Asplenia and Polysplenia Syndrome

Agenesis of the spleen is associated with malposition of the abdominal viscera and complex cyanotic congenital heart disease (Ivemark's syndrome). A combination of the following defects is usually present: L- or D-transpositions of the great vessels, pulmonary atresia or severe stenosis, large defects or absence of the atrial and ventricular septa, atrioventricular canal, total anomalous pulmonary venous return, persistence of the left superior vena cava, and absence of the coronary sinus. In the majority of cases there are bilateral trilobed lungs. Dextrocardia is present in 50 percent of cases.

The condition is extremely rare (0.1 percent of congenital heart disease) and because of the complexity of the lesions, surgical correction at present is not feasible. Males are affected more frequently, by a 2:1 ratio. Two thirds of patients die within the first 2 months of life. Survivors may be aided by palliative operation to improve pulmonary blood flow. These patients are extremely susceptible to overwhelming infection, and prophylactic antibiotics and bacterial vaccines may have to be used. Patients have Howell-Jolly bodies in the peripheral blood smear.

Polysplenia is defined as the presence of two or more spleens of nearly equal size and is nearly always associated with complex cardiac malformation. The syndrome is extremely rare. The lesions most commonly associated with polysplenia are total anomalous pulmonary venous return, absence of the hepatic portion of the inferior vena cava with azygos continuation, atrial septal defect, and situs inversus. The lungs are bilaterally bilobed. Symptoms of heart failure usually develop in infancy. Cyanosis is uncommon. The prognosis depends on the underlying defect but is in general better than in asplenia. The lesions are frequently operable. The patients do not appear to be more susceptible to infection.

Anesthetic Management. No experience with anesthesia in asplenic or polysplenic patients has been reported. The choice of technique and degree of monitoring will depend on the presentation of the dominant hemodynamic derangement and the proposed procedure. Prevention of embolization and endocarditis is essential.

Double-Outlet Right Ventricle

In double-outlet right ventricle (DORV), both great vessels arise from the morphological right ventricle. There is always an associated VSD. This malformation accounts for less than 0.5 percent of all congenital heart disease and shows no predilection for either sex or race. Prematurity is common, as is the presence of coarctation and mitral valve disease. Clinical presentation is largely determined by the location of the ventricular septal defect in relation to the great vessels and the presence or absence of pulmonic stenosis (Fig. 6–10).

Patients with subaortic VSD clinically resemble those with a large VSD and are acyanotic until pulmonary vascular disease develops. The majority of these patients, however, have associated pulmonic stenosis, and their clinical presentation is similar to that in tetralogy of Fallot. They compose the majority of patients with DORV. Patients with subpulmonic VSD and transposition of the great vessels compose the so-called Taussig-Bing group of DORV, which is rarely associated with pulmonic stenosis. They clinically resemble patients with D-transposition and are cyanotic from birth. In rare cases the VSD is either beneath both great vessels or completely remote. The latter anatomy is usu-

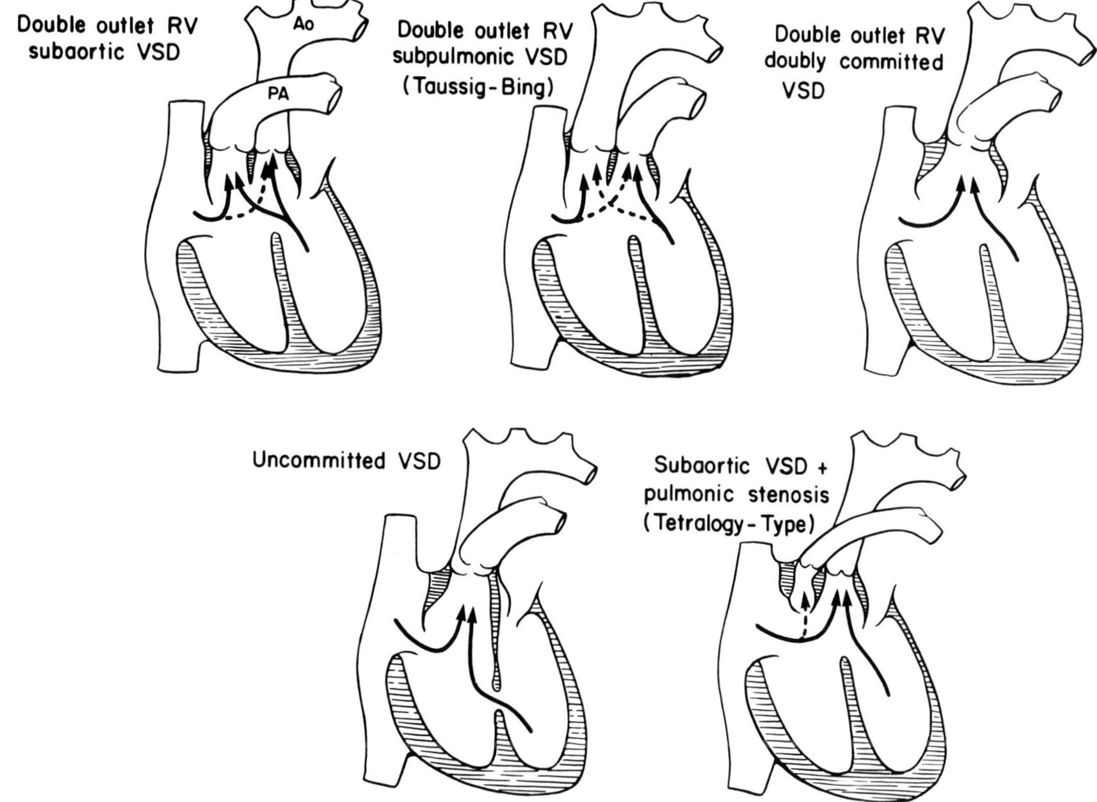

FIGURE 6–10. Double outlet ventricle. Relationship between the location of the ventricular septal defect (VSD) and the great vessels. The first diagram represents the most common form of double outlet right ventricle. Ao = Aorta; PA = pulmonary artery.

ally associated with other complex anomalies like AV canal and the asplenia syndrome.

Patients with unrestricted blood flow to the lung present with congestive heart failure or cyanosis or both in early infancy. The presence of associated coarctation (25 to 30 percent of the Taussig-Bing group) or mitral valve disease (30 percent of patients with subaortic VSD without pulmonary stenosis) is an ominous prognostic feature; mortality approaches 100 percent within the first 6 months.

Patients with pulmonic stenosis usually present later and generally have no other associated defects, appearing clinically similar to those with tetralogy of Fallot. They have the best prognosis of all groups of patients with DORV, as 75 percent survive to adulthood, whereas only 50 percent of patients with only subaortic VSD and unrestricted pulmonary blood flow and 35 percent of patients with the Taussig-Bing malformation survive early childhood.

Medical treatment in patients with volume and pressure overload consists of control of congestive heart failure by digitalis and diuretics. Because of the complex anatomy normally present, surgical correction is generally delayed until after the age of 1 year, and in many centers only palliative operations are performed in infancy. These include pulmonary artery (PA) banding to control congestive heart failure and prevent development of pulmonary vascular obstructive disease, and creation of a systemic-to-pulmonary shunt in the patient with pulmonic stenosis and insufficient pulmonary blood flows. Surgical correction consists of diverting the left ventricular output via an intracardiac tunnel to the aorta, which may necessitate enlargement of the VSD. Blood from the right ventricle flows around the tunnel to the pulmonary artery. Enlargement of the right ventricular outflow tract or interposition of a prosthesis may be necessary in patients with pulmonic stenosis. Repair of a Taussig-Bing anomaly may be achieved by arterial switch and VSD closure or by using the Damus-Kaye-Stansel operation in which the proximal pulmonary artery is anastomosed to the side of the aorta, so that both ventricles empty into the aorta, and the right atrium or the SVC (proximal and distal end) is anastomosed to the pulmonary artery (Fig. 6–11). Patients who underwent repair of a Taussig-Bing anomaly a few years ago may have had VSD closure and a Mustard or Senning procedure for atrial inversion.

Anesthetic Considerations. Cardiac function in DORV patients who have had palliative operation will be similar to that in patients who have VSD with PA banding, D-transposition with PA banding, or tetralogy of Fallot with or without a systemic-to-pulmonary shunt. Prevention of systemic embolization and endocarditis prophylaxis are important.

Myocardial depression, excessive peripheral vasodilatation, and increases in pulmonary vascular resistance should be avoided. After correction, patients may appear normal clinically, but they may exhibit reduced myocardial reserve under stress and may develop conduction disturbances in later life. Endocarditis prophylaxis is particularly important in patients with external valved conduits.

Double-Outlet Left Ventricle

In double-outlet left ventricle, both great arteries arise entirely or predominantly above the left ventricle. Fourteen different anatomical types of this malformation have been described. Patients may present signs of tetralogy of Fallot, transposition, large VSD, Ebstein anomaly, or tricuspid atresia. Surgical palliation and either anatomical or physiological correction are usually possible with acceptable risk if patients survive infancy. Anesthetic management should be guided by the predominant physiological derangement. Endocarditis prophylaxis is required pre- and postoperatively.

OBSTRUCTIVE CARDIAC LESIONS

LESIONS CAUSING LEFT VENTRICULAR OUTFLOW OBSTRUCTION

Valvular Aortic Stenosis

Valvular aortic stenosis represents one of the more common congenital defects, accounting for 3 to 6 percent of all congenital heart disease. It is much more common in males by a 4:1 ratio. Twenty percent of patients have associated defects, most commonly patent ductus arteriosus and coarctation of the aorta. A bicuspid aortic valve is present in approximately 1 percent of the population but will generally not cause aortic stenosis or insufficiency until after childhood. Thickening and increased rigidity of the valve tissue and varying degrees of commisural fusion constitute the basic malformation in valvular aortic stenosis. Only severe stenosis, usually with unicuspid valve and hypoplastic aortic valve ring, is symptomatic in infancy. Almost all children with aortic stenosis are asymptomatic.

The essential hemodynamic abnormality consists of a pressure gradient between the left ventricle and the aorta during the systolic ejection period. Blood flow is turbulent, and the pressure gradient is proportional to the square of the flow rate across the valve. The left ventricle develops concentric hypertrophy which decreases compliance and offers resistance to filling. The mean left atrial pressure does not rise, except in severe stenosis, but the left atrium develops vigorous contractions that prevent elevation of the pulmonary venous pressure while at the same time elevating left ventricular end-diastolic pressure sufficient for effective left ventricular action.

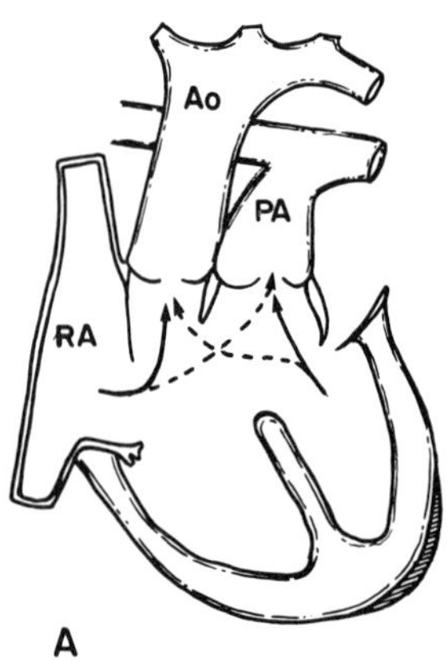

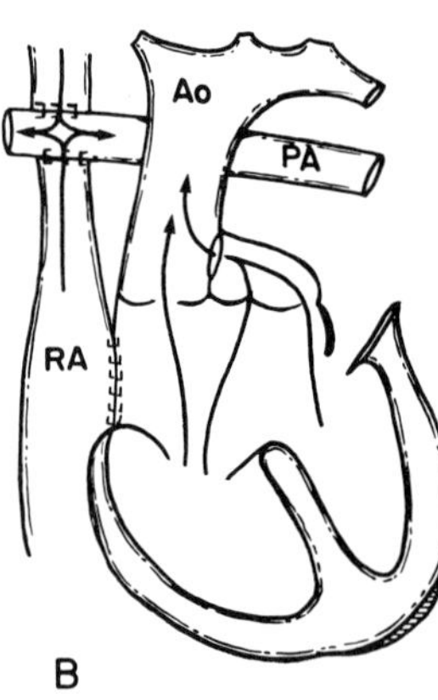

FIGURE 6–11. Damus-Kaye-Stansel modification of Fontan repair for correction of a Taussig-Bing heart.

Left ventricular myocardial fibrosis may develop over time. Left ventricular ejection is prolonged, which leads to changes in the second heart sound (narrow splitting or single). Myocardial blood supply may be compromised owing to the limited cardiac output, myocardial hypertrophy, and raised end-diastolic intracavitary pressure. Shortened diastole, as in tachycardia, will worsen this situation. Most children have only a murmur and are otherwise normal. The major threats to these children are from endocarditis and sudden death, especially with exercise. The risk of endocarditis, which may occur in more than 4 percent of patients, is unrelated to the severity of obstruction. The risk of sudden death is reported to be between 4 and 18 percent.

Critical aortic stenosis is present when the pressure gradient across the valve is greater than 75 mm Hg in the presence of a normal cardiac output, or the valve area is less than 0.5 cm^2 per m^2 of body surface area. These patients are always symptomatic and require operation or balloon valvuloplasty. Infants show dyspnea and congestive failure. Older children may show dyspnea syncope or anginal pains.

Operation consists of open valvotomy. This procedure usually can palliate the symptoms, with significant reduction in the pressure gradient. Percutaneous balloon valvuloplasty may also be used in cases of moderate-to-severe stenosis. Since the valve is malformed, however, restenosis, calcification, or aortic insufficiency may develop with time in a large number of these children. Valve replacement is usually postponed as long as possible, since it will require repeat operations to replace the valve for inadequate size or malfunction. Critical aortic stenosis in neonates and infants is frequently associated with endocardial fibroelastosis from myocardial ischemia and mitral insufficiency from papillary muscle dysfunction. Operative mortality is greater than 50 percent among these patients.

Supravalvular Aortic Stenosis. In supravalvular aortic stenosis, the aorta is locally or diffusely narrowed above the level of the coronary arteries. This is most commonly associated with Williams' syndrome—idiopathic infantile hypercalcemia. Patients are often retarded. Since the coronary arteries are located proximal to the obstruction, they are subjected to the high pressures of the left ventricle, are frequently tortuous, and may develop premature coronary arteriosclerosis. Clinical symptoms are similar to those of valvular aortic stenosis. Treatment consists of patch enlargement of the narrowed segment if localized stenosis is present.

Discrete Subvalvular Aortic Stenosis. In this lesion, a membranous diaphragm or ring encircling the left ventricular outflow tract is present. The malformation accounts for 8 to 10 percent of all cases of congenital aortic stenosis. It occurs commonly in patients with coarctation and ventricular septal defect and following pulmonary artery banding. Jet lesions of the aortic cusps occur with this type of aortic stenosis, causing valve degeneration with development of aortic insufficiency. There is a very high risk of infective endocarditis. The clinical presentation is similar to that of valvular aortic stenosis and depends on the severity of obstruction. Because of the likelihood of development of progressive obstruction and aortic insufficiency, operation is recommended even for mild-to-moderate stenosis. It consists of excision of the membranous or fibrous ridge. Because of the existing jet lesion and scarring following manipulation of the valve during operation, children with this malformation eventually may require valve replacement.

Anesthetic Considerations in Aortic Stenosis. Increases in the inotropic state of the heart or decreases in peripheral vascular resistance tend to increase the pressure gradient across the stenotic area. Tachycardia shortens the duration of diastole more than that of systole and may cause myocardial ischemia in these patients. The stroke volume is limited by the size of the aortic orifice and ejection time. Peripheral vasodilatation may lower blood pressure critically because cardiac output is fixed. This reduces myocardial perfusion dangerously.

Anesthetic agents with minimal effects on myocardial performance and heart rate should be chosen. Prevention of anxiety and stress and the resulting tachycardia are important. Low-dose inhalation anesthesia or narcotic relaxant techniques may be useful. For major operation, invasive monitoring should be established. Endocarditis prophylaxis is of utmost importance. Patients who have undergone valvuloplasty usually have a residual defect that should be assessed prior to elective operation. They are still at high risk for endocarditis. Patients with critical stenosis should not undergo elective non-cardiac surgery.

Hypoplastic Left Heart Syndrome

Atresia of the aortic valve, associated with atresia or severe stenosis of the mitral valve; hypoplasia or absence of the left ventricle and hypoplasia of the ascending aorta or interrupted aortic arch constitute the hypoplastic left heart syndrome. It is more common in males and affects 7 to 9 percent of all infants seen with cardiac disease. Systemic perfusion is maintained via a patent ductus arteriosus and an atrial septal defect. Severe heart failure is always present. Mortality approaches 95 percent within the first month of life.

Surgical palliation is possible in selected patients (Fig. 6–12). In the first-stage Norwood procedure the heart is converted physiologically to a single-ventricle system, with the proximal pulmonary artery connected to the aorta and supplying systemic perfusion. Pulmonary blood flow is supplied via an aortopulmonary graft. Eventual physiological correction (second-stage Norwood) consists of a modified Fontan procedure with redirection of systemic venous return directly into the pulmonary artery and pulmonary venous return to the right ventricle, which supplies the aorta. Surgical mortality for the first stage palliation ranges between 10 and 50 percent, with between 20 and 40 percent of patients surviving for the second stage. Complications following first-stage palliation include insufficient diameter of the ASD leading to pulmonary venous hypertension and cyanosis from insufficient mixing, coarctation of the neoaorta, and tricuspid regurgitation. A successful alternative to the Norwood procedure has been cardiac transplantation in the newborn period, which has resulted in excellent functional result in the survivors but is limited in its applicability because of a shortage of donor organs.

Anesthetic Considerations. Only palliated patients will ever be seen for noncardiac operation. They are at risk for systemic embolization and endocarditis. Patients will exhibit various degrees of cyanosis, depending on atrial mixing and pulmonary blood flow. Pulmonary venous return has to pass across an ASD to the right atrium and right ventricle to reach the aorta. Maintenance of normal pulmonary and systemic vascular resistance is essential. Hyperventilation may lead to flooding of the lungs and systemic underperfusion; arterial saturation should be maintained at between 80 and 85 percent. Most patients after first-stage Norwood exhibit various degrees of congestive heart failure and may tolerate potent inhalational anesthetic agents poorly. After physiological correction, patients need sufficient venous pressure to maintain pulmonary and hence systemic perfusion, as the right atrium becomes the systemic venous chamber.

LESIONS CAUSING RIGHT VENTRICULAR OUTFLOW OBSTRUCTION

Pulmonary Stenosis

The presence of a pressure gradient between the right ventricle and the pulmonary artery constitutes the main physiological derangement in pulmonary stenosis. It is an associated feature in 25 to 30 percent of congenital cardiac lesions but occurs as an isolated defect in about 10 percent of patients with congenital heart disease. It is the lesion most commonly associated with Noonan's syndrome. Most commonly, the stenosis is at the valve level, with fusion of the leaflets producing a dome-shaped valve with a small central opening. The severity of clinical symptoms depends on the degree of obstruction to right ventricular outflow. Patients with mild-to-moderate obstruction are generally asymptomatic, and the stenosis is usually discovered during a routine examination because of the presence of a systolic murmur.

Secondary changes include hypertrophy of the right ventricle (which may produce infundibular stenosis) and poststenotic dilatation of the pulmonary trunk.

In severe stenosis, right ventricular pressure may exceed the pressure in the left ventricle. Right atrial pressure is elevated, and right-to-left shunting occurs across a patent foramen ovale or atrial septal defect. If no communication between the right and left heart exists, syncope may occur during exercise because of inability to increase cardiac output. Right ventricular ischemic changes with myocardial fibrosis and coronary artery occlusions may develop in these patients, leading to right ventricular failure.

All symptomatic patients, or those with right ventricular–to–pulmonary artery gradients exceeding 70 mm Hg, require relief of their obstruction. Patients with gradients of less than 50 mm Hg usually do not become worse over time. Obstruction may be relieved by open or closed valvotomy or percutaneous valvuloplasty. The latter is not recommended for patients with associated infundibular stenosis. Successful valvotomy will lead to a reduction in right ventricular pressure to half of preoperative values or lower. Infundibular stenosis will usually improve with time. In the presence of a dysplastic valve, enlargement of the valve ring may be necessary, leading to postoperative pulmonary valve insufficiency.

Infants with critical pulmonic stenosis are

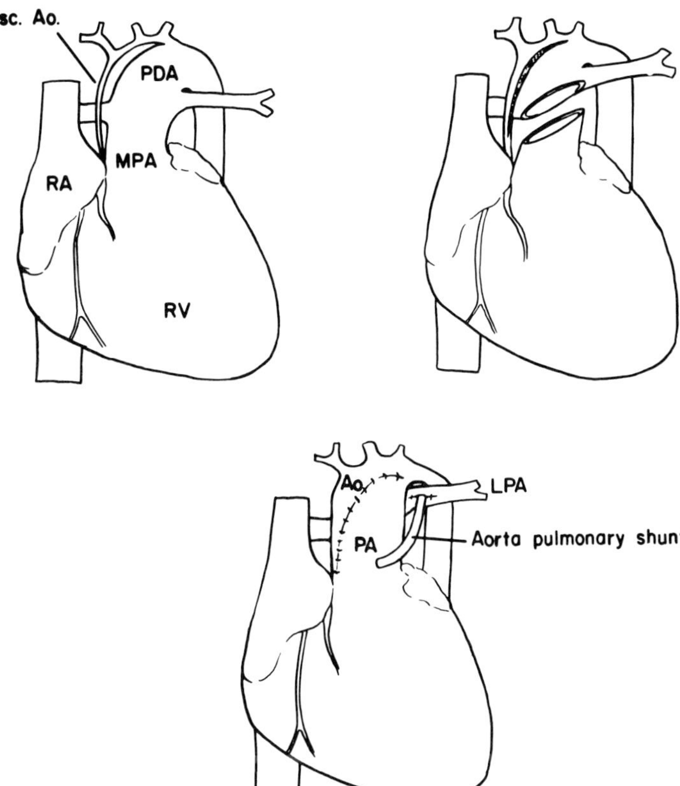

FIGURE 6–12. Palliation of hypoplastic left heart syndrome. RA = Right atrium; Ao = Aorta; RV = right ventricle; MPA = main pulmonary artery; PDA = patent ductus arteriosus. (After Norwood WI, Lang P: Physiologic repair of aortic atresia—hypoplastic left heart syndrome. N Engl J Med *308*:23, 1983. Reprinted with permission from *The New England Journal of Medicine*.)

usually seen 24 to 48 hours after birth with cyanosis and metabolic acidosis. Pulmonary blood flow is ductus dependent. The patients frequently have hypoplasia of the right ventricle associated with endomyocardial fibrosis. Relief of the right ventricular outflow obstruction has to be performed on an emergency basis, frequently combined with a systemic-to-pulmonary shunt, since pulmonary blood flow may still be insufficient. For major surgical therapy, invasive monitoring should be established. Endocarditis prophylaxis is of utmost importance. Patients who have undergone valvuloplasty usually have a residual defect that should be assessed prior to elective surgery. They are still at high risk for endocarditis. Patients with critical stenosis should not undergo elective noncardiac operation.

Primary Infundibular Stenosis. This lesion is rare as an isolated malformation. If the stenosis is discrete, immediately below the valve, the clinical symptoms are similar to those of valvular stenosis and depend on the degree of obstruction. However, if there is a long, narrow segment, the obstruction behaves more dynamically and may vary with the degree of muscular activity. It becomes worse during exercise or with positive inotropic drugs. Treatment is surgical if symptoms or significant pressure gradients exist.

Anomalous Right Ventricular Muscle Bands. Aberrant right ventricular muscle bands cause division of the right ventricle into a proximal high-pressure chamber and a distal low-pressure chamber. Clinical presentation is similar to that of valvular or infundibular stenosis. Treatment is surgical.

Peripheral Pulmonic Stenosis. Stenosis of the pulmonary arteries, either proximal or distal, occurs in 2 to 3 percent of all patients with congenital heart disease. This, and patency of the ductus arteriosus, are the lesions most commonly associated with the congenital rubella syndrome. Patients with mild-to-moderate bilateral stenosis or unilateral disease are usually asymptomatic. Patients with severe obstruction have dyspnea, fatigue, and signs of right heart failure. Treatment is surgical if the obstruction is located proximally or with balloon dilatation. Multiple distal stenoses may improve with the growth of the patient, or treatment with balloon angioplasty may be sequential. If severe peripheral stenosis cannot be relieved, death occurs during infancy or early childhood.

Anesthetic Considerations. All patients with pulmonic stenosis (pre- or postoperatively) need endocarditis prophylaxis, although endocarditis risk is low. Patients with mild degrees of obstruction should otherwise experience no anesthetic problems. Patients with moderate degrees of obstruction who appear clinically normal may have limited myocardial reserve. An increase in pulmonary vascular resistance may cause right heart failure. During stressful surgery, right heart function should be carefully monitored. Patients with infundibular stenosis may benefit from mild reduction in myocardial contractility, such as is induced by 0.5 percent halothane.

Pulmonary Atresia

Absence of the pulmonary valve, with an intact ventricular septum and varying degrees of right ventricular hypoplasia, accounts for about 1 percent of all congenital heart disease. Pulmonary blood flow is completely dependent on the ductus arteriosus, which is frequently hypoplastic.

Symptoms appear shortly after birth with cyanosis and tachypnea. Metabolic acidosis and signs of heart failure may develop rapidly. Patients require palliation or correction within the first few days of life. The patency of the ductus arteriosus is maintained with prostaglandin E_1 or E_2. For severe hypoplasia of the right ventricle or atresia of the main pulmonary artery, a systemic-to-pulmonary shunt is constructed, combined with balloon atrioseptostomy. If the right ventricle is nearly normal in size, open or closed valvotomy is performed, and the patient is maintained on a prostaglandin infusion until the right ventricle has adapted to the increasing forward flow. In patients with questionable hypoplasia, a systemic-to-pulmonary shunt in addition to valvotomy may have to be performed to maintain pulmonary perfusion and systemic oxygenation. In patients who have small right ventricles, systemic or suprasystemic pressures, and tricuspid atresia, fistulous connections occur between the right ventricular endocardium and the right, left, or rarely both coronary arterial systems. These may cause shunting of hypoxemic blood from the right ventricle to the aorta and result in left ventricular ischemia and fibrosis. Acute right ventricular decompression following valvotomy can result in reversal of flow from the sinusoid to the right ventricle, with resulting coronary steal and ischemia.

The prognosis without operation is dismal: Most patients die within the first few weeks of life. Even with operation, the patients do poorly because of their abnormal right ventricular anatomy and function. surgical mortality for the initial procedure ranges around 10 percent, with 80 percent of patients surviving the first year. In patients with a severely hypoplastic, thickened right ventricle, insufficient growth of the right ventricle occurs even after successful valvotomy. These patients are clinically similar to those with tricuspid atresia, and their pulmonary atresia may be "corrected" with a Fontan-type operation. In patients with atresia of the pulmonary trunk, a Rastelli operation can be performed in later childhood if the right ventricle is of adequate size.

Anesthetic Considerations. Candidates for elective surgical therapy should have a functioning systemic-to-pulmonary shunt or should have undergone relief of the obstruction by valvotomy, patch graft, conduit insertion, or right ventricular bypass. Endocarditis prophylaxis is necessary in all patients. Anesthetic management has to be tailored to the specific hemodynamic sequelae of the corrective or palliative procedure. The maintenance of acceptable systemic pressure, preload, and pulmonary vascular resistance is essential. The right ventricle in these patients may function abnormally permanently and may fail with surgical stress or use of myocardial depressing agents.

LESIONS CAUSING LEFT VENTRICULAR INFLOW OBSTRUCTION

Mitral Stenosis

Isolated mitral stenosis is one of the rarest forms of congenital heart disease, occurring in 0.6 percent of autopsied and 0.2 to 0.4 percent of clinically diagnosed patients with congenital heart disease. It is more common in males.

Developmental abnormalities of the mitral valve leaflets, commissures, chordae tendineae, annulus, supravalvular area, or papillary muscles may lead to obstruction of left ventricular filling. Left atrial pressure rises as a compensatory mechanism to maintain blood flow across the stenotic area. With further reduction in the valve orifice, blood flow becomes turbulent, which increases resistance to total flow and leads to a higher pressure gradient. Pulmonary venous pressure becomes secondarily elevated, eventually leading to elevation of pulmonary artery and right ventricular pressures. The vascular congestion results in a decrease in static and dynamic compliance. Bronchial venous congestion leads to edema of the bronchial mucosa and increased airway resistance. The work of breathing is increased, and abnormalities in gas exchange are common with significant disease. Pulmonary interstitial or alveolar edema occurs if pulmonary capillary hydrostatic pressures exceed plasma oncotic pressure and the maximal transport capacity of the pulmonary lymphatics.

Left ventricular filling depends on the size of the valve orifice and diastolic filling time. Tachycardia will lead to marked elevation in atrial pressure and reduction in cardiac output. Left ventricular dysfunction from ischemia and fibrosis frequently complicates severe stenosis. Approximately 50 percent of patients with congenital mitral stenosis have other congenital cardiac anomalies.

Patients commonly have exertional dyspnea and recurrent pulmonary infections. Infants may show failure to thrive, and episodes of congestive heart failure may occur. The diagnosis is frequently established late. Patients with mild-to-moderate stenosis (gradient less than 25 mm Hg across the mitral valve) are managed medically with control of failure and attention to pulmonary infections and endocarditis. Survival appears to be related mostly to the presence of associated cardiac lesions, and the median survival is 3 years.

Patients with intractable congestive failure, pulmonary edema, or pulmonary artery hypertension at the systemic level require surgical intervention. Unrelieved left atrial hypertension will lead to progressive obstructive pulmonary vascular disease. Mitral valvotomy or fenestration of the mitral valve is generally carried out in infants or small children. With severely deformed valves, radical valvuloplasty is recommended to avoid replacement. These procedures will generally provide palliation sufficiently to allow for growth and development and relief of clinical symptoms. Eventually, mitral valve replacement will become necessary in the majority of cases.

Prognosis of symptomatic infants is poor. Forty percent die within the first 6 months, irrespective of therapy. Surgical mortality is reported at between 30 and 40 percent, with 50 percent of patients surviving beyond 5 to 10 years. Presently, less than 20 percent of patients survive to adulthood.

SUPRAVALVULAR RING

Accumulation of connective tissue arising from the atrial surface of the mitral valve produces a supravalvular ring, reducing the effective mitral orifice. It rarely occurs as an isolated malformation but is usually associated with some degree of valvular mitral stenosis. The clinical presentation is indistinguishable from that of valvular stenosis. Treatment consists of surgical excision of the ring tissue.

PARACHUTE MITRAL VALVE—SHONE'S SYNDROME

Insertion of all chordae tendineae into a single papillary muscle leads to a parachute deformity of the mitral valve. Blood flow from the left atrium must pass through the interchordal spaces, and various degrees of functional mitral stenosis are the result. The lesion is commonly associated with other forms of left-sided obstruction, for example, supravalvular mitral ring, subvalvular or valvular aortic stenosis, and coarctation of the aorta. The presence of all four obstructive lesions together constitutes Shone's syndrome. Median survival approaches 10 years of age and correlates best with left ventricular size. Patients are managed medically with control of heart failure and pulmonary infections throughout childhood, since relief of the obstruction requires mitral valve replacement.

Anesthetic Considerations. Because of the rarity of the lesion and the poor prognosis, no experience with anesthesia in patients with any form of congenital mitral stenosis has been reported. Extrapolating from experience with adults, the following management suggestions could be made. All preoperative and the majority of postoperative patients will have a pressure gradient across the mitral valve. Flow though the valve occurs during diastole, and shortening diastole will decrease ventricular filling. Hypovolemia and reduction in preload may decrease left atrial pressure below the pressure necessary to pump blood across the stenotic valve. With reduction in afterload, the heart may be unable to compensate by increasing stroke volume or cardiac output, since both are limited by the amount of blood that can pass across the stenotic area. Overzealous administration of fluids or alterations in position may increase central blood volume and cause a rapid rise in left atrial pressure; this may lead to pulmonary edema, since the volume cannot be transported rapidly across the stenosis. Patients are at risk for bacterial endocarditis. Patients may have marked alterations in gas exchange due to small airway disease and maldistribution.

The anesthetic technique chosen should cause no tachycardia, minimal vasodilatation, and no depression of myocardial function. Preload must be maintained. Tachycardia, if it occurs, requires prompt treatment with digitalis, propranolol, or verapamil. Atrial fibrillation is extremely uncommon in children with mitral stenosis, as is systemic embolization. Congestive failure should be controlled but without excessive depletion of intravascular volume, since induction of anesthesia may lead to severe hypotension under these circumstances. Hypotension, if due to peripheral vasodilatation, should be treated with judicious use of a peripheral vasoconstrictor like phenylephrine.

Because of frequently seen disturbances in pulmonary gas exchange, the airway should be secured, and positive pressure ventilation, which tends to counteract pulmonary edema, should be utilized. Patients require higher inspired oxygen concentrations. Hypoxia may lead to acute right heart failure through a further increase in pulmonary vascular resistance.

Circulatory and fluid status for any major surgical therapy should be assessed by intravascular monitoring. Electrolyte abnormalities caused by diuretic therapy should be normalized prior to elective surgery. Pulmonary artery monitoring will reflect only filling status of the left atrium, with left ventricular end-diastolic pressure dependent on the gradient across the valve and the outflow resistance of the left ventricle. Acute elevations in left atrial pressure may be treated with an increase in positive-pressure ventilation and venodilatation (nitroglycerin, low-dose nitroprusside, and reverse Trendelenburg position) to promote venous pooling. Patients who suffer decompensation during operation may need inotropic support.

A narcotic-relaxant technique may be a prudent choice. Induction of anesthesia may be markedly prolonged secondary to low cardiac output. Ketamine causes less tachycardia in infants and children and will maintain vascular tone. Inhalation anesthetics may be poorly tolerated in the presence of a low, fixed cardiac output. Regional techniques may cause extensive sympathetic blockade, which will readily lead to hypotension and necessitate the use of vasopressors. Fluid therapy may cause left atrial hypertension and pulmonary edema when the sympathetic block wears off.

Cor Triatriatum

In cor triatriatum, the left atrium is abnormally portioned into two chambers: the upper one receives the pulmonary veins and the lower one contains the mitral valve. Communication between the two chambers is through fenestrations in the dividing membrane. The hemodynamic consequence is pulmonary venous obstruction similar to that in mitral stenosis. The malformation occurs in about 0.02 to 0.5 percent of all congenital heart disease. Males are slightly more affected.

In classic cor triatriatum, no communication exists between the two left atrial chambers and the right atrium. Consequent to the obstruction of pulmonary venous return, pulmonary artery hypertension develops, with right ventricular hypertrophy. The onset of symptoms is usually within the first few years of life, characterized by breathlessness and frequent respiratory infections. Patients with severe obstruction have pulmonary edema and right heart failure and are often considered to have primary pulmonary disease. Death occurs within months if the obstruction is not relieved by surgical excision of the membrane dividing the atrium. Patients who survive the operation have an excellent prognosis. The pulmonary vascular changes appear to be reversible.

Some patients with subdivided left atria have connections between the upper chamber and the right atrium via a patent foramen ovale or atrial septal defect. The clinical presentation is similar to that of total anomalous pulmonary venous return. The correct diagnosis is often established only at operation or autopsy. Treatment consists of excision of the obstructing membrane and closure of the intra-atrial communication. Surgical enlargement of the left atrium may be required.

Anesthetic Considerations. Patients with classic cor triatriatum have clinical signs and symptoms similar to those of mitral stenosis and should be normal clinically after repair but require endocarditis prophylaxis.

LESIONS CAUSING RIGHT VENTRICULAR INFLOW OBSTRUCTION

Tricuspid Atresia

Atresia of the tricuspid valve is always associated with an ASD (usually a patent foramen ovale). The mitral valve and left ventricle are hyperplastic, and the right ventricle is hypoplastic or absent. Tricuspid atresia occurs in 1.5 to 3 percent of all patients with congenital heart disease and is slightly more common in males.

Tricuspid atresia can be divided into three different types (I, II, and III), depending on the relationship of the great vessel (normal, D-transposed, or L-transposed) (Fig. 6–13). Fur-

Tricuspid Atresia With No Transposition (69 percent)

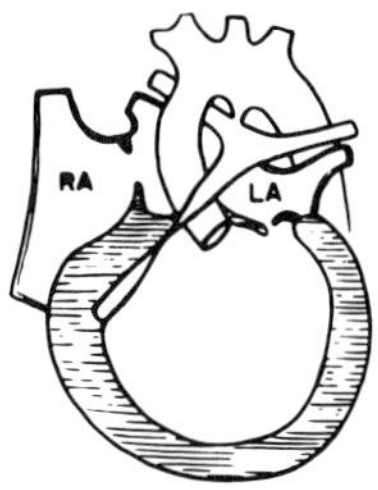

Pulmonary atresia

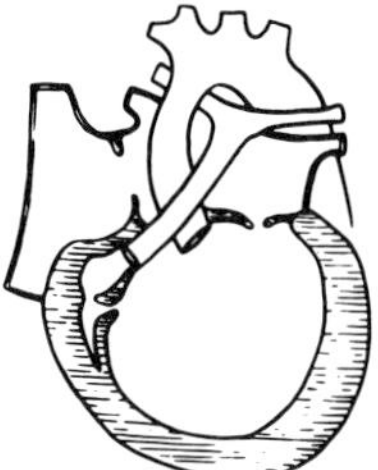
Pulmonary hypoplasia, small ventricular septal defect

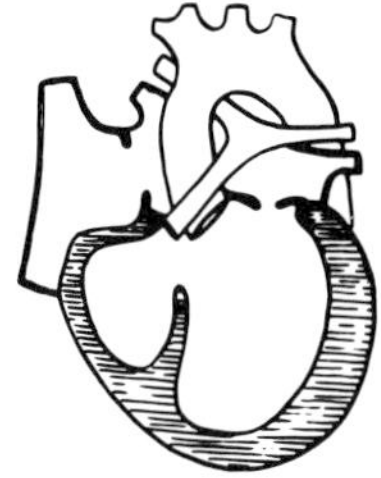
No pulmonary hypoplasia, large ventricular septal defect

Tricuspid Atresia With D Transposition (27 percent)

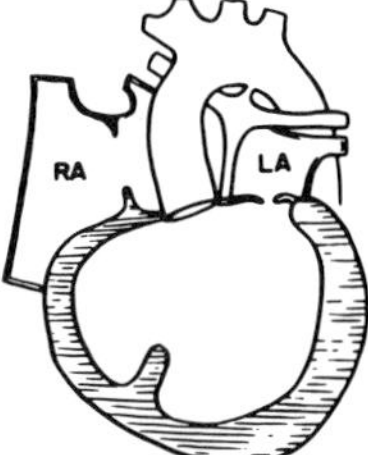

Pulmonary atresia

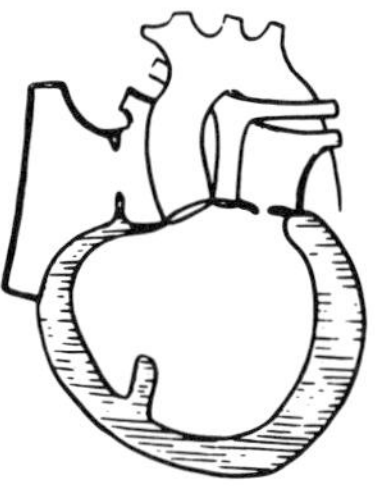
Pulmonary or subpulmonary stenosis

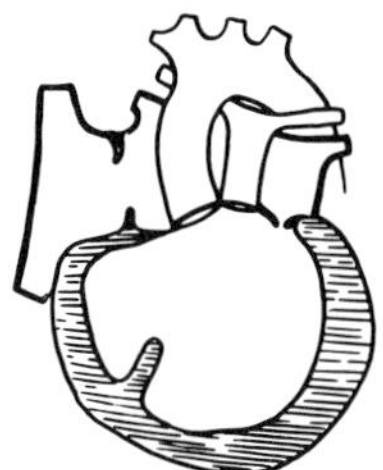
Large pulmonary artery

Tricuspid Atresia With L Transposition (3 percent)

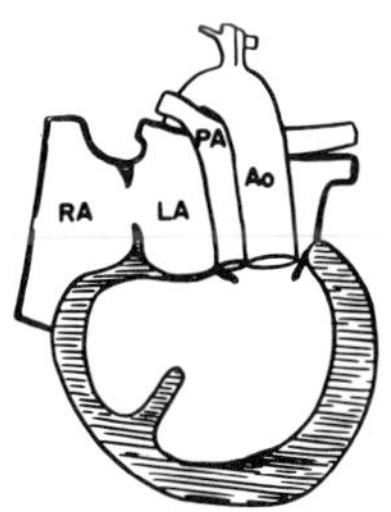

Pulmonary or subpulmonary stenosis

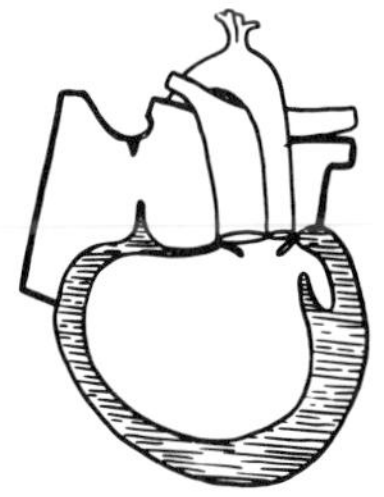
Subaortic stenosis

FIGURE 6–13. Classification of tricuspid atresia. (After Vlad P: Tricuspid atresia. *In* Keith JD, et al [eds]: Heart Disease in Infancy and Childhood. 3rd edition. New York, Macmillan, 1978.)

ther subclassification relates to the presence of pulmonic stenosis or a ventricular septal defect. Fifty percent of all patients with tricuspid atresia have normally related great vessels, a small VSD, and pulmonary atresia and stenosis. Only 10 to 15 percent have no obstruction to pulmonary blood flow.

Cyanosis occurs often on the first day of life and is due to the obligatory right-to-left shunt across the ASD. The intensity varies with the degree of pulmonary outflow obstruction and is most intense in patients with an intact septum. Patients with transposition and a large VSD may have only mild cyanosis and present with congestive heart failure in the first few months. A diagnosis of tricuspid atresia should be suspected when there is cyanosis with left axis deviation on the ECG and a left ventricular hypertrophy pattern in the precordial leads.

The prognosis without surgical intervention is poor: 50 percent of patients die within the first 6 months, and only 10 percent survive past the age of 10 years. Tricuspid atresia is an incorrectable lesion, and only palliative surgery is available. However, with surgical management, more than 50 percent of patients do survive past the second decade of life.

Patients with excessive pulmonary blood flow may develop pulmonary obstructive disease within the first year of life. Patients with a Potts' or Waterston's shunt may develop the same problem.

Patients display delayed growth. If the foramen ovale is restrictive, signs of venous conges-

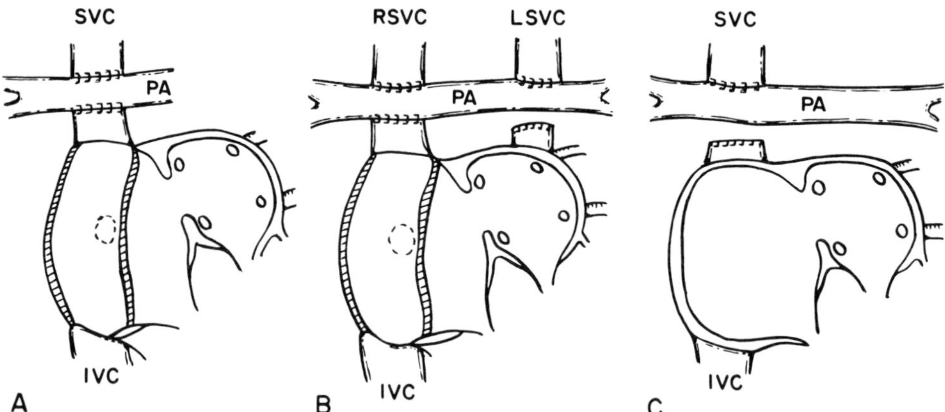

FIGURE 6–14. Modification of the Fontan procedure with caval anastomoses. *A* and *B*, Total caval anastomosis with one or two superior venae cavae. *C*, Bidirectional Glenn shunt. (Dotted circle represents fenestration for patients with borderline pulmonary vascular resistance.)

tion with a prominent "a" wave in the jugular pulse may become apparent. This is unusual in infants, more common in children and adolescents. Life-threatening atrial dysrhythmias tend to develop in older patients, probably owing to the distention of the atrium. They tend to aggravate existing heart failure and reduce pulmonary blood flow.

Severely cyanotic newborn infants whose pulmonary blood flow depends on patency of the ductus require urgent shunting. Infusion of prostaglandin E_1 may maintain oxygenation by preventing ductal closure. A Blalock-Taussig shunt has been preferred until recently, since it is rarely associated with the development of obstructive pulmonary vascular disease. A bidirectional Glenn's shunt is presently preferred as a prelude to an eventual Fontan's repair (Fig. 6–14). A venous-pulmonary arterial shunt will function only if pulmonary vascular resistance is normal or low. Patients with increased pulmonary blood flow require pulmonary artery banding in the first 6 months of life for control of failure and to protect the pulmonary vasculature. Thirty-eight percent of patients with VSDs undergo spontaneous closure of the defect, at which point cyanosis intensifies and a shunt procedure becomes necessary.

Twenty-five to thirty percent of patients with tricuspid atresia and shunts develop endocarditis. Between 1 and 5 percent develop brain abscesses.

During the past decade, physiological correction of tricuspid atresia has gained popularity. The procedures were first described by Fontan and Kreutzer and consist of connection of the right atrium to the pulmonary artery or right ventricular infundibulum and closure of the septal defects (Fig. 6–15). This separates the pulmonary and systemic circulations, with relief of cyanosis and left ventricular volume overload. The procedure can be performed only in patients with normal pulmonary vascular resistance. In some centers it is performed instead

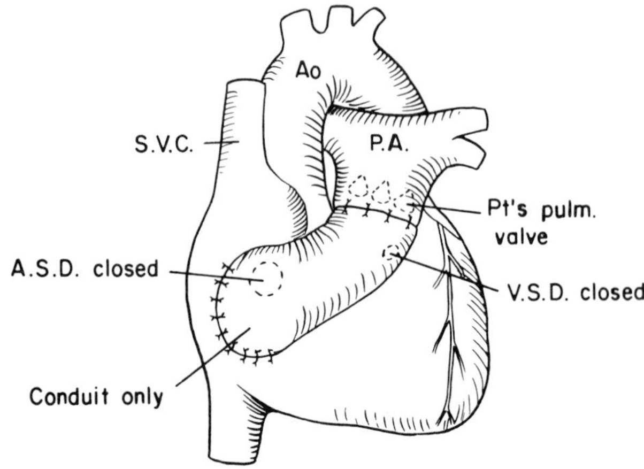

FIGURE 6–15. A modified Fontan repair for tricuspid atresia. SVC = Superior vena cava; Ao = Aorta; PA = pulmonary artery; ASD = atrial septal defect; VSD = ventricular septal defect.

of a shunting procedure in children past early infancy. Pulmonary blood flow is dependent on a pressure difference between the right atrium and the pulmonary artery. Right atrial pressures are mildly-to-moderately elevated postoperatively. Chronic liver congestion and ascites may be present, and patients demonstrate low baseline cardiac output and inability to increase cardiac output with exercise to normal levels. The maintenance of sinus rhythm is important to maintain pulmonary blood flow and low systemic venous pressures. Long-term survival after Fontan's repair for tricuspid atresia is good, with 87 percent of patients surviving for more than 5 years. Late obstruction of the right atrium to pulmonary artery anastomosis has occurred in 14 percent of patients by 10 years and 41 percent by 15 years following repair. The long-term problems with bicaval anastomoses are not yet known. These patients may develop lower lobe pulmonary arteriovenous fistulae because of maldistribution of pulmonary blood flow.

Anesthetic Considerations. Most patients with tricuspid atresia requiring anesthesia for noncardiac surgery will have a functioning systemic-to-pulmonary shunt. Anesthetic management is similar to that of patients with tetralogy of Fallot and a shunt. Rigorous endocarditis prophylaxis, prevention of systemic embolization, maintenance of cardiac output, peripheral vascular resistance, and venous return are paramount. Perioperative dehydration should be avoided to prevent an increase in blood viscosity and intravascular thrombosis. Hematocrit should not exceed 60 percent.

Patients with increased pulmonary blood flow should have the failure well controlled with digitalis and diuretics. They have a high incidence of pulmonary infections and require careful ventilatory management perioperatively. After a Fontan-type correction, patients require maintenance of right-sided filling pressures for pulmonary perfusion. Increases in pulmonary vascular resistance may lead to an acute drop in systemic cardiac output and cyanosis.

Maintenance of sinus rhythm is important, since atrial dysrhythmias also may lead to deterioration in cardiac performance. Venous pooling should be counteracted. Patients may exhibit an increase in physiological dead space. Since these patients have a single-ventricle circulatory physiology, they may be more sensitive to myocardial depression from anesthetic agents.

Ketamine may be a useful anesthetic agent for these patients, as is a narcotic-relaxant technique, whereas regional techniques causing sympathetic blockade are probably contraindicated. Cardiac filling pressures should be monitored carefully, and monitoring of saturation in the superior vena cava can be used to estimate the adequacy of cardiac output. Positive-pressure ventilation should be used cautiously, since it may interfere with venous return and pulmonary perfusion and thereby lead to a reduction in systemic cardiac output. Early re-establishment of spontaneous ventilation after major surgery is desirable to improve forward flow across the pulmonary vascular bed.

Ebstein's Anomaly of the Tricuspid Valve

Ebstein's anomaly consists of a malformation of the posterior and septal leaflets of the tricuspid valve, which are adherent to the right ventricular wall, resulting in downward displacement of the free edge of the valves into the right ventricle away from the atrioventricular junction. The portion of the right ventricle above the downwardly displaced valve is thin-walled and forms a common chamber with the right atrium. The right ventricle below the displaced valve is normal but markedly reduced in size, with a patent foramen ovale in 75 percent of cases. The malformation is rare, with an incidence of 0.5 percent of all congenital heart disease, and affects both sexes equally. Familial occurrence has been reported.

Tricuspid valve stenosis and insufficiency coexist in most cases. Cyanosis due to intra-atrial shunting may be present to various degrees and tends to become more pronounced with age. With severe tricuspid malformation, cyanosis may be present in the neonate and improves with the fall in pulmonary vascular resistance postnatally. Tachycardia causes increased cyanosis owing to impaired right ventricular filling. Atrial emptying is delayed, blood being shunted back and forth between the right atrium and the atrialized portion of the right ventricle between atrial and ventricular systole (Ping-Pong effect). Paroxysmal atrial tachycardias occur in 25 percent of patients and may lead to syncope. Death during childhood is due to congestive heart failure or cardiac arrhythmias. The majority of patients with Ebstein's disease who are relatively asymptomatic survive for many years. The mean age at death in several series was quoted as 20 years. Ten to twenty percent of symptomatic infants died within the first year of life.

If exercise intolerance, heart failure, and progressive cyanosis appear in patients with this anomaly, surgical intervention should be considered. The abnormal valve may be replaced, or plication of the atrialized portion of the ventricle together with tricuspid annuloplasty may be carried out. The latter procedure appears to have better results.

Anesthetic Management. Prevention of endocarditis and systemic embolization is important. Patients frequently are marginally compensated hemodynamically and may develop frank failure with myocardial depression or volume overload. Intravenous induction may be markedly delayed owing to pooling of blood in the right atrium. Tachycardia is very poorly tolerated, and tachyarrhythmias should be treated promptly. Intracardiac lines may trigger serious arrhythmias and are probably contraindicated, since right heart failure is the dominant feature, and measurement of central venous pressure should be an adequate guide to volume replacement. Agents producing myocardial depression or tachycardia should be avoided.

TRICUSPID STENOSIS

Isolated stenosis of the tricuspid valve is extremely rare. Usually, severe stenosis or atresia of the pulmonary valve with right ventricular hypoplasia is present. The lesion is more common in females and has a strong tendency to occur in families. Signs of right heart failure with a prominent "a" wave on the jugular pulse tracing, liver congestion, and ascites are present with severe obstruction. Cyanosis occurs through shunting via a patent foramen ovale. The clinical presentation may be indistinguishable from that of tricuspid atresia. Some cases are amenable to corrective surgery through valvuloplasty or replacement of the tricuspid valve if an adequately sized right ventricle is present and there is no pulmonary outflow obstruction. Patients without intra-atrial communications will demonstrate signs of right heart failure without cyanosis unless pulmonary blood flow is insufficient. Patients with severely deformed valves may require shunting to increase pulmonary blood flow.

Anesthetic management is similar to that for patients with tricuspid atresia and reduced pulmonary perfusion. Increases in pulmonary vascular resistance may worsen cyanosis and signs of right heart failure. Maintenance of adequate venous pressure is essential to permit flow across the stenotic area. Reduction in left ventricular outflow resistance will increase right-to-left shunting. Endocarditis prophylaxis is required pre- and postoperatively. Patients are at risk for systemic embolization if an intra-atrial communication is present.

REGURGITANT CARDIAC LESIONS

AORTIC REGURGITATION

Isolated aortic valvular insufficiency does not occur in infancy except in Marfan's syndrome, in which it is associated with annuloaortic ectasia. A variety of congenital defects, however, are associated with development of aortic insufficiency, usually during childhood. Five percent of patients with ventricular septal defects develop signs of aortic insufficiency, which is progressive unless the underlying defect is closed. The jet lesion of discrete subaortic stenosis may cause extensive damage to the aortic cusps, but aortic insufficiency generally is not recognized until after the excision of the obstruction. Patients with truncus arteriosus may show signs of truncal valve insufficiency prior to operation but can also develop truncal valve insufficiency some time after corrective surgery. There is a 6 to 14 percent incidence of mild aortic regurgitation following an arterial switch procedure. The congenital bicuspid aortic valve becomes insufficient in approximately one third of affected patients past the age of 20 years.

The main physiological derangement is left ventricular volume overload by the diastolic regurgitation of blood across the incompetent valve. The net forward blood flow is decreased, unless left ventricular stroke volume and work are increased. The left ventricle initially dilates to accommodate the regurgitated volume, and maximum force is generated by the Frank-Starling mechanism. In chronic regurgitation, left ventricular hypertrophy develops, but compliance remains high, maintaining left ventricular end-diastolic pressures. Because of the regurgitation and low peripheral vascular resistance that are commonly present, diastolic pressure is low and coronary ischemia may occur, a problem not seen in the pediatric population. Patients have a wide pulse pressure and a characteristic diastolic murmur. With severe regurgitation, particularly if acute in onset, congestive heart failure may occur. Following the onset of congestive failure, death usually occurs between 12 and 24 months. Children with mild-to-moderate degrees of regurgitation may be asymptomatic. A regurgitant aortic valve is particularly susceptible to infective endocarditis, and adequate antibiotic prophylaxis is essential.

If signs of congestive failure or angina occur,

operation becomes necessary. In infants with aortic regurgitation and failure, valvuloplasty is performed whenever possible; valve replacement is usually necessary in symptomatic children.

Aortic–Left Ventricular Tunnel

This represents an extremely rare congenital malformation, with fewer than 50 cases reported. Most of the patients are male. An endothelialized vascular tunnel arises above the right coronary ostium, traverses the right infundibular portion of the ventricular septum, and enters the left ventricle just below the right and left aortic cusps. Severe aortic regurgitation is produced, with left ventricular enlargement, congestive failure, dilatation of the aortic valve ring, and secondary valvar insufficiency occurring with time. Symptoms occur early in life, usually within the first weeks. Medical therapy of heart failure is generally ineffective. Early surgical repair is indicated to prevent deformity of the aortic valve and consists of patching of the aortic orifice of the tunnel.

Aneurysm of the Sinus of Valsalva

Congenital weakness of the tissue of one sinus of Valsalva results in gradual downward bulging of this structure, which eventually herniates into an atrium or ventricle and may rupture. It is a rare problem in infancy and childhood. Seventy-five percent of reported cases occurred in males. Aneurysms of the sinus of Valsalva are most commonly associated with ventricular septal defect. The rupture usually occurs into the right ventricle but may occur into the left ventricle or right atrium. Patients exhibit a wide pulse pressure from diastolic runoff, and there may be volume overload of the right and left ventricles. Left-to-right shunt occurs, with rupture into the right heart. There is severe aortic insufficiency, with rupture into the left ventricle. Heart failure is acute and severe. The diagnosis should be established and corrective surgery performed as soon as possible, since most patients follow a progressive downhill course if the defect is not corrected. Residual aortic insufficiency is common after surgical repair.

Anesthetic Considerations. In children with mild-to-moderate aortic insufficiency, anesthetic techniques that have minimal influence on myocardial contractility should be chosen to maintain left ventricular stroke volume. Tachycardia causes shortening of diastole, thereby decreasing regurgitant flow. High peripheral vascular resistance increases regurgitation, and the usual low peripheral vascular tone should be maintained. Isoflurane and narcotic-relaxant techniques, combined with adequate atropination, may be useful choices. Intravascular monitoring is indicated for major or traumatic operation. In patients with impaired ventricular function due to severe regurgitation, ketamine may be indicated in combination with a butyrophenone such as droperidol, which counteracts the peripheral constricting effect of ketamine. Patients will generally undergo repair of their lesions prior to elective operation. All patients require endocarditis prophylaxis. Postoperative patients with nontissue prosthetic valves are treated with anticoagulants and require reversal of anticoagulation prior to further operation.

MITRAL REGURGITATION

Congenital Mitral Regurgitation

Insufficiency of the mitral valve as an isolated defect is an extremely rare condition. It is generally associated with other congenital cardiac defects, like endocardial cushion defect, corrected transposition, or anomalous origin of the left coronary artery. Lesions causing dilatation of the left ventricle may cause dilatation of the valve ring with secondary mitral incompetence. These include patent ductus arteriosus, VSD, ASD, aortic stenosis or incompetence, endocardial fibroelastosis, and obstructive cardiomyopathy. Insufficiency of the mitral valve may accompany congenital metabolic disorders and is the most common presenting feature of Marfan's syndrome in childhood.

Isolated insufficiency is generally caused by abnormal clefting of either the anterior or posterior leaflet, anomalous chordae, or deformed valve tissue. In the complex of anomalous mitral arcade, the free margins of the valve are thickened and the chordae shortened and fused. Together they form an arcade-like structure connecting directly to the papillary muscle.

The obvious hemodynamic defect in mitral insufficiency is the regurgitation of blood into the left atrium during ventricular systole. This augments the volume of the left atrium that empties into the left ventricle during the next diastole, leading to diastolic overload. Since regurgitation occurs into a low-pressure system, left ventricular wall tension during systole is decreased. To allow for sufficient stroke output into the systemic circulation, left ventricular volume increases. The left ventricle slowly increases in size, both in systole and in diastole. The left atrium adapts to the increased volume by enlargement, but left atrial pressure is maintained close to normal. Eventually congestive heart failure due to volume overload occurs.

Infants with congenital mitral insufficiency are generally symptomatic within the first year of life, whereas older patients tend to tolerate the condition for many years. There is a history of fatigue, frequent respiratory infections, and failure to grow. Congestive heart failure is a common feature. The maximally dilated left atrium in severe regurgitation may encroach on the left mainstem bronchus, leading to signs of airway obstruction or recurrent atelectasis. Mild-to-moderate pulmonary hypertension is frequently present. In severe or rapidly occurring mitral incompetence, left atrial pressure may be markedly elevated, and pulmonary venous congestion and edema may be present. Mitral insufficiency complicating any congenital cardiac lesion considerably worsens the prognosis of the underlying defect. Mild-to-moderate degrees of central regurgitation generally can be managed medically with control of failure through childhood. The progress of the lesion has to be assessed at regular intervals. In cases with severe regurgitation or persistent congestive failure, plication or annuloplasty of the mitral valve is performed. Prosthetic replacement is delayed if at all possible because of the problems of anticoagulation, valve size, and prosthetic failure.

Anesthetic Considerations. Volume overload of the left ventricle is the major problem. Myocardial depression may cause congestive failure. Regurgitation is less with fast heart rates, and tachycardia is therefore desirable. An increase in peripheral vascular resistance will increase impedance to left ventricular output, leading to an increase in regurgitated volume and a fall in systemic cardiac output.

Agents with minimal myocardial depressant effects should be used. Maintenance of heart rate and drying of excessive secretions may be achieved by generous atropinization. Adequate oxygenation should be assured by securing the airway and controlled ventilation. Infants may show the pulmonary sequelae of congestive failure, with ventilation-perfusion inequalities, small airway disease, and pulmonary congestion. Intravascular monitoring should guide fluid replacement in all major surgical cases. A low peripheral vascular resistance should be maintained by adequate depth of anesthesia and the use of appropriate anesthetic agents (isoflurane, droperidol with narcotic, or ketamine).

Electrolyte abnormalities should be corrected preoperatively and digitalis therapy discontinued for the immediate perioperative period to avoid occurrence of digitalis toxicity. When possible, regional techniques may be reasonable alternatives to general anesthesia. Endocarditis prophylaxis is mandatory. Patients who have undergone valvuloplasty or annuloplasty generally are only palliated and still have some degree of regurgitation. Patients with nontissue prosthetic valves receive anticoagulant treatment, which must be reversed prior to further operation.

Mitral Valve Prolapse

Mitral valve prolapse, or the clinical constellation of midsystolic click and late systolic murmur, represents the most common congenital anomaly. It is present probably in from 4 to 21 percent of the population and in at least 6 percent of pediatric patients. A marked female preponderance of 2:1 is reported in adolescents and adults, but in children it is only slightly more common in females. Mitral valve prolapse may be an associated feature of various other congenital cardiac lesions, most frequently secundum ASD (up to 40 percent), Ebstein's anomaly, and corrected transposition. It is commonly associated with Marfan's syndrome.

The mitral valve contains redundant tissue and is generally markedly enlarged, and the chordae are lengthened. The leaflets show focal myxomatous degeneration. Apposition of the leaflets during ventricular systole is incomplete, with slippage and ballooning of the affected leaflet, which exposes leaflets and chordae to the full stress of ventricular contraction. During diastole, dumping of the blood-filled leaflet into the left ventricular cavity subjects the valve tissue to additional trauma. The traumatized endothelium provides a nidus for thrombi and sterile or infected vegetation.

The disease is relatively benign during childhood, with a mean age at diagnosis of 10 years. The presenting feature is generally an atypical murmur, and some patients complain of exertional chest pain. Arrhythmia or fatigue is extremely uncommon. Most patients show the characteristic electrocardiographic pattern of isolated T-wave inversion, but diagnosis is generally established by the characteristic auscultatory findings.

Serious but infrequent complications of mitral valve prolapse are infective endocarditis, development of severe mitral regurgitation, and ventricular arrhythmias with episodes of ventricular tachycardia or fibrillation or both. Cerebrovascular accidents due to embolization have been described. Long-term studies in adults, with a mean follow-up period of 14 years, have revealed a 15 percent incidence of serious complications. In children, cardiac dysrhythmias at rest or during exercise are uncommon. They generally respond to therapy with propranolol. Progressive mitral regurgitation develops in at least 2 percent of pediatric patients and can be treated with annuloplasty or valvuloplasty.

Anesthetic Considerations. Most pediatric patients with mitral valve prolapse are asymptomatic, and no particular anesthetic technique appears superior. Careful electrocardiographic monitoring in the perioperative period is indicated because of the reported tendency to ventricular ectopy in these patients, particularly under stress. Endocarditis prophylaxis is presently not recommended for patients without mitral regurgitation. Patients with signs of mitral insufficiency should be managed according to the degree of hemodynamic derangement and do require endocarditis prophylaxis.

PULMONARY REGURGITATION

Isolated pulmonary valve regurgitation is an uncommon congenital lesion, accounting for less than 1 percent of all congenital heart disease. More commonly, pulmonary outflow insufficiency is the result of pulmonary artery hypertension or of surgery to relieve pulmonary outflow obstruction. In congenital pulmonary insufficiency the pulmonary valve is hypoplastic or deformed, and the main pulmonary artery trunk is dilated.

Patients with congenital pulmonary insufficiency are generally asymptomatic. The normally low diastolic pressure in the pulmonary artery precludes the regurgitation of large volumes of blood during ventricular diastole. Patients are usually diagnosed because of the presence of harsh, early diastolic murmur and main pulmonary artery dilatation.

If, however, a patient develops secondary pulmonary hypertension as a sequela of lung disease or left heart failure, pulmonary regurgitation worsens and may lead to right ventricular volume overload and failure. This generally does not occur until the later decades of life.

A few isolated cases of neonatal pulmonary insufficiency complicated by severe heart failure have been described. The high pulmonary vascular resistance of persistent fetal circulation in these infants leads to massive regurgitation. Therapy of the heart failure and the natural regression of pulmonary vascular resistance will lead to improvement with time if the patient does not succumb in the initial stage of the disease from heart failure and hypoxia.

Anesthetic Considerations. Since patients are generally asymptomatic, no special anesthetic problems should arise. Because of the malformed pulmonary valve, patients are susceptible to infectious endocarditis, and appropriate prophylaxis is necessary. The acute elevation in pulmonary vascular resistance resulting from hypoxia or pulmonary embolization may cause massive, acute right heart failure.

ABSENT PULMONARY VALVE SYNDROME

Congenital absence of the pulmonary valve is a very rare congenital anomaly. It is nearly always associated with tetralogy of Fallot and massive dilatation of the pulmonary arteries. Branching of the pulmonary arteries is abnormal at the segmental artery level. The condition appears to be more common in males and has been reported with a variety of other congenital cardiac lesions.

Severely affected infants are seen shortly after birth with symptoms of respiratory distress due to tracheobronchial compression by the massively dilated pulmonary arteries, leading to atelectasis and obstructive emphysema. In addition, patients with little right-sided obstruction may show signs of congestive heart failure due to a large left-to-right shunt. Patients with significant right ventricular outflow tract obstruction are cyanotic and appear clinically similar to those with tetralogy of Fallot. Prognosis is related to the degree of bronchial obstruction, with the majority of severely symptomatic patients dying within the first year of life from pulmonary obstructive disease or intractable congestive failure. The bronchial obstruction may be somewhat relieved by positioning the infant prone.

Various surgical approaches have been used to correct the abnormality of the pulmonary arteries, including aneurysmectomy, plication of the pulmonary arteries, and interposition of a prosthetic valve or homograft in addition to closure of the VSD. The results of operation in infants are relatively poor and depend primarily on whether or not bronchial obstruction has been relieved. Patients who survive infancy usually improve spontaneously, probably owing to maturational changes, including stiffening and enlargement of the tracheobronchial tree, rendering it less susceptible to collapse from outside compression. In addition, pulmonary artery pressure may decrease owing to a relative increase in valve ring stenosis. Definitive repair is carried out in older children, with good results. Insertion of a valve at the pulmonary annulus appears to lead to better hemodynamic performance.

Anesthetic Considerations. Recommendations regarding anesthesia can be made only on a theoretical basis. Symptomatic infants will need meticulous respiratory care. Positive intratracheal pressure may counteract the external bronchial compression. Pulmonary vascular resistance should be kept low to avoid increases in regurgitation and right-to-left shunting. Myocardial depression may lead to worsening congestive failure. Maintenance of the heart rate is essential. A reduction in peripheral vascular resistance should benefit patients with predominant left-to-right shunt, whereas it may worsen cyanosis in patients with severe right ventricular outflow obstruction.

Infundibular spasm may occur and should be treated promptly with either morphine or propranolol. Perioperative mechanical ventilation is probably indicated. Older children may have fewer respiratory problems and should be managed according to the predominant hemodynamic presentation—ventricular septal defect with or without pulmonic stenosis or tetralogy of Fallot. Endocarditis prophylaxis is indicated in all patients, particularly in patients with prosthetic valves or conduits.

TRICUSPID INSUFFICIENCY

Isolated congenital tricuspid incompetency is extremely rare. More commonly it is associated with Ebstein's anomaly, right ventricular hypertension due to right-sided outflow obstruction, obstructive pulmonary vascular disease, or a cleft tricuspid valve due to an endocardial cushion defect. Occasionally, transient tricuspid insufficiency may follow perinatal asphyxiation. The proposed cause is myocardial ischemia leading to papillary muscle dysfunction, which is reversible.

In isolated congenital tricuspid insufficiency the valve leaflets and chordae tendineae are dysplastic. Affected patients are seen as neonates or young infants with extreme cardiomegaly, heart failure, and cyanosis. The free regurgitation across the tricuspid annulus may make it impossible for the right ventricle to generate enough pressure to open the pulmonary valve in the presence of the high perinatal pulmonary vascular resistance. With the normal fall in pulmonary vascular resistance, the tricuspid insufficiency improves.

Treatment in infancy is supportive, with judicious use of digoxin and diuretics. In older patients, tricuspid annuloplasty or replacement may be performed. Infants with severe tricuspid regurgitation and right ventricular outflow obstruction have a very poor prognosis. Mortality approaches 100 percent with or without operation.

Patients who survive infancy and still have tricuspid insufficiency will eventually develop right ventricular and atrial hypertrophy with dilatation, caused by volume overload, and signs of right ventricular failure in later life, unless the lesion is corrected surgically.

UHL'S ANOMALY

Partial or complete absence of the myocardium of the right ventricle, also known as parchment right ventricle, is an extremely rare congenital anomaly usually not recognized during life. Pulmonary atresia or stenosis and atrial septal defect can occur concurrently. The clinical presentation is similar to that of Ebstein's anomaly and tricuspid insufficiency, with signs of right heart failure, massive cardiomegaly (caused by dilation of the right atrium and ventricle), cyanosis, and growth failure, usually within the first years of life. Patients respond poorly to conservative management. Complete heart block may occur spontaneously and is unresponsive to transvenous pacing because of the lack of excitable tissue in the right ventricle, which serves only as a venous reservoir.

The characteristic catheterization findings are equal pressures in the right atrium, ventricle, and pulmonary artery. Creation of an anastomosis of the superior vena cava to the pulmonary artery has been recommended to increase pulmonary blood flow and relieve venous congestion. The majority of patients die within the first 2 years of life, although survival to late adulthood with only mild symptoms has been described.

Anesthetic Considerations. Only patients who survive infancy will be seen for elective surgical therapy. The primary physiological derangement in tricuspid insufficiency is volume overload of the right ventricle, which is usually well tolerated past infancy. Right atrial pressure remains low, since the regurgitation volume dissipates in the very compliant venous vascular bed. Right ventricular filling volume has to be high to maintain cardiac output in the presence of regurgitation. The increase in pulmonary vascular resistance may lead to a decrease in forward output of the right ventricle, increased regurgitation, and cardiovascular collapse. Tachycardia decreases regurgitation, as it does in mitral insufficiency. Induction with intravenous agents may be delayed because of pooling in a large right atrium and regurgitation from the right ventricle. Maintenance of right-sided filling volume, low pulmonary vascular resistance, and adequate heart rate should be essential and can be achieved by a variety of anesthetic techniques. Antibiotic prophylaxis is necessary.

MALFORMATIONS INVOLVING THE GREAT VESSELS

PATENT DUCTUS ARTERIOSUS (PDA)

During fetal life, 55 to 60 percent of the combined ventricular output is carried by the ductus arteriosus, which develops from the distal portion of the sixth aortic arch and connects the main pulmonary artery to the descending aorta. This avoids unnecessary perfusion of the nonventilated lung. Within 10 to 15 hours after birth, closure of the ductus occurs through contraction of medial smooth muscle and intimal protrusion. The main stimulus to ductal closure appears to be the increase in arterial oxygen tension. Permanent closure through intimal fibrosis and connective tissue formation generally is completed by 2 to 3 weeks of age.

Persistent patency of the ductus arteriosus occurs in about 1 in 2000 live, full-term births, accounting for 5 to 10 percent of all congenital heart disease. It is more common in females by a ratio of 2:1. In these infants, failure to close is due to structural abnormality. This is commonly associated with congenital rubella syndrome, together with stenosis of the peripheral pulmonary arteries and of the systemic arteries, especially the renal arteries. Persistent patency of the ductus is essential for postnatal survival in patients with congenital cardiac lesions with right ventricular outflow obstruction, or in those with aortic atresia or interrupted arch. Patency may have to be maintained by infusion of prostaglandin E_1 until surgical palliation or correction can be performed.

In premature infants, closure of the ductus arteriosus may be markedly delayed. This may be due to immature ductal musculature, which responds poorly to the constricting effect of oxygen but is very sensitive to the vasodilating effect of prostaglandins (PGE_2 and PGI_2), which are produced intramurally in the ductus. Persistent patency is inversely related to the maturity of the infants. More than 80 percent of infants with a birth weight of less than 1000 gm have a significant PDA. This frequency decreases to 15 to 45 percent in infants weighing between 1000 and 1750 gm at birth.

Clinical symptoms depend on the degree of shunting across the ductus. Because of the higher postnatal systemic vascular resistance, the systemic arterial pressure exceeds pulmonary artery pressure, and shunting occurs from left to right. The magnitude of shunting depends on the diameter of the ductus, the pressure gradient between the aorta and pulmonary artery, and the difference between systemic and pulmonary vascular resistances. With a small ductus, resistance to flow is high, and only a small shunt will occur despite a large pressure gradient. With a large ductus, pressures may become equalized, and shunting is determined by the difference in vascular resistance between systemic and pulmonary circulations.

Left-to-right shunting leads to an increased volume load for the left ventricle. Left ventricular diastolic volume is increased, leading to increased ventricular stroke volume through the Frank-Starling mechanism. In newborn infants, and particularly in premature babies, the myocardium is not fully developed; it contains fewer contractile elements, and sympathetic innervation is incomplete. Volume loads are less well tolerated than later in life, and left ventricular failure occurs readily. As a result of increased left ventricular end-diastolic pressure, left atrial pressure rises, leading to overt pulmonary edema through pulmonary venous congestion. Eventually, pulmonary hypertension and right ventricular failure may occur. With a dilated left atrium, stretching of the foramen ovale may occur, with subsequent shunting at the atrial level. Aortic diastolic pressure is low with a large ductus, owing to runoff into the low-pressure pulmonary circulation. This may lead to myocardial ischemia in the presence of elevated left ventricular end-diastolic pressures, further aggravating heart failure. Systemic perfusion and oxygen delivery may become compromised, particularly if anemia is also present together with a high percentage of fetal hemoglobin.

Symptoms of left-to-right shunting due to PDA generally appear at 3 to 5 days of age, most commonly in infants recovering from respiratory distress syndrome. Patients develop a systolic or continuous murmur, bounding pulses, and a hyperactive precordium. Tachycardia and tachypnea are signs of early left ventricular failure. Respiratory function deteriorates, with increasing oxygen requirements and elevation of arterial P_{CO_2}. Patients without lung disease may have symptoms of mild heart failure, while infants with severe lung disease present deteriorating ventilatory function and failure to wean. Diagnosis usually can be made clinically and confirmed by echocardiography.

Medical therapy with fluid restriction, maintenance of hematocrit above 45 percent, and administration of indomethacin, 0.2 mg/kg (maximum 3 doses 12 to 24 hours apart intravenously or via nasogastric tube), are usually sufficient to control symptoms and effect functional closure of the ductus. Digitalis is generally ineffective in premature infants and may cause toxicity. If symptoms persist after 48 to 72 hours of medical management, surgical ligation is performed. Indomethacin is a contraindication in patients with impaired renal function or elevated bilirubin levels.

Manifestations of PDA in term infants and older children are similar to those described for premature infants and depend on the degree of shunting. With a small ductus, patients are generally asymptomatic, and the characteristic machinery murmur is detected on routine physical examination. The main risk for this group is development of bacterial endocarditis. With a moderate-sized ductus, symptoms may include poor feeding and tachypnea. Compensatory ventricular hypertrophy develops in these patients, and symptoms improve. General physical development is usually retarded, however, and easy fatigability is noted in older children. Infants with a large ductus are always symptomatic, with failure to grow, poor feeding, sweating, tachypnea, and recurrent respiratory infections. Without operation, patients eventually develop obstructive pulmonary vascular disease with progression to Eisenmenger's syndrome.

Surgical repair of the ductus should be performed in all patients to prevent long-term complications (endocarditis with a small-to-moderate ductus, irreversible pulmonary vascular disease with a large one). Indomethacin is ineffective in term infants and children. The life expectancy of patients with PDA after the age of 17 years is half that of the general population.

Anesthetic Considerations. The presence of a small ductus does not interfere with general anesthetic management, since cardiovascular function is normal. The main risk is bacterial endocarditis. With a large ductus, chronic pulmonary congestion may be present, and heart failure may occur with rapid fluid administration or increase in pulmonary vascular resistance. The latter may cause shunt reversal and systemic embolization of air or debris. These patients generally should undergo ductus repair prior to elective surgery. The anesthetic management is similar to that of patients with a large left-to-right shunt at the ventricular level. Avoidance of agents with a myocardial depressant effect, careful ventilatory management to avoid hypoventilation and atelectasis, and monitoring of fluid administration are important. Endocarditis prophylaxis should be maintained. Premature infants have been successfully managed with narcotic-relaxant technique and air-oxygen mixtures. Prevention of the retinopathy of prematurity is an added concern in this age group.

Infants and children are normal after closure of an isolated ductus arteriosus and have no specific anesthetic requirements. Endocarditis prophylaxis is not necessary 6 months following ligation.

AORTOPULMONARY WINDOW

Failure of aortopulmonary septation during early fetal life leaves an open communication between the great arteries just above their valve origins. This lesion is exceedingly rare and is isolated in over 50 percent of cases. The clinical presentation is indistinguishable from that of a large PDA, since the defect is usually large. Congestive heart failure in infancy is generally the presenting symptom. Pulmonary and right ventricular pressures are at or near systemic levels. The prognosis without surgical repair is poor, with death occurring from congestive failure in infancy or obstructive pulmonary vascular disease developing after the first year of life. If possible, failure should be controlled medically in the newborn period, and the defect closed electively in the first 1 to 3 months of life. If medical therapy fails, surgery is performed earlier. Repair consists of transaortic closure of the defect with a patch, requiring cardiopulmonary bypass.

Less than 10 percent of patients with this anomaly have a small defect and can be treated as if they have a small ductus. Since the surgical approach is radically different for these two lesions, a definite diagnosis has to be established prior to attempts at correction.

Anesthetic considerations are similar to those that apply to patients with a large ventricular septal defect in infancy. Elective noncardiac surgery preferably should be postponed until the lesion has been repaired. Endocarditis prophylaxis is necessary pre- and postoperatively. Closure of the defect should lead to normalization of physiological parameters.

TRUNCUS ARTERIOSUS

Truncus arteriosus is an uncommon congenital anomaly in which a single great vessel arises from both ventricles above a large VSD, giving rise to the pulmonary and coronary arteries. This malformation represents 1 to 4 percent of congenital cardiac lesions. At present, three forms of truncus are differentiated (Fig. 6–16). In type I, a short pulmonary trunk arises from the truncus and divides into both pulmonary arteries; in type II, the pulmonary arteries arise separately but in close proximity to each other from the posterior aspect of the truncus; and in type III, both pulmonary arteries arise separately from the respective lateral aspects of the truncal artery.

In early infancy, patients show signs of congestive heart failure and pulmonary overperfusion. Truncal valve insufficiency may also be present. Heart failure is severe and resistant to therapy. Unless surgical correction is performed, death occurs in the first year of life in over 80 percent of patients. Survivors develop obstructive pulmonary vascular disease, after the age of 6 months, rendering them inoperable. These patients all deteriorate progressively, with signs of pulmonary hypertension and right heart failure.

Because of the dismal natural history of this disease, correction is generally performed after the first month of life and before 6 months of age. It consists of closure of the VSD, with the left ventricular output diverted to the truncal artery and positioning of a valved graft (generally a homograft) between the right ventricle and pulmonary artery (or arteries) (Fig. 6–17). Surgical mortality ranges from 9 to 25 percent. Since only a small conduit can be used during infancy, at least one other operation will become necessary with growth of the patient once the size of the conduit becomes inadequate. Up to 67 percent of patients require reoperation for conduit replacement by 2 years of age. Truncal valve insufficiency may necessitate valvuloplasty or valve replacement at either initial or subsequent surgery. Truncal valve replacement in the infant requires Kono's aortoventriculoplasty and carries a mortality of more than 50 percent.

Anesthetic Considerations. Elective surgery is unlikely to be performed prior to the correction of the cardiac lesion in the first 6 months of life. Patients with truncus arteriosus that is considered inoperable may present with this lesion and Eisenmenger's syndrome. After successful correction patients may appear asymptomatic but nevertheless have a considerable pressure gradient across the right ventricular-to-pulmonary artery conduit. Right ventricular failure and ventricular arrhythmias may develop with stress or large and rapid fluid shifts. Central venous monitoring will be essential under these circumstances to assess right ventricular function. Increases in pulmonary vascular resistance will worsen the condition of these patients, and acute preload reduction may lead to systemic cardiovascular collapse. Older patients may ex-

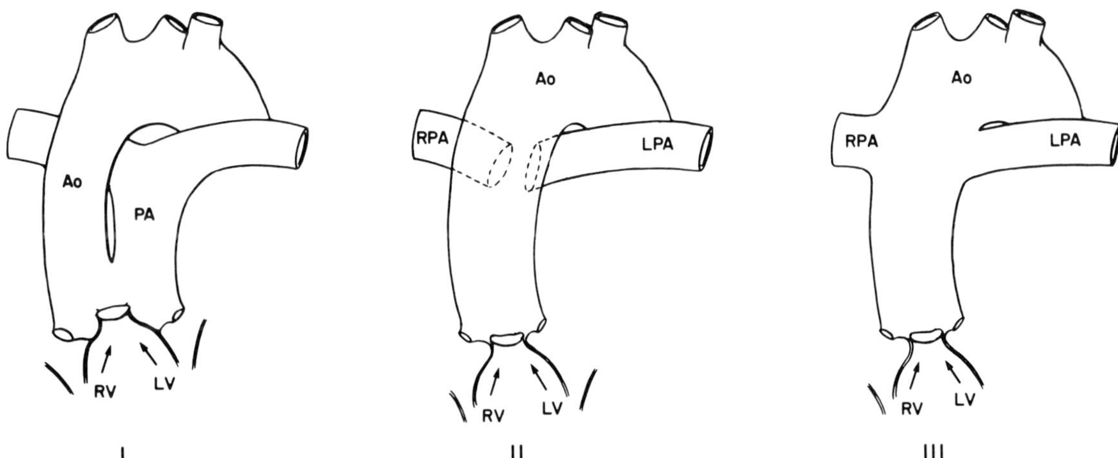

FIGURE 6–16. Truncus arteriosus. Classification according to Colett and Edwards. Ao = Aorta; PA = pulmonary artery; RPA = right pulmonary artery; LPA = left pulmonary artery; RV = right ventricle; LV = left ventricle.

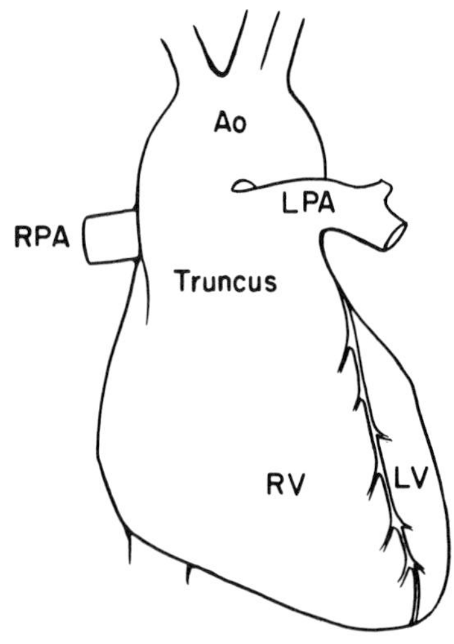

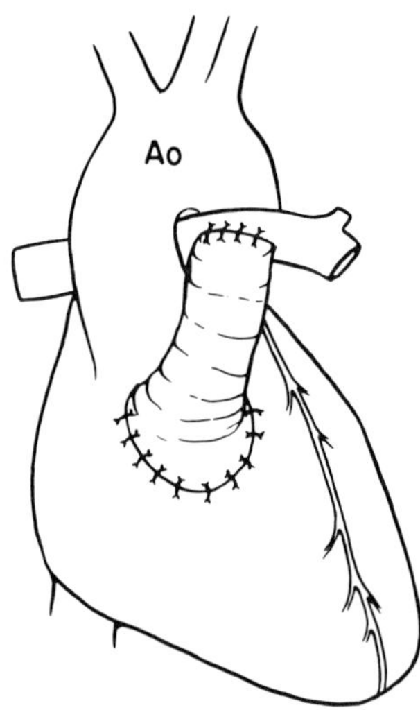

FIGURE 6–17. Truncus arteriosus before and after operation. Repair with insertion of a conduit between the right ventricle and pulmonary artery and closure of the ventricular septal defect. Ao = Aorta; RPA = right pulmonary artery; LPA = left pulmonary artery; RV = right ventricle; LV = left ventricle.

hibit various degrees of aortic insufficiency and may be at risk for ventricular ectopy from the right ventriculotomy required for conduit replacement.

The selection of anesthetic agents should center on drugs that have a minimal effect on vasomotor tone and myocardial performance. Maintenance of heart rate is essential, as is endocarditis prophylaxis. The use of invasive monitoring should be considered early for extensive surgery. Because of the presence of a prosthetic valve in the pulmonary outflow tract, use of a Swan-Ganz catheter is relatively contraindicated.

COARCTATION OF THE AORTA

Isolated coarctation of the aorta is the fifth or sixth most common congenital cardiac defect, accounting for 6 to 7 percent of all congenital heart disease and for 7.5 percent of all critically ill infants with heart disease. It affects males twice as frequently as females. It is the lesion most commonly associated with Turner's syndrome of XO karyotype. A bicuspid aortic valve is found in 50 to 80 percent of patients with coarctation.

The coarctation occurs as a constriction of the aorta, at or near the junction of the ductus arteriosus and the aortic arch and distal to the left subclavian artery. The involved segment may be discrete or of significant length. The narrowing of the aorta may occur above the entrance of the ductus (preductal or infantile type of coarctation), usually as a long, segmental narrowing, or at or below the ductus (postductal or adult type of coarctation), usually localized (Fig. 6–18). Forty percent of patients with preductal coarctation have associated severe intra-

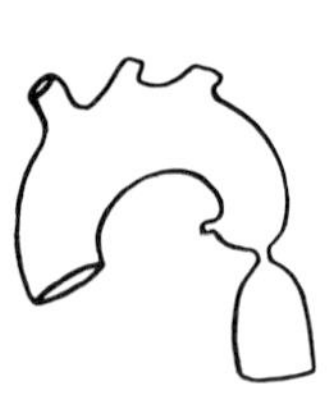

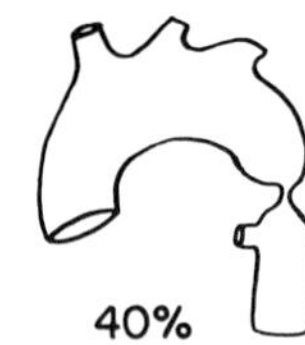

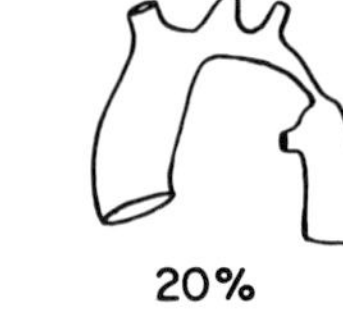

FIGURE 6–18. Coarctation of the aorta. (After Keith JD: Coarctation of the aorta. *In* Keith JD, et al [eds]: Heart Disease in Infancy and Childhood. 3rd edition. New York, Macmillan, 1978.)

cardiac anomalies, compared with only 14 percent of patients with postductal coarctation.

The physiological problem in coarctation is the maintenance of blood flow to the lower half of the body in the presence of an aortic obstruction. Adaptive mechanisms result in elevation of the systolic blood pressure in the proximal aorta to increase the pressure gradient, arteriolar constriction to maintain diastolic pressure, and development of collaterals to bypass the obstruction. In the preductal form of coarctation, blood flow to the lower half of the body occurs via a patent ductus arteriosus.

Coarctation of the aorta is the second most common cause of congestive heart failure in infancy and childhood, with more than half of patients becoming symptomatic within the first years of life. Eighty percent of these patients have an associated defect, most commonly PDA (two thirds) or VSD (30 to 35 percent). In two thirds of these infants, the coarctation is preductal.

Elevation of the systolic blood pressure in the upper extremity, particularly the right arm, above the systolic pressure in the lower extremity is generally present except in patients with a low output state or with a large ductus supplying blood flow to the lower extremity. The latter is frequently associated with a VSD and systemic pressures in the pulmonary artery.

Medical therapy is frequently unsuccessful, necessitating surgical repair of the coarctation by resection and end-to-end anastomosis, patch aortoplasty, subclavian flap, or subclavian artery transposition (Fig. 6–19). The last procedures appear to be associated with a low surgical mortality and low risk of recoarctation. Recoarctation occurs in 9 to 24 percent of patients whose lesion was repaired before 4 months of age. Gradients of higher than 25 mm Hg at rest require intervention. Balloon angioplasty may be used to dilate a native coarctation. However, long-term relief of the gradient is less than with surgical therapy, and since the dilatation results in tearing of the intima and media of the aorta, aneurysms at the coarctation site may develop. Balloon angioplasty of recurrent coarctation has better long-term results and carries less risk of late aneurysmal dilation. Reduction of left ventricular afterload following coarctation repair generally will lead to improvement in patients with associated VSD. Repair of this defect can be postponed, since 50 percent of VSDs become smaller or close spontaneously. In patients with complex lesions that could result in pulmonary hypertension and are not amenable to correction in infancy, pulmonary artery banding is carried out at the time of coarctation repair. A PDA is always divided.

The majority of patients with isolated postductal coarctation are diagnosed later in life, most commonly between 4 and 5 years of age, because of the incidental finding of a heart murmur or systolic hypertension. A systolic pressure that is higher in the upper extremity is present in 90 percent. The children are otherwise normal, without signs of congestive failure.

Surgical repair is performed during early childhood, preferably between 2 and 4 years of age if diagnosis is made that early. Repair in later childhood and adolescence is associated with a 10 to 20 percent incidence of persistent hypertension despite adequate relief of obstruction. This leads to premature death from cardiovascular disease.

Patients with coarctation have an increased incidence of cerebral aneurysm, which may lead to cerebrovascular accidents even in the presence of a normal postoperative blood pressure. The risk of endocarditis is not eliminated with coarctation repair. Infection may occur at the anastomotic site, with mycotic aneurysm formation and aortic rupture, or at the aortic or mitral valve; these valves are frequently abnormal (bicuspid aortic valve, mitral valve prolapse). Aneurysmal dilatation of the site of the coarctation repair has been described as a long-term sequela of patch aortoplasty. In childhood it has been seen only in patients with hypertension. A very rare (0.4 percent) but catastrophic sequela of coarctation repair is spinal cord injury with paraplegia. The prognosis for unrepaired coarctation is poor. Twenty percent of patients die in the second decade of life and 90 percent before the age of 50 years as a consequence of severe hypertension.

Two percent of patients with coarctation have associated coarctation of the abdominal aorta. This is most commonly seen in females. Hypertension is usually pronounced, and renal involvement is common. Corrective surgery is usually performed after childhood, with resection of the lesions or interposition of a graft.

Anesthetic Considerations. Symptomatic infants usually undergo coarctation repair prior to any elective noncardiac surgery. Heart failure should be relieved, and blood pressure should be normal postoperatively. Persistent hypertension despite relief of the obstruction is not generally seen after repair in infancy. Recurrence of a pressure gradient is indicative of recoarctation. Patients may show an exaggerated blood pressure response with stress and require sufficient anesthetic depth to prevent

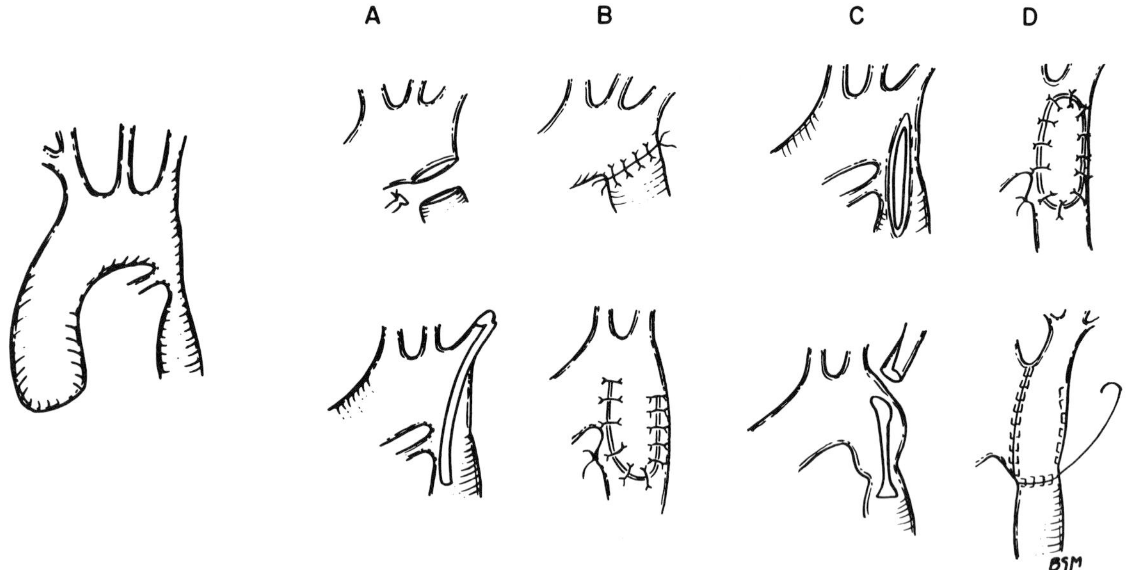

FIGURE 6–19. Methods of repair for coarctation of the aorta. *A*, Resection and end-to-end anastomosis. *B*, Patch aortoplasty. *C*, Subclavian flap repair. *D*, Subclavian flap with repositioning of the subclavian artery.

this problem. Inhalation anesthetics and muscle relaxants without sympathetic side effects appear to be wise choices. The presence of associated cardiac defects and their physiological consequences should be taken into consideration. Patients with associated Turner's syndrome may have difficulties with intubation. Hypertension is commonly seen in a considerable percentage of patients postoperatively. With stress, two thirds of patients after coarctation repair may show marked systolic hypertension. Since cerebral aneurysms are more common in these patients, subarachnoid hemorrhage may occur.

Resting hypertension should be controlled medically prior to elective surgery. Blood pressure should be monitored carefully perioperatively, and early, direct monitoring should be established for major surgical therapy. Pressure should always be measured in the right arm, since blood pressures may still differ between the upper extremities postoperatively, even if the subclavian artery was not sacrificed. A sufficient depth of anesthesia should be achieved prior to stressful manipulations. Topical anesthesia, superior laryngeal nerve block, or intravenous lidocaine should be used to attenuate the sympathetic response to laryngoscopy and intubation. Inhalation anesthesia lowers blood pressure and allows for rapid changes in anesthetic depth. Relaxants should also be chosen according to their cardiovascular side effects.

All patients require endocarditis prophylaxis pre- and postoperatively.

INTERRUPTED AORTIC ARCH

Interrupted aortic arch is an uncommon congenital lesion accounting for approximately 1.4 percent of all infants seen with congenital heart disease. A segment of the aortic arch is absent or atretic, leading to complete aortic discontinuity. The embryogenetic basis is failure of fusion of the fourth and sixth aortic arches. The defect may be located distal to the left subclavian artery (type A), between the left carotid and left subclavian arteries (type B), or distal to the innominate and proximal to the left carotid arteries (type C) (Fig. 6–20). The lesion is commonly associated with VSD and PDA, the latter supplying the blood flow to the distal aorta. A bicuspid aortic valve is present in 50 to 80 percent of patients, and as many as 48 percent of patients have associated DiGeorge's syndrome. Type B interruption is most commonly seen. Symptoms of a large left-to-right shunt with heart failure and pulmonary hyperperfusion are present shortly after birth. Physiological closure of the ductus leads to systemic underperfusion, with metabolic acidosis and renal failure. Without surgical intervention, death occurs in 90 percent of patients within the first month of life. Bypass of the interruption by using the carotid or subclavian artery, tube graft interposition, and direct anastomosis have been utilized. Pulmonary artery banding or primary repair of an associated VSD has been performed simultaneously. Surgery is carried

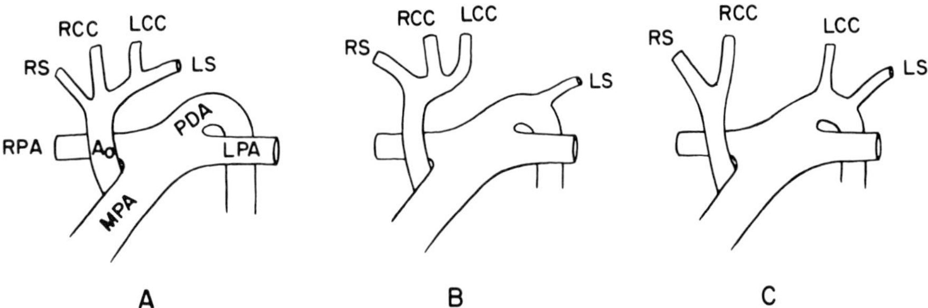

FIGURE 6–20. Interrupted aortic arch. Classification after Celoria and Patton. Ao = Aorta; MPA = main pulmonary artery; RPA = right pulmonary artery; PDA = patent ductus arteriosus; LPA = left pulmonary artery; RS = right subclavian artery; LS = left subclavian artery; RCC = right common carotid artery; LCC = left common carotid artery.

out as soon as the diagnosis is established and the patient has been medically stabilized.

Prostaglandin E_1 is used preoperatively to maintain the patency of the ductus and systemic perfusion. Serum calcium levels may be abnormally low and require treatment. A surgical mortality of between 23 and 45 percent is reported but may be as low as 10 percent in some centers. No long-term follow-up of survivors has been reported. Subaortic stenosis appears to be more common in these patients, requiring further surgery. With growth, relative coarctation at the graft site may occur, necessitating surgical revision.

Anesthetic Management. Survivors should pose problems similar to those of patients after coarctation repair. Aortic interruption may be associated with DiGeorge's syndrome and these patients may develop severe hypocalcemia. Calcium levels should be carefully monitored perioperatively. There also may be a greater susceptibility to infection because of absent or hypoplastic thymic tissue.

VASCULAR RING ANOMALIES

Anomalies in the development of the aortic arch system may lead to the formation of anomalous vascular structures compressing the trachea and/or esophagus (Fig. 6–21). The incidence of aortic arch malformation is not known. Symptomatic patients comprise approximately 1.5 percent of patients seen with congenital heart disease.

The heart is generally normal in these patients, and symptoms usually relate to the degree of respiratory obstruction. In patients with severe tracheal compression, stridor, wheezing, recurrent pneumonia, and emphysematous pulmonary changes are present within the first few months of life. Respiratory distress is aggravated by feeding and lessened by hyperextension of the head. Severely affected infants show failure to thrive. Other causes of stridor or frequent pneumonia (for example, laryngeal web, tracheomalacia, tracheoesophageal fistula, gastric reflux, Pierre-Robin anomaly, choanal atresia) have to be excluded. The airway obstruction may be life-threatening. The compressed area is frequently located in the lower trachea but may be located distally in one of the main bronchi. However, symptoms are generally less severe, and the condition may remain undiagnosed for many years.

Medical management consists of careful positioning to minimize tracheal compression, feeding with liquids or soft foods, and prompt treatment of pulmonary infections. As the infant grows, the trachea becomes stiffer and less easily compressed. In patients with severe symptoms and significant tracheal narrowing, surgery to relieve the vascular obstruction must be performed.

DOUBLE AORTIC ARCH

This is the most common vascular ring anomaly and usually occurs as an isolated entity. A right and a left aortic arch arise from the ascending aorta, encircle the trachea and esophagus, and unite to form a single descending aorta. Symptoms of tracheal compression are usually present in early infancy. Surgical treatment consists of division of the smaller of the two arches, usually in the left.

RIGHT AORTIC ARCH WITH LEFT LIGAMENTUM ARTERIOSUM

In this anomaly, a vascular ring is formed by the right aortic arch, the left subclavian artery,

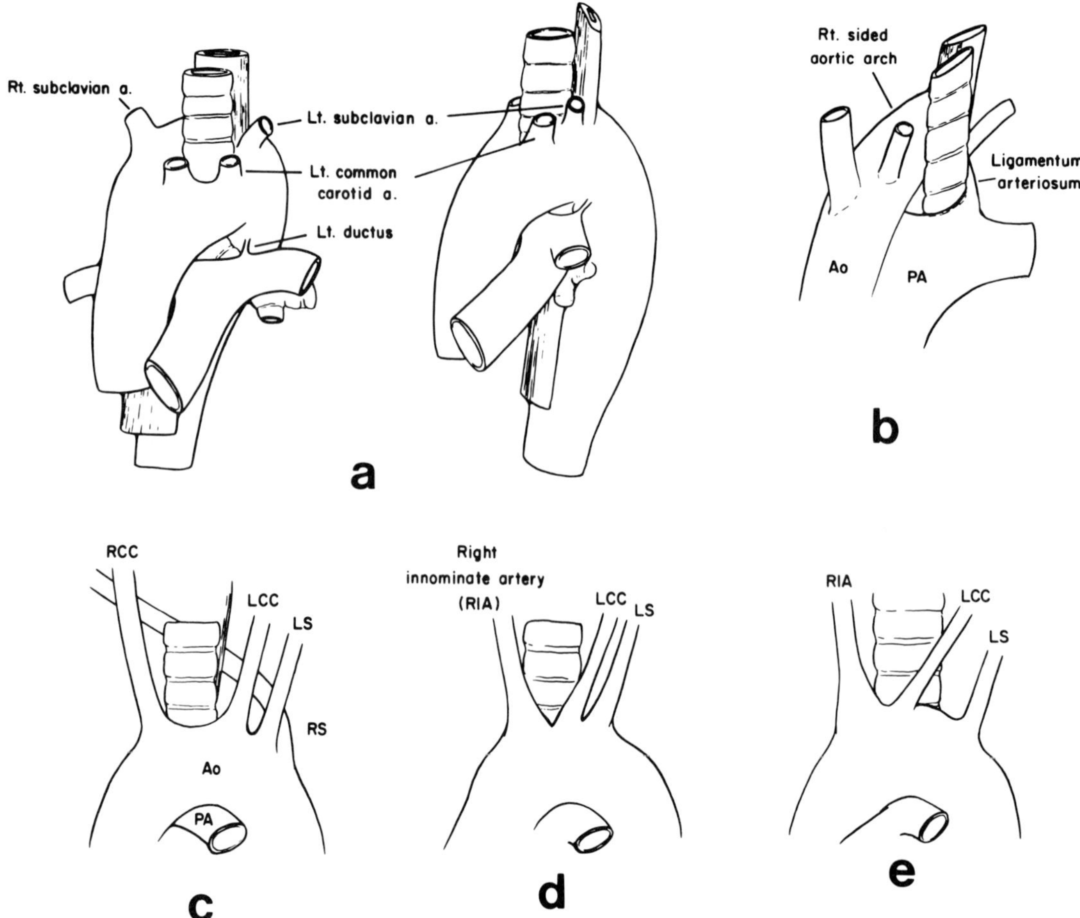

FIGURE 6–21. Vascular ring anomalies: *a*, double aortic arch; *b*, right aortic arch with left ligamentum arteriosum; *c*, anomalous right subclavian artery; *d*, anomalous right innominate artery; *e*, anomalous left common carotid. Ao = Aorta; PA = pulmonary artery; RCC = right common carotid; LCC = left common carotid; LS = left subclavian; RS = right subclavian. (Redrawn from Gross RE: The Surgery of Infancy and Childhood. Philadelphia, WB Saunders, 1953.)

and a left-sided ductus arteriosus or ligamentum arteriosum connecting the left subclavian artery to the left pulmonary artery. This anomaly is only rarely associated with intracardiac defects. In contrast with right aortic arch and mirror image branching of the brachiocephalic vessels and no vascular ring malformation, intracardiac defects are present in over 90 percent of patients. Symptoms of tracheal compression are often less severe, and surgical treatment usually is not necessary. Division of the ligamentatum arteriosum or the subclavian artery or both will relieve the obstruction.

ANOMALOUS INNOMINATE ARTERY

In this anomaly, the innominate artery arises more posteriorly and may be congenitally short. Symptoms of tracheal compression occur in early infancy and may include apneic spells. With severe symptomatology, operation is indicated, which consists of mobilizing the offending vessels and suturing them to the posterior aspect of the sternum. An anomalous left carotid artery arising more posteriorly may cause similar symptoms. Relief is provided through fixation of the vessel to the sternum.

ABERRANT RIGHT SUBCLAVIAN ARTERY

In this lesion, the right subclavian artery arises as the last branch of the aortic arch and courses to the right arm at an oblique angle behind the esophagus. It is frequently associated with tetralogy of Fallot and may be present in over one third of patients with Down's syndrome. It has been observed in 0.5 to 0.7 percent of postmortem examinations. Dysphagia lusoria has long been attributed to this lesion, whereas respiratory symptoms have only rarely been associated with it. Most patients are asymptomatic and require no treatment. In symptomatic infants, the artery can be divided surgically; however, in older patients reconstruction of the vessel is recommended to prevent ischemic changes or the subclavian steal syndrome.

ANOMALOUS ORIGIN OF THE LEFT PULMONARY ARTERY (VASCULAR SLING)

In this anomaly, the left pulmonary artery arises from the elongated main pulmonary artery on the right, encircles the right mainstem bronchus, and passes to the left between the trachea and esophagus. Constriction of the right main bronchus, the trachea, or both may occur. Congenital tracheal stenosis or tracheal rings are frequently associated. Symptoms of tracheal compression are usually severe and begin within the first few weeks of life. The prognosis without surgical intervention is extremely poor, with death occurring within the first few weeks of life. Until recently, the surgical correction consisted of detachment of the anomalous pulmonary artery and reimplantation into the main pulmonary artery anterior to the trachea. The mortality for this procedure approaches 50 percent. If tracheal stenosis is also present, symptoms may be only partially relieved, and the transplanted vessel frequently occluded. Now, however, the tracheal stenosis has been resected on cardiopulmonary bypass, which allows the left pulmonary artery to be relocated anteriorly through the gap in the trachea prior to reanastomosis, thereby alleviating the need for the reimplantation of this vessel.

Anesthetic Considerations. Various degrees of airway compromise are the prominent feature of these anomalies; securing and maintaining an adequate airway is the main anesthetic problem. Secondary pulmonary changes of atelectasis or emphysema may complicate the respiratory impairment.

The smooth induction of anesthesia, preferably with a nonirritating inhalational anesthetic like halothane, should be attempted. Struggling on induction, which increases negative intrathoracic pressure, may cause considerable worsening of the symptoms and even complete tracheal or bronchial obstruction. The head should be kept extended and continuous positive airway pressure applied, which tends to maintain the patency of the airway by passive distention. Relaxants or intravenous agents should not be given unless controlled ventilation can be performed adequately. If secondary pulmonary changes are present, higher-than-normal inspired oxygen concentrations may be necessary to insure adequate oxygenation. The smallest-diameter endotracheal tube permitting adequate ventilation should be chosen to minimize mechanical trauma to the compressed area. The adequacy of gas exchange and the ventilation of both lungs should be monitored closely throughout operation. Controlled ventilation with constant positive airway pressure should be maintained.

If no audible leak is present, worsening of the respiratory impairment should be expected postoperatively and the patient closely monitored. Mechanical ventilation may be necessary until tracheal edema subsides.

Postoperatively, the trachea may remain weakened for a considerable time, and symptoms may recur, with tracheal narrowing caused by inflammatory or reactive edema. All patients should be closely observed for signs of airway obstruction for several hours.

Except in patients who have undergone repair of pulmonary artery sling with reimplantation, the endocarditis risk is not increased in these patients unless other cardiovascular anomalies are present.

CONGENITAL SUBCLAVIAN STEAL

Obstruction of blood flow into the subclavian artery proximal to the origin of the vertebral artery may cause reversal of flow in the latter vessel, draining blood from the cerebral circulation into the arm. This is a very rare congenital anomaly, usually occurring together with either severe coarctation or interrupted aortic arch, with one or both subclavian arteries originating distal to the obstruction. The diagnosis is established angiographically. In symptomatic patients, bypassing the obstruction with a shunt or reimplantation of the subclavian artery resolves the cerebral symptomatology.

Anesthetic Considerations. Patients should pose no unusual anesthetic problems if the lesion is isolated, except that systemic blood pressure should not be monitored on the affected side. However, use of a tourniquet in the affected arm is contraindicated since the vasodilatation following tourniquet release may cause cerebral ischemia. Blood pressure should be maintained in the normal range. Since most patients have other cardiac anomalies, anesthetic management should be guided by the predominant physiological derangement.

ANOMALIES OF THE PULMONARY ARTERY TREE

Anomalous Origin of the Pulmonary Artery from the Aorta

The origin of one pulmonary artery from the ascending aorta is a rare congenital malformation usually affecting the right pulmonary artery. The anomalous vessels may originate anywhere on the aortic arch.

The pathophysiological consequences result from a large left-to-right shunt at systemic pressures, with consequent pulmonary hypertension in one or both lungs and the development of obstructive pulmonary vascular disease. Patients are uniformly symptomatic within the first few weeks of life, and most die within the first 6 months if surgical correction is not performed. The symptoms are those of congestive heart failure, respiratory distress, and poor weight gain. Early diagnosis and correction are imperative to prevent development of irreversible pulmonary vascular disease. Surgical correction consists of anastomosing the aberrant vessel to the main pulmonary artery and correcting associated defects (usually PDA). Prognosis after surgery is good.

Anesthetic Considerations. No particular anesthetic technique can be recommended. Patients should be asymptomatic but have pulmonary function abnormalities consistent with a ventilated but underperfused lung. Since patients are also prone to respiratory infections, particular attention should be paid to adequacy of ventilation and tracheobronchial toilet. In the presence of unilateral bronchiectasis, contamination of the healthy lung during surgery should be prevented by the use of endobronchial intubation or a bronchus blocker such as a Fogarty's catheter.

CONGENITAL PULMONARY ARTERIOVENOUS FISTULA OR ANEURYSM

Direct communication between branches of the pulmonary artery and pulmonary veins without interposition of capillaries is a relatively uncommon lesion. It may occur as a single or multiple communication or, extremely rarely, as a communication of an aneurysmal dilatation of the right pulmonary artery and left atrium. Both sexes are equally affected. In 60 percent of multiple fistulae, the condition is associated with hereditary hemorrhagic telangiectasia (Rendu-Osler-Weber syndrome).

The essential physiological disturbance is a shunt of venous blood from the pulmonary arteries to the pulmonary veins, producing various degrees of systemic arterial desaturation. Although between 18 and 89 percent of the right ventricular output may pass through the fistula, cardiac output is usually not increased and pulmonary pressures remain normal.

Clinical symptoms are present in childhood and consist of cyanosis and exertional dyspnea. The chest roentgenogram usually shows abnormal shadows. Neurological symptoms caused by paradoxical embolization or thrombosis from polycythemia or brain abscesses occur in at least 25 percent of patients. Hemoptysis may occur either from telangiectatic lesions of the bronchial mucosa or from rupture of the aneurysmal fistula. Because of the frequency of fatal complications past childhood, repair should be performed in all symptomatic patients. Resection of the involved lung segment or resection of the aneurysm in cases with left atrial communication is performed.

Anesthetic Considerations. Cyanosis is due to the direct pulmonary arteriovenous connection and is influenced little by the addition of oxygen. Normal arterial P_{CO_2} is maintained by hyperventilation if the shunt is large. In low flow states causing low venous saturation, systemic desaturation may worsen. Meticulous attention should be paid to the prevention of systemic air embolization from venous lines. Polycythemia should be controlled to a hematocrit of less than 60 percent perioperatively to prevent systemic thrombosis. Manipulation of the airway should be performed atraumatically to prevent bleeding from telangiectatic lesions. Patients should be protected against endocarditis.

After resection of the fistula, patients should pose no special anesthetic problems unless familial telangiectasia is also present. Since the heart is normal in these patients, no particular anesthetic technique can be recommended.

ANOMALIES OF THE PULMONARY VENOUS BED

Total Anomalous Pulmonary Venous Return

Connection of all pulmonary veins to either the right atrium or one of the systemic veins is a relatively rare congenital anomaly present in less than 1.5 percent of all patients with congenital heart disease, but it is the 12th most common lesion seen during the first year of life. It is seen more frequently in males. Four anatomical sites of anomalous vein insertion are usually differentiated: *supracardiac*, into either a left or right superior vena cava; *cardiac*, into the coronary sinus or right atrium; *infracardiac*, into the portal or hepatic veins or ductus venosus; and *mixed*, with insertion at more than one level (Fig. 6–22). Drainage into the left superior vena cava is seen most frequently. Twenty-five to thirty percent of patients have associated cardiac anomalies, particularly of the asplenia type. The presence of an intra-atrial communication is necessary for survival, and an atrial septal defect or patent foramen ovale is part of the complex.

The right heart carries an increased volume load from a large left-to-right shunt, similar to the physiology of a secundum atrial septal defect. Systemic saturation and output depend on the degree of mixing at the atrial level. Pulmonary arterial hypertension is present in the majority of supracardiac and cardiac connections and in all infradiaphragmatic connections owing to obstruction to pulmonary venous return. It may also develop in later life secondary to high pulmonary blood flow in patients without pulmonary venous obstruction but with a large intra-atrial communication, which allows survival into adulthood.

The majority of patients are symptomatic within the first month of life. If no pulmonary venous obstruction is present, signs of congestive heart failure from volume overload and

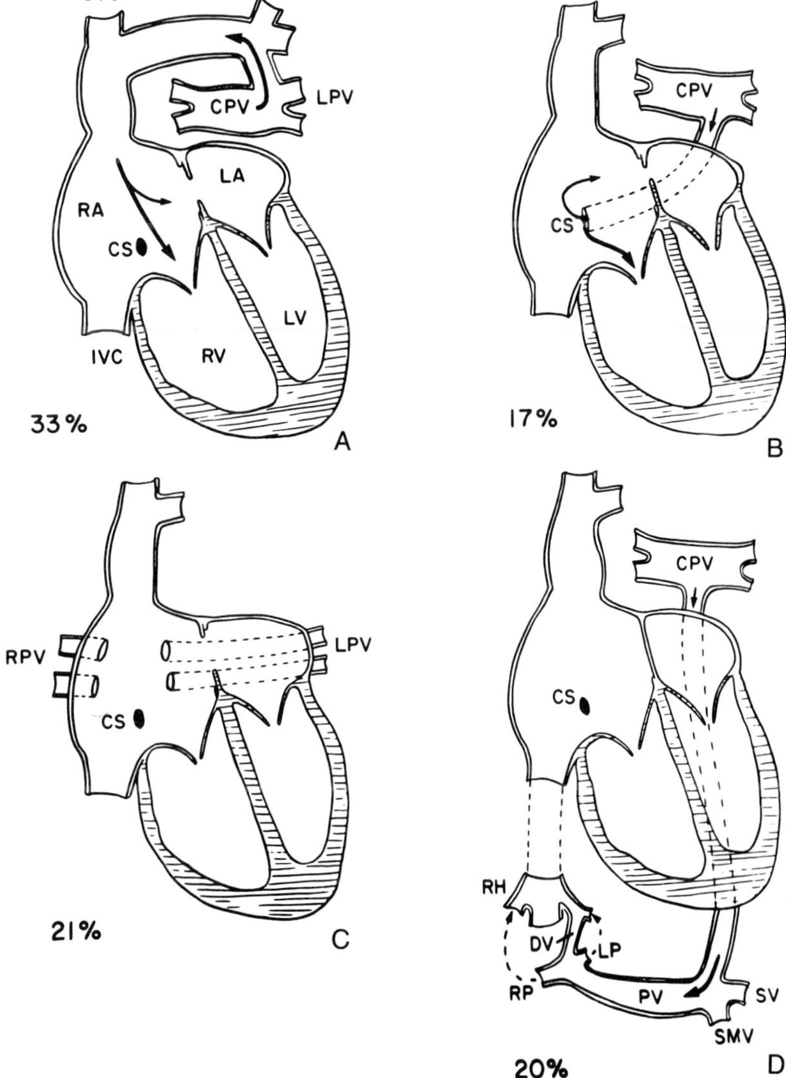

FIGURE 6–22. Total anomalous pulmonary venous return: *A*, to left innominate vein; *B*, to coronary sinus; *C*, to right atrium; *D*, infradiaphragmatic to portal vein. SVC = Superior vena cava; IVC = inferior vena cava; CPV = common pulmonary vein; LPV = left pulmonary vein; RPV = right pulmonary vein; LA = left atrium; RA = right atrium; CS = coronary sinus; RV = right ventricle; LV = left ventricle; SV = splenic vein; PV = portal vein; DV = ductus venosus; RH = right hepatic vein; SMV = superior mesenteric vein. (Redrawn from Lucas RV: Anomalous venous connections, pulmonary and systemic. *In* Adams FH, Emmanouilides GC [eds]: Heart Disease in Infants, Children, and Adolescents. 3rd edition. Baltimore, Williams and Wilkins, 1983. © 1983, the Williams & Wilkins Co., Baltimore.)

only mild cyanosis are seen. Tachypnea, frequent respiratory infections, and failure to thrive are the common presenting features. Without surgical treatment, the mortality of these infants approaches 80 percent by 1 year of age. With pulmonary venous obstruction, cyanosis and tachypnea are present at birth or appear shortly thereafter. Cardiac failure occurs from obstruction to right heart output relatively early, and patients die within days to a few months from hypoxia and pulmonary edema unless surgical relief can be achieved. Operation should be performed as soon as possible. At operation, a connection between the common pulmonary venous trunk and the left atrium is created, and the intra-atrial connection is closed. Surgical mortality ranges from 10 to 30 percent.

Anesthetic Considerations. The majority of patients with this anomaly who are seen for elective noncardiac operation will have undergone a corrective procedure. Since adequate surgical survival has occurred only in recent years, no long-term observations are yet available. In patients with pulmonary vascular disease at the time of operation, progression of the pulmonary arteriolar obstruction may occur despite repair. This is unlikely in patients operated upon in infancy. As the child grows, stenosis of the pulmonary venous–to–left atrial anastomosis may occur, leading to secondary pulmonary venous hypertension. Such patients have a clinical picture somewhat similar to that seen in patients with mitral stenosis. Patients with a widely patent intra-atrial connection, no venous obstruction, and an increase in pulmonary arteriolar resistance restricting pulmonary blood flow may have few clinical symptoms but have signs similar to those of an atrial septal defect. Endocarditis prophylaxis and prevention of systemic embolization are important anesthetic considerations.

COMMON PULMONARY VEIN ATRESIA

Complete absence of a connection between the pulmonary veins and the left atrium or any other cardiac chamber or systemic vein is an extremely rare and nearly uniformly fatal congenital cardiac lesion. Cyanosis, tachypnea, and heart failure occur shortly after birth. Pulmonary venous blood flow may be drained via the bronchopulmonary veins to the systemic venous system, albeit severely restricted, which explains survival of afflicted babies of up to 1 month of life without surgical intervention. The lesion is generally isolated. Surgical correction has been successfully performed only recently and needs to be done as soon as the diagnosis is established. It consists of anastomosis of the usually large confluence of the pulmonary veins, which is located directly behind the left atrium, to the usually adequately sized left atrium. Patients should be normal postoperatively unless stenosis of the pulmonary venous–left atrial connection occurs.

PARTIAL ANOMALOUS PULMONARY VENOUS RETURN

Connection of one or more, but not all, of the pulmonary veins to either the right atrium or a systemic vein is a fairly common condition observed in 0.7 percent of all routine postmortem examinations. It is present in 9 percent of patients with atrial septal defects. Both sexes are equally affected. Most commonly, the right pulmonary veins drain into the superior vena cava or right atrium, with an associated sinus venosus defect. The physiological consequences and clinical symptomatology are similar to those of a secundum ASD.

Drainage of the right pulmonary veins to the inferior vena cava constitutes part of the scimitar syndrome. The atrial septum is usually intact. Anomalies of the bronchial system of the right lung, including hypoplasia of the lung and right pulmonary artery, and abnormal systemic arterial connections are generally present. Respiratory infections are commonly seen, because of the abnormal pulmonary structure. The abnormal venous connection produces a crescent or scimitar-shaped shadow in the right lower lung field on the chest radiograph. The clinical presentation is similar to that seen in the patient with an ASD.

Surgical correction is recommended during childhood in all patients with partial anomalous pulmonary venous connection, to prevent development of obstructive pulmonary vascular disease. Those with the scimitar syndrome may require pulmonary resection. Redirection of the abnormal venous return to the left atrium can be a technically difficult surgical problem.

The postoperative prognosis when operation has been successful is excellent unless pulmonary vascular obstruction is present. Atrial arrhythmias and the sick sinus syndrome may follow repair of partial anomalous return of the right superior pulmonary vein with high sinus venous defect.

Anesthetic Considerations. Patients should be managed as are patients with secundum ASD.

Endocarditis prophylaxis is necessary pre- and postoperatively.

ANOMALIES OF THE SYSTEMIC VENOUS RETURN

Aberrations in the embryological development of the cardinal venous system result in either persistence of two superior venae cavae, or anomalies of the coronary sinus. They frequently are associated with other congenital cardiac anomalies, most commonly tetralogy of Fallot. These anomalies are usually important only with regard to difficulties during cardiac catheterization and cardiac surgery.

PERSISTENT LEFT SUPERIOR VENA CAVA

The most common anomaly of systemic venous return is persistence of a left superior vena cava draining into the coronary sinus and the right atrium. It is found in 0.3 percent of routine postmortems but is present in 20 percent of patients with tetralogy of Fallot and 3 to 5 percent of all patients with congenital heart disease. Since venous drainage is physiologically normal, no clinical manifestations are present. Patients with this anomaly who undergo central venous catheterization from the left may demonstrate an abnormal pathway of the catheter on the follow-up chest radiograph. This is probably the only important anesthetic implication of this syndrome.

In 8 percent of cases with persistent left superior vena cava the vessel connects directly to the left atrium. This lesion is almost always associated with other cardiac anomalies. Occasionally the right superior vena cava is absent. The anomaly results in various degrees of right-to-left shunting, depending on blood return through the abnormal vessel, from 20 to 40 percent of total venous return. Cyanosis may be prominent if no atrial communication is present, without cardiac enlargement or failure. Systemic embolization and brain abscesses may occur. Treatment is surgical, with either ligation or transposition of the abnormal vessel.

Anesthetic Considerations. The physiological consequences of the associated lesions will generally be the prominent feature guiding anesthetic management. In isolated forms, management should be similar to the management of cyanotic lesions with normal pulmonary blood flow and directed toward prevention of endocarditis, systemic embolization, and thrombosis from polycythemia. No particular anesthetic technique seems likely to be superior, since the myocardial function in these patients is normal.

ANOMALIES OF THE CORONARY SINUS

Anomalies of the coronary sinus are rare and are infrequently diagnosed during life. Complete absence of the coronary sinus is always associated with persistent left superior vena cava. The coronary sinus may be hypoplastic, stenosis of the ostium may be present, or drainage may occur to the inferior vena cava or left atrium. The latter will result in a small right-to-left shunt, which is of no clinical significance. No unusual anesthetic problems should be caused by these anomalies.

ANOMALIES OF THE INFERIOR VENA CAVA

Complete absence of the inferior vena cava, with drainage of infradiaphragmatic systemic venous return through an enlarged azygos vein, is present in close to 3 percent of patients with congenital heart disease but extremely rare in those with normal hearts. The anomaly has no physiological consequences but may cause problems during cardiac catheterization and venous cannulation for cardiac surgery.

A very rare anomaly consists of drainage of the inferior vena cava to the left atrium. It may occur as an isolated lesion or in conjunction with persistence of the sinus venosus valve or an ASD. Signs of systemic venous obstruction and a right-to-left shunt are present. Fifty percent of patients have associated cardiac defects, most commonly right ventricular outflow obstruction. Treatment of this anomaly is surgical. Its presence may complicate surgical repair of associated cardiac lesions, particularly atrial septal defects. Anesthetic implications are similar to those in patients with persistent left superior vena caval drainage into the left atrium.

ANOMALIES OF THE CORONARY ARTERIES

ANOMALOUS ORIGIN OF THE LEFT CORONARY ARTERY

Anomalous origin of the left coronary artery from the right sinus of Valsalva results in this vessel's running between the aorta and right ventricular outflow tract or pulmonary trunk. Compression of the vessel may occur during exercise and has been implicated as a cause of death in young healthy athletes. The anomaly is rare.

Origin of the left coronary artery from the pulmonary trunk is a rare but frequently lethal anomaly. It is usually referred to as Bland-White-Garland syndrome. Eighty to ninety percent of patients become symptomatic in infancy, and the majority die from congestive heart failure. The physiological derangement consists of perfusion of the left coronary artery from a low-pressure system, with reduced oxygen saturation. This occurs as pulmonary pressure falls postnatally, although pulmonary artery pressure may remain elevated subsequent to poor left ventricular output, with elevated left atrial pressures and secondary pulmonary hypertension.

Development of collateral vessels from the right coronary artery may be life-saving but results in a left-to-right shunt and volume overload of the heart with coronary steal. More commonly, endocardial and myocardial ischemia and infarction result from the decreased left myocardial perfusion, leading to papillary muscle dysfunction and mitral regurgitation. With feeding, infants may present with signs of anginal attacks. The electrocardiogram resembles that of an adult with coronary artery disease. Infants with ischemic attacks require urgent operation because of the risk of sudden death, whereas patients with heart failure may be managed conservatively in the expectation that the collateral circulation will develop and myocardial function will improve.

Eventually, all patients with this anomaly require correction to prevent sudden death. Various surgical approaches have been used. Simple ligation of the vessel in cases with left-to-right shunting and good collaterals may effect cure, but the result is unpredictable and leaves the patient with a system with one coronary artery. Presently favored are procedures that preserve a system with two coronary arteries by anastomosing either a systemic artery or a vein graft to the anomalous vessel, redirecting aortic blood flow to the anomalous coronary ostium via transpulmonary arterial baffle, or reanastomosing the vessel with a cuff of pulmonary trunk to the aorta. Surgical therapy results in the resolution of ischemic attacks and improved myocardial performance. The long-term prognosis of infants after operation is not yet known.

Anesthetic Considerations. Patients with classic Bland-White-Garland syndrome require early surgical correction. Elective noncardiac surgery should be performed only after cardiac surgery. Management will depend on the degree of residual cardiovascular abnormality. Patients may have reduced cardiac reserve owing to myocardial scarring or residual mitral insufficiency. The use of anesthetic agents causing minimal myocardial depression, maintenance of heart rate, and direct monitoring of systemic arterial and venous pressures for major surgery are indicated.

In older patients with the uncorrected anomaly, care should be taken to avoid increases in myocardial oxygen demand (tachycardia, hypertension) or decreases in myocardial oxygen supply (low diastolic pressure, high left ventricular end-diastolic pressure). A left-to-right shunt is often present but of only small-to-moderate size. Patients are at risk for bacterial endocarditis after corrective surgery.

Anomalous Origin of the Right Coronary Artery

Origin of the right coronary artery from the pulmonary artery causes no symptoms. The area supplied by the pulmonary artery is the low-pressure right ventricle, and no ischemia results. The condition is extremely rare and has usually been seen only on routine postmortem.

Anomalous Origin of Both Coronary Arteries

Origin of both coronary arteries from the pulmonary artery is extremely rare and is uniformly fatal within the first weeks of life unless associated with a lesion causing pulmonary hypertension, such as truncus arteriosus. The latter lesion requires correction in infancy.

Coronary Arteriovenous Fistula

Communication between the arterial and venous coronary vasculature can occur singly or as numerous, aneurysmically dilated loops. This anomaly is rare. Over 90 percent of fistulas drain into the right side of the heart, with the physiological consequence of a left-to-right shunt with runoff from the aorta and volume overload of the left heart and pulmonary vasculature. The presentation is similar to that of patients with PDA but with an atypical murmur. Signs of myocardial ischemia from coronary steal are very uncommon. In the presence of a large shunt, symptoms of congestive heart failure and pulmonary hyperperfusion may occur. With most fistulas, symptoms are minimal and the shunt is small. Since patients are at risk for endocarditis, secondary atherosclerotic changes with rupture, and thromboembolic phenomena, surgical correction of the lesion is recommended. Usually the fistula can be clamped and ligated without the use of cardiopulmonary bypass, with very low surgical mortality. With suitable anatomy, closure of the fistula can be achieved by transcatheter coil embolization in the catheterization laboratory. Patients should be normal postoperatively. Prior to surgical correction, patients should be managed similarly to patients with a small-to-moderate PDA. They require endocarditis prophylaxis.

CARDIOMYOPATHIES

Cardiomyopathies are diseases of the myocardium not caused by structural abnormalities of the heart. They can be divided into primary cardiomyopathies, not associated with other disease and usually of unknown etiology, and secondary cardiomyopathies, associated with other diseases or known etiological agents. Pediatric cardiomyopathies are characterized by a high degree of morbidity and mortality. Primary cardiomyopathies are relatively uncommon—2.5 percent of pediatric cardiac disease. They can be classified according to the main physiological derangement into congestive cardiomyopathy, characterized by poor systolic ejection function; restrictive, with poor ventricular compliance or reduced ventricular volume; and obstructive, with obstruction to left ventricular output or obliteration of the ventricular cavities or both (Table 6–4) (Fig. 6–23).

CONGESTIVE CARDIOMYOPATHIES

The physiological derangement in congestive cardiomyopathy is a reduction in contractile force of the heart muscle. The initial compensatory mechanism consists of increased filling volumes, which maintain stroke volume via the Frank-Starling mechanism. As the ventricle dilates, wall tension and end-diastolic pressure increase, adversely affecting myocardial oxygenation. As stroke output falls, reflex sympathetic stimulation occurs, increasing impedance to left ventricular output, which increases myocardial oxygen demand. The elevated end-diastolic pressures are transmitted to the left atrium and pulmonary vascular bed, leading to pulmonary venous engorgement, pulmonary arterial hypertension, and eventually right heart failure. The elevated pulmonary vascular pressures result in transudation of fluid, interstitial or alveolar pulmonary edema, and ventilation-perfusion abnormalities through small airway disease caused by bronchial cuffing and reduced compliance. Low cardiac output results in poor peripheral perfusion, with metabolic acidosis and salt and water retention secondary to poor renal blood flow. The nutritional status deteriorates, owing to reduced caloric intake and increased metabolic demand from respiratory distress.

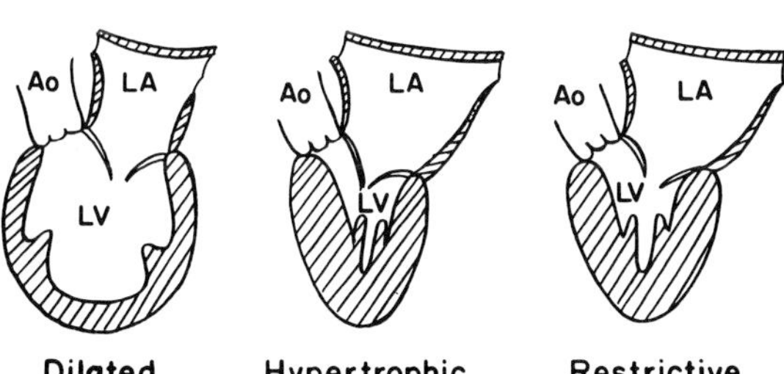

FIGURE 6–23. Various forms of cardiomyopathies.

Signs and symptoms of congestive heart failure in infancy are the same regardless of etiology. Tachycardia and tachypnea are commonly present. Patients have a history of feeding difficulties, poor weight gain, frequent respiratory infections, excessive sweating (particularly with feeding), grunting, and wheezing. Rales may be heard, and there is pallor and peripheral cyanosis secondary to poor output. Older children may have tachycardia on exertion, orthopnea, chest discomfort or abdominal pain from a distended liver, a persistent dry cough, and anorexia. Pulses may be normal or reduced with cold extremities.

Therapy consists of digitalization, fluid restriction, diuresis, and reduction of cardiac afterload with an oral vasodilator (hydralazine). In the acutely decompensated patient, intravenous inotropic support with isoproterenol or dopamine infusion may be necessary. Isoproterenol reduces afterload by peripheral vasodilatation and is a pulmonary vasodilator. Its undesirable side effects are tachycardia and ventricular dysrhythmia. It is the preferred agent in patients with pulmonary hypertension requiring afterload reduction and an increase in peripheral perfusion and in whom tachycardia or arrhythmias are not problems. Patients with arrhythmias or in whom tachycardia is undesirable should be treated with dopamine or dobutamine. Dopamine will not influence left ventricular afterload but causes renal arteriolar dilatation. Nitroprusside or nitroglycerin may be added for preload and afterload reduction. Patients unresponsive to medical therapy are candidates for cardiac transplantation. The prognosis of congestive cardiomyopathies is

Table 6–4. PEDIATRIC CARDIOMYOPATHIES

	Clinical Symptoms	Associated Features
Primary Cardiomyopathies		
Congestive nonobstructive		
Endocardial fibroelastosis of infancy Idiopathic nonobstructive cardiomyopathy	Mitral and aortic insufficiency Left ventricular thrombi Pulsus alternans	Long-term digitalis therapy
Restrictive		
Endomyocardial fibrosis Hypertrophic form with ventricular hypertrophy and small ventricular cavities	Atrial fibrillation, marked cardiomegaly, ventilation-perfusion abnormalities, restriction to cardiac filling, AV valve incompetence	Common in Africa
Loeffler endocarditis	Restriction to ventricular filling Eosinophilia	Steroid therapy
Obstructive		
Idiopathic hypertrophic subaortic stenosis	Obstruction increased by inotropic agents or reduction in preload or afterload Sudden death	Familial Uncommon in pediatric age groups
Secondary Cardiomyopathies		
Infective		
Virus *Trypanosoma*	Congestive failure	Congestive failure May progress to chronic cardiopathy
Myocardial abscess in bacterial endocarditis	Congestive failure	
Diphtheria Rheumatic carditis	Congestive failure Conduction defects common	Heart block Sensitive to digitalis
Metabolic		
Glycogenous Type II (Pompe's)	Massive cardiomegaly Outflow tract obstruction	Unremitting failure
Associated with neurological or vascular disease Friedreich's ataxia Duchenne's muscular dystrophy	Conduction defects Tachyarrhythmias	Replacement of muscle fibers by connective tissue
Collagen disorders		
Disseminated lupus erythematosus Dermatomyositis	Pericarditis and pericardial effusion	
Neoplastic		
Leiomyofibroma Lymphoma Myxoma	Mechanical obstruction	
Miscellaneous		
Radiation Phosphorus Lead Antineoplastic drugs Snake venom Scorpion venom	Myocarditis	Congestive failure

poor; 40 percent of patients die within 1 year, 50 percent within 2 years and nearly 70 percent within 5 years following onset of symptoms.

Anesthetic Considerations. Elective operation should be carried out only in compensated patients. Since myocardial reserve may be very limited, filling pressures of the right and left sides of the heart and continuous intra-arterial blood pressure should be monitored during major operation to allow better assessment of the circulatory status as well as blood gases. Electrocardiographic monitoring is essential, since arrhythmias or conduction defects may readily occur. Electrolyte abnormalities should be corrected and alkalosis avoided in these patients, since they may precipitate digitalis toxicity.

Anesthetic agents with minimal effects on myocardial contractility should be used to avoid precipitating heart failure. Inhalation anesthetics are probably best avoided. Narcotics, particularly fentanyl and ketamine, are useful alternatives. Since stroke volume is generally limited, heart rate should be maintained so that cardiac output does not decrease. The generous use of atropine and the appropriate choice of muscle relaxants are important. Because of the ventilatory impairment that is commonly present, the airway and ventilation should be controlled. Regional techniques may be a useful alternative to general anesthesia where possible.

PRIMARY ENDOCARDIAL FIBROELASTOSIS

Primary endocardial fibroelastosis occurs in approximately 2 to 4 percent of patients with congenital heart disease and constitutes the most common cause of heart failure and death in children with heart disease between 2 months and 1 year of age. It occurs equally in both sexes. It may be of viral origin and a result of interstitial myocarditis. Secondary fibroelastosis is a common complication of cardiac lesions producing left ventricular wall stress (aortic stenosis, coarctation, mitral valve disease, hypoplastic left heart, anomalous origin of the left coronary artery).

The disease affects the left ventricle and usually extends into the left atrium. The right side of the heart is only rarely affected. The heart size is markedly increased, because of enlargement of the left ventricle and left atrium. The endocardium is diffusely thickened and is of milky-white appearance. Chordae tendineae and papillary muscles are involved in the fibrotic process.

The disease typically leads to rapid cardiac decompensation in a previously healthy infant. One third of patients become symptomatic within the first 3 months and 80 percent within the first year of life, with classic signs of left ventricular failure. Thrombi may form in the dilated ventricle and cause systemic embolization. One third of patients develop mitral insufficiency in later stages of the disease.

The clinical course of patients with early onset of the disease is poor. Death commonly occurs between 2 and 6 months of age despite vigorous antifailure therapy. Patients who are seen in late infancy and early childhood may recover completely from their symptoms. The mainstay of therapy for endocardial fibroelastosis is prompt and prolonged administration of digitalis. Digitalis therapy should be maintained for a minimum of 2 years after symptoms have disappeared.

Premature discontinuation of digitalis may lead to recurrence of heart failure, which may not respond to renewed digitalis administration. If heart failure recurs on cessation of digitalis therapy, patients usually progress to chronic cardiac failure and ultimately death. Mitral insufficiency may progress and necessitate valve replacement in childhood or adolescence.

Anesthetic Considerations. Patients should be managed according to the recommendations outlined earlier for congestive failure. Maintenance of digitalis therapy is essential. Patients need close monitoring for signs of digitalis toxicity.

IDIOPATHIC NONOBSTRUCTIVE CARDIOMYOPATHY

This form of congestive cardiomyopathy is characterized by dilatation of both ventricular cavities, reduced ejection fraction, and increased end-systolic volume. This disease is very common in South Africa, accounting for 25 to 35 percent of cases of heart disease, but is rare elsewhere. The increased end-systolic volume leads to relative stasis of the blood in the apical portion of the ventricles, resulting in intracavitary thrombosis. Patients have signs of congestive failure and usually pulsus alternans. The disease may be present in infants but more commonly occurs in children and adolescents. Treatment consists of antifailure therapy and anticoagulation until symptoms resolve. The majority of patients have a slow downhill course over a number of years.

Anesthetic management should be tailored to the degree of myocardial failure.

RESTRICTIVE CARDIOMYOPATHIES

Restrictive cardiomyopathies are characterized by abnormal diastolic function while ventricular contractile function is unimpaired or even greater than normal. The resistance to diastolic filling from the nonelastic ventricles results in elevation of ventricular end-diastolic pressures, leading to elevation in atrial and systemic and pulmonary venous pressures. Pulmonary hypertension is usually observed. Left-sided filling pressures are generally higher than right-sided pressures, in contrast to constrictive pericarditis. Eventually signs of right-sided failure with systemic venous distention and hepatic congestion and ascites occur. Stroke volume may be limited and cardiac output maintained by increases in heart rate. The most common clinical symptoms are dyspnea and exercise intolerance. Atrial fibrillation may occur in patients with marked atrial enlargement and usually leads to clinical deterioration because of further impairment in left ventricular filling. Patients may respond poorly to digitalis. Diuretic therapy may control symptoms temporarily.

Anesthetic Management. Maintenance of cardiac contractility and heart rate is essential. Preload must be adequate to maintain filling pressures and cardiac output. Patients may be unable to compensate for reduction in afterload, which should be kept close to normal. Direct monitoring of filling and systemic arterial pressures should be established for all major procedures. Because pulmonary congestion is frequently present, ventilation-perfusion abnormalities should be expected and treated with higher oxygen concentrations and controlled ventilation. Reliable electrocardiographic monitoring is necessary, and every effort should be made to maintain sinus rhythm.

Patients with the hypertrophic form of restrictive myocarditis may benefit from use of an inhalational anesthetic agent, such as halothane, that causes reduction in the hypercontractile state of the left ventricular muscle unless congestive heart failure is present. All other forms of restrictive myocarditis require maintenance of myocardial contractility; narcotics and ketamine are probably better choices for anesthetic management.

Patients require endocarditis prophylaxis.

ENDOMYOCARDIAL FIBROSIS

Endomyocardial fibrosis is an unusual form of cardiomyopathy, characterized by restriction of ventricular filling and obliteration of the inflow portion of the ventricles by dense fibrosis and thrombus formation. The fibrosis involves the papillary muscles, leading to secondary AV valve incompetence. The right heart is usually more affected, and signs of right-sided obstruction are present. In addition, pleural effusion and pericardial effusion are common. Atrial fibrillation is commonly seen in advanced disease. The disease is most prevalent in tropical Africa, where it affects up to 20 percent of patients with heart disease. It is a disease of children and young adults; 70 percent of patients are under 20 years of age.

Medical therapy in symptomatic patients is generally unsuccessful, with a reported average survival of 2 years. Surgical therapy consists of pericardiectomy or pericardioperitoneal shunt in patients with recurrent massive pericardial effusion. A Glenn's shunt may be performed to improve pulmonary perfusion. Corrective surgery consists of stripping of the endocardium, with or without AV valve replacement.

LOEFFLER'S ENDOCARDITIS

This is a form of myocardiopathy similar to tropical endomyocardial fibrosis, but it is seen in temperate climates and more commonly in males. It is associated with marked eosinophilia without identifiable cause. Multiple other organs may also be affected. The disease occurs in adolescents and young adults. Concentric left ventricular wall thickening occurs, with intracavitary thrombosis and systemic embolization. In addition, scarring of the mitral valve, with adhesion of the posterior leaflet to the ventricular wall, results in mitral insufficiency. The disease causes a high morbidity and mortality, but the prognosis appears to have improved recently with corticosteroid or hydroxyurea therapy.

OBSTRUCTIVE CARDIOMYOPATHIES

Idiopathic Hypertrophic Cardiomyopathy

Hypertrophic cardiomyopathy is a primary disease of cardiac muscle characterized by a hypertrophied nondilated left ventricle. Histologically, marked disorganization of myocardial cells, particularly of the ventricular septum, is present. The disease is genetically transmitted in the majority of cases as an autosomal dominant trait and affects both sexes equally. It is rare in Africans and black Americans. It appears to be associated with lentiginosis, neurofibromatosis, pheochromocytoma, and Friedreich's ataxia.

Obstructive hypertrophic cardiomyopathy represents 0.7 percent of all congenital heart disease and 10 percent of all cases of aortic stenosis. Septal hypertrophy of at least 1.3 times the thickness of the left ventricular free wall is an invariable feature. Although the disease was originally described in the context of dynamic left ventricular outflow obstruction (idiopathic subaortic stenosis), in reality this obstruction is absent in a large proportion of patients with this disease.

Clinical manifestations are generally not present until adolescence or adulthood. The most frequent presentation is in the third or fourth decade of life. The predominant complaint is exertional dyspnea or fatigue; in childhood the usual presenting finding is a murmur. When the disease presents during infancy, which is rare, a high incidence of congestive heart failure and right and left ventricular outflow obstruction is noted. Heart failure in these infants occurs in the presence of a nondilated ventricle with normal or increased systolic function and appears to be a sign of poor prognosis. The majority of affected infants die from their congestive failure within the first year of life. Congestive heart failure is uncommon in older children and adolescents with this disease.

The major abnormality in hypertrophic cardiomyopathy is a diminution in left ventricular compliance causing increased resistance to left ventricular filling. Left ventricular outflow tract obstruction is caused by the hypertrophied septum and an abnormal forward movement of the anterior mitral leaflet during systole. The latter frequently also results in some mitral valve incompetence. The obstruction is dynamic in nature and may be reduced by increased ventricular volume, reduced contractility, and increased systemic vascular resistance. Hypovolemia, low peripheral vascular resistance, and increased contractility (as in sympathetic stimulation) will lead to worsening of the gradient across the left ventricular outflow tract. Patients with hypertrophic cardiomyopathy have a high incidence of serious ventricular arrhythmias despite lack of symptoms.

Sudden death occurs in 3 to 4 percent of affected patients and is particularly common in young patients between 12 and 30 years, frequently in association with strenuous exercise. Half these patients are asymptomatic prior to sudden death. Sudden death appears to be more common in some families.

Atrial fibrillation may occur in later stages, probably owing to left atrial enlargement caused by a poorly compliant left ventricle. It generally leads to clinical deterioration, since it interferes with left ventricular filling.

The mainstay of medical therapy for hypertrophic cardiomyopathy is beta-adrenergic blockade. Calcium channel blockers may prove beneficial by improving left ventricular filling. Excessive use of diuretics, preload and afterload reducing agents, beta-agonistic drugs, and digitalis may lead to worsening of symptoms because of an increase in subaortic obstruction. Paroxysmal atrial fibrillation may require use of digitalis to control the dysrhythmia, and patients require anticoagulation to prevent system embolization.

Surgical therapy is of only limited use. Septal myotomy or myectomy is usually recommended for patients with severe symptoms refractory to medical therapy and outflow gradients of 50 mm Hg or more. Operative mortality ranges from 5 to 10 percent. Operation usually results in relief of the obstruction when the patient is at rest, although a mild-to-moderate gradient may recur with provocation. Aortic insufficiency due to damage of the cusps at operation may develop later. The mortality for patients with hypertrophic cardiomyopathy not treated surgically ranges around 3 percent per year, but mortality appears to be somewhat lower for patients after surgery (1.9 percent).

Anesthetic Considerations. Preoperative anxiety should be reduced by generous sedation. In addition to reliable electrocardiographic monitoring, close monitoring of systemic and right or left filling pressures is indicated for all major operations. Changes in filling volume, distending pressure of the left ventricle, heart rate and rhythm, and left ventricular afterload and contractility may adversely influence left ventricular outflow obstruction and decrease cardiac output. In addition, these patients exhibit a high propensity for ventricular arrhythmias.

Hypovolemia, vasodilation, and hypotension should be prevented. Use of the Trendelenburg position and phenylephrine may be helpful for acute therapy. Tachycardia and sympathetic stimulation may accompany light anesthesia and lead to increased contractility and decreased filling, with increased obstruction. Reduction in peripheral vascular resistance, as with sympathetic blockade, may also result in an increased outflow gradient.

Inhalation anesthetics (particularly halothane) appear to be well tolerated if combined with adequate volume replacement, since they tend to decrease myocardial contractility and permit rapid changes in anesthetic depth. A smooth induction is essential. In older children, a barbiturate induction may be useful. Excessive positive-pressure ventilation should be avoided, since it interferes with venous return and may cause a decrease in left ventricular volume and subsequent worsening of the outflow gradient.

Sinus rhythm should be maintained. Tachyarrhythmias may require treatment with propranolol or verapamil. Positive inotropic agents and vasodilators should be avoided. Fentanyl, which causes mild bradycardia and has little cardiovascular effect, may prove useful, whereas ketamine is relatively contraindicated. Major regional anesthesia is probably contraindicated since it results in widespread sympathetic blockade. Peripheral vascular resistance should be maintained, if necessary, with a peripherally acting vasoconstrictor like phenylephrine. Patients require endocarditis prophylaxis.

TUMORS OF THE HEART

Primary tumors of the heart and pericardium are rare, with an incidence of between 0.001 and 0.28 percent in reported autopsy series.

In infants and children, rhabdomyoma is the most common cardiac tumor. Seventy-five percent of all cardiac tumors in infants less than 1 year old are rhabdomyomas or teratomas. In children from 1 to 15 years of age, rhabdomyomas, fibromas, and myxomas account for 80 percent of benign cardiac tumors and 60 percent of all tumors and cysts of the heart and pericardium. Malignant tumors account for less than 10 percent of all tumors and cysts in this age group.

The manifestations of cardiac tumors depend on the location of the tumor. Involvement of the conduction tissue may lead to dysrhythmia. Intracavitary tumors may result in obstruction to blood flow and filling of the affected chamber, obstruction of valves, or embolization of fragmented tumor material. Involvement of the myocardium may lead to myocardial failure.

BENIGN TUMORS

Rhabdomyoma

This is the most common tumor in infancy and childhood, occurring in 80 percent of patients with cardiac tumors who are less than 1 year old. The tumors commonly are multiple, occurring in the right and left ventricles or, less often, in the atria. The largest mass is usually located in the ventricular septum, but over half the tumors are intracavitary and lead to obstruction of blood flow. Thirty percent of patients have tuberous sclerosis and adenomas of the sebaceous glands. Presenting symptoms are arrhythmias, congestive failure, or signs of valvular obstruction, usually of the inlet type. The natural history of patients with cardiac rhabdomyoma is poor. Fifty percent die within the first 6 months and 80 percent before 1 year unless surgical excision of the tumor is performed. Survival after excision appears excellent, with resolution of cardiac symptoms.

FIBROMA

Cardiac fibromas are almost always solitary and constitute the second most common cardiac tumor in childhood. Symptoms generally occur within the first decade. The tumors compress surrounding structures because of their size. They frequently occur in the ventricular septum and invade the conduction system, leading to ventricular dysrhythmia and sudden death. With large tumors, intractable heart failure or signs of cardiac obstruction are common.

Tumors located in the free ventricular wall are usually amenable to resection; septal tumors often cannot be completely removed but can be sufficiently debulked to result in improvement in clinical symptoms. The prognosis after debulking is guarded. Patients often die from ventricular arrhythmias.

MYXOMA

Intracavitary myxomas constitute about half of all benign cardiac tumors in adults but occur rarely in children. The tumor commonly arises as a pedunculated mass from the atrial septum; 75 percent occur in the left atrium. Patients have changing signs of mitral valve disease, either stenosis or insufficiency, and a history of fainting spells. Because the tumor is soft, it fragments easily, with resulting pulmonary or systemic embolization, depending on the primary location of the myxoma. Signs of mitral stenosis in a child should lead the physician to suspect left atrial myxoma.

Therapy consists of surgical excision of the tumor and the attached atrial wall to prevent recurrence. The prognosis postoperatively is generally excellent. Patients with systemic embolization prior to surgery may develop coronary and cerebral aneurysms in later years from myxomatous degeneration at the embolic site.

TERATOMA

The majority of teratomas of the heart are extracardiac but intrapericardiac, arising from the origin of the great vessels. These tumors are very rare, are usually seen in infancy or childhood, and more commonly affect females. The tumors cause cardiac compression with dyspnea and cyanosis. Surgical excision is the only effective therapy.

MALIGNANT TUMORS

Primary malignant tumors of the heart are very uncommon in infants and children. They are most commonly malignant teratomas or rhabdomyosarcomas. The clinical presentation depends on the degree of intracavitary obstruction and the involvement of the conduction system. The cardiac valves are often invaded by the tumor in rhabdomyosarcoma. Prognosis is poor, with most patients dying within a year of diagnosis.

Anesthetic Considerations. Patients with benign lesions should undergo excision prior to elective operation. Reliable electrocardiographic monitoring is essential and should be continued postoperatively, since conduction defects may persist. Agents causing increased ventricular irritability should be avoided in patients with a known propensity for ventricular arrhythmias. Blood pressure control may be important after myxoma excision, since patients may have unrecognized cerebral aneurysms. Those with myocardial fibromas may have a residual defect similar to a restrictive cardiomyopathy with decreased diastolic function and require careful fluid management and maintenance of myocardial contractility.

CONGENITAL CONDUCTION DEFECTS

CONGENITAL COMPLETE HEART BLOCK

Congenital complete heart block is a rare anomaly, occurring in less than 1 percent of patients with congenital heart disease. It is, however, very common in children of mothers with lupus erythematosus even if the mother is clinically asymptomatic. The defect is commonly a singular one but may be associated with other congenital cardiac anomalies, particularly corrected transposition or atrial septal defects. Heart block in infancy and childhood most commonly arises following repair of intracardiac lesions.

Congenital complete heart block is characterized by complete absence of conduction between the atria and ventricles. The heart rate is usually less than 80 beats/min in infants and around 50 in children. The diagnosis may be suspected prenatally if there is a fetal heart rate of less than 100 in the absence of any etiology for fetal distress. Most patients have a block located high in the septum, between the AV node and the His bundle. The QRS complexes are narrow (less than 0.1 sec) and normally configurated. The heart rate characteristically can be increased by exercise, atropine, and sympathomimetics. In contrast to acquired complete heart block, cardiac output is maintained by an increased stroke volume. Clinically, patients exhibit bounding pulses, a low diastolic pressure from diastolic runoff with a slow heart rate, and cannon waves in the jugular pulse when the atrium contracts against the closed tricuspid valve.

A small subgroup of patients with congenital heart block have the block located distal to the bundle of His. In these patients the QRS complex is widened and abnormal, and the heart rate is usually slower; most such patients are symptomatic.

Congestive heart failure is the usual presenting symptom in infancy, whereas older children with congenital heart block who become symptomatic usually have exercise intolerance and a history of syncopal attacks, which are frequently caused by ventricular dysrhythmia and not bradycardia.

Death from congenital heart block usually occurs within the first year, generally in infants with heart rates of below 55 beats/min and wide QRS complexes. Older children tend to be asymptomatic. They may exhibit episodic supraventricular dysrhythmia without untoward side effects. Asymptomatic patients need continued follow-up to evaluate exercise tolerance and search for development of ventricular ectopy.

Symptomatic infants and children with a history of congestive failure, syncope, or marked exercise intolerance, as well as patients with block below the bundle of His and those with associated cardiac defects and heart rates below 65 to 70, require pacing. The occurrence of frequent or complex ventricular dysrhythmias also may be an indication for pacing. Permanent pacemakers in infants and children are fraught with technical problems. Small infants usually require placement of epicardial pacerleads; transvenous pacemaker insertion is used in children over 10 kg. The mortality rate for pediatric patients with pacemakers has been reported to be as high as 15 percent, with half the deaths due to pacemaker failure. Infection, erosion, and breakage or failure of leads, particularly with growth, are common problems. The average duration of pacing in one study was 20 to 30 months, with frequent reoperations to maintain pacing (at least one procedure per patient per year). With improvement in pacemaker technology, survival has become better, and patients require fewer reoperations. The intervention-free interval is generally more than 4 years.

The most common indication for implantation of a permanent pacemaker is acquired heart block below the bundle of His following repair of an intracardiac congenital lesion.

Anesthetic Considerations. Because of the relatively high risk of death from congenital heart block in infants, a temporary pacemaker should be inserted in these patients prior to any anesthetic. In older children who are asymptomatic and have a narrow QRS complex, anesthesia and operation have been carried out without problems and without temporary pacing. Adequate vagolysis and the use of anesthetic agents without negative chronotropic or inotropic side effects (atropine, ketamine, narcotics, isoflurane, pancuronium, or gallamine) are recommended. An isoproterenol infusion and temporary external or transvenous pacing should be readily available in the operating room.

Local anesthetics may be used for selected procedures if low blood levels are maintained, but high blood levels of local anesthetics may cause further slowing of ventricular conduction.

Patients with wide QRS complexes, a history of syncope or congestive heart failure, moderate-to-severe exercise intolerance, associated cardiac anomalies, or absence of chronotropic response to atropine, and all patients with acquired heart block, require at least temporary pacing prior to administration of any anesthetic, since perioperative stress may cause life-threatening dysrhythmia.

REENTRY TACHYCARDIAS

Supraventricular Tachycardia

Supraventricular tachycardia (SVT) is a common pediatric disorder. It is estimated to occur in 1 in 25,000 children and is more common in males and in the first few months of life. Recognition of the anomaly is important, since congestive heart failure develops in a significant number of infants with sustained SVT of longer than 24 hours' duration.

The etiology in most cases is unknown and may be related to abnormal postnatal development of the specialized tissue in the atrioventricular node and His bundle. Twenty-five to fifty percent of infants with SVT will manifest Wolff-Parkinson-White syndrome on their ECG after conversion. Most cases of SVT in children are due to a reentry mechanism with antegrade conduction through a slow pathway and retrograde conduction through a fast pathway. In this form of tachycardia, P waves are not visible on the surface ECG, since atrial activation and ventricular depolarization occur simultaneously.

Infants who present with SVT and fast heart rates are usually in heart failure or cardiogenic shock, either of which represents a medical emergency. Normal cardiac rhythm should be restored by direct synchronized cardioversion, ½ to 1 watt-sec/kg. Digitalization should be carried out immediately after cardioversion. In infants with less cardiac impairment, vagal stimulation by the diving reflex may be successful in converting the tachycardia. A small plastic bag filled with ice and covering the face may be used instead of dunking the face in ice water. If the diving reflex is not successful, rapid intravenous digitalization or direct current cardioversion is advocated. If these maneuvers fail, intravenous propranolol or overdrive pacing may be attempted.

The majority of infants with SVT readily respond to digoxin, have few recurrences, and may have digoxin therapy withdrawn after 1 year of age. Patients unresponsive to digoxin should be treated with propranolol. Older children who develop supraventricular tachycardia have a higher incidence of Wolff-Parkinson-White syndrome and usually do not present in heart failure. Besides vagal stimulation, treatment with verapamil, 0.1 mg/kg, as an intravenous bolus is currently recommended. Verapamil should not be given to patients on propranolol therapy or patients suspected of sick sinus syndrome. With relatively slow tachycardias, chronic digitalization should be started. All patients are maintained on digitalis to prevent recurrence of tachycardia.

Wolff-Parkinson-White Syndrome

This form of reentry tachycardia is characterized by the presence of an accessory atrioventricular conduction pathway (Kent's bundle), represented on the normal electrocardiogram with a short P-R interval, widened QRS complex, and a delta wave in the initial portion of the QRS complex.

The syndrome is probably present in 0.1 percent of unselected children but is more frequent in children with congenital heart disease. About 70 percent of patients are male. Forty percent of children with Wolff-Parkinson-White syndrome have associated congenital heart disease, most commonly Ebstein's anomaly. Corrected transposition, primary cardiomyopathies, atrial septal defect, and floppy mitral valve also have been described. Wolff-Parkinson-White syndrome may be subdivided into type A, with abnormal conduction along the left bundle, and type B, with conduction along the right bundle. Seventy percent of patients with Wolff-Parkinson-White syndrome develop premature beats and tachyarrhythmias. The episodes may be triggered by sympathetic stimulation. Digoxin is effective in controlling arrhythmias in the majority of cases. Propranolol, quinidine, and recently amiodarone have been used in refractory cases. Verapamil, esmolol, and adenosine may terminate narrow-complex tachycardia associated with this syndrome. Verapamil and digoxin are contraindicated in the management of atrial fibrillation or flutter associated with W-P-W syndrome since they accelerate the rate of conduction in the accessory pathway and may induce ventricular flutter or fibrillation under these circumstances. If no control of tachyarrhythmias can be achieved, overdrive pacing or surgical division of the accessory pathway can be performed. The latter procedure has been reported with a 90 percent success rate in infants and children. Transvenous electrical ablation or cryoablation of the abnormal pathways can be performed in older children or adolescents.

Lown-Ganong-Levine Syndrome

A rare cause of supraventricular tachycardia is the presence of an AV nodal bypass (James' fiber). The ECG is characterized by a short P-R interval and a normal QRS complex. Patients have a high incidence of atrial flutter-fibrillation. It is more common in females. Therapy is similar to that for the Wolff-Parkinson-White syndrome. Quinidine and procainamide may slow conduction through the abnormal bypass tract.

Anesthetic Considerations. Prevention of reentry tachycardias, which may lead to very rapid ventricular response and cardiovascular collapse, is the major anesthetic problem. Since sympathetic stimulation may trigger a tachyarrhythmia, adequate preoperative sedation and sufficient depth of anesthesia are important. Antiarrhythmic therapy should be continued preoperatively. Anesthetic agents without positive chronotropic or sympathomimetic side effects should be used. Halothane, although it causes sinus bradycardia, may predispose to occurrence of atrial extrasystoles, which may trigger reentry tachycardias. Enflurane and isoflurane appear to have a mild dysrhythmic effect and may be preferable. Barbiturates, narcotics, nitrous oxide, and muscle relaxants, other than pancuronium and gallamine, have been successfully used. Increased sympathetic activity, exogenous epinephrine, hypoxia, hypercapnia, and metabolic acidosis all may cause increased atrial or ventricular automaticity and trigger SVT.

If SVT occurs during anesthesia, vagal stimulation by a Valsalva maneuver, stimulation of the gag reflex, ice application to the face, or unilateral carotid massage should be tried initially. If these measures are unsuccessful, verapamil, propranolol, direct current cardioversion, or esophageal overdrive pacing can be used to restore sinus rhythm. In patients with junctional ectopic tachycardia, verapamil should not be used, since it may lead to acceleration of the ventricular rate with cardiovascular collapse. Should this problem occur, it may be treated with intravenous calcium chloride. Propranolol and verapamil should not be given concurrently, since complete heart block and severe myocardial depression may result. Patients on amiodarone may develop pulmonary fibrosis or thyroid dysfunction. Amiodarone causes beta-receptor blockade and has a half-life of 25 to 55 days. Patients on this drug need careful monitoring to prevent undue cardiovascular side effects.

PROLONGED Q-T INTERVAL

The association of a prolonged (long) Q-T interval (LQTS), congenital deafness, syncopal attacks, and a high incidence of sudden death is known as Jervell and Lange-Nielsen syndrome. It affects between 0.25 and 1 percent of children with congenital neural deafness and is transmitted as an autosomal recessive gene. An identical condition without congenital deafness is about three times more frequent and is known as Romano-Ward syndrome. It is transmitted as an autosomal dominant gene. Familial ventricular tachycardia, also transmitted as an autosomal dominant gene, is an atypical form of prolonged Q-T interval, with prolongation occurring during exercise. The syncopal attacks in all three conditions are due to paroxysmal ventricular fibrillation of the type known as torsades de pointes and are typically triggered by exercise or physical or emotional stress. All these factors result in increased sympathetic activity, and the arrhythmias appear to be caused by an imbalance of the outflows of the right and left cardiac sympathetics. The mortality in untreated cases is high, between 30 and 70 percent. Attacks usually begin in childhood and become less frequent with increasing age.

All prolonged QT syndromes are characterized by prolongation of the QT interval (QTI) when corrected for heart rate (QTc) according to Bazett's formula:

$$\text{QTc} = \frac{\text{Q-T interval}}{\text{R-R interval}}$$

The QTc interval extends from the beginning of the QRS complex to the end of the T wave. The upper limit of normal of the QTc is 0.44 sec.

The treatment of choice for LQTS consists of adequate beta-blockade, which has decreased the mortality rate from 73 to 6 percent. Complete β-adrenergic blockade should be achieved and maintained. In some cases, a combination of beta-blockade and phenytoin may be used when the dose of β-blockers has to be reduced because of side effects. Phenytoin shortens the QTc. In addition to phenytoin, primidone, phenobarbital, bretylium, and calcium channel blockers have been used in combination with β-blockade to control symptoms of LQTS. If medical treatment fails, left stellate ganglionectomy should be performed, which generally results in complete suppression of the attacks although thc Q-T intcrval may not bc normalized. Left stellate ganglion block may also result in shortening of the Q-T interval and abolition of the arrhythmia. Right-sided stellate ganglion block results in worsening of the condition.

Anesthetic Management. The key to successful anesthetic management is recognition of the syndrome and adequate β-blockade preoperatively. Children with deafness, seizure history, or family history of sudden death must have preoperative electrocardiographic evaluation. Reliable electrocardiographic monitoring is essential during anesthesia and recovery. A defibrillator needs to be immediately available. All conditions causing excitement and anxiety should be avoided. Patients should be well premedicated to reduce anxiety and sympathetic stress. Adequate perioperative pain relief is essential. Bradycardia should be avoided, since it may lead to escape beats and trigger a ventricular arrhythmia in these susceptible patients. Adequate β-blockade needs to be maintained or established, if necessary with a rapid acting intravenous β-blocker like esmolol. Anesthetic agents that sensitize the myocardium to endogenous catecholamines or have sympathomimetic side effects should be avoided, and a relatively deep level of anesthesia needs to be maintained to prevent sympathetic stimulation.

Drugs causing prolongation of the Q-T interval are contraindicated. These include phenothiazine, quinidine, lidocaine, and procainamide. Hypokalemia, hypomagnesemia, and hypocalcemia have the same undesirable effect as has hypothermia. Barbiturates, narcotics, enflurane, and isoflurane have all been used successfully in combination with nitrous oxide in patients with prolonged Q-T interval. Halothane is a poor choice in LQTS, as are pancuronium and gallamine, since they may trigger dysrhythmia.

DISEASES OF THE PERICARDIUM

ABSENT PERICARDIUM

Partial or complete absence of the pericardium is an extremely rare congenital defect. The defect is usually left-sided. Most patients have no symptoms but may demonstrate an abnormal shift of the heart on x-ray. Complete absence of the pericardium does not interfere with a normal life if no other malformations are present. Partial absence may allow herniation, followed by strangulation of the atria or part of the ventricles, which can cause death. Patients with defects large enough to allow herniation require pericardioplasty or enlargement of the defect to prevent strangulation. Small defects require no treatment.

PERICARDIAL CYST

Pericardial cysts usually are solitary and lie against the parietal pericardium; they rarely communicate with the pericardial sac. They may be confused with cardiac tumors. They commonly are located at the costophrenic angles, usually on the right. They generally are asymptomatic but give rise to a tremendously enlarged heart on radiological examination, without evidence of heart failure or electrocardiographic changes. Treatment consists of surgical removal.

PERICARDITIS

Except for the two conditions already discussed, pericardial disease is a manifestation of some other systemic disease that leads either to fluid accumulation in the pericardial sac, resulting in cardiac tamponade, or to scarring and fibrosis of the pericardium, leading to constrictive pericarditis. The latter condition is extremely rare in pediatric patients.

The most common manifestation of pericarditis in children is rheumatic pericarditis. Pericarditis otherwise can be due to pyogenic organisms, rheumatoid arthritis, or viral, uremic, or neoplastic disease, or it can be part of the postpericardiotomy syndrome. Lupus, tuberculosis, congenital hypoplastic anemia, Mediterranean anemia, Friedreich's ataxia, ulcerative colitis, and radiation are rare causes of pericardial disease in children.

The physiological disturbance in pericardial disease is due to impairment of cardiac filling, caused by either compression from accumulated fluid or restriction of myocardial movement. The restriction of cardiac filling leads to elevation of the venous pressure and a fall in stroke volume and cardiac output. Compensatory mechanisms include increases in heart rate, contractility, and peripheral vasoconstriction. Decreased renal perfusion leads to aldosterone secretion and salt and fluid retention. Coronary perfusion may be decreased secondary to reduced diastolic time and increased intraventricular pressure. Myocardial dysfunction is more commonly seen with pericardial tamponade. The raised diastolic pressure in both ventricles results in equality of all filling pressures. Right atrial, pulmonary artery diastolic, and left atrial pressures are equal. The normal respiratory variation in systemic blood pressure resulting from pooling of blood in the pulmonary vascular bed is markedly increased with the restriction of cardiac filling, leading to pulsus paradoxus (a fall of greater than 10 mm Hg in systolic blood pressure with inspiration).

Most patients with acute pericardial disease respond to medical management. Anti-inflammatory agents, steroids, or antibiotics are used, depending on the etiology. Patients with cardiac tamponade may require pericardiocentesis under local anesthesia to improve cardiac performance. With recurrent fluid accumulation, a pericardial window may have to be constructed. Patients with symptomatic constrictive pericarditis require surgical pericardiectomy.

Anesthetic Considerations. Patients with acute pericarditis will be seen only on an emergency basis for relief of cardiac tamponade. Patients with mild constrictive pericarditis not requiring surgical intervention should be treated as are patients with restrictive cardiomyopathy. Electrocardiographic monitoring and direct measurement of filling and systemic pressure are indicated for most procedures. Right-sided pressures and volume are more seriously affected in pericardial effusion, and central venous pressure measurements are usually sufficient. Patients require maintenance of adequate filling pressures and heart rate. Anesthetic agents causing minimal myocardial depression should be used. Peripheral vascular resistance should be maintained. Positive-pressure ventilation may seriously interfere with cardiac filling, and spontaneous ventilation should be maintained if possible. Ketamine, narcotics, and relaxants with sympathomimetic side effects may be advantageous.

MALPOSITIONS OF THE HEART

The heart may be located on the right, on the left with the viscera inverted, in the middle of the thorax, or outside the thorax.

DEXTROCARDIA

Dextrocardia is the most common malposition of the heart. It may occur with or without situs inversus and is commonly associated with asplenia or polysplenia syndrome. In most cases other cardiac anomalies are present, most commonly transposition and septation defects. Isolated dextrocardia is usually associated with other congenital malformations, particularly hypoplasia or aplasia of the right lung. In patients with dextrocardia and asplenia syndrome, complex cardiac malformations are the rule. Fifty to eighty percent of patients with dextrocardia and situs inversus, however, have normal hearts. In Kartagener syndrome, situs inversus totalis with dextrocardia is associated with bronchiectasis and sinusitis.

LEVOCARDIA

Levocardia is associated with either asplenia or polysplenia and visceral heterotaxia in 80 percent of cases and with situs inversus in only 20 percent. Complex cyanotic heart disease is frequently present, and the majority of patients die in infancy.

MESOCARDIA

Mesocardia is extremely rare, and congenital cardiac lesions are present in 75 percent of patients.

Anesthetic Considerations for the Preceding Malpositions. The associated cardiac defects and the physiological derangement caused thereby will generally influence the anesthetic management. Patients with asplenia syndrome need prophylaxis against encapsulated bacteria like *Klebsiella, Escherichia*, and *Haemophilus* with either amoxicillin or ampicillin. Patients with isolated dextrocardia may have marked ventilatory impairment owing to reduced lung tissue and tracheal compression from the aortic arch. Bronchiectasis may be present in patients with "mirror image" dextrocardia (dextrocardia and situs inversus).

ECTOPIA CORDIS

The position of the heart partially or completely outside the thorax represents ectopia cordis, an extremely rare malformation. The classic form of ectopia cordis is the thoracic type with a sternal defect; absence of the parietal pericardium; cephalic orientation of the apex, which beats against the infant's chin; epigastric omphalocele or diastasis recti; and a small thoracic cavity. Other cardiac lesions are usually present. Patients require immediate operation to correct their cardiac lesion and reconstruct the chest wall defect. Initially the heart usually cannot be positioned inside the small thoracic cavity without causing kinking of the vessels or tamponade, and various plastic procedures for reconstruction of the anterior thoracic wall have been utilized to effect closure.

Thoracoabdominal Ectopia Cordis (Cantrell's Syndrome). The heart is displaced inferiorly through an anterior diaphragmatic defect into the epigastrium. A partial cleft of the lower sternum, a defect of the diaphragmatic pericardium, and omphalocele or diastasis recti are always present. Most patients have congenital heart disease. Repair has been achieved by closure of the diaphragmatic defect and repair of the abdominal wall defect. Thoracic ectopia has a high mortality with or without operation. Survival into adulthood with abdominal ectopia cordis without surgical intervention has been described.

ACQUIRED HEART DISEASE

RHEUMATIC HEART DISEASE

Acute rheumatic fever remains the leading cause of acquired pediatric heart disease worldwide, although rheumatic fever and rheumatic heart disease have sharply declined in the developed countries.

Rheumatic fever is closely associated with group A beta-hemolytic streptococcal infections of the upper respiratory tract. Approximately 3 percent of infected patients will develop acute rheumatic fever within 7 to 35 days. The disease used to occur in the young school-age child from a low socioeconomic group in winter or spring but is now commonly seen in warmer climates. The pathogenetic basis of the disease is still not fully understood but may involve hypersensitivity reactions, an autoimmune process, direct toxic effects of bacterial lysins, or direct bacterial infection.

Rheumatic heart disease is present in approximately 0.7 to 1.6 per 1000 school children in the United States. The fatality rate is estimated to be 2 to 3 percent. The disease is by nature recurrent, and chronic disability and death are related to recurrent attacks. Recurrence is invariably preceded by streptococcal infection, with the highest risk of recurrence in the first few years after the initial event. Adequate prolonged penicillin treatment and continuous sulfadiazine or low-dose penicillin prophylaxis is highly effective in protecting from recurrent attacks. The most effective form of prophylaxis appears to be benzathine penicillin G, 1.2 million units intramuscularly once a month, which should be continued throughout childhood.

The diagnosis of acute rheumatic fever is still based on the Jones' criteria. The major criteria are fever, polyarthritis, carditis, Sydenham's chorea, erythema marginatum, and subcutaneous nodules. Evidence of preceding streptococcal infection (antistreptolysin titer) strengthens the diagnosis. Carditis may be silent in its appearance until heart failure or a murmur appears or a pericardial effusion is manifested. It is noted in 50 to 75 percent of cases within the first week of onset of the disease.

Aspirin and corticosteroids are dramatically effective in suppressing the acute manifestations of rheumatic fever. Aspirin does not appear to alter the frequency of residual rheumatic heart disease. Steroids appear to improve the prognosis of patients with moderate-to-severe carditis, but their dosage should be tapered as soon as the acute disease is under control and the patient is changed over to aspirin therapy. Aspirin in daily doses of 90 to 120 mg/kg is usually sufficient to achieve therapeutic blood levels of 20 to 25 mg/dl. Higher doses may produce hepatic injury. Residual streptococcal infection is eradicated with therapeutic doses of penicillin, with prophylaxis started subsequently. Patients with carditis may require prolonged bed rest and should not be ambulatory until all signs of heart failure have disappeared. Heart failure may be treated with digitalis and diuretics.

The patient with severe carditis or frequent recurrences may develop rheumatic heart disease. This complication occurs with high frequency in economically underprivileged areas, particularly in Africa and Asia, and most often in childhood. In 85 percent of cases the mitral valve is involved, in 54 percent the aortic valve, and in less than 5 percent the tricuspid or pulmonary valve.

Rheumatic carditis may heal, with residual interstitial fibrosis and some fibrosis of the endocardium. These lesions do not appear to be progressive and produce no hemodynamic abnormalities, but predispose patients to endocarditis. The interstitial fibrosis may lead to intensified myocardial dilatation resulting from valvular defects.

MITRAL INSUFFICIENCY

Valvular rheumatic heart disease in childhood and adolescence is most commonly present as mitral insufficiency. Because the left ventricle is subject only to diastolic volume overload, most defects are well tolerated for many years. The pressure and volume of the left atrium are elevated, and chronic pulmonary congestion, pulmonary hypertension, and right ventricular hypertrophy and dilatation develop with time. In most children and adolescents the lesion is mild, with absence of symptoms and only a murmur of mitral regurgitation. The main emphasis is placed on long-term prophylaxis. Patients with signs of heart failure should be managed conservatively. Operation is seldom indicated for children and adolescents. If one is necessary, an annuloplasty or valvuloplasty is performed, if possible, to avoid the long-term problems of prosthetic valves.

MITRAL STENOSIS

Many years are usually necessary for narrowing of the mitral orifice to develop enough to produce symptoms. For this reason, significant rheumatic mitral stenosis is extremely uncommon in the pediatric age group. However, in some parts of the world, particularly Asia and Africa, tight mitral stenosis occurs relatively frequently in children less than 15 years old. Mitral stenosis is more common in females.

The physiological derangement, as described in the discussion of congenital mitral stenosis earlier, consists of an obstruction to ventricular filling at the mitral valve. To overcome the obstruction, left atrial pressure is raised and a gradient is established between left atrial mean and left ventricular end-diastolic pressures. Filling depends on orifice size, pressure gradient, and diastolic interval. With a fast heart rate, diastolic filling time is reduced, and cardiac output may fall. Elevated left atrial pressure leads to pulmonary venous congestion and secondary pulmonary hypertension. Pulmonary edema may occur. With progressive disease, pulmonary function becomes markedly abnormal, with decreased total lung volume and vital capacity, reduced compliance, and increased work of breathing.

Mitral stenosis in children is generally asymptomatic except for the characteristic middiastolic-presystolic murmur. In rare instances affected children show some exertional dyspnea or fatigue. If cardiac symptoms occur, acute carditis should be suspected.

The management of children with rheumatic mitral stenosis centers on prevention of recurrent attacks of rheumatic fever and prevention of bacterial endocarditis. In the rare child with progressive severe mitral stenosis, mitral commissurotomy may have to be performed to palliate the obstruction. Calcific mitral stenosis is extremely rare in children. Mitral valve replacement is avoided if at all possible because of the long-term problems with prosthetic valves in this age group.

Anesthetic Management. Anesthetic considerations have been discussed in the section on congenital mitral stenosis. Prevention of tachycardia, maintenance of cardiac contractility, avoidance of peripheral vasodilatation, and careful ventilation and fluid management are essential. Endocarditis prophylaxis is indicated.

AORTIC INSUFFICIENCY

Rheumatic aortic valve disease presents as isolated or dominant aortic insufficiency with mild or moderate aortic stenosis. Males are more commonly affected.

The physiological derangement of aortic insufficiency consists of volume overload of the left ventricle with resultant dilatation of the chambers. Stroke volume is increased, but end-diastolic pressure is maintained near normal. Aortic impedance is usually low because peripheral vasodilatation reduces regurgitation, resulting in a wide pulse pressure. Regurgitation occurs during diastole and is reduced with fast heart rates. The characteristic finding is an early, blowing diastolic murmur.

Aortic regurgitation is less common than mitral regurgitation with rheumatic fever but may also occur early in the disease. It is generally well tolerated throughout childhood, since the left ventricle is able to compensate well. The average life expectancy in patients with aortic insufficiency is 20 to 30 years after the onset of the disease. Death usually occurs suddenly and is due to arrhythmias or heart failure.

Treatment of rheumatic aortic insufficiency in children consists mostly of prevention of recurrence of rheumatic carditis. If signs of congestive heart failure, ventricular arrhythmias, or anginal attacks occur, surgical therapy is indicated. Surgery should be performed before serious left ventricular dysfunction occurs. Aortic valve replacement is usually required, with the inherent problems of anticoagulation, thromboembolism, and valve dysfunction. Patients are high endocarditis risks after operation and continue to require prophylaxis against rheumatic fever.

Anesthetic Considerations. Anesthetic management of aortic insufficiency is discussed earlier in this chapter. Regurgitation is decreased by fast heart rates and low peripheral vascular resistance. Vasodilatation and tachycardia are desirable and can be achieved by various anesthetic techniques. Depression of myocardial contractility should be avoided. Children with rheumatic aortic insufficiency usually have adequate cardiac reserve. They require endocarditis prophylaxis. After valve replacement, patients should be asymptomatic but require reversal of anticoagulation if they are being treated with vitamin K antagonists.

KAWASAKI DISEASE

Mucocutaneous lymph node syndrome, or Kawasaki disease, is an acute febrile illness characterized by nonexudative conjunctivitis, erythema of the lips and oral mucosa, and nonsuppurative cervical lymphadenitis, accompanied by myocarditis in 25 to 50 percent of cases. The disease is most common in children between 6 months and 5 years of age, with a median age of 2.3 years; it occurs primarily in children of Japanese descent with a male: female ratio of 1.5:1. The syndrome, however, has been observed in children of all races worldwide. It can occur in community-wide epidemics and is a leading cause of acquired heart disease in children in the United States.

The pathological basis for the disease consists of widespread microvasculitis. Involvement of the coronary vessels results in development of coronary aneurysms, coronary artery stenoses, thromboses, or rupture. Coronary artery aneurysms or ectasia occurs in about 15 to 25 percent of affected patients, particularly in infants less than 6 months of age. Involvement of the heart accounts for the 0.3 percent mortality reported for this disease. The coronary arteritis is usually silent until infarction or angina occurs.

Treatment consists of therapy with aspirin, 80 to 100 mg/kg/day until the acute symptoms have subsided. The addition of high-dose intravenous γ-globulin therapy reduces the incidence of coronary artery abnormalities between three- and fivefold. After approximately 2 weeks, the aspirin dose is reduced to 3 to 5 mg/kg/day and continued until all signs of inflammation have resolved. In patients with coronary aneurysms, aspirin therapy should be continued indefinitely or until the coronary artery aneurysms have regressed spontaneously. Dipyridamole may be added to prevent coronary thrombosis. If no improvement occurs and severe coronary artery disease persists, bypass grafting or coronary aneurysmectomy must be performed. The prognosis for patency of venous bypass grafts is poor below the age of 8 years; however, the use of internal mammary artery grafts increases the patency rate to more than 80 percent.

Anesthetic Considerations. Anesthetic management should take into consideration the predominant cardiac derangement. Heart failure or dysrhythmia may be present. With significant coronary artery disease, maintenance of myocardial oxygen balance is essential, as well as prevention of coronary thrombosis. Patients should be monitored for arrhythmias and myocardial ischemia. For major surgical therapy, direct monitoring of systemic and filling pressures and cardiac function is indicated. Vasoactive and antiarrhythmic drugs should be readily available. In case of systemic arterial involvement with distal vascular insufficiency, peripheral blood flow may be improved with repeated sympathetic blocks of the upper or lower extremities.

TAKAYASU DISEASE (PULSELESS DISEASE)

Takayasu disease is a relatively rare form of arteritis that predominately occurs in Japanese and Korean females in their second and third decades. It involves the aorta and the proximal segments of its branches, leading to progressive destruction and occlusion. The disease may begin during childhood. Symptoms in this age group include hypertension, dyspnea, cardiomegaly, and absent pulses. Treatment with steroids and cytotoxic drugs is recommended, but the disease is nevertheless slowly progressive. Survival has ranged from 1 to 20 years after the onset of symptoms.

Patients are at high risk for cerebral and coronary ischemia and frequently have poorly controlled hypertension. Because of the involvement of the proximal aortic branches, monitoring of blood pressure may be difficult. Maintenance of adequate blood volume and blood pressure are essential to prevent ischemia of vital organ systems. Adrenal suppression due to chronic steroid therapy may aggravate cardiovascular instability, and steroid supplementation should be provided. With involvement of both carotid arteries, monitoring of cerebral function may be helpful for major surgical procedures in addition to monitoring for coronary ischemia. Monitoring mixed venous oxygen content and pH may help gauge the adequacy of organ perfusion.

REFERENCES

CONGENITAL HEART DISEASE: INCIDENCE, ETIOLOGY, CLASSIFICATION

Child JS, Perloff JK: Natural survival patterns. *In* Perloff JK, Child JS (eds): Congenital Heart Disease in Adults. Philadelphia, WB Saunders, 1991.

Clarke CT, Beall MH, Perloff JK: Genetics, epidemiology counseling, and prevention. *In* Perloff JK, Child JS (eds): Congenital Heart Disease in Adults. Philadelphia, WB Saunders, 1991.

Editorial: Congenital heart disease: Incidence and etiology. Lancet *2:*692, 1975.

Fyler DC: Trends. *In* Fyler DC (ed): Nadas' Pediatric Cardiology. Philadelphia, Hanley and Belfus, 1992.

Fyler DC, Buckley LP, Hellenbrand WE, et al: Report of the New England Regional Infant Cardiac Program. Pediatrics *65*(suppl): 376, 1980.

Kaplan S, Perloff JK: Survival patterns after surgery or interventional catheterization. *In* Perloff JK, Child JS (eds): Congenital Heart Disease in Adults. Philadelphia, WB Saunders, 1991.

Keith JD: Congenital heart disease: Prevalence, incidence and epidemiology. *In* Keith JD, Rowe RD, Vlad P (eds): Heart Disease in Infancy and Childhood. New York, Macmillan, 1978.

Mitchell SC, Korones SB, Berendes HW: Congenital heart disease in 56,109 births. Circulation *63:*323, 1971.

Mitchell SC, Sellman RH, Westphal MC, et al: Etiologic correlates in a study of congenital heart disease in 56,109 births. Am J Cardiol *28:*653, 1971.

Morgan BC: Incidence, etiology and classification of congenital heart disease. Pediatr Clin North Am *25:*721, 1978.

Noonan JA: Association of congenital heart disease with syndromes of other defects. Pediatr Clin North Am *25:*797, 1978.

Nora JJ: Etiologic aspects of heart disease. *In* Adams FH, Emmanouilides GC, Riemenschneider TA (eds): Moss' Heart Disease in Infants, Children, and Adolescents. 4th edition. Baltimore, Williams and Wilkins, 1983.

Roberts WC: Congenital cardiovascular anomalies usually silent until adulthood. Cardiovasc Clin *10:*407, 1979.

Steinberg AG, Bearn AG, Motulsky AG, et al: Progress in Medical Genetics. Volume V: Genetics of Cardiovascular Disease. Philadelphia, WB Saunders, 1983.

Van Mierop LHS, Gessner IH: Pathogenetic mechanisms in congenital cardiovascular malformations. Prog Cardiovasc Dis *15:*67, 1972.

Wagner HR: Cardiac disease in congenital infections. Clin Perinatol *8:*481, 1981.

CONGENITAL HEART DISEASE: LONG-TERM PROGNOSIS

Child JS, Perloff JK: Natural survival patterns. *In* Perloff JK, Child JS (eds): Congenital Heart Disease in Adults. Philadelphia, WB Saunders, 1991.

Fyler DC, Rothmann KJ, Buckley LP, et al: The determinants of five-year survival of infants with critical congenital heart disease. Cardiovasc Clin *12:*393, 1981.

Kidd LS, Rowe RD (eds): The Child with Congenital Heart Disease After Surgery. Mount Kisco, NY, Futura Publishing Company, 1976.

McNamara DG, Latson LA: Long-term follow-up of patients with malformations for which definite surgical repair has been available for 25 years or more. Am J Cardiol *50:*560, 1982.

Pacifico AD, McKay R: Advances in the surgical management of congenital heart disease in infants and children. Cardiovasc Clin *12:*127, 1981.

Roberts WC (ed): Congenital heart disease in the adult. Cardiovasc Clin *10:*1, 1979.

Stevenson WG, Klitzner T, Perloff JK: Electrophysiologic abnormalities. *In* Perloff JK, Child JS (eds): Congenital Heart Disease in Adults. Philadelphia, WB Saunders, 1991.

Wilkinson JJ: Changing patterns of congenital heart disease. J Roy Soc Med *72:*432, 1979.

ANESTHESIA AND CONGENITAL HEART DISEASE

Allen HD: Anesthesia and congenital heart disease. *In* Brown B (ed): Contemporary Anesthesia Practice. Volume 2. Philadelphia, FA Davis, 1980.

Beynen FM, Tarhan S: Anesthesia for the surgical repair of congenital heart defects in children. *In* Tarhan S (ed): Cardiovascular Anesthesia and Postoperative Care. 2nd edition. Chicago, Year Book Medical Publishers, 1989.

Bull AP: The anesthetic evaluation and management of the surgical patient with heart disease. Surg Clin North Am *63:*1035, 1983.

Campbell FW, Schwartz AJ: Problems in anesthetic management of children with congenital heart disease for noncardiac surgery. *In* Kirby RR, Brown DL (eds): Problems in Anesthesia. Philadelphia, JB Lippincott, 1987.

Cooper JR: Septal and endocardial cushion defects. *In* Lake CL (ed): Pediatric Cardiac Anesthesia. Norwalk, Conn, Appleton Lange, 1988.

Crean P, Goresky G, Koren G, et al: Fentanyl pharmacokinetics in children with congenital heart disease. Anesthesiology *59:*A448, 1983.

Davis PJ, Cook DR, Stiller RL, Davis-Robinson KA: Pharmacodynamics and pharmacokinetics of high-dose sufentanil in infants and children undergoing cardiac surgery. Anesth Analg *66:*203, 1987.

Duncan PG: Anesthesia for patients with congenital heart disease. Can Anesth Soc J *30:*S20, 1983.

Eger EI: Effect of shunting on alveolar anesthetic rise. *In* Eger EI: Anesthetic Uptake and Action. Baltimore, Williams and Wilkins, 1974.

Fyman PN, Goodman K, Casthely PA, et al: Anesthetic management of patients undergoing Fontan procedure. Anesth Analg *65:*516, 1986.

Greeley WJ, Bushman GA, Davis DP, Reves JG: Comparative effects of halothane and ketamine on systemic arterial oxygen saturation in children with cyanotic heart disease. Anesthesiology *65:*666, 1986.

Hansen DD, Hickey PR: Anesthesia for hypoplastic left heart syndromes. Anesth Analg *65:*127, 1986.

Hickey PR: Anesthesia for the reconstructed heart. *In* Stoelting RK (ed): Advances in Anesthesia. Volume 111. Chicago, Year Book Medical Publishers, 1991.

Hickey PR, Hansen DD: Fentanyl- and sufentanil-oxygen-pancuronium anesthesia for cardiac surgery in infants. Anesth Analg *63:*117, 1983.

Hickey PR, Hansen DD, Cranolini GM: Pulmonary and systemic hemodynamic responses to ketamine in infants with normal and elevated pulmonary vascular resistance. Anesthesiology *61:*438, 1984.

Hickey PR, Hansen DD, Norwood WI, Castaneda AR: Anesthetic complications in surgery for congenital heart disease. Anesth Analg *63:*657, 1984.

Hickey PR, Hansen DD, Strafford M, et al: Pulmonary and systemic hemodynamic effects of nitrous oxide in infants with normal elevated pulmonary vascular resistance. Anesthesiology *65:*374, 1986.

Hickey PR, Hansen DD, Wessel D: Response to high-dose fentanyl in infants. Anesthesiology *61:*A445, 1984.

Hickey PR, Streitz S: Preoperative assessment of the patient with congenital heart disease. *In* Mangano DT (ed): Preoperative Cardiac Assessment. Philadelphia, JB Lippincott, 1990.

Hickey PR, Wessel DL: Anesthesia for congenital heart disease. *In* Gregory GA (ed): Pediatric Anesthesia. 2nd edition. New York, Churchill Livingstone, 1989.

Hickey PR, Wessel DL: Anesthesia for the treatment of congenital heart disease. *In* Kaplan JA (ed): Cardiac Anesthesia. Volume 2, 2nd edition. New York, Grune and Stratton, 1987.

Hoskin MP, Beynen F: Repair of coarctation of the aorta in a child after modified Fontan's operation. Anesthetic implications and management. Anesthesiology *71:*312, 1989.

Karl HW, Hensley FA, Cyran SE, et al: Hypoplastic left heart syndrome: Anesthesia for elective non-cardiac surgery. Anesthesiology *72:*753, 1990.

Laishley RS, Burrows FA, Lerman J, et al: Effect of anesthetic induction regimens on oxygen saturation in cyanotic congenital heart disease. Anesthesiology *65:*673, 1986.

Lowenstein E, Walker HL, Zaroff LI: The effect of a standard cyanotic circulatory lesion on the induction dose of methohexital in the dog. Anesthesiology *26:*254, 1965.

Morgan P, Lynn AM, Parrot C, Morray JP: Hemodynamic and metabolic effects of two anesthetic techniques in children undergoing surgical repair of acyanotic congenital heart disease. Anesth Analg *66:*1028, 1987.

Radnay PA, Nagashima H (eds): Anesthetic considerations for pediatric cardiac surgery. Int Anesthesiol Clin *18:*1, 1980.

Ramez-Salem M, Hall SC, Motoyama EK: Anesthesia for thoracic and cardiovascular surgery. *In* Motoyama EK, Davis PJ (eds): Smith's Anesthesia for Infants and Children. 5th edition. St. Louis, CV Mosby, 1990.

Schwartz AJ, Campbell FW: Pathophysiological approach to congenital heart disease. *In* Lake CL (ed): Pediatric Cardiac Anesthesia. Norwalk, Conn, Appleton Lange, 1988.

Stolting RK, Longnecker DE: The effect of right-to-left shunt on the rate of increase of arterial anesthetic concentration. Anesthesiology *36:*352, 1972.

Tanner GE, Anger DG, Barash PG, et al: Effects of left-to-right, mixed left-to-right and right-to-left shunts on inhalational anesthetic induction in children. Anesth Analg *64:*101, 1985.

Werner JC, Fripp RR, Whitman V: Evaluation of the pediatric surgical patient with congenital heart disease. Surg Clin North Am *63:*1003, 1983.

Wolfe RR, Loehr JP, Schaffer MS, Wiggins JW: Hemodynamic effects of ketamine, hypoxia and hyperoxia in children with surgically treated congenital heart disease residing ≥ 1200 meters above sea level. Am J Cardiol *67:*84, 1991.

VENTILATORY FUNCTION IN CONGENITAL HEART DISEASE

Bancalari E, Jesse MJ, Gelband H, et al: Lung mechanics in congenital heart disease with increased and decreased pulmonary blood flow. J Pediatr *90:*192, 1977.

Baraka AS, Taka SK, El-Khatib RA: Is hypoxic pulmonary vasoconstriction exaggerated during one-lung ventilation in patients with patent ductus arteriosus? Anesth Analg *72:*238, 1991.

Blesa MI, Lahiria S, Rashkind WT, et al: Normalization of the blunted ventilatory response to acute hypoxia in congenital cyanotic heart disease. N Engl J Med *296:*237, 1977.

Fletcher R: Carbon dioxide production in cyanotic children during anaesthesia with controlled ventilation. Br J Anaesth *61:*743, 1988.

Hoffman JI, Rudolph AM, Heymann MA: Pulmonary vascular disease with congenital heart lesions: Pathologic features and causes. Circulation *64:*873, 1981.

Jenkins J, Lynn A, Edmonds J, et al: Effects of mechanical ventilation on cardiopulmonary function in children after open-heart surgery. Crit Care Med *13:*77, 1985.

Lazzell V, Burrows FA: Stability of the intraoperative arterial to end-tidal carbon dioxide partial pressure difference in children with congenital heart disease. Can J Anaesth *38:*859, 1991.

Lister G, Pitt BR: Cardiopulmonary interactions in the infant with congenital cardiac disease. Clin Chest Med *4:*219, 1983.

Oleson K, Lindahl SGE: Spontaneous versus controlled ventilation in anaesthetized children with congenital malformations. Acta Anaesthesiol Scand *31:*87, 1987.

Shannon DC, Kazemi H: Distribution of lung function in patients with anomalies of the pulmonary circulation. J Thorac Cardiovasc Surg *64:*26, 1972.

Thorsteinsson A, Jonmarker C, Larsson A, et al: Functional residual capacity in anesthetized children: Normal values and values in children with cardiac anomalies. Anesthesiology *73:*876, 1990.

INTRACARDIAC DEFECTS PRODUCING PREDOMINANT LEFT-TO-RIGHT SHUNT

Feldt AH, Porter J, Edwards WD, Riemenschneider TA, et al: Atrial septal defects and atrioventricular canal. *In*

Adams FH, Emmanouilides GC (eds): Moss' Heart Disease in Infants, Children, and Adolescents. 4th edition. Baltimore, Williams and Wilkins, 1983.

Fyler DC: Atrial septal defect. *In* Fyler DC (ed): Nadas' Pediatric Cardiology. Philadelphia, Hanley and Belfus, 1992.

Fyler DC: Endocardial cushion defect. *In* Fyler DC (ed): Nadas' Pediatric Cardiology. Philadelphia, Hanley and Belfus, 1992.

Fyler DC: Ventricular septal defect. *In* Fyler DC (ed): Nadas' Pediatric Cardiology. Philadelphia, Hanley and Belfus, 1992.

Graham TP, Bender HW: Preoperative diagnosis and management of infants with critical congenital heart disease. Ann Thorac Surg *29:*272, 1980.

Graham TP, Bender HW, Spach MS: Ventricular septal defect. *In* Adams FH, Emmanouilides GC: Heart Disease in Infants, Children and Adolescents. 3rd edition. Baltimore, Williams and Wilkins, 1983.

Gronert GA, Messick JM, Cucchiara RF, et al: Paradoxical air embolism from a patent foramen ovale. Anesthesiology *50:*548, 1979.

Keith JD: Ventricular septal defect and atrial septal defect. *In* Keith JD, Rowe RD, Vlad P (eds): Heart Disease in Infancy and Childhood. 3rd edition. New York, Macmillan, 1978.

Kidd LBS: Single ventricle. *In* Keith JD, Rowe RD, Vlad P (eds): Heart Disease in Infancy and Childhood. 3rd edition. New York, Macmillan, 1978.

Murphy JG, Gersh BJ, McGoon MD, et al: Long-term outcome after surgical repair of isolated atrial septal defect. N Engl J Med *323:*1645, 1990.

Nadas AS, Fyler DC: Communications between systemic and pulmonary circuits with predominantly left to right shunt. *In* Nadas AS, Fyler DC: Pediatric Cardiology. Philadelphia, WB Saunders, 1972.

Pacifico AD: Surgical treatment of complex atrioventricular septal defect. Cardiol Clin *7:*399, 1989.

Rao TLK, Mathou M, Azad C, et al: Bronchoscopy and reversal of intracardiac shunt. Anesthesiology *51:*558, 1979.

Riemenschneider TA: Left ventricular–right atrial communication. *In* Adams FH, Emmanouilides GC: Heart Disease in Infants, Children, and Adolescents. 3rd edition. Baltimore, Williams and Wilkins, 1983.

Rudolph AM: Atrial septal defect: Partial anomalous drainage of pulmonary veins. *In* Rudolph AM: Congenital Diseases of the Heart. Chicago, Year Book Medical Publishers, 1974.

Rudolph AM: Endocardial cushion defect. *In* Rudolph AM: Congenital Diseases of the Heart. Chicago, Year Book Medical Pubishers, 1974.

Rudolph AM: Ventricular septal defect. *In* Rudolph AM: Congenital Diseases of the Heart. Chicago, Year Book Medical Publishers, 1974.

Stevenson GJ: Acyanotic lesions with increased pulmonary blood flow. Pediatr Clin North Am *25:*743, 1978.

EISENMENGER'S COMPLEX AND SYNDROME

Bird TM, Strybyb L: Anesthesia for a patient with Down's syndrome and Eisenmenger's complex. Anaesthesia *39:*48, 1984.

Graham TP: The Eisenmenger reaction and its management. Cardiovasc Clin *10:*531, 1979.

Grossman W, Braunwald E: Eisenmenger syndrome. *In* Braunwald E (ed): Heart Disease. 3rd edition. Philadelphia, WB Saunders, 1988.

Lumley J, Whitwan JG, Morgan M: General anesthesia in the presence of Eisenmenger's syndrome. Anesth Analg *56:*543, 1977.

MacArthur CGC, Hunter D, Gibson GJ: Ventilatory function in the Eisenmenger syndrome. Thorax *34:*348, 1979.

Rabinovitch M: Pulmonary hypertension. *In* Adams FH, Emmanouilides GH, Riemenschneider TA: Moss' Heart Disease in Infants, Children, and Adolescents. 4th edition. Baltimore, Williams and Wilkins, 1989.

Weber RK, Buda AJ, Levene DL: General anesthesia in Eisenmenger's syndrome. Can Med Assoc J *117:*1413, 1977.

Young D, Mark H: Fate of the patient with Eisenmenger syndrome. Am J Cardiol *28:*653, 1971.

INTRACARDIAC LESIONS PRODUCING PREDOMINANT RIGHT-TO-LEFT SHUNT WITH CYANOSIS

Arciniegas E, Farokin ZR, Hakimi M, et al: Classic shunting operations for congenital cyanotic heart defects. J Thorac Cardiovasc Surg *85:*88, 1982.

Balaji S, Gevillig M, Bull C, et al: Arrhythmias after the Fontan procedure. Circulation *84*(Suppl III):162, 1991.

Calza G, Panizzon G, Rovida S, et al: Incidence of residual defects determining the clinical outcome after correction of tetralogy of Fallot. Ann Thorac Surg *47:*428, 1989.

Castaneda AR, Mayer JE Jr, Jonas RA, et al: Transposition of the great arteries: The arterial switch operation. Cardiol Clin *7:*369, 1989.

DeLeon SY, Iebawi MN, Idriss FS, et al: Fontan-type operation for complex lesions. J Thorac Cardiovasc Surg *92:*1029, 1986.

DiDonato RM, Wernowsky G, Jonas RA, et al: Corrected transposition in situs inversus. Circulation *84*(Suppl III):193, 1991.

Elliot LP, Anderson RH, Bargeron LM, et al: Single ventricle or univentricular heart. *In* Adams FH, Emmanouilides GC, Riemenschneider TA (eds): Moss' Heart Disease in Infants, Children, and Adolescents. 4th edition. Baltimore, Williams and Wilkins, 1989.

Freed MD, Heyman MA, Lewis AB, et al: Prostaglandin E_1 in infants with ductus arteriosus–dependent congenital heart disease. Circulation *64:*899, 1981.

Fyler DC: "Corrected" transposition. *In* Fyler DC: Nadas' Pediatric Cardiology. Philadelphia, Hanley and Belfus, 1992.

Fyler DC: Double-outlet right ventricle. *In* Fyler DC: Nadas' Pediatric Cardiology. Philadelphia, Hanley and Belfus, 1991.

Fyler DC: D-transposition of the great arteries. *In* Fyler DC: Nadas' Pediatric Cardiology. Philadelphia, Hanley and Belfus, 1992.

Fyler DC: Single ventricle. *In* Fyler DC: Nadas' Pediatric Cardiology. Philadelphia, Hanley and Belfus, 1992.

Garson A, Randall DC, Gillette PC, et al: Prevention of sudden death after repair of tetralogy of Fallot: Treatment of ventricular arrhythmias. J Am Coll Cardiol *6:*221, 1985.

Gevillig M, Cullen S, Mertus B, et al: Risk factors for arrhythmia and death after Mustard operation for simple transposition of the great arteries. Circulation *84*(Suppl III):187, 1991.

Graham TP, Bender HW: Preoperative diagnosis and management of infants with critical congenital heart disease. Ann Thorac Surg *29:*272, 1980.

Greeley WJ, Stanley TE, Ungerleider RM, Kisslo JH: Intraoperative hypoxemia spells in tetralogy of Fallot. Anesth Analg *68:*815, 1989.

Groh MA, Melioues JN, Bore EL, et al: Repair of tetralogy of Fallot in infancy. Circulation *84*(Suppl III):206, 1991.

Gunteroth WG, Kawabori J, Baun D: Tetralogy of Fallot. *In* Adams FH, Emmanouilides GC (eds): Heart Disease in Infants, Children, and Adolescents. 3rd edition. Baltimore, Williams and Wilkins, 1983.

Gutgesell HP, Garson A, McNamara DG: Prognosis for the newborn with transposition of the great arteries. Am J Cardiol *44:*96, 1979.

Hagler DJ, Ritter DG, Puga FJ: Double outlet right ventricle. *In* Adams FH, Emmanouilides GC, Riemenschneider TA (eds): Heart Disease in Infants, Children, and Adolescents. 4th edition. Baltimore, Williams and Wilkins, 1989.

Hastreiter A, Van der Hosser L: Hemodynamics of neonatal cyanotic heart disease. Crit Care Med *5:*23, 1977.

Jatene AD, Iontes VF, Paulista PP: Anatomical correction of transposition of the great vessels. J Thorac Cardiovasc Surg *72:*364, 1976.

Jenkins KJ, Hanley FL, Colan SD: Function of the anatomic pulmonary valve in the systemic circulation. Circulation *84*(Suppl III):173, 1991.

Kam CA: Infundibular spasm in Fallot's tetralogy. An account and its management in anesthesia. Anaesth Intens Care *6:*138, 1978.

Kidd BSL: Single ventricle. *In* Keith JD, Rowe RD, Vlad P (eds): Heart Disease in Infancy and Childhood. 3rd edition. New York, Macmillan, 1978.

Kidd BSL: Transpositions of the great arteries. *In* Keith JD, Rowe RD, Vlad P: Heart Disease in Infancy and Childhood. 3rd edition. New York, Macmillan, 1978.

Kirklin JK, Blackstone EH, Kirlin JW, et al: The Fontan operation. J Thorac Cardiovasc Surg *92:*1049, 1986.

Lev M, Bharati S, Meng CCL, et al: A concept of double outlet right ventricle. J Thorac Cardiovasc Surg *44:*271, 1972.

Losay J, Planche C, Gerardine B, et al: Mid-term surgical results of arterial switch operations for transposition of the great arteries with intact septum. Circulation *82*(Suppl IV):146, 1990.

Mair DD, Edwards WD, Julsond PR, et al: Pulmonary atresia and ventricular septal defect. *In* Adams FH, Emmanouilides GC, Riemenschneider TA (eds): Heart Disease in Infants, Children, and Adolescents. 4th edition. Baltimore, Williams and Wilkins, 1989.

Mayer JE, Helgason H, Jonas RA, et al: Extending the limits for modified Fontan procedures. J Thorac Cardiovasc Surg *92:*1021, 1986.

Nadas AS, Fyler DC: The transpositions. *In* Nadas AS, Fyler DC: Pediatric Cardiology. Philadelphia, WB Saunders, 1972.

Nadas AS, Fyler DC: Valvular and vascular lesions with a right to left shunt or no shunt at all. *In* Nadas AS, Fyler DC: Pediatric Cardiology. Philadelphia, WB Saunders, 1972.

Norwood WI, Dobell AR, Freed MO, et al: Intermediate results of the arterial switch repair. J Thorac Cardiovasc Surg *96:*854, 1988.

Paul MH: Complete transposition of the great arteries. *In* Adams FH, Emmanouilides GC, Riemenschneider TA (eds): Heart Disease in Infants, Children, and Adolescents. 4th edition. Baltimore, Williams and Wilkins, 1989.

Puga FJ, Chiavarelli M, Hagler DJ: Modifications of the Fontan operation applicable to patients with left atrioventricular valve atresia or single atrioventricular valve. Circulation *76*(Suppl III):53, 1987.

Robicsek F, Riopel DA, Robicsek LK: Long-term results after cavopulmonary anastomosis. J Thorac Cardiovasc Surg *101:*740, 1991.

Rosenthal A, Nathan J, Marty AT, et al: Acute hemodynamic effects of red cell volume reduction in polycythemia of cyanotic congenital heart disease. Circulation *42:*297, 1970.

Rowe RD: Tetralogy of Fallot. *In* Keith JD, Rowe RD, Vlad P (eds): Heart Disease in Infancy and Childhood. 3rd edition. New York, Macmillan, 1978.

Rudolph AM: Pulmonic stenosis with ventricular septal defect and aortopulmonary transposition. *In* Rudolph AM: Congenital Diseases of the Heart. Chicago, Year Book Medical Publishers, 1974.

Ruttenberg HD: Corrected transposition of the great arteries and splenic syndromes. *In* Adams FH, Emmanouilides GC, Riemenschneider TA (eds): Heart Disease in Infants, Children, and Adolescents. 4th edition. Baltimore, Williams and Wilkins, 1989.

Sammuelson PN, Lell WA: Tetralogy of Fallot. *In* Lake CL. Pediatric Cardiac Anesthesia. Norwalk, Conn, Appleton Lange, 1988.

Sietsema KE, Perloff JK: Cyanotic congenital heart disease: Dynamics of oxygen uptake and control of ventilation during exercise. *In* Perloff JK, Child JS (eds): Congenital Heart Disease in Adults. Philadelphia, WB Saunders, 1991.

Sondheimer HM, Freedom RM, Olley PM: Double outlet right ventricle. *In* Keith JD, Rowe RD, Vlad P (eds): Heart Disease in Infancy and Childhood. 3rd edition. New York, Macmillan, 1978.

Strafford M: Transposition of the great vessels. *In* Lake CL: Pediatric Cardiac Anesthesia. Norwalk, Conn, Appleton Lange, 1988.

Sullivan ID, Wren C, Stark J, et al: Surgical unifocalization in pulmonary atresia and ventricular septal defect—a realistic goal. Circulation *78*(Suppl III):5, 1988.

Territo MC, Rosore MH, Perloff JK: Cyanotic congenital heart disease: Hematologic management, renal function and urate metabolism. *In* Perloff JK, Child JS (eds): Congenital Heart Disease in Adults. Philadelphia, WB Saunders, 1991.

Trusler GA, Williams WG, Cohen AJ, et al: The cavopulmonary shunt. Circulation *82*(Suppl IV):131, 1990.

Turnia MI, Siebenmann RV, Segesser L, et al: Late functional deterioration after atrial correction for transposition of the great arteries. Circulation *80*(Suppl I):162, 1989.

Van Praagh R, Weinberg PM: Double outlet left ventricle. *In* Adams FH, Emmanouilides GC: Heart Disease in Infants, Children, and Adolescents. 3rd edition. Baltimore, Williams and Wilkins, 1983.

Zahka K, Horneffer P, Rowe S, et al: Long-term valvular function after total repair of tetralogy of Fallot; Relation to ventricular arrhythmias. Circulation *78*(Suppl II):14, 1988.

Zuberbuhler JR: Tetralogy of Fallot. *In* Adams FH, Emmanouilides GC, Riemenschneider TA: Moss' Heart Disease in Infants, Children, and Adolescents. 4th edition. Baltimore, Williams and Wilkins, 1989.

VALVULAR LESIONS

Baylen BG, Waldhausen JA: Diseases of the mitral valve. *In* Adams FH, Emmanouilides GC, Riemenschneider TA (eds): Moss' Heart Disease in Infants, Children, and Adolescents. 4th edition. Baltimore, Williams and Wilkins, 1989.

Beekman RH, Rocchini AP, Rosenthal A: Therapeutic catheterization for pulmonary valve and pulmonary artery stenosis. Cardiol Clin *7:*331, 1989.

Bisset GS, Schwartz DC, Meyer RA, et al: Clinical spectrum and long-term follow up of isolated mitral valve prolapse in 119 children. Circulation *62:*423, 1980.

Bloom KR: Mitral valve and tricuspid valve stenosis. *In* Keith JD, Rowe RD, Vlad P (eds): Heart Disease in Infancy and Childhood. 3rd edition. New York, Macmillan, 1978.

Bohn D: Anomalies of the pulmonary valve and pulmonary circulation. *In* Lake CL (ed): Pediatric Cardiac Anesthesia. Norwalk, Conn, Appleton Lange, 1988.

Braunwald E: Mitral regurgitation. N Engl J Med *281:*425, 1969.

Brooks JL, Kaplan JA: Valvular lesions. *In* Katz J, Benumof J, Kadis LB (eds): Anesthesia and Uncommon Diseases. 2nd edition. Philadelphia, WB Saunders Co., 1981.

Brown LM: Mitral valve prolapse in children. Adv Pediatr *25:*327, 1978.

Collins-Nakai RL, Rosenthal A, Castaneda AR, et al: Congenital mitral stenosis. Circulation *56:*1039, 1977.

Dobell ARC, Bloss RS, Gibbons JE, et al: Congenital valvular aortic stenosis. J Thorac Cardiovasc Surg *81:*916, 1981.

Elsten JL, Kim YD, Hanowell JT, et al: Prolonged induction with exaggerated chamber enlargement in Ebstein's anomaly. Anesth Analg *60:*909, 1981.

Emmanouilides GC, Baylen BG: Congenital absence of the pulmonary valve, pulmonary stenosis and pulmonary atresia with intact ventricular septum. *In* Adams FH, Emmanouilides GC (eds): Heart Disease in Infants, Children, and Adolescents. 3rd edition. Baltimore, Williams and Wilkins, 1983.

Emmanouilides GC, Doroshow RW: Congenital absence of the pulmonary valve. *In* Adams FH, Emmanouilides GC, Riemenschneider TA (eds): Moss' Heart Disease in Infants, Children, and Adolescents. 4th edition. Baltimore, Williams and Wilkins, 1989.

Freedom RM: Congenital valvar regurgitation. *In* Keith JD, Rowe RD, Vlad P (eds): Heart Disease in Infancy and Childhood. 3rd edition. New York, Macmillan, 1978.

Freedom RM: Hypoplastic left heart syndrome. *In* Adams FH, Emmanouilides GC, Riemenschneider TA (eds): Heart Disease in Infants, Children, and Adolescents. 4th edition. Baltimore, Williams and Wilkins, 1989.

Freedom RM, Keith JD: Pulmonary atresia. Aortic atresia. *In* Keith JD, Rowe RD, Vlad P (eds): Heart Disease in Infancy and Childhood. 3rd edition. New York, Macmillan, 1978.

Friedman WF, Benson LN: Aortic stenosis. *In* Adams FH, Emmanouilides GC (eds): Heart Disease in Infants, Children, and Adolescents. 3rd edition. Baltimore, Williams and Wilkins, 1983.

Frommelt PC, Rocchini AP, Bove EL: Natural history of apical left ventricular to aortic conduits in pediatric patients. Circulation *84*(Suppl III):213, 1991.

Fulton DR, Hongen TJ, Keane JF, et al: Repeat aortic valvotomy in children. Am Heart J *106:*60, 1983.

Fyler DC: Mitral valve and left atrial lesions. *In* Fyler DC (ed): Nadas' Pediatric Cardiology. Philadelphia, Hanley and Belfus, 1992.

Fyler DC: Tricuspid atresia. *In* Fyler DC (ed): Nadas' Pediatric Cardiology. Philadelphia, Hanley and Belfus, 1992.

Fyler DC: Tricuspid valve problems. *In* Fyler DC (ed): Nadas' Pediatric Cardiology. Philadelphia, Hanley and Belfus, 1992.

Gardner TJ, Roland JM, Neill CA, et al: Valve replacement in children. J Thorac Cardiovasc Surg *83:*178, 1982.

Guigell RL, Vlad P: Mitral valve prolapse. *In* Keith JD, Rowe RD, Vlad P (eds): Heart Disease in Infancy and Childhood. New York, Macmillan 1978.

Hansen DD, Hickey PR: Anesthesia for hypoplastic left heart syndrome. Anesth Analg *65:*127, 1986.

Ishikawa T, Neutze JM, Brandt PWT, et al: Hemodynamics following the Kreutzer procedure for tricuspid atresia in patients under two years of age. J Thorac Cardiovasc Surg *88:*373, 1984.

Jackson JM, Thomas SJ: Valvular heart disease. *In* Kaplan JA (ed): Cardiac Anesthesia. 2nd edition. Orlando, Fla, Grune and Stratton, 1982.

Kare HW, Hensley FA, Cyran SE, et al: Hypoplastic left heart syndrome: Anesthesia for elective non-cardiac surgery. Anesthesiology *72:*753, 1990.

Keith JD: Bicuspid aortic valve. *In* Keith JD, Rowe RD, Vlad P (eds): Heart Disease in Infancy and Childhood. 3rd edition. New York, Macmillan, 1978.

Keith JD: Congenital mitral atresia. *In* Keith JD, Rowe RD, Vlad P (eds): Heart Disease in Infancy and Childhood. 3rd edition. New York, Macmillan, 1978.

Keith JD: Ebstein's disease. *In* Keith JD, Rowe RD, Vlad P (eds): Heart Disease in Infancy and Childhood. 3rd edition. New York, Macmillan, 1978.

Laks H, Billingsley AM: Advances in the treatment of pulmonary atresia with intact ventricular septum: Palliative and definite repair. Cardiol Clin *7:*387, 1989.

Lang P, Fyler DC: Hypoplastic left heart syndrome, mitral atresia, aortic atresia. *In* Fyler DC (ed): Nadas' Pediatric Cardiology. Philadelphia, Hanley and Belfus, 1992.

Leung MP, McKay R, Smith A, et al: Critical aortic stenosis in early infancy. J Thorac Cardiovasc Surg *101:*526, 1991.

Levy MJ, Schachner A, Blieden LC: Aortico-left ventricular tunnel. J Thorac Cardiovasc Surg *84:*102, 1982.

Lone DA: Abnormalities of the atrioventricular valves. *In* Lake CL (ed): Pediatric Cardiac Anesthesia. Norwalk, Conn, Appleton Lange, 1988.

Marino JP, Mihaileanu S, El Asumar B, et al: Echocardiography and color flow mapping; Evaluation of a new reconstructive surgical technique for Ebstein's anomaly. Circulation *80*(Suppl I):197, 1989.

Marvin WJ, Mahoney LT: Pulmonary atresia with intact ventricular septum. *In* Adams FH, Emmanouilides GC, Riemenschneider TA (eds): Moss' Heart Disease in Infants, Children, and Adolescents. Baltimore, Williams and Wilkins, 1989.

McGriffin DC, O'Brien MF, Strafford EG, et al: Long-term results of the viable cryopreserved allograft aortic valve. Continuing evidence for superior valve durability. J Cardiovasc Surg *3:*289, 1988.

Meliones JN, Snider AR, Bove EL, et al: Longitudinal results after first-stage palliation for hypoplastic left heart syndrome. Circulation *82*(Suppl IV):151, 1990.

Molina JE, Edwards J, Bianco R, et al: Growth of fresh frozen pulmonary allograft conduit in growing lambs. Circulation *80*(Suppl I):183, 1989.

Murdison KA, Baffa JM, Farrell PE, et al: Hypoplastic left heart syndrome—outcome after initial reconstruction and before modified Fontan procedure. Circulation *82*(Suppl IV): 1990.

Nadas AS, Fyler DC: Valvular and vascular lesions with a right-to-left shunt or no shunt at all. *In* Nadas AS, Fyler DC: Pediatric Cardiology. 3rd edition. Philadelphia, WB Saunders, 1972.

Nicholson SC, Jobes DR: Hypoplastic left heart syndrome. *In* Lake CL (ed): Pediatric cardiac anesthesia. Norwalk, Conn, Appleton Lange, 1988.

Norwood WI: Hypoplastic left heart syndrome. Cardiol Clin *7:*377, 1989.

Norwood WI, Lang P, Hansen DD: Physiologic repair of aortic atresia–hypoplastic left heart syndrome. N Engl J Med *308:*23, 1983.

Olley PM, Bloom KR, Rowe RD: Aortic stenosis. *In* Keith JD, Rowe RD, Vlad P (eds): Heart Disease in Infancy and Childhood. 3rd edition. New York, Macmillan 1978.

Perez Diaz L, Wuero Jimenez M, Moreno Granados F, et

al: Congenital absence of myocardium of right ventricle: Uhl's anomaly. Br Heart J *35*:570, 1973.

Perry SP, Zeevi B, Kean JF, Lock JE: Interventional catheterization of left heart lesions, including aortic and mitral valve stenosis and coarctation of the aorta. Cardiol Clin *7*:341, 1989.

Pigott JD, Murphy JD, Barber G, Norwood WI: Palliative reconstruction surgery for hypoplastic left heart syndrome. Ann Thorac Surg *45*:122, 1988.

Rastan H, Koncz J: Aortoventriculoplasty: A new method for the treatment of left ventricular outflow tract obstruction. J Thorac Cardiovasc Surg *71*:920, 1976.

Reich DL, Brooks JL, Kaplan JA: Uncommon cardiac disease. *In* Katz J, Benumof JL, Kadis LB: Anesthesia and Uncommon Diseases. 3rd edition. Philadelphia, WB Saunders, 1990.

Richardson JV, Doty DB, Siewers RD, et al: Cor triatriatum. J Thorac Cardiovasc Surg *81*:232, 1981.

Rocchini AP, Emmanouilides GC: Pulmonary stenosis. *In* Adams FH, Emmanouilides GC, Riemenschneider TA (eds): Moss' Heart Disease in Infants, Children, and Adolescents. Baltimore, Williams and Wilkins, 1989.

Rosenthal H, Dick M: Tricuspid atresia. *In* Adams FH, Emmanouilides GC (eds): Heart Disease in Infants, Children, and Adolescents. 3rd edition. Baltimore, Williams and Wilkins, 1983.

Roth SL, Thomas SJ, Tunick P, et al: Mitral valve prolapse: Risk of dysrhythmias in the perioperative period. Anesthesiology *55*:A57, 1981.

Rowe RD: Pulmonary stenosis and pulmonary arterial stenosis. *In* Keith JD, Rowe RD, Vlad P (eds): Heart Disease in Infancy and Childhood. 3rd edition. New York, Macmillan, 1978.

Rudolph AM: Aortic atresia, mitral atresia and hypoplastic left ventricle. *In* Rudolph AM: Congenital Disease of the Heart. Chicago, Year Book Medical Publishers, 1974.

Rudolph AM: Aortic stenosis. *In* Rudolph AM: Congenital Diseases of the Heart. Chicago, Year Book Medical Publishers, 1974.

Rudolph AM: Pulmonary stenosis and atresia with intact ventricular septum. *In* Rudolph AM: Congenital Diseases of the Heart. Chicago, Year Book Medical Publishers, 1974.

Rudolph AM: Tricuspid atresia and hypoplastic right ventricle. *In* Rudolph AM: Congenital Diseases of the Heart. Chicago, Year Book Medical Publishers, 1974.

Sanders SP, Wright GB, Keane JF, et al: Clinical and hemodynamic results of the Fontan operation for tricuspid atresia. Am J Cardiol *49*:1733, 1982.

Saner U, Gittenberger de Groot A, Geishauser M, et al: Coronary arteries in the hypoplastic left heart syndromes. Circulation *80*(Suppl 1):168, 1989.

Schaff HV, DiDonato RM, Danielson GK, et al: Reoperation for obstructed pulmonary ventricle–pulmonary artery conduits. J Thorac Cardiovasc Surg *88*:334, 1984.

Shaddy RE, Sturtevant JE, Judd VE, McGough EC: Right ventricular growth after transventricular pulmonary valvotomy and central aortopulmonary shunt for pulmonary atresia with intact ventricular septum. Circulation *82*(Suppl IV):157, 1990.

Shone JD, Sellers RD, Anderson RC, et al: The developmental complex of parachute mitral valve, supravalvular ring of left atrium, subaortic stenosis and coarctation of aorta. Am J Cardiol *11*:714, 1963.

Stuhlmuller JE, Perloff JK, Skorton DJ: Valvular residual and sequelae after cardiac surgery or interventional cardiac catheterization. *In* Perloff JK, Child JS: Congenital Heart Disease in the Adult. Philadelphia, WB Saunders, 1991.

Taylor SP: Aortic valve and aortic arch anomalies. *In* Lake CL (ed): Pediatric Cardiac Anesthesia. Norwalk, Conn, Appleton Lange, 1988.

Thomas SJ, Lowenstein E: Anesthetic management of the patient with valvular heart disease. Int Anesthesiol Clin *17*:67, 1979.

Uhl HS: A previously undescribed congenital malformation of the heart: Almost total absence of the myocardium of the right ventricle. Bull Johns Hopkins Hosp *91*:197, 1952.

Van Mierop LHS, Rutsche LM, Victorica BE: Ebstein anomaly. *In* Adams FH, Emmanouilides GC, Riemenschneider TA (eds): Heart Disease in Infants, Children, and Adolescents. 4th edition. Baltimore, Williams and Wilkins, 1989.

Vlad P: Tricuspid atresia. *In* Keith JD, Rowe RD, Vlad P (eds): Heart Disease in Infancy and Childhood. 3rd edition. New York, Macmillan, 1978.

MALFORMATIONS INVOLVING THE GREAT VESSELS, CORONARY ARTERIES AND PULMONARY VASCULAR BED

Abe T, Kuribayashi R, Sato M, et al: Direct communication of the right pulmonary artery with the left atrium. J Thorac Cardiovasc Surg *64*:38, 1972.

Ardito JM, Tucker GF, Ossoff RH, DeLeon S: Innominate artery compression of the trachea in infants with reflex apnea. Ann Otol Rhinol Laryngol *89*:401, 1980.

Arensman FW, Schwartz DC, Kaplan S: Multiple coronary arteriocameral fistulas associated with D-transposition of the great vessels. Am Heart J *105*:517, 1983.

Asch AJ: Turner's syndrome, occurring with Horner's syndrome, seen with coarctation of the aorta and aortic aneurysm. Am J Dis Child *133*:817, 1979.

Aytac A, Ozme S, Sarikayalar F, Saylan A: Pulmonary artery sling. Ann Thorac Surg *22*:596, 1976.

Bergdahl LAL, Blackstone EH, Kirklin JW, et al: Determinants of early success in repair of aortic coarctation in infants. J Thorac Cardiovasc Surg *83*:736, 1982.

Bhat R, Fisher E, Raju TNK, et al: Patent ductus arteriosus: Recent advances in diagnosis and management. Pediatr Clin North Am *29*:1117, 1982.

Breckenridge IM, deLeval M, Stark J, et al: Correction of total anomalous pulmonary venous drainage in infancy. J Thorac Cardiovasc Surg *66*:447, 1973.

Culham JAG: Congenital anomalies of the coronary arteries. *In* Keith JD, Rowe RD, Vlad P (eds): Heart Disease in Infancy and Childhood. 3rd edition. New York, Macmillan, 1978.

Dala FY, Bennett EJ, Salen MR, et al: Anesthesia for coarctation. Anaesthesia *29*:704, 1974.

DiSersa TG, Child JS, Perloff JK, et al: Systemic venous and pulmonary arterial flow patterns after Fontan's procedure for tricuspid atresia or single ventricle. Circulation *70*:898, 1984.

Editorial: Patent ductus arteriosus: Current clinical status. Arch Dis Child *55*:106, 1980.

Emmanouilides GC, Doroshow RW: Congenital absence of the pulmonary valve. *In* Adams FH, Emmanouilides GC, Riemenschneider TA, (eds): Moss' Heart Disease in Infants, Children, and Adolescents. 4th edition. Baltimore, Williams and Wilkins, 1989.

Ergin MA, Jayaram N, La Corte M: Left aortic arch and right descending aorta: Diagnostic and therapeutic implications of a rare type of vascular ring. Ann Thorac Surg *31*:82, 1981.

Fishman NH, Bronstein MH, Berman W, et al: Surgical management of severe aortic coarctation and interrupted aortic arch in neonates. J Thorac Cardiovasc Surg *71*:35, 1976.

Friedman WF, Fitzpatrick KM, Merritt TA, et al: The patent ductus arteriosus. Clin Perinatol *5*:283, 1978.

Fyler DC: Anomalous origin of the left coronary artery. *In* Fyler DC (ed): Nadas' Pediatric Cardiology. Philadelphia, Hanley and Belfus, 1992.

Fyler DC: Aortopulmonary window. *In* Fyler DC: Nadas' Pediatric Cardiology. Philadelphia, Hanley and Belfus, 1992.

Fyler DC: Coarctation of the aorta. *In* Fyler DC: Nadas' Pediatric Cardiology. Philadelphia, Hanley and Belfus, 1992.

Fyler DC: Congenital vascular fistulas. *In* Fyler DC (ed): Nadas' Pediatric Cardiology. Philadelphia, Hanley and Belfus, 1992.

Fyler DC: Origin of a right pulmonary artery from the aorta (hemitruncus). *In* Fyler DC (ed): Nadas' Pediatric Cardiology. Philadelphia, Hanley and Belfus, 1992.

Fyler DC: Total anomalous pulmonary venous return. *In* Fyler DC: Nadas' Pediatric Cardiology. Philadelphia, Hanley and Belfus, 1992.

Fyler DC: Truncus arteriosus. *In* Fyler DC (ed): Nadas' Pediatric Cardiology. Philadelphia, Hanley and Belfus, 1992.

Garcia OL, Hernandez FA, Tamer O, et al: Congenital bilateral subclavian steal. Am J Cardiol *44*:101, 1979.

Gersony WM: Coarctation of the aorta. *In* Adams FH, Emmanouilides GC, Riemenschneider TA (eds): Moss' Heart Disease in Infants, Children, and Adolescents. 4th edition. Baltimore, Williams and Wilkins, 1989.

Goldstein JD, Rabinovitch M, Van Praagh R, Reid L: Unusual vascular anomalies causing persistent pulmonary hypotension in a newborn. Am J Cardiol *43*:962, 1979.

Gutgesell HP: Myocardial and coronary artery anomalies. *In* Lake CL (ed): Pediatric Cardiac Anesthesia. Norwalk, Conn, Appleton Lange, 1988.

Haas G, Laks H, Perloff JK: The selection, use and long-term effects of prosthetic materials. *In* Perloff JK, Child JS: Congenital Heart Disease in Adults. Philadelphia, WB Saunders, 1991.

Hayward RH, Martt JM, Brewer LM, et al: Surgical correction of the vena cava bronchovascular complex. J Thorac Cardiovasc Surg *64*:203, 1972.

Hickey PR: Intraoperative tension pneumopericardium with tamponade after ligation of patent ductus arteriosus in a premature. Neonate Anesthesiol *64*:641, 1986.

Jimenez MQ, Guillen FA: Arteriovenous fistulas. *In* Adams FH, Emmanouilides GC, Riemenschneider TA (eds): Moss' Heart Disease in Infants, Children, and Adolescents. 4th edition. Baltimore, Williams and Wilkins, 1989.

Jonas RA, Spevak PJ, Casteneda AR: Pulmonary artery sling: Primary repair by tracheal resection in infancy. J Thorac Cardiovasc Surg *97*:548, 1989.

Keith JD: Coarctation of the aorta. *In* Keith JD, Rowe RD, Vlad P (eds): Heart Disease in Infancy and Childhood. 3rd edition. New York, Macmillan, 1978.

Keith JD: Congenital pulmonary arteriovenous aneurysm. *In* Keith JD, Rowe RD, Vlad P (eds): Heart Disease in Infancy and Childhood. 3rd edition. New York, Macmillan, 1978.

Khonsari B, Saunders PW, Lees MH, et al: Common pulmonary vein atresia. J Thorac Cardiovasc Surg *83*:443, 1982.

Lee CN, Schaff HV, Danielson GK, et al: Comparison of atriopulmonary versus atrioventricular connections for modified Fontan/Kreutzer repair of tricuspid valve atresia. J Thorac Cardiovasc Surg *92*:1038, 1986.

Lin AE, Laks H, Barber G, et al: Subaortic obstruction in complex congenital heart disease: Management by proximal pulmonary artery to ascending aorta end-to-side anastomosis. J Am Coll Cardiol *7*:617, 1986.

Lucas RV, Krabill K: Anomalous venous connections, pulmonary and systemic. *In* Adams FH, Emmanouilides GC, Riemenschneider TA (eds): Moss' Heart Disease in Infants, Children, and Adolescents. 4th edition. Baltimore, Williams and Wilkins, 1989.

Lurie PR, Takahashi M: Abnormalities and diseases of the coronary vessels. *In* Adams FH, Emmanouilides GC (eds): Heart Disease in Infants, Children, and Adolescents. 3rd edition. Baltimore, Williams and Wilkins, 1983.

Mair DD, Edwards WD, Tulsrud PR, et al: Truncus arteriosus. *In* Adams FH, Emmanouilides GC, Riemenschneider TA (eds): Moss' Heart Disease in Infants, Children, and Adolescents. 4th edition. Baltimore, Williams and Wilkins, 1989.

Mair DD, Hagler DJ, Puga FJ, et al: Fontan operation in 176 patients with tricuspid atresia. Circulation *82*(Suppl IV):164, 1990.

Mandell VS, Braverman RM: Vascular rings and slings. *In* Fyler DC (ed): Nadas' Pediatric Cardiology. Philadelphia, Hanley and Belfus, 1992.

McLeskey CH, Martin WE: Anesthesia for repair of a pulmonary artery sling in an infant with severe tracheal stenosis. Anesthesiology *46*:368, 1977.

Meier MA, Lucchese FA, Jazbik W, et al: A new technique for repair of aortic coarctation. J Thorac Cardiovasc Surg *92*:1005, 1986.

Moes CAF: Vascular rings and anomalies of the aortic arch. *In* Keith JD, Rowe RD, Vlad P (eds): Heart Disease in Infancy and Childhood. 3rd edition. New York, Macmillan, 1978.

Moodie DS, Fyfe D, Gill GC, et al: Anomalous origin of the left coronary artery from the pulmonary artery (Bland-White-Garland syndrome) in adult patients: Long-term follow-up after surgery. Am Heart J *100*:381, 1983.

Neuman GG, Handen DD: The anesthetic management of preterm infants undergoing ligation of a patent ductus arteriosus. Can Anaesth Soc J *27*:248, 1980.

Norwood WI, Lang P, Castaneda AR, et al: Reparative operations for interrupted aortic arch with ventricular septal defect. J Thorac Cardiovasc Surg *86*:832, 1983.

Robinson S, Gregory GA: Fentanyl-air-oxygen anesthesia for ligation of patent ductus arteriosus in preterm infants. Anesth Analg *60*:331, 1981.

Rosenthal A, Dick M: Tricuspid atresia. *In* Adams FH, Emmanouilides GC, Riemenschneider TA (eds): Moss' Heart Disease in Infants, Children, and Adolescents. Baltimore, Williams and Wilkins, 1989.

Rowe RD: Anomalies of venous return. *In* Keith JD, Rowe RD, Vlad P (eds): Heart Disease in Infancy and Childhood. 3rd edition. New York, Macmillan, 1978.

Ruckman RN: Anomalies of the aortic arch complex. *In* Adams FH, Emmanouilides GC, Riemenschneider TA (eds): Moss' Heart Disease in Infants, Children, and Adolescents. 4th edition. Baltimore, Williams and Wilkins, 1989.

Rudolph AM: Aortic coarctation and isthmus narrowing. *In* Rudolph AM: Congenital Diseases of the Heart. Chicago, Year Book Medical Publishers, 1974.

Rudolph AM: The ductus arteriosus and persistent patency of the ductus arteriosus. *In* Rudolph AM: Congenital Diseases of the Heart. Chicago, Year Book Medical Publishers, 1974.

Rudolph AM: Truncus arteriosus. *In* Rudolph AM: Congenital Diseases of the Heart. Chicago, Year Book Medical Publishers, 1974.

Seraf A, Bruniaux J, Lacour-Gayet F, et al: Obstructed total anomalous pulmonary venous return. J Thorac Cardiovasc Surg *101*:601, 1991.

Stellin G, Jonas RA, Goh TH, et al: Surgical treatment of absent pulmonary valve syndrome in infants: Relief of bronchial obstruction. Ann Thorac Surg *34*:468, 1983.

Van Meter C, LeBlanc J, Culpepper WS, Ochsner JL: Partial anomalous pulmonary venous return. Circulation *82*(Suppl IV): 195, 1990.

Welz A, Reichert B, Wienhold C, et al: Innominate artery compression of the trachea in infancy and childhood: Is surgical therapy justified? J Thorac Cardiovasc Surg *32*:85, 1984.

CARDIOMYOPATHIES

Artman M, Graham TP: Congestive heart failure in infancy. Am Heart J *103*:1040, 1982.

Artman M, Parrish MD, Graham TP: Congestive heart failure in childhood and adolescence. Am Heart J *105*:471, 1983.

Bell CF, Kelly JM, Jones RE: Anesthesia for Friedreich's ataxia. Anaesthesia *41*:296, 1986.

Bowers JR: Anesthesia and cardiomyopathies. Anesth Analg *50*:1013, 1971.

Brooks JL, Kaplan JA: Cardiac diseases. *In* Katz J, Benumof J, Kadis LB (eds): Anesthesia and Uncommon Diseases. 2nd edition. Philadelphia, WB Saunders, 1981.

Cherian G, Vijayaragharan G, Krishnaswami S, et al: Endomyocardial fibrosis. Am Heart J *105*:659, 1983.

Child JS, Perloff JK: The restrictive cardiomyopathies. Cardiol Clin *8*:289, 1988.

Child JS, Perloff JK, Bach PM, et al: Cardiac involvement in Friedreich's ataxia. J Am Coll Cardiol *7*:1370, 1986.

Colan SD, Spevak PJ, Parness JA, Nadas AS: Cardiomyopathies. *In* Fyler DC (ed): Nadas' Pediatric Cardiology. Philadelphia, Hanley and Belfus, 1992.

Epstein SE, Maron BJ: Hypertrophic cardiomyopathy. Clin Invest Med *3*:185, 1980.

Harris LC, Ngheim RX: Cardiomyopathies in infants and children. Prog Cardiovasc Dis *15*:255, 1972.

Hirota Y, Furubayashi K, Kaku K, et al: Hypertrophic nonobstructive cardiomyopathy. Am J Cardiol *50*:990, 1982.

Jaiyesimi F: Controversies and advances in endomyocardial fibrosis. Afr J Med Sci *11*:37, 1982.

Keith JD, Rose V, Manning JA: Endocardial fibroelastosis. *In* Keith JD, Rowe RD, Vlad P (eds): Heart Disease in Infancy and Childhood. 3rd edition. New York, Macmillan, 1978.

Kowey PR, Eisenberg R, Engle TR: Sustained arrhythmias in hypertrophic obstructive cardiomyopathy. N Engl J Med *310*:1566, 1984.

Kubal K, Pasricha SK, Bliargava M: Spinal anesthesia in a patient with Friedreich's ataxia. Anesth Analg *72*:257, 1991.

Maron BJ: Cardiomyopathies. In Adams TH, Emmanouilides GC, Riemenschneider TA (eds.): Heart Disease in Infants, Children and Adolescents. 3rd edition. Baltimore, Williams and Wilkins, 1983.

Maron B, Epstein SE: Hypertrophic cardiomyopathy. Am J Cardiol *45*:141, 1980.

Maron BJ, Tajik AJ, Ruttenberg HD, et al: Hypertrophic cardiomyopathy in infants. Circulation *65*:7, 1982.

Mohr R, Schaff HV, Puga FJ, Danielson GK: Results of operation for hypertrophic obstructive cardiomyopathy in children and adults less than 40 years of age. Circulation *80*(Suppl I):191, 1989.

Nadas AS, Fyler DC: Myocardial diseases. *In* Nadas AS, Fyler DC: Pediatric Cardiology. 3rd edition. Philadelphia, WB Saunders, 1972.

Pereira Barretto AC, Lemos da Luz P, Almeida de Oliveira S, et al: Determinants of survival in endomyocardial fibrosis. Circulation *80*(Suppl I):177, 1989.

Perloff JK: The cardiomyopathies. Cardiol Clin *6*:185, 1988.

Reich DL, Brooks JL, Kaplan JA: Uncommon cardiac diseases. *In* Katz J, Benumof J, Kadis L (eds): Anesthesia and Uncommon Diseases. 3rd edition. Philadelphia, WB Saunders, 1990.

Reitan JA, Wright RG: The use of halothane in a patient with asymmetric septal hypertrophy. Can Anaesth Soc J *29*:154, 1982.

Sasson Z, Rakowski H, Wigle EO: Hypertrophic cardiomyopathy. Cardiol Clin *6*:233, 1988.

Seward JB, Tajik AJ: Primary cardiomyopathies: Classification, pathophysiology, clinical recognition and management. Cardiovasc Clin *10*:199, 1980.

Stevenson LW, Perloff JK: The dilated cardiomyopathies: Clinical aspects. Cardiol Clin *6*:187, 1988.

Werner JC, Sicard RE, Hansen TW, et al: Hypertrophic cardiomyopathy associated with dexamethasone therapy for broncho-pulmonary dysplasia. J Pediatr *120*:286, 1992.

Wilberg-Jorgensen F, Skovsted P, Fischer Hansen J, et al: Cardiovascular haemodynamics during fluroxene anaesthesia in patients with muscular subaortic stenosis. Acta Anaesth Scand *17*:142, 1973.

TUMORS OF THE HEART

Becker RC, Loeffler JS, Leopold KA, et al: Primary tumors of the heart: A review with emphasis on diagnosis and potential treatment modalities. Surg Oncol *1*:161, 1985.

Bharati S, Lev M: Cardiac tumors. *In* Adams FH, Emmanouilides GC, Riemenschneider TA (eds): Moss' Heart Disease in Infants, Children, and Adolescents. 4th edition. Baltimore, Williams and Wilkins, 1989.

Corno A, de Simone G, Catena G, Marcelleti C: Cardiac rhabdomyoma: Surgical treatment in the neonate. J Thorac Surg *87*:725, 1984.

Edwards JE: Cardiac tumors. *In* Adams FH, Emmanouilides GC (eds): Heart Disease in Infants, Children, and Adolescents. 3rd edition. Baltimore, Williams and Wilkins, 1978.

Fowler RS, Keith JD: Cardiac tumors. *In* Keith JD, Rowe RD, Vlad P (eds): Heart Disease in Infancy and Childhood. 3rd edition. New York, Macmillan, 1978.

Fyler DC: Cardiac tumors. *In* Fyler DC (ed): Nadas' Pediatric Cardiology. Philadelphia, Hanley and Belfus, 1992.

Hanson EC, Gill CL, Razzivi M, et al: The surgical treatment of atrial myxomas. J Thorac Cardiovasc Surg *89*:298, 1985.

Legler DC: Uncommon diseases and cardiac anesthesia. *In* Kaplan JA: Cardiac Anesthesia. 2nd edition. Orlando, Fla, Grune and Stratton, 1987.

McAllister HA: Primary tumors and cysts of the heart. Curr Probl Cardiol *4*:1, 1979.

Reece IJ, Cooley DA, Frazier OH, et al: Cardiac tumors. J Thorac Cardiovasc Surg *88*:439, 1984.

Semb BKH: Surgical considerations in the treatment of cardiac myxoma. J Thorac Cardiovasc Surg *87*:251, 1984.

CONGENITAL CONDUCTION DEFECTS

Bazett HC: An analysis of the time-relations of electrocardiograms. Heart *7*:353, 1920.

Brown M, Liberthson RR, Ali HH, Lowenstein E: Perioperative anesthetic management of a patient with long Q-T syndrome (LQTS). Anesthesiology *55*:586, 1981.

Burchell HB: The QT interval historically treated. Pediatr Cardiol *4*:139, 1983.

Callaghan ML, Nichols AB, Sweet RD: Anaesthetic management of prolonged QT interval syndrome. Anesthesiology *47*:67, 1977.

Carlock FJ, Brown M, Brown EM: Isoflurane anaesthesia for a patient with long QT syndrome. Can Anaesth Soc J *31*:83, 1984.

Diaz JH, Friesen RH: Anesthetic management of congenital complete heart block in childhood. Anesth Analg *58*:334, 1979.

Duffy BL: Congenital complete heart block. Anaesthesia *36*:956, 1981.

Dunn CM, Gunter JB, Quattromani A, Bruns PK: Esmolol in the anaesthetic management of a boy with Romano-Ward syndrome. Paediatr Anaesthesia *1*:129, 1991.

Galloway PA, Glass PSA: Anesthetic implications of prolonged QT interval syndromes. Anesth Analg *64*:612, 1985.

Garson A Jr: Medicolegal problems in the management of cardiac arrhythmias in children. Pediatrics *79*:84, 1987.

Garson A, Moak JP, Friedman RA, et al: Surgical treatment of cardiac arrhythmias in children. Cardiol Clin *7*:319, 1989.

Gillette PC: Advances in the diagnosis and treatment of tachydysrhythmias in children. Am Heart J *102*:111, 1981.

Gillette PC, Carson A, Crawford F, et al: Dysrhythmias. *In* Adams FH, Emmanouilides GC, Riemenschneider TA (eds): Moss' Heart Disease in Infants, Children, and Adolescents. 4th edition. Baltimore, Williams and Wilkins, 1989.

Jones RM, Broadbent MP, Adams P: Anaesthetic considerations in patients with paroxysmal supraventricular tachycardia. Anaesthesia *39*:307, 1984.

Klitzner TS, Friedman WF: Cardiac arrhythmias: The role of pharmacological intervention. Cardiol Clin *7*:299, 1989.

Moss AJ, Schwartz PJ: Sudden death and idiopathic long QT syndrome. Am J Med *66*:6, 1979.

O'Callaghan AC, Normandale JP, Morgan M: The prolonged QT syndrome. A review with anaesthetic implications. Anaesth Intens Care *10*:50, 1982.

O'Gara JP, Edelman JD: Anesthesia and the patient with complete congenital heart block. Anesth Analg *60*:906, 1981.

Olley PM: Cardiac arrhythmias. *In* Keith JD, Rowe RD, Vlad P (eds): Heart Disease in Infancy and Childhood. 3rd edition. New York, Macmillan, 1978.

Owitz S, Pratilas V, Pratila MG, Dimich L: Anaesthetic considerations in the prolonged QT interval syndrome (LQTS): A case report. Can Anaesth Soc J *26*:50, 1979.

Pickoff AS, Wolff GS, Tamer D, et al: Arrhythmias and conduction system disturbances in infants and children. Cardiovasc Clin *11*:203, 1980.

Richmond MN, Connoy PT: Anesthetic management of a neonate born prematurely with Wolff-Parkinson-White syndrome. Anesth Analg *67*:477, 1988.

Sadowski AR, Moyers JR: Anesthetic management of the Wolff-Parkinson-White syndrome. Anesthesiology *51*:553, 1979.

Scheffer GJ, Jonges R, Holley H, et al: Effects of halothane on the conduction system of the heart. Anesth Analg *69*:721, 1989.

Schmeling WT, Warltier DC, McDonald DJ, et al: Prolongation of the Q-T interval by enflurane, isoflurane and halothane in humans. Anesth Analg *72*:137, 1991.

Schwartz PJ, Periti M, Malliani A: The long QT syndrome. Am Heart J *89*:378, 1975.

Stevenson GW, Schuster J, Kress J, Hall SC: Transesophageal pacing for perioperative control of neonatal paroxysmal supraventricular tachycardia. Can J Anaesth *37*:672, 1990.

Steward DJ, Izukawa T: Congenital complete heart block. Anesth Analg *59*:81, 1980.

Van der Starre PJ: Wolff-Parkinson-White syndrome during anesthesia. Anesthesiology *48*:369, 1978.

Vetter VL, Rashkind WJ: Congenital complete heart block and connective tissue disease. N Engl J Med *309*:236, 1983.

Walsh EP, Saul JP: Cardiac arrhythmias. *In* Fyler DC: Nadas' Pediatric Cardiology. Philadelphia, Hanley and Belfus, 1992.

White SE, Frison LM, Brown SE: Hypoglycemia associated with supraventricular tachycardia in an infant. Anesthesiology *69*:944, 1988.

Yanagida H, Kemi C, Suwa K: The effects of stellate ganglion block on idiopathic prolongation of the Q-T interval with cardiac arrhythmia (the Roman-Ward syndrome). Anesth Analg *55*:782, 1976.

DISEASES OF THE PERICARDIUM

Fyler DC: Pericardial disease. *In* Fyler DC: Nadas' Pediatric Cardiology. Philadelphia, Hanley and Belfus, 1992.

Keith JD: Pericarditis. *In* Keith JD, Rowe RD, Vlad P (eds): Heart Disease in Infancy and Childhood. 3rd edition. New York, Macmillan, 1978.

Lake CL: Anesthesia and pericardial disease. Anesth Analg *62*:431, 1983.

Reich DL, Brooks JL, Kaplan JA: Uncommon cardiac diseases. *In* Katz J, Benumof J, Kadis LB (eds): Anesthesia and Uncommon Diseases. 3rd edition. Philadelphia, WB Saunders, 1990.

Shabetai R: Diseases of the pericardium. Cardiol Clin *8*:4, 1990.

MALPOSITIONS OF THE HEART

Keith JD: Ectopia cordis. *In* Keith JD, Rowe RD, Vlad P (eds): Heart Disease in Infancy and Childhood. 3rd edition. New York, Macmillan, 1978.

Rao PS: Dextrocardia. Am Heart J *102*:389, 1981.

Van Praagh R, Santini F, Sanders SP: Cardiac malposition with special emphasis on visceral heterotaxy. *In* Fyler DC: Nadas' Pediatric Cardiology. Philadelphia, Hanley and Belfus, 1992.

Van Praagh R, Weinberg PM, Smith SD, et al: Malpositions of the heart. *In* Adams FH, Emmanouilides GC, Riemenschneider TA (eds): Heart Disease in Infants, Children, and Adolescents. 4th edition. Baltimore, Williams and Wilkins, 1989.

ACQUIRED HEART DISEASE

Ayoub EM: Acute rheumatic fever. *In* Adams FH, Emmanouilides GC, Riemenschneider TA (eds): Moss' Heart Disease in Infants, Children, and Adolescents. 4th edition. Balimore, Williams and Wilkins, 1989.

Bell DM, Moorens DM, Holman RC, et al: Kawasaki syndrome in the United States. Am J Dis Child *137*:211, 1983.

Dajani AS, Bisno AL, Chung KJ, et al: Prevention of bacterial endocarditis: Recommendations by the American Heart Association. JAMA *264*:2919, 1990.

Edwards WT, Burney RG: Use of repeated nerve blocks in management of an infant with Kawasaki's disease. Anesth Analg *67*:1008, 1988.

Fyler DC: Rheumatic fever. *In* Fyler DC: Nadas' Pediatric Cardiology. Philadelphia, Hanley and Belfus, 1992.

Kaplan E, Shulman ST: Endocarditis. *In* Adams FH, Emmanouilides GC, Riemenschneider TA (eds): Moss' Heart Disease in Infants, Children, and Adolescents. 3rd edition. Baltimore, Williams and Wilkins, 1989.

Kaplan EL: Acute rheumatic fever. Pediatr Clin North Am *25*:817, 1978.

Kaplan S: Chronic rheumatic heart disease. *In* Adams FH, Emmanouilides GC, Riemenschneider TA (eds): Moss' Heart Disease in Infants, Children, and Adolescents. 4th edition. Baltimore, Williams and Wilkins, 1989.

Keith JD: Rheumatic fever and rheumatic heart disease. *In* Keith JD, Rowe RD, Vlad P (eds): Heart Disease in Infancy and Childhood. 3rd edition. New York, Macmillan, 1978.

McKay RS, Dillasel SR: Management of epidural anesthesia in a patient with Takayasu disease. Anesth Analg *74*:297, 1992.

McNieve WL, Krishna G: Kawasaki disease. A disease with anesthetic implications. Anesthesiology *58*:269, 1983.

Newburger JW: Infective endocarditis. *In* Fyler DC: Nadas' Pediatric Cardiology. Philadelphia, Hanley and Belfus, 1992.

Newburger JW: Kawasaki syndrome. *In* Fyler DC: Nadas' Pediatric Cardiology. Philadelphia, Hanley and Belfus, 1992.

Newburger JW, Burus JC: Kawasaki syndrome. Cardiol Clin *7*:453, 1989.

Ramanathan S, Gupta U, Chalou J, Turndorf H: Anesthetic considerations in Takayasu arteritis. Anesth Analg *58*:247, 1979.

Shulman ST, Amren DP, Bisno AL, et al: Prevention of rheumatic fever. Circulation *70*:1118A, 1984.

Stinson EB: Surgical treatment of infective endocarditis. Prog Cardiovasc Dis *22*:145, 1979.

Sum K, Takeuchi Y, Shiroma K, et al: Early and late postoperative studies in coronary arterial lesions resulting from Kawasaki's disease in children. J Thorac Cardiovasc Surg *84*:224, 1982.

Takahashi M, Lurie PR: Abnormalities and diseases of the coronary vessels. *In* Adams TH, Emmanouilides GC, Riemenschneider TA (eds): Moss' Heart Disease in Infants, Children, and Adolescents. 4th edition. Baltimore, Williams and Wilkins, 1989.

Warner MA, Hughes DR, Resnick JM: Anesthetic management of a patient with pulseless disease. Anesth Analg *62*:532, 1983.

INTERVENTIONAL CARDIOLOGY

Beekman RH, Rocchini AP, Rosenthal A: Therapeutic cardiac catheterization for pulmonary valve and pulmonary artery stenosis. Cardiol Clin *7*:331, 1989.

Greenberg MA, Menegus MA, Issenberg H, Spindola-Franco H: Advances in interventional cardiology: Endomyocardial biopsy, valvuloplasty and pediatric interventional cardiology. Curr Opinions Radiol *2*:616, 1990.

Hellenbrand WE, Mullins CE: Catheter closure of congenital heart defects. Cardiol Clin *7*:351, 1989.

Hickey PR, Wessel DL, Streitz SL, et al: Transcatheter closure of atrial septal defects: Hemodynamic complications and anesthetic management. Anesth Analg *74*:44, 1992.

Issenberg HI: Transcatheter coil closure of congenital coronary artery fistula. Am Heart J *120*:1441, 1990.

Jamarkami JM, Isabel-Jones JB: Cardiac catheterization as a therapeutic intervention. *In* Perloff JK, Child JS (eds): Congenital Heart Disease in Adults. Philadelphia, WB Saunders, 1991.

Malviya S, Burrows FA, Jonston AE, Beuson LN: Anaesthetic experience with paediatric interventional cardiology. Can J Anaesth *36*:320, 1989.

Meretoja OA, Rantiainen P: Alfentanil and fentanyl sedation in infants and small children during cardiac catheterization. Can J Anaesth *37*:624, 1990.

Mullins CE: Therapeutic cardiac catheterization. *In* Adams FH, Emmanouilides GC, Riemenschneider TA (eds): Moss' Heart Disease in Infants, Children, and Adolescents. 4th edition. Baltimore, Williams and Wilkins, 1989.

Perry SB, Radthe W, Fellows KE, et al: Coil embolization to occlude aortopulmonary collateral vessels and shunts in patients with congenital heart disease. J Am Coll Cardiol *13*:100, 1989.

Rhenban KS, Carpenter MA: Diagnostic cardiac catheterization, angiography and interventional catheterization. *In* Lake CL (ed): Pediatric Cardiac Anesthesia. Norwalk, Conn, Appleton Lange, 1988.

APPENDIX A

ANTIBIOTIC PROPHYLAXIS FOR PREVENTION OF BACTERIAL ENDOCARDITIS

Antimicrobial prophylaxis is at present recommended for all children with structural heart disease or a history of previous infective endocarditis who undergo procedures that may cause gingival bleeding or involve the respiratory, gastrointestinal, urinary, or genital tracts. Exceptions to this rule are patients with uncomplicated secundum atrial septal defect (ASD) or patients who have undergone surgical repair (without residual) of secundum ASD, patent ductus arteriosus, or ventricular septal defect more than 6 months previously. In addition, patients with mitral valve prolapse without valve dysfunction, with previous Kawasaki's syndrome without valve dysfunction, with pacemakers or defibrillators, and with ventriculoatrial shunts do not require antimicrobial prophylaxis. Patients at higher risk for the development of infective endocarditis are those with prosthetic valves, surgically constructed systemic pulmonary shunts, conduits, and a previous history of endocarditis.

Prophylaxis against recurrence of acute rheumatic fever is insufficient for the prevention of bacterial endocarditis. These patients have to be treated with recommended antibiotic therapy for prevention of bacterial endocarditis. However, since these patients may harbor penicillin-resistant strains of *Streptococcus viridans*, they should be treated with the antibiotic regimens recommended for penicillin-allergic patients. Endocarditis prophylaxis should be initiated shortly (1 to 2 hours) before the procedure and should not be prolonged beyond 6 to 8 hours, to prevent selection of resistant bacterial flora.

ANTIBIOTIC REGIMEN (AMERICAN HEART ASSOCIATION RECOMMENDATIONS)

	Drug	Route	Dose
Standard regimen for dental, oral, or upper respiratory tract procedures	Amoxicillin	Oral	50 mg/kg orally 1 hour before the procedure, then 25 mg/kg 6 hours later (max dose: 3000 mg) **Simplified:** <15 kg = 750 mg 15–30 kg = 1500 mg >50 kg = 3000 mg
For patients allergic to amoxicillin/penicillin	Erythromycin	Oral	20 mg/kg orally 2 hours before the procedure, followed by 10 mg/kg 6 hours later
	OR		
	Clindamycin		10 mg/kg 1 hour before the procedure, followed by 5 mg/kg 6 hours later
	Ampicillin	Parenteral	50 mg/kg IV or IM 30 minutes before the procedure; repeat half the dose 6 hours later (max dose: 2000 mg)
Patients allergic to amoxicillin, ampicillin, penicillin	Clindamycin	Parenteral	10 mg/kg IV 30 minutes before the procedure; repeat half the dose 6 hours later (max dose: 300 mg)
Recommendations for high-risk patients (prosthetic valve, systemic-pulmonary shunt, previous endocarditis) **ALSO** Special regimen for genitourinary or gastrointestinal procedures	Ampicillin, gentamicin, and amoxicillin	Parenteral	IV or IM administration of ampicillin, 50 mg/kg (max dose: 2.0 g) **plus** gentamicin,* 1.5 mg/kg (max dose: 80 mg) 30 minutes before the procedure, followed by the **same** dose 8 hours later, or followed by amoxicillin, 25 mg/kg (max dose: 1.5 g) orally 6 hours later
Patients allergic to penicillin and high-risk	Vancomycin	Parenteral	20 mg/kg IV over 1 hour, started 1 hour before the procedure. No repeat dose necessary
Patients allergic to penicillin	Vancomycin, gentamicin	Parenteral	20 mg/kg IV (max dose: 1.0 g) over 1 hour and gentamicin, 1.5 mg/kg (max dose: 80 mg) IV or IM 1 hour before the procedure. May be repeated once after 8 hours*
Alternative low-risk patient regimen	Amoxicillin	Oral	50 mg/kg (max dose: 3 g) orally 1 hour before the procedure and 25 mg/kg (max dose: 1.5 g) 6 hours later

*In patients with impaired renal function, the second dose of vancomycin or gentamicin may have to be modified or eliminated.

APPENDIX B

COMMONLY USED PEDIATRIC CARDIAC DRUGS

Drug	Route	Dose	Onset of Action	Indications (I), Precautions (P), and Complications (C)
Digoxin	PO	*Initial:* <2 yr: 0.03–0.04 mg/kg >2 yr: 0.02–0.04 mg/kg	1–2 hr	I: Congestive failure, supraventricular arrhythmias
	PO	*Maintenance:* ¼–⅓ initial dose divided in 2 doses		C: Toxicity may appear with fluid shifts and hypokalemia perioperatively
	IM IV	75% of PO dose	15–60 min 5–30 min	P: Give 50% of total digitalizing dose, then 2 doses of 25% q 6–8 hr
Furosemide	IV PO	1–2 mg/kg 1–4 mg/kg/day	5–15 min	I: Congestive failure with fluid retention C: Causes hypokalemia and metabolic alkalosis
Propranolol	IV	0.01–0.015 mg/kg over 10 min, repeat q 6–8 min 0.1–0.2 mg/kg maximum, repeat q 6–8 hr	2–5 min	I: Hypertrophic myopathy, beta-blockade, atrial arrhythmias
	PO	0.5–1.0 mg/kg q 6 hr	30–60 min	I: Hypercyanotic spells C: May cause failure and heart block
Lidocaine	IV IV cont. infusion	0.5–1.0 mg/kg 0.01–0.05 mg/kg/min	15–90 sec	I: Ventricular dysrhythmia C: Causes heart block, hypotension, convulsion
Dopamine	IV cont. infusion	5–25 μg/kg/min	Minutes	I: Hypotension due to reduced contractility P: Low dose improves renal perfusion C: May cause tachyarrhythmias, tissue necrosis
Dobutamine	IV cont. infusion	5–20 μg/kg/min	Minutes	I: Heart failure, cardiogenic shock
Epinephrine	IV IV cont. infusion	10 μg/kg 0.1–1 μg/kg/min, start with 0.1 μg/kg/min	Seconds	I: Cardiac arrest, bradycardia, hypotension C: Causes ventricular arrhythmias
Phenylephrine	IV	5–10 μg/kg		I: To counteract sudden decrease in peripheral vascular resistance in cyanotic lesion; paroxysmal tachycardia C: May cause bradycardia and hypertension
Norepinephrine	IV cont. infusion	0.1 μg/kg/min, titrate to desired effect		I: Hypotension without peripheral vasoconstriction C: May cause hypertension and tissue necrosis
Calcium chloride	IV	10–15 mg/kg		I: Slow and weak cardiac action C: May cause cardiac arrest and tissue necrosis
Isoproterenol	IV cont. infusion	0.05–0.4 μg/kg/min, titrate to desired effect	30–60 sec	I: Bradycardia and failure C: Causes ventricular irritability
Sodium nitroprusside	IV cont. infusion	0.5–0.8 μg/kg/min	Minutes	I: Afterload reduction, lowering of blood pressure C: Hypotension, cyanide toxicity
Tolazoline	IV	1–2 mg/kg over 15–20 min, then 2.0 mg/kg/hr	Minutes	I: Pulmonary vasodilation C: Systemic hypotension
Prostaglandin E_1	IV cont. infusion	0.01–0.1 μg/kg/min	Minutes	I: Prevention of ductal closure C: Apnea, fever, hypotension
Nitroglycerin	IV cont. infusion	0.2–0.6 μg/kg/min, titrate to desired effect	Minutes	I: Preload reduction C: Hypotension tachycardia

APPENDIX C

REVERSAL OF ANTICOAGULATION

In order to avoid bleeding problems during surgery, anticoagulation with vitamin K antagonists is generally discontinued 36 hours prior to elective surgery; anticoagulation is then maintained with intravenous heparin, which can be more readily reversed if necessary. For emergency procedures, 10 ml/kg of fresh frozen plasma is administered pre- and postoperatively along with vitamin K_1, 10 mg IM or slowly IV, as soon as possible preoperatively to reverse the effect of warfarin (Coumadin).

CHAPTER

7 Diseases of the Renal System

G. MARK CRAMOLINI, M.D.

Normal renal physiology in the preterm, full-term, and older infant differs significantly from that of the normal adult. Differences in total body water content and distribution, glomerular filtration rate, electrolyte and solute excretion, concentrating ability, and drug distribution and clearance are well known to the anesthesiologist caring for children, and are thoroughly discussed elsewhere.[1, 2] Likewise, the effect of anesthesia on renal function is a topic unto itself and will be discussed here only in the context of interactions with specific renal diseases.

Many hereditary, congenital, and acquired diseases affect the kidney, ureter, bladder, urethra, and genitalia in infants and children. Structural abnormalities often require early surgical intervention for correction. Functional abnormalities may be intrinsic or the result of structural abnormalities or other diseases. The resulting pathophysiological manifestations have important implications for anesthesia.

Many of these disorders lead to chronic renal failure and ultimately to end-stage renal disease. The manifestations of uremia are widespread, involving almost every organ system, and have a myriad of anesthetic implications. An understanding of the pathophysiological changes in renal failure and the resulting anesthetic considerations forms the basis for the detailed anesthetic management of these complex patients. It also provides a background against which the anesthetic implications of specific, less severe renal and genitourinary abnormalities can be readily discussed. We begin, therefore, with a discussion of renal failure in pediatric patients and the consequent anesthetic implications for diagnostic, palliative, and therapeutic surgical interventions, including pediatric renal transplantation.

CHRONIC RENAL FAILURE

Adequate renal function is essential for the functional integrity of the other organ systems. The neonate is provided with approximately 1 million nephrons per kidney. Symptoms of chronic renal failure do not appear until there is destruction of almost 80 percent of the nephrons, and survival is possible with only 2 to 3 percent.[3, 4] Thus renal homeostasis may not be threatened until genitourinary disease is well advanced; on the other hand, by preventing the appearance of symptoms, this adaptive capability may cause treatment to be delayed until significant loss has occurred.

INCIDENCE AND CAUSES

More than 50 different renal diseases may progress to renal failure over time spans of months to decades.[3] The incidence of renal failure in adults shows a striking racial difference, with an incidence of 188 per million blacks and 44 per million whites.[5, 6] Table 7–1 shows the causes of chronic renal failure (CRF) in adults in the United States according to race. Fewer data exist on the incidence and causes of chronic renal failure in children.[7] The entry rate of children into chronic renal failure treatment programs ranges from 1 to 2.4 per million total population per year; of new children entering such programs, 5 percent are under 5 years of age, 26 percent between 5 and 10 years of age, and 69 percent between 10 and 15 years of age.[8] These data reflect only those children who enter a treatment program; those who die without undergoing dialysis are not included. In particular, very few data exist on the mortality from chronic renal failure in children under 5 years of age.[9] Table 7–2 shows the distribution of underlying renal diseases in children entering renal failure treatment programs in Europe in 1978. More recent data show little change in the distribution of etiologies of pediatric chronic renal failure.[7] When the underlying cause is glomerular disease, renal failure in children may progress very rapidly, whereas CRF resulting from urological abnormalities tends to have a more prolonged course. The progression of CRF in infants and children is difficult to predict, but a plot of their glomerular filtration rate (GFR) versus age can give some indication of this rate. Table 7–3 lists the clinical status and need for intervention at different degrees of renal failure as assessed by the GFR.[9] When evaluating plasma creatinine and GFR in infants and children, one must recall that normal values vary with age, as shown in Figure 7–1 and Table 7–4. An empirical approximation for the normal predicted GFR for different-sized patients[10, 11] is given by:

$$GFR = K \frac{L}{P_{creat}}$$

where GFR = glomerular filtration rate in ml/min per 1.73 m^2, L = length (height) in cm, P_{creat} = plasma creatinine in mg/dl, and K = 0.55 in children (aged 1 year and older) or 0.45 in infants (full-term to 1 year).[10] It is important to note that this empirical formula is for patients who are not growth-retarded.

Table 7–1. CAUSES OF CHRONIC RENAL FAILURE IN ADULTS IN THE UNITED STATES

Disease	White (%)	Black (%)	Total (%)
Glomerulonephritis	36	26	31
Hypertension	10	46	28
Diabetes	13	12	13
Interstitial nephropathy	17	5	11
Polycystic disease	9	2	6
Undetermined	7	4	6
Collagen disorders	4	3	4
Others*	4	2	1

*Hereditary disease, neoplasms, other cystic diseases, congenital diseases, gout, amyloidosis, sickle cell disease, radiation, cortical necrosis, trauma.

Reprinted with permission from Kuruvila KC, Schrier RW: Chronic renal failure. Int Anesthesiol Clin *22*:101, 1984.

Table 7–2. PRIMARY RENAL DISEASE IN CHILDREN ENTERING RENAL FAILURE PROGRAMS IN EUROPE, 1978

Disease	Incidence (%)
Glomerulonephritis	34
Pyelonephritis	22
Cystic disease	8
Hereditary nephropathy	8
Renal hypoplasia/dysplasia	11
Renal vascular disease	2
Cortical/tubular necrosis	1
Other*	14

*Principally kidney tumors and the hemolytic-uremic syndrome.

From Barratt TM, Baillod RA: Chronic renal failure and regular dialysis. *In* Williams DI, Johnston JH (Eds.): Paediatric Urology. London, Butterworth Scientific, 1982.

PHYSIOLOGICAL ADAPTATION TO RENAL FAILURE

As there is progressive renal destruction, each remaining nephron must assume a larger workload in order to maintain homeostasis. In the "intact nephron" hypothesis, as nephrons are destroyed, surviving nephrons continue to function normally or "supranormally."[12] The renal function as a whole resembles that of a normal kidney, but with an increased requirement of solute and water diuresis. As a result, the kidney demonstrates a diminished ability to adapt to changes in plasma volume and composition.[13]

The "trade-off" hypothesis proposes that the

Table 7–3. GFR VERSUS CRF STATUS AND INTERVENTION

GFR (ml/min/1.73 m²)	CRF Status	Intervention
80 to 40	Mild, asymptomatic	Follow growth status Detect and treat hypertension
40 to 20	Moderately severe, growth failure probable, risk of osteodystrophy	Careful medical supervision Initiate dietary management
20 to 10	Severe, uremic symptomatology	Tight dietary management to optimize growth Control infection, hypertension, edema, cardiac failure Psychological, social, medical preparation for dialysis and/or transplant
10 or less	Extreme	Need for dialysis or transplantation is imminent

Data from Barratt TM, Baillod RA: Chronic renal failure and regular dialysis. *In* Williams DI, Johnston JH (Eds.): Paediatric urology. London, Butterworth Scientific, 1982.

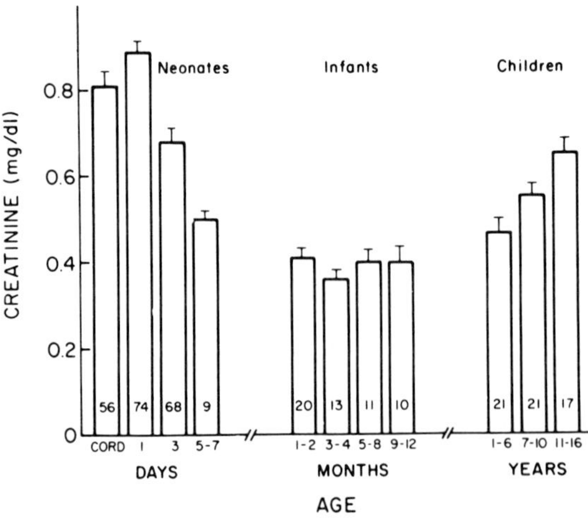

FIGURE 7–1. Normal plasma creatinine concentrations in neonates, infants, and children. Mean plasma creatinine concentration on the ordinate is plotted for the specific age group denoted on the abscissa. Figures within each bar represent numbers of patients studied. Length of the vertical line above the bar corresponds to 1 standard error. (From Schwartz GJ, Feld LG, Langford DJ: A simple estimate of glomerular filtration rate in full-term infants during the first year of life. J Pediatr *104*:849, 1984.)

Table 7–4. NORMAL GLOMERULAR FILTRATION RATE BY AGE

Age	GFR *Mean*	GFR *Range ± 2 SD*
Premature	47	29–65
2–8 days	38	26–60
4–28 days	48	28–68
35–95 days	58	30–86
1–5.9 months	77	41–103
6–11.9 months	103	49–157
12–19 months	127	63–191
2–12 years	127	89–165
Adult male	131	88–174
Adult female	117	87–147

GFR measured in ml/min/1.73 m².

From Barratt TM: Renal function. *In* Williams DJ, Johnston JH (Eds.): Paediatric Urology. London, Butterworth Scientific, 1982.

improved efficiency of individual surviving nephrons comes only at a cost.[14] This cost expresses itself as the clinical manifestations of uremia and renal failure. Examples are raised plasma urea levels, which rise until excretion again matches production; hypertension, which results from an overexpansion of extracellular fluid needed to drive sodium excretion; and hyperparathyroid bone disease, which is a result of increased secretion of parathyroid hormone needed to decrease tubular reabsorption of phosphate.[14]

ANESTHETIC IMPLICATIONS OF THE PATHOPHYSIOLOGICAL MANIFESTATIONS OF RENAL FAILURE

The clinical manifestations of renal failure involve almost every organ system (Table 7–5).

Table 7–5. FEATURES OF CHRONIC RENAL FAILURE AND UREMIA IN CHILDREN

Fatigue, lethargy, somnolence, coma
Anorexia, nausea, vomiting, hematemesis, gastric ulcers
Uremic colitis, diarrhea, melena
Pericarditis, myocardiopathy, cardiac failure
Pleuritis, pulmonary edema, pulmonary hemorrhage
Anemia, thrombasthenia, purpura
Edema, hypertension
Rickets/osteomalacia, osteitis fibrosa, hyperphosphatemia, hypocalcemia, hyperparathyroidism, pruritus
Hyperkalemia, metabolic acidosis, hyperuricemia
Glucose intolerance
Peripheral neuropathy
Impaired immunological competence
Retardation of growth and maturation

From Lewy PR, Hurley JK: Chronic renal insufficiency. Pediatr Clin North Am *23*:829, 1976.

Since most of these manifestations have implications for anesthesia, we will detail them individually and follow with the anesthetic considerations for each.

SODIUM AND WATER EXCRETION

As GFR decreases, less sodium and water are filtered and available for excretion. To compensate for this, the fractional excretion (the portion filtered that is excreted) of sodium and water increases. This occurs because of Na^+ and H_2O retention leading to an expanded extracellular fluid (ECF) volume and effective arterial volume. Volume receptors that modulate Na^+ reabsorption then cause a decrease in reabsorption of the filtered Na^+ and thus an increase in Na^+ excretion. The detector and effector mechanisms involved in this natriuresis include the juxtaglomerular apparatus and the renin-angiotensin-aldosterone system,[15, 16] redistribution of renal blood flow and glomerular filtrate,[16, 17] intrarenal hemodynamic changes,[18] and a "natriuretic hormone,"[19–21] which is now known to be secreted by the atrium ("atrial natriuretic factor" or "atrial natriuretic peptide").[22–24] In fact, plasma atrial natriuretic peptide (ANP) levels have been found to be elevated in volume-overloaded children with chronic renal failure.[25] Volume-mediated hypertension may result as a "trade-off" for this adaption.[26, 27]

Several patterns of abnormal sodium and water excretion exist in infants and children in renal failure, and these are somewhat characteristic for the underlying renal lesion.[28] In congenital renal dysplasia and urinary obstructive diseases, the renal medullary concentrating mechanism may be poorly developed or damaged. A state resembling nephrogenic diabetes insipidus may ensue in which there is excretion of large volumes of dilute urine low in sodium content. Affected infants will often cry until provided fluids, but since babies are generally assumed to be frequently "wet," their large volumes of urinary output may not be obvious unless measured. If fluid intake is decreased owing to illness, these infants are at high risk for severe dehydration. Routine NPO orders preoperatively may be particularly dangerous. Recent studies have reappraised the need for long periods of preoperative oral fluid restriction. In normal children, drinking clear liquids up to 2 hours prior to anesthetic induction did not substantially change the volume or pH of gastric fluid content.[29, 30] This additional fluid intake may be significantly beneficial to those children with obligate urinary fluid losses. If significant uremia exists, however, gastric emptying may be prolonged[31] and routine NPO regimens with preoperative intravenous fluid supplementation are indicated. Serial weights and accurate intake and output measurements are necessary to manage fluids properly in these children.

In chronic glomerulonephritis, there may be a greater reduction in glomerular filtration than in tubular reabsorption, causing glomerulotubular imbalance.[28] Sodium and water retention may lead to hypertension, congestive failure, and pulmonary edema. Peripheral edema may be exacerbated by hypoproteinemia secondary to marked proteinuria. The volume of urinary production may be normal but with a fixed osmolality that may be equal to (isosthenuria) or, in advanced renal failure, less than (hyposthenuria) plasma osmolality.[32] Sodium restriction, diuretics, and antihypertensives are useful in limiting edema and ameliorating hypertension.[33]

A third pattern of abnormal salt and water excretion is that of salt wasting, accompanied by an inability to concentrate or dilute the urine. This is seen in some children with chronic pyelonephritis, sickle cell nephropathy, hydronephrosis, or medullary cystic disease.[28] Sodium reabsorption is defective primarily in the distal nephron, resulting in large volumes of urine high in sodium content (60 to 120 mEq/L). These children will spontaneously ingest large amounts of sodium, and sodium restriction can quickly lead to severe hyponatremic dehydration. Proper fluid management is based on careful measurement of the obligatory urinary loss and urine sodium content.

With end-stage renal disease, GFR has decreased to the point that excretion of normal sodium and water loads is not possible. Sodium and water retention leads to edema and vascular congestion and may result in pulmonary edema, hypertension, and congestive heart failure. These symptoms can be controlled with careful water and sodium restriction. When problems in fluid management are severe, peritoneal dialysis or hemodialysis may be necessary. Special attention to the management of sodium intake is needed in all these patients. Even in end-stage renal failure, if there is urine output, then there is an obligate urinary sodium loss. This is attributable to the increased filtered load of sulfates and phosphates, which require excretion of Na^+ as the primary accompanying cation, and to the osmotic diuresis of solutes per remaining nephron.[34] Because of edema and hypertension, the diagnosis of excessive sodium intake is easily made. Inadequate sodium intake, on the other hand, results in symptoms that are subtle and may be overlooked without a high index of suspicion. This diagnosis is important to make, however, since overzealous sodium restriction or sudden sodium losses may result in a contracted extracellular fluid volume, a decreased GFR, and an exacerbation of uremia.[35] The relative hypovolemia that exists represents an unexpected hazard at the time of anesthetic induction.

The pathophysiological abnormalities of sodium and water homeostasis just described hold several implications for the anesthetic management of these children. They cannot compensate for incorrect sodium and water administration pre-, intra-, or postoperatively. The preoperative evaluation of volume status is essential. Edema and hypertension are signs of sodium and water overload that will require preoperative sodium and fluid restriction, diuretics, antihypertensives, and/or dialysis. As noted, a high index of suspicion is needed to detect a state of sodium depletion. Clues to this are a worsening in uremic symptoms and signs of hypovolemia, such as orthostatic changes in pulse and blood pressure or a decreased requirement for antihypertensives. Children with obligate urinary losses due to renal disease, who present with an acute illness preventing intake or causing large sodium and water losses (for example, bowel obstruction or gastroenteritis) may suffer profound hypovolemia. They will require preoperative fluid resuscitation, based on clinical signs (as given in Table 7–6) or a knowledge of the magnitude of an acute weight loss. This may be accomplished with normal saline[36] or Ringer's lactate, but a solution of the following composition has been suggested as being one that simulates ECF more exactly: isotonic sodium chloride, 800 ml, plus 22 mEq of sodium bicarbonate, plus 5 percent dextrose in water to a total volume of 1 liter (Na^+ = 140 mEq/L, Cl^- = 118 mEq/L, HCO_3 = 22 mEq/L).[35] Careful monitoring during ECF expansion is necessary to avoid fluid overload.

Table 7–6. CLINICAL ESTIMATES OF VOLUME DEFICITS IN INFANTS AND YOUNG CHILDREN

Sign	Percent Deficit	Volume of Deficit per Kilogram of Body Weight
Dry oral mucous membranes Absent tears	5	50 ml
Decreased skin turgor ("tenting") Depressed fontanelle	10	100 ml
Shock	15	150 ml

Reprinted with permission from Nash MA: Water and solute homeostasis. *In* Edelmann CM Jr (Ed.): Pediatric Kidney Disease. Boston, Little, Brown, 1978.

Even if volume status is normal, it is important to determine which pattern of abnormal sodium and water excretion the child demonstrates, since this will influence perioperative fluid management. The underlying lesion causing renal failure may provide a clue to the pattern of sodium and water excretion, but a more accurate method is to assess ongoing intake and output, urine and serum osmolalities and electrolytes, and serial weights. If an obligate large urinary water and/or sodium loss exists, then an intravenous fluid and electrolyte regimen based on the foregoing assessment should be instituted prior to making the patient NPO preoperatively. One such regimen, which is useful for most situations, including anuria, is as follows: Insensible losses (based on 45 ml per 100 kcal metabolized[37] or approximately 30 ml/kg/day for infants up to 1 year of age and 20 ml/kg/day to a maximum of 500 ml in older children[28]) are replaced IV with 10 percent dextrose in water. (Caloric expenditure may be calculated as 100 kcal/kg for the first 10 kg, 50 kcal/kg for the next 10 kg, and 20 kcal/kg for each additional kilogram.)[37] "Piggy-backed" into this is an IV solution that is equal in electrolyte composition to the urine produced and is run milliliter for milliliter to replace urinary losses. Important to remember when utilizing this regimen is that any other fluid losses (such as NG, CSF, or stool) must also be quantified in volume and electrolyte composition and replaced. Adjustment to the rate for insensible losses may need to be made, based on whether inspired gases are dry (increasing the losses) or humidified (decreasing the losses), as well as for other variables shown in Table 7–7. Serial determinations of serum and urine electrolytes and osmolality, with appropriate modification of IV therapy, are a cornerstone of fluid management of these patients while NPO pre-, intra-, and postoperatively. Intraoperative blood losses and fluid shifts may further complicate fluid management. It is imperative to remember that when urinary output is obligatory, it is *not* a reflection of the child's volume status. For this reason, central venous pressure assessment of volume status is frequently a useful tool perioperatively.

Table 7–7. MODIFICATION OF FLUID REQUIREMENT DUE TO PHYSIOLOGICAL ALTERATIONS

Reason for Modification	Modification Required
Altered Metabolic Rate	
Fever	Increase water allowance by 12% per °C increase in body temperature
Hypermetabolic states	Increase water allowance by 25–75%
Decreased Metabolic Rate	
Hypothermia	Decrease water allowance by 12% per °C decrease in body temperature
Hypometabolic states	Decrease water allowance by 10–25%
Sweating	
Mild-to-moderate sweating	Add 10–25 ml/100 kcal for water loss and an additional 0.5–1.0 mEq sodium and chloride per 100 kcal
Sweating in cystic fibrosis	Increase water allowance by same amount as in normal subjects but allow 1–2 mEq/100 kcal additional sodium and chloride

Modified and reprinted with permission from Nash MA: Water and solute homeostasis. *In* Edelmann CM Jr (Ed.): Pediatric Kidney Disease. Boston, Little, Brown, 1978. Adapted from Winters RW: Principles of Pediatric Fluid Therapy. North Chicago, Abbott Laboratories, 1975.

HYPERKALEMIA

The chronically failing kidney has the capacity to increase K^+ secretion by the distal tubule, decrease fractional reabsorption of K^+, and thereby increase K^+ excretion per nephron as much as sixfold.[28] This, coupled with increased fecal loss of K^+, makes hyperkalemia rare until very late in chronic renal failure. Hyperkalemia in a child with renal failure with a usual GFR of more than 10 ml/min/1.73 m^2 should alert one to an acute deterioration. Alternatively, hyperkalemia could be due to increased catabolism, metabolic acidosis, dietary K^+ excess, GI hemorrhage with absorption of K^+, potassium-sparing diuretics, angiotensin antagonists, converting enzyme inhibitors that decrease aldosterone availability, suppression of aldosterone production by heparin (even at low doses),[38] K^+ salts of drugs (such as penicillin), constipation due to phosphate binders that decrease fecal K^+ excretion, and so forth.[4, 34]

With anuria, potassium accumulates at a rate of 0.4 to 0.8 mEq/L/day, and the rate may be increased by acidosis, infection, hemolysis, and malnutrition.[39] The major concern with hyperkalemia is its effects on cardiac rhythm and function. These are mediated by the effect of the intra- to extracellular concentration gradient of K^+ ions on transmembrane potential and may occur at different serum K^+ levels, depending on the rate of potassium accumulation. For this reason, different researchers recommend different serum K^+ levels at which to be concerned (serum K^+ = 7.0 mEq/L,[39] serum K^+ = 6.5 mEq/L,[28] serum K^+ = 5.5 mEq/L[40]). All agree, however, that ECG monitoring provides insight into the status of the transmembrane potential, and that ECG changes are an indication for aggressive therapy. Figure 7–2 shows the ECG changes associated with progressive hyperkalemia,[41] and Table 7–8 lists the therapeutic regimens used to treat hyperkalemia in children aggressively. In treating children,

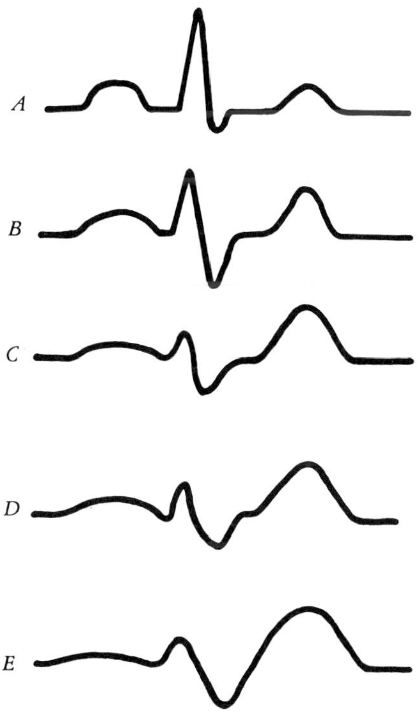

FIGURE 7–2. Electrocardiographic changes associated with progressive hyperkalemia. *A,* Normal pattern. *B,* Slight prolongation of P wave, decrease in R wave, and increase in amplitude and peaking of T wave. *C,* Flattening of P wave, widening of QRS, and further increase in T-wave amplitude. *D,* Marked flattening and prolongation of P wave; wide, low-voltage QRS; and wide, tall T wave. *E,* Sine wave pattern due to marked widening and slowing of QRS, depression of S-T segment, and increased amplitude of T wave. (Reprinted with permission from Rudolph AM: Disturbances of the cardiovascular system. *In* Edelmann CM Jr [Ed.]: Pediatric Kidney Disease. Boston, Little, Brown, 1978.)

Table 7–8. REGIMENS FOR THE TREATMENT OF HYPERKALEMIA

Regimen	Dosage and Route	Onset and Duration	Mode of Action	Comments
Calcium gluconate 10% (100 mg/ml = 9 mg elemental Ca/ml) Calcium chloride 10% (100 mg/ml = 27 mg elemental Ca/ml)	5 to 10 mg elemental Ca/kg IV slowly	Immediate onset Transient duration	Stabilizes myocardial membrane, no change in serum K^+	Monitor ECG May cause bradycardia if given as bolus Tissue damage with extravasation Precipitates with $NaHCO_3$
$NaHCO_3$ 8.4% (1 mEq HCO_3^-/ml)	1–3 mEq/kg IV bolus (Dilute 1:1 with sterile water and give slowly in prematures and neonates)	Rapid onset Short-term duration	K^+ enters cells in exchange for H^+	Monitor ECG Large osmotic shift with IV bolus associated with intraventricular hemorrhage in prematures Tissue damage with extravasation Precipitates with CA^{++}
Regular insulin and glucose	Give 3 g glucose/L of ECF to lower K^+ by 1 mEq/L Insulin:glucose ratio of 1 unit:3 grams. Give ½ dose to achieve desired serum K^+ IV over 10 min or by infusion	Moderate onset Longer duration	Promotes K^+ entry into cells with glucose	Monitor ECG Monitor for hypoglycemia with serial glucoses Monitor serial serum K^+ Adjust insulin:glucose ratio based on serum glucose
Sodium polystyrene sulfonate (Kayexalate) Mix 1 g/4 ml of 70% sorbitol for oral use (nonconstipating) and 1 g/4 ml of $D_{10}W$ for rectal use	1 g/kg (each gram will exchange ~ 1 mEq K^+). (Warm the enemas, especially in small infants)	Slow onset Enema needs to be retained at least 50 min, the longer the better Initial results in 2–4 h, may repeat q4h	Na^+ on resin is exchanged for K^+ in large bowel	1–2 mEq Na^+ absorbed/g of resin. Observe for overload Also exchanges Ca^{++} and Mg^{++} Constipating (sorbitol 70% helps) Concretions with aluminum hydroxide may cause intestinal obstruction Monitor serum K^+, Ca^{++}, Mg^{++}, Na^+ Total body depletion of K^+ may not be reflected in serum K^+. Observe for weakness, ECG changes of prolonged QT, wide, flat or inverted T, prominent U waves, with prolonged use
Dialysis (peritoneal dialysis and hemodialysis)		May take time to arrange, especially if peritoneal catheter or hemodialysis access sites are not already available	Ion exchange across peritoneal membrane or dialysis membrane	BP, ECG, electrolyte monitors Done under supervision of pediatric nephrologist and experienced nursing and technical personnel Most effective means of decreasing total body K^+ Serum K^+ may not reflect total body K^+ immediately post dialysis Monitor ECG

Data from Lewy and Hurley,[28] Trainin and Spitzer,[39] and Jordan and Lemire.[468]

one must be careful not to be misled by false elevations in serum K^+. This is not an uncommon occurrence, because of the difficulty in obtaining blood samples, and may result from hemolysis induced by small sampling needles or from tissue breakdown products contaminating "heel-stick" samples.

Most workers recommend preoperative treatment of serum K^+ in excess of 5.5 mEq/L.[40, 42] This conservative value is chosen out of a concern about intraoperative rises in serum K^+ due to tissue catabolism, further intraoperative renal deterioration (due to hypovolemia, hypotension, or surgical misadventure), transfusion, acidosis, or infection. Succinylcholine will raise serum K^+ by 0.5 to 0.7 mEq/L in normal subjects when given as a bolus dose of 1 mg/kg, and this increase is not ameliorated by pretreatment with curare.[43, 44] This increase is not made larger by the presence of renal failure, and for this reason a single dose of succinylcholine in patients in renal failure whose serum K^+ is less than 5.5 mEq/L has been considered safe.[45, 46] On the other hand, increases by as much as 2.4 mEq/L have been reported with repeated doses of succinylcholine.[43, 47] Although one controlled study could demonstrate only a rise of less than 0.6 mEq/L in serum K^+,[48] the safety of multiple doses of succinylcholine is debated. The effects of succinylcholine on serum K^+ in patients with uremic neuropathy are unpredictable, and perhaps this explains the difference in these observations. It has been suggested that in the presence of uremic neuropathy succinylcholine should be avoided altogether.[45, 49]

ACIDOSIS

Children produce 1.5 to 2.0 mEq/kg/day of acid (almost twice that of adults[50, 51]), and 20 mEq of hydrogen ion is released for each gram of calcium deposition in new bone.[52] With a decrease in the GFR to about 20 ml/min/1.73 m^2, retention of fixed acid occurs,[53] resulting in a fall in serum HCO_3 by as much as 1 to 2 mEq/L/day.[54] Renal compensatory mechanisms include tubular hydrogen ion secretion and urinary acidification, proximal and distal tubular reabsorption of HCO_3^-, excretion of titratable acid, and ammonium production and excretion.[55–57] All of these may be defective in CRF. The primary cause of metabolic acidosis, however, is thought to be a deficiency in total production of urinary ammonia, which decreases in proportion to the fall in GFR even though each remaining nephron secretes more than normally.[53, 55] In a few children with CRF, bicarbonate wasting may also add to acidosis.[58] Other compensatory mechanisms that come into play are buffering by calcium phosphate of bone, resulting in bone dissolution and increased urinary excretion of Ca^{++};[59] secondary hyperparathyroidism, which increases the tubular excretion of titratable acids and mobilizes extrarenal buffer in bone;[60] and respiratory alkalosis. Large anion gap metabolic acidosis is seen with retention of sulfates and phosphates. Hyperchloremic acidosis may also be seen, especially if a sodium deficit has been corrected with sodium chloride alone (see earlier section on Sodium and Water Excretion). Chronic acidosis has been shown to be deleterious in children, especially retarding growth.[61]

For the anesthesiologist, the major concern is that a child with a low P_{CO_2} and serum HCO_3^- is extremely vulnerable to any further metabolic insult. Diarrhea with HCO_3^- loss, catabolic states, hypoglycemia, cold and hypotension with poor tissue perfusion, as well as lactic acidosis, may cause a precipitous and life-threatening fall in arterial pH.[4] Hyperkalemia may also be seriously increased by acidosis.[62] Serum levels of bicarbonate of less than 15 should be corrected preoperatively by dialysis if time allows,[60] or by administration of sodium bicarbonate, in which 1 mEq/kg of HCO_3 can be expected to raise the serum HCO_3 acutely by approximately 2 mEq/L.[39] It has been recommended that the same degree of hyperventilation should be maintained intraoperatively as was present preoperatively.[64]

HYPOCALCEMIA, HYPERPHOSPHATEMIA, AND RENAL OSTEODYSTROPHY

The normal homeostasis of serum calcium, phosphate, and bone metabolism depends on a complex interplay of many factors: dietary intake; gastrointestinal and renal reabsorption and secretion; acid-base balance; parathyroid hormone; calcitonin; vitamin D intake and metabolic conversion in skin, liver, and kidney; and the influence of other hormones such as somatomedin, thyroid hormone, estrogens, and androgens.[60, 65] The interaction and feedback control in this complex system are only partially understood, but it is known that the kidney plays a central role as a primary controller of calcium and phosphate excretion and reabsorption, as a target organ for endocrine control systems, as a metabolic activator of vitamin D, and as the site of degradation of parathyroid hormone and calcitonin. It is not surprising, therefore, that renal failure has a profound effect on calcium, phosphate, and bone metabolism. It is a tribute to the feedback control mechanism, given the central role of Ca^{++} in so many processes essential to life, that a fatal outcome is delayed.

It is also not surprising that in growing children renal osteodystrophy occurs more frequently than in adults. In one study, almost half the children receiving hemodialysis in preparation for transplantation met radiological criteria for renal osteodystrophy—twice the figure for adults.[66] Renal osteodystrophy is more frequent and severe in children whose renal failure has occurred early in life as a result of congenital nephropathies or obstructive uropathies and has persisted many years before treatment of the bone disease. Abnormalities in renal osteodystrophy include osteopenia or generalized demineralization, osteitis fibrosa, osteosclerosis, rickets, and metastatic calcification. Secondary hyperparathyroidism may occur when GFR falls to 45 ml/min/1.73 m^2.[67] Although symptoms may appear at any age, the peak incidence is in the 5- to 10-year age range.[60]

The pathogenesis of renal osteodystrophy is as complex as the normal homeostatic mechanisms outlined earlier; a simplified overview is shown in Figure 7–3. As the filtered load of phosphate falls, remaining nephrons are unable to increase their fractional excretion of phosphate adequately, and hyperphosphatemia occurs. Serum calcium falls in a reciprocal manner, causing increased parathyroid hormone secretion. Concomitantly, the conversion of 25-hydroxy vitamin D to 1,25-hydroxy vitamin D in the kidney is impaired by renal disease and possibly by metabolic acidosis in renal failure.[68] The result is hypocalcemia, hyperphosphatemia, and renal osteodystrophy.

The first step in treatment is to lower serum phosphate. Dietary restriction and oral administration of aluminum hydroxide (60 mg/kg/day) is effective,[69] although there is some evidence that aluminum toxicity may be contributory in renal osteodystrophy.[70] Calcium administration in the face of hyperphosphatemia is ineffective and may cause metastatic calcification.[39] Once serum phosphate is in an acceptable range (3 to 5 mg/dl), dietary supplementation with calcium carbonate not only supplies additional calcium but aids in correcting acidosis.[60] Vitamin D therapy may then be instituted, with careful monitoring of serum Ca^{++} levels. 1,25-Hydroxy vitamin D_3 is frequently used, not only because lower doses of this end-product are needed but also because of the very rapid turnover, which allows more rapid resolution of hypercalcemic toxicity when overdose occurs.[65] If these measures fail to lower parathyroid hormone, subtotal parathyroidectomy is considered.[71] With renal transplantation, vitamin D metabolism, parathyroid hormone, and somatomedin levels normalize and osteodystrophy heals, but growth may continue to be impaired owing to immunosuppressive steroid therapy,[60] which may also weaken bone.

For the anesthesiologist, the foregoing problems have several implications. Hypocalcemia may be present, although it is usually not symptomatic. Treatment should be directed at lowering serum phosphorus, and if this is urgent, dialysis is indicated. In emergency cases in which symptoms of hypocalcemia are present, or when it is difficult to rule out hypocalcemia as a cause of seizures, intravenous calcium may be given slowly, although its effectiveness may be short-term and repeated doses may result in metastatic calcification.[39] Hypocalcemia has been reported to prolong postoperative neuromuscular relaxation,[72] but there are many other reasons why this might occur in renal failure patients (see later).

Anesthesia for parathyroidectomy must include consideration of the manifestations of the

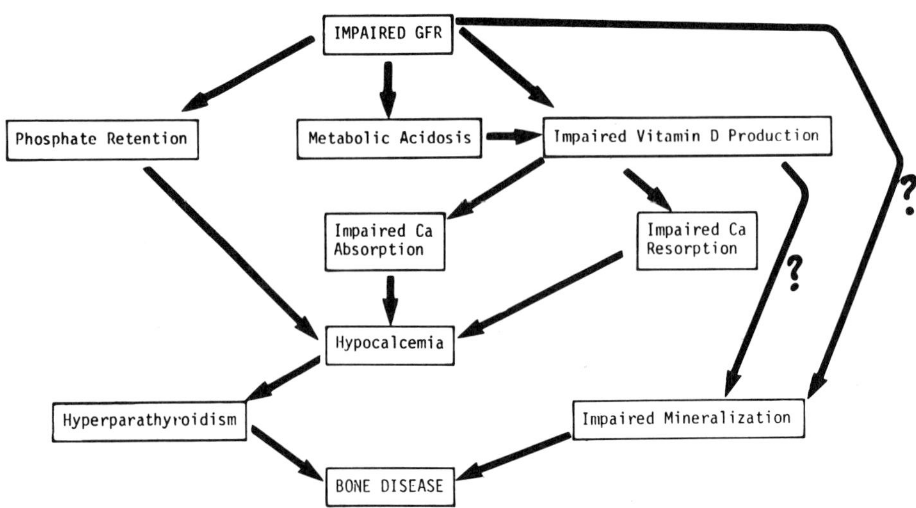

FIGURE 7–3. Pathogenic factors in renal osteodystrophy. (From Norman ME: Vitamin D in bone disease. Pediatr Clin North Am *29*:947, 1982.)

renal disease as well as consideration of surgery in the region of the airway.[73] Hypocalcemic seizures and tetany may occur postoperatively if serum Ca^{++} is not closely followed. Hypocalcemia is treated with Ca^{++} supplements and vitamin D.[4] In children with severe osteodystrophy or a history of chronic steroid therapy (see Chapter 12), care must be taken with intraoperative positioning to avoid fractures.

HYPERMAGNESEMIA

Infants and children with chronic renal failure usually have serum magnesium levels in the normal range (1.9 to 2.5 mg/dl). Hypermagnesemia is a rare finding,[41] but it may occur when the GFR falls below 10 ml/min/1.73 m^2, especially if the patient is receiving magnesium-containing antacids.[74] Very high magnesium levels may lead to neuromuscular weakness, respiratory depression, refractory hypotension, and coma[75] and will potentiate the neuromuscular blockade of both depolarizing and nondepolarizing muscle relaxants.[76] Dialysis will effectively lower serum magnesium, and intravenous calcium administration will acutely antagonize the neuromuscular effects.[63]

ANEMIA

Anemia is a consistent finding in CRF when the serum creatinine rises above 3 mg/dl[77] and is poorly correlated to the degree of uremia.[78] The degree of anemia varies, with hemoglobin levels ranging from 5 to 10 gm/dl. It is usually a normocytic and normochromic anemia with a normal reticulocyte count.[79] Slowed erythropoiesis is attributed to decreased renal production of erythropoietin,[80] to operation at a lower setpoint of the tissue oxygenation-erythropoietin-hematocrit feedback mechanism,[81] and to circulating inhibitors that may be removed by dialysis.[82, 83]

Red cell survival is also decreased.[84] In vitro autohemolysis studies[85] and human cross-transfusion studies show that it is the uremic plasma and not a defect of the red blood cell that causes the short survival.[86] Several byproducts of the urea cycle (for example, guanidines) are elevated in uremia and have been implicated as toxins, possibly inhibiting normal red blood cell enzymes (such as transketolase and various glucolytic enzymes needed for energy production).[87–90] The acquired abnormalities of the pentose phosphate pathway put these patients at risk for increased hemolysis when exposed to oxidizing drugs such as quinidine, primaquine, and sulfonamides.[4]

Microangiopathic changes are seen only when CRF is severe.[91] It is important to remember that anemia from blood loss (gastrointestinal, frequent venipuncture, dialysis) and from nutritional deficiencies (due to anorexia or removal by dialysis) may be superimposed on the chronic anemia in growing children. These additional factors should be diagnosed and treated with iron, folate, and vitamin B_6 supplementation.[28]

Compensatory mechanisms for anemia include an increased cardiac output and a shift in the oxygen-hemoglobin dissociation curve to improve tissue O_2 delivery. 2,3-Diphosphoglycerate (2,3-DPG) levels do increase in CRF, but not to the degree expected for the anemia present.[92] This may be because metabolic acidosis, although directly shifting the oxygen-hemoglobin dissociation curve to the right by the Bohr effect, also decreases 2,3-DPG levels.[63] A study of the hemoglobin P_{50} values in anemic, dialyzed patients showed no significant difference from normals.[93]

Infants and children with CRF tolerate their anemia remarkably well, and routine transfusions are rarely required.[79] It was once feared that transfusion would cause sensitization to histocompatibility antigens and threaten future graft survival. The opposite has now been shown to be true.[94] Repeated pretransplant transfusions improve graft survival slightly with frozen washed cells, significantly with packed red blood cells (from 50 to 68 percent), and remarkably with whole blood (from 49 to 89 percent).[95, 96]

Therapy for anemia in chronic renal failure includes dialysis and treatment of deficiencies in iron, folate, and vitamin B_6.[97] Recombinant human erythropoietin is now available for use, although studies suggest that the erythropoietic response is subnormal and dependent on the severity of uremia.[98–100] Renal transplantation dramatically raises serum erythropoietin, reticulocytes, and hemoglobin.[101] In addition, restoration of renal function markedly improves the response to erythropoietin, such that slight increases in endogenous erythropoietin levels induce erythropoiesis to the same magnitude as large doses of recombinant exogenous erythropoietin in uremic patients.[100]

Except for pretransplantation, multiple transfusions are not advisable because of risks of hemosiderosis, suppression of erythropoiesis, development of anti–red blood cell antibodies, hemolytic reactions, volume overload, and blood-borne infection. If transfusion is urgently required to raise the hematocrit, packed red blood cells (pRBCs) achieve this with the lowest volume. Frozen pRBCs have the lowest potassium content (1 to 2 mEq/L for frozen pRBCs as opposed to 18 to 26 mEq/L in citrated pRBCs).[102] Citrated cells may also further lower serum Ca^{++} in an already hypocalcemic patient. The decision to transfuse preoperatively depends on the child's overall condition, associated problems, such as the presence of cardiac or pulmonary disease, and the anticipated risk of surgical blood loss. It has been suggested that no patient with a hemoglobin level of less than 5 g/dl should be anesthetized.[42]

It is also important to remember that anemic children with CRF appear pale rather than cyanotic when hypoxemic, because of their low hemoglobin levels. Arterial blood gas measurement and pulse oximetry are the best ways to document adequate arterial oxygenation. Increased inspired O_2 concentrations will help guard against subtle hypoxemia in anemic children whose O_2 transport capability is diminished.

The blood gas partition coefficient of halothane is decreased by 15 to 25 percent with anemia, and alveolar concentrations approach inspired concentrations more quickly, leading to more rapid induction and emergence.[103] The need to maintain an increased cardiac output to compensate for the decreased oxygen-carrying capacity, as well as impaired myocardial function in chronic renal failure, contraindicates the use of high inspired halothane concentration and controlled ventilation during a mask induction. Spontaneous ventilation with gradual titration of halothane concentration will help preserve venous return and cardiac output if this induction technique is chosen. Frequently, concerns about regurgitation and aspiration call for an intravenous induction (see later). Regardless of the technique chosen, anesthetics and positive-pressure ventilation should be utilized in a manner that ensures adequate venous return and cardiac output.

Coagulopathy

Bleeding in chronic renal failure may be a result of capillary fragility caused by malnutrition or steroid therapy, irritation of mucosal and serosal surfaces by uremic toxins, and abnormal platelet number and function. Depression of specific clotting factors and prolongation of prothrombin time (PT) and partial thromboplastin times (PTTs) have been reported but are rare.[79] Prolongation of coagulation times preoperatively should alert one to the possibility of residual or rebound heparinization, which can occur up to 10 hours after dialysis.[104] The incidence of this may be greatly reduced with regional heparinization, and any residual heparin effect may be reversed with protamine.[105]

Platelets are sometimes decreased in number, but rarely below 50,000/μl, and platelet survival is normal, indicating that the problem is reduced production.[106] The most significant hemostatic defect, however, is a reversible platelet malfunction attributed to dialyzable uremic compounds. Guanidinosuccinic acid concentrations are elevated enough in uremia to inhibit ADP-induced activation of platelet factor III, which normally promotes platelet adhesion.[107] Phenol and phenolic acids have also been implicated.[108] Defects of clot retraction, decreased adhesiveness, impaired aggregation, and diminished platelet factor III have all been demonstrated[109, 110] and fortunately seem to be induced by plasma factors that are removable by hemodialysis or peritoneal dialysis.[111]

Patients with creatinine levels that are still below 6 mg/dl usually have normal platelet function.[112] However, if the child is dialyzed, it is wise to check coagulation studies for platelet function and heparin effect. If the PT and PTT are elevated, the thrombin time is a more specific test to elucidate residual heparin effect.[113] This may be reversed with protamine. The bleeding time correlates well with the danger of hemorrhage and should be measured preoperatively.

Dialysis reverses the platelet dysfunction and is advisable preoperatively. Platelet transfusions should be reserved for the treatment of symptomatic deficits, since they otherwise produce only transient improvement.[114] This is not surprising, since the plasma factors causing the reversible platelet dysfunction persist and presumably have a similar pathological effect on the freshly transfused platelets. On the other hand, transfusion of cryoprecipitate has been shown to shorten the bleeding time for about 12 hours, with return to original prolonged times by 24 to 36 hours.[115]

Infusion of deamino-8-D-arginine vasopressin (DDAVP), at a rate of 0.3 μg/kg in normal saline over 30 minutes, has been shown to shorten the bleeding time. The effect occurs 90 minutes after infusion and lasts about 4 hours.[116, 117] DDAVP given by nasal insufflation is also being studied for this effect.[4] In emergency cases when preoperative dialysis is not possible, these measures may be helpful. More study of the mode of action, the time course and efficacy, and side effects of vasopressin is needed before its routine use can be recommended. If major intraoperative bleeding is anticipated, then warmed platelet concentrate, packed red cells and fresh frozen plasma, or fresh whole blood should be available. Adequate intravenous lines should be established to administer these products; in the infant or small child this may require a saphenous or antecubital cut-down.

Regional anesthesia, spinal or epidural, has been advocated for adults with renal failure, including those undergoing transplantation.[118–120] Regional techniques are being increasingly used in children and, if contemplated, must raise consideration of the risk of bleeding, as well as of possible infection.

INFECTION

Infection and sepsis are serious problems in patients with renal failure and may lead to death.[121, 122] In vitro studies demonstrate an impaired immunological status in uremia.[123] Infection may increase caloric requirements and worsen azotemia, hyperkalemia, hyperphosphatemia, and acidosis. It may delay wound healing, lead to pyelonephritis, and further impair renal function. Septic shock may decrease renal perfusion and GFR with grave consequences. The most common site of infection is the urinary tract, followed by the lungs, surgical wounds, and blood. The organisms most often isolated are *Staphylococcus aureus* and various gram-negative bacilli. Treatment may be hampered by poor urinary excretion of bactericidal drugs and because of drug resistance.[39, 124] Care must be taken to use aseptic technique when placing intravenous cannulae or invasive monitors in these children.

Up to 55 percent of patients on hemodialysis are hepatitis B antigen carriers.[125] This appears to be caused not only by their frequent exposure to dialysis equipment and blood products but also by depressed interferon production, which predisposes them to becoming chronic carriers.[126] Because transmission can occur with mucosal as well as percutaneous exposure to infected secretions or blood, anesthesiologists should protect themselves appropriately and treat needle sticks seriously.[127] Hepatitis B immune globulin is effective for protection after known inoculation. Because the hepatitis B risk to anesthesiologists is five to eight times that of the general population and similar to that of other medical personnel frequently exposed to blood, vaccination against hepatitis B has been recommended.[128, 129] Hepatitis B vaccination has also been tried in chronic dialysis patients, with 80 percent developing antibodies after a booster dose 6 months later (as compared with 98 percent in persons not on dialysis).[130]

CARDIOVASCULAR MANIFESTATIONS

Hypertension. A major manifestation of renal failure is hypertension, which affects many children with advanced CRF.[131, 132] Eight separate but interacting mechanisms for the autoregulation of blood pressure have been proposed: baroreceptors (in the aorta and carotid sinus), chemoreceptors (carotid and aortic arteries), the CNS (the vasomotor center), the renin-angiotensin-aldosterone system (involving kidney, plasma, liver, adrenals, and lung), a stretch receptor mechanism (in arteriolar muscle), a capillary transudation mechanism (with transudation decreasing circulating volume), the renal-ECF mechanism (involving renal water and salt retention, independent of aldosterone effects), and a vasodilation mechanism (an ill-defined blood pressure–lowering role of the kidney).[133] Although hypertension may involve any of these interacting control mechanisms to some degree, it has been attributed primarily to abnormalities in renal-ECF regulation. Fluid overload, the renin-angiotensin-aldosterone system (Fig. 7–4), and perhaps the deficiency of a vasodilator substance released by normal kidneys may also be involved.[134–136]

Diagnosis of hypertension (BP > 95th percentile) is important in children with renal failure. Treatment is effective in preventing cerebral and cardiac involvement and in slowing the progression of renal failure due to hypertension, independent of the original disease.[132, 137, 138]

Figures 7–5, 7–6, and 7–7 show normal blood pressures and percentile ranges in neonates, infants, children, and adolescents.[139–141] The report of the second Task Force on Blood Pressure Control in Children was published in 1987 and further refines the above blood pressure guidelines.[142] Proper equipment and technique are required for reliable measurements. The cuff should be appropriate for the size of the child's arm, covering two thirds of the length of the upper arm. The bladder should encircle more than half the arm over the brachial artery.[138, 139, 141] In infants, flush pressure (the cuff pressure at which capillary refilling occurs) approximates mean arterial pressure,[143] but Doppler ultrasound provides systolic pressure more accurately and reproducibly.[144, 145] If blood pressure is measured using Korotkoff's sounds, the best index of diastolic pressure in children is the

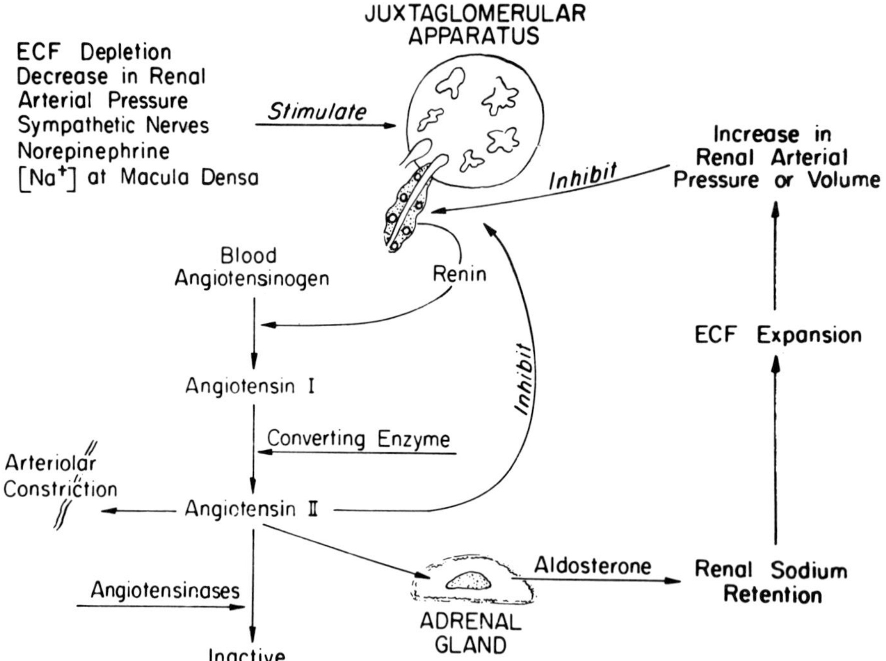

FIGURE 7–4. The juxtaglomerular apparatus and control of renin secretion. (Reprinted with permission from Mulrow PJ, Siegel NJ: Mechanisms in hypertension. *In* Edelmann CM Jr [Ed.]: Pediatric Kidney Disease. Boston, Little, Brown, 1978.)

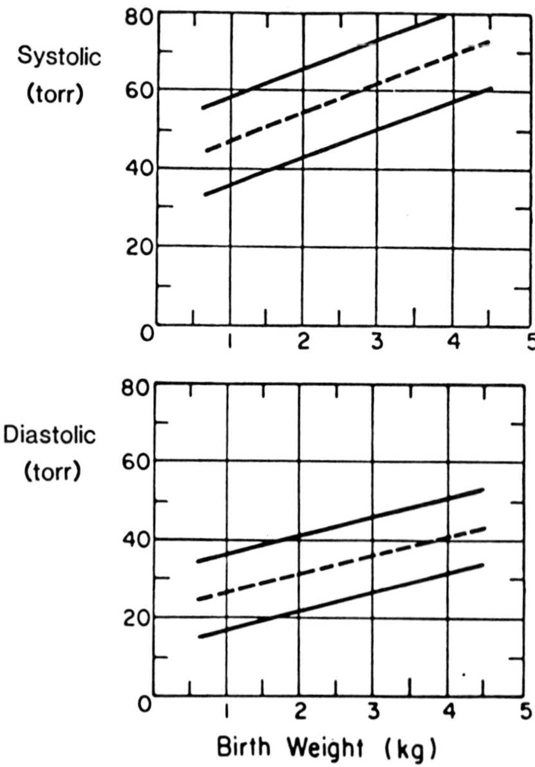

FIGURE 7–5. Linear regressions *(broken lines)* and 95 percent confidence limits *(solid lines)* of systolic and diastolic aortic blood pressures on birth weight in 61 healthy newborn infants during the first 12 hours after birth. For systolic pressure, $y = 7.13x + 40.45$; $r = 0.79$. For diastolic pressure, $y = 4.81x + 22.18$; $r = 0.71$. For both, $n = 413$ and $p < .001$. (From Versmold HT, Kitterman JA, Phibbs RH, et al: Aortic blood pressure during the first 12 hours of life in infants with birth weight 610 to 4,220 grams. Pediatrics *67*:607, 1981. Reproduced by permission of Pediatrics.)

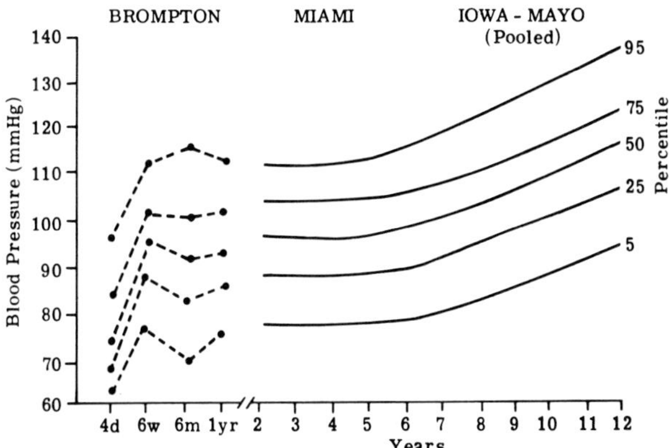

FIGURE 7–6. Percentiles of systolic blood pressure in awake infants (both sexes pooled) at age 4 days to 1 year (Brompton study). At age 6 weeks, the percentile values were calculated from the 594 boys and 538 girls who were awake at the time of BP measurement. At ages 6 months and 1 year, all infants were awake. At age 4 days, only 174 infants were awake at the time of BP measurement, and the percentile values were therefore taken from measurements made on sleeping infants and corrected for wakefulness. The percentiles for ages 2 to 14 years have been taken from the values for 29 to 45 boys from the Miami study and from 453 to 592 boys from the Muscatine and Rochester studies (Iowa-Mayo pool), as summarized by the Task Force for Blood Pressure Control in Children. (From DeSwiet M, Fayers P, Shinebourne EA: Systolic blood pressure in a population of infants in the first years of life: The Brompton study. Pediatrics *65*:1028, 1980. Reproduced by permission of Pediatrics.)

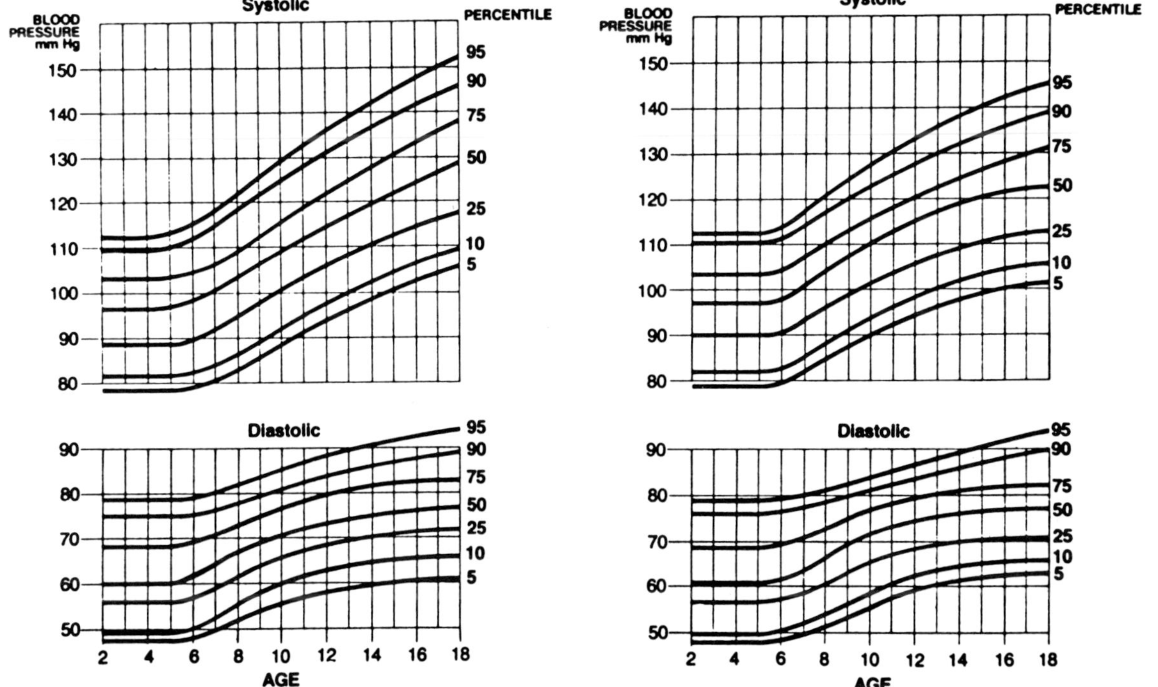

Percentiles of blood pressure measurement in boys (right arm, seated).

Percentiles of blood pressure measurement in girls (right arm, seated).

FIGURE 7–7. Systolic and diastolic blood pressure in children and adolescents. (From Report of the Task Force on Blood Pressure Control in Children. Pediatrics *59*[Suppl]:803, 1977. Reproduced by permission of Pediatrics.)

onset of muffling rather than the disappearance of sounds, which is the index used in monitoring adults.[141, 146] Provided appropriate techniques and equipment are used, blood pressure measurements made on the thigh, lower leg, and forearm approximate upper arm measurement fairly well.[147]

Treatment of hypertension is directed at the pathophysiological mechanism that predominates. ECF sodium and water overload is the most common problem and is thought to increase cardiac output and peripheral vascular resistance.[136] It is often successfully treated with salt restriction (taking care not to overrestrict and decrease GFR; see earlier section on Sodium and Water Excretion), diuretics, and dialysis.[132, 137, 138] Those who do not respond have a major component of vasoconstriction mediated by increased autonomic tone, circulating catecholamines, and angiotensin II.[132, 136, 138] These children are treated with antihypertensive medication. These are vasodilators or have an anti–renin-angiotensin effect. Care must be exercised to eliminate foods and drugs (for example, licorice or decongestants) that can exacerbate hypertension.[134, 148] When these measures fail to control the hypertension even with dialysis, determination of elevated plasma renin activity may distinguish those children whose blood pressure will improve with bilateral nephrectomy.[149, 150]

As mentioned earlier, evidence exists for an antihypertensive renal function that has been variously attributed to renal production of prostaglandins,[151, 152] a nonprostaglandin neutral lipid,[153] and/or kallidin—an active kinin produced by renal kallikrein.[154] It is hypothesized that these may become deficient, but too little is known to provide a basis for speculation about therapeutic replacement.

Table 7–9 lists the medications commonly employed for treatment of hypertension in children with renal disease.[138] Several caveats and specifics should be mentioned. The pharmacokinetics of renal excretion of many drugs (for example, methyldopa) are altered in CRF, so that their dosage and dosing interval must be adjusted accordingly, and their elimination may be delayed when they are discontinued (see Drug Pharmacokinetics and Pharmacodynamics later in this chapter). Conversely, the pharmacodynamics of some of these drugs are such that abrupt discontinuation may cause severe rebound hypertension (for example, minoxidil[155] and clonidine[156]) or tachycardia (for example, propranolol[157]).

The most commonly used drugs are the thiazide diuretics (chlorothiazide and hydrochlorothiazide), which are effective in mild hypertension. They work initially by diuretic and natriuretic effects, and volume, salt, and potassium depletion must be anticipated. Their sustained antihypertensive effect is most likely a result of decreased peripheral vascular resistance.[158] In severe renal failure, the thiazide diuretics are usually ineffective and may actually be harmful since they may decrease GFR and increase the level of azotemia and hyperuricemia.[138] The potent "loop" diuretics, furosemide and ethacrynic acid, are more effective in severe renal failure, although they may also cause hypokalemia, volume depletion, and hyperuricemia. Furosemide has been shown to increase renal blood flow and GFR transiently in acute glomerulonephritis and is especially indicated for this condition.[159] The doses required in severe renal failure may be very large and have been associated with transient hearing loss. Ethacrynic acid has been associated with permanent nerve deafness.[138]

Vasodilators are frequently added to diuretic therapy to control hypertension in children with CRF. Even though mental status changes and a possible association with breast cancer have limited the use of reserpine in children,[132, 138] some nephrologists feel that it is more effective at controlling hypertension in children than in adults.[160] Anesthesiologists may still encounter children on this drug. Bradycardia and nasal congestion may occur with use of reserpine; this drug is contraindicated in infants whose cardiac output is very rate-dependent and who are obligate nasal breathers.[138] Reserpine, like guanethidine, acts by depleting catecholamine stores. Treatment of intraoperative hypotension with directly acting pressor amines (such as norepinephrine, phenylephrine, methoxamine, or metaraminol) may evoke a greatly exaggerated increase in blood pressure. Indirectly acting pressor amines, which rely in part on the secondary release of norepinephrine from nerve terminals (such as ephedrine), may have a disappointingly small effect.[161] In addition to catecholamine depletion, guanethidine causes alpha-adrenergic block with resultant symptomatic postural hypotension. A decrease in cardiac output occurs, leading to a decrease in renal blood flow and GFR, with possible worsening of azotemia.[138] Methyldopa, a "false neurotransmitter," is thought to have no deleterious effects on renal blood flow or GFR and lowers serum renin levels.[162]

Propranolol, a nonspecific beta-blocker, is useful for its antirenin effects[163] as well as direct

Table 7—9. ORAL MEDICATIONS USED IN THE MANAGEMENT OF HYPERTENSION IN CHILDREN AND ADOLESCENTS WITH RENAL DISEASE*

Drug	Oral Dose: Initial (per kg/day)	Oral Dose: Maximum (per kg/day)	Action	Comment
Propranolol	1–2 mg	15 mg	Beta-blocker	Drug of choice; contraindicated in asthma and cardiac failure
Metoprolol	2–4 mg	8 mg	Beta-blocker	
Atenolol	1–2 mg	2 mg	Beta-blocker	
Hydralazine	1–2 mg	8 mg	Direct vasodilator	Drug of choice; occasionally causes reversible lupus syndrome; reflex tachycardia is avoided by use of a beta-blocker as well
Hydrochlorothiazide	1–2 mg	4 mg	Diuretic	Useful for mild hypertension; may need potassium supplementation
Chlorothiazide	10 mg	40 mg	Diuretic	
Chlorthalidone	0.5–2 mg	2 mg	Diuretic	
Furosemide	0.5–1.0 mg	15 mg	Diuretic	Often necessary with vasodilator drugs and in renal failure; potassium supplementation necessary
Triamterene	1–2 mg	4 mg	Diuretic	
Prazosin	0.05–0.1 mg	0.4 mg	Direct vasodilator and alpha-blocker	Well tolerated; introduce carefully since hypotension can occur with a large initial dose
Minoxidil	0.1–0.2 mg	1–2 mg	Direct vasodilator	Extremely effective for refractory hypertension; side effects are hirsutism and saline retention
Captopril	<6 mo: 0.05–0.5 mg >6 mo: 0.5–2.0 mg	6 mg	Converting enzyme inhibitor	Remarkably effective in renin-dependent hypertension
Methyldopa	5–10 mg	40 mg	Central alpha-adrenergic stimulator	Main problems are sedation and depression
Bethanidine	0.4 mg	10 mg	Postganglionic adrenergic blocker	Marked postural hypotension
Clonidine	5 μg	30 μg	Central alpha-adrenergic stimulator	Depression; reflex hypertension on withdrawal
Phenoxybenzamine	1 mg	4 mg	Alpha-sympathetic blocker	Useful for oral control of blood pressure in pheochromocytoma before surgery; often needs a beta-blocker because of reflex tachycardia
Spironolactone	1–2 mg	4 mg	Competitive aldosterone antagonist	Potassium retention and gynecomastia

*Do not exceed usual adult daily dosage with any of these drugs.

Modified from Dillon MJ: Hypertension. *In* Williams DI, Johnston JH (Eds.): Paediatric Urology. London, Butterworth Scientific, 1982; and reproduced by permission from Report of the Second Task Force on Blood Pressure Control in Children—1987. Pediatrics *79*:1–25, 1987.

effects on the central vasomotor center.[164] Beta-adrenergic blocking agents may reduce cardiac output, renal blood flow, and GFR and should be used with caution in heart failure, asthma, and diabetes. Patients receiving up to 7 mg/kg/day of propranolol show a normal increase in heart rate with atropine administration, but those receiving larger doses in the treatment of renal hypertension have an impaired chronotropic response and may require large doses of isoproterenol to overcome bradycardia due to beta-blockade.[165] Severe bradycardia following administration of neostigmine to patients on propranolol has been reported.[165, 166] This may be much less responsive to atropine administration. Excessive negative inotropic effects of propranolol may be overcome without resorting to beta-agonists by using intravenous calcium or glucagon, which bypass the beta-receptor mechanism.[167]

Hydralazine directly relaxes arteriolar smooth muscle, thereby decreasing peripheral vascular resistance and blood pressure.[168] Tolerance to its antihypertensive effects occurs less frequently in children, in whom the side effect of tachycardia is well tolerated and easily controlled with propranolol. Parenteral administration can cause nausea, vomiting, flushing, and headache, and this may be confusing when the possibility of hypertensive encephalopathy exists.[138]

Minoxidil, also a peripheral vasodilator, is extremely potent and reserved for severe hypertension resistant to usual drug therapy. It causes sodium and water retention, necessitating concurrent use of diuretics or dialysis, and may lead to pericardial effusions and severe rebound hypertension if abruptly discontinued.[155, 169] It has been used with success in children with severe, uncontrollable hypertension.[170]

Clonidine (a central alpha-agonist) and prazosin (a direct peripheral vasodilator with alpha-blockade properties) do not seem to have any major advantages in children over the aforementioned drugs and are rarely used.[137] Abrupt withdrawal of clonidine may cause severe rebound hypertension,[153] and this can be treated with combined alpha- and beta-receptor blockade or nonspecific arterial vasodilators.[171]

Captopril reduces blood pressure by inhibiting angiotensin I–converting enzyme and thus blocking the conversion of angiotensin I to angiotensin II, as well as by indirectly elevating bradykinin and suppressing aldosterone secretion.[172] It has also been used effectively in children with severe, resistant hypertension and is currently reserved for this use, with major side effects being hyperkalemia, leukopenia, proteinuria, and rashes.[173]

The treatment of a hypertensive crisis is an emergency in which anesthesiologists may be involved, either in the perioperative period or in the ICU setting. Diazoxide given as an IV bolus at a dose of 5 mg/kg (up to 300 mg) has a rapid onset of action and a dramatic and predictable vasodilator effect with prompt lowering of blood pressure.[174, 175] Care must be taken to avoid extravasation, which may result in tissue necrosis, but otherwise a single bolus dose is relatively safe and rarely results in hypotension.[176] Its effect may be expected in seconds to minutes, and a dose may be repeated in 60 minutes if the desired effect has not been achieved. Once controlled, the blood pressure will usually stay down for several hours to a day, during which time other antihypertensives may be instituted.[138] Repeated doses may be associated with sodium and water retention requiring diuretic therapy and may also lead to severe hyperglycemia and elevation of serum amylase.[176]

Sodium nitroprusside is a potent vasodilator familiar to anesthesiologists. It acts rapidly and is a very effective parenterally administered antihypertensive.[177, 178] Its rapid onset and cessation of action allow a continuous infusion to be readily titrated to the desired effect. This offers advantages in the perioperative setting, when other factors (volume status, anesthetics) may rapidly alter blood pressure. Continuous infusion in the 0.5 to 8 μg/kg/min range is almost always effective and usually avoids cumulative cyanide toxicity.[179] The renal clearance of thiocyanate is normally low (2.2 ml/min) and is reduced by almost half in patients with renal disease (1.3 ml/min).[180] Thiocyanate levels should be measured during prolonged nitroprusside administration in patients with renal failure. At levels of 10 mg/dl, weakness, nausea, tinnitus, and behavioral changes are manifest.[138, 179, 180] Excessive levels can be lowered by discontinuing nitroprusside and by peritoneal dialysis or hemodialysis.[180] Intraoperatively, adding or increasing the concentration of halothane or isoflurane may effectively reduce the nitroprusside dose requirement.[181] It is interesting that cyanide toxicity is rarely a problem in renal failure patients, probably because decreased renal excretion of thiosulfate provides additional substrate for the conversion of cyanide to thiocyanate, which then accumulates as described earlier. An increased resistance to nitroprusside-induced cyanide toxicity has been demonstrated in anuric dogs.[182]

Labetalol, an alpha- and beta-blocker given by infusion, may replace diazoxide as the drug of choice in hypertensive crises.[183–185a] Table 7–10 lists the dosages and routes of administration of drugs used in hypertensive crises.[142, 184–186]

Congestive Heart Failure and Pericarditis. Children with marked hypertension due to renal failure may develop left ventricular failure. Mitral valve insufficiency (due to cardiac distention), dyspnea, rales, and later right ventricular failure with hepatomegaly, venous congestion, and worsening edema may occur.[4] Volume overload, anemia, hypoproteinemia, shunting through arteriovenous connections, negative inotropic effects of electrolyte disturbances, and acidosis may all contribute to congestive cardiac failure.[4, 187] Echocardiographic assessment of cardiac function in children with chronic renal failure suggests that while only a minority of children with advanced CRF develop severe congestive heart failure, this is probably a result of a cardiodepressant substance in uremia.[188] Hemodialysis transiently improves this cardiac dysfunction, whereas successful transplantation reverses it.[188] Immediate therapy is directed at the control of hypertension, volume overload, and anemia and the correction of acidosis and electrolyte abnormalities. Dialysis is the most effective means of achieving these ends.

Table 7–10. DRUGS USED IN THE TREATMENT OF ACUTE HYPERTENSIVE CRISES

Drug	Dose	Action	Comment
Labetalol	1–3 mg/kg per h IV (total 5.0 mg/kg)	Alpha-blocker and beta-blocker	Use alone; stop infusate when blood pressure is controlled; effective 4–6 hours. May also be given by bolus
Sodium nitroprusside	0.5–8 μg/kg per min IV	Direct vasodilator	Very short duration of action; possible cyanide toxicity with prolonged use
Diazoxide	2–10 mg/kg IV bolus	Direct vasodilator	Can cause hyperglycemia, hypotension, and salt and water retention
Hydralazine	1–5 mg/kg IV or IM	Direct vasodilator	Can cause tachycardia, headache, and flushing
Minoxidil	0.1–0.2 mg/kg PO	Direct vasodilator	Rapidly effective even though orally administered
Furosemide	1–2 mg/kg IV	Diuretic	Avoid unless saline overload is obvious
Phentolamine	0.1–0.2 mg/kg IV	Alpha-blocker	Hypertensive crisis of pheochromocytomas

Modified from Dillon MJ: Hypertension. *In* Williams DI, Johnston JH (Eds.): Paediatric Urology. London, Butterworth Scientific, 1982; and from Report of the Second Task Force on Blood Pressure Control in Children—1987. Pediatrics *79*:1–25, 1987. See also references 185, 185a, and 186.

Digitalis therapy in children with renal disease may be difficult to regulate, because of electrolyte abnormalities and markedly reduced urinary excretion.[41] Inotropic support with dopamine (up to 15 μg/kg/min) in infants does not lead to a reduction in GFR.[189] This may be preferred to digitalis in the rare case when control of hypertension and fluid overload does not improve cardiac output.

The possibility of pericardial effusion and tamponade must be considered.[41] Up to 60 percent of patients with untreated uremia may develop pericardial disease.[187] Twenty percent may develop pericarditis in spite of hemodialysis,[190] and 30 percent of these may develop cardiac tamponade.[191] Although dialysis, steroids, and indomethacin are beneficial, surgical intervention with pericardiocentesis, pericardiotomy, or pericardiectomy may be necessary.[192] Although it has been reported that chronic percutaneous pericardial drainage in children is safe,[193] past experience in uremic patients has shown that pericardiocentesis carries a significant mortality.[192] Repeated pericardiocentesis increases the subsequent operative risk substantially[194]; therefore it should be reserved for the emergency relief of acute tamponade. The use of local anesthesia for subxiphoid pericardiotomy has been recommended as safe,[194, 195] and this may be acceptable in older, cooperative children. In such cases, intra-arterial and central venous pressure lines are useful to monitor blood pressure and to insure optimal volume status and cardiac preload. Sedative premedicants are contraindicated.[63] However, anticholinergics are indicated to prevent vagally induced bradycardia upon induction and laryngoscopy, since cardiac output may be critically dependent on heart rate (because of a restricted stroke volume). This is especially important in infants and small children. Extreme caution should be exercised with inhalational agents, which may lead to vasodilatation, decreased preload and afterload, hypotension, bradycardia, and even cardiac arrest.[196]

Positive-pressure ventilation may decrease venous return, cardiac output, and blood pressure. Spontaneous ventilation preserves venous return and obviates these concerns. Controlled ventilation can be safely accomplished with shortened inspiratory times, low peak pressures, avoidance of PEEP, and slower rates. This will decrease mean intrathoracic pressure and minimize effects on venous return.

In adults with uremic pericardial effusions undergoing pericardiectomy, ketamine has been recommended because of its effects of preserving peripheral vascular resistance and increasing heart rate and cardiac output.[197] It is also very useful for children, although in children the salutary effects of ketamine on heart rate and cardiac output may not be present.[198]

PULMONARY MANIFESTATIONS

Fluid may accumulate in the lungs of children with renal failure as a result of congestive failure and fluid overload, hypoproteinemia (resulting in decreased intravascular oncotic pressure), and increased pulmonary vascular permeability.[4] Decreased vital capacity and diffusion capacity and mild restrictive defects may be the result.[199] Pleuritis and both transudative and exudative pleural effusions may occur, and organizing fibrous exudates can cause adhesions and restrictive pleuritis.[199] Although acute exacerbations of pulmonary edema may be palliated with positive airway pressure and ventilation, forced diuresis and dialysis are the most effective treatments. Metabolic acidosis, which induces pulmonary vasoconstriction and may exacerbate cardiac failure and contribute to pulmonary edema, can be concomitantly corrected with dialysis.

NEUROLOGICAL MANIFESTATIONS

Many neurological complications may occur in children with chronic renal failure. These include uremic encephalopathy, hypertensive encephalopathy, seizures, peripheral neuropathy, autonomic nervous system dysfunction, and neurological complications of dialysis (dialysis disequilibrium syndrome).[200–202] Uremic encephalopathy is characterized by a global depression of cerebral function, although focal neurological signs may occur. These include transient loss of vision (uremic amaurosis), abducens nerve palsy, hearing loss, cerebellar ataxia, transient monoplegia, and hemiplegia.[200, 203] Focal neurological deficits and EEG changes are more commonly characteristic of hypertensive encephalopathy and may include focal weakness, asymmetrical reflexes, unilateral Babinski's sign, nystagmus, oculomotor palsies, and visual disturbances that may progress to cortical blindness.[204] Acute funduscopic changes with a hypertensive crisis are rarer in children than in adults,[160] and children may have seizures without manifesting papilledema, retinal hemorrhages, or exudates. Subarachnoid or intracerebral hemorrhage or other rapidly expanding mass lesions must also be considered in the differential diagnosis of hypertensive encephalopathy.

The management of uremic encephalopathy consists of adequate dialysis. Hypertensive encephalopathy requires urgent reduction of blood pressure (as detailed earlier) and, if severe, the institution of measures aimed at the reduction of cerebral edema and increased intracranial pressure. In patients with renal failure and oliguria or anuria, the use of hyperosmotic agents to achieve this must be controlled as determined by continual assessment of their effects on intravascular volume and electrolytes.[205, 206, 215, 216]

Generalized seizures occur frequently in renal failure, sometimes as a result of uremic or hypertensive encephalopathy, but more frequently owing to rapid changes in pH, calcium, and electrolytes. Hyponatremia may occur due to water overload or to transient cerebral edema and SIADH in association with the dialysis disequilibrium syndrome.[200] While correction of the inciting etiology of the seizure is essential, intravenous benzodiazepine (lorazepam, midazolam, or diazepam) is used for its initial control. Subsequent seizure control is maintained with longer-acting anticonvulsants, such as phenobarbital or phenytoin.[200] A significant portion of administered phenobarbital is normally excreted unchanged in the urine,[207] and dosage modification may be required in renal failure.[208] The initial loading dose of phenobarbital in children is 10 mg/kg IV slowly, with a maintenance dose of 5 mg/day divided BID, striving for a therapeutic level of 20 to 40 μg/ml. Twenty to 40 percent of phenobarbital is bound to plasma protein,[208] but in renal failure the ratio of free to bound barbiturate may be increased. Thus sensitivity is increased compared with that in normals at the same serum levels.[200] This is also true of phenytoin. Only 5 percent is excreted in the urine, and the half-life is actually shortened in end-stage renal disease,[208] yet renal failure has a marked influence on effective plasma levels.[200, 209] Ninety percent of phenytoin is protein-bound, and the remaining 10 percent is pharmacologically active.[208, 209] In uremia, protein binding is markedly diminished[210, 211] so that the effective plasma level is less than the normal of 10 to 20 μg/ml.[202] The loading dose of phenytoin is 10 to 15 mg/kg IV slowly, followed by lower maintenance doses of 3 to 5 mg/kg/day divided BID. Measurement and proper interpretation of plasma levels are necessary for control of therapy.

Peripheral neuropathy is a common manifestation of chronic renal failure with which the anesthesiologist should be familiar. The pathological lesion is axonal degeneration with segmental demyelination, which may be caused by uremic inhibition of the enzyme transketolase.[212] This is often reversible with dialysis or transplantation.[200, 213] The common peroneal and median nerves are frequently involved,[214] and distal, symmetrical lesions first involving the lower, then the upper extremities are usually seen.[200] The "restless leg syndrome" and the "burning feet syndrome" are initial manifestations that may herald progressive sensory, motor, and sympathetic neuropathy, which may progress to paraplegia. Unilateral pressure palsies, secondary to sensory neuropathy, may occur.[200] Sensory and motor deficits, such as foot drop, should be carefully documented preoperatively, especially if positioning (stirrups for GU surgery) or operation (such as the creation of a shunt in an arm or leg) will involve an affected extremity.

The possibility of progression to paraplegia may influence the anesthesiologist's choice of conduction versus general anesthesia. Diagnosis of overt clinical neuropathy is rare under 10 years of age, yet prolonged nerve conduction velocities in young children[213] suggest that in this group the lesions are simply not recognized until advanced.[200] When uremic neuropathy has led to immobilization, succinylcholine has unpredictable effects on serum K^+ and is best avoided.[45, 49]

Children with end-stage renal failure may also develop an autonomic neuropathy with impairment of sweating and baroreceptor activity. Hypotension that is unresponsive to volume but responds to norepinephrine infusion may occur during dialysis.[217, 218] This possibility should be kept in mind intraoperatively when unexplained hypotension unresponsive to volume is encountered.[63]

Finally, "dialysis dementia" has been attributed to chronic aluminum intoxication in adults on chronic dialysis.[219, 220] This is characterized by progressive dementia, speech disturbances, bizarre involuntary movements, facial grimacing, and myoclonic seizures, and sometimes progresses to coma and death.[221] This syndrome has been described in children,[222, 223] and elevated serum and bone aluminum levels have been documented in those undergoing continuous ambulatory peritoneal dialysis who were taking aluminum hydroxide.[224]

Gastrointestinal Manifestations

Anorexia, nausea, vomiting, hiccoughs, gastrointestinal bleeding, diarrhea, and constipation may all accompany chronic renal failure and uremia.[225] Autonomic neuropathy as described earlier may account for delayed gastric emptying in renal failure, and this may double in association with hemodialysis.[31] Metoclopramide (0.1 mg/kg) has been suggested to improve gastric motility, although caution must be exercised when it is used in children. Extrapyramidal side effects occur more frequently in children than in adults, and are especially common in patients with known seizure disorders.

Despite earlier suggestions of decreased gastric acid secretions in uremia,[4, 226] gastric acid hypersecretion, thought to be due to decreased renal removal of gastrin in renal failure,[227, 228] is known to occur.[229] It is suggested as the cause of peptic ulceration in renal failure.[228, 230] Cimetidine (5 mg/kg every 12 hours in severe renal failure) may be given preoperatively.[214, 231]

Persistent hiccoughs may be a particularly distressing gastrointestinal symptom that may not always yield to treatment with vagal maneuvers, nasopharyngeal stimulations, or phenothiazines.[4] Profound neuromuscular blockade may be required intraoperatively to eliminate bothersome movement during intra-abdominal surgery.

Endocrine, Nutritional, and Psychological Manifestations

Chronic renal failure in children leads to a myriad of abnormalities in endocrine control systems.[232] Disturbances of nitrogen, carbohydrate, and lipid metabolism[233] may occur and affect growth and development.[234] Peptide hormones, such as vasopressin, prolactin, growth hormone, calcitonin, somatostatin, parathyroid hormone, glucagon, and insulin, all tend to be elevated, although the end-organ effects are variable.[235] Other hormones are decreased, such as erythropoietin and 1,25-dihydroxycholecalciferol, resulting in some of the common clinical manifestations of renal disease, such as anemia and renal osteodystrophy. Carbohydrate metabolism is altered in end-stage renal failure. Some patients develop hypoglycemia, but most have a mildly elevated fasting glucose and abnormal glucose tolerance test.[234, 236] It is interesting that while diabetic patients tend to require less insulin as renal failure progresses, the nondiabetic patient with CRF develops peripheral insulin resistances and glucose intolerance.[236] In addition, exogenously administered corticosteroids may further contribute to endocrine, carbohydrate metabolism, and growth disturbances. Because of potential adrenal insufficiency, perioperative steroid coverage is recommended.[214]

Finally, the impairment of growth, development, and sexual maturation coupled with the psychological stress of a limiting, chronic illness may lead to severe psychological disturbance in children with CRF and in their family members.[237] Extra time and effort will be required of the anesthesiologist in order to establish optimal communication and understanding during the perioperative period.

Drug Pharmacokinetics and Pharmacodynamics

The pharmacokinetics and pharmacodynamics of most drugs are altered in chronic renal failure. This results from decreased renal excretion of the drug and its metabolites, decreased renal metabolism, altered volume of distribution, altered protein binding, altered lipid solubility, and altered end-organ sensitivity and response.[238, 239] The effects of these pharmacological alterations on drugs used in the treatment of the specific clinical manifestations of renal failure have already been discussed. For additional information about the use of specific drugs in the presence of renal failure, readers are referred to the excellent reviews available in the literature.[208, 238–240]

Anesthetic drugs also are altered in their pharmacokinetics and pharmacodynamics by renal failure and have significant effects on renal function.

The use of succinylcholine in renal failure is well studied[43–49] and has been discussed in detail earlier in the section on hyperkalemia. Concern over lowered plasma cholinesterase levels with the older cellophane-type dialysis membrane no longer exists with current hemodialysis membrane materials.[241]

Reduced muscle mass, reduced renal blood flow, and alterations in the distribution volume of nondepolarizing muscle relaxants may result in a lower dosage requirement.[214, 242] Furthermore, neuromuscular blockade may be potentiated in renal failure by acidosis, hypokalemia, hypocalcemia, hypermagnesemia, diuretics, and antibiotics (Table 7–11).[76, 214, 243, 244] Gallamine is excreted exclusively by the kidney.[63, 214]

Renal excretion plays a major role in the excretion of pancuronium and metocurine, although biliary and other routes of elimination may increase in the face of renal failure.[242, 245] D-Tubocurarine used to be the nondepolarizing drug of choice because its protein binding and potency are unchanged in renal failure,[246, 247] and hepatic excretion appears to be significantly increased.[247, 248] Curare may cause hypotension through ganglionic blockade and vasodilatation due to histamine release.[214]

Atracurium and vecuronium are newer nondepolarizing muscle relaxants, which are the drugs of choice for use in renal failure.[250–255, 260–262] Atracurium is cleared by Hoffman elimination (a form of spontaneous ester hydrolysis) and by nonspecific esterases and is not dependent on renal excretion.[249] Concerns have been raised about accumulation of the degradation products laudanosine[256] and acrylates,[257] especially in renal failure, in which uremia may predispose to an abnormal blood-brain barrier[258] and seizures. Vecuronium relies primarily on biliary elimination,[259] and has been studied in patients with end-stage renal failure,[260, 261] and in infants and children.[262] "Re-curarization" should not be a problem with either of these agents. Both pipecuronium and doxacurium have been found to have a variable and unpredictable duration of action in renal failure patients, and therefore their use in this setting is not recommended.[263, 264] Reversal of nondepolarizing neuromuscular blockade may be accomplished with pyridostigmine or neostigmine, the elimination times of which are prolonged with renal failure to the same degree as that of D-tubocurarine.[265, 266]

Inhalational agents are taken up and eliminated rapidly via the lungs, independent of renal

Table 7–11. INTERACTION OF ANTIBIOTICS, MUSCLE RELAXANTS, NEOSTIGMINE, AND CALCIUM

	Neuromuscular Block from Antibiotic Alone Antagonized by		Increase in Neuromuscular Block of		Neuromuscular Block from Antibiotic-dTc Antagonized by	
Antibiotic	***Neostigmine***	***Calcium***	***dTc***	***SCh***	***Neostigmine***	***Calcium***
neomycin	Sometimes	Sometimes	Yes	Yes	Usually	Usually
streptomycin	Sometimes	Sometimes	Yes	Yes	Yes	Usually
gentamicin	Sometimes	Yes	Yes	*	Sometimes	Yes
kanamycin	Sometimes	Sometimes	Yes	Yes	Sometimes	Sometimes
paromomycin	Yes	Yes	Yes	*	Yes	Yes
viomycin	Yes	Yes	Yes	*	Yes	Yes
polymyxin A	No	No	Yes	*	No	No
polymyxin B	No†	No	Yes	Yes	No†	No
colistin	No	Sometimes	Yes	Yes	No	Sometimes
tetracycline	No	*	Yes	No	Partially	Partially
lincomycin	Partially	Partially	Yes	*	Partially	Partially
clindamycin	Partially	Partially	Yes	*	Partially	Partially

dTc, D-tubocurarine; SCh, succinylcholine.
*Not studied.
†Block augmented by neostigmine.
From Miller RD: Reversal of Muscle Relaxants. 32nd Annual Refresher Course Lectures, American Society of Anesthesiologists, Lecture 222, pp 1–6, Oct 1981.

function. This, in addition to their usefulness in potentiating neuromuscular relaxation and controlling hypertension, has made them popular agents for anesthesia in patients with renal failure.[214] All potent inhalational agents may depress renal function if cardiovascular depression leads to a reduction in renal blood flow and glomerular filtration rate.[267] Metabolism of these agents and release of inorganic fluoride with resultant nephrotoxicity is another problem. At a GFR below 16 ml/min/m^2, normal excretion of inorganic fluoride is impaired,[268] and accumulation will depend on the degree of metabolic degradation versus the rate of elimination. Methoxyflurane is no longer used as a result of these concerns.[269] Enflurane is metabolized less than methoxyflurane,[270] but there have been several reports of renal failure associated with elevated inorganic fluoride levels.[271–273] For this reason, enflurane is generally not used in patients with renal failure.[63, 214] In one study, however, enflurane administered in the presence of mild renal failure (serum creatinine of 1.5 to 3.0 mg/dl) was associated with a slight improvement in postoperative renal function.[274] In the total absence of renal function, the question of nephrotoxicity is moot. Enflurane has been used in this setting without excessive serum fluoride accumulation because of deposition of fluoride in bone.[275] The availability of isoflurane, which is less metabolized[276] and results in lower fluoride levels,[277] or halothane generally obviates the need to use enflurane. Studies with desflurane have shown no increase in serum or urinary inorganic fluoride or urinary nonvolatile organic fluoride in normal volunteers,[278, 279] indicating promise for the use of this new inhalational anesthetic in patients with impaired renal function.

Narcotics should be used with caution in renal failure. Increased secretion of ADH and decreased urine output were originally thought to be direct effects of morphine[280] but are now thought to be a result of surgical stimulation.[281] Although narcotics are metabolized in the liver, urinary output can markedly influence the duration of their effect.[282] Prolonged respiratory depression has been reported in anuric patients.[283] Renal failure does not alter the elimination of unchanged morphine but has been shown to result in the accumulation of active morphine metabolites, resulting in a prolongation of narcotic effect.[284] Likewise, the repeated use of meperidine may lead to the accumulation of the active metabolite normeperidine and can result in seizures.[285] Unlike the case with other plasma protein–bound drugs, the magnitude of change in the free fraction of fentanyl found in uremic patients is not clinically significant.[286] In high doses, fentanyl significantly attenuates the catecholamine response to operation and preserves renal function.[287] Fentanyl in combination with droperidol for "neuroleptanalgesia" has been used with success in patients with renal failure.[288, 289] Neuroleptanalgesia causes minimal hemodynamic changes and has little effect on renal function.[290, 291] Droperidol, when given alone to patients with renal failure, causes a small decrement in blood pressure and an increased cardiac output.[292]

The pharmacokinetics of alfentanil in chronic renal failure has been studied in adults and children, and the dosage need not be altered in renal failure.[293, 294] Likewise, sufentanil pharmacokinetics (rate of clearance, half-life, and apparent volume of distribution) is statistically unchanged in adolescent patients with chronic renal failure when compared with age-matched controls, although the clearance and half-life are more widely variable among patients with renal failure.[295]

Pentothal is normally 75 percent plasma protein–bound, but in uremia the free fraction increases significantly owing to reduced albumin levels and to displacement by uremic products.[296] Clinically, the required induction dose may be significantly decreased (as much as 75 percent) and the duration of action prolonged, depending on the severity of the azotemia.[297] This also may be due to an abnormal blood-brain barrier in uremia.[258]

Ketamine is largely metabolized in the liver. Following intravenous administration, only 4 percent is recoverable in the urine either unchanged or as norketamine, and 16 percent as hydroxylated derivatives.[298] Animal studies suggest that ketamine causes little or no change in renal blood flow and urine output.[299, 300] It has been used in pediatric patients for intramuscular induction, but caution must be exercised in the presence of uncontrolled hypertension.[301]

Little is known about the effect of renal failure on the pharmacokinetics and pharmacodynamics of local anesthetics in infants and children. Lack of acceptance, along with concerns about coagulopathy, peripheral and autonomic uremic neuropathy, uncertain volume status, poor acid-base status, and alterations of the blood-brain barrier in uremia, has limited the experience with regional techniques in uremic children. Epidural and spinal anesthesia have been used successfully in adults with renal failure.[118–120, 302] It has been shown in patients with normal renal function that if blood pressure is maintained, GFR and renal hemodynamics are only minimally altered.[303, 304] Brachial plexus block has been considered a useful anesthetic for the creation of an arteriovenous fistula in the arm because of the attendant sympathetic blockade.[289, 305] It is also a technique used with success in children.[306] The duration of the block in renal failure patients has been noted to be significantly shorter (38 percent), and this has been attributed to faster tissue washout because of an increased cardiac output.[305] One study in adults showed that plasma levels of etidocaine after axillary block were significantly higher in renal failure patients.[307] This, in connection with a report of bupivacaine cardiotoxicity with regional anesthesia in a patient with renal failure,[308] suggests that the ratio of effective-to-toxic dose may be decreased and dosage of regional anesthetics should be reduced in patients with renal failure.

ANESTHESIA FOR CHILDREN WITH RENAL FAILURE

Multiple reviews describing various successful anesthetic techniques in renal failure have been published,[40, 42, 63, 118–120, 214, 289, 309, 310] demonstrating that no particular technique is best.[63] The foregoing discussion details the anesthetic implications of the manifestations of renal failure in children. This information provides the basis for the preoperative evaluation and design of an anesthetic tailored to the individual needs of the uremic child and the particular operation planned. Although surgery of any kind may be necessary, an operation in the child with renal failure will usually be related to the child's renal disease. Renal biopsy, diagnostic or radiotherapeutic procedures, peritoneal catheter insertion, arteriovenous fistula creation, parathyroidectomy, pericardial drainage or pericardiectomy, nephrectomy, or renal transplantation may be indicated. The best method of anesthesia for a child having a particular procedure will depend on the child's status, age, and state of cooperation and the procedure contemplated. Techniques may include local or regional blocks, intramuscular or intravenous sedation, or general anesthesia requiring invasive monitoring. Comments on appropriate monitoring and anesthetic choices for given problems have been included earlier in this chapter in the discussions of the anesthetic implications of the manifestations of renal failure.

RENAL TRANSPLANTATION IN INFANTS AND CHILDREN

Renal transplantation is the ultimate therapeutic procedure for end-stage renal failure. This operation is being undertaken with increasing frequency in infants and children.[94, 311–315] It presents an anesthetic challenge in which all the problems of renal failure may complicate the usual concerns about anesthesia in seriously ill infants and small children. Many reviews of anesthesia for renal transplantation with a focus on adults have been published,[119, 120, 316–322] and the considerations presented are equally relevant when a child is the kidney recipient. The usual retroperitoneal approach and right iliac fossa placement of the kidney graft may be satisfactory in children over 20 kg in body weight.[315] However, in infants and smaller children (under 20 kg) the operation needs to be modified. In these small patients, a long midline incision and a transperitoneal approach are necessary. This large exposure necessitates special consideration of heat loss and fluid balance.

A large kidney placed in a small infant's abdomen may require maximal abdominal relaxation to facilitate closure. Nasogastric tube decompression of the bowel and discontinuation of nitrous oxide to reduce intestinal distention are helpful. Increased intra-abdominal pressure may result in respiratory compromise, necessitating prolonged postoperative assisted ventilation, particularly in infants, in whom much of the respiratory excursion is diaphragmatic. Other problems arising from the transperitoneal approach and tight abdominal closure are prolonged ileus, compromised venous return, and kinking of vascular anastomoses, which may threaten graft survival.[311, 315]

Because of the discrepancy in size between the donor graft (often an adult kidney) and the recipient's small vasculature, anastomoses to the bifurcations of the aorta and inferior vena cava, rather than to the iliac vessels, are used (Fig. 7–8).[311] As a result, there is the potential for major hemorrhage and the need for cross-clamping of the aorta and inferior vena cava. Large-bore intravenous catheters must be placed in the upper body so that transfused volume may reach the heart via the patent superior vena cava. A central venous catheter, placed from an antecubital fossa or an external jugular vein, is useful to evaluate trends in central venous pressure and volume status. If these lines are long, the additional resistance may make rapid transfusion of viscous blood products through them difficult. Percutaneous

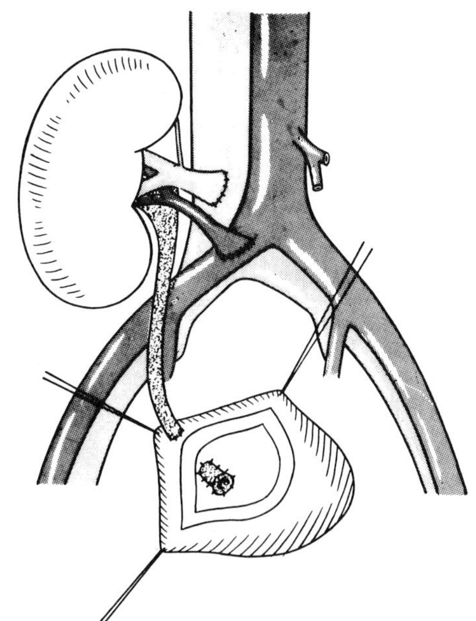

FIGURE 7–8. Placement of a large donor kidney in a small recipient. (From Fernando ON: Renal transplantation in children. *In* Williams DI, Johnston JH [Eds.]: London, Butterworth Scientific, 1982.)

placement of internal jugular and subclavian lines is difficult in infants and carries the attendant risk of pneumothorax and occult bleeding, especially if clotting parameters are abnormal. In the very small child destined to receive a large kidney, it is not unreasonable as a first step to place a large-bore central venous line surgically. This may then be used intraoperatively for assessment of volume status, blood transfusion, and administration of medications, and postoperatively for hyperalimentation if required. Infection is always a concern in uremic patients who will receive immunosuppressive therapy, and all lines must be placed aseptically.

An arterial line is necessary for continuous blood pressure monitoring, as well as for serial blood gas, hematocrit, and electrolyte determinations. Concern about graft failure and the future need for hemodialysis has led some to discourage strongly the use of any artery at a potential shunt site.[323] This has led others to recommend cannulation of the dorsalis pedis or temporal artery.[63, 289] In small children in whom the need to cross-clamp the abdominal aorta is likely, lower extremity arterial lines are of limited value. Furthermore, temporal artery cannulation in infants has been shown to carry a high risk of retrograde cerebral embolization.[324–326] Studies of radial artery cannulation in adults[327] have suggested that the risk of arterial obstruction increases with increasing catheter size, decreasing patient age, duration of cannulation, and cut-down versus percutaneous insertion. In a study of 53 cannulations in 47 pediatric patients, radial artery obstruction occurred in 27 cases (51 percent), but all obstructed vessels eventually became patent again, most within 1 to 2 weeks.[328] The placement of a small, nontapered catheter, preferably percutaneously, into a radial artery for as short a period as possible would seem to be justified. For the child who presents with Scribner's dialysis shunt already in place in an upper extremity (Fig. 7–9), an excellent solution is to remove the external connecting catheter, as is routinely done at the time of dialysis. The venous end can then be used to infuse blood, plasma, or fluids, and the arterial end to monitor blood pressure and arterial blood gases and electrolytes.[315] Subcutaneous arteriovenous fistulae have been used for infusions and for blood gas sampling,[323, 329] but this should probably be reserved for extreme access problems and emergencies. When not in use the fistula should be padded, and one should refrain from taking blood pressures in that extremity, if possible. Fistula patency may be continuously monitored with an overlying Doppler flow probe.[214]

A final problem associated with a large kidney in a small child is the volume of blood "stolen" from the circulation to fill the new kidney,[315] and the considerable proportion of the patient's cardiac output that is diverted to the new organ.[311] Cardiac arrest has been reported following anastomosis and release of the arterial clamp in the potassium-preserved kidney and upon unclamping of the iliac artery in adults.[330, 331] This has been attributed to hyperkalemia from the graft preservative and acidosis from the ischemic leg. This is exacerbated in the small child, in whom the volume of preservative relative to the patient's size is larger, and aortic cross-clamping causes the whole lower body to become ischemic and acidotic. It has been recommended to transfuse 75 to 100 ml of blood prior to releasing the vascular clamps in order to accommodate the increased vascular volume and flow required by the new graft.[315] Also, it has been shown that aggressive administration of intravenous colloids to increase the central venous pressure to 16 to 20 mm Hg prior to renal reperfusion can decrease the incidence of acute tubular necrosis in adult kidneys transplanted into infants.[315a] However, this may result in an increased incidence of pulmonary edema, requiring anticipation of the need for postoperative ventilatory support.[315a] Likewise, it is

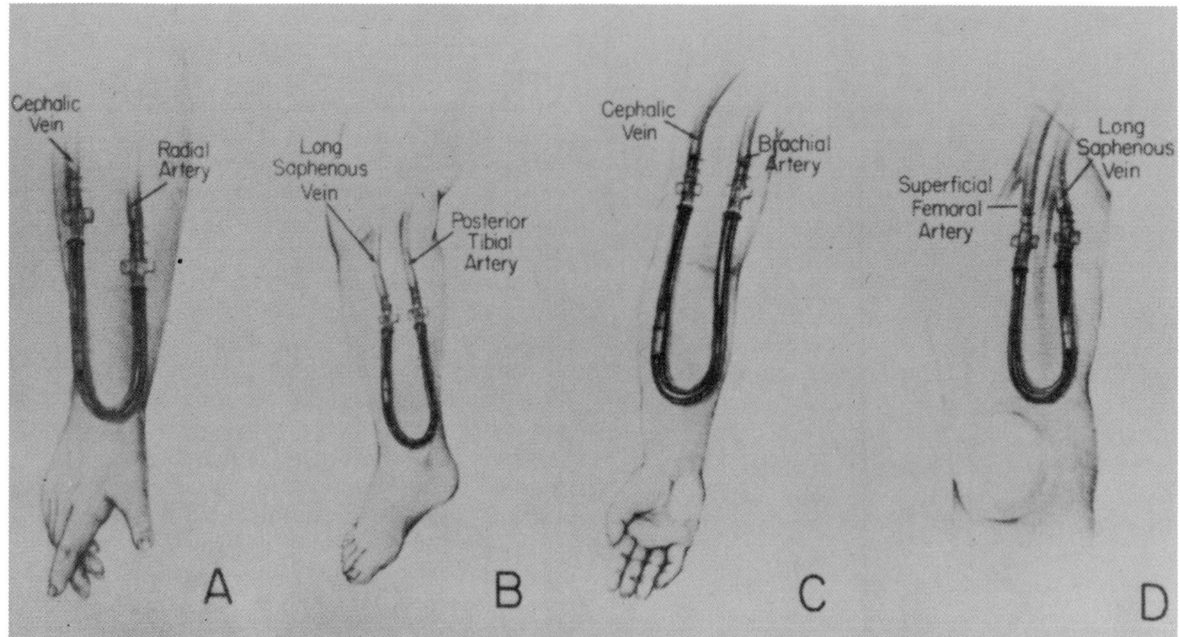

FIGURE 7–9. The Scribner shunt and various locations of placement. (From Buselmeier TJ, Kjellstrand CM: A-V shunts and fistulas for hemodialysis in neonates, infants, and small children. Proc E.D.T.A. *10*:511–515, 1973, with permission.)

advisable to administer 1 mEq/kg of sodium bicarbonate prior to release of the vascular clamp, in order to combat the predictable lactic acidosis and hyperkalemia.[315] Hypotension occurring intraoperatively or immediately postoperatively may be a result of poor cardiac output and depressed myocardial performance from acidosis or hyperkalemia. However, in small uremic patients with potential coagulopathies, immunosuppression, and high ventilatory pressures due to a tight abdominal closure, other complications that must be considered include hemorrhage, hypocalcemia, sepsis, adrenal insufficiency, pericardial effusion with tamponade, and pneumothorax.

A late complication following renal transplantation may be the development of severe hypoglycemia, manifesting as diaphoresis, lethargy, stupor, and seizures. Post-transplant hypoglycemia developed in children 1.7 to 7.5 years of age as late as 5 to 45 months post-transplantation, with serum glucose levels ranging from 36 mg/dl down to 14 mg/dl.[332] Hypoglycemia was associated with the use of beta-blockers in most, but not all, patients manifesting hypoglycemia and was precipitated by prolonged fasting in a significant number.[332] Preoperative fasting, therefore, may be harmful in these children, and beta-blockers used to control hypertension, as well as general anesthesia itself, may mask the symptoms of this potentially devastating complication of pediatric renal transplantation. In children postrenal transplantation who present for operation, perioperative intravenous infusion of glucose-containing solutions and frequent evaluation of serum glucose levels should be instituted to evaluate and control hypoglycemia.

ACUTE RENAL FAILURE

INCIDENCE AND CAUSES

A major intra- and postoperative concern in transplant recipients or other children with marginal renal function is the onset of an acute deterioration in renal function. Even in children without prior renal disease, trauma, operation (especially cardiac), intraoperative hemoglobinuria or myoglobinuria, drug toxicity, and the use of radiocontrast media are significant causes of perioperative acute renal failure.[333–337] Trauma, infection, muscle ischemia, succinylcholine administration, and malignant hyperthermia may all lead to rhabdomyolysis,[54, 338, 339] and at serum concentrations of 0.15 g/L, myoglobin appears in the urine.[340] Likewise, inborn errors of metabolism, such as congenital carnitine palmityl transferase deficiency, which may cause renal tubular acidosis,[340a] may also result in severe intraoperative rhabdomyolysis, myoglobinuria, and acute renal failure.[341] Hemolysis and transfusion reactions (which may be delayed up to several days after transfusion) may cause serum levels of hemoglobin as high as 0.5 to 1.4 g/L, at which time it appears in urine.[342] Up to 12 percent of patients undergoing radiocontrast procedures may develop signs of renal injury, and the incidence is higher after angiography than after other contrast studies, probably because the occurrence is dose-dependent.[336, 343] Excretory urography can be a low-yield and high-risk procedure in the infant or child with oliguria, and therefore ultrasonography and radionuclide studies are preferred.[344–346]

Table 7–12 lists the multitude of causes of acute renal failure (ARF) in infants and children.[39, 333, 347, 348] Some of these, such as renovascular defects and obstructive uropathies, are amenable to surgical intervention, and the implications for anesthesia for these entities are discussed later.

PROGNOSIS

Despite early institution of dialysis and parenteral hyperalimentation, the mortality rate of postsurgical patients with ARF remains 25 to 65 percent.[333, 334, 348] Although the underlying illness is a major determinant of mortality in ARF, infection accounts for one third to two thirds of all deaths.[349–351] Gastrointestinal hemorrhage is also a frequent complication and can contribute significantly to mortality.[350, 352] Use of antacids for prophylaxis against gastritis and peptic ulcer may be difficult because of the danger of magnesium toxicity.[333] Mental confusion may result from cimetidine therapy in renal failure.[353] There is encouraging evidence in children, however, that when the underlying cause of ARF is reversible and appropriate treatment is instituted early, the child has an excellent chance of survival and recovery of renal function.[354] Hence, early recognition and treatment of ARF are essential.

DIAGNOSIS

Oliguria is usually the first sign of ARF. However, azotemia and signs of tubular dysfunction may be present in spite of a normal urine output or even polyuria, particularly in burn patients or when ARF is induced by toxins.[355, 356] Fortunately, this insidious form of "nonoliguric" ARF is easier to manage and is associated with a more favorable prognosis.[356–358]

It should be noted that up to 16 percent of neonates, regardless of gestational age, will not void for 16 hours postnatally, but that all should void by 24 hours of age.[359] After that time, oliguria is variably defined as a urine output of less than 1.5 to 1 ml/kg/h.[360–362] Glomerulogenesis occurs up to the 36th week of gestation,[363] and infants of low birth weight normally have higher plasma creatinine levels than term neonates or older children.[364–367] Likewise, normal GFR and renal blood flow measurements vary for term infants, healthy premature infants, and premature infants with respiratory distress syndrome and are lower than for older children.[363, 364, 366, 368] Evaluation of parameters of renal function must take into consideration these age and developmental differences. Figure 7–1 and Table 7–4 give normal values for plasma creatinine and GFR by age.

The evaluation of the acute onset of oliguria and azotemia should proceed in a rapid but organized fashion to eliminate the possibilities of "prerenal" (renal hypoperfusion) or "postrenal" (urinary obstructive) causes. One systematic approach is shown in Figure 7–10.[333] Underlying, insidious, chronic renal failure exacerbated by an acute deterioration will usually be diagnosed by a careful review of the child's history, physical findings, and laboratory examinations prior to and during the acute deterioration.[333] A cause for the acute exacerbation must be aggressively sought and treated, in order to preserve maximal residual renal function. Physical examination and imaging techniques (preferably ultrasound, radionuclide scans, and computed tomography scans rather than radiocontrast studies, as discussed earlier) are usually successful at ruling out obstructive uropathy.[333, 344] Acute obstruction causes intratubular backflow pressure, which diminishes GFR and leads to decreased urine flow and increased sodium and water reabsorption by functional tubules.[369] This may yield a concentrated urine low in sodium, similar to the urine produced with diminished renal blood flow. On the other hand, prolonged partial obstruction in which the GFR is maintained and tubular function fails may yield an isotonic or hypotonic urine. This is high in sodium, with low potassium and hydrogen ion content suggestive of nonoliguric acute parenchymal renal failure.[333, 369]

In addition to oliguria and azotemia due to obstructive lesions, "prerenal" or "functional" renal failure arising from inadequate renal perfusion needs to be ruled out. This should begin

Table 7–12. CAUSES OF ACUTE RENAL FAILURE IN INFANTS AND CHILDREN

Renal Ischemia

- Hypovolemia
  - Hemorrhage
  - Dehydration
  - Burns
  - Hypoproteinemia
  - Peritonitis
  - Sepsis
- Cardiogenic shock
  - Cardiomyopathy
  - Myocarditis
  - Congenital heart disease
  - Cardiac surgery
- Renovascular
  - Bilateral renal artery thrombosis (rare, usually associated with umbilical artery lines)
  - Renal artery stenosis/dysplasia and hypertension
  - Renal vein thrombosis (associated with birth asphyxia, maternal diabetes mellitus, cyanotic congenital heart disease, hyperosmolar dehydration, trauma, nephrotic syndrome)
  - Microvascular occlusion (DIC, sickle cell disease, thrombotic thrombocytopenic purpura, hemolytic-uremic syndrome, Shwartzman's reaction—endotoxic cortical necrosis)
  - Prolonged use of vasoconstrictive drugs
  - Malignant hypertension
  - Prolonged aortic cross-clamping (coarctation repair)

Inflammatory and Immunological Processes

- Infectious
  - Pyelonephritis
  - Bacterial endocarditis
  - Shwartzman's reaction—endotoxic cortical necrosis
- Immune-related
  - Postinfectious glomerulonephritis (including poststreptococcal)
  - Idiopathic crescentic glomerulonephritis
  - Membranoproliferative glomerulonephritis
  - Tubulointerstitial nephritis
  - Membranous nephropathy
  - IgA-IgG (Berger's) nephropathy
  - Henoch-Schönlein purpura (anaphylactoid purpura)
  - Systemic lupus erythematosus
  - Wegener's granulomatosis
  - Periarteritis nodosa, scleroderma
- Specifically directed autoimmunity
  - Anti–glomerular basement membrane disease
  - Goodpasture's syndrome
  - Renal transplant rejection
- Hypersensitivity reactions
  - Penicillins, sulfonamides, cephalosporins, rifampin
  - Anticonvulsants

Direct Nephrotoxicity

- Uricosuric or hyperuricemic agents
  - Antineoplastic agents
  - Radiographic contrast media
  - Salicylates
  - Furosemide, ethacrynic acid
  - Pancreatic enzymes
- Other medications
  - Aminoglycosides
  - Amphotericin B
  - Cyclosporin A
  - Salicylates
  - Methoxyflurane, enflurane
- Heavy metals
  - Mercurials, lead, bismuth, gold, iron, copper, arsenic, thallium, cadmium, uranium
- Glycols and organic solvents
  - Carbon tetrachloride
  - Turpentine
  - Methanol
- Organic toxins
  - Mushrooms *(Amanita phalloides)*
  - Snakebites (especially sea snakes)
  - Phosphorus
- Hemoglobinuria, myoglobinuria
  - Burns
  - Crush injury
  - Myonecrosis (electrical shock, snakebites)
  - Hemolysis

Obstructive Uropathy

- Ureteral obstruction
  - Retroperitoneal masses or fibrosis
  - Solitary kidney with obstruction
  - Renal calculi
  - Ureteral debris
  - Bilateral ureteral pelvic junction obstruction
- Urethral obstruction
  - Posterior urethral valves
  - Urethral stenosis
  - Periurethral abscess
  - Pelvic hematoma
  - Neoplasm
  - Trauma

Hepatorenal Syndrome

Data from Trainin and Spitzer,[39] Ruley and Bock,[333] Oken,[347] and Ellis et al.[348]

with an accurate assessment of the child's volume status and effective cardiac output and may require central venous pressure measurement and Doppler echocardiography or invasive assessment of cardiac function, in addition to clinical examination. If the volume status is normal or has been returned to normal, and there is no evidence for fluid overload or congestive failure, then urine and serum samples should be obtained for analysis, and a diagnostic challenge with 20 ml/kg of saline or lactated Ringer's solution should be administered.[39, 370] If this does not increase urine output, then examination of urinary sediment and laboratory tests to assess tubular function, as outlined in Table 7–13, are helpful in distinguishing prerenal azotemia from acute parenchymal renal failure.[348] Early in prerenal oliguria, tubular function remains intact, and increased tubular reabsorption of urea, sodium, and water occurs

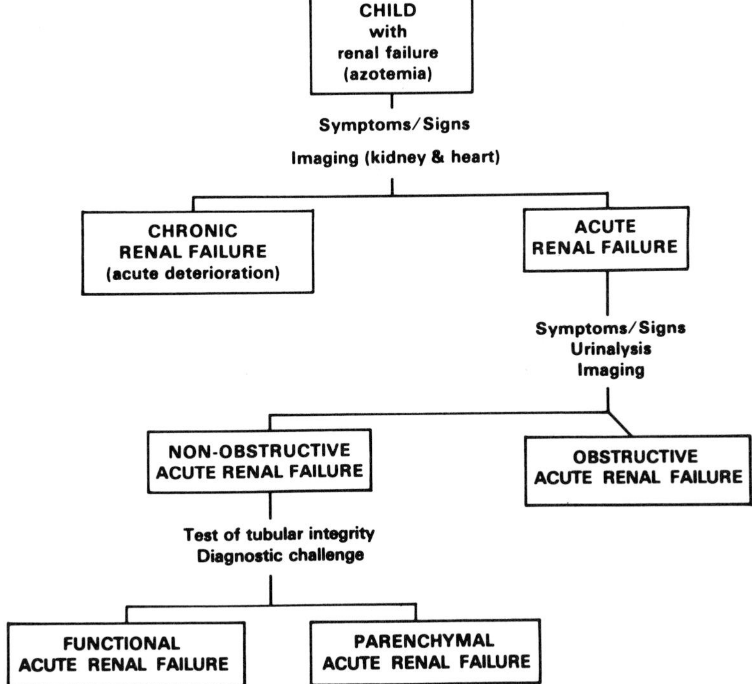

FIGURE 7–10. Systematic approach to the child with renal failure. (From Ruley EJ, Bock GH: Acute renal failure in infants and children. *In* Shoemaker WC, Thompson WL, Holbrook PR [Eds]: The Society of Critical Care Medicine: Textbook of Critical Care. Philadelphia, WB Saunders, 1984.)

in the face of diminished glomerular filtration and reduced tubular flow.[333] All the indices in Table 7–13 make use of these facts to assess tubular function. The single best test appears to be the fractional excretion of sodium (FE_{Na}), which is 90 percent accurate.[360, 361, 371, 372] In the newborn infant, the ratio of urine to plasma osmolality is also a good index.[361]

Table 7–13. LABORATORY STUDIES USED TO DIFFERENTIATE PRERENAL AZOTEMIA FROM PARENCHYMAL ACUTE RENAL FAILURE IN CHILDREN AND NEONATES

	Study	Prerenal Azotemia	ARF	Comment
Children	FE_{Na} (%)	<1	>3	FE_{Na} may be low in acute glomerulonephritis and in cases of early obstructive uropathy
	RFI	<1	>1	
	U_{Na} (mEq/L)	<20	>40	Considerable overlap exists; for patients with in-between values for U_{Na}, use U osmolarity, U/P creatinine, or U/P urea
	U osmolarity (mOsm/kg H_2O)	>500	<350	
	U/P creatinine	>40	<20	
	U/P urea	>8	<3	
	U/P osmolarity	>1.3	<1.3	Unreliable in malnourished children
Neonates	FE_{Na} (%)	<2.5	>2.5	
	RFI	<2.5	>2.5	
		<3	>3	
	U/P osmolarity	>1	<1	As good as FE_{Na} in newborn infants
	U/P urea	>4.8	<4.8	
	U/P creatinine	Variable	Variable	Not reliable

Indices should not be obtained after a sodium load or after administration of diuretic agents. Indices are more reliable in oliguric patients. They are not valid in infants less than 32 weeks' gestational age.

FE_{Na} = fractional excretion of filtered sodium = (U/P)Na/(U/P) creatinine × 100.

U = urinary; P = plasma.

RFI = renal failure index = U_{Na}(U/P) creatinine.

Modified from Ellis D, Gartner JC, Galvis AG: Acute renal failure in infants and children: Diagnosis, complications, and treatment. Crit Care Med 9:607, 1981.

A challenge with mannitol or potent loop diuretics has also been used in an effort to distinguish prerenal from parenchymal acute renal failure,[373–377] but this particular diagnostic maneuver may be fraught with several hazards. First, this challenge yields confounding information if obstruction has not been ruled out. Likewise, it may exacerbate renal ischemia and azotemia if an adequate volume status has not been established prior to the challenge, and significant hypotension may result.[348, 376, 378] Also, if parenchymal renal failure is present, an increased urine output may be falsely reassuring, since it may represent only a conversion from oliguric to nonoliguric renal failure.[357, 377, 378] Although this may be favorable from the standpoint of prognosis and ease of management, it may not obviate the problem of ongoing azotemia and should not be interpreted as signalling resolution of renal decompensation.[356] Finally, the administration of diuretic agents, by impairing tubular reabsorption in the normal kidney, invalidates subsequent urinary index studies, as outlined in Table 7–13, for at least 6 to 8 hours.[348] It is important to remember that if obstructive or prerenal insults are prolonged, renal parenchymal injury will ensue, and amelioration of the extrarenal factors at that point will not result in the rapid restoration of renal function.[333, 348]

PATHOPHYSIOLOGY

The pathophysiology of acute parenchymal renal failure remains controversial, but important concepts have emerged.[379, 380] Several of the theories of the pathogenesis of acute parenchymal renal failure are incorporated into Figure 7–11.[348] Renal ischemia is a consistent finding even in toxin-induced models of ARF,[381] and may initiate ARF by lowering glomerular capillary pressure to such a degree that filtration ceases. Ischemia also may injure tubular cells, which swell and cause further ischemia, which contributes to the continuation of ARF.[54, 382] The term *vasomotor nephropathy* refers to this pathogenetic sequence of events.[347] Likewise, tubular injury, with functional and often morphological changes, is a hallmark of ARF and may be a primary event.[54, 383] The term *acute tubular necrosis* is used to describe this pathogenetic theory.[379] As indicated by the bidirectional arrows in Figure 7–11, tubular injury, tubular obstruction, and renal ischemia may all interrelate, regardless of the initial insult, and contribute to the initiation and maintenance of acute parenchymal renal failure.[339]

A unifying hypothesis has recently evolved from an understanding of the role of mitochondria and calcium ions in ischemic and toxic cellular injury.[384, 385] An ischemic or toxic insult may lead to decreased cellular energy production and increased calcium entry into the cellular cytoplasm and mitochondria. The resulting arteriolar vasoconstriction and vascular endothelial swelling perpetuate the ischemia and alter glomerular permeability. Likewise, tubular cellular metabolism is impaired, leading to tubular swelling, dysfunction, back-leak, and obstruction.[54] The end-result of both is the clinical

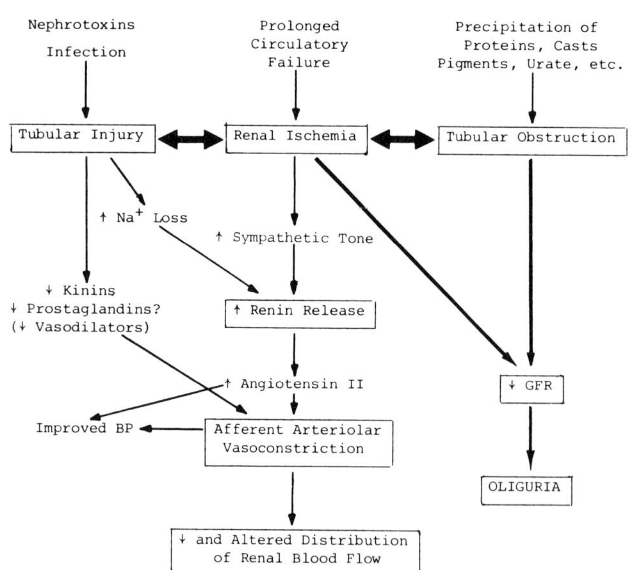

FIGURE 7–11. Pathogenesis of acute parenchymal renal failure. According to this schema, renal ischemia is the central event but *bidirectional arrows* indicate important interaction among tubular obstruction, tubular injury, and renal ischemia in the development of renal insufficiency and oliguria. Note that renal ischemia may continue despite correction of prerenal events that initiated ARF, owing to persistence of tubular damage, tubular obstruction, or altered intrarenal hemodynamics. Undernutrition (not shown) may prolong the oliguric phase by contributing to hypoperfusion and delayed healing of damaged tissue. (From Ellis D, Gartner JC, Galvis AG: Acute renal failure in infants and children: Diagnosis, complications and treatment. Crit Care Med 9:607, 1981. © 1981, The Williams and Wilkins Co., Baltimore.)

manifestation of acute parenchymal renal failure.

PREVENTION AND TREATMENT

The theories of the mechanism of renal injury have led to several proposals for the prevention of acute parenchymal renal failure. Postischemic infusion of adenine nucleotide energy substrate and magnesium chloride as a calcium antagonist results in significant renal protection in experimental models.[386] The administration of verapamil at the time of hypoxemia or norepinephrine-induced renal ischemia protects the glomerular filtration rate and prevents the morphological changes usually seen in the proximal tubular cells.[54, 387] Interruption of the renin-angiotensin-aldosterone cascade with captopril, an inhibitor of angiotensin-converting enzyme, improves systemic and renal hemodynamics, renal blood flow, and GFR in adults with azotemia and heart failure.[388, 389] Likewise, hydralazine and nitroprusside have been shown to improve renal perfusion in the face of severely depressed left ventricular function, provided filling pressures are optimized and the decrease in systemic arterial pressure is not excessive.[390, 391] Propranolol has been shown to attenuate experimentally induced postischemic renal failure, perhaps as a result of depression of renin release.[392] Thus, this is not in apparent contradiction to the salutary effects seen with administration of low-dose dopamine in acute parenchymal renal failure.[393, 394]

Dopamine at low doses (<5 μg/kg/min) is primarily a dopaminergic receptor stimulant that causes selective renal arteriolar dilatation plus inhibition of aldosterone secretion to increase renal blood flow, GFR, sodium excretion, and total urine output.[395–397] In addition, low-dose dopamine may well have direct diuretic and natriuretic effects and may inhibit norepinephrine release and norepinephrine-induced vasoconstriction.[398, 399] Finally, low-dose dopamine has been experimentally shown to increase renal blood flow, GFR, and urinary flow in transplanted kidneys despite beta-receptor blockade, when a constant cardiac output, heart rate, and mean arterial pressure are maintained.[400] Certainly, decreased cardiac output and hypotension induced by beta-blockers or calcium channel blockers would be extremely deleterious, and much more clinical work needs to be done before these experimental findings will become clinically applicable. Other experimentally successful regimens that fall into this category include infusions of acetylcholine, prostaglandin E, and bradykinin as renal vasodilators.[401–403]

Recently, atrial natriuretic peptide (ANP) infusion has been investigated as a preventive measure, as well as for "rescue" therapy, in experimental ARF induced by gentamicin or norepinephrine.[404, 405] ANP infusion has been found as effective as mannitol in the prevention of superimposed ARF in patients in chronic renal failure undergoing radiocontrast studies.[406]

Simple volume loading with optimization of preload is known to help prevent parenchymal ARF in high-risk patients.[407, 408] In addition to improving cardiac output, this may result because left atrial hypotension is a potent stimulus of renal vasoconstriction, whereas left atrial hypertension causes renal vasodilatation.[409–411] This effect occurs independently of the volume-induced decrease in renin secretion.[412]

Mannitol (0.25 to 0.5 g/kg) has been used to prevent or attenuate parenchymal ARF in almost every setting but has been especially useful with post-traumatic, hemoglobinuric, and myoglobinuric renal insults.[374, 375, 413–415] By acting as an intratubular osmotic agent, mannitol may maintain GFR at or above control values in the hypoperfused kidney.[416] It may also prevent cellular swelling and continued ischemia while the forced osmotic tubular diuresis may prevent tubular obstruction.[414, 416, 417] Renal arteriolar vasodilatation has also been shown,[418, 419] and the volume expansion accompanying administration may also be beneficial.[420] The risks of excessive mannitol administration include the possibility of decreased renal perfusion if volume is not replaced during vigorous diuresis, or if volume overload and ventricular failure ensue. Hyponatremia, acidosis, and hyperkalemia may also be exacerbated.[205, 206, 215, 216]

Furosemide has also been used in parenchymal ARF in moderate (1 to 2 mg/kg) to large (8 to 10 mg/kg) doses.[421, 422] Several beneficial effects of potent diuretics in ARF have been documented. They are renal arteriolar vasodilatation and an increase in renal blood flow,[377, 423] an increase in urinary flow,[421] a conversion from oliguric to nonoliguric parenchymal ARF,[357, 377, 424] and a decrease in the need for dialysis.[421, 425] Furosemide appears to be particularly useful in parenchymal ARF of acute childhood glomerulonephritis.[159] On the other hand, prospective controlled studies have shown a questionable value in preventing parenchymal ARF,[378] no benefit in established parenchymal ARF in medical patients,[422] and no change in duration of ARF or in overall mortality.[422, 425, 426] The timing of diuretic therapy seems to be important. Administration just prior to the insult is twice as effective as just after, and mannitol alone is ineffective after a renal insult, as is furosemide once parenchymal ARF is established.[422, 427] Combinations of drug therapy may be more effective, as shown by the synergistic protection afforded by dopamine in combination with furosemide in experimental nephrotoxic ARF.[394]

Although conversion to nonoliguric ARF and a decreased need for dialysis are important benefits, the use of furosemide or ethacrynic acid in the doses required is not without risk. These risks include causing hypovolemic cardiac instability, exacerbating renal failure, and producing ototoxicity, especially if acidosis or other ototoxins (for example, aminoglycosides) are present.[348, 428–430]

ANESTHETIC IMPLICATIONS

A practical approach for the anesthesiologist faced with a child with early, acute parenchymal renal failure is to eliminate all potential nephrotoxins and to ameliorate renal ischemia by optimizing preload and cardiac output. This may require invasive monitoring (arterial and central venous lines and, rarely, pulmonary artery catheter and cardiac output thermistor) in order to diagnose and treat hypovolemia, septic shock, or cardiac failure. When administering dopamine to infants to optimize hemodynamics, one must recall that significantly higher doses may be required than those needed in the adult, presumably owing to catecholamine receptor immaturity or deficiency.[431] Fortunately, at these higher doses (15 μg/kg/min as compared with 5 μg/kg/min in the adult), there seem to be no adverse effects on GFR or urinary output.[189] Following hemodynamic optimization, mannitol and/or furosemide may be administered in an attempt to prevent tubular obstruction and to convert oliguric ARF to nonoliguric parenchymal ARF. Diuretic administration should never be a substitute for hemodynamic optimization, and great care should be taken to avoid worsening the hemodynamic status. This means that careful monitoring and replacement of obligatory urinary fluid and electrolyte losses are mandatory.[427]

Once ARF is established, the major pathophysiological changes are impaired fluid and electrolyte balance, abnormal acid-base status, altered excretion of protein catabolites and drugs, the appearance of hypertension, bleeding diatheses and anemia, and decreased resistance to infection.[347, 348, 432] The anesthetic implications and management of these problems are discussed in detail earlier in this chapter (see Anesthetic Implications of the Pathophysiological Manifestations of Renal Failure). Caloric and nutritional balance seems to be an important factor in acute renal failure, and aggressive enteral or parenteral alimentation has been shown to be one of the few interventions that may hasten the recovery of renal function and improve the prognosis of ARF.[433–437] The beneficial effects seem to accrue from a decrease in urea nitrogen production,[438, 439] from a decreased incidence of and improved recovery from infection,[433, 434, 438] and from direct enhancement of tubular regeneration.[440] Because infection is a frequent life-threatening occurrence in ARF, meticulous care must be exercised in handling hyperalimentation and all other intravascular lines in these children.

Finally, dialysis during the course of ARF may become necessary to allow adequate volume for hyperalimentation, to treat acute volume overload resulting in intractable hypertension or congestive failure, to treat hyperkalemia unresponsive to other treatment regimens, to correct acidosis, and to remove nitrogenous wastes, which may rise suddenly during times of metabolic stress and result in encephalopathy.[39, 348, 432] Early institution of dialysis has been reported to reduce the overall incidence of serious complications, such as gastrointestinal hemorrhage and infection.[350, 352, 441–443] In patients requiring open heart surgery who in addition present in renal failure, intraoperative hemodialysis has been utilized in conjunction with cardiopulmonary bypass.[444, 445]

Because children have a high ratio of peritoneal to total body surface area, peritoneal dialysis achieves 50 percent of the efficiency of hemodialysis. This is in contrast to adults, in whom peritoneal dialysis is only 20 percent as efficient.[446] In addition, peritoneal dialysis is immediately available after catheter placement (often done under local anesthesia), is easier for ICU staff to administer, and requires no heparinization. It can be administered continuously and is less hemodynamically destabilizing, especially in infants, in whom a hemodialysis machine's volume may be large compared with the total blood volume of the infant and thus may require priming with blood. It also does not require large vessels for access, sparing them for other uses.[348, 447–449] On the other hand, peritoneal dialysis may not be as rapidly effective as hemodialysis in the removal of potassium and certain toxins and drugs,[348, 442] and it is not

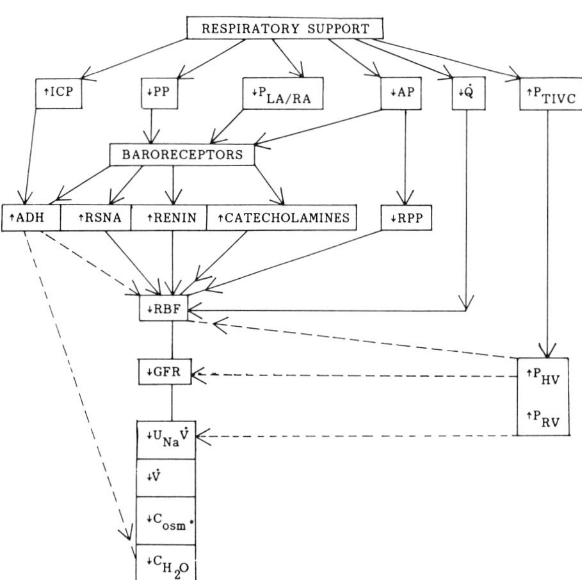

FIGURE 7–12. Mechanisms involved in the pathogenesis of renal dysfunction during respiratory support. ICP = intracranial pressure; PP = pulse pressure; $P_{LA/RA}$ = transmural left and right atrial pressures; AP = systemic arterial pressure; $\dot{Q}$ = cardiac output; P_{TIVC} = thoracic inferior vena caval pressure; ADH = antidiuretic hormone; RSNA = renal sympathetic nerve activity; RPP = renal perfusion pressure; RBF = renal blood flow; GFR = glomerular filtration rate; P_{HV} = hepatic venous pressure; P_{RV} = renal venous pressure; $U_{NA}\dot{V}$ = urinary sodium excretion; $\dot{V}$ = urinary output; C_{Osm} = osmolal clearance; C_{H_2O} = free water clearance. Dotted lines indicate that the mechanism is unlikely to be of significance. (Reprinted with permission from Priebe HJ, Hedley-White J: Respiratory support and renal function. Int Anesthesiol Clin *22*:203, 1984.)

without its own risks. These include hemorrhage, infection (peritonitis, pneumonia, sepsis), respiratory compromise (from subdiaphragmatic pressure or acute hydrothorax), hollow viscus perforation, increased protein loss, and a reduction in exchange efficiency if splanchnic blood flow is compromised.[450]

Anesthesiologists called upon to anesthetize children who are also undergoing peritoneal dialysis need to be aware of these potential hazards. It is also important to recognize that when hypertonic dialysate is used to remove excess intravascular volume, what appears to be only a moderate amount of peritoneal volume at the beginning may increase to the point of compromising ventilation, venous return, and cardiac output by the end of the dwell period. Positioning that might improve venous return (Trendelenburg positioning) may then further impair ventilation, and vice versa. Positive-pressure ventilation in and of itself may decrease renal blood flow and GFR, and this effect may be augmented if higher ventilatory pressures are required (Fig. 7–12).[451, 452] These considerations, along with the increased risks of regurgitation and aspiration associated with intra-abdominal distention, are strong arguments for the anesthesiologist to resist the suggestion that an intraoperative peritoneal dialysate dwell would optimize the patient's intraoperative and postoperative metabolic status. When possible, preoperative dialysis should be completed and the dialysate drained from the peritoneal cavity (except for a small, isotonic volume to help prevent catheter adherence to omentum or bowel) before the patient is brought to the operating room.

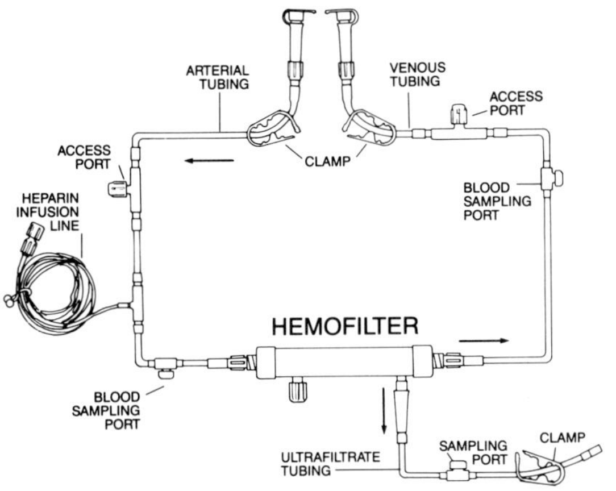

FIGURE 7–13. Continuous arteriovenous hemofiltration apparatus for use in pediatric patients. (Courtesy of Amicon Division, W.R. Grace & Company, Conn.)

A third alternative in the treatment of ARF is continuous arteriovenous hemofiltration (CAVH).[453–456] CAVH requires less and simpler equipment than does hemodialysis (Fig. 7–13). CAVH most commonly utilizes the child's own blood pressure to provide blood flow, as well as to generate the hemofiltration pressure across the selective membrane. In some cases (for example, in hypotensive patients), a simple roller pump may be added and suction applied to the distal side of the filter to increase the transmembrane pressure gradient.[456, 457] The blood diverted through the extracorporeal hemofilter is cleansed of nonprotein-bound solutes smaller than 10,000 daltons by convective mass transport, in a slow and continuous manner, providing a creatinine clearance of up to 10 ml/min (depending on multiple variables, including flow and pressure gradient).[453, 458] A major advantage includes gradual and controllable fluid and solute removal, which avoids the risk of hypotension or disequilibrium syndrome.[453, 456]

CAVH has been employed successfully in critically ill children and neonates, including premature infants.[455, 457, 459, 460] An advantage over hemodialysis in the neonate is the relatively smaller extracorporeal blood volume required,[457] although efficacy may vary significantly depending on the characteristics of the catheters used for arterial and venous access.[461] CAVH still requires anticoagulation and vascular access and runs the risk of infection from indwelling vascular lines. The precision and stability with which the ultrafiltration rate can be controlled and electrolyte balance maintained (independently of therapeutic volume changes) exceed those of peritoneal dialysis, making CAVH an attractive alternative modality in critically ill children.

CAVH can be utilized intraoperatively to remove excess crystalloid, to control serum electrolyte levels, and to provide hemoconcentration as needed, although continued heparinization is required. It can most conveniently be utilized in parallel with cardiopulmonary bypass, in open heart cases. If hemofiltration is discontinued during operation, the indwelling arterial and venous lines may be utilized for drug, fluid, and blood product administration, for blood sampling, and for pressure transduction.

Many drugs utilized intraoperatively or in an intensive care unit (such as antibiotics, theophylline, and barbiturates) have a limited but potentially clinically significant clearance during CAVH.[458, 462] Clearance of a particular compound depends on the rate of ultrafiltration and the compound's sieving coefficient (the ability to permeate the hemofiltration membrane, a characteristic highly influenced by protein binding).[458] The serum level of highly protein- or tissue-bound drugs should be minimally affected by CAVH. However, because these variables may be unpredictable in a particular setting, continuous monitoring and titration of anesthetic medications to the desired clinical effect is required.

DISEASES OF RENAL PARENCHYMA

As noted previously, there are multitudes of congenital, hereditary, and acquired renal diseases, as well as systemic illnesses not usually considered primarily renal, that may result in renal parenchymal injury and failure (see Tables 7–1, 7–2, and 7–12). As shown in Table 7–14, classification of these illnesses is further complicated by the fact that each distinct histopathological finding on renal biopsy may be associated with many very different clinical entities and syndromes.[463–466] Conversely, distinct clinical syndromes (such as acute nephritis or the nephrotic syndrome) may demonstrate many different histopathological findings and have many etiologies (Table 7–15). Because of these difficulties in classification, information about etiology, epidemiology, and prognosis is often conflicting and confusing. From the standpoint of anesthetic care, it is therefore more important to evaluate each of the particular clinical components of renal impairment that an individual child demonstrates than just to know the clinical or histopathological diagnosis. With this understanding, we will now consider some of the more distinct clinical syndromes of parenchymal renal disease and the extrarenal manifestations with which the anesthesiologist should be familiar. Little has been published with regard to anesthetic recommendations for these entities, and especially for specific rare conditions in children. Anesthetic evaluation and care, therefore, must follow from theoretical considerations with regard to pathophysiology, and from anecdotal anesthetic experience with some of the rarer pediatric renal diseases.

GLOMERULONEPHRITIS

As first described, *acute glomerulonephritis (Bright's disease)* was any acute inflammatory process of the glomerulus and nephron resulting in hematuria and proteinuria.[467] It is now recognized to be a collection of many diseases (Tables 7–14 and 7–15) with varying presentations.[463, 468] Acute glomerulonephritis is thought to result from immunological injury to the kidney due to anti–glomerular basement membrane disease, tubulointerstitial disease, and immune complex deposition.[469–471] The antigen involved may be renal or nonrenal endogenous antigen, exogenous antigen, or foreign material that is haptogenic combining with endogenous protein to form the antigen (Table 7–16).[468, 472, 473] The immune complexes may be deposited from the circulation during glomerular filtration or may form in situ, or both.[468, 470, 471] Complement activation and platelet aggregation also seem to be involved in the mechanism of injury and have led to trials of anticoagulant and

Table 7–14. HETEROGENEITY OF CLINICAL SYNDROMES WITHIN DISTINCT HISTOPATHOLOGICAL CATEGORIES

Proliferative Glomerulonephritis
- Nephrotic syndrome
- Acute glomerulonephritis
- Rapidly progressive (oliguric) glomerulonephritis
- Chronic glomerulonephritis
- Persistent hematuria and proteinuria
- Schönlein-Henoch purpura
- Systemic lupus erythematosus
- Periarteritis nodosa and hypersensitivity angiitis
- Bacterial endocarditis
- Mixed essential cryoglobulinemia
- Rheumatic fever
- Narcotic abuse
- Hereditary progressive nephritis (Alport's syndrome)
- Hereditary deficiency of complement
- Tumor-associated nephropathy
- Sarcoidosis
- Bee-sting nephrotic syndrome

Necrotizing and Crescentic Glomerulonephritis
- Acute glomerulonephritis
- Rapidly progressive glomerulonephritis
- Membranoproliferative glomerulonephritis
- Chronic glomerulonephritis
- Schönlein-Henoch purpura
- Periarteritis nodosa and hypersensitivity angiitis
- Goodpasture's syndrome
- Wegener's granulomatosis
- Systemic lupus erythematosus
- Mixed essential cryoglobulinemia
- Bacterial endocarditis
- Hereditary progressive nephritis (Alport's syndrome)

Membranous Glomerulonephropathy
- Nephrotic syndrome
- Chronic glomerulonephritis
- Renal vein thrombosis
- Systemic lupus erythematosus
- Diabetes mellitus
- Tumor-associated nephropathy
- Sarcoidosis
- Rheumatoid arthritis
- Bullous dermatoses
- Chronic infection
  - Syphilis, schistosomiasis
  - Filariasis, Guillain-Barré
  - Hepatitis B antigenemia
- Drug-associated nephrotic syndrome
  - Trimethadione, D-penicillamine
  - Gold, mercury
- Slowly progressive glomerulonephritis

Membranoproliferative Glomerulonephritis
- Nephrotic syndrome
- Acute glomerulonephritis
- Rapidly progressive (oliguric) glomerulonephritis
- Chronic glomerulonephritis
- Slowly progressive glomerulonephritis
- Persistent hematuria and proteinuria
- Schönlein-Henoch purpura
- Systemic lupus erythematosus
- Allograft rejection
- Progressive and partial lipodystrophy
- Sickle cell disease
- Hereditary deficiency of complement
- Hepatic cirrhosis and chronic hepatitis
- Quartan malaria
- Chronic staphylococcal bacteremia ("shunt nephritis")

Focal Glomerulonephritis
- Nephrotic syndrome
- Acute glomerulonephritis
- Chronic glomerulonephritis
- Chronic hematuria
- Bacterial endocarditis
- Schönlein-Henoch purpura
- Systemic lupus erythematosus
- Goodpasture's syndrome
- Periarteritis nodosa and hypersensitivity angiitis
- Wegener's granulomatosis
- Hereditary deficiency of complement

Focal Segmental Glomerulosclerosis
- Nephrotic syndrome
- Chronic glomerulonephritis
- Persistent hematuria
- Asymptomatic proteinuria
- Rheumatoid arthritis
- Narcotic abuse (heroin)
- Hereditary progressive nephritis (Alport's and nail-patella syndromes)
- Sickle cell disease
- Massive obesity
- Allograft rejection

Reprinted with permission from Bernstein J, Barnett HL, Edelmann CM Jr: Glomerular diseases: Introduction and classification. *In* Edelmann CM Jr (Ed.): Pediatric Kidney Disease. Boston, Little, Brown, 1978.

platelet inhibitory therapy.[474–477] Children with glomerulonephritis may also be treated with glucocorticoids and cytotoxic agents such as cyclophosphamide, and so in addition to having an induced abnormality in clotting, they may be relatively immunosuppressed and may require perioperative "stress" coverage with glucocorticoids. The inflammation and injury of acute glomerulonephritis manifest themselves clinically as an acute nephritic episode, the nephrotic syndrome, or interstitial nephritis.[478] Although it frequently completely resolves, acute glomerulonephritis may progress to cause permanent damage and chronic renal failure.

Table 7–15. CLINICAL SYNDROMES OF RENAL PARENCHYMAL DISEASE AND THEIR MULTIPLE ETIOLOGIES

Persistent Microscopic and Recurrent Gross Hematuria	Nephrotic Syndrome
Benign recurrent hematuria	Corticosteroid-sensitive minimal change nephrotic syndrome
Hereditary progressive nephritis (Alport's)	Corticosteroid-resistant nephrotic syndrome with focal segmental glomerulosclerosis
IgA nephropathy (Berger's)	Corticosteroid-resistant nephrotic syndrome with membranous glomerulonephropathy
Schönlein-Henoch purpura	Corticosteroid-resistant nephrotic syndome with membranoproliferative glomerulonephritis
Systemic lupus erythematosus	Congenital nephrotic syndrome
Membranoproliferative glomerulonephritis	Acute postinfectious glomerulonephritis
Postinfectious glomerulonephritis	Schönlein-Henoch purpura
Chronic glomerulonephritis	Systemic lupus erythematosus
Sickle cell disease	Narcotic addiction
Acute Glomerulonephritis	Sickle cell disease
Acute postinfectious glomerulonephritis	Familial nephritis (Alport's)
Following streptococcal infection	Diabetes mellitus
Following other infections (staphylococcal, viral)	Amyloidosis
Membranoproliferative glomerulonephritis	Renal vein thrombosis
Exacerbation of persistent glomerulonephritis	Quartan malaria
Recurrent hematuria and IgA nephropathy	Congenital syphilis
Schönlein-Henoch purpura	Drug reaction
Systemic lupus erythematosus	Neoplasia
Familial nephritis (Alport's)	Bee stings
Rapidly Progressive Glomerulonephritis	Poison oak dermatitis
Idiopathic crescentic and necrotizing glomerulonephritis	Bullous dermatoses
Acute postinfectious glomerulonephritis	
Membranoproliferative glomerulonephritis	
Goodpasture's syndrome	
Hemolytic-uremic syndrome	
Schönlein-Henoch purpura	
Systemic lupus erythematosus	
Hypersensitivity angiitis	

Reprinted with permission from Bernstein J, Barnett HL, Edelmann CM Jr.: Glomerular diseases: Introduction and classification. *In* Edelmann CM Jr (Ed.): Pediatric Kidney Disease. Boston, Little, Brown, 1978.

Acute Nephritic Syndrome

The acute nephritic syndrome is characterized by the sudden onset of hematuria, frequently accompanied by proteinuria, hypertension, oliguria, and edema.[478]

Acute poststreptococcal glomerulonephritis is a prime example of this syndrome. It is the most common form of glomerulonephritis in children and follows a skin or upper respiratory tract infection with group A beta-hemolytic streptococci.[468, 479] The true incidence is unknown since the majority of cases are subclinical.[480, 481] It is most prevalent during the school-age years, with an average onset at ages 6 to 7 years, although cases have been described during infancy and it may occur during adolescence or adulthood.[468, 482] Most series report a prevalence in males of twice that in females, although this has been attributed to the tendency to misdiagnose mild cases in females as cystitis.[468] Analysis of the male-to-female ratio during epidemics shows no sex predilection.[468] A latent period of 8 to 21 days following infection usually precedes the onset of clinical glomerulonephritis, although cases with shorter or longer latency have been described.[469] In symptomatic patients, the common presenting features are those of the acute nephritic syndrome: hematuria, proteinuria, hypertension, edema, and oliguria. Frequently there may also be circulatory congestion with pulmonary edema, exacerbated by mild anemia that is partially dilutional. In severe cases, hypertensive encephalopathy and seizures may occur, and rarely renal impairment may progress to anuria.[468] Treatment follows the principles detailed earlier under Acute Renal Failure, and as mentioned previously, furosemide appears particularly useful in the management of fluid overload and hypertension in these children.[159] The development of poststreptococcal glomerulonephritis does not seem to be decreased with early antibiotic treatment of the streptococcal infection, but the severity of the disease may be attenuated.[468, 483] Improvement following immunosuppressive therapy in severe proliferative glomerulonephritis following streptococcal infection has been reported, but a cause-and-effect relationship between the treatment and the improvement has not been established.[479] In

Table 7–16. ANTIGENIC FACTORS ASSOCIATED WITH ACUTE IMMUNE COMPLEX–MEDIATED GLOMERULONEPHRITIS

1. Glomerulonephritis mediated by anti-GBM antibodies. Also includes anti-GBM antibody nephritis with pulmonary hemorrhage (Goodpasture's syndrome).
2. Glomerulonephritis mediated by immune complexes deposited from the circulation or possibly formed in situ.
3. Infectious agents associated with AICGN:
   - Bacterial
     - Group A β-hemolytic streptococci
     - *Streptococcus viridans*
     - *Diplococcus pneumoniae*
     - *Staphylococcus aureus*
     - *Treponema pallidum*
     - Leptospirosis
     - *Salmonella typhosa*
     - *Staphylococcus epidermidis*
   - Viral
     - Hepatitis B
     - Cytomegalovirus
     - Enteroviral infections
     - Measles
     - Guillain-Barré syndrome
     - Oncornavirus
     - Mumps virus
   - Parasitic
     - *Plasmodium malariae* and *falciparum*
     - Toxoplasmosis
     - Schistosomiasis
     - Filariasis
     - Trypanosomiasis
   - Rickettsial
     - Scrub typhus
   - Fungal
     - *Coccidioides immitis*
4. Drugs, toxins, and antisera
   - Vaccinations, excessive DPT
   - Antivenoms and antitoxins
   - Organic gold compounds
   - D-Penicillamine
   - Organic and inorganic mercurials
   - Sulfonamides
   - Captopril
5. Endogenous antigens
   - Tumor-associated antigens
   - Thyroglobulin
   - Autologous immunoglobulin
   - DNA

GBM = Glomerular basement membrane; AICGN = acute immune complex–mediated glomerulonephritis; DPT = diphtheria, pertussis, tetanus toxoid vaccine.

From Jordan SC, Lemire JM: Acute glomerulonephritis: Diagnosis and treatment. Pediatr Clin North Am *29*:857, 1982.

general, corticosteroids and immunosuppressive drugs are not routinely used in acute poststreptococcal glomerulonephritis.[479, 483] The prognosis is remarkably good, with all but 2 to 5 percent of children recovering completely.[471] Sporadic rather than epidemic cases, as well as cases in the older child, seem to have a worse prognosis, with residual renal impairment.[468] Recurrence of poststreptococcal glomerulonephritis is fortunately rare.[471]

Differentiation of acute poststreptococcal glomerulonephritis from other causes of the nephritic syndrome is important from a treatment and prognostic standpoint. Detection of rising antibody titers to various streptococcal antigens (most commonly antistreptolysin O titers), together with a depression in complement C_3 levels, aids greatly in the diagnosis.[468, 483] Included in the differential diagnosis are the infectious agents and disease entities listed in Tables 7–14 to 7–16. Although clinical presentation, clinical course, and response to treatment may distinguish among different entities, renal biopsy may be necessary.[471]

Chronic glomerulonephritis, made apparent by an acute exacerbation, *membranoproliferative glomerulonephritis, membranous or epimembranous glomerulonephritis,* and *rapidly progressive glomerulonephritis* are all primary renal diseases that may present with the nephrotic syndrome (see later), the acute nephritic syndrome, or both. These may be even further subcategorized according to histopathological findings, rate of progression, response to immunosuppressants, and prognosis.[463, 471] Major manifestations are those of nephritis, nephrosis, and ARF.

Benign recurrent hematuria (familial and nonfamilial), *focal nephritis,* and *Berger's disease (IgG-IgA mesangial nephropathy)* are benign diseases that are characterized by recurrent hematuria, which may be gross.[468, 484] Usually the occurrence of benign hematuria coincides with a febrile illness or exercise, but it may also occur with the stress of operation and be unnecessarily alarming. In Berger's disease, gross hematuria and moderate proteinuria occur simultaneously with a febrile illness, usually a nonstreptococcal rhinopharyngeal infection.[471]

Hereditary progressive nephritis is characterized by recurrent hematuria, progressive renal failure, and a frequent association with high-frequency neurosensory hearing loss and lenticular ocular abnormalities.[468, 471, 485] The distinction between *Alport's disease* (hereditary nephritis with deafness) and *Guthrie's disease* (hereditary nephritis alone) has no medical or historical basis, since these contemporary investigators studied and reported on the same family.[485] The disease is thought to be due to an autosomally inherited defect in glomerular basement membrane, and immunofluorescent staining for immunocomplexes is negative.[463] Variable expression and penetrance are required to explain all patterns of inheritance, and one fifth of affected neonates may represent new mutations.[486] The prevalence of the disease is unknown, but men are affected more than women and blacks are rarely affected. It is estimated that Alport's disease accounts for 3 percent of chronic renal failure in childhood.[485] Variants of Alport's disease may have associated polyneuropathy, severe ichthyosis, diabetes, myopathy, or thrombocytopenia with giant platelets.[485] Each patient must be individually evaluated for these associated problems, which may affect anesthetic care. The presence of the nephrotic syndrome may also influence anesthetic management (see later).

Hereditary onycho-osteodysplasia, or *nail-patella syndrome,* is characterized by dystrophic and hypoplastic nails, iliac horns, malformed radial heads, and hypoplastic patellae.[485] Abnormal pigmentation of the iris and cutaneous manifestations also may occur. Forty percent of patients have renal disease, which progresses to renal failure in 25 percent. An abnormality of basement membrane is transmitted with an autosomal dominant inheritance, linked to the gene locus for ABO blood groups, and distinct from Alport's disease.[485, 487]

Prolonged bacteremia associated with infected ventriculoatrial shunts or bacterial endocarditis may produce immune complex glomerulonephritis presenting as a persistent nephritic syndrome (*"endocarditis nephritis"* and *"shunt nephritis"*).[471, 488, 489] Antibiotic therapy may often be ineffective, requiring surgical removal of the infected shunt or valve.[471] The anesthesiologist is then faced with anesthetizing a child with ongoing nephritis and bacteremia, as well as the problems associated with either a malfunctioning ventriculoatrial shunt or an infected heart valve.

Henoch-Schönlein purpura (Schönlein-Henoch syndrome, anaphylactoid purpura, allergic purpura, purpura rheumatica) is a serious cause of nephritis and may account for up to 15 percent of glomerular nephropathies in children.[471] Males are more commonly affected than females. The age of onset is usually between 6 months and 6 years of age, more severe renal involvement occurs in older children, and recurrent episodes are common.[471, 490, 491] It is a disease of unknown etiology, which usually presents 1 to 3 weeks after a nonspecific upper respiratory tract infection. A characteristic purpuric and symmetrical rash invariably appears over the lateral malleoli and is frequently distributed over the extensor surfaces of the lower legs, arms, and buttocks.[490, 491] Painful edema of the scalp, hands, and feet, along with ankle and knee joint pain, may occur independently of the degree of renal involvement. Subcutaneous bleeding may occur in the conjunctiva, eyelids, scrotum (mimicking torsion of the testicle), and calves (mimicking deep venous thrombosis). Colicky abdominal pain is common, suggesting an acute abdominal emergency, and indeed may be accompanied by hematemesis, melena, and rarely intussusception, requiring surgical intervention.[490, 492] Other extrarenal manifestations of importance to the anesthesiologist are severe nosebleeds, hepatomegaly, and rare neuronal involvement, including facial palsy, chorea, encephalopathy, and convulsions.[490] Hematological studies reveal an elevated white cell count and erythrocyte sedimentation rate, and a hemoglobin concentration normal or depressed in proportion to the degree of prior bleeding. Clotting studies, platelet count, and bleeding time are all normal. The bleeding, purpura, edema, and renal and gastrointestinal manifestations are all thought to be vascular in origin.[490] This may be particularly frustrating to the anesthesiologist and surgeon faced with diffuse intraoperative bleeding unresponsive to replacement therapy. The renal involvement usually begins within 4 weeks of onset of the illness, may be quite variable, and markedly influences the prognosis.[493, 494] Although the combination is fortunately uncommon, of those children who manifest both an acute nephritic syndrome and nephrosis, 50 percent at 10-year follow-up will demonstrate, or have died of, severe renal insufficiency.[490, 493, 495] Treatment has been attempted with corticosteroids, immunosuppressive drugs (such as cyclophosphamide and azathioprine), oral anticoagulants, and platelet inhibitors (dipyridamole). The anesthesiologist may encounter children on any one or combination of these drugs, with their attendant side effects. Although spectacular recoveries have been reported, there are no data from adequately controlled studies that this treatment favorably alters the course of either the disease or the renal involvement,[490, 491] and institution of such therapy represents a desperate effort in the severely affected child. Fortunately, most children have mild-to-moderate disease and require only symptomatic care. More severe illness may require supportive treatment according to the degree of renal failure and complications. Secondary nephrotic syndrome may become manifest, with the attendant implications for anesthetic care (see later).

Goodpasture's syndrome (hemorrhagic pulmonary-renal syndrome, lung purpura with nephritis, pulmonary hemosiderosis with glomer-

ulonephritis, hemorrhagic and interstitial pneumonitis with nephritis) is a combination of pulmonary hemorrhage and glomerulonephritis, most commonly occurring in adolescent males.[496, 497] Most patients present with hemoptysis, which ranges from scant to massive and fatal. Extensive alveolar hemorrhage causes a decrease in pulmonary compliance, impaired gas exchange, and arterial hypoxemia. Compensatory hyperpnea may result in respiratory alkalosis.[496] Microcytic and hypochromic anemia results from the large quantity of blood chronically lost into the lung.[497] Glomerulonephritis causing hematuria, proteinuria, and hypertension may rarely precede the pulmonary symptoms but usually occurs concomitantly or following pulmonary involvement by up to several months.[496, 498] Kidney biopsies antedating clinical signs of renal involvement will still show immunofluorescent and electron microscopic abnormalities. These are characteristic of the anti–basement membrane lesions that cause both the renal and pulmonary injury.[496, 498, 499]

The prognosis of Goodpasture's syndrome is poor, with the usual acute, fulminant onset leading to pulmonary or renal failure within months of presentation. Reports of prolonged survival and spontaneous remission emphasize the unpredictability of the illness in any given patient, however, and make reports of apparent responses to therapy difficult to interpret.[496] Steroids and immunosuppressive drugs (such as azathioprine, 6-mercaptopurine, cyclophosphamide, and nitrogen mustard) have all been tried, with the pulmonary manifestations seemingly responding better than the renal lesions.[496, 498] Because of the pulmonary hemorrhage, anticoagulants have not been used. Plasmapheresis (undertaken to decrease anti–glomerular basement membrane antibody titers), in combination with steroid and alkylating agent therapy, has shown promise.[494] The most aggressive and radical intervention has been bilateral nephrectomy, which has been associated with dramatic cessation of massive pulmonary hemorrhage.[500, 501] This treatment is not always effective, however.[498, 502] Advanced renal failure has been treated with transplantation, with a surprisingly low incidence of recurrence of anti–glomerular basement membrane lesions in the kidney allograft.[498, 503]

Considerations for anesthesia in these very ill patients include those for acute or chronic renal failure and renal transplantation as discussed previously. The severe pulmonary involvement, coupled with anemia, may result in severe hypoxemia, pulmonary hypertension, and a reduced oxygen-carrying capacity. This places further demands on a cardiovascular system already compromised by systemic hypertension, fluid overload, electrolyte imbalance, and azotemia. When possible, these problems should be corrected preoperatively with dialysis, antihypertensive agents, and transfusion. Because of the severe pulmonary involvement and oliguria, intraoperative volume assessment necessitates the use of pulmonary capillary wedge pressures to estimate left atrial filling pressures.

The *hemolytic-uremic syndrome* (HUS) is characterized by acute renal failure, hemolytic anemia (with fragmented erythrocytes), and thrombocytopenia.[504–506] The syndrome occurs mainly in white infants and children, and rarely in neonates; there is no sex predilection.[506] Cases have also been reported in adults, often in association with pregnancy, and the similarity to *thrombotic thrombocytopenic purpura* has led to the suggestion that these syndromes are essentially the same, but occurring in different age groups.[504, 507] Recognition that the triad of acute renal failure, hemolytic anemia, and thrombocytopenia is a syndrome and not a distinct clinicopathological entity helps in understanding the geographical differences in reported incidence and age of onset. It has also been observed that there is a mild form, a severe acute form, a severe progressive form, and two distinct forms of familial involvement, one autosomal recessive, the other autosomal dominant, both with incomplete penetrance.[504, 506, 508, 509] Severity and prognosis vary among these groups.

Many infectious agents (viral and bacterial) have been implicated as precipitating factors in epidemics and individual cases of HUS, including an association with *Shigella* and *Salmonella* infections.[504, 510] Several epidemiological studies have shown a strong association between HUS and direct or immunological evidence of infection with *Escherichia coli,* serotype O 157:H7.[511–513] This has led to the suggestion that the development of a vaccine may become a preventive strategy for HUS.[514]

A universal finding is injury to the epithelial lining or arterioles in the kidney and elsewhere, leading to deposition of platelet and fibrin thrombi, which cause vascular occlusion.[515] A composite theory of the pathogenesis of the vascular endothelial injury is that bacterial neuraminidase, *Shigella* toxin, or circulating endotoxin precipitates localized intravascular coagulation and microangiopathic changes. This occurs in individuals genetically predisposed to microvascular thrombosis because of a congenital prostacyclin deficiency, increased thromboxane production, or antithrombin-III deficiency.[504, 516]

Widespread occlusion of arterioles is responsible for the acute renal deterioration and may lead to bilateral renal cortical necrosis. These microvascular lesions are not restricted to the kidneys. Microangiopathic hemolytic anemia and platelet consumption occur diffusely and may involve other organ systems, most notably the central nervous system, heart, and gastrointestinal tract.[504, 517]

A prodromal illness usually precedes the onset of the hemolytic-uremic syndrome by a few days or weeks. This prodrome may consist of diarrhea, which may be frankly bloody, and vomiting, with occasional hematemesis. Otherwise it may consist of an upper respiratory tract infection, urinary tract infection, varicella, or measles.[504, 505]

The onset of the full-blown syndrome may be heralded by any one or combination of severe gastrointestinal pain, oliguria, petechiae, striking pallor due to anemia, hypertension, volume overload, congestive heart failure, and convulsions.[504–506] In 20 percent of cases the symptoms may mimic an abdominal emergency. In a few, intestinal ulceration, obstruction, gangrene, perforation, or intussusception may require emergency surgery.[504] The liver may also be involved, with hepatosplenomegaly and elevation of liver enzymes, but jaundice is rare. The anemia may be acute and severe, with hemoglobin concentrations falling by 2 g/dl/h, resulting in hemoglobin levels as low as 2 g/dl on admission.[505] This degree of anemia, coupled with hypervolemia, azotemia, hypertension, and electrolyte abnormalities, as well as direct myocardial involvement, may lead to severe congestive heart failure.[505, 517, 518] Central nervous system involvement may occur, with drowsiness, irritability, coma, seizures, and hemiparesis. This may result from hypertensive or uremic encephalopathy, hyponatremia or hypocalcemia, hemorrhage due to thrombocytopenia or anticoagulant therapy, or direct microvascular involvement.[506, 519, 520] Thrombotic microangiopathy of the optic nerve and retina, resulting in blindness, has been described,[521] and rarely large vessel thrombotic stroke may occur, resulting in severe neurological sequelae or death.[522] The majority of patients recover from the central nervous system involvement, although some suffer permanent neurological impairment, and a few infants may die as a result.[505]

The renal involvement in HUS is acute in onset and always present. It may vary from a transient decrease in urinary volume and renal function to fulminant acute renal failure with bilateral cortical necrosis, anuria, and progression to chronic renal failure.[505, 523] All the systemic manifestations of renal failure may appear. Early diagnosis and aggressive treatment, including dialysis, have reduced the mortality to 4 to 7 percent in endemic areas, and revealed the importance of the nonrenal disease processes in the prognosis of HUS.[504, 506, 517]

In addition to therapy for renal failure, treatment of the anemia and thrombocytopenia may be necessary, especially in the event of bleeding or in preparation for operation. Attempts to raise the platelet count may fail owing to ongoing consumption and may cause further microvascular occlusion. Therefore, platelet transfusion is usually reserved for extreme thrombocytopenia (platelet counts of less than 20,000 per μl) or to treat active bleeding.[505, 506] Transfusion of packed red blood cells to treat anemia must be carefully monitored, since the infusion of even a small volume of blood may induce, or severely exacerbate, hypertension or congestive heart failure.[506] There is also speculation that the hemolysis of relatively older transfused cells may release large amounts of adenosine disphosphate. This is a potent stimulant of platelet aggregation, resulting in increased microvascular thrombosis.[504]

Attempts have been made to interrupt the microvascular thrombosis with aspirin, dipyridamole, heparin, and streptokinase. The results are mixed, and all the attendant risks of anticoagulant therapy are present.[504, 524–526] Other interventions have been directed at removing increased plasma thrombogenic factors (such as thromboxane) by exchange transfusion or plasmapheresis.[527–529] Replacement of deficient plasma inhibitors of platelet aggregation and coagulation by infusions of prostacyclin, antithrombin III, or fresh-frozen plasma has also been tried.[504, 530–533] Bilateral nephrectomy has resulted in a prompt return of the platelet count to normal.[504] Successful subsequent renal homotransplantation has been reported in infants, children, and adults, despite the occasional recurrence of HUS lesions in the transplanted kidney.[534, 535] Fortunately, HUS very rarely requires such aggressive intervention.

Anesthetic considerations for surgery in an infant or child with HUS primarily involve the presence of acute renal failure. The child's condition should be optimized with preoperative dialysis, and treatment of hypertension and anemia is desirable. This is frequently impossible when these children require exploratory laparotomy for a suspected intra-abdominal emergency. This contraindicates peritoneal dialysis. The anticipation of oliguria, a large operative blood loss, and dramatic hemodynamic responses to even small blood volume changes justifies invasive monitoring. Intra-arterial and central venous pressure lines, as well as large-bore intravenous catheters, should be inserted by surgical placement if necessary. In small infants, large intraoperative blood loss requires diligent replacement with blood components or fresh whole blood and platelets, as well as careful monitoring and treatment of plasma calcium levels. The anesthesiologist may take solace in the knowledge that incidental intraoperative exchange transfusion may be beneficial to the patient.[527]

Nephrotic Syndrome

The nephrotic syndrome, as defined, consists of massive proteinuria, hypoalbuminemia, hyperlipidemia, and edema.[536–538] In children this means a urinary protein loss exceeding 0.05 g/kg/day and serum albumin levels of less than 2.5 g/dl.[536] Like the acute nephritic syndrome, it represents a particular pattern of response of the kidney to one of many different insults and diseases. Many diseases that cause nephritis may also result in the nephrotic syndrome (see Table 7–15). Although varying with etiology, age, and subtype, the overall incidence of the nephrotic syndrome in children under 16 years of age is 2 in 100,000.[536] It results from primary glomerular disease in 90 percent of affected children, whereas in the remaining 10 percent the nephrotic syndrome arises secondary to a systemic disease.[537] The primary or "idiopathic" nephrotic syndrome may be divided into subtypes according to histopathological appearance.

Minimal change nephrotic syndrome (minimal lesion, nil lesion, lipoid nephrosis, foot process disease, or *idiopathic primary nephrotic syndrome)* is the most common lesion in children, accounting for up to 75 percent of cases, whereas it is associated with only 30 percent of adult nephrotic syndrome.[539] The onset is usually between 2 and 7 years of age, with a male-to-female predilection of 2 to 1.[539, 540] The course of the disease may vary with the initial response to treatment and the success of treating relapses, intercurrent infections, and complications, but in general the prognosis is excellent for the minimal change lesion.[541–543] Acute renal failure may appear during the course of minimal change nephrotic syndrome, although this is even rarer in children than in adults.[544, 545] Causes include severe intravascular volume depletion resulting in prerenal azotemia and progressing to acute tubular necrosis, nephrotoxic injury, or acute bilateral renal vein thrombosis, although most often no inciting etiology can be found.[545]

Focal segmental glomerulosclerosis (focal glomerular sclerosis) is found in about 10 percent of children with nephrotic syndrome. Clinical onset may be at any age, and there is no sex predilection.[546] It should be distinguished from *focal global glomerulosclerosis* or *congenital glomerulosclerosis,* which can be seen normally in kidneys during the first year of life and in which fewer than 1 percent of glomeruli are involved by total sclerosis. This probably represents an error in nephrogenesis and is of little consequence to overall renal function.[546] The finding of focal *segmental* glomerulosclerosis is far more ominous, because a significant proportion of children with this condition are resistant to therapy and progress to end-stage renal disease.[537, 547] Therapy with high-dose steroids, azathioprine, cyclophosphamide, and chlorambucil has yielded occasional success but a poor overall response rate.[537] Preliminary trials with aspirin and dipyridamole have shown some success.[548, 549]

Diffuse proliferative glomerulonephritis can be divided into *membranoproliferative glomerulonephritis (mesangiocapillary, persistent hypocomplementemic,* or *lobular glomerulonephritis)* and *mesangial proliferative glomerulonephritis (pure endocapillary, endocapillary,* or *extracapillary proliferative glomerulonephritis).*[536] Mesangial proliferation occurs in 2 to 5 percent of children with the nephrotic syndrome.[537] The response to treatment and prognosis are difficult to determine because of confusion about classification of these lesions, but overall, the mesangial proliferative lesion carries a good prognosis. Nonresponders are subsequently found to have had, or to have developed, focal segmental glomerulosclerosis.[537] Membranoproliferative glomerulonephritis, on the other hand, has a poor long-term prognosis, with no evidence of therapeutic benefit from corticosteroids, anticoagulants, or cytotoxic drugs.[550] In fact, administration of corticosteroids in high daily doses is associated with rapid deterioration of renal function and severe hypertension.[538, 550] Massive perioperative steroid coverage is not indicated and may be detrimental. Children who present with the acute nephritic syndrome and never develop nephrosis may have a better prognosis, but most children with membranoproliferative glomerulonephritis progress to end-stage renal failure over 8 to 15 years and are then candidates for renal transplantation.[550]

Membranous nephropathy (membranous glomerulonephropathy; epimembranous nephropathy; extramembranous, perimembranous, transmembranous glomerulonephritis) may occur at any age from infancy to adulthood and shows a predilection for males.[551] The clinical course is extremely variable and is characterized by spontaneous remissions that have confused the evaluation of response to therapy. Steroids, anticoagulants, and immunosuppressive agents have all been used, but in one study remissions were most frequent in untreated patients.[551] The presence or persistence of the nephrotic syndrome is a poor prognostic sign and usually occurs in the 10 percent of children who progress to end-stage renal failure.[551]

Congenital nephrotic syndrome, presenting at birth or shortly thereafter, is usually secondary to congenital infection (syphilis, toxoplasmosis, cytomegalovirus), renal vein thrombosis (due to perinatal trauma, asphyxia, or shock), renal tumors, or toxins.[552]

Primary or *"idiopathic" congenital nephrotic syndrome* is usually a familial disease, inherited in an autosomal recessive pattern, and designated as *congenital nephrotic syndrome of the Finnish type.* It has been reported in various ethnic groups and races from many different geographical locations but occurs most commonly in Finland, where the incidence is 10 per 100,000 births (five times the incidence of nephrosis from all causes in children below the age of 16 years in the United States).[536, 552] Affected infants are often nephrotic at birth, with edema and abdominal ascites, and do not respond to therapy. The disease is invariably fatal, with few patients surviving beyond 2 years of age. The immediate cause of death is usually gastrointestinal or pulmonary infection.[552] Idiopathic congenital nephrotic syndrome may present initially as pyloric stenosis in as many as 12 percent of affected infants.[553, 554] The etiology of this association is unknown but may relate to bowel edema further compromising a narrowed pyloric lumen.

Other idiopathic congenital nephrotic syndromes have been reported, one being an autosomal recessive familial form *(diffuse mesangial sclerosis)* that sometimes responds to corticosteroid therapy but invariably progresses to renal failure and death at an age of 1 to 3 years.[552] It is important to remember that focal segmental glomerulosclerosis, minimal change nephrotic syndrome, and nephrotic syndrome secondary to infectious causes may all occur in the first year of life and are amenable to therapeutic intervention.[536, 555] The incidence and prognosis depend on the underlying cause.

Regardless of the cause, the pathophysiology of the nephrotic syndrome appears to result uniformly from an increase in glomerular permeability to plasma protein.[536–538] Selective permeability is a remarkable attribute of normal glomerular capillary membrane that allows it to distinguish macromolecules on the basis of size, shape, and molecular charge.[556–558] Structural damage to the basement membrane may result in passage of high molecular weight proteins. This occurs in acute and chronic nephritis and focal segmental glomerulosclerosis.[537, 559] The disruption of selective permeability may be much more subtle, however. It has been proposed that in minimal change nephrotic syndrome the selectively increased permeability to low molecular weight polyanionic proteins, such as albumin, occurs solely because of a loss of fixed negative ions situated in the glomerular capillary membrane.[560, 561] The relative resistance to therapy of focal segmental glomerulosclerosis, as compared with the responsiveness of minimal change nephrosis, may represent a clinical correlation of the major structural damage in the former lesion versus the minor electrostatic changes in the latter.[537]

Once glomerular permeability has been altered, the clinical manifestations of the nephrotic syndrome appear as a result of the pathophysiological mechanisms illustrated in Figure 7–14.[536] Hypoproteinemia and edema lead to other complications with implications for anesthesia. In spite of the edema and appearance of fluid overload, these children usually have depleted intravascular volume, especially when salt intake is restricted.[536, 562] Diuretics may induce severe volume contraction, hypokalemia, and azotemia, and induction of anesthesia may be associated with a marked fall in blood pressure.[536, 538, 562] Central venous pressure monitoring may be necessary for accurate volume assessment. Gastrointestinal disturbances are common, and diarrhea, attributed to edema of the intestinal mucosa, may further add to volume depletion.[536, 537] Ascites and abdominal distention may result in the appearance of umbilical or inguinal hernias. Scrotal edema may become so severe as to result in perforation requiring surgical repair.[563]

Respiratory compromise may occur from increased intra-abdominal pressure or from pleural effusions, which further confuse the question of fluid overload.[536, 537] Respiratory distress may increase in the supine position, and

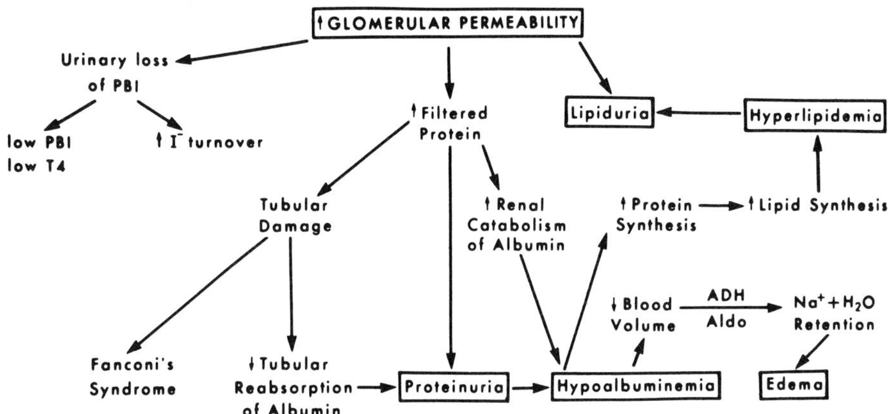

FIGURE 7–14. Pathophysiology of clinical manifestations of the nephrotic syndrome. PBI = protein-bound iodine; ADH = antidiuretic hormone; Aldo = aldosterone. (From Rance CP, Arbus GS, Balfe JW: Management of the nephrotic syndrome in children. Pediatr Clin North Am *23*:735, 1976. Modified from Earley LE, Havel RJ, Hopper J, et al: Nephrotic syndrome. Calif Med *115*:23, 1971.)

the risk of passive regurgitation from increased intra-abdominal pressure is always present.

In such cases, it is reasonable to delay operation and administer salt-poor albumin intravenously in a dose of 0.5 to 1.0 g/kg over 30 minutes while the patient is carefully monitored for hemodynamic changes. This will usually mobilize pleural, peritoneal, and peripheral edema fluid and often result in a diuresis.[564] If a diuresis has not occurred after 30 to 60 minutes and intravascular volume is judged to be adequate, then a dose of furosemide, 1 to 2 mg/kg, may be given intravenously, with continued hemodynamic monitoring. This almost always results in diuresis and symptomatic improvement.[538] If necessary, the same regimen can be employed intraoperatively. This emphasizes the need for invasive monitoring to assess volume and hemodynamic status accurately.

An increased susceptibility to infection in the nephrotic child has been attributed to low immunoglobulin levels, generalized protein and nutritional deficiency, decreased bactericidal activity of leukocytes, and immunosuppressive therapy.[538] Pneumonia, peritonitis, and septicemia due to pneumococcus, *E. coli, Pseudomonas,* and *Serratia* can be life-threatening.[565, 566] Sterile technique during placement of invasive lines should be carefully observed.

An increased incidence of vascular thrombosis is observed in the nephrotic syndrome. It is known that renal vein or inferior vena caval thrombosis may cause nephrosis, but in children the nephrotic syndrome is usually the primary event.[538, 567, 568] Thromboses have occurred in the pulmonary, coronary, and mesenteric arteries. They are not infrequent in the femoral artery following femoral puncture and have occurred in axillary and subclavian veins.[538, 568–570] Pulmonary embolism may also occur,[571] with an incidence in one study as high as 28 percent of children with nephrotic syndrome.[572] The hypercoagulability has been attributed to hemoconcentration (due to intravascular volume depletion), thrombocytosis, increased platelet aggregation, elevated levels of coagulation factors V and VII, and low plasma levels of antithrombin III and plasminogen.[573, 574] Prophylactic anticoagulant therapy has not been adequately assessed and is not currently recommended.[538] It would seem prudent to be particularly vigilant of intravascular lines and to remove them as soon as they are no longer necessary or at the first signs of possible vascular compromise.

Preoperative laboratory assessment of renal function in nephrotic children will often show elevations of BUN and creatinine. This is presumably due to intravascular volume depletion and decreased GFR, since these tests normalize following resolution of proteinuria.[537, 541] Preservation of maximal renal function requires the restoration and maintenance of intravascular volume. In addition to albumin, whole blood, plasma, and dextran have been used and have resulted in diuresis.[538] With a normal volume status and GFR, creatinine and urea clearance actually may be increased, possibly from leakage and loss into tubular fluid.[536, 575] Preoperative electrolyte studies may demonstrate hypokalemia from aggressive diuretic and corticosteroid therapy, and the patient may require replacement therapy. Hypocalcemia is usually attributable to hypoproteinemia, but low ionized calcium levels may occur in chronically nephrotic patients owing to loss of vitamin D metabolites in the urine.[576]

Immunosuppressant, antihypertensive, and corticosteroid therapy should be continued in the perioperative period, with an increase in steroid dosage to provide "stress" coverage. The acute illness or surgical stress nevertheless may exacerbate the nephrotic syndrome, and children in remission may begin to spill protein intraoperatively. Urine should be monitored for protein content, and, if the surgery is prolonged or the proteinuria massive, replacement with albumin will help prevent postoperative edema. Intraoperative steroids may also be given. Continued monitoring of hemodynamics and urine for protein in the postoperative period is necessary to detect sudden resolution of the albuminuria and to avoid fluid overload from continued infusion of albumin. Finally, the dosage of highly protein-bound drugs, such as thiopental, may have to be reduced in the presence of hypoproteinemia.[296] Children with nephrotic syndrome and progressive renal disease may develop increasing degrees of renal failure, and their anesthetic management must also be tailored to these concerns.

INTERSTITIAL NEPHRITIS, PYELONEPHRITIS, AND FOCAL RENAL SCARRING

Interstitial nephritis (interstitial renal inflammation) is another type of renal response to injury. It is characterized by inflammation in the interstitial space between nephrons and the renal vasculature. This leads to interstitial scarring, resulting in atrophy and loss of renal tubules.[577] Table 7–17 lists the many causes of interstitial renal inflammation. The incidence and population at risk vary with each cause. Frank *papillary necrosis* is associated with diseases that cause renal papillary ischemia (shock, dehydration, aplastic and sickle cell anemia, diabetes mellitus, renal vascular compromise, and urinary obstruction), and a similar mechanism may be associated with the renal lesions of analgesic abuse.[578, 579]

Acute pyelonephritis and *chronic recurrent pyelonephritis* have been implicated as major causes of interstitial renal inflammation. Whether the infection, associated reflux, or a combination of both is the primary cause of renal injury is still debated.[577, 580–582] The degree of renal damage appears to depend on the presence of obstruction, age (younger children suffer greater injury), delay in therapy, individual susceptibility, and bacterial virulence.[583, 584]

Table 7–17. CAUSES OF INTERSTITIAL NEPHRITIS

Group 1. Immunologic Reactions
- Transplantation rejection
- Drug hypersensitivity
  - Methicillin
  - Rifampin
  - Penicillin
  - Ampicillin
  - Other antibiotics
  - Anticonvulsant drugs
  - Glafenine
  - Diuretics
  - Phenindione
  - Allopurinol
- Lupus erythematosus
- Glomerulonephritis
- Sjögren's syndrome
- Sarcoidosis
- Granulomatous disease, unknown etiology

Group 2. Congenital Lesions
- Cystinosis
- Oxalosis
- Wilson's disease
- Alport's syndrome
- ? Ask-Upmark kidney
- Medullary cystic disease and/or nephronophthisis
- Other congenital lesions

Group 3. Association with Papillary Damage
- A. Papillary necrosis
  - Urinary obstruction
  - Vesicoureteral reflux
  - Diabetes mellitus
  - Vascular disease of the kidney
  - Sickle cell disorders
  - Aplastic anemia
  - Hemorrhagic fever
  - Balkan nephropathy
  - Analgesic mixture abuse—phenacetin, phenylbutazone, other
  - Transplantation rejection
  - Aging
  - Alcoholism
  - Unilateral xanthogranulomatous change with pyelonephritis
- B. Papillary injury
  - Uric acid deposition
  - Gout
  - Lesch-Nyhan syndrome
  - Nephrocalcinosis
  - Potassium depletion
  - Hyperphosphatemia
  - Sulfonamides
  - Heavy metal poisoning
  - Amyloidosis

Group 4. Miscellaneous Causes
- Choline deficiency
- Irradiation
- Disseminated intravascular coagulation
- Systemic infection
  - Scarlet fever
  - Typhoid fever
  - Toxoplasmosis
  - Leptospirosis
  - Brucellosis
  - Bacterial sepsis
  - Viral infection
  - ? Syphilis
- Heat stroke
- Acute tubular necrosis

Group 5. Bacterial Infection of the Kidney

Reprinted with permission from Freedman LR: The interstitial nephritides. *In* Edelman CM Jr (Ed.): Pediatric Kidney Disease. Boston, Little, Brown, 1978.

A recent hypothesis of renal damage proposes that there are specific epithelial cell surface receptors to which pyelonephritogenic *E. coli* adhere.[583] Ascending ureteral infection occurs with transport of bacteria by turbulent flow and reflux, while ureteral receptors facilitate local bacterial replication. Structural damage to the ureter and endotoxic inhibition of peristalsis cause pyelorenal backflow at low pressure. Finally, bacterial attachment to tubular epithelial receptors results in acute interstitial inflammation.[583]

Children with interstitial nephritis may show oliguria, hypertension, and renal insufficiency. Presenting symptoms may also be those of the underlying illness, such as urinary tract infection, pyelonephritis with flank pain and fever, diabetes, or sepsis. Damage to renal tubules may result in impairment of the ability to concentrate urine and cause tubular loss of bicarbonate, sodium, and potassium.[577] Medical management is directed at treatment of the underlying disease and the manifestations of renal failure. Discontinuation of analgesics is essential in nephropathy due to these drugs.

Sterilization of the urine is of great importance, because interstitial nephritis with persistent infection may precipitate acute papillary necrosis, leading to life-threatening sepsis or renal insufficiency.[577]

Although sterile pyuria may result during the recovery phase of papillary necrosis and persist for weeks or months after antibiotic treatment, *renal tuberculosis* should be considered in children with persistent sterile pyuria.[577] Bloodborne extension from a primary focus establishes renal cortical tubercles, which, if untreated, may pass into the tubules, renal papillae, renal pelvis, ureter, and ultimately the bladder.[585] The ureteral orifice may become rigid and open, allowing vesicoureteral reflux, and exacerbate the interstitial nephritis. Inflammatory strictures may form at the pelviureteral junction, while severe scarring and contraction of the bladder may occur, requiring surgical intervention.[585]

Viral infections, such as infectious mononucleosis, may also cause interstitial nephritis with foci of tubular necrosis and result in sterile pyuria.[586] Though rare, many bacterial, rickettsial, viral, fungal, and parasitic agents have been identified as causing nephritis, sometimes by direct renal involvement but more commonly through immunological mechanisms.[587] Proper diagnosis may require recognition of the systemic manifestation of the underlying illness.

Regardless of etiology, the manifestations of interstitial nephritis important to the anesthesiologist are those of impairment of renal function. Preoperative evaluation should determine the child's pattern of obligate urine output and bicarbonate and electrolyte loss, so that appropriate preoperative replacement can be accomplished. Severely ill children who have been unable to maintain oral intake may require volume replacement prior to anesthetic induction. Those children with hypertension, oliguria, and renal insufficiency merit the anesthetic considerations for acute renal failure detailed previously.

RENAL TUBULAR DISORDERS

Disorders of tubular function may arise secondary to generalized renal parenchymal disease or may be present as inherited or acquired defects.[588]

Renal Tubular Acidosis

Renal tubular acidosis (RTA) is perhaps the prime example of disorders of renal tubular function. It may be broadly classified as proximal or distal. Table 7–18 details this classification together with some of the causes and characteristics of renal tubular acidosis.[340a, 589] Renal tubular acidosis may be further subdivided on the basis of serum electrolyte findings and the response to mineralocorticoids, and the incidence, prognosis, and pattern of presentation vary according to subtype.[588, 589] Some children share features of both proximal and distal RTA and are considered to have *hybrid renal tubular acidosis.* All forms, however, are characterized by renal tubular inability adequately to reabsorb bicarbonate, excrete hydrogen ions, or both.[589]

Normally almost all filtered bicarbonate is reabsorbed in the proximal tubule and appears in the urine only when plasma bicarbonate levels exceed the renal threshold. In adults, this occurs at plasma bicarbonate concentrations above 25 mmol/L, but in normal infants the threshold is as low as 22 mmol/L.[590] In *proximal renal tubular acidosis,* the threshold is depressed to as low as 16 mmol/L.[591] A distinguishing feature of proximal renal tubular acidosis is the continued ability of the distal tubule to excrete hydrogen ion and acidify the urine.[589] This prevents nephrocalcinosis. Biochemical manifestations are limited to a hyperchloremic metabolic acidosis, hypokalemia, and a decreased ability to concentrate the urine, and symptoms may be limited to excessive vomiting in early infancy and

Table 7–18. CLASSIFICATION, CAUSES, AND CHARACTERISTICS OF RENAL TUBULAR ACIDOSIS

Etiology, Diagnosis, and Treatment	Renal Tubular Acidosis	
	Proximal	*Distal*
Etiology		
Primary	Permanent Familial Isolated (vitamin D deficiency?) Transient Infantile	Permanent Classic adult type Incomplete RTA With bicarbonate wasting With nerve deafness Transient (in infancy?)
Secondary	Fanconi's syndrome Cystinosis Lowe's syndrome Hereditary fructose intolerance Primary and secondary hyperparathyroidism Vitamin D deficiency Medullary cystic disease Renal transplantation Osteopetrosis Cyanotic congenital heart disease Leigh's syndrome Mineralocorticoid deficiency	Primary hyperthyroidism with nephrocalcinosis Primary hyperparathyroidism with nephrocalcinosis Idiopathic hypercalcemia Vitamin D intoxication Idiopathic hypercalciuria with nephrocalcinosis Amphotericin B nephropathy Toxicity to lithium Hepatic cirrhosis Hyperglobulinemic states Hereditary fructose intolerance with nephrocalcinosis Carnitine palmitoyl transferase type 1 deficiency[340a] Ehlers-Danlos syndrome Elliptocytosis Medullary sponge kidney Renal transplantation
Diagnosis		
Urine pH	4.5 to 7.8 depending on level of plasma bicarbonate	Always above 6.0 regardless of level of plasma bicarbonate
Bicarbonate threshold	Decreased	Normal
Hydrogen ion excretion	Normal, below bicarbonate threshold	Impaired, below bicarbonate threshold
Therapy	Resistant to alkali therapy; diuretics have effect	Sensitive to alkali therapy; no effect of diuretics

Reprinted with permission from Rodriguez-Soriano J: Renal tubular acidosis. *In* Edelmann CM Jr (Ed.): Pediatric Kidney Disease. Boston, Little, Brown, 1978; and Falik-Borenstein ZC, Jordan SC, Saudubray J, et al: Brief report: Renal tubular acidosis in carnitine palmitoyl transferase type 1 deficiency. N Engl J Med *327*:24, 1992.

growth retardation.[588] Rickets and osteomalacia may occur with time. As opposed to the transient infantile proximal RTA, the permanent, hereditary infantile form may be associated with cataracts and mental retardation.[588, 592]

Therapy for proximal RTA requires frequent replacement of lost bicarbonate with 10 mEq/kg/day, or more, of bicarbonate. Potassium replacement is frequently necessary, especially when potassium loss increases with correction of acidosis and diuretic therapy.[593] In severe proximal RTA, the administration of hydrochlorothiazide, 1 to 3 mg/kg/day, increases the bicarbonate threshold and reduces the required dose of replacement bicarbonate.[594] Thiazide diuretics may produce this effect by increasing tubular reabsorption of phosphate and decreasing urinary calcium excretion, thereby decreasing parathyroid hormone levels and its bicarbonate wasting effect on the tubule.[589] This leads to improvement in osteomalacic lesions and would explain why thiazides, which decrease calcium excretion, raise the serum bicarbonate threshold, whereas furosemide, which increases calcium excretion, does not.[589] On the other hand, increased tubular reabsorption of bicarbonate occasionally may be achieved with sodium chloride restriction.[588] In both cases, the mechanism of action may be related to contraction of the extracellular fluid volume.[595] This explains why pre- or intraoperative expansion of a chronically reduced extracellular volume in some of these children may paradoxically induce acidosis.[588] Conversely, obligatory urine output, sodium wasting, and diuretic therapy may produce significant hypovolemia. Since urinary output and metabolic acidosis may not reflect volume status, pre- and intraoperative measurement of central venous pressure is extremely useful. Restriction of oral intake preoperatively requires ongoing intravenous replacement of fluids, electrolytes, and diuretics.

In *distal renal tubular acidosis,* the primary defect is the diminished ability to excrete hydrogen ions as ammonium and titratable acid in the distal tubule, despite a low plasma bicarbonate concentration.[588] Acidosis results primarily from the inability to excrete the full endogenous load of nonvolatile acid, and loss of bicarbonate is minimal. Correction with exogenously administered alkali must meet or exceed the rate of endogenous fixed acid production, which is 1 mEq/kg/day in adults and 2 to 3 mEq/kg/day in infants and children.[589] Clinical manifestations of distal RTA are more severe than those of proximal RTA and result from the inability to acidify the urine (Fig. 7–15).[589]

Permanent, primary distal renal tubular acidosis (Butler-Albright syndrome, adult-type distal RTA) is inherited in an autosomal dominant fashion but frequently occurs sporadically. There is a slight predominance in females, and onset usually occurs after 2 years of age. It is distinguished from *transient, primary distal renal tubular acidosis (Lightwood's syndrome, infantile-type distal RTA),* which is mild, transient, and observed only within the first year of life.[589] Permanent distal RTA varies considerably in its degree of severity but usually presents with anorexia, vomiting, constipation, polyuria, dehydration, and growth retardation. Nephrocalcinosis is almost a constant finding and may lead to interstitial nephritis and renal failure.[588] If treatment is delayed, nephrolithiasis, urolithiasis, osteomalacia, and pathological fractures may occur with advancing age. Potassium loss and hypokalemia may be so severe as to cause weakness and periodic paralysis. Severe polyuria, hypokalemia, acidosis, and vomiting may combine to cause life-threatening dehydration, respiratory difficulty, flaccid paralysis, coma, cardiac arrhythmias, and circulatory collapse.[588, 589]

Despite the potential severity of symptoms, the prognosis of permanent distal RTA is good, provided that diagnosis and treatment are established early enough to prevent severe nephrocalcinosis, interstitial nephritis, and renal damage.[589] Because the proximal tubule is able to reabsorb bicarbonate avidly, sustained correction of acidosis may be achieved with less than 3 mEq/kg/day of bicarbonate and results in reversal of bony lesions and arrest of renal injury.[596] Potassium administration may also be necessary. It should begin prior to correction of acidosis if severe hypokalemia is present, in

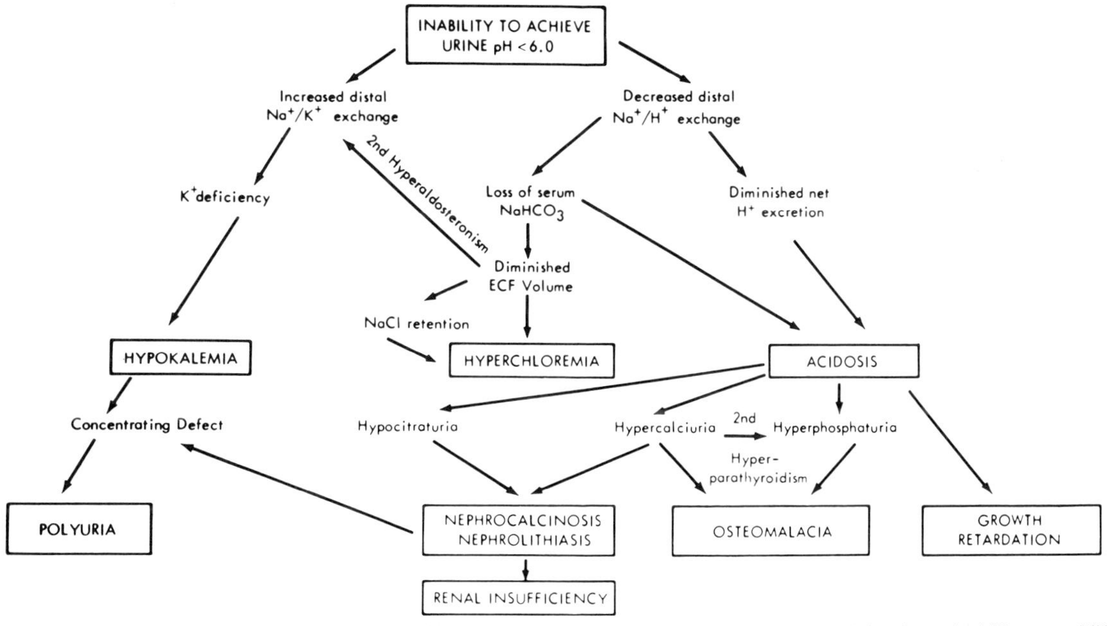

FIGURE 7–15. Pathophysiology of clinical manifestations of distal renal tubular acidosis resulting from inability to acidify urine. (From Rodriquez-Soriano J, Edelmann CM Jr: Renal tubular acidosis. Annu Rev Med *20*:363, 1969. Reproduced with permission from the Annual Review of Medicine. © 1969 by Annual Reviews Inc.)

order to prevent a further fall in serum potassium. Administration of thiazide diuretics is of limited benefit and may aggravate the hypokalemia. As the name indicates, the distal tubular defect is permanent, and interruption or attempts to withdraw therapy result in reappearance of metabolic acidosis and other clinical manifestations.[589] Any intercurrent illness that limits oral intake demands prompt intravenous replacement. Preanesthetic care requires evaluation of the adequacy of therapy and correction of volume, acid-base, and electrolyte abnormalities. Children with inadequate therapy over long periods of time may have varying degrees of nephrocalcinosis and renal failure. A central venous line is useful not only for evaluation of volume status but also as a secure port for perioperative administration of irritating electrolyte solutions. The usual precautions when delivering concentrated potassium solutions must be observed.

Finally, *hyperkalemic distal renal tubular acidosis (RTA type 4)* may result from aldosterone deficiency, from reduced tubular responsiveness to aldosterone, or from obstructive uropathy.[597–599] A primary defect in tubular secretion of potassium is the cause of acidosis in the *Spitzer-Weinstein syndrome.*[599–601] It is interesting that unilateral renal disease may induce a generalized state of tubular aldosterone unresponsiveness in both kidneys, amenable to oral bicarbonate and diuretic therapy and resolving with nephrectomy of the diseased kidney.[588, 598] *Pseudohypoaldosteronism* is a similar aldosterone-resistant lesion, characterized by renal salt wasting, and effectively treated by sodium supplementation.[601, 602]

Table 7–19. CAUSES OF THE FANCONI SYNDROME

1. Heritable disorders
   - Cystinosis
   - Idiopathic
   - Lowe's syndrome (oculocerebrorenal syndrome)
   - Tyrosinemia, type 1
   - Familial nephrosis
   - Galactosemia
   - Glycogen storage disease
   - Hereditary fructose intolerance
   - Wilson's disease
2. Other disorders
   - Kidney transplantation
   - Myeloma or Bence Jones proteinuria
   - Amyloidosis
   - Sjögren's syndrome
   - Nephrotic syndrome
   - Pancreatic carcinoma
   - Hyperparathyroidism
3. Exogenous toxins
   - Heavy metals (especially lead, mercury; including organic mercurials)
   - Nonmetals (Lysol, maleic acid, methyl-3-chromone, outdated tetracycline, streptozotocin, vitamin D)

From Shulman JD, Schneider JA: Cystinosis and the Fanconi syndrome. Pediatr Clin North Am *23*:779, 1976.

FANCONI'S SYNDROME

Fanconi's syndrome (de Toni-Debré-Fanconi syndrome) is characterized by impaired tubular reabsorption of glucose, amino acids, phosphate, bicarbonate, uric acid, and potassium.[588] It is a generalized disorder of renal tubular transport, which may be congenital or acquired, either primary or secondary, as indicated in Table 7–19.[603] Children with Fanconi's syndrome show metabolic acidosis, hypokalemia, hypophosphatemia, hypercalciuria, glucosuria, aminoaciduria, and polyuria. Rickets, osteomalacia, and pathological fractures may result, as well as the other aforementioned clinical manifestations of renal tubular acidosis.[588] Children with primary Fanconi's syndrome progress slowly to chronic renal failure; the progression and prognosis of secondary Fanconi's syndrome depend on the response of the underlying illness to specific therapy.

Symptomatic treatment consists of correction of acidosis and hypokalemia by bicarbonate, hydrochlorothiazide, and potassium therapy, together with supplementation with neutral phosphate and high-dose vitamin D to treat the bony involvement.[588, 604] Indomethacin has improved tubular function in patients with Fanconi's syndrome caused by *cystinosis (cystine storage disease),* and renal transplantation has been successful in these patients.[588] Anesthetic recommendations for Fanconi's syndrome have emphasized consideration of the characteristic fluid and electrolyte disorders and are essentially the same as those for renal tubular acidosis discussed earlier.[605] Frequently, anesthetic management is also influenced by the systemic manifestations of the precipitating illness. For example, children with Fanconi's syndrome due to cystinosis may also suffer from recurrent epistaxis, portal hypertension, esophageal varices, hypothyroidism, and diabetes mellitus.[588] Finally, patients with end-stage illness with renal failure may have any or all of the problems associated with azotemia, including cardiovascular impairment.[605]

PRIMARY HYPOPHOSPHATEMIC RICKETS

Primary hypophosphatemic rickets (vitamin D–resistant rickets) is characterized by reduced tubular reabsorption of phosphate, leading to profound hypophosphatemia (less than 0.6 mEq/L), with normocalcemia, short stature, rickets, and osteomalacia.[588] It is usually transmitted via an X-linked dominant gene, although sporadic autosomal dominant and recessive patterns have been reported.[606] Clinical features appear at the end of the first year of life, and, aside from the hyperphosphaturia, renal function is normal.[588] Treatment with inorganic phosphate supplementation and high-dose vitamin D (used to suppress parathyroid hormone hypersecretion) usually is able to achieve the therapeutic goal of raising serum phosphate levels to greater than 1.8 mEq/L (normals in growing children may be as high as 6 mEq/L).[589, 606, 607] Overzealous treatment can result in hypercalcemia, hypercalciuria, and nephrocalcinosis resulting in renal injury.[608] Appropriate early treatment may result in normal growth rates and avoidance of bony deformities.[606, 608] Anesthetic care should include preoperative evaluation of serum calcium levels and the degree of bony involvement. Precautions should be taken with positioning and intraoperative manipulation to avoid fractures in older children with severe osteomalacia.

NEPHROGENIC DIABETES INSIPIDUS

Nephrogenic diabetes insipidus is characterized by persistent hyposthenuria due to a partial or complete inability of the renal tubules to respond to antidiuretic hormone.[588] The primary disorder is X-linked, with variable expression in females. More commonly, nephrogenic diabetes insipidus occurs secondary to a systemic disease (for example, *Sjögren's syndrome* or *amyloidosis*) or drug therapy (lithium, propoxyphene, demeclocycline).[588, 609] ADH normally binds tubular receptors to activate adenylate cyclase, increasing intracellular cyclic AMP.[610, 611] This leads to a cascade of enzymatic processes that results in increased tubular free water absorption along the medullary concentration gradient.[609, 612] Hypokalemia and hypercalcemia may interfere with tubular cellular cyclic-AMP production in response to ADH, and any disorder leading to hypokalemia or hypercalcemia may lead to renal concentrating defects.[609, 611, 613, 614]

Likewise, disorders that reduce the medullary concentration gradient will interfere with tubular reabsorption of water and urinary concentration, independent of ADH. Such disorders may include any osmotic diuresis, acute and chronic renal failure, obstructive nephropathy, interstitial nephritis, medullary cystic disease, polycystic renal disease, sickle cell anemia, and others.[609] Clinical manifestations are polydipsia, nocturia, and polyuria, all of which may go unnoticed in infants. Inadequate hydration may lead rapidly to severe hypernatremic dehydration, seizures, and coma.[588] Treatment consists of providing adequate fluids, reducing dietary solute intake, and administering thiazide diuretics (which increase proximal tubular fluid reabsorption by causing extracellular volume contraction).[615] Aspirin and indomethacin inhibition of prostaglandin synthetase may also help reduce urine output.[616] Anesthetic management must include preoperative evaluation of volume status, electrolyte abnormalities (hypokalemia and hypercalcemia may be induced by diuretics and contribute to the urinary concentrating abnormality), and platelet function (for children on aspirin or indomethacin). Intraoperative evaluation of the volume status should be made independently of the large, obligate urinary output.

LIDDLE'S SYNDROME

Liddle's syndrome (pseudohyperaldosteronism) is an autosomal dominant disorder appearing as early as 10 months of age and characterized by hypertension, hypokalemic alkalosis, and hyperkaluria, with low aldosterone levels.[601] Hypertension, retinopathy, headaches, paresthesias, epigastric cramping, polyuria, weakness, acute paralysis, and occasionally tetany may occur. Apart from the failure to conserve potassium, renal function is normal. Spironolactone and aldosterone synthesis inhibitors have no effect on the disease, but triamterene (8 to 10 mg/kg/day) normalizes serum potassium and blood pressure by inhibiting the excessive distal tubular ion transport. This is aided by potassium supplementation and sodium restriction.[601]

BARTTER'S SYNDROME

Bartter's syndrome is characterized by juxtaglomerular and renomedullary cell hyperplasia, hyperreninemia, hyperaldosteronemia, and hypokalemic metabolic alkalosis. Blood pressure is normal, however, and there is no hypertensive response to infused angiotensin II or norepinephrine.[617] The recent finding of elevated *atrial natriuretic peptide* plasma levels in patients with Bartter's syndrome has raised the possibility that excess or uncontrolled secretion of ANP may be a cause of this syndrome.[618, 619] Clinical features appearing in infancy or childhood include anorexia, failure to thrive, polyuria, polydipsia, and muscle weakness. Rarely, hypercalcemia, hypophosphatemia, rickets, tetany, seizures, and distal renal tubular acidosis may be present. Renal failure may develop in a few patients.[601, 620] Elevated production of prostaglandins has been linked to the disease and has led to effective therapy with prostaglandin synthetase inhibitors such as aspirin, indomethacin, and ibuprofen.[621, 622] Treatment may also include potassium supplementation, spironolactone as an aldosterone antagonist, propranolol to block renin secretion, captopril to block angiotensin-converting enzyme, and triamterene as a potassium-sparing diuretic. It is not yet known whether early detection and aggressive treatment will prevent development of the mental retardation seen in one third of patients.[588] Anesthetic considerations for patients with Bartter's syndrome must focus on the status of renal function, the intravascular volume, serum electrolytes, and the side effects of medications used to treat the syndrome.[623] Hyperventilation and consequent respiratory alkalosis should be avoided in the presence of hypokalemic metabolic alkalosis. The diminished response to angiotensin and norepinephrine, the use of diuretics, and the presence of hypovolemia and beta-blockade all may predispose the patient to hypotension and a reduced response to vasopressors. Prostaglandin synthetase inhibitors may impair platelet function. If renal impairment is significant, systemic manifestations of azotemia may also influence anesthetic care.

IDIOPATHIC HYPOMAGNESEMIA

Renal wasting of magnesium, an autosomal recessive trait, occurs as an isolated defect or in association with renal potassium wasting and hypokalemia.[624] Tremor, fasciculations, tetany, and seizures may accompany irritability, apathy, weakness, nausea, and osteochondrosis. All these signs and symptoms resolve with magnesium supplementation of 1 to 2 mEq/kg/day, with additional potassium supplementation in hypokalemic patients.[601] Theoretical anesthetic concerns in these patients would be the potential for interaction between hypomagnesemia and neuronal function, muscular function, and neuromuscular blockade.

CYSTIC DISEASES OF THE KIDNEY

THE SPECTRUM OF CYSTIC DISEASES

Many diseases may result in renal parenchymal cysts, which in turn may cause varying degrees of renal dysfunction. In some of these diseases, the renal lesion may be the most significant; in others, renal involvement is mild and the other systemic manifestations of the illness are by far the most significant, from a clinical and anesthetic point of view. For example, the medullary cystic dilatations in *medullary sponge kidney (precalyceal canalicular ectasia, cystic dilatation of renal collecting tubules)* are the only lesions seen and are associated with only mild renal dysfunction, usually as a result of recurrent pyelonephritis or nephrolithiasis.[625] In contrast, the cystic renal involvement in *Ehlers-Danlos syndrome* and *tuberous sclerosis* may present prior to the other diagnostic stigmata and may cause severe renal disease.[626, 627] Other syndromes, such as *Jeune's asphyxiating thoracic dysplasia* or *Zellweger's cerebrohepatorenal syndrome,* occasionally may be associated with significant cystic renal disease, but this is usually overshadowed by the other, more serious clinical features of the syndromes.[626, 628] Anesthetic considerations will usually be directed at the most significant pathophysiological features, as determined during preoperative evaluation.[629] The many types of renal parenchymal cysts are shown in Table 7–20, and Table 7–21 lists the various malformation syndromes associated with renal cortical cysts.[626] In addition, there is evidence that reversible renal cyst formation may accompany chronic hypokalemia (as occurs in primary renal potassium wasting or primary aldosteronism) and, if untreated, it may progress to interstitial scarring and renal insufficiency.[630]

INFANTILE POLYCYSTIC DISEASE

Although termed infantile polycystic disease, this diffuse, bilateral, autosomal recessive illness may be first recognized in adolescence and adulthood. It is characterized by dilation of distal tubules and collecting ducts and takes on several forms that vary in severity and presentation.[626] In the perinatal form, the cysts may be enormous and cause oliguria, which may result in oligohydramnios and pulmonary hypoplasia in utero. Abdominal distention may interfere with delivery; if not stillborn, the newborn infant may suffer from life-threatening renal failure and pulmonary insufficiency.[626, 631] Interstitial pulmonary emphysema and pneumothorax may occur during resuscitative efforts. Malformations other than renal and hepatic cysts are rare and may suggest the presence of a different syndrome.[626] When the disease presents in older children, renal enlargement is less

Table 7–20. CLASSIFICATION OF RENAL PARENCHYMAL CYSTS

Polycystic disease
- Infantile polycystic disease:
  - Polycystic disease of the newborn infant
  - Polycystic disease of infancy and childhood
  - Congenital hepatic fibrosis
- Adult polycystic disease

Renal cysts in hereditary syndromes
- Diffuse cystic involvement in tuberous sclerosis
- Diffuse cystic involvement in von Hippel–Lindau disease
- Cystic dysplasia in Zellweger's cerebrohepatorenal syndrome and Jeune's asphyxiating thoracic dysplasia
- Severe cystic involvement in Ehlers-Danlos syndrome
- Cortical microcysts in syndromes of multiple malformation

Renal cortical cysts
- Diffuse glomerular cystic disease
- Juxtamedullary cortical microcysts (Finnish-type congenital nephrotic syndrome)
- Solitary and multiple simple cysts
- Segmental and unilateral cystic disease

Renal medullary cysts
- Uremic medullary cystic disease complex:
  - Familial juvenile nephronophthisis
  - Medullary cystic disease
  - Renal-retinal dysplasia
- Medullary sponge kidney

Renal dysplasia
- Cystic dysplasia associated with lower urinary tract obstruction
- Multicystic and aplastic dysplasia
- Hereditary cystic dysplasia
- Focal and segmental cystic dysplasia

Reprinted with permission from Bernstein J: Polycystic disease. *In* Edelmann CM Jr (Ed.): Pediatric Kidney Disease. Boston, Little, Brown, 1978. Modified from Bernstein J, Gardner KD Jr: Cystic diseases of the kidney and renal dysplasia. *In* Harrison JH, Gittes RF, Perlmutter AD, et al (Eds.): Campbell's Urology. 4th edition. Philadelphia, WB Saunders, 1978.

severe, and renal insufficiency progresses at a variable rate. Severe systemic hypertension develops in many children and hepatic cysts are usually present, although hepatocellular dysfunction is rare.[632] In a few children, systemic and portal hypertension may coexist and result in congestive heart failure, chronic renal failure, and bleeding esophageal varices.[626] As opposed to the oliguria of the neonate, in older children there is typically an impaired tubular ability to concentrate or acidify the urine (renal tubular acidosis).[633]

Infantile polycystic disease is usually progressive and is often fatal in childhood, although the prognosis seems to improve if the patient survives the neonatal period.[634] Medical management is supportive.[622, 635] Appropriate fluid and electrolyte therapy may vary from severe restriction in oliguric neonates to generous salt and water administration in polyuric children. Severe systemic hypertension often requires aggressive medical intervention with its attendant problems, and congestive heart failure may require chronic inotropic support with digitalis. Chronic hemodialysis prolongs survival and allows successful renal transplantation. Portal hypertension may require a portacaval shunt in a few children. Anesthetic considerations are determined by the degree and type of renal involvement and resulting systemic manifestations. Congestive heart failure, hepatic involvement, and esophageal variceal bleeding may further influence anesthetic management.

Adult Polycystic Disease in Childhood

A diffuse, bilateral, autosomal dominant disease appearing most frequently in adulthood, adult polycystic disease may present at any age.[631, 636] When it is seen in infancy, the disease may be quite severe, perhaps as a result of the presence of two dominant genes (homozygous disease) in these unfortunate infants.[626] It is relatively uncommon in blacks and may occur rarely in association with other hereditary conditions such as *spherocytosis, Peutz-Jeghers syndrome, lobster-claw deformity of the feet, orodigitofacial syndrome,* and *myotonic dystrophy.*[626] In older children and adults, the presenting symptom may be flank pain, but in infants palpable flank masses or renal impairment may appear first. Hematuria, proteinuria, and an inability to concentrate the urine precede increasingly severe renal impairment. Renal hemorrhage, lithiasis, and infection complicate

Table 7–21. SYNDROMES OF MULTIPLE MALFORMATION ASSOCIATED WITH RENAL CORTICAL CYSTS

- Zellweger's cerebrohepatorenal syndrome
- Jeune's asphyxiating thoracic dysplasia syndrome
- Autosomal trisomy syndromes, D and E
- Orodigitofacial syndrome
- Lissencephaly syndrome
- Goldenhar's syndrome
- Marden-Walker (Schwartz-Jampel) syndrome
- Ehlers-Danlos syndrome
- Congenital cutis laxa syndrome
- Short rib–polydactyly syndrome
- DiGeorge's syndrome
- Noonan's syndrome
- Turner's syndrome
- Chromosomal translocation syndromes

Reprinted with permission from Bernstein J: Polycystic disease. *In* Edelmann CM Jr (Ed.): Pediatric Kidney Disease. Boston, Little, Brown, 1978.

the illness and accelerate renal injury. Focal hepatic involvement affects one third of adults with adult polycystic disease; berry aneurysms of the cerebral arteries affect 10 percent and may lead to life-threatening intracranial hemorrhage. Both are infrequent in children.[626] Renal parenchymal ischemia, caused by cyst expansion, may stimulate renin release and activate the renin-angiotensin-aldosterone system.[637] This contributes to the development of severe systemic hypertension, which is present early in the course of autosomal dominant polycystic kidney disease in up to 75 percent of patients.[637] This hypertension requires aggressive therapeutic intervention to prevent accelerated renal deterioration. Secondary congestive heart failure may require digitalization, and renal infection requires prompt recognition and antibiotic therapy. Dialysis prolongs survival in anticipation of renal transplantation. Anesthetic considerations are the same as those for the infantile form, with the exception that the potential presence of cerebral artery aneurysms makes control of blood pressure even more critical.

Familial Juvenile Nephronophthisis and Medullary Cystic Disease

Familial juvenile nephronophthisis is an autosomal recessive disorder with onset in childhood, characterized by polyuria and progressive renal failure. *Medullary cystic disease* is an adult-onset, autosomal dominant disease with a urinary concentrating defect and progressive azotemia. Morphologically, they are quite similar, which has led to nosological confusion and a variety of descriptions that have been applied to one or the other or both: *cystic disease of the renal medulla, uremic medullary cystic disease, Fanconi nephronophthisis, salt-losing nephritis, uremic sponge kidney,* and *polycystic disease of medullary type.*[638] Variants of familial juvenile nephronophthisis may show ocular, cerebellar, skeletal, and hepatic abnormalities, and the characteristic medullary cystic lesions may be seen with rare syndromes such as *Alström's syndrome* (obesity, diabetes mellitus, blindness, and deafness), *Laurence-Moon-Bardet-Biedl syndrome,* and *renal-retinal dysplasia.*[638]

The initial clinical features of familial juvenile nephronophthisis and medullary cystic disease are similar: polydipsia, polyuria, sodium and potassium wasting, azotemia, mild hypertension, anemia out of proportion to the degree of renal failure, and weakness. Both diseases progress inexorably to renal failure over a period of years, culminating in chronic dialysis, transplantation, or death. Treatment is nonspecific and supportive, and anesthetic considerations relate to the individual child's pattern of fluid and electrolyte excretion and degree of renal failure.

RENAL DYSPLASIA, APLASIA, AND HYPOPLASIA

Renal Dysplasia and Aplasia

Renal dysplasia is a condition of abnormal renal development resulting in abnormal nephronic structural organization.[628] It is often associated with obstructive urinary tract malformations, a probable pathogenetic relationship. It may also occur on a hereditary basis and may be associated with varying degrees of structural and functional impairment.

Hereditary cystic dysplasia is a bilateral, diffuse cystic lesion unassociated with urinary tract obstruction. It usually occurs sporadically but may follow an autosomal recessive pattern of occurrence. The degree of renal impairment is variable, but severely affected infants may have suffered from oligohydramnios and may present with life-threatening pulmonary hypoplasia and renal failure. Association with other malformations is common, such as occurs in *Meckel's syndrome,* which consists of cystic renal dysplasia, posterior encephalocele, microcephaly, polydactyly, and cleft lip and palate. In addition to the less significant renal cortical cysts mentioned previously, infants with *Jeune's asphyxiating thoracic dysplasia* and *Zellweger's cerebrohepatorenal syndrome* may occasionally demonstrate severe cystic renal dysplasia.[628] Infants with *Beckwith-Wiedemann syndrome* (omphalocele, macroglossia, hypoglycemia, and hyperplastic visceromegaly) may demonstrate medullary renal dysplasia, but this is rarely cystic.[628, 639]

Obstructive renal dysplasia, as the name implies, is thought to result from early urinary obstruction causing back pressure and affecting normal renal development.[640, 641] Obstructive renal dysplasia may be associated with any form of congenital urinary tract obstruction and has occurred with *bladder dysfunction due to meningomyelocele, prune belly syndrome, ectopic ureterocele, anterior urethral diverticulum,* and severely obstructive *posterior urethral valves.*[628] Concomitant ureteral reflux may exacerbate the formation of renal dysplasia, and reflux and obstruction may occur asymmetrically, accounting for asymmetrical and unilateral renal dysplasia.[628, 642]

Severe forms of obstructive renal dysplasia are *multicystic* and *aplastic renal dysplasia,* in which the involved kidney is severely malformed and nonfunctioning. Both types are associated with ureteropelvic occlusion, which causes the severe dysplasia. Bilateral aplastic or multicystic kidneys are lethal malformations associated with oligohydramnios and stillbirth, or neonatal death from renal failure, pulmonary hypoplasia, or their complications.[628] Unilateral involvement may be silent until recurrent infection, flank pain, or hypertension occurs. Because of the difficulty of differentiating the abnormal kidney from one with malignant degeneration, treatment is by surgical removal, which also achieves control of hypertension. The outcome depends on the functional viability of the contralateral kidney and the presence of associated contralateral abnormalities, such as renal or ureteral ectopia and ureteral reflux.

Renal Hypoplasia

Renal hypoplasia, as opposed to dysplasia, is characterized by a diminished number of normally developed nephrons.[643] Most cases are sporadic, but some may occur in association with other malformations. *Unilateral hypoplasia* is a common incidental finding often referred to as a *miniature kidney, doll's kidney,* or *vest pocket kidney.*[628] These small kidneys are prone to infection, lithiasis, and vascular disease causing hypertension.

Segmental hypoplasia (Ask-Upmark kidney) is a form of renal hypoplasia more frequently associated with hypertension due to segmental hypersecretion of renin.[644, 645] Although segmental hypoplasia is considered a congenital abnormality by some, infantile vesicoureteral reflux or local vascular injury may account for the segmental renal hypoplasia and scarring.[628] Infection, lithiasis, and severe hypertension, which is difficult to control, are indications for surgical removal of the abnormal segment or whole kidney.

Bilateral renal hypoplasia is an important cause of chronic renal failure in childhood.[628] *Simple bilateral hypoplasia* is rare and is characterized by salt and water wasting, renal tubular acidosis, and refractory hypokalemia.[643] *Oligomeganephronia* is a much more common form of bilateral renal hypoplasia and is characterized by marked hypertrophy of individual nephrons.[646] The cause is unknown, it occurs more frequently in males than females, and cases are sporadic. Clinical manifestations are polyuria, salt wasting, hyperchloremic metabolic acidosis, proteinuria, and slowly progressive azotemia. Hypertension is uncommon. Treatment is supportive and may include dialysis in anticipation of renal transplantation.[628] Anesthetic considerations for all these lesions are governed by the type and extent of renal impairment.

SYSTEMIC DISEASES AFFECTING RENAL PARENCHYMA

As indicated in Tables 7–12, 7–14, 7–15, and 7–17, many systemic diseases may impair renal function and injure the kidney. The renal response to injury in any given disease may be manifested as any combination of interstitial nephritis, glomerulonephritis, the nephrotic syndrome, tubular dysfunction, acute renal failure, and progressive chronic renal failure, depending on the stage of the disease and the extent of renal involvement. For example, extrarenal neoplasms may directly invade renal parenchyma, blood vessels, or ureters; they may cause abnormalities in tubular function resulting in disturbances in excretion of water, sodium, potassium, calcium, and uric acid, or induce membranous glomerulopathy, minimal change nephrotic syndrome, or amyloidosis.[647]

Amyloidosis of the kidney may also result from chronic inflammatory conditions (tuberculosis, osteomyelitis, endocarditis, bronchiectasis, ulcerative colitis, regional ileitis, rheumatoid arthritis), multiple myeloma, and *familial Mediterranean fever,* and it may lead to end-stage renal failure.[648]

Hyperuricemia from chemotherapy of myeloproliferative disorders, genetically abnormal purine metabolism *(Lesch-Nyhan syndrome),* or decreased urate excretion may lead to urolithiasis, urinary obstruction, and acute oliguric renal failure as well as renal interstitial inflammation, scarring, and chronic renal failure *(urate nephropathy).*[649] Allopurinol, adequate hydration, and maintenance of an alkaline urine all help prevent intrarenal deposition of urate crystals and should be continued in the perioperative period.

The *lysosomal storage diseases*—recessive hereditary disorders of glycogen, glycosphingolipid, glycoprotein, and mucopolysaccharide metabolism—may all manifest renal involvement. The most dramatic of these is *Fabry's disease* (defective alpha-galactosidase A activity), which in addition to cardiac and cerebral vascular disease may cause renal disease presenting as proteinuria, polyuria, tubular dysfunction, and progressive azotemia.[650] Renal transplantation not only treats renal failure but also provides genetically normal kidneys with normal alpha-galactosidase A activity to metabolize substrate.[651]

Dysglobulinemia, cryoglobulinemia, and *macroglobulinemia* (including *Waldenström's macroglobulinemia*) may all cause renal impairment ranging from focal tubular atrophy to the nephrotic syndrome, to rapidly progressive, diffuse, proliferative glomerulonephritis with hypertension, hematuria, and proteinuria.[652, 653]

Cirrhosis of the liver may be associated with severe and progressive renal failure, known as the *hepatorenal syndrome.* Decreased plasma volume, renal blood flow, and GFR, as well as renal vasoconstriction, have been proposed as pathogenetic mechanisms, but therapeutic measures such as plasma volume expansion, paracentesis, vasodilators, and portacaval anastomosis provide only transient renal improvement.[654–656]

Radiation, drugs, toxins, and heavy metals all may cause renal injury and functional impairment. *Acute lead poisoning* leads characteristically to proximal tubular dysfunction and occasionally the full-blown *Fanconi syndrome,* whereas *chronic lead poisoning* has been associated with the subsequent development of chronic renal failure.[657] *Wilson's disease (hepatolenticular degeneration)* is a hereditary disorder of copper metabolism resulting in elevated serum and renal copper levels and aminoaciduria or generalized Fanconi's syndrome.[658] Gold remains a useful therapeutic agent in severe *juvenile rheumatoid arthritis* and may cause nephrotoxicity (with proteinuria, hematuria, and tubular dysfunction, and rarely acute tubular necrosis) or a hypersensitivity reaction resulting in the nephrotic syndrome.[657] In addition to amyloidosis and gold therapy, the systemic inflammatory process of *juvenile rheumatoid arthritis* may directly involve the kidney and result in interstitial nephritis, renal papillary necrosis, and focal mesangial proliferative glomerulonephritis.[659] Tubular dysfunction may cause obligatory salt and water loss, hypertension may require aggressive medical therapy, aspirin therapy may cause platelet malfunction, and chronic glucocorticoid therapy may require perioperative steroid coverage.

Scleroderma (progressive systemic sclerosis), in addition to myocardial, pericardial, and pulmonary fibrosis, may involve the kidneys in 45 percent of patients, with a mortality of 60 percent.[660, 661] Proteinuria, progressive azotemia, and severe hypertension may all occur. Transplantation has been successful, and subsequent immunosuppression with azathioprine and corticosteroids can improve the systemic manifestations of the disease.[661, 662] *Dermatomyositis (polymyositis)* rarely involves the kidneys, causing focal glomerulosclerosis or membranoproliferative glomerulonephritis and the nephrotic syndrome.[659, 663] Cardiac conduction defects and pulmonary interstitial fibrosis are extrarenal manifestations of concern to the anesthesiologist.[664, 665] Interstitial nephritis, proliferative glomerulonephritis, and membranous glomerulonephropathy have all been reported in children with *mixed connective tissue disease,* and respond well to corticosteroid and immunosuppressive therapy.[666] Although renal disease is reported in only 10 percent of patients, one half of the deaths from mixed connective tissue disease are due to renal failure.[659]

Polyarteritis nodosa (periarteritis nodosa) occurs in an *infantile form* with hematuria, proteinuria, and hypertension but is rapidly fatal owing to coronary artery involvement and heart failure.[667] The *adult form,* occurring in adolescent males twice as frequently as in females, has an 80 percent incidence of renal involvement, with hematuria, proteinuria, hypertension, acute nephritic syndrome, and occasionally acute renal failure. Pulmonary involvement and granulomatous lesions of the upper respiratory tract and ears may precede renal involvement in some types of adult-form polyarteritis nodosa (such as *Wegener's granulomatosis, allergic granulomatosis, allergic angiitis,* and *Löffler's syndrome*) and may dominate anesthetic considerations.[667] Cyclophosphamide, azathioprine, corticosteroids, and heparin all have been used in different combinations and have prevented the previously unchecked progression to death from renal failure.[667]

Renal involvement in children with *systemic lupus erythematosus* may occur in up to 80 percent and may present as mesangial, focal or diffuse proliferative, or membranous lupus nephritis.[668] Without adequate therapy, nephrosis, hypertension, uremia, and progressive renal failure may ensue. Cardiopulmonary and central nervous system involvement are frequent and must influence anesthetic care. Treatment with corticosteroids, supplemented with immunosuppressive agents, has greatly improved the course and prognosis of childhood systemic lupus erythematosus.[669, 670]

Sickle cell nephropathy may occur with homozygous (SS) disease or heterozygous (AS) sickle cell trait, as well as in sickle cell—thalassemia or SC disease.[671, 672] Polymerization of hemoglobin S and sickling of red blood cells occur with hypoxemia, hyperosmolarity, acidosis, and increased prostaglandin E_2 levels, all of which may occur in the renal medulla.[672, 673] There are several clinical manifestations of sickle cell nephropathy. Hematuria may be the presenting sign of a sickle cell crisis but may also occur with sickle trait. It often originates unilaterally from the left kidney.[672, 674] Hyposthenuria resulting from an inability to concentrate the urine is an early and chronic finding, unrelated to changes in GFR or RBF. In the early stage it is reversible by transfusion of normal erythrocytes.[671, 672] The ability to concentrate urine decreases with age, and the large obligate urine output may lead to dehydration, especially if children with sickle cell nephropathy remain NPO without intravenous hydration. A defect of urinary acidification exists in both sickle cell disease and trait, and this, together with the concentrating defect, has led some to describe the functional lesion as a mild form of distal renal tubular acidosis.[671, 672] Membranoproliferative and minimal change glomerulonephritis have been reported in sickle cell patients with the nephrotic syndrome.[672] Renal vein thrombosis also occurs, often in association with the nephrotic syndrome, but whether the primary event is the sickling, thrombosis, or nephrosis is not clear.[675] Pyelonephritis may occur more frequently with sickle cell disease, and unchecked renal infection, as well as an acute vaso-occlusive crisis, may cause renal papillary necrosis and acute renal failure.[672] Renal failure is otherwise rare among children with sickle cell disease, and end-stage renal failure with the need for dialysis or transplantation occurs primarily in adulthood.[676]

Anesthetic care for patients with sickle cell nephropathy requires a recognition of their large obligate urine output. Fluid replacement should err on the generous side, because the ability to produce dilute urine is usually unaffected.[671, 677] Other general principles for anesthesia in patients with sickle cell disease, such as avoidance of hyperosmolarity, dehydration, hypoxia, ischemia, hypothermia, stasis, and extreme anemia, will also help avoid intrarenal sickling and prevent further renal damage.

Renal disease in diabetes mellitus may include a tendency toward bacteriuria, chronic pyelonephritis and renal papillary necrosis, an enhanced susceptibility to contrast media–induced nephropathy, toxin-induced nephropathy and interstitial nephritis, bladder atony and hydronephrosis from diabetic neuropathy, arteriolar nephrosclerosis, and diabetic glomerulosclerosis.[678] *Nodular intercapillary glomerulosclerosis (Kimmelstiel-Wilson nodules)* is a specific lesion present in over 50 percent of patients with diabetes mellitus and is considered pathognomonic of *diabetic nephropathy*.[678, 679] Microvasculopathy affecting the glomerulus (and other microvasculature such as the retina) is a serious threat to longevity in juvenile diabetes mellitus.[678, 679] Proteinuria, once fixed, is an ominous sign, with subsequent decline in GFR by 11 ml/min each year.[680] Without dialysis or transplantation, survival after the establishment of uremia is usually less than 2 years.[679] Because diabetic nephropathy and glomerulosclerosis are asymptomatic and slowly progressive over 13 to 18 years, it is uncommon for these problems to present prior to adolescence or early adulthood.[678] The initial sign is usually proteinuria, which later progresses to frank nephrotic syndrome and then to relentless renal failure, although nephrotic syndrome may appear in children with diabetes mellitus of recent onset.[681] Hypertension is common and may appear concomitantly with proteinuria. Although the treatment is unproved, tight control of hypertension and serum glucose may slow the progression to renal failure.[679]

Anesthesia for nephrotic diabetics should follow the principles outlined earlier for nephrotic children, with the understanding that the diabetic patient may have marginal cardiac reserve and will tolerate intravascular volume changes poorly.[678] One third of each insulin dose is metabolized by the kidney, and as renal function is lost and renal catabolism of exogenous insulin diminishes, juvenile diabetic patients may suffer hypoglycemic episodes if their insulin is not decreased appropriately.[678] This makes perioperative insulin management more difficult and requires frequent monitoring of serum glucose levels. Finally, with end-stage renal failure treated with hemodialysis in juvenile diabetic patients, the leading cause of death is myocardial infarction or failure.[682] The anesthetic care of these young adults must address this major potential complication.

NEPHROLITHIASIS AND EXTRACORPOREAL SHOCK WAVE LITHOTRIPSY

Nephrocalcinosis, nephrolithiasis, and *urolithiasis* leading to obstruction and severe renal impairment may result not only from *Proteus* urinary tract infections, but also from hypercalcemia and hypercalciuria due to thyroid disease, hyperparathyroidism, vitamin D intoxication, fat necrosis, sarcoidosis, renal tubular acidosis, immobilization, and *idiopathic hypercalcemia.*[683] The association of mental retardation, elfin facies, and supravalvular aortic stenosis *(Williams's triad)* occurs with *idiopathic hypercalcemia,*[684] in which pulmonary stenosis and seizures have also been observed. Other causes of nephrolithiasis include metabolic diseases (such as von Gierke's disease or Type I glycogen storage disease),[685] obstructive lesions (such as ureteropelvic junction obstruction or posterior urethral valves),[686] and inherited defects (such as X-linked recessive nephrolithiasis with renal failure),[687] as well as iatrogenic causes (such as renal stone formation in preterm infants with chronic lung disease receiving loop diuretics, especially furosemide).[688] Regardless of etiology, renal calcification can lead to obstructive uropathy, recurrent infections, renal scarring, and ultimately renal failure. Surgical removal of renal calculi may be required, and in addition to open removal, shock wave lithotripsy may be employed. Anesthetic considerations for these procedures depend on the type and degree of renal impairment demonstrated by the affected child, ranging from tubular dysfunction with an inability to concentrate urine and an obligatory urinary loss, to uremia and anuria. Hemoptysis due to shock wave damage to the lungs in a child undergoing extracorporeal shock wave lithotripsy has been described.[685] Because of the closer proximity of the lung bases to the kidneys in children, the potential for pulmonary damage is greater in children than in adults. Recommendations to avoid this complication include shielding the lung bases with a 1-cm-thick Styrofoam sheet (a 0.3-cm thickness has been shown to block the shock waves completely), observing the lung bases on fluoroscopy when this modality is being used to target the stone, and providing ventilation only between episodes of shock wave application to prevent inspiratory excursion of the lungs into the shock wave field.[685, 689]

RETROPERITONEAL AND RENAL TUMORS

The systemic manifestations of nonrenal tumors and their therapy may induce renal impairment, as discussed earlier. Nonrenal, retroperitoneal tumors may in addition affect renal function by virtue of their location and size. *Neuroblastoma* is the most common retroperitoneal tumor in children, occurring in about 1 in 30,000 children, usually before the age of 4 years. It is more common in females than in males.[690] Over 75 percent of patients secrete catecholamines detectable in the urine, and hypertension may be present. Neuroblastoma may also occur in association with *neurofibromatosis (von Recklinghausen's disease).* Neurofibromas may cause renal artery stenosis and renal hypertension and may be associated with pheochromocytomas, which have many features of importance to the anesthesiologist[691] (see Chapter 12). *Ganglioneuroma* is considered a fully differentiated, benign extreme of neuroblastoma. Levels of catecholamine secretion are lower, and renal impairment is limited to that produced by local pressure effects.[690]

Nephroblastoma (Wilms' tumor) is the most common abdominal tumor in children, with a reported incidence of from 1 in 100,000 to 1 in 13,500.[692] It is usually diagnosed between 6 months and 5 years of age, and may be bilateral in 8 to 12 percent of cases.[692] Congenital absence of the iris (aniridia), in a familial or a sporadic form, and hemihypertrophy of the body may be associated.[692, 693] Wilms' tumor may occur in conjunction with horseshoe kidneys, duplication of the urinary tract, solitary kidney, hypospadias, or with nephritis and male pseudohermaphroditism to form a distinct syndrome described by Barakat and colleagues.[694] The tumor may extend into the renal vein or inferior vena cava, may cause renovascular distortion and hypertension, and may produce renin with resulting hypertension.[695, 696] An enlarged abdomen or an expanding abdominal mass is the usual presenting symptom, and vomiting, abdominal pain, hematuria, proteinuria, and metastases to para-aortic nodes, liver, and lungs may be present.[692, 697] Mild fever occurs in as many as 30 percent of patients and may accompany hemorrhage into the tumor.[692] It is not a reason to delay surgery. The associated anemia may be treated either preoperatively or by transfusion during surgery to maintain volume and hemoglobin concentration.[698]

Treatment is by surgical resection, radiation therapy, and chemotherapy. Actinomycin D and vincristine are the most commonly employed chemotherapeutic agents. Vomiting and thrombocytopenia may occur with actinomycin D. Neurotoxicity may accompany vincristine therapy in the form of paresthesias, ptosis, muscular weakness, and rarely convulsions, associated with inappropriate secretion of ADH.[692]

In more advanced stages of the disease, cyclophosphamide and doxorubicin (Adriamycin) may be used. Nausea, vomiting, bone marrow suppression, and hemorrhagic cystitis may occur with cyclophosphamide. Cardiotoxicity with severe, intractable heart failure may occur when total Adriamycin doses exceed 300 mg/m^2.[692] Chest radiograph and electrocardiogram are usually not helpful in detecting early cardiac involvement, but serial echocardiograms may be more useful.[692]

The prognosis in Wilms' tumor depends on the age of the child and stage of the disease. Almost 90 percent of children under 2 years of age with an encapsulated tumor and no evidence of spread of disease have no recurrence after 4 years.

Anesthetic considerations for the resection of a Wilms' tumor are those of major transabdominal, retroperitoneal surgery in the small child. The large, intra-abdominal tumor may predispose the patient to regurgitation on induction. Ventilation may be compromised by the size of the tumor, abdominal retraction, or pulmonary involvement with metastases. Blood loss may be massive. Manipulation of tumor extending into the renal vein and inferior vena cava may require caval cross-clamping and introduces the danger of pulmonary embolism. Large-bore intravenous access must be secured in the upper body.[698] Central venous access via the arms or the subclavian or internal or external jugular veins serves not only as a secure route for transfusion but also to assess volume status. If a large line is to be placed surgically for postoperative chemotherapy, it is helpful to have this done first, immediately followed by the tumor resection. An arterial line is helpful to monitor respiratory and acid-base status, as well as to provide rapid evaluation of the effects of manipulation and volume changes on blood pressure. The large abdominal exposure may cause significant loss of fluid to the "third space," and great care must be taken to provide adequate replacement to preserve optimal renal function in the remaining kidney, especially in the occasional case in which there is bilateral renal involvement. Baseline preoperative studies provide a guideline for postoperative evaluation of renal function. The large exposure also predisposes to significant heat loss, and all the usual procedures to maintain a normal body temperature are required.

Anesthesiologists may also become involved with Wilms' tumor patients for repeated surgery (for example, for venous access for chemotherapy) or for radiation therapy. Particular attention then should be paid to the potential neurological, hematological, immunological, and cardiac impairment caused by chemotherapy.

Sedation for radiation therapy in the uncooperative child usually may be achieved with intramuscular ketamine or rectal methohexital, although the rectal route should probably not be utilized if immunosuppression or mucosal breakdown is present. If venous access is available, intravenous sedation of short duration (as with propofol, ketamine, pentothal, or Brevital) is also effective.

Congenital mesoblastic nephroma, at times referred to as *neonatal Wilms' tumor,* is a relatively benign tumor that causes renal impairment because of location and size. Treatment is by elective nephrectomy at a time when the infant's general condition is stable.[692] These tumors may be so large as to replace the whole kidney, and anesthetic considerations are similar to those cited earlier.

CONGENITAL ABNORMALITIES OF THE URINARY SYSTEM

DEVELOPMENTAL ABNORMALITIES AND ASSOCIATED ANOMALIES

Many neonates demonstrate anomalies of the urinary tract, and as much as 30 percent of pediatric surgery is dedicated to the correction of these lesions.[698] Some of these infants may also have other congenital anomalies. When these involve the musculoskeletal system, the ears, or facial development, they are usually obvious. More subtle, but significant, anomalies may be present in the gastrointestinal, pulmonary, and cardiovascular systems and may escape preoperative detection. An awareness of these associated defects will help in their preoperative detection. Any unexplained cardiovascular or pulmonary response to anesthesia should rekindle the suspicion that other anomalies may coexist.

Cardiovascular malformations (CVMs) are variably associated with anomalies of the urinary system and may easily escape detection in the neonatal period.[699] *Horseshoe kidney* may frequently have an associated CVM, with ventricular septal defect (VSD) and endocardial cushion defect being the most common.[699] *Bilateral renal agenesis* is associated with a 75 percent incidence of CVM, while *unilateral renal agenesis* has a 17 percent association, with VSD being the most common lesion. Patients with *ectopic kidneys* and *cystic kidneys* have associated CVM in 1 in 7 cases, whereas in *renal dysplasia* the rate of CVM is 1 in 20. Fortunately, the more common congenital urinary malformations requiring surgical intervention, such as *hypospadias, cryptorchidism, urinary duplications, ureteropelvic* and *ureterovesical junction obstructions, exstrophy, urethral valves, genital anomalies,* and *Wilms' tumor,* are very rarely associated with CVM.[699, 700]

While the cause for the association of cardiovascular malformations with urinary tract anomalies has not been defined, the etiological relationship between urinary tract anomalies leading to *oligohydramnios* and *pulmonary maldevelopment* has been established. Fetal urinary production contributes significantly to the production of amniotic fluid, which is essential for normal pulmonary development.[701] Oligohydramnios may also result in fetal compression, causing limb defects and characteristic *Potter's facies.* Severe involvement may lead to the florid *Potter's syndrome,* characterized by bilateral renal agenesis (or severe cystic dysplasia) with hypoplastic lungs, the characteristic facies, skeletal anomalies, and gastrointestinal malformations.[702] The renal agenesis may be primary, or, as discussed previously, intrauterine urinary obstruction, if bilateral and severe, may lead to bilateral cystic renal dysplasia.[640, 641] Less severe degrees of obstruction may lead to varying degrees of renal and extrarenal involvement.

If the obstruction is distal, it may lead to the *prune belly syndrome (Eagle-Barrett syndrome)* or variations of what has come to be called the *urethral obstruction malformation complex.*[703, 704] Figure 7–16 shows the developmental pathology of the urethral obstruction malformation complex. In addition to pulmonary hypoplasia and deformities due to oligohydramnios, the severely distended bladder is thought to interfere mechanically with the development of surrounding tissues, resulting in other characteristics of the prune belly syndrome: renal dysplasia, abdominal muscular deficiency, excess abdominal skin, cryptorchidism, colonic malrotation, and lower limb deficiency.[704] Figure 7–17 is a picture of an infant with prune belly syndrome, showing his lax abdominal musculature, protuberant abdomen, and small thorax.

The prune belly syndrome occurs in 1 in 40,000 births, with a male-to-female ratio of 20:1. Females may demonstrate only the abdominal wall involvement.[705] X-linked transmission, association with chromosomal aberration, and sporadic occurrences have all been described, as well as a familial occurrence associated with pulmonic stenosis, mental retardation, and deafness.[706] There is no racial predilection. Survival depends on the severity of the renal and pulmonary involvement, with 20 percent of patients being stillborn or dying within the first month and 50 percent dying within 2 years.[707] Although the pathogenesis of the prune belly syndrome is still debated, recent reports have confirmed nonspecific distal urinary tract obstruction as an etiology, and in utero ultrasonic diagnosis by 21 weeks' gestation has become possible.[708–710] Furthermore, it has been suggested that early fetal surgical decompression of urinary tract obstruction may prevent the prune belly phenotype. Although such intervention at 21 weeks' gestation has resulted in improvement in the abdominal wall laxity, it did not prevent severe pulmonary and renal involvement.[710] Infants and children with prune belly syndrome

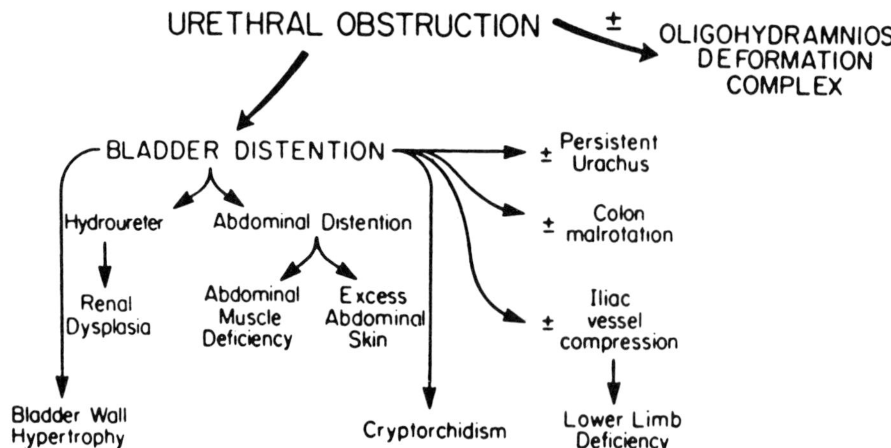

FIGURE 7–16. Pathogenesis of the urethral obstruction malformation complex. The pathogenesis of the more severe degrees of this complex is interpreted as the secondary effect of bladder distention on surrounding tissues. (From Pagon RA, Smith DW, Shepard TH: Urethral obstruction malformation complex: A cause of abdominal muscle deficiency and the "prune belly." J Pediatr *94*:900, 1979.)

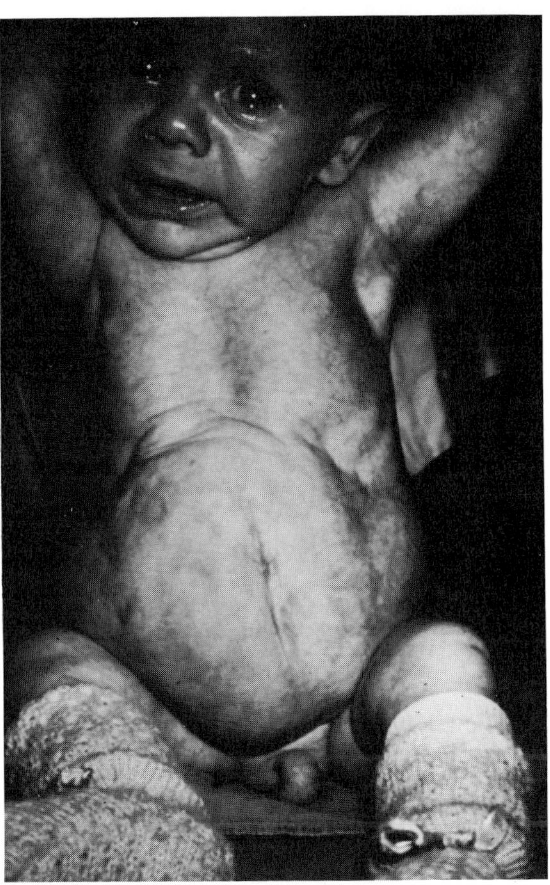

FIGURE 7–17. Prune belly syndrome. (Photograph courtesy of Dr. Babu Koka, The Children's Hospital, Boston.)

come to operation mainly for genitourinary procedures ranging from cystoscopy to ureteric reconstruction or renal transplantation.

Anesthetic considerations for children with the prune belly syndrome must focus on the compromised renal and pulmonary status.[707, 711, 712] Pulmonary hypoplasia may be complicated by atelectasis, recurrent respiratory infection, and reduced expiratory effort and cough as a result of abdominal muscular deficiency. Preoperative antibiotic treatment of pneumonia and chest physiotherapy have been recommended to optimize the pulmonary status. The use of preoperative sedation has been discouraged for fear of respiratory depression.[713] Rapid-sequence induction with cricoid pressure to avoid regurgitation and gain rapid control of ventilation, as well as routine nasotracheal intubation in anticipation of prolonged postoperative ventilation, has also been suggested.[711, 712] Others have utilized awake intubation or, failing this, have proceeded with a mask induction with assisted ventilation.[707] Controlled intraoperative ventilation, with monitoring of airway pressures, tidal volume, end-tidal P_{CO_2}, transcutaneous hemoglobin saturation, and/or serial blood gases, helps safeguard the respiratory status. Muscle relaxants are rarely needed, even for extensive intra-abdominal operation, because of the lax abdominal musculature. Avoiding muscle relaxants eliminates one variable when assessing postoperative hypoventilation. Depending on the surgical procedure, the exposure may be large, predisposing to heat and fluid loss. Preoperative evaluation of renal function dictates fluid and electrolyte therapy and the possible need for central venous pressure monitoring. Extubation postoperatively is delayed until the patient is vigorous and demonstrates adequate ventilatory exchange, as indicated by spirometry and blood gases.[707, 711, 713] Postoperative chest physiotherapy has been recommended.[707]

OBSTRUCTIVE UROPATHY

The pathophysiology of acute and chronic obstruction in the developed kidney varies with each individual lesion. The degree and duration of obstruction, the time of onset, and the presence or absence of infection are important factors.[714] Acute ureteral obstruction initially results in an increase in afferent arteriolar blood flow and glomerular capillary pressure to compensate for the rise in tubular pressure.[715] Subsequently, the activation of the renin-aldosterone-angiotensin system may contribute to vasoconstriction and a lowered GFR.[716] The production from arachidonic acid of vasodilator prostaglandins and vasoconstrictor thromboxanes is increased, perhaps as a result of invasion of the renal cortex by macrophages and fibroblasts.[716] The level of GFR in the obstructed kidney is greatly influenced by these vasoactive metabolites.[716] After 24 hours of complete obstruction, however, glomerular capillary pressure and renal blood flow are depressed and GFR is markedly reduced.[715] Parenchymal renal injury may rapidly ensue (see Acute Renal Failure earlier in this chapter).

The pathophysiological changes during partial obstruction (as in *chronic obstructive nephropathy*) differ considerably.[717] Outer cortical nephrons are relatively spared and maintain their GFR, while juxtamedullary nephrons suffer markedly. The ability to concentrate urine may be lost, and an obligate urinary flow results. Alterations in renal function due to partial obstruction may remain unchanged for weeks to years.[714]

Recovery of GFR after *complete* obstruction is rapid if the obstruction is relieved within an hour, but otherwise recovery may be delayed or absent.[714] With *partial* obstruction, improvement following relief of obstruction is variable and is related to the presence of hydronephrosis.[714, 717] It is generally felt that the outcome for an individual child with chronic obstructive uropathy is improved with early correction, and in infants with subnormal GFR, intervention within the first year of life appears essential to preserve the capacity to improve glomerular function.[718, 719] Even after early release of partial obstruction, the urinary concentrating capacity may remain diminished.[719] Complications arising from chronic obstruction and urinary stasis include recurrent infection and the tendency to form calculi, both of which may contribute to the progression of renal injury.[720]

RENAL ANOMALIES AND ANOMALIES OF THE COLLECTING SYSTEM AND THE LOWER URINARY TRACT

It is because of renal injury, and complications associated with urinary obstruction, that many of the anomalies of the kidney, the collecting system, and the lower urinary tract are significant to thc urologist and ancsthcsiologist. In one prospective study using real-time ultrasound to screen 437 asymptomatic infants, 1.37 percent, or 1 of every 73 babies, was found to have a uropathological finding severe enough to warrant operation.[721]

Renovascular anomalies include renal arterial narrowing due to *fibromuscular dysplasia* or *intrarenal aneurysm* and may result in marked hypertension.[722, 723] Treatment is by segmental or total nephrectomy, percutaneous transluminal angioplasty, or segmental arterial embolization.[137, 723, 724] *Anomalous renal vessels* may become clinically significant because they obstruct ureteral flow.[720, 725] *Supernumerary kidneys, malrotation, renal fusion,* and *renal ectopia (simple ectopia* or *crossed ectopia* in which the ureter enters the bladder on the contralateral side) all may be associated with ureteral obstruction. This may be due to bands, aberrant vessels, or tortuous ureteral pathways from kidney to bladder.[726] *Hydronephrosis, ureteral strictures* and *duplications,* and associated skeletal, central nervous system, cardiovascular, and gastrointestinal tract anomalies may be present.[698] *Fused* and *ectopic kidneys* also may be more vulnerable to traumatic injury because of their location and fixation.[726]

The ureter may also be the site of developmental anomalies that cause urinary obstruction. The *ureteropelvic junction* is the most common site of supravesical obstruction in children. Such obstruction occurs as a result of intrinsic narrowing or angulation due to aberrant vessels to the lower pole of the kidney or fibrous bands.[720] Obstetrical ultrasound occasionally may detect the lesion in utero. Twenty-five percent of such lesions are detected in the first year of life because of a palpable mass, abdominal pain, hematuria, or urinary tract infection. Isosthenuria may occur, but renal insufficiency occurs only late in bilateral obstruction or obstruction of a solitary system.[720] *Ureteral stricture, valves, polyps, retrocaval ureter,* and *idiopathic retroperitoneal fibrosis*[727] all may cause ureteral obstruction.

The second most common site of ureteral obstruction is at the *ureterovesical junction.* The most frequently encountered problem resulting from obstruction at this location is *megaureter.*[720] Although any ureter greater than 1 cm in diameter, regardless of cause, has nonspecifically been called megaureter, *primary megaureter* refers to the condition in which the distal ureteral segment is aperistaltic and acts as a functional obstruction.[720] There is a male preponderance, the left side is more frequently involved, and it may be bilateral in 20 percent of children. The usual mode of presentation is with hematuria or urinary tract infection.[728] Treatment is by surgical resection of the aperistaltic segment, tailoring of the dilated ureter, and reimplantation.

Ureteral ectopia, ureteroceles, ureteropelvic and *ureteral duplications (complete, partial, or blind-ending),* and *bladder diverticuli* are other developmental anomalies of the urinary collecting system that may cause ureteral obstruction.[720, 726] *Ureteropelvic duplication* is a common anomaly occurring in 1 in 160 individuals, and patients are usually asymptomatic,[698] although obstruction and recurrent infection may occur.

A further major concern in these lesions is *reflux. Ureteroureteral reflux* may occur in proximal partial ureteropelvic duplications but more frequently occurs with *complete ureteral duplications* and *ectopic ureteral implantation.*[726]

Vesicoureteral reflux may occur as a result of these developmental anomalies or secondary to primary incompetence of the functional, interdigitating ureteral-bladder wall valve; elevated intravesical voiding pressures due to bladder malfunction; fixation of the orifice by bladder wall trabeculation; a neurogenic bladder; or even transient, acute inflammation due to infection.[714, 729, 730] The long-term consequences of reflux depend on the cause, severity, age, and degree of renal injury at presentation, the presence of infection, the degree of compliance with medical therapy, and probably many other unknown factors.[714, 731, 732] Normal renal function at presentation favors a good prognosis, whereas existing renal impairment represents a poor prognostic sign regardless of medical or surgical intervention.[714]

Because of the heterogeneity of causes and the complexity of factors influencing outcome, controversy persists as to the proper therapeutic approach and the timing of surgery.[729, 730] It is clear that even if vesicoureteral reflux is not in itself intrinsically injurious and one half to two thirds of children may outgrow primary vesicoureteral reflux, ascending bacterial infection is severely damaging, especially in younger children.[729] Bilateral vesicoureteral reflux and recurrent infection may cause severe, atrophic parenchymal scarring and renal insufficiency. Unilateral disease may be associated with hypertension and systemic infection, which are risks to long-term well-being.[714] Antireflux surgery has been shown to be effective with respect to resolution of reflux and prevention of upper urinary tract infection.[733–735] Such operation obviates the need for long-term antibiotic therapy and repeated radiological investigations. It is clearly indicated for severe reflux, for reflux that is not resolving with age, and for children in families in which compliance with chronic medication and continued medical follow-up is a problem.[714]

Ureteroneocystostomy (ureteral reimplantation) is the usual surgical procedure in primary reflux. A new, relatively long ureteral submucosal tunnel is created and effectively functions as a valve, preventing reflux.[736] Reflux secondary to bladder abnormalities may require urinary diversion.

Anesthetic considerations for operation for ureteral obstruction or reflux focus primarily on the type and degree of renal involvement. Hypertension may be present in as many as 25 percent of children with reflux and renal scarring, independent of the degree of azotemia. Antihypertensive agents may need to be continued perioperatively. Preoperative evaluation should determine whether chronic obstruction has led to a concentrating defect with an obligatory urine output and whether a degree of azotemia exists. Pre- and intraoperative fluid therapy should be managed accordingly. Intraoperative volume assessment may be complicated by the inability to collect and measure urine output because of drainage into the surgical field. An experienced surgeon may be able to estimate the amount of urine flow, or be willing to collect and measure urine in the field; for example, an open ureter may be placed in a sterile glove while not being manipulated. In children with significant renal impairment and/or hypertension, invasive monitoring with an arterial and a central venous pressure catheter will aid in fluid and anesthetic management. All the anesthetic considerations for renal failure discussed previously may need to be observed.

The surgical approach will vary with the procedure and the size of the patient. A lateral decubitus position, flank incision, and retroperitoneal approach may be preferred in older children to avoid bowel manipulation, adhesions, and obstruction. Care must be taken to provide appropriate and adequate padding, and ventilation and blood pressure should be carefully monitored during positioning. Extremes in angulation and tilting may significantly alter pulmonary and cardiovascular dynamics, decrease venous return, and result in hypotension. Smaller infants, and certain procedures, may require a transperitoneal approach. This demands greater abdominal muscular relaxation, and on occasion the avoidance of nitrous oxide to prevent gaseous bowel distention from interfering in the surgical field. A large surgical exposure will predispose to significant heat and fluid loss in small children.

Congenital anomalies of the bladder and urethra such as *duplications, cysts, strictures, polyps, stenoses,* and *valves* may cause urinary obstruction and stasis. The most significant of these lesions is *posterior urethral valves.* The degree of obstruction is variable, and if minor obstruction is included, it is the most common obstructive anomaly in male children.[737] Severe in utero obstruction may lead to the *urethral obstruction malformation complex* as described earlier. Male neonates may present with flank masses or a palpable bladder. Hydronephrosis, renal dysplasia, and azotemia may be complicated by acidosis, hyperkalemia, hyponatremia, and sepsis, requiring fluid and electrolyte resuscitation, antibiotic therapy, and emergent urinary drainage.[720] This is usually accomplished with the placement of a small urethral catheter but may sometimes require a suprapubic vesicostomy or urinary diversion.[720] Older children have less severe obstruction, and symptoms may be limited to urinary hesitancy, frequency, and incontinence. Cystoscopy, voiding cystourethrography, and urodynamic studies will confirm the diagnosis. Transurethral resection is usually possible, but occasionally urethral reconstruction is required.

A *neuropathic bladder* may also cause urinary stasis and obstruction and lead to infection, reflux, and renal parenchymal injury.[738] Myelomeningocele is the most common cause in children, but neuropathic bladder may also result from diastematomyelia, tethered cord syndrome, sacral agenesis or dysgenesis, spinal tumors, pelvic surgery, trauma, transverse myelitis, and osteomyelitis of the vertebral column.[738] Cystoscopy, voiding cystourethrography, and urodynamic studies are used in the evaluation of the lesion and response to treatment. Aggressive antibiotic therapy, manual expression of the bladder (Credé's maneuver), intermittent catheterization, drug therapy, and implantation of artificial sphincters are all designed to prevent the complications of urinary stasis and provide acceptable forms of urinary drainage.[739]

Several pharmacological agents have been employed in an attempt to alter the parasympathetic and sympathetic influence on bladder and urethral sphincter tone. Imipramine, a tricyclic antidepressant that blocks reuptake of norepinephrine in nerve terminals and has prominent anticholinergic effects, increases bladder outlet resistance and decreases bladder contractility. This sometimes leads to continence.[740] Phenoxybenzamine, an alpha-adrenergic blocker, has been used to decrease bladder outlet resistance and allow more complete bladder emptying in children who are able to void voluntarily.[741] On the other hand, ephedrine and phenylpropanolamine have been used as alpha-adrenergic agonists to increase bladder outlet resistance in children on intermittent catheterization programs in whom incontinence has been a problem.[738, 739] Likewise, when incontinence is felt to be due to bladder contraction, anticholinergic agents such as propantheline and oxybutynin have been used to reduce bladder (detrusor muscle) tone. By contrast, bladder contraction has been stimulated with cholinergic agents such as bethanechol and carbachol in cases of transient retention following spinal cord surgery.[738] Finally, diazepam and dantrolene have been used in an attempt to relieve external (voluntary) sphincter spasm,[739, 742] but surgical division by urethrotomy is often required for this problem.[738]

Which drugs are employed in a given child will depend on whether voluntary voiding or catheterization is the goal, whether incontinence is due to increased bladder tone or decreased internal sphincter tone, or whether a large residual urine volume is the principal problem. These drugs have significant interactions with anesthetic, adrenergic, anticholinergic, and neuromuscular blocking and reversal agents commonly employed during anesthesia. In addition, they may interact with antihypertensive medications that the patient may be taking. It is therefore important for the anesthesiologist to determine which, if any, of these drugs the patient is taking, and what interactions might be expected.

Cystoscopy, voiding cystourethrography, and urodynamic studies are important procedures in the urological evaluation of bladder abnormalities. In pediatric practice these studies are usually performed with the patient under anesthesia. Just as the drugs described earlier may affect bladder and sphincter tone, so also may anesthetics and other drugs commonly employed during anesthesia. As a result, anesthesia for cystoscopy and urodynamic studies must not only address the issues of patient safety but also attempt to provide conditions under which the results of the urodynamic studies are valid. For example, laryngospasm upon urethral instrumentation (the Breuer-Luckhardt reflex) may occur if the depth of anesthesia is inadequate, whereas a very light anesthetic, almost to the point of awakening, is required to allow voiding to occur for a voiding cystourethrogram.[698] Bladder activity and sphincter tone may be suppressed for up to 10 minutes following the use of thiopental or potent inhalational agents, and reliable results during urodynamic measurement require the use of only nitrous oxide and oxygen.[743] Atropine is commonly used in children to dry secretions, to decrease the potential for laryngospasm, and to counteract bradycardia. Unfortunately, it also relaxes bladder tone and invalidates the results of urodynamic studies.[698] It has been suggested that the risks of regurgitation and laryngospasm, which may accompany the rapid changes required in anesthetic depth, may be diminished if intravenous lidocaine (1 to 1.5 mg/kg, repeatable after 5 minutes) is used to smooth out these transitions.[744]

Many congenital anomalies of the bladder and lower genitourinary tract do not lead to obstruction and consequent renal involvement but do require surgical intervention. Perhaps the most dramatic of these are the *exstrophic anomalies,* which may range from *epispadias* to complete *cloacal exstrophy.* The cleft may be so large as to extend up the abdomen to the thorax. Associated anomalies are usually genitourinary and gastrointestinal but may include cleft palate, chromosomal abnormalities, and cardiac malformations.[698]

Bladder exstrophy has an incidence of 1 in 10,000 to 50,000 live births, with twice as many males affected as females.[745] Exstrophy of the bladder has been reported in twins and siblings, but familial inheritance is rare and sporadic occurrence is the rule.[746] The problems associated with bladder exstrophy include incontinence, with subsequent discomfort and social ostracism, squamous metaplasia of bladder mucosa, and a predisposition many years later to malignancy, most commonly adenocarcinoma.[746] Following bladder reconstruction or urinary diversion, the problems of upper urinary tract deterioration, obstruction, formation of calculi, infection, and reflux may lead to renal impairment.[745, 746] Although the timing and staging of surgical repair remain controversial, several investigators suggest that it may be advantageous to perform the repair on an urgent basis.[745, 746] Early closure may decrease inflammatory changes in the bladder and limit perimuscular fibrosis.[745] Possibly because of the persistent influence of the maternal hormone relaxin, approximation of the pubes may be accomplished without iliac osteotomies in the first day or two of life.[745, 746] After this time it is often necessary to divide the bony pelvic ring to relieve tension at the pubic symphysis. This requires bilateral iliac osteotomies, a major and time-consuming procedure that is done with the patient in the prone position prior to attempted bladder reconstruction and may add significantly to the operative risk.[746] A further advantage to early operative intervention is that if bladder closure can be accomplished prior to bacterial colonization of the gastrointestinal tract, sterility of the urinary system may be more readily preserved.

Many *anomalies of the urethra and genitalia,* including *malposition, dorsal or ventral duplications,* and *diverticuli,* as well as acquired lesions, are of functional and cosmetic significance.[747–749] The most common of these anomalies is *hypospadias,* which has an incidence of 8 per 1000 male births and varies in severity from the mild coronal variety to the severe penoscrotal type.[747] There is some evidence to suggest that maternal ingestion of synthetic progestins may be a cause of hypospadias,[750] and there have been reports of a familial incidence.[751] Associated anomalies are usually restricted to the lower genitourinary system (hernia, hydrocele, cryptorchidism), but major anomalies of the upper urinary tract may also occur.[749] Although the timing of operation is still debated, repair may begin by 6 months of age; even with a severe lesion requiring multiple stages, the repair is usually concluded by 4 to 5 years of age.[747, 749]

Almost any form of anesthesia may be used for hypospadias repair, as long as the anesthesiologist takes care to meet the special needs of small infants being anesthetized, such as limitation of heat loss and maintenance of fluid balance. Nitrous oxide plus narcotic anesthesia or light volatile anesthesia may be associated with penile erection, which is bothersome to the surgeon. This is usually easily resolved by deepening the anesthetic with a volatile agent or with intravenous ketamine.[747, 752–754] This problem may also be corrected by the surgeon manually forcing drainage of the corpora cavernosa and applying a rubber band tourniquet to prevent reinflation. It is important to take note and advise the surgeon of the elapsed tourniquet time in this instance.

Recent anesthetic reports have focused on the use of regional techniques (dorsal penile nerve block versus caudal anesthesia) to provide postoperative analgesia after hypospadias repair or circumcision.[755–758] Although most of these blocks have been performed at the conclusion of the procedure, some have suggested placing caudal blocks immediately after the induction of anesthesia to reduce general anesthetic requirements.[759] Spinal anesthesia has been used as the sole anesthetic in high-risk infants for cystoscopy with fulguration of urethral valves and for circumcision.[760] An advantage of caudal and spinal anesthesia is that penile erection is blocked.[747] The techniques of nerve block and caudal and spinal anesthesia in infants are described in detail elsewhere.[306]

It is important to differentiate penile erection during light anesthesia from pathological *priapism,* which is associated with obstructed venous drainage in *sickle cell anemia, leukemia, trauma,* and *Fabry's disease* (a glycosphingolipid storage disease).[747, 761] Regional anesthesia, topical nitroglycerin,[762] inhalation of amyl nitrate,[763] benzodiazepines,[764] terbutaline,[765] ephedrine,[766] and ketamine[754] are ineffective in these mechanical, obstructive causes and treatment is directed at the underlying illness (oxygenation and hypertransfusion in sickle cell disease, radiation and chemotherapy in leukemia, plasma transfusion in Fabry's disease, and surgical drainage in trauma and for other failed therapies).[747, 752, 753]

There are many congenital and acquired lesions of the scrotum and testes, some of which require urgent surgical intervention, such as *torsion of the testicle.*[767, 768] *Cryptorchidism (undescended testes)* is the most common anomaly, with an incidence of 1 percent in term infants and much more frequent occurrence in premature infants, the incidence increasing with decreasing gestational age.[749, 768] The chance of complete spontaneous testicular descent after infancy is small, with the testis suffering degenerative changes proportionate to its delay in reaching the scrotum.[768] Problems associated with cryptorchidism include inguinal hernia, torsion, trauma, malignancy, and infertility.[767, 768] Hormonal treatment to induce descent is only partially successful and is associated with side effects, including premature puberty. Orchiopexy is therefore usually performed at an early age in an effort to improve fertility, prevent testicular malignancy (and make it more readily detectable should it occur), and repair the associated hernia. Anesthesia for orchiopexy includes the same considerations as those for genital and inguinal hernia operation in infants, and regional techniques for postoperative analgesia (ilioinguinal and iliohypogastric nerve blocks and caudal anesthesia) have been effective.[759] Traction on the testicle and/or peritoneum may induce a marked vagal response in infants, for which anticholinergic blockade with atropine is helpful. On occasion, the search for an undescended testicle may extend into an intra-abdominal, retroperitoneal exploration. In this case, endotracheal intubation and controlled ventilation may be advisable, and abdominal muscular relaxation may be helpful.

ENDOCRINE FUNCTION AND GENITOURINARY ABNORMALITIES

Renal function and genitourinary development are intimately related to endocrine function. The kidney is not only the target organ for such hormones as atrial natriuretic peptide, aldosterone, and antidiuretic hormone but also the endocrine source of renin and erythropoietin and a significant site of metabolism of hormones (for example, gastrin and insulin). As noted previously, an excess of plasma atrial natriuretic peptide may be a cause of Bartter's syndrome, whereas an impaired responsiveness to ANP may be the cause of Gordon's syndrome, a syndrome characterized by plasma volume overexpansion.[618, 619] The effects of renal injury and failure on some of these interactions have already been discussed.

Much has been learned about atrial natriuretic peptide (ANP) in the last several years. Released in response to atrial distention, even small elevations can result in natriuresis, diuresis, and vasodilatation.[24] Endogenous ANP has been detected in the fetus and in premature neonates and may provide an important endocrine system for the control of sodium balance.[769, 770] Ventilated premature neonates with respiratory distress syndrome have been found to have elevated plasma ANP levels.[771] Decreased secretion of ANP with positive airway pressure ventilation, PEEP, and CPAP has been postulated to be one cause of antidiuresis during positive-pressure ventilation,[772–774] although this has been disputed.[775] Elevated levels of ANP have been detected in ARDS,[776] and in high-altitude pulmonary edema.[777] ANP causes a relatively larger degree of relaxation in the pulmonary arterial vascular bed than elsewhere,[778] raising the possibility of selective pulmonary vascular vasodilatation.[783] ANP also induces an extravascular shift of fluid, perhaps by increasing capillary leakiness.[780] However, a clear pathogenic role for ANP in ARDS and high-altitude pulmonary edema has not been defined. ANP has also demonstrated bronchodilatory effects.[779]

ANP levels have been found to be elevated in normotensive children with chronic renal failure, but this is related to hypervolemia and resolves with appropriate hemodialysis and decrease in body weight.[25, 781] Likewise, ANP levels are elevated in children with congenital heart disease whose cardiac lesions have caused left atrial enlargement.[782]

More significant for the anesthesiologist is that ANP is beginning to be investigated as a potent, short-acting diuretic and therapeutic agent to help preserve renal blood flow. In animal models, ANP has been used to prevent acute renal failure, or even as a "rescue" therapy after onset of acute renal failure induced by norepinephrine or gentamicin.[404, 405] In humans with chronic renal failure undergoing radiocontrast infusion for cardiac catheterization, ANP has been compared with mannitol for the preservation of renal blood flow and prevention of superimposed acute renal failure.[406] In both the mannitol and ANP groups, renal blood flow was maintained or increased in spite of the administration of diatrizoate contrast, a known renal vasoconstrictor. It is interesting that plasma ANP levels also rose significantly in the mannitol infusion group, suggesting that mannitol may induce ANP release, perhaps accounting for a portion of mannitol's beneficial effect.

Several studies have looked at the effects of

anesthetics on the secretion of ANP. Studies in experimental animals have shown an increase in ANP release with halothane and morphine,[784, 786] as well as an increased natriuretic response to ANP with pentobarbital anesthesia.[785] Fentanyl anesthesia in animals[784] and in humans[786] did not alter ANP release or responsiveness, nor did muscle relaxants, diazepam, or initiation of cardiopulmonary bypass in humans.[787] Unlike experimental animals, humans demonstrate little or no ANP response to opiates, halothane, or surgical stimulation of the sympathetic nervous system.[788] This suggests that in humans, ANP secretion and response, even with anesthesia and surgical therapy, remain volume-mediated and responsive. Pressor agents, especially alpha-agonists such as norepinephrine, have been shown to cause ANP release, but this is most likely mediated by changes in atrial pressure.[789]

The *syndrome of inappropriate antidiuretic hormone secretion (SIADH)* is an example of a disease state in which normal renal function may lead to a dangerously pathological condition: severe hyponatremia and hypoosmolarity.[790] Excessive secretion of antidiuretic hormone (due to a neurological insult or other causes) promotes tubular reabsorption of water. Although definitive treatment must be directed at the underlying cause of ADH secretion, it may be necessary to impose conditions that make the excessive ADH secretion and the normal renal response appropriate; this is accomplished by severe fluid restriction. Another temporizing solution is to interfere with normal tubular function in order to prevent the detrimental effects of water reabsorption. This may be accomplished by the administration of diuretics, ethanol, or lithium, with careful attention to the electrolyte disturbances that may result.[790] In children with convulsions or coma due to hyponatremia, the infusion of hypertonic saline results in transient improvement. (A sodium dose of 6 mEq/kg will transiently raise the serum sodium by 10 mEq/L.[790]) The associated risk is that the hypertonic saline will contribute to the already expanded extracellular volume, inducing circulatory overload.[790] Anesthesia in such children requires careful attention to volume and electrolyte status and therapy.

Adrenogenital syndrome (congenital adrenal hyperplasia) is an example of a disease state in which the development of the genitourinary system is affected. Deficiency of adrenal C-21-hydroxylase activity results in virilization of females, with occasional severe salt wasting. C-11-hydroxylase deficiency may be associated with severe hypertension.[698, 791] These defects are thought to be autosomal recessive and vary in incidence from 1 in 50,000 live births to 1 in 500 live births among natives of southwestern Alaska.[791] Treatment with exogenous cortisone inhibits ACTH secretion and provides the deficient adrenal end-product. This decreases the accumulation of intermediate products of cortisol synthesis that cause virilization and helps reverse electrolyte abnormalities, such as hyponatremia and hyperkalemia.[698, 791] Females will often present for surgical correction of malformed genitalia between 2 and 4 years of age. However, undiagnosed newborn males with dehydration, electrolyte abnormalities, and vomiting may present for surgical therapy with a misdiagnosis of pyloric stenosis or intestinal obstruction.[791]

Anesthetic care in these children requires careful preoperative evaluation of their volume and electrolyte status and a continuation of their steroid therapy. The acute stress of operation or illness may require an increase in their steroid coverage by one and a half times to three times their normal dosage, although excessive administration may lead to sodium retention and hypertension.[744, 791] Since these children are often placed in an extreme lithotomy or knee-to-chest position, endotracheal intubation and controlled ventilation are recommended.[791] Because of the potential for partial recovery from pancuronium neuromuscular blockade following hydrocortisone administration, intraoperative monitoring of neuromuscular blockade is useful.[792, 793]

RENAL AND GENITOURINARY TRAUMA

Blunt or penetrating trauma to the back, abdomen, pelvis, or perineum may result in injury to the kidneys, ureters, bladder, urethra, or genitalia.[794, 795] Up to 7 percent of all childhood injuries may involve the genitourinary system and require urgent surgical intervention.[794] Injury may be obvious, or it may be occult, resulting in retroperitoneal, intrapelvic, or intra-abdominal urinary leakage or bleeding. In up to 40 percent of children, trauma sufficient to cause renal injury is accompanied by cerebral, spinal, bony, pulmonary, abdominal visceral, and vascular trauma, which may dictate the initial emergency management.[796] Adequate resuscitation and stabilization should precede radiological investigation, surgical exploration, and operative repair. Complications of renal injury include secondary hemorrhage, persistent urinary extravasation, perinephric abscess, hypertension secondary to segmental ischemia, renal stones, renal scarring, renal atrophy, and renal failure.[794] Anesthetic considerations are those for resuscitation and major trauma, along with the principles of management of patients with impending acute renal failure, as discussed previously.

PSYCHOLOGICAL CONSIDERATIONS

Whether a child suffers from chronic renal failure, requiring frequent medical intervention, or a disfiguring genitourinary malformation, requiring extensive surgical repair, the psychological and social impacts on the child and family are profound.[237] In severe, untreated, or unsuccessfully treated bladder exstrophy, for example, there is a high pubertal incidence of psychiatric problems, including a significant incidence of suicide.[745] Children made dependent on others by their illness may demonstrate behavior inappropriate to their chronological age, especially in the hospital setting. Additional time, effort, and empathy are required of the anesthesiologist to communicate with the child and the family and to allay anxieties associated with anesthesia and operation. Time invested preoperatively in gaining a child's understanding and trust is invaluable to the child. It may also be invaluable to the anesthesiologist when soliciting the child's cooperation during difficult venipuncture prior to induction of anesthesia, or for other unpleasant but necessary interventions.

Original chapter supported in part by the Children's Hospital Medical Center Anesthesia Foundation, Inc., Boston, Massachusetts.

REFERENCES

1. Berry FA: The renal system. *In* Gregory GA (Ed): Pediatric Anesthesia. New York, Churchill Livingstone, 1983, pp 63–128.
2. Spitzer A: Renal physiology and functional development. *In* Edelmann CM Jr (Ed.): Pediatric Kidney Disease. Boston, Little, Brown, 1978, pp 25–128.
3. Bricker NS, Bourgoignie JJ, Licht AA, et al: Pathophysiology of chronic renal failure. *In* Edelmann CM Jr (Ed.): Pediatric Kidney Disease. Boston, Little, Brown, 1978, pp 205–212.
4. Kuruvila KC, Schrier RW: Chronic renal failure. Int Anesthesiol Clin *22*:101, 1984.
5. Easterling RE: Racial factors in the incidence and causation of end-stage renal disease. Trans Am Soc Artif Intern Organs *23*:28, 1977.
6. Rostand SG, Kirk KA, Rutsky EA, et al: Racial differences in the incidence of treatment for end-stage renal disease. N Engl J Med *306*:1276, 1982.
7. Foreman JW, Chan JCM: Chronic renal failure in infants and children. J Pediatr *113*:793, 1988.
8. Chantler C, Carter JE, Bewick M, et al: Ten years' experience with regular haemodialysis and renal transplantation. Arch Dis Child *55*:435, 1980.
9. Barratt TM, Baillod RA: Chronic renal failure and regular dialysis. *In* Williams DI, Johnston JH (Eds.): Paediatric Urology. London, Butterworth Scientific, 1982, pp 37–47.
10. Schwartz GJ, Feld LG, Langford DJ: A simple estimate of glomerular filtration rate in full-term infants during the first year of life. J Pediatr *104*:849, 1984.
11. Schwartz GJ, Haycock GB, Edelmann CM Jr, et al: A simple estimate of glomerular filtration rate in children derived from body length and plasma creatinine. Pediatrics *58*:259, 1976.
12. Barratt TM: Renal function. *In* Williams DI, Johnston JH (Eds.): Paediatric Urology. London, Butterworth Scientific, 1982, pp 1–10.
13. Platt R: Structural and functional adaption in renal failure. Br Med J *1*:1313, 1372, 1952.
14. Bricker NS: The pathogenesis of the uremic state: The "trade-off" hypothesis. N Engl J Med *286*:1093, 1972.
15. Schrier RW, Regal EM: Influence of aldosterone on sodium, water and potassium metabolism in chronic renal disease. Kidney Int *1*:156, 1972.
16. Wilkinson R, Luetcher JA, Dowdy AS, et al: Studies on the mechanism of sodium excretion in uremia. Clin Sci *42*:685, 1972.
17. Carriere S, Wong NLM, Kirks JH: Redistribution of renal blood flow in acute and chronic reduction of renal mass. Kidney Int *3*:364, 1973.
18. Kahn T, Mohammad G, Stein RM: Alterations in renal tubular sodium and water reabsorption in chronic renal disease in man. Kidney Int *2*:164, 1972.
19. Bourgoignie JJ, Hwang KH, Espinel C, et al: A natriuretic factor in the serum of patients with chronic uremia. J Clin Invest *51*:1514, 1972.
20. Bricker NS, Klahr S, Lubowitz H, et al: On the biology of sodium excretion: The search for a natriuretic hormone. Yale J Biol Med *48*:293, 1975.
21. Fine LG, Bourgoignie JJ, Weber H, et al: Enhanced end-organ responsiveness of the uremic kidney to the natriuretic factor. Kidney Int *10*:364, 1976.
22. Cogan MG: Atrial natriuretic factor. West J Med *144*:591, 1986.
23. Stephenson TJ, Broughton-Pipkin F: Atrial natriuretic factor: The heart as an endocrine organ. Arch Dis Child *65*:1293, 1990.
24. Richards AM, Nicholls MG, Ikram H, et al: Renal, haemodynamic, and hormonal effects of human alpha-atrial natriuretic peptide in healthy volunteers. Lancet *1*:545, 1985.
25. Rascher W, Tullassay T, Lang RE: Atrial natriuretic peptide in plasma of volume-overloaded children with chronic renal failure. Lancet *2*:303, 1985.
26. Bricker NS: Sodium homeostasis in chronic renal disease. Kidney Int *21*:886, 1982.
27. Bourgoignie JJ, Jacob AI, Sollman L, et al: Water, electrolyte and acid base abnormalities in chronic renal failure. Semin Nephrol *1*:91, 1981.
28. Lewy PR, Hurley JK: Chronic renal insufficiency. Pediatr Clin North Am *23*:829, 1976.
29. Schreiner MS, Triebwasser A, Keon TP: Ingestion of liquids compared with preoperative fasting in pediatric outpatients. Anesthesiology *72*:593, 1990.

30. Coté CJ: NPO after midnight for children—a reappraisal. Anesthesiology *72*:589, 1990.
31. Grodstein G, Harrison A, Roberts C, et al: Impaired gastric emptying in hemodialysis patients (abstract). Annual Meeting, Am Soc Nephrol 182A, 1979.
32. Berl T, Schrier RW: Water metabolism and the hypo-osmolar syndromes. *In* Brenner B, Stein J (Eds.): Chronic Renal Failure. New York, Churchill Livingstone, 1981.
33. Blaufox MD: Systemic arterial hypertension in pediatric practice. Pediatr Clin North Am *18*:577, 1971.
34. Kurtzmann NA: Chronic renal failure: Metabolic and clinical consequences. Hosp Pract *17*:107, 1982.
35. Fine LG, Kaplan M, Bricker NS: Disturbances of salt and water metabolism in chronic renal failure. *In* Edelmann CM Jr (Ed.): Pediatric Kidney Disease. Boston, Little, Brown, 1978, pp 348–356.
36. Tasker PRW, MacGregor GA, de Wardener HE: Prophylactic use of intravenous saline in patients with chronic renal failure undergoing major surgery. Lancet *2*:911, 1974.
37. Nash MA: Water and solute homeostasis. *In* Edelmann CM Jr (Ed.): Pediatric Kidney Disease. Boston, Little, Brown, 1978, pp 290–305.
38. Sherman RA: Suppression of aldosterone production by low-dose heparin. Am J Nephrol *6*:165, 1986.
39. Trainin EB, Spitzer A: Treatment of acute renal failure. *In* Edelmann CM Jr (Ed.): Pediatric Kidney Disease. Boston, Little, Brown, 1978, pp 466–474.
40. Bastron RD, Deutsch S: Anesthesia for the functionally anephric patient. *In* Bastron RD, Deutsch S (Eds.): Anesthesia and the Kidney—The Scientific Basis of Clinical Anesthesia. New York, Grune & Stratton, 1976.
41. Rudolph AM: Disturbances of the cardiovascular system. *In* Edelmann CM Jr (Ed.): Pediatric Kidney Disease. Boston, Little, Brown, 1978, pp 429–432.
42. Zauder HL: Anesthesia for patients who have terminal renal disease. *In* Hershey SG (Ed.): Refresher Courses in Anesthesiology. Vol 4, Chapter 14. Park Ridge, Ill, American Society of Anesthesiologists, 1976.
43. Koide M, Waud BE: Serum potassium concentrations after succinylcholine in patients with renal failure. Anesthesiology *36*:142, 1972.
44. Tammisto T, Leikkonen P, Airaksinen M: The inhibitory effect of D-tubocurarine on the increase of serum creatinine kinase activity produced by intermittent suxamethonium administration during halothane anesthesia. Acta Anaesthesiol Scand *11*:333, 1967.
45. Miller RD, Way WL, Hamilton WK, et al: Succinylcholine-induced hyperkalemia in patients with renal failure. Anesthesiology *36*:138, 1972.
46. Walton JD, Farman JV: Suxamethonium, potassium and renal failure. Anaesthesia *28*:626, 1973.
47. Roth F, Wüthrich H: The clinical importance of hyperkalemia following suxamethonium administration. Br J Anaesth *41*:311, 1969.
48. Powell DR, Miller R: The effect of repeated doses of succinylcholine on serum potassium in patients with renal failure. Anesth Analg *54*:746, 1975.
49. Walton JD, Farman JV: Suxamethonium hyperkalaemia in uraemic neuropathy. Anaesthesia *28*:666, 1973.
50. Kildeberg P, Engel K, Winter RW: Balance of net acid in growing infants. Acta Paediatr Scand *58*:321, 1969.
51. Salcedo JR, Jackson ML, Coleman TN, et al: Endogenous net acid production in infants, children and adults. Pediatr Res *10*:443, 1976.
52. Winters RW, Chan JC, Klenk EL, et al: Net acid balance in metabolic acidosis. Pediatr Res *5*:395, 1971.
53. Lockhart E, Edelmann CM Jr: Acid-base disturbances in renal failure. *In* Edelmann CM Jr (Ed.): Pediatric Kidney Disease. Boston, Little, Brown, 1978, pp 357–365.
54. de Torrenté A: Acute renal failure. Int Anesthesiol Clin *22*:83, 1984.
55. Wrong O, Davies HEF: The excretion of acid in renal disease. QJ Med *28*:259, 1959.
56. Arruda JAL: Acidosis of renal failure. Semin Nephrol *1*:275, 1982.
57. Dubose TD Jr: Acid-base physiology in uremia. Artif Organs *6*:363, 1982.
58. Schwarz WB, Hall PW, Hays RM, et al: On the mechanism of acidosis in chronic renal disease. QJ Clin Invest *38*:39, 1956.
59. Litzow J, Lemann J, Lennon E: The effect of treatment of acidosis on calcium balance in patients with chronic azotemic renal disease. J Clin Invest *46*:280, 1967.
60. Avioli LV, Teitelbaum SL: Renal osteodystrophy. *In* Edelmann CM Jr (Ed.): Pediatric Renal Disease. Boston, Little, Brown, 1978, pp 366–400.
61. Cooke RE, Boyden DG, Haller E: The relationship of acidosis and growth retardation. J Pediatr *57*:326, 1960.
62. Burnell S, Villamil M, Vyero B, et al: Effect in humans of extracellular pH on the relationship between serum potassium concentration and intracellular potassium. J Clin Invest *35*:935, 1956.
63. Müller MC: Anesthesia for the patient with renal dysfunction. Int Anesthesiol Clin *22*:169, 1984.
64. Goggin MJ, Joekes AM: Gas exchange in renal failure. Dangers of hyperkalemia during anesthesia. Br J Med *2*:244, 1971.
65. Norman ME: Vitamin D in bone disease. Pediatr Clin North Am *29*:947, 1982.
66. Fine RN, Isaacson AS, Payne V, et al: Renal osteodystrophy in children: The effect of hemodialysis and renal transplantation. J Pediatr *80*:243, 1972.
67. Norman ME, Mazur AT, Borden S, et al: Early diagnosis of juvenile renal osteodystrophy. J Pediatr *97*:226, 1980.
68. Cunningham J, Avioli LV: Systemic acidosis and the bioactivation of vitamin D. *In* Abstracts of the Fifth Workshop on Vitamin D. Williamsburg, Va, Feb 14–19, 1982.
69. Boischis H, Winterborn MH: Acute renal failure in childhood. Pediatr Ann *3*:58, 1974.
70. Ott SM, Coburn JW, Alfrey AC, et al: The prevalence of bone aluminum deposition in renal osteodystrophy and its relation to the response to calcitriol therapy. N Engl J Med *307*:709, 1982.
71. Firor HV, Moore ES, Levitsky LL, et al: Parathyroidectomy in children with chronic renal failure. J Pediatr Surg *7*:565, 1972.
72. McKie BD: Hypocalcaemia and prolonged curarization. Br J Anaesth *41*:1091, 1969.
73. Pender JW, Basso LV: Diseases of the endocrine system. *In* Katz J, Benumof J, Kadis LB (Eds.): Anesthesia and Uncommon Diseases. Philadelphia, WB Saunders, 1981, pp 155–220.
74. Steele TH, Wen SF, Evenson MA, et al: The contribution of the chronically diseased kidney to magnesium homeostasis in man. J Lab Clin Med *71*:455, 1968.
75. Ferdinandus J, Pederson JA, Whang R: Hypermagnesemia as a cause of refractory hypotension, respiratory depression and coma. Arch Intern Med *141*:669, 1981.
76. Ghoneim MM, Long JP: The interaction between magnesium and other neuromuscular blocking agents. Anesthesiology *32*:23, 1970.

77. Fried W: Hematologic abnormalities in chronic renal failure. Semin Nephrol *1*:176, 1981.
78. Kasanen A, Kalliomaki JL: Correlation of some kidney function tests with hemoglobin in chronic nephropathies. Acta Med Scand *158*:213, 1957.
79. O'Brien RT, Pearson HA: Hematologic disturbances in uremia. *In* Edelmann CM Jr (Ed.): Pediatric Renal Disease. Boston, Little, Brown 1978, pp 401–407.
80. Brown R: Plasma erythropoietin in chronic uremia. Br Med J *2*:1036, 1965.
81. Chandra M, Clemons GK, McVicar MI: Relation of serum erythropoietin levels to renal excretory function: Evidence for lowered set point for erythropoietin production in chronic renal failure. J Pediatr *113*:1015, 1988.
82. Fisher JW, Hatch FE, Roh BL, et al: Erythropoietin inhibitors in kidney extracts and plasma from anemic uremic human subjects. Blood *31*:440, 1968.
83. Radtke HW, Rege AB, LaMarche MB, et al: Identification of spermine as an inhibitor of erythropoiesis in patients with chronic renal failure. J Clin Invest *67*:1623, 1981.
84. Shaw AB: Hemolysis in chronic renal failure. Br Med J *2*:213, 1967.
85. Giovannetti S, Balestri PL, Cioni L: Spontaneous in vitro auto-haemolysis of blood from chronic uremic patients. Clin Sci *29*:407, 1965.
86. Joske RA, McAlister JM, Prankerd TAJ: Isotope investigations of red cell production and destruction in chronic renal disease. Clin Sci *15*:511, 1956.
87. Giovannetti S, Cioni L, Balestri PL, et al: Evidence that guanidines and some related compounds cause haemolysis in chronic uremia. Clin Sci *34*:141, 1968.
88. Shainkin R, Giatt Y, Berlyne G: The presence and toxicity of guanidino-propionic acid in uremia. Kidney Int *7*:S302, 1975.
89. Merrill JP: Uremia. N Engl J Med *282*:1014, 1970.
90. Lonergan ET, Semar M, Sterzel RB, et al: Erythrocyte transketolase activity in dialyzed patients. N Engl J Med *284*:1399, 1971.
91. Aherne WA: The "burr" red cell and azotemia. J Clin Pathol *10*:252, 1957.
92. Lichtman MA, Miller DR, Abel V, et al: Erythrocyte glycolysis, 2,3-diphosphoglycerate and adenosine triphosphate concentration in uremic subjects: Relationship to extracellular phosphate concentration. J Lab Clin Med *76*:267, 1970.
93. Lichtman MA, Murphy MS, Byer BJ, et al: Hemoglobin affinity for oxygen in chronic renal disease: Effect of hemodialysis. Blood *43*:417, 1974.
94. Potter D, Feduska N, Melzer J, et al: Twenty years of renal transplantation in children. Pediatrics *77*:465, 1986.
95. Vincenti F, Duca RM, Amend W, et al: Immunologic factors determining survival of cadaver kidney transplants: Effect of HLA serotyping, cytotoxic antibodies and blood transfusions on graft survival. N Engl J Med *299*:793, 1978.
96. Opelz G, Terasaki PI: Improvement of kidney graft survival with increased number of transfusions. N Engl J Med *299*:799, 1978.
97. Eschbach JW, Funk D, Adamson J, et al: Erythropoiesis in patients with renal failure undergoing chronic dialysis. N Engl J Med *276*:653, 1967.
98. Bozzini EE, Devoto FC, Tomio JM: Decreased responsiveness of hematopoietic tissue to erythropoietin in acutely uremic rats. J Lab Clin Med *68*:411, 1966.
99. Eschbach JW, Kelly MR, Haley NR, et al: Treatment of the anemia of progressive renal failure with recombinant human erythropoietin. N Engl J Med *321*:158, 1989.
99a. Pinevich AJ, Petersen J: Erythropoietin therapy in patients with chronic renal failure. West J Med *157*:154, 1992.
100. Sun CH, Ward HJ, Paul WL, et al: Serum erythropoietin levels after renal transplantation. N Engl J Med *321*:151, 1989.
101. Hoffman GS: Human erythropoiesis following kidney transplantation. Ann NY Acad Sci *149*:504, 1968.
102. Miller RD: Complications of massive blood transfusions. Anesthesiology *39*:82, 1973.
103. Ellis DE, Stoelting RK: Individual variations in fluroxene, halothane, and methoxyflurane blood-gas partition coefficients and the effect of anemia. Anesthesiology *42*:748, 1975.
104. Hampers CL, Blaufox MD, Merrill JP: Anticoagulation rebound after hemodialysis. N Engl J Med *275*:776, 1966.
105. Kjellstrand CM, Buselmeier TJ: A simple method for anticoagulation during pre- and post-operative hemodialysis, avoiding rebound phenomena. Surgery *72*:630, 1972.
106. Stewart JH: Platelet numbers and life span in acute and chronic renal failure. Thromb Diath Haemorrh *17*:532, 1967.
107. Horowitz HI, Stein IM, Cohen BD, et al: Further studies on the platelet inhibitory effect of guanidinosuccinic acid and its role in uremic bleeding. Am J Med *49*:336, 1970.
108. Rabiner SF, Molinas F: The role of phenol and phenolic acids on the thrombocytopathy and defective platelet aggregation of patients with renal failure. Am J Med *49*:346, 1970.
109. Eknoyan G, Wacksman SJ, Glueck HI, et al: Platelet function in renal failure. N Engl J Med *280*:667, 1969.
110. Rabiner SF, Hrodek O: Platelet factor 3 in normal subjects and patients with renal failure. J Clin Invest *47*:901, 1968.
111. Stewart JH, Castaldi PA: Uremic bleeding: A reversible platelet defect corrected by dialysis. QJ Med *36*:409, 1967.
112. Lindsay RM, Moorthy AV, Koens F, et al: Platelet function in dialyzed and non-dialyzed patients with chronic renal failure. Clin Nephrol *4*:52, 1975.
113. Fischback DP, Fogdall RP: Coagulation: The Essentials. Baltimore, William & Wilkins, 1981.
114. Carvalho ACA: Bleeding in uremia—a clinical challenge. N Engl J Med *308*:38, 1983.
115. Janson PA, Jubelirer SJ, Weinstein MJ, et al: Treatment of the bleeding tendency in uremia with cryoprecipitate. N Engl J Med *303*:1318, 1980.
116. Watson AJS, Keough JAB: Effect of 1-deamino-8-D-arginine vasopressin on the prolonged bleeding time in chronic renal failure. Nephron *32*:49, 1982.
117. Mannucci PM, Remuzzi G, Pusineri F, et al: Deamino-8-D-arginine vasopressin shortens the bleeding time in uremia. N Engl J Med *308*:8, 1983.
118. Deutsch S: Anesthetic management of patients with chronic renal disease. South Med J *68*:65, 1975.
119. Linke CL, Merin RG: A regional anesthetic approach for renal transplantation. Anesth Analg *55*:69, 1976.
120. Merin RG, Linke CL: Regional anesthesia for renal transplantation. Reg Anaesth *4*:13, 1979.
121. Montgomerie JZ, Kalmanson GM, Guze LB: Renal failure and infection. Medicine *47*:1, 1968.
122. Kennedy AC, Burton JA, Luke RG, et al: Factors affecting the prognosis in acute renal failure. QJ Med *42*:73, 1973.
123. Kunori T, Fehrman I, Ringdon O, et al: In vitro characterization of immunological responsiveness of uremic patients. Nephron *26*:234, 1980.

124. Fergus EB: Infection as a cause and complication of renal disease. J Chron Dis *15*:647, 1962.
125. Soulier JP, Jungers P, Zingraff J: Virus B hepatitis in hemodialysis centers. Adv Nephrol *6*:383, 1976.
126. Greenberg HB, Pollard RB, Lutwick LI, et al: Human leukocyte interferon and hepatitis B virus infection. N Engl J Med *295*:517, 1976.
127. du Moulin GC, Hedley-Whyte J: Hospital-associated viral infection and the anesthesiologist. Anesthesiology *59*:51, 1983.
128. Berry AJ, Isaacson IJ, Hunt D, et al: The prevalence of hepatitis B viral markers in anesthesia personnel. Anesthesiology *60*:6, 1984.
129. Oxman MN: Hepatitis B vaccination of high-risk hospital personnel (editorial views). Anesthesiology *60*:1, 1984.
130. Stevens E, Szmuness W, Goodman AI, et al: Hepatitis B vaccine: Immune responses in haemodialysis patients. Lancet *2*:1211, 1980.
131. Acosta JH: Hypertension in chronic renal disease. Kidney Int *22*:702, 1982.
132. Schoeneman M: Dietary and pharmacologic treatment of chronic renal failure. *In* Edelmann CM Jr (Ed.): Pediatric Kidney Disease. Boston, Little, Brown, 1978, pp 475–486.
133. Guyton AC, Coleman TG, Cowley AW, et al: Arterial pressure regulation. *In* Laragh JH (Ed.): Hypertension Manual. New York, Yorke Medical Books, 1974.
134. Laragh JH: Vasoconstriction-volume analysis for understanding and treating hypertension: The use of renin and aldosterone profiles. Am J Med *55*:261, 1973.
135. Weidman P, Maxwell MH, Lupu AN: Plasma renin activity and blood pressure in terminal renal failure. N Engl J Med *285*:757, 1971.
136. Mulrow PJ, Siegel NJ: Mechanisms in hypertension. *In* Edelmann CM Jr (Ed.): Pediatric Kidney Disease. Boston, Little, Brown, 1978, pp 325–331.
137. Menster M: Diagnosis and treatment of hypertension in children. Pediatr Clin North Am *29*:933, 1982.
138. Siegel NJ, Mulrow PJ: The management of hypertension. *In* Edelmann CM Jr (Ed.): Pediatric Kidney Disease. Boston, Little, Brown, 1978, pp 457–465.
139. Versmold HT, Kitterman JA, Phibbs RH, et al: Aortic blood pressure during the first 12 hours of life in infants with birth weight of 610 to 4220 grams. Pediatrics *67*:607, 1981.
140. de Swiet M, Fayers P, Shinebourne EA: Systolic blood pressure in a population of infants in the first year of life: The Brompton study. Pediatrics *65*:1028, 1980.
141. Report of the Task Force on Blood Pressure Control in Children. Pediatrics *59*(Suppl):797, 1977.
142. Report of the Second Task Force on Blood Pressure Control in Children–1987. Pediatrics *79*:1, 1987.
143. Moss AJ, Liebling W, Austin WO, et al: An evaluation of the flush method for determining blood pressure in infants. Pediatrics *20*:53, 1957.
144. Kirkland RT, Kirkland JL: Systolic blood pressure measurements in the newborn infant with the transcutaneous Doppler method. J Pediatr *80*:52, 1972.
145. Whyte RK, Elseed AM, Fraser CB, et al: Assessment of Doppler ultrasound to measure systolic pressures in infants and young children. Arch Dis Child *50*:542, 1975.
146. American Heart Association: Recommendations for Human Blood Pressure Determination by Sphygmomanometer. 1981.
147. Pascarelli EF, Bertrand CA: Comparison of blood pressures in the arms and legs. N Engl J Med *270*:693, 1964.
148. Koster M, David GK: Reversible severe hypertension due to licorice ingestion. N Engl J Med *278*:1381, 1968.
149. Wilkinson R, Scott DF, Uldall PR, et al: Plasma renin and exchangeable sodium in the hypertension of chronic renal failure: The effect of bilateral nephrectomy. QJ Med *39*:377, 1970.
150. Schiff M, Brown RS, Lytton B: The role of bilateral nephrectomy in the treatment of hypertension of chronic renal failure. J Urol *109*:152, 1973.
151. Lee JB: Anti-hypertensive activity of the kidney: The renomedullary prostaglandins. N Engl J Med *277*:1073, 1967.
152. Tan SY, Mulrow PJ: Impaired renal prostaglandin E production: A newly identified lesion in hypertensives. Clin Res *25*:450A, 1977.
153. Muirhead EE, Germain G, Leach B, et al: Blood pressure regulation and control. Circ Res (Suppl II) *31*:161, 1972.
154. Margolius HS, Horowitz D, Pisano JJ, et al: Urinary kallikrein excretion in hypertensive man. Circ Res *35*:820, 1974.
155. Makker SP, Moorthy B: Rebound hypertension following minoxidil withdrawal. J Pediatr *96*:762, 1980.
156. Bruce DL, Croley TF, Lee JS: Pre-operative clonidine withdrawal syndrome. Anesthesiology *51*:90, 1979.
157. Maling TJB, Dollery CT: Changes in blood pressure, heart rate and plasma noradrenaline concentration after sudden withdrawal of propranolol. Br Med J *2*:366, 1979.
158. Conway J, Lauwers P: Hemodynamic and hypotensive effects of long-term therapy with chlorothiazide. Circulation *21*:21, 1960.
159. Repetto HA, Lewy JE, Brando JL, et al: Furosemide in acute glomerulonephritis. J Pediatr *80*:660, 1972.
160. Loggie JMH: Hypertension in children and adolescents. II. Drug therapy. J Pediatr *74*:640, 1969.
161. Prys-Roberts C, Meloche R: Management of anesthesia in patients with hypertension or ischemic heart disease. Int Anesthesiol Clin *18*:181, 1980.
162. Mohammed S, Hanenson IB, Magenheim HG, et al: The effects of alpha-methyldopa on renal function in hypertensive patients. Am Heart J *76*:21, 1968.
163. Potter DE, Schambelan M, Salvatierra O, et al: Treatment of high renin hypertension with propranolol in children after renal transplantation. J Pediatr *90*:307, 1977.
164. Holland OB, Kaplan NM: Propranolol in the treatment of hypertension. N Engl J Med *294*:930, 1976.
165. Prys-Roberts C: Hemodynamic effects of anesthesia and surgery in renal hypertensive patients receiving large doses of beta-receptor antagonists. Anesthesiology *51*(Suppl):122, 1979.
166. Sprague DH: Severe bradycardia after neostigmine in a patient taking propranolol to control paroxysmal atrial tachycardia. Anesthesiology *42*:208, 1975.
167. Prys-Roberts C: Adrenergic mechanisms, agonists and antagonist drugs. *In* Prys-Roberts C (Ed.): The Circulation in Anesthesia. Oxford, Blackwell, 1979.
168. Koch-Weser J: Drug therapy: Hydralazine. N Engl J Med *295*:320, 1976.
169. Linas SL, Nies AS: Minoxidil. Ann Intern Med *94*:61, 1981.
170. Pennisi AJ, Takahashi M, Bernstein BH, et al: Minoxidil therapy in children with severe hypertension. J Pediatr *90*:813, 1977.
171. Hansson LM, Hunyor SN: Blood pressure over-shoot due to acute clonidine (Catapres) withdrawal: Studies on arterial and urinary catecholamines and suggestions for management of the crisis. Clin Sci Mol Med *45*:181s, 1973.

172. Heel RC, Brogden RN, Speight TM, et al: Captopril: A review of its pharmacologic properties and therapeutic efficacy. Drugs *20*:409, 1980.
173. Friedman A, Chesney RW, Ball D, et al: Effective use of captopril (angiotensin I–converting enzyme inhibitor) in severe childhood hypertension. J Pediatr *97*:664, 1980.
174. McLaine PN, Drummond KN: Intravenous diazoxide for severe hypertension in childhood. J Pediatr *79*:829, 1971.
175. McLain LG: Drugs in the management of hypertensive emergencies in children. Clin Pediatr *15*:85, 1976.
176. Olson DL, Lieberman E: Renal hypertension in children. Pediatr Clin North Am *23*:795, 1976.
177. Tinker JH, Michenfelder JD: Sodium nitroprusside: Pharmacology, toxicology and therapeutics. Anesthesiology *45*:340, 1976.
178. Davies DW, Greiss L, Kadar D, et al: Sodium nitroprusside in children: Observations on metabolism during normal and abnormal responses. Can Anaesth Soc J *22*:553, 1975.
179. Ivankovich AD, Miletich DJ, Tinker JH: Sodium nitroprusside: Metabolism and general considerations. Int Anesthesiol Clin *16*:1978.
180. Danzig LE: Dynamics of thiocyanate dialysis: The artificial kidney in the therapy of thiocyanate intoxication. N Engl J Med *252*:49, 1955.
181. Bedford RF: Increasing halothane concentrations reduce nitroprusside dose requirement. Anesth Analg *57*:457, 1978.
182. Tinker JH, Michenfelder JD: Increased resistance to nitroprusside-induced cyanide toxicity in anuric dogs. Anesthesiology *52*:40, 1980.
183. Cumming AMM, Davies DL: Intravenous labetalol in hypertensive emergency. Lancet *1*:929, 1979.
184. Dillon MJ: Hypertension. *In* Williams DI, Johnston JH (Eds.): Paediatric Urology. London, Butterworth Scientific, 1982, pp 57–72.
185. Ferguson RK, Vlasses PH: Hypertensive emergencies and urgencies. JAMA *255*:1607, 1986.
185a. Bunchman TE, Lynch RE, Wood EG: Intravenously administered labetalol for treatment of hypertension in children. J Pediatr *120*:140, 1992.
186. Calhoun DA, Oparil S: Treatment of hypertensive crisis. N Engl J Med *17*:1177, 1990.
187. Agus JC, Frommer JP, Young JB: Cardiac and circulatory abnormalities in chronic renal failure. Semin Nephrol *1*:112, 1981.
188. O'Regan S, Matina D, Ducharme G, et al: Echocardiographic assessment of cardiac function in children with chronic renal failure. Kidney Int *24*:S77, 1983.
189. Outwater KM, Treves S, Lang P, et al: Renal and hemodynamic effects of dopamine in infants following corrective cardiac surgery. Anesthesiology *61*:A130, 1984.
190. Kumar S, Lesch M: Pericarditis in renal disease. Prog Cardiovasc Dis *22*:357, 1980.
191. Uraemic pericarditis (editorial). Lancet *1*:941, 1977.
192. Movin JE, Hollomby D, Gonda A, et al: Management of uremic pericarditis: A report of 11 patients with cardiac tamponade and review of the literature. Ann Thorac Surg *22*:588, 1976.
193. Lock JE, Bass JL, Kulik TJ, et al: Chronic percutaneous pericardial drainage with modified pigtail catheters in children. Am J Cardiol *53*:1179, 1984.
194. Wray TM, Humphreys J, Perry JM, et al: Pericardiectomy for treatment of uremic pericarditis. Circulation *50*(Suppl 2):268, 1974.
195. Stanley TH, Weidauer HE: Anesthesia for the patient with cardiac tamponade. Anesth Analg *52*:110, 1973.
196. Kaplan JA, Bland JW, Dunbar RW: The perioperative management of pericardial tamponade. South Med J *69*:417, 1976.
197. Konchigeri HN, Levitsky S: Anesthetic considerations for pericardiectomy in uremic pericardial effusion. Anesth Analg *55*:378, 1976.
198. Hickey PR, Hansen DD, Cramolini GM, et al: Pulmonary and systemic hemodynamic responses to ketamine in infants with normal and elevated pulmonary vascular resistance. Anesthesiology *62*:287, 1985.
199. Brigham KL, Bernard G: Pulmonary complications of chronic renal failure. Semin Nephrol *1*:188, 1981.
200. Martinez WC, Rapin I, Moore CL: Neurologic complications of renal failure. *In* Edelmann CM Jr (Ed.): Pediatric Kidney Disease. Boston, Little, Brown, 1978, pp 408–420.
201. Alfrey AC: Dialysis encephalopathy syndrome. Annu Rev Med *29*:93, 1978.
202. Reese GN, Appel SH: Neurologic complications of renal failure. Semin Nephrol *1*:137, 1981.
203. Mitschke H, Schmidt P, Kopsa H, et al: Reversible uremic deafness after successful renal transplantation. N Engl J Med *292*:1062, 1975.
204. Jellinek EH, Painter M, Prineas J, et al: Hypertensive encephalopathy with cortical disorders of vision. QJ Med *33*:239, 1964.
205. Berry AJ, Peterson ML: Hyponatremia after mannitol administration in the presence of renal failure. Anesth Analg (Cleve) *60*:165, 1981.
206. Borges HF, Hocks J, Kjellstrand CM: Mannitol intoxication in patients with renal failure. Arch Intern Med *142*:63, 1982.
207. Maynert EW: Phenobarbital, mephobarbital and metharbital: Absorption, distribution and excretion. *In* Woodbury DM, Penry JK, Schmidt RP (Eds.): Antiepileptic Drugs. New York, Raven Press, 1972.
208. Bennett WM, Singer I, Golper T, et al: Guidelines for drug therapy in renal failure. Ann Intern Med *86*:754, 1977.
209. Woodbury DM, Swinyard E: Diphenylhydantoin: Absorption, distribution and excretion. *In* Woodbury DM, Penry JK, Schmidt RP (Eds.): Antiepileptic Drugs. New York, Raven Press, 1972.
210. Letteri JM, Mellk H, Louis S, et al: Diphenylhydantoin metabolism in uremia. N Engl J Med *285*:648, 1971.
211. Reidenberg MM, Odar-Cederlöf J, Von Bahr ML, et al: Protein binding of diphenylhydantoin and desmethylimipramine in plasma from patients with poor renal function. N Engl J Med *285*:264, 1971.
212. Stenzel RB, Semar M, Lonergan ET, et al: Relationship of nervous tissue transketolase to the neuropathy in chronic uremia. J Clin Invest *50*:2295, 1971.
213. Arbus GS, Barnor NA, Hsu AC, et al: Effect of chronic renal failure, dialysis and transplantation on motor nerve conduction velocity in children. Can Med Assoc J *113*:517, 1975.
214. Weir PHC, Chung FF: Anaesthesia for patients with chronic renal disease. Can Anaesth Soc J *31*:468, 1984.
215. Warren SE, Blantz RC: Mannitol. Arch Intern Med *141*:493, 1981.
216. Makoff DL, DaSilva JA, Rosenbaum BJ, et al: Hypertonic expansion: Acid base and electrolyte changes. Am J Physiol *218*:1201, 1970.
217. Kersh ES, Kronfield SJ, Unger A, et al: Autonomic insufficiency in uremia as a cause of hemodialysis-induced hypotension. N Engl J Med *290*:650, 1974.
218. Campese VM, Romoff MS, Levitan D, et al: Mechanisms of autonomic nervous system dysfunctions in uremia. Kidney Int *20*:246, 1981.

219. Alfrey AC, Legendre GR, Kaehny WD: The dialysis encephalopathy syndrome. N Engl J Med *294*:184, 1976.
220. McDermott JR, Smith AI, Wark MK, et al: Brain aluminum concentrations in dialysis encephalopathy. Lancet *1*:901, 1978.
221. Mahurkar SD, Dhar SK, Salta R, et al: Dialysis dementia. Lancet *1*:1412, 1973.
222. Sedman AB, Wilkening GN, Warady BA, et al: Encephalopathy in childhood secondary to aluminum toxicity. J Pediatr *105*:836, 1984.
223. Polinsky MS, Gruskin AB: Aluminum toxicity in children with chronic renal failure. J Pediatr *105*:758, 1984.
224. Salusky IB, Coburn JW, Paunier L, et al: Role of aluminum hydroxide in raising serum aluminum levels in children undergoing continuous ambulatory peritoneal dialysis. J Pediatr *105*:717, 1984.
225. Zelnic EB, Goyal RK: Gastrointestinal manifestations of chronic renal failure. Semin Nephrol *1*:124, 1981.
226. Leiber CS, Lefevre A: Ammonia as a source of gastric hypoacidity in patients with uremia. J Clin Invest *38*:1271, 1959.
227. Sullivan SN, Tustanoff E, Slaughter DN, et al: Hypergastrinemia and gastric acid hypersecretion in uremia. Clin Nephrol *5*:25, 1976.
228. Black M: Disturbances of the gastrointestinal system. *In* Edelmann CM Jr (Ed.): Pediatric Kidney Disease. Boston, Little, Brown, 1978, pp 421–428.
229. Goldstein H, Murphy D, Sokol A, et al: Gastric acid secretion in patients undergoing chronic dialysis. Arch Intern Med *120*:645, 1967.
230. Shepherd AMM, Stewart WK, Wormsley KG: Peptic ulceration in chronic renal failure. Lancet *1*:1357, 1973.
231. Manchikanti L, Kraus JW, Edds SP: Cimetidine and related drugs in anesthesia. Anesth Analg *61*:595, 1982.
232. Avioli LV: Endocrine disturbances in uremia. *In* Edelmann CM Jr (Ed.): Pediatric Kidney Disease. Boston, Little, Brown, 1978, pp 442–447.
233. Cohen BD: Disturbances of nitrogen, carbohydrate, and lipid metabolism. *In* Edelmann CM Jr (Ed.): Pediatric Kidney Disease. Boston, Little, Brown, 1978, pp 432–491.
234. Holliday MA: Growth retardation in children with renal disease. *In* Edelmann CM Jr (Ed.): Pediatric Kidney Disease. Boston, Little, Brown, 1978, pp 331–341.
235. Emmanouel DS, Lindheimer MD, Katz AI: Endocrine abnormalities in chronic renal failure. Pathogenetic principles and clinical implications. Semin Nephrol *1*:151, 1981.
236. Rubenfeld S, Garber AJ: Abnormal carbohydrate metabolism in chronic renal failure. J Clin Invest *62*:20, 1978.
237. Korsch BM: Psychological complications of renal disease in childhood. *In* Edelmann CM Jr (Ed.): Pediatric Kidney Disease. Boston, Little, Brown, 1978, pp 342–347.
238. Anderson RJ: Drug prescribing for patients in renal failure. Hosp Pract *18*:145, 1983.
239. Anderson RJ, Schrier RW: Clinical Use of Drugs in Patients with Kidney and Liver Disease. Philadelphia, WB Saunders, 1981.
240. Bennet WM, Muther RS: Drug metabolism in renal failure. *In* Brenner B, Stein J (Eds.): Chronic Renal Failure. New York, Churchill Livingstone, 1981, p 287.
241. Ryan DW: Preoperative serum cholinesterase concentration in chronic renal failure. Br J Anaesth *49*:945, 1977.
242. McLeod K, Watson MJ, Rawlins MD: Pharmacokinetics of pancuronium in patients with normal and impaired renal function. Br J Anaesth *48*:341, 1976.
243. Miller RD, Sohn YJ, Matteo RS: Enhancement of D-tubocurarine neuromuscular blockage by diuretics in man. Anesthesiology *45*:442, 1976.
244. Miller RD: Reversal of muscle relaxants. American Society of Anesthesiologists. ASA Refresher Course Lectures. *32*:222, 1981.
245. Brotherton WP, Matteo RS: Pharmacokinetics and pharmacodynamics of metocurine in humans with and without renal failure. Anesthesiology *55*:273, 1981.
246. Ghoneim MM, Kramer SE, Bannow R, et al: Binding of D-tubocurarine to plasma proteins in normal patients with hepatic or renal disease. Anesthesiology *39*:410, 1973.
247. Miller RD, Matteo RS, Benet LZ, et al: The pharmacokinetics of D-tubocurarine in man with and without renal failure. J Pharmacol Exp Ther *202*:1, 1977.
248. Cohen EN, Brewer HW, Smith D: The metabolism and elimination of D-tubocurarine-H^3. Anesthesiology *28*:309, 1967.
249. Hughes R, Chapple DJ: The pharmacology of atracurium: A new competitive neuromuscular blocking agent. Br J Anaesth *53*:31, 1981.
250. Fahey MR, Rupp SM, Fisher DM, et al: Pharmacokinetics and pharmacodynamics of atracurium in normal and renal failure patients. Anesthesiology *59*:A263, 1983.
251. Hunter JM, Jones RS, Utting JE: Use of the muscle relaxant atracurium in anephric patients: Preliminary communication. J R Soc Med *75*:336, 1982.
252. Brandom BW, Rudd GD, Cook DR: Clinical pharmacology of atracurium in paediatric patients. Br J Anaesth *55*:175, 1983.
253. Goudsouzian NG, Liu LMP, Cote CJ, et al: Safety and efficacy of atracurium in adolescents and children anesthetized with halothane. Anesthesiology *59*:459, 1983.
254. Brandom BW, Woelfel SK, Cook DR, et al: Clinical pharmacology of atracurium in infants. Anesth Analg *63*:309, 1984.
255. Ved SA, Chen J, Reed M, Fleming N: Intubation with low-dose atracurium in children. Anesth Analg *68*:609, 1989.
256. Hennis PJ, Fahey MR, Miller RD, et al: Pharmacology of laudanosine in dogs. Anesthesiology *61*:A305, 1984.
257. Nigrovic V, Koechel DA: Atracurium—additional information needed. Anesthesiology *60*:606, 1984.
258. Freeman RB, Sheff MF, Maher JF, et al: The blood–cerebrospinal fluid barrier in uremia. Ann Intern Med *56*:233, 1962.
259. Upton RA, Nguyen TL, Miller RD, et al: Renal and biliary elimination of vecuronium (Org NC45) and pancuronium in rats. Anesth Analg *61*:313, 1982.
260. Meistelman C, Lienhart A, Leveque C, et al: Pharmacology of vecuronium in patients with end-stage renal failure. Anesthesiology *59*:293, 1983.
261. Lynam DP, Cronnelly R, Castagnolli KP, et al: The pharmacodynamics and pharmacokinetics of vecuronium in patients anesthetized with isoflurane with normal renal function or with renal failure. Anesthesiology *69*:227, 1988.
262. Fisher DM, Miller RD: Neuromuscular effects of vecuronium (Org NC45) in infants and children during N_2O, halothane anesthesia. Anesthesiology *58*:519, 1983.
263. Caldwell JE, Claver Canfell P, Castagnolli KP, et al: The influence of renal failure on the pharmacokinetics and duration of action of pipecuronium bromide in

patients anesthetized with halothane and nitrous oxide. Anesthesiology *70*:7, 1989.

264. Cook DR, Freeman JA, Lai AA, et al: Pharmacokinetics and pharmacodynamics of doxacurium in normal patients and in those with hepatic or renal failure. Anesth Analg *72*:145, 1991.
265. Cronnelly R, Stanski DR, Miller RD, et al: Renal function and the pharmacokinetics of neostigmine in anesthetized man. Anesthesiology *51*:222, 1979.
266. Cronnelly R, Stanski DR, Miller RD, et al: Pyridostigmine kinetics with and without renal function. Clin Pharmacol Ther *28*:78, 1980.
267. Everett GB, Allen GD, Kennedy WF, et al: Renal hemodynamic effects of general anesthesia in outpatients. Anesth Analg *52*:470, 1973.
268. Parsons V, Choudhury AA, Wass JAH, et al: Renal excretion of fluoride in renal failure and after renal transplantation. Br Med J *1*:128, 1975.
269. Cousins MJ, Mazze RI: Methoxyflurane nephrotoxicity. A study on dose response in man. JAMA *225*:1611, 1973.
270. Cousins MJ, Greenstein LR, Hitt BA, et al: Metabolism and renal effects of enflurane in man. Anesthesiology *44*:44, 1976.
271. Loehming R, Mazze RI: Possible nephrotoxicity from enflurane in a patient with severe renal disease. Anesthesiology *40*:203, 1974.
272. Harnett MN, Lane W, Bennett WM: Non-oliguric renal failure and enflurane. Ann Intern Med *81*:560, 1974.
273. Eichhorn JH, Hedley-Whyte J, Steinman TI, et al: Renal failure following enflurane anesthesia. Anesthesiology *45*:557, 1976.
274. Mazze RI, Sievenpiper TS, Stevenson J: Renal effects of enflurane and halothane in patients with abnormal renal function. Anesthesiology *60*:161, 1984.
275. Carter R, Heerdt M, Acchiardo S: Fluoride kinetics after enflurane anesthesia in healthy and anephric patients and in patients with poor renal function. Clin Pharmacol Ther *20*:565, 1977.
276. Mazze RI, Cousins MJ, Barr GA: Renal effects and metabolism of isoflurane in man. Anesthesiology *40*:536, 1974.
277. Cousins MJ, Mazze RI, Barr GA, et al: A comparison of the renal effects of isoflurane and methoxyflurane in Fischer 344 rats. Anesthesiology *38*:557, 1973.
278. Jones RM, Koblin DD, Cashman JN, et al: Biotransformation and hepatorenal function in volunteers after exposure to desflurane (I-653). Br J Anaesth *64*:482, 1990.
279. Sutton TS, Koblin DD, Gruenke LD, et al: Fluoride metabolites after prolonged exposure of volunteers and patients to desflurane. Anesth Analg *73*:180, 1991.
280. Deutsch S, Bastron RD, Pierce EC, et al: The effects of anaesthesia with thiopentone, nitrous oxide, narcotics and neuromuscular blocking drugs on renal function in normal man. Br J Anaesth *41*:807, 1969.
281. Philbin DM, Coggins CH: Plasma antidiuretic hormone levels in cardiac surgical patients during morphine and halothane anesthesia. Anesthesiology *49*:95, 1978.
282. Stanley TH, Lathrop GD: Urinary excretion of morphine during and after valvular and coronary artery surgery. Anesthesiology *46*:166, 1977.
283. Don HF, Dieppa RA, Taylor P: Narcotic analgesics in anuric patients. Anesthesiology *42*:745, 1975.
284. Chauvin M, Sandouk P, Scherrmann JM, et al: Morphine pharmacokinetics in renal failure. Anesthesiology *66*:327, 1987.
285. Drayes DE: Active drug metabolites and renal failure. Am J Med *62*:486, 1977.
286. Bower S: Plasma protein binding of fentanyl: The effect of hyperlipoproteinaemia and chronic renal failure. J Pharm Pharmacol *34*:102, 1982.
287. Kono K, Philbin DM, Coggins CH, et al: Renal function and stress response during halothane or fentanyl anesthesia. Anesth Analg *60*:552, 1981.
288. Trudnowski RJ, Mostert JW, Hobika GH, et al: Neuroleptanalgesia for patients with kidney malfunction. Anesth Analg *50*:679, 1971.
289. Morgan M, Lumley J: Anaesthetic considerations in chronic renal failure. Anaesth Intens Care *3*:218, 1975.
290. Gorman HM, Graythorne NWB: The effect of a new neuroleptic analgesic agent (Innovar) on renal function in man. Acta Anaesthesiol Scand (Suppl 24) *10*:111, 1966.
291. Järnberg PO, Santesson J, Eklund J: Renal function during neuroleptanaesthesia. Acta Anaesthesiol Scand *22*:167, 1978.
292. Mostert JW, Evers JL, Hobika GH, et al: Circulatory effects of analgesic and neuroleptic drugs in patients with chronic renal failure undergoing maintenance dialysis. Br J Anaesth *42*:501, 1970.
293. Chauvin M, Lebrault C, Levron JC, Duvaldestin P: Pharmacokinetics of alfentanil in chronic renal failure. Anesth Analg *66*:53, 1987.
294. Davis PJ, Stiller RL, Cook DR, et al: Effects of cholestatic hepatic disease and chronic renal failure on alfentanil pharmacokinetics in children. Anesth Analg *68*:579, 1989.
295. Davis PJ, Stiller RL, Cook DR, et al: Pharmacokinetics of sufentanil in adolescent patients with chronic renal failure. Anesth Analg *67*:268, 1988.
296. Ghoneim MM, Pandya H: Plasma protein binding of thiopental in patients with impaired renal or hepatic function. Anesthesiology *42*:545, 1975.
297. Dundee JW, Richards RK: Effect of azotemia upon the action of intravenous barbiturate anesthesia. Anesthesiology *15*:333, 1954.
298. Wieber J, Gugler R, Hengstman JH, et al: Pharmacokinetics of ketamine in man. Anaesthesist *24*:260, 1975.
299. Bevan DR, Budhu R: The effect of ketamine on renal blood flow in greyhounds. Br J Anaesth *47*:634, 1975.
300. Hirasawa H, Yonezawa T: The effects of ketamine and Innovar on the renal cortical and medullary blood flow of the dog. Anaesthesist *24*:349, 1975.
301. White PF, Way WL, Trevor AJ: Ketamine—its pharmacology and therapeutic uses. Anesthesiology *56*:119, 1982.
302. Wyant GM: The anaesthetist looks at tissue transplantation: Three years' experience with kidney transplants. Can Anaesth Soc J *14*:255, 1967.
303. Kennedy WF, Sawyer TK, Gerbershagen HU, et al: Systemic cardiovascular and renal hemodynamic alterations during peridural anesthesia in normal man. Anesthesiology *31*:414, 1969.
304. Kennedy WF, Sawyer TK, Gerbershagen HU, et al: Simultaneous systemic cardiovascular and renal hemodynamic measurements during high spinal anaesthesia in normal man. Acta Anaesthesiol Scand (Suppl) *37*:163, 1970.
305. Bromage PR, Gertel M: Brachial plexus anesthesia in chronic renal failure. Anesthesiology *36*:488, 1972.
306. Singler RC: Pediatric regional anesthesia. *In* Gregory GA (Ed.): Pediatric Anesthesia. New York, Churchill Livingstone, 1983, pp 481–518.
307. Strasser K, Abel J, Breuhmann M, et al: Plasmakonzentration von Etidocain in den erster zwei Stunden nach axillärer Blockade bei Gesunden und bei Patienten mit Niereninsuffizienz. Anaesthesist *30*:14, 1981.

308. Gould DB, Aldrete JA: Bupivacaine cardiotoxicity in a patient with renal failure. Acta Anaesthesiol Scand *27*:18, 1983.
309. Mazze RI: Critical care of the patient with acute renal failure. Anesthesiology *47*:138, 1977.
310. Slawson KB: Anaesthesia for the patient in renal failure. Br J Anaesth *44*:277, 1972.
311. Fernando ON: Renal transplantation in children. *In* Williams DI, Johnston JH (Eds.): Paediatric Urology. London, Butterworth Scientific, 1982, pp 49–56.
312. Fine RN, Malekzadeh MH, Pennisi AJ, et al: Long-term results of renal transplantation in children. Pediatrics *61*:641, 1978.
313. Ingelfinger JR, Grupe WE, Harmon WE, et al: Growth acceleration following renal transplantation in children less than 7 years of age. Pediatrics *68*:255, 1981.
314. Avner ED, Harmon WE, Grupe WE, et al: Mortality of chronic hemodialysis and renal transplantation in pediatric end-stage renal disease. Pediatrics *67*:412, 1981.
315. Mauer SM, Howard RJ: Renal transplantation in children. *In* Edelmann CM Jr (Ed.): Pediatric Kidney Disease. Boston, Little, Brown, 1978, pp 503–530.
315a. Beebe DS, Belani KG, Mergens P, et al: Anesthetic management of infants receiving an adult kidney transplant. Anesth Analg *73*:725, 1991.
316. Vandam LD, Harrison JH, Murray JE, et al: Anesthesia aspects of renal homotransplantation in man. Anesthesiology *23*:783, 1962.
317. Strunin L: Some aspects of anesthesia for renal homotransplantation. Br J Anaesth *38*:662, 1966.
318. Samuel JR, Powell D: Renal transplantation: Anaesthetic experience of 100 cases. Anaesthesia *25*:165, 1970.
319. Aldrette JH, Daniel W, O'Higgins JW, et al: Analysis of anesthetic-related morbidity in human recipients of renal homografts. Anesth Analg *50*:321, 1971.
320. Levine DS, Virtue RW: Anaesthetic agents and techniques for renal homotransplants. Can Anaesth Soc J *20*:259, 1973.
321. Logan DH, Howie HB, Crawford J: Anaesthesia and renal transplantation: 56 cases. Br J Anaesth *46*:69, 1974.
322. Strunin L, Davies JM, Filshie JJ: Anesthesia for renal transplantation. Anesthesiol Clin *22*:189, 1984.
323. Mauer SM, Lynch RE: Hemodialysis techniques for infants and children. Pediatr Clin North Am *23*:843, 1976.
324. Simmons MA, Levine RL, Lubchenco LO, et al: Warning: Serious sequelae of temporal artery catheterization. J Pediatr *92*:284, 1978.
325. Prian GW, Wright GB, Rumack CM, et al: Apparent cerebral embolization after temporal artery catheterization. J Pediatr *93*:115, 1978.
326. Bull MJ, Schreiner RL, Garg BP, et al: Neurologic complications following temporal artery catheterization. J Pediatr *96*:1071, 1980.
327. Downs JB, Rackstein AD, Klein EF Jr, et al: Hazards of radial artery catheterization. Anesthesiology *38*:283, 1973.
328. Miyasaka K, Edmonds JF, Conn AW: Complications of radial artery lines in the paediatric patient. Can Anaesth Soc J *23*:9, 1976.
329. Santiago-Delphin EA, Buselmeier TJ, Simmons RL: Blood gases and pH in patients with artificial arteriovenous fistulas. Kidney Int *1*:131, 1972.
330. Hirschman CA, Edelstein G: Intraoperative hyperkalemia and cardiac arrest during renal transplantation in an insulin-dependent diabetic patient. Anesthesiology *51*:161, 1979.
331. Hirschman CA, Leon D, Edelstein G, et al: Risk of hyperkalemia in recipients of kidneys preserved with an intra-cellular electrolyte solution. Anesth Analg *59*:283, 1980.
332. Wells TG, Ulstrom RA, Nevins TE: Hypoglycemia in pediatric renal allograft recipients. J Pediatr *113*:1002, 1988.
333. Ruley EJ, Bock GH: Acute renal failure in infants and children. *In* Shoemaker WC, Thompson WL, Holbrook PR (Eds.): Society of Critical Care Medicine: Textbook of Critical Care. Philadelphia, WB Saunders, 1984, pp 604–614.
334. Chesney RW, Kaplan BS, Freedom RM, et al: Acute renal failure: An important complication of cardiac surgery in infants. J Pediatr *87*:381, 1975.
335. Halperin BD, Feeley TW: The effect of anesthesia and surgery on renal function. Int Anesthesiol Clin *22*:157, 1984.
336. Byrd L, Sherman RL: Radio-contrast induced acute renal failure: A clinical and pathophysiologic review. Medicine *58*:270, 1979.
337. Schreiner SE, Maher JF: Toxic nephropathy. Am J Med *38*:409, 1965.
338. Koffler A, Friedler RM, Massry SG: Acute renal failure due to non-traumatic rhabdomyolysis. Ann Intern Med *85*:23, 1976.
339. Knochel JP: Rhabdomyolysis and myoglobinuria. Semin Nephrol *1*:75, 1981.
340. Rowland LP, Penn AS: Myoglobinuria. Med Clin North Am *56*:1233, 1972.
340a. Falik-Borenstein ZC, Jordan SC, Saudubray J, et al: Brief report: Renal tubular acidosis in carnitine palmitoyltransferase type 1 deficiency. N Engl J Med *327*:24, 1992.
341. Katsuya H, Misumi M, Ohtani Y, Miike T: Postanesthetic acute renal failure due to carnitine palmitoyl transferase deficiency. Anesthesiology *68*:945, 1988.
342. Schmidt PJ, Holland PV: Pathogenesis of the acute renal failure associated with incompatible transfusions. Lancet *2*:1169, 1967.
343. Nicot GS, Merle LJ, Charmes JP, et al: Transient glomerular proteinuria, enzymuria and nephrotoxic reaction induced by radiocontrast media. JAMA *252*:2432, 1984.
344. Mattern W, Staab EV: Imaging studies in renal failure: Emphasis on selection and sequencing in the clinical setting. CRC Rad Nuc Med *6*:459, 1975.
345. Schleigel JV, Lang EK: Computed radionuclide urogram for assessing acute renal failure. AJR *134*:129, 1980.
346. Sanders RC, Menon S, Saunders AD: The complementary uses of nuclear medicine and ultrasound in the kidney. J Urol *120*:521, 1978.
347. Oken DE: Clinical aspects of acute renal failure (vasomotor nephropathy). *In* Edelmann CM Jr (Ed.): Pediatric Kidney Disease. Boston, Little, Brown, 1978, pp 1108–1122.
348. Ellis D, Gartner JC, Galvis AG: Acute renal failure in infants and children: Diagnosis, complications and treatment. Crit Care Med *9*:607, 1981.
349. Hodson EM, Kjellstrand CM, Maurer SM: Acute renal failure in infants and children: Outcome of 53 patients requiring hemodialysis treatment. J Pediatr *93*:756, 1978.
350. Kleinknecht D, Junges P, Chanard J, et al: Factors influencing immediate prognosis in acute renal failure, with special reference to prophylactic hemodialysis. Adv Nephrol *1*:207, 1971.
351. Zech P, Bouletreau R, Moscoutchenko JR, et al: Infection in acute renal failure. Adv Nephrol *1*:231, 1971.

352. Kennedy AC, Burton JA, Luke RG, et al: Factors affecting the prognosis of acute renal failure. QJ Med *42*:73, 1973.
353. Schentag JJ, Cerra FB, Calleri G, et al: Pharmacokinetic and clinical studies in patients with cimetidine-associated mental confusion. Lancet *1*:177, 1979.
354. Counahan R, Cameron JS, Ogg CS, et al: Presentation, management complications and outcome of acute renal failure in childhood: Five years' experience. Br Med J *1*:599, 1977.
355. Vertel RM, Knochel JP: Nonoliguric acute renal failure. JAMA *200*:118, 1967.
356. Anderson RJ, Linas SL, Berns AS, et al: Nonoliguric renal failure. N Engl J Med *296*:1134, 1977.
357. Shin B, Mackenzie CF, McAslan TC, et al: Postoperative renal failure in trauma patients. Anesthesiology *51*:218, 1979.
358. Chevalier RL, Campbell F, Brembridge AN: Prognostic factors in neonatal acute renal failure. Pediatrics *74*:265, 1984.
359. Clark DA: Times of first void and first stool in 500 newborns. Pediatrics *60*:457, 1977.
360. Mathew OP, Jones AJ, James E, et al: Neonatal renal failure: Usefulness of diagnostic indices. Pediatrics *65*:57, 1980.
361. Norman ME, Farahnak KA: A prospective study of acute renal failure in the newborn infant. Pediatrics *63*:475, 1979.
362. Anand SK, Northway JD, Crussi FG: Acute renal failure in newborn infants. J Pediatr *92*:985, 1978.
363. Arant BS Jr: Developmental patterns of renal functional maturation compared in the human neonate. J Pediatr *92*:705, 1978.
364. Guignard JP, Torrado A, Da Cunha O, et al: Glomerular filtration rate in the first three weeks of life. J Pediatr *87*:268, 1975.
365. Stonestreet BS, Oh W: Plasma creatinine levels in low birth weight infants during the first three months of life. Pediatrics *61*:788, 1978.
366. Sertel H, Scopes J: Rates of creatinine clearance in babies less than one week of age. Arch Dis Child *48*:717, 1973.
367. Schwartz GJ, Haycock GB, Spitzer A: Plasma creatinine and urea concentrations in children: Normal values for age and sex. J Pediatr *88*:828, 1976.
368. Guignard JP, Torrado A, Mazouni SM, et al: Renal function in respiratory distress syndrome. J Pediatr *88*:845, 1976.
369. Suki W, Eknoyan G, Rector FC, et al: Patterns of nephron perfusion in acute and chronic hydronephrosis. J Clin Invest *45*:122, 1966.
370. Boichis H, Winterborn MH: Acute renal failure in childhood. Pediatr Ann *3*:58, 1974.
371. Espinel CH: The FE_{NA} test. Use in the differential diagnosis of acute renal failure. JAMA *236*:579, 1976.
372. Miller TR, Anderson RJ, Linas SL, et al: Urinary diagnostic indices in acute renal failure. A prospective study. Ann Intern Med *89*:47, 1978.
373. Gordillo-Paniagua G, Velasquez-Jones L: Acute renal failure. Pediatr Clin North Am *23*:817, 1976.
374. Barry KG, Malloy JP: Oliguric renal failure. Evaluation and therapy by the intravenous infusion of mannitol. JAMA *179*:510, 1962.
375. Luke RG, Briggs JD, Allison ME, et al: Factors determining the response to mannitol in acute renal failure. Am J Med Sci *259*:168, 1971.
376. Stone AM, Stahl WM: Effect of ethacrynic acid and furosemide on renal function in hypovolemia. Ann Surg *174*:1, 1971.
377. Birtch AG, Zakheim RM, Jones LG, et al: Redistribution of renal blood flow produced by furosemide and ethacrynic acid. Circ Res *21*:869, 1967.
378. Lucas CE, Zito JG, Carver KM, et al: Questionable value of furosemide in preventing renal failure. Surgery *82*:314, 1977.
379. Levinsky NG: Pathophysiology of acute renal failure. N Engl J Med *296*:1453, 1977.
380. Flamenbaum W: Pathophysiology of acute renal failure. Arch Intern Med *131*:191, 1973.
381. Huguenin M, Thiel G, Brunner FP: Mercuric bichloride–induced acute renal failure studied by split drop micropuncture technique in the rat. Nephron *20*:147, 1978.
382. Flores J, DiBona DR, Beck CH, et al: The role of cell swelling in ischemic renal damage and the protective effect of hypertonic solute. J Clin Invest *51*:118, 1972.
383. Myers BD, Hilberman M, Spence RJ, et al: Glomerular and tubular function in non-oliguric renal failure. Am J Med *72*:642, 1982.
384. Jennings RB, Ganote CE: Mitochondrial structure and function in acute myocardial ischemic injury. Circ Res *38*(Suppl 1):80, 1976.
385. Schanne FAX, Kane AB, Young EE, et al: Calcium dependence of toxic cell death: A final common pathway. Science *206*:700, 1979.
386. Siegel NJ, Glazier W, Chandry IH, et al: Enhanced recovery from acute renal failure by the postischemic infusion of adenine nucleotides and magnesium chloride in rats. Kidney Int *17*:338, 1980.
387. Guignard JP, Wallimann C, Gautier E: Prevention by verapamil of the hypoxaemia-induced renal vasoconstriction. Kidney Int *20*:139, 1981.
388. Creager MA, Halperin JL, Bernard DB, et al: Acute regional circulatory and renal hemodynamic effects of converting enzyme inhibition in patients with congestive heart failure. Circulation *61*:316, 1980.
389. Dzan VJ, Colvucci WS, Williams GH, et al: Sustained effectiveness of converting enzyme inhibition in patients with severe congestive failure. N Engl J Med *302*:1373, 1980.
390. Maseda J, Hilberman M, Derry DC, et al: The renal effects of sodium nitroprusside in post-operative cardiac surgical patients. Anesthesiology *54*:284, 1981.
391. Cogan J, Humphreys M, Carlson J, et al: Renal effects of nitroprusside and hydralazine in patients with congestive heart failure. Circulation *61*:316, 1980.
392. Stowe N, Emma J, Magnusson M, et al: Protective effect of propranolol in the treatment of ischemically damaged canine kidneys prior to transplantation. Surgery *84*:265, 1978.
393. Henderson IS, Beattie TJ, Kennedy AC: Dopamine hydrochloride in oliguric states. Lancet *2*:827, 1980.
394. Lidner A, Cutler RE, Goodman WG, et al: Synergism of dopamine plus furosemide in preventing acute renal failure in the dog. Kidney Int *16*:158, 1979.
395. Noth RH, McCallum RW, Contino C, et al: Tonic dopaminergic suppression of plasma aldosterone. J Clin Endocrinol Metab *51*:64, 1980.
396. Chernow B: Hormonal and metabolic considerations in critical care medicine. *In* Shoemaker WC, Thompson WL, Holbrook PR (Eds.): Society of Critical Care Medicine: Textbook of Critical Care. Philadelphia, WB Saunders, 1984, pp 646–664.
397. Hilberman M, Maseda J, Stinson EB, et al: The diuretic properties of dopamine in patients after open-heart operation. Anesthesiology *61*:489, 1984.
398. Miller ED Jr: Renal effects of dopamine. Anesthesiology *61*:487, 1984.
399. Kebabian JW, Calne DB: Multiple receptors for dopamine. Nature *277*:93, 1979.

400. Grodin W, Scantlebury V, Warmington N: Dopaminergic stimulation of renal blood flow and renal function after transplantation. Anesthesiology *61*:A129, 1984.
401. deTorrenté A, Miller PD, Cronin RE, et al: Effects of furosemide and acetylcholine in norepinephine-induced acute renal failure. Am J Physiol *235*:F131, 1978.
402. Mauk RH, Patak RV, Dadem SZ, et al: Effect of prostaglandin E administration in a nephrotoxic and a vasoconstrictor model of acute renal failure. Kidney Int *12*:122, 1978.
403. Patak RV, Faden SZ, Lifschitz MD, et al: Study of factors which modify the development of norepinephrine-induced acute renal failure in the dog. Kidney Int *15*:227, 1979.
404. Schafferhaus K, Heidbreder E, Grimm D, et al: Norepinephrine-induced acute renal failure: Beneficial effects of atrial natriuretic factor. Nephron *44*:240, 1986.
405. Davis AL: Atrial natriuretic factor. Adv Pediatr *36*:137, 1989.
406. Kurnick BRC, et al: Effects of atrial natriuretic peptide versus mannitol on renal blood flow during radiocontrast infusion in chronic renal failure. J Lab Clin Med *116*:27, 1990.
407. Berry KG, Mazze RI, Schwartz FD: Prevention of surgical oliguria and renal hemodynamic suppression by sustained hydration. N Engl J Med *270*:1371, 1964.
408. Bush HL, Huse JB, Johnson WC, et al: Prevention of renal insufficiency after abdominal aortic aneurysm resection by optimal volume loading. Arch Surg *116*:1517, 1981.
409. Kahl FR, Flint JF, Szidon JP: Influence of left atrial distention on renal vasomotor tone. Am J Physiol *226*:240, 1974.
410. Mason JM, Ledsome JR: Effects of obstruction of the mitral orifice or distention of the pulmonary vein–atrial junctions on renal and hind-limb vascular resistance in the dog. Circ Res *35*:24, 1974.
411. Brosnihan KB, Bravo EL: Graded reductions of atrial pressure and renin release. Am J Physiol *235*:H175, 1978.
412. Bidani A, Churchill P, Fleischmann L: Sodium chloride–induced protection in nephrotoxic acute renal failure: Independence from renin. Kidney Int *16*:481, 1979.
413. Barry KG, Cohen A, Knochel JP, et al: Mannitol infusion. II. The prevention of acute functional renal failure during resection of an aneurysm of the abdominal aorta. N Engl J Med *264*:967, 1961.
414. Burke TS, Cronin RE, Duchin KL, et al: Ischemia and tubule obstruction during acute renal failure in dogs. Role of mannitol in protection. Am J Physiol *238*:F305, 1980.
415. Barry KG: Post-traumatic renal shutdown in humans: Its prevention and treatment by the intravenous infusion of mannitol. Milit Med *128*:224, 1963.
416. Morris CR, Alexander EA, Burns SJ, et al: Restoration and maintenance of glomerular filtration by mannitol during hypoperfusion of the kidney. J Clin Invest *51*:1555, 1972.
417. Eneas JF, Schoenfeld PY, Humphreys MH: The effect of infusion of mannitol-sodium bicarbonate on the clinical course of myoglobinuria. Arch Intern Med *139*:801, 1979.
418. Stahl WM: Effect of mannitol on the kidney. Changes in intrarenal hemodynamics. N Engl J Med *272*:381, 1965.
419. Johnston PA, Bernard DB, Levinsky NG: Mechanism of vasodilatory effect of mannitol in the hypoperfused rat kidney: Role of renal hormones. Kidney Int *16*:774, 1979.
420. Barry KG, Berman AR: Mannitol infusion. III. The acute effect of the intravenous infusion of mannitol on blood and plasma volumes. N Engl J Med *264*:1085, 1961.
421. Cantarovich R, Locatelli A, Fernandez JC, et al: Furosemide in high doses in the treatment of acute renal failure. Postgrad Med J *47*:13, 1971.
422. Brown CB, Ogg CS, Cameron JS: High-dose furosemide in acute renal failure: A controlled trial. Clin Nephrol *15*:90, 1981.
423. Epstein M, Schneider NS, Befeler B: Effect of intrarenal furosemide on renal function and intrarenal hemodynamics in acute renal failure. Am J Med *58*:510, 1975.
424. Bailey RR, Natale R, Turnbull DI, et al: Protective effect of furosemide in acute tubular necrosis and acute renal failure. Clin Sci *45*:1, 1973.
425. Minuth AN, Terrell JB, Suki WN: Acute renal failure: A study of the course and prognosis of 104 patients and of the role of furosemide. Am J Med Sci *271*:317, 1976.
426. Kleinknecht D, Ganeval D, Gonzalez-Duque LA, et al: Furosemide in acute oliguric renal failure. A controlled trial. Nephron *17*:51, 1976.
427. Hilberman M: Renal protection. *In* Shoemaker WC, Thompson WL, Holbrook PR (Eds.): Society of Critical Care Medicine: Textbook of Critical Care. Philadelphia, WB Saunders, 1984, pp 597–604.
428. Gallagher KL, Jones JK: Furosemide-induced ototoxicity. Ann Intern Med *91*:744, 1979.
429. Cooperman LB, Rubin IL: Toxicity of ethacrynic acid and furosemide. Am Heart J *85*:831, 1973.
430. Pillay VKG, Schwartz FD, Aimi K, et al: Transient and permanent deafness following treatment with ethacrynic acid in renal failure. Lancet *1*:77, 1969.
431. Kelly KJ, Outwater KM, Crone RK: Vasoactive amines in infants and children. Clin Anaesthesiol *2*:427, 1984.
432. Lieberman E: Management of acute renal failure in infants and children. Nephron *11*:193, 1973.
433. Abel RM, Beck CH, Abbott WM, et al: Improved survival from acute renal failure after treatment with intravenous essential L-amino acids and glucose. N Engl J Med *288*:695, 1973.
434. Baek SM, Makabali GG, Bryan-Brown CW, et al: The influence of parenteral nutrition on the course of acute renal failure. Surg Gynecol Obstet *141*:405, 1975.
435. Abitol CL, Holliday MA: Total parenteral nutrition in anuric children. Clin Nephrol *5*:153, 1976.
436. Blumenkrantz MJ, Kopple JD, Koffler A, et al: Total parenteral nutrition in the management of acute renal failure. Am J Clin Nutr *31*:1831, 1978.
437. Ellis D, Knappenberger W: Fluid and caloric intake in infants with acute renal failure (abstract). Pediatr Res *14*:1017, 1980.
438. Giordano C, DeSanto NG, Senatore R: Effects of catabolic stress in acute and chronic renal failure. Am J Clin Nutr *31*:1561, 1978.
439. Feinstein EI, Blumenkrantz MJ, Healy M, et al: Clinical and metabolic responses to parenteral nutrition in acute renal failure. Medicine *60*:124, 1981.
440. Toback FG, Teergarden DE, Havener LJ: Amino acid–mediated stimulation of renal phospholipid biosynthesis after acute tubular necrosis. Kidney Int *15*:542, 1979.
441. Conger JD: A controlled evaluation of prophylactic dialysis in post-traumatic acute renal failure. J Trauma *15*:1056, 1975.
442. Kleinknecht D, Jungers P, Chanard J, et al: Uremic and nonuremic complications in acute renal failure:

Evaluation of early and frequent dialysis on prognosis. Kidney Int *1*:190, 1972.
443. Parsons FM, Blagg CR, Hobson SM, et al: Optimum time for dialysis in acute reversible renal failure. Lancet *1*:129, 1961.
444. Soffer O, MacDonnel RC, Finlayson DC, et al: Intraoperative hemodialysis during cardiopulmonary bypass in chronic renal failure. J Thorac Cardiovasc Surg *77*:789, 1979.
445. Intoni F, Alquati P, Schiavello R, et al: Ultrafiltration during open heart surgery in chronic renal failure. Scand J Thorac Cardiovasc Surg *15*:217, 1981.
446. Esperanca MJ, Collins DL: Peritoneal dialysis efficiency in relation to body weight. J Pediatr Surg *1*:162, 1966.
447. Potter DE: Comparison of peritoneal dialysis and hemodialysis in children. Dial Transplant 7:800, 1978.
448. Day RE, White RH: Peritoneal dialysis in children. Arch Dis Child *52*:56, 1977.
449. Fine RN: Peritoneal dialysis update. J Pediatr *100*:1, 1982.
450. Vaamonde CA, Michael UF, Metzger RA, et al: Complications of acute peritoneal dialysis. J Chron Dis *28*:637, 1975.
451. Berry AJ: Respiratory support and renal function. Anesthesiology *55*:655, 1981.
452. Priebe HJ, Hedley-White J: Respiratory support and renal function. Int Anesthesiol Clin *22*:203, 1984.
453. Horton MW, Godley PJ: Continuous arteriovenous hemofiltration: An alternative to hemodialysis. Am J Hosp Pharm *45*:1361, 1988.
454. Bartlett RH, Bosch J, Geronemus R, et al: Continuous arteriovenous hemofiltration for acute renal failure. ASAIO Trans *34*:67, 1988.
455. Lieberman KV: Continuous arteriovenous hemofiltration in children. Pediatr Nephrol *1*:330, 1987.
456. Nahman NS Jr, Middendorf DF: Continuous arteriovenous hemofiltration. Med Clin North Am *74*:975, 1990.
457. Lieberman KV, Nardi L, Bosch JP: Treatment of acute renal failure in an infant using continuous arteriovenous hemofiltration. J Pediatr *106*:646, 1985.
458. Bickley SK: Drug dosing during continuous arteriovenous hemofiltration. Clin Pharm 7:198, 1988.
459. Ronco C, Brendolan A, Bragantini L, et al: Treatment of acute renal failure in newborns by continuous arteriovenous hemofiltration. Kidney Int *29*:908, 1986.
460. Leone MR, Jenkins RD, Golper TA, Alexander SR: Early experience with continuous arteriovenous hemofiltration in critically ill pediatric patients. Crit Care Med *14*:1053, 1986.
461. Jenkins RD, Kuhn RJ, Funk JE: Clinical implications of catheter variability on neonatal continuous arteriovenous hemofiltration. ASAIO Trans *34*:108, 1988.
462. Keller E: Drug therapy during continuous arteriovenous hemofiltration. Adv Exp Med Biol *260*:117, 1989.
463. Bernstein J, Barnett HL, Edelmann CM Jr.: Glomerular diseases: introduction and classification. *In* Edelmann CM Jr (Ed.): Pediatric Kidney Disease. Boston, Little, Brown, 1978, pp 586–592.
464. Hayslett JP, Siegel NJ, Kashgarian M: Glomerulonephropathy. Adv Intern Med *20*:215, 1975.
465. Hyman LR, Walker PF: Progressive renal failure and nephrotic syndrome in children: A spectrum of glomerulonephropathies. Milit Med *140*:608, 1975.
466. McClusky RT, Klassen J: Immunologically mediated glomerular, tubular and interstitial renal disease. N Engl J Med *288*:564, 1973.
467. Bright R: Cases and observations illustrative of renal disease accompanied by the secretion of albuminous urine. Guy's Hospital Reports *1*:338, 1836.
468. Jordan SC, Lemire JM: Acute glomerulonephritis: Diagnosis and treatment. Pediatr Clin North Am *29*:857, 1982.
469. Cochrane CG, Koffler D: Immune complex disease in experimental animals and man. Adv Immunol *16*:185, 1973.
470. Couser WG, Salant DJ: In situ immune complex formation and glomerular injury. Kidney Int *17*:1, 1980.
471. McDonald BM, McEnery PT: Glomerulonephritis in children: Clinical and morphologic characteristics and mechanisms of glomerular injury. Pediatr Clin North Am *23*:691, 1976.
472. Jordan SC, Buckingham B, Sakai R, et al: Studies of immune complex glomerulonephritis mediated by human thyroglobulin. N Engl J Med *304*:1212, 1981.
473. Kaplan BS, Klassen J, Gault MH: Glomerular injury in patients with neoplasia. Ann Rev Med *27*:117, 1976.
474. George CRP, Clark WF, Cameron JS: The role of platelets in glomerulonephritis. Adv Nephrol *5*:19, 1975.
475. Zimmerman SW, Moorthy AV, Dreher WH, et al: Prospective trial of warfarin and dipyridamole in patients with membranoproliferative glomerulonephritis. Am J Med *75*:920, 1983.
476. Hayslett JP: Role of platelets in glomerulonephritis. N Engl J Med *310*:1457, 1984.
477. Donadio JV Jr, Anderson CF, Mitchell JC III, et al: Membranoproliferative glomerulonephritis: A prospective clinical trial of platelet-inhibitor therapy. N Engl J Med *310*:1421, 1984.
478. Barralt TM: Glomerular disease and haematuria. *In* Williams DI, Johnston JH (Eds.): Paediatric Urology. London, Butterworth Scientific, 1982, pp 79–88.
479. Lewy JE: Acute post-streptoccocal glomerulonephritis. Pediatr Clin North Am *23*:751, 1976.
480. Dodge WF, Spargo BH, Travis LB: Occurrence of acute glomerulonephritis in sibling contacts of children with sporadic acute glomerulonephritis. Pediatrics *40*:1029, 1967.
481. Kaplan EL, Anthony BF, Chapman SS, et al: Epidemic acute glomerulonephritis associated with type 49 streptococcal pyoderma. Am J Med *48*:9, 1970.
482. Dodge WF, Spargo BH, Travis LB, et al: Poststreptococcal glomerulonephritis: A prospective study in children. N Engl J Med *286*:273, 1972.
483. Travis LB: Acute postinfectious glomerulonephritis. *In* Edelmann CM Jr (Ed.): Pediatric Kidney Disease. Boston, Little, Brown, 1978, pp 611–630.
484. McConville JM, West CD, McAdams AJ: Familial and nonfamilial benign hematuria. J Pediatr *69*:207, 1966.
485. Bernstein J, Kissane JM: Hereditary nephritis. *In* Edelmann CM Jr (Ed.): Pediatric Kidney Disease. Boston, Little, Brown, 1978, pp 571–579.
486. Shaw RF, Kallen RJ: Population genetics of Alport's syndrome: Hypothesis of abnormal segregation and the necessary existence of mutation. Nephron *16*:427, 1976.
487. Simila S, Vesa L, Wasz-Hockert O: Hereditary onychoosteodysplasia (the nail-patella syndrome) with nephrosis-like renal disease in a newborn boy. Pediatrics *46*:61, 1970.
488. Boulton-Jones JM, Sissons JG, Evans DJ, et al: Renal lesions of subacute infective endocarditis. Br Med J *2*:11, 1974.
489. Dobrin RS, Day NK, Quie PG, et al: The role of complement, immunoglobulin and bacterial antigen in coagulase-negative staphylococcal shunt nephritis. Am J Med *59*:660, 1975.
490. Meadow SR: Schönlein-Henoch syndrome. *In* Edel-

mann CM Jr (Ed.): Pediatric Kidney Disease. Boston, Little, Brown, 1978, pp 788–795.

491. Meadow SR, Glasgow EF, White RHR, et al: Schönlein-Henoch nephritis. QJ Med *41*:241, 1972.
492. Goldbloom RB, Drummond KN: Anaphylactoid purpura with massive gastrointestinal hemorrhage and glomerulonephritis. Am J Dis Child *116*:97, 1968.
493. Counahan R, Winterborn MH, Meadow SR, et al: The prognosis of Schönlein-Henoch nephritis. Br Med J *2*:11, 1977.
494. Hurley RM, Drummond KN: Anaphylactoid purpura nephritis: Clinopathological correlations. J Pediatr *81*:904, 1972.
495. Glasgow EF: Renal changes in Henoch-Schönlein purpura. Arch Dis Child *45*:151, 1970.
496. Lewis EJ: Pulmonary hemorrhage and glomerulonephritis (Goodpasture's syndrome). *In* Edelmann CM Jr (Ed.): Pediatric Kidney Disease. Boston, Little, Brown, 1978, pp 736–744.
497. Proskey AJ, Weatherbee L, Easterling RE, et al: Goodpasture's syndrome: A report of five cases and review of the literature. Am J Med *48*:162, 1970.
498. Wilson CB, Dixon FJ: Anti-glomerular basement membrane antibody-induced glomerulonephritis. Kidney Int *3*:74, 1973.
499. Beirne GJ, Octaviano GN, Kopp WL, et al: Immunohistology of the lung in Goodpasture's syndrome. Ann Intern Med *69*:1207, 1968.
500. Maddock RK, Stevens LE, Reetsma K, et al: Goodpasture's syndrome: Cessation of pulmonary hemorrhage after bilateral nephrectomy. Ann Intern Med *67*:1258, 1967.
501. Siegel RR: The basis of pulmonary disease resolution after nephrectomy in Goodpasture's syndrome. Am J Med Sci *259*:201, 1970.
502. Eisinger AJ: Goodpasture's syndrome: Failure of nephrectomy to cure pulmonary hemorrhage. Am J Med *55*:565, 1973.
503. Couser WG, Wallace A, Monaco AP, et al: Successful renal transplantation in patients with circulating antibody to glomerular basement membrane: Report of 2 cases. Clin Nephrol *1*:381, 1973.
504. Fong JSC, deChadarevian JP, Kaplan BS: Hemolytic-uremic syndrome: Current concepts and management. Pediatr Clin North Am *29*:835, 1982.
505. Gianantonia CA: Hemolytic-uremic syndrome. *In* Edelmann CM Jr (Ed.): Pediatric Kidney Disease. Boston, Little, Brown, 1978, pp 724–735.
506. Kaplan BS, Thomson PD, deChadarevian JP: The hemolytic-uremic syndrome. Pediatr Clin North Am *23*:761, 1976.
507. Hellman RM, Jackson DV, Buss DH: Thrombotic thrombocytopenic purpura and hemolytic-uremic syndrome in HLA-identical siblings. Ann Intern Med *93*:283, 1980.
508. Kaplan BS, Drummond KN: The hemolytic uremic syndrome is a syndrome. N Engl J Med *298*:964, 1978.
509. Mattoo TK, Mahmood MA, Al-Harbi MS, Mikail I: Familial, recurrent hemolytic-uremic syndrome. J Pediatr *114*:814, 1989.
510. Koster F, Levin J, Walker L, et al: Hemolytic-uremic syndrome after shigellosis: Relation to endotoxemia and circulating immune complexes. N Engl J Med *298*:927, 1978.
511. Neill MA, Tarr PI, Clausen CR, et al: *Escherichia coli* O157:H7 as the predominant pathogen associated with the hemolytic uremic syndrome: A prospective study in the Pacific Northwest. Pediatrics *80*:37, 1987.
512. Martin DL, MacDonald KL, White KE, et al: The epidemiology and clinical aspects of the hemolytic uremic syndrome in Minnesota. N Engl J Med *323*:1161, 1990.
513. Rowe PC, Orrbine E, Wells GA, et al: Epidemiology of hemolytic-uremic syndrome in Canadian children from 1986 to 1988. J Pediatr *119*:218, 1991.
514. Bitzan M, Moebius E, Ludwig K, et al: High incidence of serum antibodies to *Escherichia coli* O157 lipopolysaccharide in children with hemolytic-uremic syndrome. J Pediatr *119*:380, 1991.
515. Katz J, Krawitz S, Sacks PV, et al: Platelet, erythrocyte and fibrinogen kinetics in the hemolytic-uremic syndrome of infancy. J Pediatr *83*:739, 1973.
516. Remuzzi G, Misiani R, Marchesi D, et al: Hemolytic uremic syndrome: Deficiency of plasma factors regulating prostacyclin activity. Lancet *2*:871, 1978.
517. Upadhyaya K, Barwick K, Fishaut M, et al: The importance of non-renal involvement in hemolytic-uremic syndrome. Pediatrics *65*:115, 1980.
518. Ray CG, Portman JN, Stamm SJ, et al: Hemolytic-uremic syndrome and myocarditis: Association with coxsackievirus B infection. Am J Dis Child *122*:418, 1971.
519. Bale JF, Brasher C, Siegler RL: CNS manifestations of the hemolytic-uremic syndrome: Relationship to metabolic alterations and prognosis. Am J Dis Child *134*:869, 1980.
520. Rooney JC, Anderson RM, Hopking IH: Clinical and pathological aspects of central nervous system involvement in the haemolytic-uraemic syndrome. Aust Paediatr J *7*:28, 1971.
521. Siegler RL, Brewer ED, Swartz M: Ocular involvement in hemolytic-uremic syndrome. J Pediatr *112*:594, 1988.
522. Trevathan E, Dooling EC: Large thrombotic strokes in hemolytic-uremic syndrome. J Pediatr *111*:863, 1987.
523. Dolislager D, Tune B: The hemolytic-uremic syndrome. Spectrum of severity and significance of prodrome. Am J Dis Child *132*:55, 1978.
524. O'Regan S, Chesney RW, Mongeau J, et al: Aspirin and dipyridamole therapy in the hemolytic-uremic syndrome. J Pediatr *97*:473, 1980.
525. Vitacco M, Sanchez-Avalos J, Gianantonio CA: Heparin therapy in the hemolytic-uremic syndrome. J Pediatr *83*:271, 1973.
526. Van Damme-Lombaerts R, Proesmans W, Van Damme B, et al: Heparin plus dipyridamole in childhood hemolytic-uremic syndrome: A prospective, randomized study. J Pediatr *113*:913, 1988.
527. Harden LB, Gluck RS, Salcedo JR: Simultaneous hemodialysis and exchange transfusion in hemolytic uremic syndrome. Clin Pediatr *10*:640, 1980.
528. Denneberg T, Friedberg M, Holmberg L, et al: Combined plasmapheresis and hemodialysis treatment for severe hemolytic-uremic syndrome following *Campylobacter* colitis. Acta Paediatr Scand *71*:243, 1982.
529. Beattie TJ, Murphy AV, Willoughby MLN, et al: Plasmapheresis in the haemolytic-uraemic syndrome in children. Br Med J *282*:1667, 1981.
530. Brandt P, Jesperson J, Gregersen G: Post partum haemolytic-uraemic syndrome treated with antithrombin-III. Nephron *27*:15, 1981.
531. Remuzzi G, Misiani R, Marchesi D, et al: Treatment of the hemolytic-uremic syndrome with plasma. Clin Nephrol *12*:279, 1979.
532. Rizzoni G, Claris-Appiani A, Edefonti A, et al: Plasma infusion for hemolytic-uremic syndrome in children: Results of a multicenter controlled trial. J Pediatr *112*:284, 1988.
533. Siegler RL: Management of hemolytic-uremic syndrome. J Pediatr *112*:1014, 1988.

534. Cerilli CJ, Nelson C, Dorfmann L: Renal homotransplantation in infants and children with the hemolytic-uremic syndrome. Surgery *71*:66, 1972.
535. Howard EJ, Mauer SM, Miller K, et al: Biopsy-proven recurrence of hemolytic uremic syndrome early after kidney transplantation with a favorable outcome. Kidney Int *10*:544, 1976.
536. Rance CP, Arbus GS, Balfe JW: Management of the nephrotic syndrome in children. Pediatr Clin North Am *23*:735, 1976.
537. McEnery PT, Strife CF: Nephrotic syndrome in childhood: Management and treatment in patients with minimal change disease, mesangial proliferation, or focal glomerulosclerosis. Pediatr Clin North Am *89*:875, 1982.
538. Barnett HL, Schoeneman M, Bernstein J, et al: The nephrotic syndrome. *In* Edelmann CM Jr (Ed.): Pediatric Kidney Disease. Boston, Little, Brown, 1978, pp 679–694.
539. International Study of Kidney Disease in Children: The nephrotic syndrome in children. Prediction of histopathology from clinical and laboratory characteristics at the time of diagnosis. Kidney Int *13*:159, 1978.
540. Heymann W, Makker S, Post R: The preponderance of males in the idiopathic nephrotic syndrome. Pediatrics *50*:814, 1972.
541. International Study of Kidney Disease in Children: The primary nephrotic syndrome in children. Identification of patients with minimal change nephrotic syndrome from initial response to prednisone. J Pediatr *98*:561, 1981.
542. Barnett HL, Schoeneman M, Bernstein J, et al: Minimal change nephrotic syndrome. *In* Edelmann CM Jr (Ed.): Pediatric Kidney Disease. Boston, Little, Brown, 1978, pp 695–710.
543. International Study of Kidney Disease in Children: Minimal change nephrotic syndrome in children: Deaths during the first 5 to 15 years' observation. Pediatrics *73*:497, 1984.
544. Lowenstein J, Schacht RG, Baldwin DS: Renal failure in minimal change nephrotic syndrome. Am J Med *70*:227, 1981.
545. Springate JE, Coyne JF, Karp MP, Feld LG: Acute renal failure in minimal change nephrotic syndrome. Pediatrics *80*:946, 1987.
546. Nash MA: Focal segmental glomerulosclerosis. *In* Edelmann CM Jr (Ed.): Pediatric Kidney Disease. Boston, Little, Brown, 1978, pp 718–724.
547. Cameron JS, Turner DR, Ogg CS, et al: The long-term prognosis of patients with focal segmental glomerulosclerosis. Clin Nephrol *10*:213, 1978.
548. Futrakul P, Poshyachinda M, Mitrakul C: Focal sclerosing glomerulonephritis: A kinetic evaluation of hemostasis and the effect of anticoagulant therapy: A controlled study. Clin Nephrol *10*:180, 1978.
549. Futrakul P: A new therapeutic approach to nephrotic syndrome associated with focal segmental glomerulosclerosis. Int J Pediatr Nephrol *1*:18, 1980.
550. White RHR: Membranoproliferative glomerulonephritis. *In* Edelmann CM Jr (Ed.): Pediatric Kidney Disease. Boston, Little, Brown, 1978, pp 660–678.
551. Habib R, Kleinknecht C, Gübler MC, et al: Membranous glomerulopathy in children. *In* Edelmann CM Jr (Ed.): Pediatric Kidney Disease. Boston, Little, Brown, 1978, pp 646–659.
552. Hallman N, Rapola J: Congenital nephrotic syndrome. *In* Edelmann CM Jr (Ed.): Pediatric Kidney Disease. Boston, Little, Brown, 1978, pp 711–717.
553. Mahan JD, Mauer SM, Sibley RK, Vernier RL: Congenital nephrotic syndrome: Evolution of medical management and results of renal transplantation. J Pediatr *105*:549, 1984.
554. Grahame-Smith HN, Ward PS, Jones RD, Lind J: Finnish-type congenital nephrotic syndrome in twins: Presentation with pyloric stenosis. J R Soc Med *81*:358, 1988.
555. Kaplan BS, Bureau MA, Drummond KN: The nephrotic syndrome in the first year of life: Is a pathologic classification possible? J Pediatr *85*:615, 1974.
556. Bohrer MP, Dean WM, Robertson CR, et al: Influence of molecular configuration in the glomerular filtration of macromolecules. Kidney Int *14*:751, 1978.
557. Chang RLS, Deen WM, Robertson CR, et al: Permselectivity of the glomerular capillary wall. Restricted transport of polyanions. Kidney Int *8*:212, 1975.
558. Rennke HC, Venkatachalam MA: Glomerular permeability: In vivo tracer studies with polyanionic and polycationic ferritins. Kidney Int *11*:94, 1977.
559. Hulme B, Hardwicke J: Human glomerular permeability to macromolecules in health and disease. Clin Sci *34*:515, 1968.
560. Blau EB, Haas DE: Glomerular sialic acid and proteinuria in human renal disease. Lab Invest *28*:477, 1973.
561. Carrie BJ, Salyer WR, Myers BD: Minimal change nephropathy: An electrochemical disorder of the glomerular membrane. Am J Med *70*:262, 1981.
562. Egan TJ, Kenny FM, Jarrah A, et al: Shock as a complication of the nephrotic syndrome. Am J Dis Child *113*:364, 1967.
563. Welch TR, Gianis J, Sheldon CA: Perforation of the scrotum complicating nephrotic syndrome. J Pediatr *113*:336, 1988.
564. Davison AM, Lambie AT, Verth AH, et al: Salt-poor albumin in the management of nephrotic syndrome. Br Med J *1*:481, 1974.
565. Wilfert CM, Katz SL: Etiology of bacterial sepsis in nephrotic children. Pediatrics *42*:841, 1968.
566. Gorensek MJ, Lebel MH, Nelson JD: Peritonitis in children with nephrotic syndrome. Pediatrics *81*:849, 1988.
567. Kendall AG, Lohmann RC, Dossetor JB: Nephrotic syndrome—a hypercoagulable state. Arch Intern Med *127*:1021, 1971.
568. Lieberman E, Heuser E, Gilchrist GS, et al: Thrombosis, nephrosis and corticosteroid therapy. J Pediatr *73*:320, 1968.
569. Goldbloom RB, Hillman DA, Santulli TV: Arterial thrombosis following femoral venipuncture in edematous nephrotic children. Pediatrics *40*:450, 1967.
570. Levin SE, Zamit R, Schmaman A: Thrombosis of the pulmonary arteries and the nephrotic syndrome. Br Med J *1*:153, 1967.
571. Mehls O, Andrassy K, Koderisch J, et al: Hemostasis and thromboembolism in children with nephrotic syndrome: Differences from adults. J Pediatr *110*:862, 1987.
572. Hoyer PF, Gonda S, Barthels M, et al: Thromboembolic complications in children with nephrotic syndrome: Risk and incidence. Acta Paediatr Scand *75*:804, 1986.
573. Adler AJ, Lundlin AP, Feinroth MV, et al: Beta-thromboglobulin levels in the nephrotic syndrome. Am J Med *69*:551, 1980.
574. Lau SO, Tkachuck JY, Hasegawa DK, et al: Plasminogen and antithrombin III deficiencies in the childhood nephrotic syndrome associated with plasminogenuria and antithrombinuria. J Pediatr *96*:390, 1980.
575. Anderson CF, Jaecks DM, Ballon HS, et al: Renal handling of creatinine in nephrotic and non-nephrotic patients. Clin Sci *38*:555, 1970.

576. Goldstein DA, Haldimann B, Sherman D, et al: Vitamin D metabolites and calcium metabolism in patients with nephrotic syndrome and normal renal function. J Clin Endocrinol Metab *52*:116, 1981.
577. Freedman LR: The interstitial nephritides (interstitial renal inflammation). *In* Edelmann CM Jr (Ed.): Pediatric Kidney Disease. Boston, Little, Brown, 1978, pp 879–889.
578. Murray T, Goldberg MD: Etiologies of chronic interstitial nephritis. Ann Intern Med *82*:453, 1975.
579. Nanra RS, Chirawong P, Kincaid-Smith P: Medullary ischaemia in experimental analgesic nephropathy—the pathogenesis of renal papillary necrosis. Aust NZ J Med *3*:580, 1973.
580. Kunin CM: The natural history of recurrent bacteriuria in school-girls. N Engl J Med *282*:1443, 1970.
581. Amar AD: Colicotubular backflow with vesico-ureteral reflux. Relation to pyelonephritis. JAMA *213*:293, 1970.
582. Hodson CJ: Vesico-ureteric reflux and renal scarring—with and without infection. Kidney Int *5*:308, 1974.
583. Winberg J, Bollgren I, Kallenius G, et al: Clinical pyelonephritis and focal renal scarring. A selected review of pathogenesis, prevention and prognosis. Pediatr Clin North Am *29*:801, 1982.
584. Miller T, Phillips S: Pyelonephritis: The relationship between infection, renal scarring, and antimicrobial therapy. Kidney Int *19*:654, 1981.
585. Johnston JH: Urinary tract infection: Tuberculosis and other specific infections. *In* Williams DI, Johnston JH (Eds.): Paediatric Urology. London, Butterworth Scientific, 1982, pp 121–127.
586. Woodroffe AJ, Row PG, Meadows R, et al: Nephritis in infectious mononucleosis. QJ Med *43*:451, 1974.
587. Kim Y, Michael AF: Infection and nephritis. *In* Edelmann CM Jr (Ed.): Pediatric Kidney Disease. Boston, Little, Brown, 1978, pp 828–836.
588. Donckerwolcke RA: Diagnosis and treatment of renal tubular disorders in children. Pediatr Clin North Am *29*:895, 1982.
589. Rodriguez Soriano J: Renal tubular acidosis. *In* Edelmann CM Jr (Ed.): Pediatric Kidney Disease. Boston, Little, Brown, 1978, pp 995–1011.
590. Edelmann CM Jr, Rodriguez Soriano J, Boichis H, et al: Bicarbonate reabsorption and hydrogen ion excretion in normal infants. J Clin Invest *46*:1309, 1967.
591. Rodriguez Soriano J, Boichis H, Edelmann CM Jr: Bicarbonate reabsorption and hydrogen ion excretion in children with renal tubular acidosis. J Pediatr *71*:802, 1967.
592. Brenes LG, Brenes JN, Hernandez MM: Familial proximal renal tubular acidosis. A distinct clinical entity. Am J Med *63*:244, 1977.
593. Sebastian A, McSherry E, Morris RC Jr: Renal potassium wasting in renal tubular acidosis (RTA): Its occurrence in types 1 and 2 RTA despite sustained correction of systemic acidosis. J Clin Invest *50*:667, 1971.
594. Donckerwolcke RA, van Stekelenburg GJ, Tiddens HA: Therapy of bicarbonate losing renal tubular acidosis. Arch Dis Child *45*:774, 1970.
595. Oetliker O, Rossi E: The influence of extracellular fluid volume on the renal bicarbonate threshold: A study of two children with Lowe's syndrome. Pediatr Res *3*:140, 1969.
596. McSherry E, Morris RC: Attainment and maintenance of normal stature with alkali therapy in infants and children with classic renal tubular acidosis. J Clin Invest *61*:501, 1978.
597. Battle CD, Arruda JAL, Kurkman HA: Hyperkalemic distal renal tubular acidosis associated with obstructive uropathy. N Engl J Med *304*:373, 1981.
598. Alon U, Kodroff MB, Broecker BH, et al: Renal tubular acidosis type 4 in neonatal unilateral kidney diseases. J Pediatr *104*:855, 1984.
599. Weinstein SF, Allan DME, Mendoza SA: Hyperkalemia, acidosis and short stature associated with a defect in renal potassium excretion. J Pediatr *85*:355, 1974.
600. Spitzer A, Edelmann CM Jr, Goldberg LD, et al: Short stature, hyperkalemia and acidosis: A defect in renal transport of potassium. Kidney Int *3*:251, 1973.
601. Schwartz GJ, Spitzer A: Disorders of renal transport of sodium, potassium and magnesium. *In* Edelmann CM Jr (Ed.): Pediatric Kidney Disease. Boston, Little, Brown, 1978, pp 1079–1093.
602. Dillon MJ, Leonard JV, Buckler JM, et al: Pseudohypoaldosteronism. Arch Dis Child *55*:427, 1980.
603. Schulman JD, Schneider JA: Cystinosis and the Fanconi syndrome. Pediatr Clin North Am *23*:779, 1976.
604. Brodehl J: The Fanconi syndrome. *In* Edelmann CM Jr (Ed.): Pediatric Kidney Disease. Boston, Little, Brown, 1978, pp 955–987.
605. Joel M, Rosales JK: Fanconi syndrome and anesthesia. Anesthesiology *55*:455, 1981.
606. Glorieux FH, Marie PF, Pettifor JM, et al: Bone response to phosphate salts, ergocalciferol, and calcitriol in hypophosphatemic vitamin-D–resistant rickets. N Engl J Med *303*:1023, 1980.
607. Avioli LV: Clinical syndromes characterized by disturbances in phosphate transport and excretion. *In* Edelmann CM Jr (Ed.): Pediatric Kidney Disease. Boston, Little, Brown, 1978, pp 1012–1035.
608. Rasmussen H, Pechet M, Anast C, et al: Long-term treatment of familial hypophosphatemic rickets with oral phosphate and 1-alpha-hydroxyvitamin D3. J Pediatr *99*:16, 1981.
609. Stern P: Nephrogenic defects of urinary concentration. *In* Edelmann CM Jr (Ed.): Pediatric Kidney Disease. Boston, Little, Brown, 1978, pp 987–995.
610. Dousa TP, Valtin H: Cellular actions of vasopressin in the mammalian kidney. Kidney Int *10*:46, 1976.
611. Marumo F, Edelman IS: Effects of calcium and prostaglandin E-1 on vasopressin activation of renal adenyl cyclase. J Clin Invest *50*:1613, 1971.
612. Jamison RL, Maffly RH: The urinary concentrating mechanism. N Engl J Med *295*:1059, 1976.
613. Bennett CM: Urine concentration and dilution in hypokalemic and hypercalcemic dogs. J Clin Invest *49*:1447, 1970.
614. Dousa TP: Cellular action of antidiuretic hormone in nephrogenic diabetes insipidus. Mayo Clin Proc *49*:188, 1974.
615. Earley LE, Orloff J: The mechanism of antidiuresis associated with the administration of hydrochlorothiazide to patients with vasopressin-resistant diabetes insipidus. J Clin Invest *41*:1988, 1962.
616. Blachar Y, Zadik A, Shemesh M, et al: The effect of inhibition of prostaglandin synthesis on free water and osmolar clearances in patients with hereditary nephrogenic diabetes insipidus. Int J Pediatr Nephrol *1*:48, 1980.
617. Bourke E, Delaney V: Bartter's syndrome—a dilemma of cause and effect. Nephron *27*:177, 1981.
618. Davis A: Atrial natriuretic factor in the pediatric intensive care unit. Crit Care Clin *4*:803, 1988.
619. Tunny TJ, Gordon RD: Plasma atrial natriuretic peptide in primary aldosteronism (before and after treatment) and in Bartter's and Gordon's syndromes (letter). Lancet *1*:272, 1986.
620. Arant BS, Brackett NC, Young RB, et al: Case studies

of siblings with juxtamedullary hyperplasia and secondary aldosteronism associated with severe azotemia and renal rickets—Bartter's syndrome or disease? Pediatrics *46*:344, 1970.
621. Littlewood JM, Lee HR, Medow SR: Treatment of Bartter's syndrome in early childhood with prostaglandin synthetase inhibitors. Arch Dis Child *53*:43, 1978.
622. Lechaz G, Arbus GS, Balfe JW, et al: Effect of ibuprofen on growth in a child with Bartter's syndrome. J Pediatr *95*:319, 1979.
623. Abston PA, Priano LL: Bartter's syndrome: Anesthetic implications based on pathophysiology and treatment. Anesth Analg *60*:764, 1981.
624. Booth BE, Johanson A: Hypomagnesemia due to renal tubular defect in reabsorption of magnesium. J Pediatr *84*:350, 1974.
625. Hayslett JP: Medullary sponge kidney. *In* Edelmann CM Jr (Ed.): Pediatric Kidney Disease. Boston, Little, Brown, 1978, pp 889–893.
626. Bernstein J: Polycystic disease. *In* Edelmann CM Jr (Ed.): Pediatric Kidney Disease. Boston, Little, Brown, 1978, pp 557–570.
627. Stapleton FB, Johnson DL, Kaplan GW, et al: The cystic renal lesion in tuberous sclerosis. J Pediatr *97*:574, 1980.
628. Bernstein J: Renal hypoplasia and dysplasia. *In* Edelmann CM Jr (Ed.): Pediatric Kidney Disease. Boston, Little, Brown, pp 541–557.
629. Borland LM: Anesthesia for children with Jeune's syndrome (asphyxiating thoracic dystrophy). Anesthesiology *66*:86, 1987.
630. Torres VE, Young WF, Offord KP, Hattery RR: Association of hypokalemia, aldosteronism and renal cysts. N Engl J Med *322*:345, 1990.
631. Guignard JP: Renal function in the newborn infant. Pediatr Clin North Am *29*:777, 1982.
632. Lieberman E, Salinas-Madrigal L, Gwinn JL, et al: Infantile polycystic disease of the kidneys and liver: Clinical, pathological, and radiological correlations and comparison with congenital hepatic fibrosis. Medicine *50*:277, 1971.
633. Anand SK, Chan JC, Lieberman E: Polycystic disease and hepatic fibrosis in children. Renal function studies. Am J Dis Child *129*:810, 1975.
634. Cole BR, Conley SB, Stapleton FB: Polycystic kidney disease in the first year of life. J Pediatr *111*:693, 1987.
635. Vuthibhagdee A, Singleton EB: Infantile polycystic disease of the kidney. Am J Dis Child *125*:167, 1973.
636. Ross DG, Travers H: Infantile presentation of adult-type polycystic kidney disease in a large kindred. J Pediatr *87*:760, 1975.
637. Chapman AB, Johnson A, Gabow PA, Schrier RW: The renin-angiotensin-aldosterone system and autosomal dominant polycystic kidney disease. N Engl J Med *323*:1091, 1990.
638. Bernstein J, Gardner KD Jr: Familial juvenile nephronophthisis—medullary cystic disease. *In* Edelmann CM Jr (Ed.): Pediatric Kidney Disease. Boston, Little, Brown, 1978, pp 580–586.
639. Sotelo-Veila C, Singer DB: Syndrome of hyperplastic fetal visceromegaly and neonatal hypoglycemia (Beckwith's syndrome): A report of seven cases. Pediatrics *46*:240, 1970.
640. Beck DA: The effect of intrauterine urinary obstruction upon the development of the fetal kidney. J Urol *105*:784, 1971.
641. Bernstein J: The morphogenesis of renal parenchymal maldevelopment (renal dysplasia). Pediatr Clin North Am *18*:395, 1971.
642. Cussen JJ: Cystic kidneys in children with congenital urethral obstruction. J Urol *106*:939, 1971.
643. Bernstein J, Meyer R: Some speculations on the nature and significance of developmentally small kidneys (renal hypoplasia). Nephron *1*:137, 1964.
644. Royer P, Habib R, Broyer M, et al: Segmental hypoplasia of the kidney in children. Adv Nephrol *1*:145, 1971.
645. Fay R, Winer R, Cohen A, et al: Segmental renal hypoplasia and hypertension. J Urol *113*:561, 1975.
646. Carter JE, Lirenman DS: Bilateral renal hypoplasia with oligomeganephronia. Oligomeganephronic renal hypoplasia. Am J Dis Child *120*:537, 1970.
647. Moorthy AV, Zimmerman SW, Burkholder PM: Effects of extra-renal neoplasms on the kidney. *In* Edelmann CM Jr (Ed.): Pediatric Kidney Disease. Boston, Little, Brown, 1978, pp 811–827.
648. Trainin EB: Renal involvement in amyloidosis. *In* Edelmann CM Jr (Ed.): Pediatric Kidney Disease. Boston, Little, Brown, 1978, pp 799–811.
649. Nyhan WL: Urate nephropathy. *In* Edelmann CM Jr (Ed.): Pediatric Kidney Disease. Boston, Little, Brown, 1978, pp 894–906.
650. Pabico RC, Atanacio BC, McKenna BA, et al: Renal pathologic lesions and functional alterations in man with Fabry's disease. Am J Med *55*:415, 1973.
651. Dresnick RJ, Allen KY, Simmons RL, et al: Correction of enzymatic deficiencies by renal transplantation: Fabry's disease. Surgery *72*:203, 1972.
652. Morel-Maroger L, Basch A, Dannon F, et al: Pathology of the kidney in Waldenström's macroglobulinemia. N Engl J Med *283*:123, 1970.
653. Kaplan NG, Kaplan KC: Monoclonal gammopathy, glomerulonephritis, and the nephrotic syndrome. Arch Intern Med *125*:696, 1970.
654. Kew MC, Brunt PW, Varma RR: Renal and intrarenal blood flow in cirrhosis of the liver. Lancet *2*:504, 1971.
655. Epstein M, Berk DP, Hollenberg NK, et al: Renal failure in the patient with cirrhosis: The role of active vasoconstriction. Am J Med *49*:175, 1970.
656. Conn HO: A rational approach to the hepatorenal syndrome. Gastroenterology *65*:321, 1973.
657. Schwartz GJ, Spitzer A: Metal nephropathy. *In* Edelmann CM Jr (Ed.): Pediatric Kidney Disease. Boston, Little, Brown, 1978, pp 940–952.
658. Elsas LJ, Hayslett JP, Spargo BH, et al: Wilson's disease with reversible renal tubular dysfunction: Correlation with proximal tubular ultrastructure. Ann Intern Med *75*:427, 1971.
659. Resnick JS, Michael AF: Renal manifestations in connective tissue disease. *In* Edelmann CM Jr (Ed.): Pediatric Kidney Disease. Boston, Little, Brown, 1978, pp 768–776.
660. Dabich L, Sullivan DB, Cassidy JT: Scleroderma in the child. J Pediatr *85*:770, 1974.
661. Cannon PJ, Hassar M, Case DB, et al: The relationship of hypertension and renal failure in scleroderma (progressive systemic sclerosis) to structural and functional abnormalities of the renal cortical circulation. Medicine *55*:1, 1974.
662. Keane WF, Danielson B, Ray L: Successful renal transplantation in progressive systemic sclerosis. Ann Intern Med *85*:199, 1976.
663. Moutsopolous H, Fye KH: Lipoid nephrosis and focal glomerulosclerosis in a patient with polymyositis. Lancet *1*:1039, 1975.
664. Singsen B, Goldreyen B, Stanton R, et al: Childhood polymyositis with cardiac conduction defects. Am J Dis Child *130*:72, 1976.
665. Park S, Nyhan WL: Fatal pulmonary involvement in dermatomyositis. Am J Dis Child *129*:723, 1975.
666. Singsen BH, Bernstein BH, Kornreich HK, et al:

Mixed connective tissue disease in childhood: A clinical and serologic survey. J Pediatr *90*:893, 1977.
667. Meadow R: Polyarteritis nodosa (periarteritis nodosa). *In* Edelmann CM Jr (Ed.): Pediatric Kidney Disease. Boston, Little, Brown, 1978, pp 796–799.
668. Fish AJ, Blau EB, Westberg NG, et al: SLE within the first two decades of life. Am J Med *62*:99, 1977.
669. Walravens PA, Chase HP: The prognosis of childhood systemic lupus erythematosus. Am J Dis Child *130*:929, 1976.
670. Fish AJ, Vernier RL, Michael AF: Systemic lupus erythematosus. *In* Edelmann CM Jr (Ed.): Pediatric Kidney Disease. Boston, Little, Brown, 1978, pp 745–767.
671. Alleyene GAO, Statius-Van-Eps LW, Addae SK, et al: The kidney in sickle cell anemia. Kidney Int 7:731, 1975.
672. Strauss J, McIntosh RM: Sickle cell nephropathy. *In* Edelmann CM Jr (Ed.): Pediatric Kidney Disease. Boston, Little, Brown, 1978, pp 776–788.
673. Johnson M, Rabinowitz I, Willis AL, et al: Detection of prostaglandin induction of erythrocyte sickling. Clin Chem *19*:23, 1973.
674. Berman LB: Sickle cell nephropathy. JAMA *228*:1279, 1974.
675. Strom T, Muehrcke RC, Smith RD: Sickle cell anemia with the nephrotic syndrome and renal vein obstruction. Arch Intern Med *129*:104, 1972.
676. Friedman EA, Sreepada TK, Sprung CL, et al: Uremia in sickle cell anemia treated by maintenance hemodialysis. N Engl J Med *291*:431, 1974.
677. Hatch FE, Culbertson JW, Diggs LW: Nature of the renal concentrating defect in sickle cell disease. J Clin Invest *46*:336, 1967.
678. Beyer MM: Diabetic nephropathy. Pediatr Clin North Am *31*:635, 1984.
679. Knowles HC Jr: Renal disease in juvenile diabetes. *In* Edelmann CM Jr (Ed.): Pediatric Kidney Disease. Boston, Little, Brown, 1978, pp 806–811.
680. Mogensen CE: Renal function changes in diabetes. Diabetes *25*:872, 1976.
681. Urizar RE, Schwartz A, Top F Jr, et al: The nephrotic syndrome in children with diabetes mellitus of recent onset. N Engl J Med *281*:173, 1969.
682. Goldstein DA, Massry SG: Diabetic nephropathy—clinical course and effect of hemodialysis. Nephron *20*:286, 1978.
683. Barratt TM: Urolithiasis: Medical aspects. *In* Williams DI, Johnston JH (Eds.): Paediatric Urology. London, Butterworth Scientific, 1982, pp 351–360.
684. Garcia RE, Friedman WF, Kaback MM, et al: Idiopathic hypercalcemia and supravalvular aortic stenosis. N Engl J Med *271*:117, 1964.
685. Malhotra V, Gomillion MC, Artusio JF: Hemoptysis in a child during extracorporeal shock wave lithotripsy. Anesth Analg *69*:526, 1989.
686. Parrott TS: Summary of annual meeting of the Section on Pediatric Urology. Pediatrics *83*:591, 1989.
687. Frymoyer PA, Scheinman SJ, Dunham PB, et al: X-linked recessive nephrolithiasis with renal failure. N Engl J Med *325*:681, 1991.
688. Ezzedeen F, Adelman RD, Ahlfors CE: Renal calcification in preterm infants: Pathophysiology and long-term sequelae. J Pediatr *113*:532, 1988.
689. Tredrea CR, Pathak D, From RP, Grucza J: Lung protection in children during extracorporeal shock wave lithotripsy. Anesth Analg *66*:S-178, 1987.
690. Johnston JH: Neuroblastoma, teratoma and other retroperitoneal tumours. *In* Williams DI, Johnston JH (Eds.): Paediatric Urology. London, Butterworth Scientific, 1982, pp 401–409.
691. Krishna G: Neurofibromatosis, renal hypertension and cardiac dysrhythmias. Anesth Analg *54*:542, 1975.
692. Williams DI, Martin J: Renal tumours. *In* Williams DI, Johnston JH (Eds.): Paediatric Urology. London, Butterworth Scientific, 1982, pp 381–399.
693. Pilling GP: Wilms' tumor in seven children with congenital aniridia. J Pediatr Surg *10*:87, 1975.
694. Barakat AY, Papadoulou ZL, Chandra RS: Pseudohermaphroditism, nephron disorder and Wilms' tumor. Pediatrics *54*:366, 1974.
695. Sukarochana K, Tolentino W, Kiesewetter WB: Wilms' tumor and hypertension. J Pediatr Surg *7*:573, 1972.
696. Spahr J, Demers LM, Shochat SJ: Renin-producing Wilms' tumor. J Pediatr Surg *16*:32, 1981.
697. Martin J, Rickham PP: Pulmonary metastases in Wilms' tumor. Arch Dis Childhood *45*:805, 1970.
698. Stehling LC, Furman EB: Anesthesia for congenital anomalies of the genito-urinary system. *In* Stehling LC, Zauder HL (Eds.): Anesthetic Implications of Congenital Anomalies in Children. New York, Appleton-Century-Crofts, 1980, pp 145–165.
699. Greenwood RD, Rosenthal A, Nadas AS: Cardiovascular malformations associated with congenital anomalies of the urinary system. Observations in a series of 453 infants and children with urinary malformations. Clin Pediatr *15*:1101, 1976.
700. Greenwood RD: Cardiovascular malformations associated with extracardiac anomalies and malformation syndromes: Patterns for diagnosis. Clin Pediatr *23*:145, 1984.
701. Inselman LS, Mellins RB: Growth and development of the lung. J Pediatr *98*:1, 1981.
702. Thomas IT, Smith DW: Oligohydramnios, cause of the nonrenal features of Potter's syndrome, including pulmonary hypoplasia. J Pediatr *84*:811, 1974.
703. Pramanik AK, Altshuler G, Light IJ, et al: Prune-belly syndrome associated with Potter (renal nonfunction) syndrome. Am J Dis Child *131*:672, 1977.
704. Pagon RA, Smith DW, Shepard TH: Urethral obstruction malformation complex: A cause of abdominal muscle deficiency and the "prune belly." J Pediatr *94*:900, 1974.
705. Belman AB, Kaplan GW: Prune belly syndrome. *In* Genitourinary Problems in Pediatrics. Philadelphia, WB Saunders, 1981, pp 254–260.
706. Lockhart JL, Reeve HR, Bredael JJ, et al: Siblings with prune belly syndrome and associated pulmonic stenosis, mental retardation, and deafness. Urology *14*:140, 1979.
707. Chinyanga HM: Cystoscopy and prune-belly syndrome. *In* Stehling LC (Ed.): Common Problems in Pediatric Anesthesia. Chicago, Year Book Medical Publishers, 1982, pp 77–82.
708. Bovicelli L, Rizzo N, Orsini LF, et al: Prenatal diagnosis of the prune belly syndrome. Clin Genet *18*:79, 1980.
709. Moerman P, Fryns JP, Goddeeris P, et al: Pathogenesis of the prune-belly syndrome: A functional urethral obstruction caused by prostatic hypoplasia. Pediatrics *73*:470, 1984.
710. Nakayama DK, Harrison MR, Chinn DH, et al: The pathogenesis of prune belly. Am J Dis Child *138*:834, 1984.
711. Karamanian A, Kravath B, Nagashima H, et al: Anaesthetic management of "prune-belly" syndrome: Case report. Br J Anaesth *46*:897, 1974.
712. Jones AEP, Pelton DA: An index of syndromes and their anaesthetic implications. Can Anaesth Soc J *23*:207, 1976.

713. Hannington-Kiff JG: Prune-belly syndrome and general anaesthesia. Br J Anaesth *42*:649, 1970.
714. Warshaw BL, Hymes LC, Woodward JR: Long-term outcome of patients with obstructive uropathy. Pediatr Clin North Am *29*:815, 1982.
715. Dal Canton A, Corradi A, Stanziale R, et al: Glomerular hemodynamics before and after release of 24-hour bilateral ureteral obstruction. Kidney Int *17*:491, 1980.
716. Awazu M, Barakat AY, Chevalier RL, Ichikawa I: The cause of uremia in obstructed kidneys. J Pediatr *114*:179, 1989.
717. Wilson DR: Micropuncture study of chronic obstructive nephropathy before and after release of obstruction. Kidney Int *2*:119, 1972.
718. Mayor G, Genton N, Torrado A, et al: Renal function in obstructive nephropathy: Long-term effect of reconstructive surgery. Pediatrics *56*:740, 1975.
719. McCrory WM, Shibuya M, Leumann E, et al: Studies of renal function in children with chronic hydronephrosis. Pediatr Clin North Am *18*:445, 1971.
720. Belman AB, Kaplan GW: Obstructive uropathy. *In* Genitourinary Problems in Pediatrics. Philadelphia, WB Saunders, 1981, pp 92–117.
721. Steinhart JM, Kuhn JP, Eisenberg B, et al: Ultrasound screening of healthy infants for urinary tract abnormalities. Pediatrics *82*:609, 1988.
722. Daniels SR, Loggie JMH, McEnery PT, Towbin RB: Clinical spectrum of intrinsic renovascular hypertension in children. Pediatrics *80*:698, 1987.
723. Lorentz WB Jr, Browning MC, D'Souza VJ, et al: Intrarenal aneurysm of the renal artery in children. Am J Dis Child *138*:751, 1984.
724. McCook TA, Mills SR, Kirks DR, et al: Percutaneous transluminal renal artery angioplasty in a 3½ year old hypertensive girl. J Pediatr *97*:958, 1980.
725. Fraley EE: Vascular obstruction of superior infundibulum causing nephralgia: A new syndrome. N Engl J Med *275*:1403, 1966.
726. Belman AB, Kaplan GW: Developmental abnormalities of the kidney and urinary collecting system. *In* Genitourinary Problems in Pediatrics. Philadelphia, WB Saunders, 1981, pp 225–237.
727. Chan SL, Johnson HW, McLoughlin MG: Idiopathic retroperitoneal fibrosis in children. J Urol *122*:103, 1979.
728. Williams DI, Hulme-Moir I: Primary obstructive megaureter. Br J Urol *42*:140, 1970.
729. Belman AB: The clinical significance of vesicoureteral reflux. Pediatr Clin North Am *23*:707, 1976.
730. Ehrlich RM: Vesicoureteral reflux: A surgeon's perspective. Pediatr Clin North Am *29*:827, 1982.
731. Lenaghan D, Whitaker JG, Jensen F, et al: The natural history of reflux and the long-term effects of reflux on the kidney. J Urol *115*:728, 1976.
732. Edwards D, Normand ICS, Prescod N, et al: Disappearance of vesicoureteral reflux during long-term prophylaxis of urinary tract infection in children. Br Med J *2*:285, 1977.
733. Levitt SB, Duckett J, Spitzer A, et al: Report of the International Reflux Study Committee. Medical versus surgical treatment of primary vesico-ureteral reflux. Pediatrics *67*:392, 1981.
734. Willscher MK, Bauer SB, Zammuto PJ, et al: Infection of the urinary tract after anti-reflux surgery. J Pediatr *89*:743, 1976.
735. Lyon RP, Marshall SK, Scott MP: Treatment of vesicoureteral reflux. Urology *16*:38, 1980.
736. Belman AB, Kaplan GW: Vesicoureteral reflux. *In* Genitourinary Problems in Pediatrics. Philadelphia, WB Saunders, 1981, pp 67–90.
737. Hendren WH: Posterior urethral valves in boys: A broad clinical spectrum. J Urol *106*:298, 1971.
738. Eckstein HB, Williams DI: The Neuropathic Bladder. *In* Williams DI, Johnston JH (Eds.): Paediatric Urology. London, Butterworth Scientific, 1982, pp 325–336.
739. Belman AB, Kaplan GW: Neurogenic bladder. *In* Genitourinary Problems in Pediatrics. Philadelphia, WB Saunders, 1981, pp 130–147.
740. Cole AT, Fried FA: Favorable experiences with imipramine in the treatment of neurogenic bladder. J Urol *107*:44, 1972.
741. Krane RJ, Olsson CA: Phenoxybenzamine in neurogenic bladder dysfunction. I. A theory of micturition. J Urol *110*:650, 1973.
742. Murdock M, Sax D, Krane RJ: The use of dantrolene sodium in external sphincter spasm. Urology *8*:133, 1976.
743. Stehling LC, Patil U, Patil V: Anesthesia for urodynamic studies in children. Anesthesiol Rev *6*:13, 1979.
744. Berry FA: Anesthesia for genitourinary surgery. *In* Gregory GA (Ed.): Pediatric Anesthesia. New York, Churchill Livingstone, 1983, pp 727–771.
745. Belman AB, Kaplan GW: Bladder exstrophy, cloacal exstrophy, and imperforate anus. *In* Genitourinary Problems in Pediatrics. Philadelphia, WB Saunders, 1981, pp 238–254.
746. Johnston JH: The exstrophic anomalies. *In* Williams DI, Johnston JH (Eds.): Paediatric Urology. London, Butterworth Scientific, 1982, pp 299–316.
747. Belman AB, Kaplan GW: Genital abnormalities in the male. *In* Genitourinary Problems in Pediatrics. Philadelphia, WB Saunders, 1981, pp 160–198.
748. Williams DI: Male urethral anomalies. *In* Williams DI, Johnston JH (Eds.): Paediatric Urology. London, Butterworth Scientific, 1982, pp 239–250.
749. Johnston JH: Abnormalities of the penis. *In* Williams DI, Johnston JH (Eds.): Paediatric Urology. London, Butterworth Scientific, 1982, pp 435–449.
750. Aarskog D: Maternal progestins as a possible cause of hypospadias. N Engl J Med *300*:75, 1979.
751. Page LA: Inheritance of uncomplicated hypospadias. Pediatrics *63*:788, 1979.
752. Benzon HT, Leventhal JB, Ovassapian A: Ketamine treatment of penile erection in the operating room. Anesth Analg *62*:457, 1983.
753. Villalonga A, Beltran, J, Gomar C, et al: Ketamine for treatment of priapism. Anesth Analg *64*:1033, 1986.
754. Pietras JR, Cromie WJ, Duckett JM: Ketamine as a detumescence agent during hypospadias repair. J Urol *121*:654, 1979.
755. Kay B: Caudal block for post-operative pain relief in children. Anaesthesia *29*:610, 1974.
756. Blaise G, Roy WL: Post-operative pain relief after hypospadias repair in pediatric patients: Regional analgesia versus systemic analgesics. Anesthesiology *61*:A430, 1984.
757. Soliman MG, Tremblay NA: Nerve block of the penis for postoperative pain relief in children. Anesth Analg *57*:495, 1978.
758. Kirya C, Werthmann MW Jr: Neonatal circumcision and penile dorsal nerve block—a painless procedure. J Pediatr *92*:998, 1978.
759. Hannallah RS, Broadman LM, Belman AB, et al: Control of post-orchiopexy pain in pediatric outpatients: Comparison of two regional techniques. Anesthesiology *61*:A429, 1984.
760. Abajian JC, Mellish RWP, Browne AF, et al: Spinal anesthesia for surgery in the high-risk infant. Anesth Analg *63*:359, 1984.

761. Maconochie IK, Scopes JW: Priapism in a 6½-year-old boy with sickle cell disease. J R Soc Med *81*:606, 1988.
762. Snyder AR, Ilko R: Topical nitroglycerin for intraoperative penile turgescence. Anesth Analg *66*:1022, 1987.
763. Welti RS, Brodsky JB: Treatment of intraoperative penile tumescence. J Urol *124*:925, 1980.
764. Baraka A, Sibai AN: Benzodiazepine treatment of penile erection under general anesthesia. Anesth Analg *67*:596, 1988.
765. Santha TR: Intraoperative management of penile erection by using terbutaline. Anesthesiology *70*:707, 1989.
766. Miyabe M, Namiki A: Ephedrine for treatment of penile erection during spinal anesthesia. Anesth Analg *67*:1019, 1988.
767. Johnston JH: Abnormalities of the scrotum and the testes. *In* Williams DI, Johnston JH (Eds.): Paediatric Urology. London, Butterworth Scientific, 1982, pp 451–465.
768. Johnston JH: Acquired lesions of the penis, the scrotum and the testes. *In* Williams DI, Johnston JH (Eds.): Paediatric Urology. London, Butterworth Scientific, 1982, pp 467–475.
769. Tulassay T, Rascher W, Seyberth HW, et al: Role of atrial natriuretic peptide in sodium homeostasis in premature infants. J Pediatr *109*:1023, 1986.
770. Datta S, Murphy MT, Carr DB, et al: Maternal and fetal plasma atrial natriuretic peptide concentrations during elective caesarean section. Acta Anaesthesiol Scand *35*:93, 1991.
771. Shaffer SG, Geer PG, Goetz KL: Elevated atrial natriuretic factor in neonates with respiratory distress syndrome. J Pediatr *109*:1028, 1986.
772. Leithner C, Frass M, Pacher R, et al: Mechanical ventilation with positive end-expiratory pressure decreases release of alpha-atrial natriuretic peptide. Crit Care Med *15*:484, 1987.
773. Frass M, Popovic R, Hartter E, et al: Atrial natriuretic peptide decrease during spontaneous breathing with continuous positive airway pressure in volume-expanded healthy volunteers. Crit Care Med *16*:831, 1988.
774. Kharasch ED, Yeo K, Kenny MA, Buffington CW: Atrial natriuretic factor may mediate the renal effects of PEEP ventilation. Anesthesiology *69*:862, 1988.
775. Fratacci MD, Greck E, Froidevaux R, et al: Antidiuresis during PEEP is not mediated by an inhibition of atrial natriuretic factor release. Anesthesiology *69*:A184, 1988.
776. Eison HB, Rosen MJ, Phillips RA, Krakoff LR: Determinants of atrial natriuretic factor in the adult respiratory distress syndrome. Chest *94*:1040, 1988.
777. Cosby RL, Sophocles AM, Durr JA, et al: Elevated plasma atrial natriuretic factor and vasopressin in high-altitude pulmonary edema. Ann Intern Med *109*:796, 1988.
778. Ishikawa N, Hayakawa A, Uematsu T, Nakashima M: Heterogeneity in vasorelaxant effects of alpha-human atrial natriuretic polypeptide in the dog. Jpn J Pharmacol *44*:515, 1987.
779. Hulks G, Jardine A, Connell JMC, Thomson NC: Bronchodilator effect of atrial natriuretic peptide in asthma. Br Med J *299*:1081, 1989.
780. Huxley VH, Tucker VL, Verburg KM, Freeman RH: Increased capillary hydraulic conductivity induced by atrial natriuretic peptide. Circ Res *60*:304, 1987.
781. Davis AL, Goldstein DS, Salcedo JR, et al: Atrial natriuretic peptide: The relationship with volume overload, atrial tachycardia, and critical illness (abstract). Crit Care Med *15*:417, 1987.
782. Matsuoka S, Kurahashi Y, Miki Y, et al: Plasma atrial natriuretic peptide in patients with congenital heart disease. Pediatrics *82*:639, 1988.
783. Adnot S, Chabrier PE, Brun-Buisson C, et al: Atrial natriuretic factor attenuates the pulmonary pressor response to hypoxia. J Appl Physiol *65*:1975, 1988.
784. Hoffman WE, Phillips MI, Kimura B: Plasma atrial natriuretic polypeptide and angiotensin II in rats during anesthesia and volume loading. Anesth Analg *68*:40, 1989.
785. Madwed JB, Wang BC: Pentobarbital anesthesia alters renal actions of alpha-hANP in dogs. Am J Physiol *258*:R616, 1990.
786. Gutkowska J, Racz K, Garcia ER, et al: The morphine effect on plasma ANF. Eur J Pharmacol *131*:91, 1986.
787. Hedner J, Towle A, Saltzman L, et al: Changes in plasma atrial natriuretic peptide immunoreactivity in patients undergoing coronary artery bypass graft placements. Regul Pept *17*:151, 1987.
788. Kidd JE, Gilchrist NL, Utley RJ, et al: Effect of opiate, general anaesthesia and surgery on plasma atrial natriuretic peptide levels in man. Clin Exp Pharmacol Physiol *14*:755, 1987.
789. Barkermann BJ, Brenner BM: Biologically active atrial peptides. J Clin Invest *76*:2041, 1985.
790. Mendoza SA: Syndrome of inappropriate antidiuretic hormone secretion (SIADH). Pediatr Clin North Am *23*:681, 1976.
791. Crumrine RS: Adrenogenital syndrome. *In* Stehling LC (Ed.): Common Problems in Pediatric Anesthesia. Chicago, Year Book Medical Publishers, 1982, pp 119–122.
792. Laflin MJ: Interaction of pancuronium and corticosteroids. Anesthesiology *47*:471, 1977.
793. Meyers EF: Partial recovery from pancuronium neuromuscular blockade following hydrocortisone administration. Anesthesiology *46*:148, 1977.
794. Belman AB, Kaplan GW: Trauma. *In* Genitourinary Problems in Pediatrics. Philadelphia, WB Saunders, 1981, pp 319–329.
795. Johnston JH: Urinary tract injuries. *In* Williams DI, Johnston JH (Eds.): Paediatric Urology. London, Butterworth Scientific, 1982, pp 369–380.
796. Morse TS, Smith JP, Howard WHR, et al: Kidney injuries in children. J Urol *98*:539, 1967.

CHAPTER

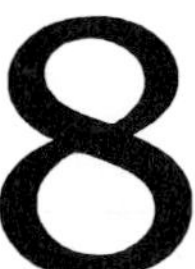

8 Diseases of the Gastrointestinal System

DAVID J. STEWARD, M.B.

A knowledge of the normal physiology of the gastrointestinal system is essential to anesthesiologists if they are to plan for the safe management of their patients. In addition, the pediatric anesthesiologist should appreciate the special features of the gastrointestinal physiology of infants and children, and also those changes that may accompany childhood diseases.

The many disorders of the gastrointestinal system during infancy and childhood are varied and may require surgical treatment. Some disorders may be present in patients who require anesthesia for operation on an unrelated lesion. Hence, the anesthesiologist must recognize the pathophysiological changes that may accompany pediatric gastrointestinal disease. Some lesions may demand special attention because of their potential to complicate the course of anesthesia. Some diseases that are relatively common in pediatric practice will be discussed because they are not frequently seen by anesthesiologists but have important anesthetic implications.

DEVELOPMENT OF GASTROINTESTINAL FUNCTION

After birth, the infant becomes dependent upon the gastrointestinal tract to provide nutrients, not only to provide for immediate energy requirements but also to sustain a period of rapid growth. The gastrointestinal tract, which has been relatively inactive in utero, must therefore rapidly assume its roles of digestion and absorption.

Intestinal motor activity is evident in the fetus. Swallowing movements begin during the second trimester, and swallowing is an important mechanism in the regulation of amniotic fluid volume. Maternal polyhydramnios frequently accompanies diseases that impair fetal swallowing (for example, esophageal atresia). Gastric emptying and small intestine motor activity develop in parallel, and by the time the infant is able to suck, coordinated gastric and small bowel movements are evident.[1] Delayed gastric emptying may accompany respiratory or cardiovascular disease in infants, especially in preterm infants.[2, 3]

Gastric secretions are present during the second trimester of intrauterine life but are not markedly acidic. The pH of gastric contents at birth is approximately 6 but falls rapidly during the first day of life.[4] Pepsin activity develops during the third trimester, hence small preterm infants may have limited ability to digest protein.[5] The weight-corrected rate of secretion of both acid and pepsinogen is below 50 percent of adult levels for the first 3 months of life.

The digestive enzymes of the pancreas and small bowel appear in a recognized sequence during intrauterine development. The newborn infant is able to digest protein much better than starch or triglycerides. The level of trypsin activity is similar to that of the adult at 1 month of age, but the levels of lipase and amylase are very low. This sequence has important implications for the feeding of infants, especially the preterm baby,[6, 7] and formulas should be prepared accordingly.

The ability of the large intestine to conserve water and electrolytes is reduced in infants; this predisposes to the dehydration and electrolyte disturbance that accompany diarrhea.

The ability of the newborn infant to suck and swallow is a very important prerequisite for normal gastrointestinal function. The mature term neonate develops in a few days a suck-swallow pattern of feeding associated with effective esophageal peristalsis.[7] The small preterm infant may have an ineffective, immature suck-swallow pattern that will persist for weeks and will seriously compromise feeding. In the absence of effective oral intake, or when contraindications to normal feeding exist (e.g., esophageal disorders, persistent aspiration), tube feeding will be required. In these circumstances a nasogastric or gastrostomy tube is usually preferred as this will permit a more normal action of gastric acid and digestive enzymes and gastric hormonal responses. In patients at high risk of aspiration, however, the tube may be advanced through the pylorus into the jejunum. Gastric emptying times have been found to be similar in preterm infants whether they are fed by mouth or by nasogastric tube.[8]

COMMON SYMPTOMS OF GASTROINTESTINAL DISEASE

VOMITING AND REGURGITATION

Vomiting and regurgitation are common in infants up to 1 year of age. Regurgitation is often a result of faulty feeding technique, but if persistent it should suggest the possibility of a gastrointestinal disease. Vomiting in babies may result from many diseases but is especially common with infections and central nervous system disease. Mechanical obstruction of the digestive tract may result from congenital lesions such as duodenal atresia or congenital hypertrophic pyloric stenosis.

Vomiting in infants, if persistent, results in progressive fluid and electrolyte depletion. The high rate of fluid turnover in infancy dictates that these losses and the accompanying limited intake will rapidly lead to serious dehydration.

Prolonged vomiting leads to several changes in the extracellular fluid.[9] There is a metabolic alkalosis with a varying degree of compensation accompanied by low plasma chloride and potassium concentrations. In addition to these changes in composition, the extracellular fluid may be severely depleted in volume. It is most important that the volume and composition of the extracellular fluid be restored to near normal before induction of general anesthesia in infants. This will require administration of sodium chloride solution, together with appropriate amounts of added potassium chloride when a good urine flow is established. The withholding of oral feeding is also important in the treatment of a child who is vomiting. This decreases the stimulus for gastric secretions and thus decreases fluid and electrolyte losses.

DIARRHEA

Diarrhea is a common problem in infancy. The extent of fluid and electrolyte depletion will vary with the cause of the diarrhea and the extent to which fluid intake is also compromised.[10]

The electrolyte content of fluid losses resulting from diarrhea is lower with viral infections (for example, rotavirus infection) than with bacterial infections. Patients with diarrhea also lose potassium in the urine. The net result of diarrhea is a dehydration, which may be hypotonic, isotonic, or hypertonic, depending upon the extent of electrolyte losses. This dehydration is accompanied by acidosis caused by loss of fixed cations and bicarbonate. Hypertonic dehydration is of particular concern, as it may be accompanied by major fluid shifts affecting the brain and leading to serious neurological complications.

The treatment may require several days to complete. Hypertonic dehydration and acidosis must be corrected gradually if further serious complications are to be avoided.

MALNUTRITION AND GROWTH FAILURE

Infants and children with gastrointestinal disease may demonstrate varying degrees of nutritional deprivation. Diseases may cause anorexia, leading to inadequate intake, or may affect absorption of nutrients from the bowel. The normal term infant has a decreased capacity for digestive and absorptive functions, and the preterm infant has an even more limited capacity. Diseases that might affect gastrointestinal function are thus very significant in infancy, and the impact of malnutrition is most obvious at this stage.

The growing infant or child is an anabolic organism that cannot easily cope with starvation and catabolic states.[11] Parenteral nutrition, therefore, is necessary unless adequate nutrition can be maintained by nasogastric, jejunal, or duodenal feeding.

Malnutrition is common in many underdeveloped countries and may occur in developed countries among poor populations or as a result of diet fads[12] or parental neglect. Serious malnutrition may compromise recovery from a surgical procedure: wound healing is impaired[13] and the resistance to infection is decreased.[14] The ability of the pediatric patient to survive a critical surgical illness may be severely affected by malnutrition.[15] In North America, a population of pediatric surgical patients may include a significant percentage of malnourished children.[16] It has been suggested that a nutritional assessment should be included in the preoperative evaluation of all pediatric surgical patients.[17]

The advent of intravenous hyperalimentation techniques has made it possible to avoid many of the problems of severe nutritional depletion in pediatric surgical patients.

SEVERE MALNUTRITION (KWASHIORKOR)

Kwashiorkor usually appears soon after weaning and is due to an inadequate protein diet. This disease is common in underdeveloped and tropical countries, but cases also have occurred in North America.[18] The early clinical signs are lethargy and irritability. Anorexia, vomiting, and diarrhea are common. Later there is loss of muscle tissue and edema, with increased susceptibility to infection. The edema may conceal a failure of true weight gain. All children with kwashiorkor have a degree of anemia, but this is seldom severe. In late stages of the disease, hepatic enlargement with fatty infiltration is common. Mild hypoglycemia may occur secondary to impaired gluconeogenesis. The cardiovascular effects of kwashiorkor range from nonspecific electrocardiographic changes to congestive cardiac failure. Renal function is characterized by reduced renal blood flow, low glomerular filtration rate, and poor tubular function. Hyponatremia is commonly seen as a result of overhydration, and hypokalemia may result from diminished body stores of potassium. Mental changes of apathy, progressing to stupor, coma, and death, occur in the late stages of the disease. The principles of treatment of kwashiorkor are supplementation of nonprotein calories and the gradual restoration of an adequate protein intake. An initial high-protein diet may result in liver enlargement, hypoglycemia, and less rapid recovery.

The important considerations for the anesthesiologist in managing children with kwashiorkor are the reduced plasma protein levels, altered fluid and electrolyte status, reduced muscle mass, and impaired cardiovascular function. Patients with severe disease may be markedly hypovolemic despite overhydration. Drugs that are normally extensively protein-bound in the plasma (for example, barbiturates and muscle relaxants) should be given very cautiously in reduced dosage.

Although kwashiorkor demonstrates all the features of malnutrition from inadequate dietary intake, similar changes may also occur as a result of defective alimentary tract function.

GASTROINTESTINAL BLEEDING

Bleeding from the gastrointestinal tract in infants and children has many causes. In the neonate, the most common cause of upper gastrointestinal bleeding is gastroduodenitis, often as a result of salicylate therapy.[19] Another cause in the newborn infant is stress ulcers, which may be related to the relatively high gastric acidity in the first few days of life. Neonates with upper gastrointestinal bleeding very rarely require operation.

Other causes of gastrointestinal bleeding in the infant include hemorrhagic disease of the newborn, for which vitamin K therapy is indicated. In addition, necrotizing enterocolitis (see page 303), midgut volvulus, and infectious diarrhea may cause bleeding. Anal fissure is a very common cause of bleeding in infants under 1 year of age and may require surgical excision.[20] Intussusception results in loss of blood and mucus in feces (red currant jelly stool) and usually occurs in patients under 2 years of age.

In older children, vomited blood may have been previously swallowed (for example, during a nosebleed) or may be a result of peptic ulceration or, more rarely, esophageal varices. Lower gastrointestinal bleeding may occur from Meckel's diverticulum, intestinal duplication, or polyp. Hemangiomas of the gastrointestinal tract may result in major blood loss and are often associated with cutaneous lesions, as in Osler-Rendu-Weber disease or Klippel-Trenaunay syndrome.

Stress ulceration may be a cause of bleeding seen in both the neonatal and the pediatric intensive care units. It is particularly common in pediatric burn patients (Curling's ulcer) and in association with lesions of the central nervous system (Cushing's ulcer). Prophylaxis against stress ulceration is important for all patients at risk. It may consist of cimetidine, 2.5 mg/kg every 6 hours,[21] or antacids (e.g., Maalox, Gelusil), or a combination of both. Gastric pH should be monitored and maintained at 5 or above. Massive gastric bleeding due to a stress ulcer may require surgical exploration or radiographic embolization.[22] In such patients regurgitation of blood during induction of anesthesia is a major concern. Large-bore intravenous cannulation and a large volume of blood for transfusion must be provided. All blood should be warmed, and the coagulation indices should be regularly monitored during the procedure. Dilutional thrombocytopenia should be anticipated and preparations to obtain platelet concentrates made prior to surgery.

DISEASES OF THE ESOPHAGUS

The esophagus is 3 to 5.5 inches in length in the full-term newborn infant, and its lumen is 4 to 6 mm in diameter. The development of effective peristaltic waves in the wall of the esophagus normally occurs as the infant acquires a normal sucking pattern. The lower esophageal sphincter is relatively incompetent in infants.[23] The sphincter tone is poor and relaxation is prolonged during swallowing, thus gastroesophageal reflux is common.

ESOPHAGEAL ATRESIA

The problems of tracheoesophageal fistula are considered in Chapter 5. When esophageal atresia occurs without a fistulous connection with the trachea, the segment of atretic esophagus is often too long to permit primary anastomosis.[24] The usual management is to perform a gastrostomy for feeding and to attempt to lengthen the upper segment by bougienage. Alternatively, circular myotomies to lengthen the esophageal segments may be performed. Some infants lacking a long segment of esophagus will require a replacement procedure, using a gastric tube or colon interposition. Such a procedure is usually delayed until the child is 1 or more years of age.

ESOPHAGEAL DUPLICATIONS

Duplication cysts of the esophagus usually present as an expanding mass originating in the posterior mediastinum. Because of their proximity to the airway, cyanosis and dyspnea may occur together with dysphagia and sometimes vomiting. Cysts that do not communicate with the esophagus contain clear, thick fluid and may grow to a large size. Communicating cysts may contain gastric mucosa and discharge into the esophagus, causing esophagitis and erosion, which may lead to hematemesis. Esophageal duplication may be associated with cervical spine anomalies, including Klippel-Feil syndrome. The treatment of esophageal duplication is by surgical excision. During the operation the anesthesiologist must be alert to the possibility of surgical retraction causing obstruction of the airway and must continuously monitor ventilation.

GASTROESOPHAGEAL REFLUX

A large percentage of infants regurgitate, possibly as a result of poorly coordinated responses to swallowing and a low lower esophageal sphincter (LES) pressure.[25] As the child grows, the LES pressure normally increases, and regurgitation of stomach contents lessens. Some infants and children, however, have persistent gastroesophageal reflux (GER), which results in serious illness.[26] Many children with GER also have a hiatus hernia, but GER is not an inevitable consequence of hiatus hernia, and serious GER may occur without it.

Older children with GER will complain of symptoms of chest pain and heartburn. Young infants demonstrate regurgitation that is effortless, in contrast to the active vomiting that occurs with pyloric stenosis. Persistent and copious regurgitation results in failure to thrive. The low pH of regurgitated material causes esophagitis, which may lead to bleeding with consequent hematemesis and iron deficiency anemia; eventually stricture may ensue. Gastroesophageal reflux may also lead to pulmonary disease; recurrent aspiration pneumonia and chronic cough and wheezing may be present. GER has also been implicated in neonatal apnea and sudden infant death syndrome.[27]

The medical management of the patient with GER consists of frequent feeding with thickened food, and maintenance of the semiupright posture for a period after each feed. Metoclopramide may be used to increase the LES pressure, and antacids or cimetidine may reduce gastric acidity. Failure of medical therapy to control the serious effects of GER or the presence of a major anatomical abnormality of the gastroesophageal junction is considered to be an indication for operation.

Nissen's fundoplication, which is commonly performed for this condition, consists of encircling the lower esophagus with the fundus of the stomach. The indications for this procedure are failure to thrive with medical management as outlined earlier, esophagitis or stricture, and apneic episodes or pulmonary problems secondary to GER. The anesthesiologist managing patients for this procedure should be aware of the possibility of reflux and aspiration during induction of anesthesia. Preoperatively, cimetidine and antacids should be administered. A rapid sequence induction with cricoid pressure should be performed to secure the airway. Many of the children presenting for this operation also have cerebral palsy (CP), but succinylcholine may safely be used in the child with CP.[28]

During the operation a nasogastric tube is passed before the repair and left in for postoperative management. This should be very carefully secured as it will be very difficult to reintroduce after the fundoplication operation if it should be accidentally removed. In patients who are suspected of having associated delayed gastric emptying, a pyloroplasty is also performed. Some patients with severe pulmonary problems associated with repeated aspiration may benefit from a period of postoperative ventilation and respiratory intensive care.

After operation some patients may suffer gastric distention and inability to vomit or burp. This problem may persist for 2 to 3 months after operation and may require gastric aspiration.[29]

HIATUS HERNIA

Hiatus hernia in infants and children is most commonly of the "sliding" type, in which the upper portion of the stomach is drawn into the thoracic cavity by what appears to be a short esophagus. The theory of the "congenital short esophagus" is no longer accepted, but the shortening may be acquired as a result of esophagitis or stricture. Hiatus hernia may be more common in children with cerebral palsy. Sandifer's syndrome consists of hiatus hernia and torticollis. The rumination syndrome, characterized by regurgitation of gastric contents into the mouth and subsequent reswallowing after chewing, may occur with hiatus hernia.

Paraesophageal hiatus hernia with an abnormally situated gastroesophageal junction is much rarer and produces abdominal pain and distention. Operation is indicated because of the risk of strangulation of the herniated stomach.

Anesthetic management for hiatus hernia is the same as for gastroesophageal reflux (see earlier).

ACHALASIA OF THE CARDIA

Achalasia, or cardiospasm, may occur in children,[30] but it is not usually associated with the voluminous dilation of the esophagus that is seen in adults. There is, however, some dilation of the proximal esophagus and a narrow distal segment. Esophageal motility studies show an absence of peristalsis and a failure of the lower esophageal sphincter to relax on swallowing. Achalasia in childhood produces severe growth retardation, and the extent of pulmonary symptoms due to aspiration is more severe than in adults.[31] The treatment of this condition is by operative myotomy (Heller's operation) or by intraesophageal balloon disruption of the constricted cardia. Myotomy is generally preferred in younger children. Gastroesophageal reflux may follow operation.

The anesthetic management of the patient with achalasia should consider the possibility of retained food and secretions within the dilated esophagus. A rapid sequence induction following a careful period of fasting is recommended.

Opitz-Frias syndrome (G syndrome, hypospadias-dysphagia syndrome) includes achalasia of the cardia plus craniofacial and genital anomalies.[32] Repeated episodes of pulmonary aspiration occur and may be fatal. Endotracheal intubation may be difficult owing to the craniofacial deformity, and thus a rapid sequence induction is not possible. It should also be noted that children with this condition have laryngeal hypoplasia[33] and may accept only a very small endotracheal tube.[32] Anesthetic management must include careful preoperative fasting, antacid and cimetidine therapy, and preoperative gastric and esophageal aspiration with a nasogastric tube, followed by a careful inhalation induction of anesthesia. A selection of endotracheal tube sizes should be available. By this means the danger of regurgitation and aspiration can be minimized when applying a technique that is appropriate to a patient with a difficult airway problem.

DISEASES OF THE STOMACH AND DUODENUM

VOLVULUS OF THE STOMACH

Gastric volvulus is a rare condition, usually occurring in the neonatal period, but it may occur throughout childhood. It is due to laxity or absence of the gastric ligaments.[34] The volvulus may be along the axis of the stomach (organoaxial type) or involve the mesentery of that organ (mesenterioaxial type). In either case the disease may progress to gangrene and perforation of the stomach. If there is an associated defect in the diaphragm, the gastric volvulus may be intrathoracic. Acute and subacute or chronic cases are reported.

In acute volvulus, the presenting symptoms are persistent regurgitation and vomiting, but respiratory distress may also be prominent.[31] The inability to pass a nasogastric tube or resistance to its advancement is characteristic of the condition. Bleeding may accompany the volvulus as an early symptom.

It is most important that the diagnosis of gastric volvulus be established rapidly. Operation is urgent, to reduce the volvulus and anchor the stomach before ischemic damage occurs. Appropriate fluid resuscitation should be achieved prior to induction of anesthesia, and precautions should be taken to prevent the possibility of regurgitation and aspiration during induction. Awake intubation or a rapid sequence induction is recommended.

In older children, gastric volvulus may present as a chronic recurring disease with episodes of intermittent abdominal pain related to eating.[35]

RUPTURE OF THE STOMACH

Rupture of the stomach is most common in the neonatal period and is usually iatrogenic, though it may occur spontaneously.[36] The cause of spontaneous rupture is unknown, but the condition may be related to birth asphyxia, hypoxia, and stress. The usual site of perforation is near the greater curvature on the fundus of the stomach. Boys appear to be affected more commonly than girls.

Perforation of the stomach due to necrotizing gastritis may also occur in infancy. The etiology of this condition is unknown, but it is speculated that gastric ischemia complicating severe septic shock may result in damage to the gastric mucosa, which is followed by necrosis and perforation.[37]

The clinical presentation is usually with lassitude, poor feeding, and abdominal distention. In addition, the infant may show respiratory distress. Radiological studies demonstrate pneumoperitoneum and absence of the normal gastric air bubble. The infant may progress rapidly to a state of severe shock; the mortality rate for this condition is high. Prompt, efficient resuscitation and early operation are required. Nitrous oxide should not be used for general anesthesia in these infants, as there may be considerable free air in the peritoneal cavity. Pncumomcdiastinum has also been reported in association with acute gastric rupture.[36]

HYPERTROPHIC PYLORIC STENOSIS

Congenital hypertrophic pyloric stenosis is one of the common gastrointestinal defects of infancy. First-born male patients are most commonly affected, and the incidence is much higher in children of affected parents. The overall incidence may approach 1 in 300 live births, but there are considerable regional variations.

The symptoms usually commence at 2 to 3 weeks of age. Bile-free vomiting occurs, which progresses to become projectile and occurs after every feeding. On examination the infant displays a degree of dehydration that is related to the severity and duration of the symptoms. Visible peristalsis across the left upper quadrant and palpation of a pyloric mass are diagnostic of the disease.[38] Associated anomalies of the renal system may be present in a small percentage of patients.[39] Elevated levels of unconjugated bilirubin may occur in up to 17 percent of patients. This is thought to be due to decreased glucuronyl transferase activity in the liver.[40] Serum bilirubin levels fall rapidly after pyloromyotomy.

Management of the infant with hypertrophic

pyloric stenosis begins with correction of fluid and biochemical derangements. There is never an indication for urgent or emergency operation.[38] Serum electrolyte determinations will demonstrate a hypochloremic metabolic alkalosis secondary to the loss of chloride and hydrogen ions. Hypokalemia may also be present because of an intracellular shift of potassium with alkalosis. As the condition of alkalosis persists, potassium may also be lost via the kidneys, and severe hypokalemia may result.[41]

Optimal preparation of the child with pyloric stenosis for operation may take several days. Oral feeding should be stopped and a nasogastric tube inserted and connected to gentle suction. Discontinuing oral feeding will decrease secretion of gastric juices and thus decrease electrolyte losses. The management of fluid and electrolyte replacement therapy is based on the extent of the deficit. In general, the greater the deficit, the greater the role for sodium chloride in replacement fluids. In a patient with only a mild deficit, rehydration may be carried out with maintenance fluid and electrolytes. Moderate dehydration requires the use of a solution of 5 percent dextrose with half-normal saline infused at 1.5 times normal maintenance rates. Severe dehydration requires the rapid infusion of normal saline (20 ml/kg) followed by an infusion of 5 percent dextrose with normal saline at 1.5 times maintenance rates. Potassium chloride, 3 to 5 mEq/kg/day, should be added to these fluids once adequate urine flow is established (1 ml/kg/h or more). The fluid therapy must be reassessed as the patient's condition improves. Dextrose infusions must be continued until oral feeding is established postoperatively, or serious hypoglycemia may result.[42]

Prior to accepting the patient for general anesthesia, the anesthesiologist should check to ensure that the fluid and electrolyte status is fully corrected. There should be no clinical signs of dehydration, a good urine output, and serum electrolytes and acid base values within normal values. Vitamin K should be given intravenously, as some infants with pyloric stenosis have been demonstrated to have prolonged prothrombin times as a result of impaired uptake of vitamin K from the bowel.

Anesthetic management should commence with preoxygenation, followed by passage of a soft gastric tube to empty the stomach. This should be done even if a nasogastric tube has been in place and will often reveal additional stomach fluid content. Lavage of the stomach with normal saline has been recommended but is not usually necessary. A rapid sequence induction is recommended to secure the airway. At the end of the operation the infant should be awake and vigorous prior to extubation, which should be performed with the patient in a lateral position.

The patient usually can be fed on the first postoperative day. Hypoglycemia may occur 2 to 3 hours postoperatively,[42] because of depletion of liver glycogen stores. Hence intravenous fluids should be continued until oral intake is established. Respiratory depression in the postoperative period has also been described.[43] This may be a result of alterations in cerebrospinal fluid pH. The child should therefore be in a closely supervised nursing area.

DUODENAL OBSTRUCTION

Duodenal obstruction may result from an intrinsic block or from extrinsic compression. Intrinsic obstruction may be due to duodenal atresia or stenosis, the latter often due to a web. There is a high incidence of duodenal atresia in Down's syndrome. Extrinsic causes of duodenal compression and obstruction include malrotation, Ladd's bands, or an annular pancreas.[44]

Infants with duodenal atresia present early in life with bile-stained vomiting and little or no abdominal distention. Duodenal atresia is treated by duodenoduodenostomy.

Malrotation of the intestines predisposes to midgut volvulus. The infant with this condition commonly presents with abdominal distention, bloody stools, and peritonitis, with hypovolemic shock. Such patients require fluid resuscitation prior to urgent laparotomy. Awake intubation or a rapid sequence induction should be performed because of the danger of regurgitation. If there is doubt about the viability of the bowel, the abdomen may be closed and a "second look" procedure planned for 24 or 48 hours later. In this case the infant may require intensive medical support between operations.

DISEASES OF THE SMALL BOWEL

MECONIUM ILEUS

In this condition the small bowel is blocked by thick, inspissated meconium. This condition is almost always associated with cystic fibrosis, but it may very rarely occur as an isolated lesion.[45] The disease is thought to be due to abnormally viscid secretions of intestinal glands.[46] The infant presents with abdominal distention and a failure to pass meconium. The intestines may be palpable through the abdominal wall, and a radiograph demonstrates a granular appearance of the bowel. A sweat chloride determination will determine the presence of cystic fibrosis. Meconium ileus may be complicated by the presence of ileal atresia, perforation, or meconium peritonitis.

The treatment of uncomplicated meconium ileus may be medical, using a diatrizoate meglumine (Gastrografin) enema.[47] This may be successful in producing disimpaction in up to 50 percent of patients. Other patients require laparotomy, in which case enterostomy and irrigation of the bowel lumen with acetylcysteine solution may be effective. Hypernatremia has been reported with the use of this technique in a small preterm infant, probably secondary to the high sodium content of the acetylcysteine preparation.[48] Alternatively, bowel resection may be required. The anesthetic management of these infants must recognize the potential for postoperative pulmonary problems. A rapid sequence induction or awake intubation should be performed to safeguard the airway. Warmed, humidified anesthetic gases should be used with careful aseptic technique in suctioning the endotracheal tube.

Postoperative problems to be anticipated in the child with meconium ileus include pneumonia, septicemia, and prolonged bowel dysfunction. Intensive respiratory care and chest physiotherapy must be commenced early, together with appropriate antibiotic therapy for infection.

INTESTINAL DUPLICATION

This most commonly occurs in the region of the small intestine. The infant presents with abdominal distention, a mass, and possible signs of gastrointestinal bleeding. The diagnosis may be difficult to confirm prior to exploratory operation. The treatment is excision of the duplicate segment, which may involve resection of adjacent bowel.

NEONATAL NECROTIZING ENTEROCOLITIS

Necrotizing enterocolitis (NEC) is a major cause of mortality and morbidity of preterm and small for gestational age (SGA) infants and is occasionally fatal in term infants as well.[49, 49a] The incidence varies considerably between different units, and this may be related to feeding practices or other factors. The mortality rate from NEC is 30 to 50 percent.[50]

Patients with NEC often have a history of intrauterine fetal distress or birth asphyxia or both,[51] or maternal exposure to cocaine. A history of respiratory distress syndrome, apnea of prematurity, umbilical artery catheterization, or patent ductus arteriosus may be obtained. The role of all these factors in the etiology of NEC is thought to be due to their potential to reduce the mesenteric flow of oxygenated blood.[52]

The method of feeding and diet may also influence the disease.[52] The presence of a feeding tube and the enteral food may cause mechanical trauma and favor the multiplication and colonization by pathogens. In addition, the type of food may promote the growth of specific bacteria. The fermentation of lactose may produce gas and acidosis. Eventually, the combination of an ischemic bowel injury and bacterial infection permits endotoxins to pass into the bloodstream. Finally, intestinal perforation or infarction may result.

The epidemiology of the disease and the initial septic manifestations strongly suggest an infective etiology for NEC. Attempts to identify a specific bacterial pathogen for NEC have been unsuccessful, but the fact that the gas present in the bowel wall has a high percentage of hydrogen favors an infective component to the etiology.[53] Cultures from the intestinal contents of affected infants have grown many different organisms, including gas-forming bacilli such as *Clostridium perfringens*. However, this organism is also a normal bowel inhabitant in healthy infants.[54, 55] It is possible that many organisms that are cultured from NEC patients are not, in fact, the principal pathogen but are opportunistic colonizers of the diseased bowel. It is suspected that the absence of a "normal" bowel flora might also be an important etiological factor. In summary, the etiology of NEC is thought to involve intestinal ischemia leading to mucosal injury, plus infection, and possibly the effect of enteral feeding, in the presence of immature intestinal function.

The clinical signs of NEC include gastric retention of food, thermal instability, and abdominal distention, often with loose, blood-streaked stools. These signs usually appear in the first few days of life and 2 to 3 days after the initiation of feeding. In addition, the infant may appear pale and lethargic and may suffer apnea if not on intermittent positive-pressure ventilation. Later in the disease the infant may show evidence of septic shock and disseminated intravascular coagulation (DIC). Early radiological examination of the abdomen demonstrates distended, gas-filled loops of bowel and later the appearance of pneumatosis intestinalis, gas in the wall of the intestine.

The medical treatment of NEC must be initiated promptly. At the first sign of the disease, oral feeding is discontinued and a nasogastric tube is inserted to provide continuous suction. Fluids, electrolytes, and calories must be provided intravenously. Antibiotics effective against gram-negative enteric organisms should be administered via the nasogastric tube. Gentamicin and colistin are the most commonly used drugs.[49] The drug selected is given every 4 hours, and the nasogastric tube is clamped for 1 hour following each dose. If the disease progresses and signs of sepsis appear, blood cultures are often positive.[56] The patients require systemic antibiotic therapy, and because their humoral immune response is inadequate, they should also receive fresh plasma. Septic shock must be treated by restoration of the intravascular volume, corticosteroids (hydrocortisone, 35 to 50 mg/kg), and inotropic drugs. DIC is common and usually requires exchange transfusion.

The indications for surgical intervention have been a matter of some controversy, but there is some general agreement that bowel perforation evidenced by pneumoperitoneum demands operation.[57] Additional indications include a paracentesis positive for gangrene (0.5 ml or more of fluid that is brown or contains bacteria), abdominal wall erythema, a fixed abdominal mass, or a persistently dilated loop of bowel on serial radiographs.[56] Some very small and unstable infants may be treated by simply inserting a peritoneal drain under local analgesia in the neonatal ICU.[58]

The successful anesthetic management of the patient with NEC must begin with a thorough preoperative evaluation, followed by appropriate therapy to optimize the status of the infant. Many such patients may already be receiving respiratory support, and this must be carefully maintained. Fluid resuscitation is required to correct hypovolemic shock, and fresh blood and platelet concentrates must be administered to restore coagulation mechanisms.

If the infant is not yet intubated, induction of anesthesia and endotracheal intubation should be planned to avoid the possibility of regurgitation and aspiration, as well as to minimize the physiological response to intubation. Awake endotracheal intubation of newborn infants has been demonstrated to result in a large increase in intracranial pressure.[59] In the very sick preterm infant, this might well lead to intracranial hemorrhage. Intubation should preferably be facilited by a relaxant drug and preceded by a very small dose of intravenous barbiturate (for example, thiopentone, 2 to 3 mg/kg). Anesthesia should be maintained using fentanyl or low concentrations of isoflurane, with a nondepolarizing neuromuscular blocking drug. Appropriate concentrations of oxygen in air should be delivered to maintain an arterial saturation of 90 to 95 percent.[60] Nitrous oxide should not be given, as this may increase the size of gas bubbles in the submucosa and porta hepatis.[61] Once the abdomen is opened, the patient may become hypotensive and require large volumes of intravenous fluid to maintain the blood pressure. This is presumably associated with the passage of large volumes of fluid into the diseased bowel.

INTUSSUSCEPTION

An intussusception consists of a segment of bowel that has entered the lumen of the adjacent distal bowel and produced an obstruction. This is the most common cause of obstruction after infancy until the age of 5 years. The obstructing segment of bowel may pass for some distance into the distal bowel and may become ischemic and gangrenous. Viral infection, often with adenovirus, is frequently found in association with intussusception, and enlarged Peyer's patches are thought to provide the lead point.

The clinical presentation is usually with sudden onset of abdominal pain, vomiting, and passing of blood and mucus in the stool. Frequently a sausage-shaped mass can be palpated in the abdomen. Though most cases are idiopathic, intussusception may also occur secondary to Meckel's diverticulum, tumors, suture lines, and duplications and may be associated with cystic fibrosis and Henoch-Schönlein purpura.

The diagnosis of intussusception is confirmed by radiological study of a contrast enema, which may also serve to reduce the intussusception. If this fails, a second attempt at hydrostatic reduction under anesthesia may be successful.[62] Inhalation anesthetics may aid in this process by decreasing smooth muscle activity in the bowel, relaxing abdominal wall muscles, and decreasing splanchnic blood flow.[62] Pneumatic pressure enemas have also been used to reduce intussusception. Air or oxygen is introduced under controlled pressure into the lower bowel and is successful in a high percentage of patients.[63]

This treatment has often been carried out under general anesthesia, and though it raises concerns for the possibility of gas embolism, this complication apparently has not been a problem. Nitrous oxide, however, should be avoided as it may certainly affect the volume of gas in the bowel, and it is contraindicated in the presence of even a remote risk of air embolism.

Indications for laparotomy[64] include signs of peritonitis, obstruction, and failed reduction by enema. Repeated intussusception is also treated surgically after the third episode.

The anesthesiologist must critically analyze the state of hydration of the child prior to operation. However, it may be necessary to proceed with an emergency laparotomy immediately if the viability of the affected bowel is in doubt. In such a case, vigorous fluid resuscitation must accompany the anesthetic. A rapid sequence induction is indicated to avoid the danger of aspiration.[65] If gangrenous bowel is present, this will require resection. Blood and fluid replacement must be carefully managed during the operation to correct losses.

MECKEL'S DIVERTICULUM AND PERSISTENT OMPHALOMESENTERIC DUCT

The omphalomesenteric duct extends from the embryo into the yolk sac. This duct normally undergoes complete degeneration but may persist in part or very rarely in toto. Partial persistence is seen as a Meckel's diverticulum or as a cystic remnant in the abdominal wall. Total persistence presents in the newborn infant as an omphalomesenteric duct, with fecal discharge at the umbilicus. An obliterated but persistent omphalomesenteric duct may precipitate a volvulus. A persistent omphalomesenteric duct must be surgically excised from the abdominal wall to the bowel.

Meckel's diverticulum is the most common remnant to persist and may be present in 2 percent of the population. The diverticulum produces symptoms only if complications occur. These include bleeding, intestinal obstruction, or perforation.[66] The incidence of major complications of Meckel's diverticulum is equal to that of appendicitis in infants under 2 years of age. Bleeding from Meckel's diverticulum can be very profuse and lead to serious hypovolemic shock. The bleeding originates in ectopic gastric mucosa occurring in the diverticulum. Obstruction may be due to intussusception of the diverticulum or to volvulus around it. Perforation of a Meckel's diverticulum is usually at the site of a peptic ulcer in the ectopic gastric mucosa.

The anesthesiologist should carefully assess the fluid status of the child preoperatively. Blood losses may lead to anemia and in some cases to significant hypovolemia. Peritonitis may be present and lead to further fluid deficit. Restoration of an adequate circulating blood volume and hematocrit must precede induction of anesthesia. In all patients with an acute abdomen, the airway should be rapidly secured at induction of anesthesia.

MAJOR ABDOMINAL WALL DEFECTS

OMPHALOCELE AND GASTROSCHISIS

Omphalocele (or exomphalos) is a congenital herniation of abdominal contents at the umbilicus. The contents are usually covered by a thin membrane that is composed of the fused layers of the amnion and the peritoneum. This membrane may rupture prior to or at birth. The omphalocele, if small, may contain only small bowel. If large, it may contain the liver, spleen, stomach, and other abdominal organs. Omphalocele occurs in approximately 1 in 6000 live births, and in 30 percent of cases it will be associated with other congenital anomalies. These most commonly affect the gastrointestinal, cardiovascular, genitourinary, or central nervous system.

The Beckwith-Wiedemann syndrome consists of omphalocele, macroglossia, and visceromegaly.[67] Thirty to fifty percent of infants with this syndrome may develop hypoglycemia, which has been demonstrated to be secondary to islet call hyperplasia and resultant hyperinsulinemia.[68] The danger of hypoglycemia may persist beyond the neonatal period into the first years of life. In addition to hyperinsulinism, patients with this syndrome may show an excessive insulin response to intravenous glucose, resulting in severe rebound hypoglycemia. Glucose should therefore be administered by constant infusion (6 to 8 mg/kg/min) and not by bolus injection. Blood glucose determinations should be repeated regularly. Infants with Beckwith-Wiedemann syndrome usually lose the tendency to hypoglycemia as they grow older, but in some patients persistent symptoms may require partial or subtotal pancreatectomy.

Gastroschisis is a full-thickness abdominal wall defect usually situated to the right of a normal umbilical cord. The herniated abdominal contents are not covered by a membrane. Gastroschisis is frequently an isolated lesion with no other congenital defects. Because omphalocele and gastroschisis pose similar problems and require similar treatment, they are usually considered together.

Infants with major abdominal wall defects may suffer significant heat loss and major fluid shifts into exposed bowel. Intestinal function is often slow to become established, and prolonged periods of intravenous alimentation may be required. The initial treatment of these lesions consists of covering the exposed bowel with sterile moist gauze and a plastic sheet. This will prevent further infection and limit heat and fluid loss from exposed viscera. A nasogastric tube should be inserted to prevent intestinal distention. Warmed intravenous fluids (clear and colloid) should be administered to restore deficits. The volumes of fluid required may be high because of evaporative loss from exposed bowel and third-space losses into the intestines.[69] The possibility of Beckwith-Wiedemann syndrome should be recognized and a blood glucose estimation performed if any signs of the syndrome or of clinical hypoglycemia are apparent. An infusion of 10 percent dextrose to provide 6 to 8 mg of dextrose/kg/min should be commenced, supplemented by administration of balanced salt solution to replace third-space losses. The volume administered must be judged by the responses seen in the patient's vital signs.

The optimal surgical management of abdominal wall defects is still the subject of some controversy. Primary closure is favored by many surgeons,[70] whereas some prefer staged closures[71] using a prosthetic sac as a temporary cover for the viscera. If primary closure is planned, the patient usually will require continued paralysis and mechanical ventilation into the postoperative period for 24 to 48 hours or more. The proponents of primary closure suggest that this procedure leads to reduced complications of sepsis, sac dehiscence, and prolonged ileus. Primary closure is usually preceded by intraoperative manual stretching of the abdominal wall. The proponents of staged closure suggest that this technique avoids subjecting abdominal viscera to compression and removes the need for prolonged ventilation. In fact, reported results show little difference in overall outcome between the two methods.[70, 71] The overall improvement in survival for infants with abdominal wall defects is considered to be due to improved surgical techniques, the use of intravenous alimentation, and progress in neonatal intensive care.[71] Broad-spectrum antibiotics are usually administered prior to operation.

The decision as to whether the infant will tolerate primary closure may be assisted by measuring intragastric pressure (IGP) during closure. If the defect can be closed with a resulting IGP of 20 mm Hg or lower, primary closure is likely possible. If higher IGP results after closure, abdominal organ blood flow will be compromised, leading to intestinal ischemia and oliguria or anuria.[72] Increased intra-abdominal pressure also compromises hepatic blood flow and results in impaired clearance of narcotic analgesics and other drugs metabolized in the liver.[73]

Prior to induction of anesthesia, the anesthesiologist should ensure that the patient has received optimal fluid replacement. A secure airway should be rapidly established, either by awake intubation or a rapid sequence induction, since regurgitation and aspiration are a danger. Nitrous oxide should not be used, but air and oxygen is provided in proportions to assure optimal PaO_2 or oxygen saturation. Low concentrations of volatile general anesthetic agents and full doses of relaxant drugs should be administered. Ventilation must be carefully controlled and adjusted as required during closure to compensate for increased intra-abdominal pressure. At the end of the procedure, after primary closure, a nasotracheal tube is left in place and controlled ventilation is continued.

PRUNE BELLY SYNDROME

This syndrome almost exclusively affects boys and consists of congenital deficiency of abdominal muscles, urinary tract dilation, and undescended testicles. Other congenital defects may occur in association with the syndrome, including malrotation of the gut, pulmonary hypoplasia, cardiac defects, dislocation of the hip, and club feet. Infants are divided into three groups according to the severity of the disease.[74] Group I infants have severe renal and pulmonary defects that are incompatible with survival. Those in group II have very severe uropathy and will require extensive reconstructive surgery. Infants in group III are healthy as neonates and will require little surgical therapy.

The diagnosis is usually obvious at birth as a result of the lax, wrinkled abdominal wall and bilateral cryptorchidism. Patients in group II have poor renal function and grossly dilated ureters. These infants have disordered micturition and easily acquire renal tract infections.

Early high diversion of urine by pyelostomy or ureterostomy is frequently required. Renal function may be significantly impaired.

Group III patients are usually well at birth and demonstrate problems later, usually in association with renal tract infection.

In management of patients with prune belly syndrome, the anesthesiologist must recognize that these patients may have renal failure.[75] They also have a relatively poor cough mechanism owing to absent abdominal muscles and are prone to respiratory infections. Laryngeal atresia has been described in association with prune belly syndrome.[76] The airway should be rapidly secured with an endotracheal tube, as these patients may regurgitate stomach contents. Muscle relaxants are unnecessary for abdominal operation, but ventilation should be controlled, as spontaneous ventilation may be seriously impaired during anesthesia. Drugs excreted by the kidneys should be avoided. Postoperatively, the patient must be carefully managed to detect and treat impending pulmonary complications, which are a potential cause of mortality and morbidity.[77, 78]

NEONATAL CHOLESTATIC JAUNDICE

Defective bile excretion (cholestasis) in the newborn infant may result from hepatocellular disease or obstruction of the bile ducts.[79] Hepatocellular causes of neonatal cholestasis include infections (hepatitis B, cytomegalovirus, rubella, herpes, and so forth), metabolic diseases, endocrine diseases, drug toxicity, and miscellaneous other congenital and acquired defects. Obstruction of the bile ducts may result from atresia, stenosis, or hypoplasia of the ducts or from external compression (as in intestinal duplication). The clinical picture of persistent jaundice, hepatomegaly, pale stools, and dark urine is similar, whichever is the etiology. Also similar regardless of etiology are the biochemical features, which will include conjugated bilirubinemia (over 15 percent of total bilirubin), elevated total bilirubin, and elevated alkaline phosphatase and aspartate transaminase levels.

Jaundice is common in the newborn period and indeed is considered physiological. However, if this jaundice persists for more than 2 weeks, or if conjugated bilirubin levels are found to be elevated, the infant must be urgently investigated. Those infants whose cholestasis has an obstructive component require early surgical intervention if the best long-term outcome is to be obtained. The problem is to distinguish the infant with extrahepatic biliary obstruction from one with hepatocellular disease.[80] At present, there is no single ideal test to diagnose these conditions accurately, and even with multiple studies the diagnosis may be difficult to confirm. Some help in diagnosis may be obtained from the general medical history and the family history. Genetic disorders and metabolic diseases associated with specific syndromes may thus be detected. Ultrasound examination is used to define or exclude mass lesions (for example, choledochal cyst).

Radioisotope scanning using ^{99m}technetium with iminodiacetic acid (^{99m}Tc-IDA) after 5 days of phenobarbital pretreatment is a most valuable test. If the isotope appears in the intestine, the bile ducts are patent; however, failure of the isotope to appear is not conclusive evidence of biliary obstruction, as severe hepatocellular disease may also cause this. Percutaneous liver biopsy is therefore required as a complementary test. Fibrosis, bile duct proliferation, and canalicular bile stasis are consistent with a diagnosis of biliary obstruction.[80] The combined use of radioisotope excretion studies and percutaneous liver biopsy should permit identification of 95 percent of cases of extrahepatic biliary atresia.

BILIARY ATRESIA

The extent of obliteration of the bile ducts is variable. This led to division of patients into two groups, "surgically correctable" and "noncorrectable." Such a definitive classification is no longer accepted. It is now recognized that obliteration of the biliary system commences in the extrahepatic ducts and spreads to involve the whole system.[81] Intrahepatic ducts are usually patent during the first weeks of life but progressively become obliterated. The etiology of the disease remains unknown, but viral infection, metabolic abnormalities, and toxic effects of bile acids have been suggested as possible causes. The progressive nature of the disease explains why early operation is most effective.

The surgical treatment of biliary atresia (Kasai's operation) is to resect the extrahepatic bile ducts, including a fibrous mass at the porta hepatis when this is present. The liver at the porta hepatis is dissected to a depth of 2 to 3 mm, and a Roux-en-Y jejunal anastomosis to the porta hepatis is performed.[82] There is now general agreement that the earlier the age at operation, the greater is the chance of success.

The anesthetic management of the infant with

biliary atresia must include all measures that are normally followed for the sick neonate having major abdominal surgical treatment. In addition, the possibility of preexisting coagulopathy must be recognized, as must the fact that major blood losses may be caused by the surgical procedure. Absence of normal biliary function leads to impaired absorption of fat-soluble vitamins, including vitamin K; hence, prothrombin time may be prolonged. The infant should be treated with intramuscular vitamin K preoperatively, and fresh-frozen plasma should be available for the operation. Large-bore intravenous lines should be inserted into the upper limbs or neck for blood replacement during operation. All blood and intravenous fluids must be warmed. During exploration of the porta hepatis, retraction of the liver may restrict flow in the inferior vena cava and cause acute hypotension. The infant must be carefully monitored, therefore, to detect sudden changes in blood pressure. Positioning the patient in a slight Trendelenburg position may facilitate surgery and also optimize venous return via the inferior vena cava. The choice of anesthetic technique may include low concentrations of volatile agents, together with a nondepolarizing neuromuscular blocking drug. Halothane has been widely used in infants with biliary atresia without any apparent adverse effects. Curare or atracurium, may be used to provide relaxation.

The postoperative course of the infant with biliary atresia may be complicated.[83] Ascending cholangitis is common, particularly for the first few years after operation. Portal hypertension is a frequent sequela and may cause serious bleeding. Fifty to eighty percent of survivors may develop esophageal varices, but only five to ten percent have episodes of bleeding. The use of aspirin in these children may be very dangerous.[80] Recently injection of varices with sclerosing solutions has become the treatment of choice. Malabsorption from lack of bile may lead to poor growth, osteomalacia, and osteoporosis.

The overall results of Kasai's operation are rather dissappointing. It is suggested that only 20 to 30 percent of patients will be cured, and that many will develop chronic liver disease even if the initial bile flow via the portoenterostomy was good. This being so, and as many of these patients with a failed Kasai's operation will later be candidates for liver transplantation, it has been suggested that early transplantation might be a reasonable alternative to Kasai's procedure. It has been suggested that liver transplantation is more difficult and risky in the child who has had a previous Kasai's procedure. However, the number of suitable-sized donor livers is extremely limited. The consensus at present is that portoenterostomy and transplantation should be considered as complementary procedures, both of which may eventually have a place in each patient with biliary atresia.[84]

LIVER TRANSPLANTATION

The major advances in the control of rejection and in the techniques of liver transplantation over the past decade have made this treatment option acceptable for use in infants and children. A principal limiting factor is the shortage of suitable-sized donor organs, and it is suggested that all physicians who are involved with pediatric acute care have a vital role to play in identifying potential donors and in the procurement of suitable organs.[85]

The most common indication for liver transplantation in pediatric patients is biliary atresia, but transplantation may also be considered for metabolic diseases (including alpha$_1$-antitrypsin deficiency, glycogen storage diseases and so on), hepatitis, and liver tumors. Children with an unsuccessful Kasai's procedure and those who develop complications of recurrent cholangitis or gastrointestinal bleeding are candidates for transplantation. The patient with chronic liver disease should be seriously considered for transplantation when evidence of decreased hepatic synthetic function is present (e.g., low prothrombin level, low serum albumin). Supportive medical therapy should be provided to allow infants to grow to at least 1 year of age, if possible, prior to transplantation. The results are significantly better in patients of over 1 year who weigh more than 10 kg.[85]

The preoperative evaluation must determine the patient's suitability for transplantation. Serious infections, malignant disease, or significant pulmonary disease is a common contraindication. Pulmonary arteriovenous shunts with cyanosis are a rare complication of pediatric liver disease. The presence of any other chronic disease that will compromise the possibility of a successful transplant or the life expectancy of the child is also usually considered to be a contraindication. Angiography of the vascular connections of the liver is performed to determine the precise anatomy and detect any anomalies that may complicate the operation. The psychosocial factors that exist for the child and the family must be considered and appropriate support programs provided. In most centers, a specialized committee representing medical, nursing, social, administrative, and other fields is charged with the responsibility of assigning the current priority of individual patients for transplantation.

The preparation of the recipient for the operation must include the appropriate treatment of any existing coagulopathy, bowel preparation, and initiation of immunosuppression; high-dose steroid therapy is commenced before operation, and cyclosporine A is usually started either before or during operation. It should be noted that the absorption of oral cyclosporine appears to be delayed by general anesthesia, hence preoperative doses should be given several hours before induction if possible.

The major intraoperative anesthesia problems relate to blood volume replacement and cardiovascular instability, coagulation defects, metabolic derangements, and hypothermia.[86]

The blood losses may be very high (4 to 5 blood volumes or more), and are increased in young patients (less than 2.5 years) and those with elevated prothrombin time, acute liver disease, bleeding varices, or encephalopathy.[87] Adequate supplies of blood must be available. If the transplanted liver is from a donor of a different ABO blood type, exchange transfusion with plasma of the donor ABO group and cells of the recipient type may be given to decrease postoperative hemolysis.[88] Large-bore peripheral intravenous cannulae should be inserted into the upper extremities. An arterial line and a central venous pressure (CVP) line are essential, as are facilities to warm infused blood efficiently and very rapidly. A urinary catheter is inserted to monitor renal function. Frequent biochemical and hematological studies are required throughout the procedure, the results of which must be immediately available.

Anesthesia with isoflurane in oxygen and air is most commonly employed.[86] An atracurium infusion has been found to provide stable neuromuscular block during all phases of the operation. If pancuronium or vecuronium is given, the amount required is significantly decreased after removal of the liver.[89] In fact, as the procedure will be long and postoperative ventilation is planned, the choice of relaxant is not crucial, and the extended effect of pancuronium may be desirable. It is not surprising that the pharmacokinetics of the narcotic analgesics are altered after replacement of a diseased liver, but fentanyl and morphine are commonly used intraoperatively and postoperatively.

The operation can be divided into three stages. In the first stage, the diseased liver is mobilized to its vascular pedicle prior to removal. Secondly, there is an anhepatic stage from the time the circulation is interrupted until the donor liver is inserted. Finally, the neohepatic stage commences when the donor liver is reperfused.

In the first stage, the amount of bleeding is related to the patient's preoperative coagulation status and the extent of intra-abdominal adhesions from previous operation. The intravascular volume should be replaced as necessary to maintain the CVP, arterial blood pressure, and urine flow. The need to treat coagulopathy intraoperatively is not based simply on regular coagulation studies but should be coupled with observation of the surgical field; if oozing occurs, replacement therapy may be commenced.[86] Otherwise, surgical blood losses should simply be replaced as needed. Caution is advised in factor replacement, as vascular thrombosis of the transplanted liver is a common complication, especially in small children. Hence platelet infusions should be deferred, especially until the donor liver is revascularized. Cardiovascular instability may also occur during the first stage owing to surgical manipulation of the liver and consequent compression of the inferior vena cava, or to a low level of serum ionized calcium.

Maintenance of normal body temperature during the operation is very difficult. All the normal problems of the small child are compounded by the need for a large volume of transfusion fluid and the open abdomen. All usual measures to prevent heat losses should be carefully applied.

During the anhepatic phase, the inferior vena cava is clamped, and venous return to the heart from the lower body depends upon anastomotic channels, unless a venovenous bypass system is used. Such a system can maintain near normal circulatory hemodynamics and may reduce blood loss but may also introduce hazards of thromboembolism, air embolism, and increased heat loss. The value of venovenous bypass in small children is uncertain.

The metabolic changes that might occur during the anhepatic phase must be considered. Hypoglycemia was considered a danger but is seldom seen. Hyperglycemia is more common and may be due to several factors, including the glucose content of the large volume of infused blood together with decreased utilization. Blood glucose levels should be monitored and the use of glucose-containing intravenous fluids carefully controlled. Metabolic acidosis may occur as a result of peripheral circulatory changes and impaired metabolism of citrate, lactate, and other acids, together with the acid load of infused blood. Severe degrees of metabolic acidosis causing cardiovascular compromise should be corrected, using sodium bicarbonate, but caution is required as severe degrees of metabolic acidosis may occur postoperatively. This is largely a result of the metabolism of the citrate load accompanying massive blood transfusion.

On reperfusion of the donor liver, marked circulatory changes may occur. These are a result of the reintroduction into the circulation of the large hepatic vascular bed and accompanying infusion from the liver of vasoactive and cardiotoxic substances. Hypotension, bradycardia, atrial or ventricular arrhythmias, heart block, or cardiac arrest may occur. Hyperkalemia, hypocalcemia, and metabolic acidosis must be anticipated. Administration of sodium bicarbonate and calcium chloride prior to reperfusion of the donor liver, together with careful adjustment of preload, may minimize these changes, but other active measures, including vasopressors, may be required, especially in the first few minutes of reperfusion.

Hypertension commonly develops during the third stage of the procedure or in the early postoperative phase. The cause is thought to be multifactorial: a result of volume overload, combined with impaired renal function, associated with cyclosporine and steroid therapy.[90] Treatment is with salt restriction, diuretics, and angiotensin-converting enzyme inhibitors if there is a low creatinine excretion index.[90]

Impaired renal function following liver transplantation is common and is associated with a high mortality. Etiological factors include preexisting renal dysfunction, acute intraoperative fluctuations in renal perfusion due to changes in arterial and venous pressures, hemolysis, and drug effects. Optimal fluid therapy, together with mannitol or furosemide diuresis, may help preserve renal function, as may a low-dose dopamine infusion.[91]

Postoperatively, controlled ventilation is maintained for at least the first 12 hours. Pulmonary problems are common and demand aggressive therapy. Acid-base and coagulation abnormalities must be corrected and renal function optimized. Hypertension is a continuing problem. Early complications that may require reoperation include continued bleeding, impaired liver perfusion, and obstruction to bile drainage.

The patient is at very high risk of infection, due to preexisting debility, immunosuppression, massive transfusion, and invasive monitoring procedures. Viral infections (cytomegalovirus, Epstein-Barr, HIV), bacterial infections (pneumonia, cholangitis, peritoneal abcesses), and fungal infections are described; great care must be taken to ensure careful asepsis.

Neurological complications are also common following liver transplantation and may manifest as seizures. These may result from vascular changes, infection, metabolic derangements, or drug therapy.

Acute rejection may present in 7 to 14 days and is accompanied by nonspecific signs of headache, fever, malaise, nausea, and abdominal pain. Jaundice may increase, and the liver is tender. Liver enzyme levels may increase and synthetic functions diminish as evidenced by increased prothrombin time. Modification of the immunosuppressive drug regimen will be required, with possibly the addition of antilymphocyte globulin (ALG) or monoclonal antibody (e.g., OKT3).

Chronic rejection is more difficult to reverse and is heralded by the vanishing bile duct (VBD) syndrome. The liver becomes hard and fibrotic, and retransplantation is usually considered to be indicated.

CHOLEDOCHAL CYST

Choledochal cysts are most common in female infants and in Oriental races. The clinical presentation is usually with recurrent pain, fever, and sometimes jaundice, and usually the diagnosis is made in children under 10 years of age. In infants, jaundice may be the principal sign. Diagnosis is usually confirmed by ultrasound imaging or computed tomography. The "cyst" is most commonly a fusiform dilatation of the common bile duct.[92] If the condition has been undiagnosed until older childhood, the patient may have developed portal hypertension and cirrhosis. The surgical treatment is usually directed at total excision of the bile duct cyst, as there is a high risk of malignancy in remnant cyst wall. The implication of this for the anesthesiologist is that the operation may entail extensive dissection and commensurate blood loss. Large-bore intravenous routes via the upper limbs or neck veins should be established prior to the operation.

CHOLELITHIASIS

Infants who develop cholelithiasis often have a history of erythroblastosis fetalis, hyperbilirubinemia, parenteral nutrition, or furosemide therapy. The combination of intravenous hyperalimentation with furosemide therapy is particularly likely to result in cholelithiasis. It is thought that furosemide diminishes bile flow and promotes stasis. Older children with gallstones commonly have a history of hemoglobinopathy or cystic fibrosis.

DISEASES OF THE COLON AND RECTUM

HIRSCHSPRUNG'S DISEASE

Hirschsprung's disease is a congenital abnormality characterized by an absence of parasympathetic ganglion cells in a portion of the sigmoid colon and rectum.[93] Failure of peristalsis in the affected segment leads to functional obstruction, with dilatation and hypertrophy of the proximal colon.[1] There is a family history of the disease in up to 30 percent of patients. Associated conditions include Down's syndrome and other forms of mental retardation.

The diagnosis may be made in the neonatal period if the infant does not pass meconium but is often delayed until the child is several months of age. A history is obtained of chronic constipation, including anal fissure; hypothyroidism; adrenal insufficiency; and other endocrine and nutritional disorders. Confirmation of the diagnosis is by rectal biopsy, which will demonstrate aganglionosis in Hirschsprung's disease.

The surgical management of Hirschsprung's disease is by means of an initial colostomy, followed by a definitive repair when the child is about 1 year of age. This definitive operation consists of one or another form of a "pull-through" procedure.

ANORECTAL ANOMALIES

Agenesis or atresia of the anal canal may affect the entire canal or high, intermediate, or low segments of the canal. Anorectal malformations occur in 1 in 4500 births, with a slight preponderance in boys. The more serious types, involving a fistula from the colon to the genitourinary tract, are also more common in boys. In girls, imperforate anus may be associated with rectovaginal or rectocloacal fistula. Though there are many types of anorectal anomalies,[94] these tend to fall into two main groups based on the location of the blind end of the bowel: the high (supralevator) imperforate anus and the low (translevator) imperforate anus. In either group the rectal pouch may end blindly or communicate via a fistula with an adjacent viscus or the perineal surface.

Sixty percent of patients with anorectal anomalies also have other associated malformations. These most commonly affect the vertebral column (28 percent), the central nervous system (18 percent), the heart (9 percent), and other parts of the gastrointestinal tract (9 percent). Infants with imperforate anus are frequently born prematurely.

The surgical treatment of imperforate anus depends upon the type of anomaly. Low imperforate anus is treated by surgical incision into the pouch. A colostomy is unnecessary, and the outlook for bowel continence is very good. High imperforate anus is more difficult to treat, and the outlook for bowel continence is much less certain. A preliminary colostomy is usually performed and a definitive repair attempted when the infant is 6 to 12 months of age.

Correction of high imperforate anus, especially when this is associated with fistulous connections, requires a major surgical procedure, which may be associated with considerable blood loss. Recently the surgical approach has been by posterior sagittal anorectoplasty.[95] For this procedure, the patient is placed in a prone "jackknife" position. An electrostimulator may be used transcutaneously and within the operative wound to map the appropriate anal course by observation of contractions of sphincteric musculature. Though the electrostimulation is primarily direct to the muscle fibers, a clearer response may be seen if neuromuscular blocking drugs are withheld.

CONSIDERATIONS FOR THE ANESTHESIOLOGIST

ASSESSMENT OF HYDRATION

It has been stressed that it is most important for the anesthesiologist to assess accurately the degree of dehydration and/or the success of volume replacement when reviewing a patient prior to anesthesia. The fluid and electrolyte status should be determined by consideration of the clinical history, physical examination, and appropriate biochemical studies.[96]

The clinical history will provide some information on the duration of symptoms and the volumes of fluid losses from the gastrointestinal tract. It may also provide valuable information concerning recent weight loss, as each kilogram lost is approximately equal to 1 liter of fluid. A reduction in urine volume is an important sign of dehydration. The older child with dehydration may complain of severe thirst.

The physical examination is most important and can reveal much information concerning fluid status. In the infant, reliable signs of dehydration are a sunken fontanelle and loss of skin turgor. These signs will be evident after a 5 percent weight loss has occurred. More severe dehydration (10 percent weight loss) is accompanied by increased manifestation of these signs plus hypotension, sunken eyes, and loss of ocular tension. Very severe dehydration is accompanied by marked peripheral vasoconstriction, which produces a mottled appearance of the skin. Hyperpyrexia may also occur. A dry tongue may be a sign of dehydration but may also result from prolonged mouth breathing.

Biochemical studies are essential to confirm the extent of dehydration and to determine the associated electrolyte and acid-base disturbance.

FLUID THERAPY FOR GASTROINTESTINAL DISEASE

Intravenous therapy to correct dehydration must be planned to restore the existing deficits progressively, while also providing for maintenance fluid plus electrolyte requirements and the replacement of ongoing losses.

Dehydration due to persistent vomiting requires the replacement of sodium, potassium, chloride, and water.[97] The usual regimen is to replace the estimated deficit with 5 percent dextrose in saline solution. In less severe dehydration, 5 percent dextrose in one third or one half normal saline is used. Fifty percent of the deficit (estimated from weight loss) may be replaced in the first 24 hours and the remainder in the second 24 hours. Severe disturbances may take longer than 48 hours to correct. In the presence of very severe dehydration due to vomiting, an infusion of normal saline may be required to restore volume rapidly and correct hypotension. As urine output becomes established and increases in volume, potassium chloride should be added to the intravenous infusion at a rate of 3 mEq/kg/24 hours. While replacing deficits, maintenance fluid of 3.5 percent dextrose in 0.3 percent sodium chloride should be infused at a daily rate appropriate for the child. Further losses due to vomiting should be replaced volume for volume with isotonic saline.

Dehydration due to persistent diarrhea must be treated according to the proportional losses of water and electrolytes that have occurred. The fluid and electrolyte status will also be influenced by the initial fluid therapy that has been instituted since the onset of diarrhea. The majority of patients will have isonatremic dehydration (serum sodium, 130 to 150 mEq/L), but a minority may have hyponatremic dehydration (serum sodium less than 130 mEq/L) or hypernatremic dehydration (serum sodium more than 150 mEq/L). Many patients with diarrhea may be treated with oral carbohydrate and electrolyte solutions, and in all but a few this will maintain or restore hydration.[98, 99] The hydration state is monitored by assessing the child's level of activity, body weight, and urine output. If these indicators fail to show improvement, intravenous fluid therapy is required. Infant diarrheal fluid contains approximately 60 mEq/L of sodium, 30 mEq/L of potassium, and 45 mEq/L of chloride. Thus, replacement of fluid deficits with a solution of 5 percent dextrose in water, with one third normal saline plus 20 mEq of potassium chloride and 20 mEq of sodium bicarbonate added to each liter, is suitable for most infants.[100] Patients with very severe dehydration may require blood or albumin transfusion to treat persisting hypotension.

Some infants and children may develop hypertonic hypernatremic dehydration with diarrhea, especially if high-solute feedings are initially used as therapy. The treatment of hypertonic dehydration consists of administration of more fluid than solute to restore hydration. This treatment, however, must be applied over an extended period (48 to 72 hours). Too rapid administration of hypotonic solutions may lead to movement of excessive fluid to the intracellular compartment and the possibility of seizures. A replacement fluid containing approximately 50 mEq/L of sodium is commonly used.

Hyponatremic dehydration is treated by administration of isotonic solutions over a period of a few days. Added sodium may be administered, but hypertonic saline is unnecessary unless frank signs of water intoxication (for example, convulsions) are present. Hypotonic solutions must be avoided for patients with hyponatremic dehydration, as they may cause further hyponatremia.

In the assessment of the patient who has been treated for dehydration from any cause, the anesthesiologist should look for evidence of signs of good replacement of deficits. The most important indicators are a normal, flat fontanelle, well-filled veins, normal skin turgor, a good urine output, and a normal sensorium. Biochemical indices should be within normal limits.

INTRAVENOUS ALIMENTATION

Total parenteral nutrition (TPN) has become refined as a technique to the point where nutrition can be maintained despite very severe gastrointestinal disease. Principal gastrointestinal indications for the use of TPN in pediatric patients are short bowel syndrome, intractable diarrhea, and conditions in which normal bowel function is compromised for a prolonged period (such as following omphalocele repair). TPN may also be used for infants with respiratory distress syndrome, sepsis, and other medical conditions, to maintain nutrition during intensive medical therapy.

Short bowel syndrome following massive intestinal resection was associated with a high incidence of morbidity and mortality prior to the introduction of TPN. A length of small bowel of not less than 30 cm was considered essential for survival.[101] Since the advent of TPN, a length of less than 15 cm is compatible with survival.[102] Many infants who are supported with TPN for short bowel syndrome ultimately will develop adequate bowel function.[103] Solutions for TPN contain amino acids, glucose, electrolytes and trace metals, lipids and carnitine, biotin, vitamins, and iron. They may be delivered by a peripheral intravenous route but are usually delivered via a central venous line.[104] A two-line system is used to mix lipid and amino acid solutions close to the infusion site. Each patient must be stabilized on a regimen that will provide energy requirements, electrolyte replacements, and other essentials suitable to his or her individual needs. The process of stabilization on TPN may require 2 to 3 days, during which frequent blood and urine glucose estimations must be performed. Once the child is stable, glucose and electrolyte levels are monitored every second or third day.

The most common complication of TPN is sepsis. The central line may become infected by improper handling but more often becomes secondarily infected by organisms entering elsewhere.[105] Thus, every child on TPN should be managed with meticulous attention to asepsis in all invasive maneuvers (endotracheal intubation, vascular cannulation, and so forth).

Whenever possible, if a child on TPN is to receive anesthesia, the TPN line should be left totally undisturbed. Injections should not be made into the line, and the line should not be used as a central venous pressure monitor. Obviously, there will be exceptions to these principles when desperately sick infants require care but have limited routes for venous access. Some drugs are compatible with intravenous hyperalimentation amino acid solutions.[106] These include many antibiotics, cimetidine, furosemide, heparin, hydrocortisone, and phenobarbital. Drugs that are not compatible with TPN solutions include pentobarbital and thiopental, diazepam, morphine, sodium bicarbonate, and digoxin. Since the lipid solutions are unstable with most drugs, these must be temporarily discontinued if any drugs are infused via a TPN solution line.

MANAGEMENT OF THE PEDIATRIC "FULL-STOMACH" PATIENT

Many patients with gastrointestinal disease may present to the anesthesiologist the challenge of providing safe anesthesia in the presence of the risk of regurgitation and aspiration of stomach contents. Some special considerations for infants and children should be recognized by the anesthesiologist when meeting this problem.

If time permits, pretreatment of the patient with drugs may reduce the volume and acidity of the gastric contents. Glycopyrrolate has been demonstrated to be the most effective of the anticholinergic drugs in reducing acid secretions.[107] It should be given in a dose of 0.01 mg/kg intramuscularly at least 30 minutes prior to induction of anesthesia. Cimetidine has also been shown to reduce gastric acidity in pediatric patients.[108] It should be given in an oral dose of 7.5 mg/kg 1 to 3 hours before anesthesia.[108] Sodium citrate may be administered to increase the pH of the stomach contents. Metoclopramide is a dopamine antagonist that has central antiemetic properties and also promotes gastric emptying into the small bowel.[109] Metoclopramide increases the tone of the lower esophageal sphincter.[110] It should be given in a dose of 0.1 to 0.2 mg/kg intravenously 30 minutes prior to induction of anesthesia. Anticholinergic drugs interfere with the action of metoclopramide and should be withheld until induction of anesthesia.

Awake intubation has been advocated for the management of infants with a potentially full stomach. This is a relatively simple procedure to perform in the neonate and has been considered a very safe approach. The airway protective reflexes are intact up to the moment of intubation. In addition, if intubation fails for any reason, the infant will maintain the airway and continue to ventilate spontaneously. More recently, however, there are concerns that the physiological response to awake intubation, and particularly any associated increase in cerebral intravascular pressure, might predispose some preterm infants to intracranial hemorrhage. It is recognized that the stressed preterm infant has impaired autoregulation of cerebral blood flow;[111] cerebral blood flow is related directly to mean arterial blood pressure. A surge in mean arterial pressure, such as might accompany intubation, will be transmitted directly to fine cerebral vessels. Thus, it might be concluded that the stressed preterm infant should be as carefully managed during intubation as is the adult with an intracranial aneurysm.

Awake intubation of preterm infants has been widely practiced, both in the operating room and in the neonatal intensive care unit. This approach should be reviewed, especially in the sick, hypoxic, preterm infant. Induction of anesthesia with a small dose of barbiturate (such as thiopental, 2 to 3 mg/kg), fentanyl (20 to 30 μg/kg), neuromuscular blockade, and the administration of lidocaine intravenously (1 mg/kg) all may diminish the increase in blood pressure associated with intubation. When practical, a suitable combination of these methods should be applied before intubation. Awake intubation of the term neonate may still be the method of choice in some situations, such as in the presence of a tracheoesophageal fistula. The use of topical lidocaine (4 percent) around the mouth and over the tongue and gums of the infant prior to intubation is a useful adjunct to awake intubation.

Awake intubation has not been widely practiced in older children. They become very upset and vigorously oppose efforts to intubate them awake, unless they are moribund. Such older patients will require another technique to establish a safe airway rapidly. For many years an inhalation induction of anesthesia with the child in a lateral position was advocated as an acceptable technique for the full-stomach patient. Today most authorities would suggest that the pediatric patient should be managed like the adult, with a rapid sequence induction and cricoid pressure.

A rapid sequence induction in infants and children must be undertaken with some considerations similar to those in adults. Hypovolemia should be first corrected, the drugs should be rapidly injected after a period of preoxygenation, and cricoid pressure should be initiated as soon as sleep intervenes. A suitable endotracheal tube should be inserted as soon as adequate relaxation is present. Some considerations are different in infants and young children. Little is to be gained by elevation of the head of the table; the vertical height gained is insufficient to diminish significantly the risk of passive regurgitation.[112] Succinylcholine does not increase intragastric pressure in young patients (under 10 years);[113] therefore, pretreatment with a nondepolarizing relaxant is unnecessary.

Cuffed endotracheal tubes are not routinely used for infants and small children, because the added bulk of the cuff limits the internal diameter of the tube. Despite this, there are few reports of significant aspiration once the endotracheal tube is in place. This might be a problem if large volumes of fluid regurgitate into the pharynx because of surgical manipulation.[114] If such a situation is anticipated, a large gastric tube should be inserted and connected to continuous suction, and in older children a cuffed endotracheal tube should be inserted.

The risk of regurgitation and aspiration during emergence from anesthesia must be recognized. All patients with a potentially full stomach should be allowed to awaken completely prior to extubation, which should be performed with the patient in a lateral position.

The foregoing recommendations for the management of the "full-stomach" patient must, of course, be modified if other disease is present. A standard "crash induction" is not recommended in a hypovolemic patient or in one with an airway abnormality that may render intubation difficult. Ketamine is a useful induction agent for the patient who cannot be fully volume-restored prior to induction. Following preoxygenation, 2 to 4 mg/kg of ketamine with 0.02 mg/kg of atropine intravenously and 1 to 2 mg/kg of succinylcholine intravenously may be used for a rapid sequence induction. Cricoid pressure should be applied as soon as the patient loses consciousness.

The patient with a possible full stomach who also has an abnormality of the airway presents special problems. A crash induction is unsafe if any doubt exists as to the ease of laryngoscopy and intubation. Awake direct laryngoscopy in such a patient is unlikely to be successful and will be very distressing for the patient. Awake flexible laryngoscopy may be practical, but many pediatric patients would find this distressing also.

If possible, the child with a difficult airway should be prepared by appropriate fasting, continuous gastric aspiration, and administration of cimetidine, glycopyrrolate, and sodium citrate. Anesthesia should then be induced by inhalation of halothane and oxygen, and the anesthetic level should be rapidly deepened while spontaneous ventilation is maintained.

When the patient is deeply anesthetized, laryngoscopy (direct or flexible) may be attempted and intubation performed if possible. Lidocaine, 2 mg/kg administered intravenously 2 to 3 minutes prior to attempts at laryngoscopy, will minimize the risk of coughing or breath-holding.

When the operation is over, the child with a difficult airway should be allowed to awaken completely and should be placed in a lateral position before extubation.

SEDATION FOR PEDIATRIC GASTROINTESTINAL ENDOSCOPY

The effective treatment of pediatric gastrointestinal disease is very dependent upon accurate diagnosis. Endoscopic examination of the gastrointestinal tract, together with biopsies as are necessary, has become a routine part of the evaluation of many patients. Most children will not lie still for such procedures and find them quite distressing. Hence a need has arisen for suitable regimens to manage these patients during their examination.

A variety of sedation regimens have been suggested, most including a benzodiazepine drug,[115] sometimes with a narcotic analgesic.[116] A combination of diazepam, 0.1 mg/kg intravenously, and meperidine, 2 mg/kg intravenously, has been recommended as safe and effective for pediatric endoscopy.[116] Midazolam has been widely used and is suggested to be superior to diazepam, as it provides better amnesia.[115, 117] Children metabolize and excrete midazolam more rapidly than do adults.[118] However, a dose of 0.1 to 0.15 mg/kg of midazolam administered slowly intravenously to the point of slurred speech and conscious sedation resulted in good-to-excellent conditions for endoscopy in only 39 percent of children. Sedation regimens as described earlier may certainly result in hypoventilation and hypoxemia.[119] These disturbances may be due to the central depressant effects of the drugs together with direct obstruction of reflexes triggered by the endoscope.[119] Desaturation to 90 percent or less has been described to occur in 37.5 percent of patients, especially those with cardiopulmonary disease.[120] Pulse oximetry should be used in all patients who are sedated and will indicate the need either for supplemental oxygen or to remove the endoscope.[121]

In fact, for upper gastrointestinal endoscopy, quite heavy sedation will be required if the child is to lie quietly and tolerate the passage of an esophagogastroscope. Though this can be achieved with various combinations of drugs, the child will then frequently be so sedated that protective reflexes are lost and ventilatory depression may occur. The child passes readily from a state of conscious sedation to that of deep sedation. Recovery may also be prolonged, which is very undesirable especially for the outpatient. In such instances, a well-conducted general endotracheal inhalation anesthetic will certainly provide better conditions for endoscopy, increased patient safety, and a much more rapid recovery. It is therefore not surprising that there is a preference for general anesthesia, especially for infants and young children.[122, 123] The myth that performing the procedure "with just a little sedation" can avoid the risks of a general anesthetic must be corrected.

When sedation regimens are used in the hospital, the anesthesiology department must assume some responsibility for their supervision. Guidelines were produced by the American Academy of Pediatrics in association with the American Society of Anesthesiologists, published in 1985[124] and revised in 1992,[125] to provide a basis for the development of safe protocols for sedation of children. These guidelines define conscious sedation, deep sedation, and general anesthesia and dictate the process that should be employed for the monitoring and management of pediatric patients before, during, and following sedation for diagnostic, dental, and therapeutic procedures. It is recommended that these guidelines be used to develop standard protocols for use in all medical departments in which sedation is employed.

REFERENCES

1. Milla PJ: Development of intestinal structure and function. *In* Tanner MS, Stocks RJ (eds): Neonatal Gastroenterology: Contemporary Issues. Newcastle on Tyne, Intercept Ltd, 1984, p 6.
2. Cavell B: Gastric emptying in preterm infants. Acta Paediatr Scand *68*:725, 1979.
3. Cavell B: Gastric emptying in infants with congenital heart disease. Acta Paediatr Scand *70*:517, 1981.
4. Ebers DW, Smith DI, Gibbs GE: Gastric acidity on the first day of life. Pediatrics *18*:800, 1956.
5. Werner B: Peptic and tryptic capacity of the digestive tract of newborns. Acta Paediatr Scand *35* (Suppl 70):1, 1948.
6. Lebenthal E, Lee PC, Heitlinger LA: Impact of development of the gastrointestinal tract on infant feeding. J Pediatr *102*:1, 1983.
7. Lebenthal E, Leung YK: Feeding the premature and compromised infant: Gastrointestinal considerations. Pediatr Clin North Am *35*:215, 1988.
8. Szabo JS, Hillemeier AC, Oh W: Effect of nonnutritive and nutritive suck on gastric emptying in preterm infants. J Pediatr Gastroenterol Nutr *4*:348, 1985.

9. Winters RW: The Body Fluids in Pediatrics. Boston, Little, Brown, 1973, pp 412–413.
10. Chandra M: Dehydration and acidosis. *In* Lifshitz F (ed): Common Pediatric Disorders. New York, Marcel Dekker, 1984, p 106.
11. Barltrop D, Wharton BA, Arneil GC, et al: Nutrition and nutritional disorders. *In* Forfar JO, Arneil GC (eds): Textbook of Pediatrics. 3rd edition. New York, Churchill-Livingstone, 1984.
12. Shull MW, Reed RB, Valadian I, et al: Velocities of growth in vegetarian preschool children. Pediatrics *60*:410, 1977.
13. Muller JL, Gertner MH, Buzby G, et al: Implications of malnutrition in the surgical patient. Arch Surg *114*:121, 1979.
14. Katz M, Striehm ER: Host defense in malnutrition. Pediatrics *59*:490, 1977.
15. Pollace MM, Wiley JS, Yeh TS, et al: Effect of nutritional depletion on physiologic stability (abstract). Crit Care Med *10*:205, 1982.
16. Merritt RJ, Suskind RM: Nutritional survey of hospitalized pediatric patients. Am J Clin Nutr *32*:1320, 1979.
17. Cooper A, Jakobowski D, Spiker J, et al: Nutritional assessment: An integral part of the preoperative pediatric surgical evaluation. J Pediatr Surg *16*:554, 1981.
18. Berlin CM Jr, Tinker DE: Kwashiorkor in a child in central Pennsylvania. A seven year follow-up. Am J Dis Child *136*:822, 1982.
19. Stevenson RJ: Gastrointestinal bleeding in children. Surg Clin North Am *65*:1455, 1985.
20. Raffensperger JG, Luck SR: Gastrointestinal bleeding in children. Surg Clin North Am *56*:413, 1976.
21. Chattriwalla Y, Colon AR, Scanlon JW: The use of cimetidine in the newborn. Pediatrics *65*:301, 1980.
22. Morden RS, Schullinger JN, Mollitt DL, et al: Operative management of stress ulcers in children. Ann Surg *196*:18, 1982.
23. Strawczinski H, Beck I, McKenna R, et al: The behavior of the lower esophageal sphincter in infants and its relationship to gastroesophageal regurgitation. J Pediatr *64*:17, 1964.
24. Vaage S, Levorstad F, Efskind L: Congenital atresia of the esophagus. Scand J Thorac Cardiovasc Surg *9*:68, 1975.
25. Moroz SP, Espinza J, Cumming WA, et al: Lower esophageal sphincter function in children with and without gastroesophageal reflux. Gastroenterology *71*:236, 1976.
26. Euler AR, Ament ME: Gastroesophageal reflux in children: Clinical manifestations, diagnosis, pathophysiology and therapy. Pediatr Ann *5*:678, 1976.
27. Walsh JK, Farrell MK, Keenan WJ, et al: Gastroesophageal reflux in infants: Relation to apnea. J Pediatr *99*:196, 1981.
28. Dierdorf SF, McNiece WL, Rao CC, et al: Effect of succinylcholine on plasma potassium in children with cerebral palsy. Anesthesiology *62*:88, 1985.
29. Nissen R: The treatment of hiatal hernia and esophageal reflux by fundoplication. *In* Nyhus LM, Harkins HN (eds): Hernia. Philadelphia, JB Lippincott, 1964, p 488.
30. Payne W, Ellis F, Olson AM: Treatment of cardiospasm (achalasia of the esophagus) in children. Surgery *50*:731, 1961.
31. Azizkhan RG, Tapper D, Eraklis A: Achalasia in childhood: A 20-year experience. J Pediatr Surg *15*:452, 1980.
32. Bolsin SN, Gillbe C: Opitz-Frias syndrome: A case with potentially hazardous anaesthetic implications. Anaesthesia *40*:1189, 1985.
33. Little JR, Opitz JM: The G syndrome. Am J Dis Child *121*:505, 1971.
34. Idowu J, Aitken DR, Georgeson KE: Gastric volvulus in the newborn. Arch Surg *115*:1046, 1980.
35. Asch MJ, Sherman NH: Gastric volvulus in children: Report of two cases. J Pediatr Surg *12*:1059, 1977.
36. Rosser SB, Clark CH, Elechi EN: Spontaneous neonatal gastric perforation. J Pediatr Surg *17*:390, 1982.
37. Bilik R, Freud N, Sheinfeld Y, et al: Subtotal gastrectomy in infancy for perforating necrotizing gastritis. J Pediatr Surg *25*:1244, 1990.
38. Stevenson RJ: Non-neonatal intestinal obstruction in children. Surg Clin North Am *65*:1225, 1985.
39. Atwell JD, Levick P: Congenital hypertrophic pyloric stenosis and associated anomalies in the genitourinary tract. J Pediatr Surg *16*:1029, 1982.
40. Wooley MM, Felsher BF, Asch MJ, et al: Jaundice, hypertrophic pyloric stenosis and glucuronyl transferase. J Pediatr Surg *9*:359, 1974.
41. Winters RW: Metabolic alkalosis of pyloric stenosis. *In* Winters RW (ed): The Body Fluids in Pediatrics. Boston, Little, Brown, 1973, p 402.
42. Shumake LB: Post-operative hypoglycemia in congenital hypertrophic pyloric stenosis. South Med J *68*:223, 1975.
43. Daly AM, Conn AW: Anaesthesia for pyloromyotomy: A review. Can Anaesth Soc J *16*:316, 1969.
44. Ghory MJ, Sheldon CA: Newborn surgical emergencies of the gastrointestinal tract. Surg Clin North Am *65*:1083, 1985.
45. Rickham PP, Boeckmann CR: Neonatal meconium obstruction in the absence of mucoviscidosis. Am J Surg *106*:173, 1965.
46. Kalayoglu M, Sieber WK, Rodman JB, et al: Meconium ileus: A critical review of treatment and eventual prognosis. J Pediatr Surg *6*:290, 1971.
47. Mabogunje OE, Wang CI, Mahour GH: Improved survival of neonates with meconium ileus. Arch Surg *117*:37, 1982.
48. Langer JC, Paes BM, Gray S: Hypernatremia associated with *N*-acetylcysteine therapy for meconium ileus in a premature infant. Can Med Assoc J *143*:202, 1990.
49. Brown EG, Sweet AY: Neonatal necrotizing enterocolitis. Pediatr Clin North Am *29*:1149, 1982.
49a. Sweet AY: Epidemiology. *In* Brown EG, Sweet AY (eds): Neonatal Necrotizing Enterocolitis. New York, Grune and Stratton, 1980, p 13.
50. Brady P, Garite T, German JC: Fetal heart rate patterns in infants in whom necrotizing enterocolitis develops. Arch Surg *115*:1050, 1980.
51. Touloukian RJ: Etiologic role of the circulation. *In* Brown EG, Sweet Y (eds): Neonatal Necrotizing Enterocolitis. New York, Grune and Stratton, 1980, p 41.
52. Goldman HI: Feeding and necrotizing enterocolitis. Am J Dis Child *134*:553, 1980.
53. Engel RR, Vernig ML, Hunt CE, et al: Origin of gas in necrotizing enterocolitis. Pediatr Res *7*:292, 1973.
54. Holdman LV, Moore WEC: Anaerobic Laboratory Manual. Blacksburg, Va, Virginia Polytechnic Institute, 1972.
55. Kleigman RM: Neonatal necrotizing enterocolitis: Implications for an infectious disease. Pediatr Clin North Am *26*:327, 1979.
56. Rowe MI, Marchildon MB: Surgical management. *In* Brown EG, Sweet AY (eds): Neonatal Necrotizing Enterocolitis. New York, Grune and Stratton, 1980, p 167.
57. Kosloske A, Papile LA, Burstein J: Indications for operation in acute necrotizing enterocolitis of the neonate. J Pediatr Surg *87*:502, 1980.

58. Ein SH, Shandling B, Wesson D, Filler RM: A 13-year experience with peritoneal drainage under local anesthesia for necrotising enterocolitis perforation. J Pediatr Surg *25*:1034, 1990.
59. Raju TNK, Vidyasager D, Torres C, et al: Intracranial pressure during intubation and anesthesia in infants. J Pediatr *96*:860, 1980.
60. Deckhart R, Steward DJ: Noninvasive arterial hemoglobin oxygen saturation versus transcutaneous oxygen tension monitoring in the preterm infant. Crit Care Med *12*:935, 1984.
61. Dierdorf SF, Krisna G: Anesthetic management of neonatal surgical emergencies. Anesth Analg *60*:204, 1981.
62. Collins DL, Pinckney LE, Miller KE, et al: Hydrostatic reduction of ileocolic intussusception: A second attempt in the operating room with general anesthesia. J Pediatr *115*:204, 1989.
63. Guo J, Ma X, Zhou Q: Results of air pressure enema reduction in intussusception: 6396 cases in 13 years. J Pediatr Surg *21*:1201, 1986.
64. Rosenkrantz JG, Cox JA, Silverman FN, et al: Intussusception in the 1970's: Indications for operation. J Pediatr Surg *12*:367, 1977.
65. Evrard M: Anesthesia problems in the infant with acute intestinal intussusception. Anesth Analg (Paris) *30*:1085, 1973.
66. Meguid M, Canty T, Eraklis AJ: Complications of Meckel's diverticulum in infants. Surg Gynecol Obstet *139*:541, 1974.
67. Filippi G, McKusick VA: The Beckwith-Wiedemann syndrome. Medicine *49*:279, 1970.
68. Schiff D, Colle E, Wells D, et al: Metabolic aspects of the Beckwith-Wiedemann syndrome. J Pediatr *82*:258, 1973.
69. Philippart Al, Cantry TG, Filler RM: Acute fluid volume requirements in infants with anterior abdominal wall defects. J Pediatr Surg *7*:553, 1972.
70. Canty TG, Collins DL: Primary fascial closure in infants with gastroschisis and omphalocele: A superior approach. J Pediatr Surg *8*:707, 1983.
71. Schwartz MZ, Tyson KRT, Milliorn K, et al: Staged reduction using a Silastic sac is the treatment of choice for large congenital abdominal wall defects. J Pediatr Surg *18*:713, 1983.
72. Yaster M, Buck J, Dudgeon DL: Hemodynamic effects of primary closure of omphalocele/gastroschisis in human newborns. Anesthesiology *69*:84, 1988.
73. Koehntop DE, Rodman JH, Brundage DM, et al: Pharmacokinetics of fentanyl in neonates. Anesth Analg *65*:227, 1986.
74. Woodhouse CRJ, Ransley PG, Innes-Williams D: Prune belly syndrome—report of 47 cases. Arch Dis Child *57*:856, 1982.
75. Hannington-Kiff JG: Prune belly syndrome and general anaesthesia: Case report. Br J Anaesth *42*:649, 1970.
76. Lyon AJ: Congenital atresia of the larynx in association with prune belly syndrome. J Army Med Corps *129*:118, 1983.
77. Hendren WH: Prune belly syndrome. *In* Devine C, Stecker JF (eds): Urology in Practice. Boston, Little, Brown, 1978, p 361.
78. Chinyanga HM: Cystoscopy and prune belly syndrome. *In* Stehling LC (ed): Common Problems in Pediatric Anesthesia. Chicago, Year Book Medical Publishers, 1982, p 77.
79. Johnston DI: Neonatal cholestatic jaundice. *In* Tanner MS, Stocks RJ (eds): Neonatal Gastroenterology: Contemporary Issues. Newcastle on Tyne, Intercept Ltd, 1984, pp 139–153.
80. Altman RP, Stolar CJH: Pediatric hepatobiliary disease. Surg Clin North Am *65*:1245, 1985.
81. Howard ER: Extrahepatic biliary atresia: A review of current management. Br J Surg *70*:193, 1983.
82. deVries PA, Cox KL: Surgical treatment of congenital and neonatal biliary obstruction. Surg Clin North Am *61*:987, 1981.
83. Barkin RM, Lilly JR: Biliary atresia and the Kasai operation: Continuing care. J Pediatr *96*:1015, 1980.
84. Wood RP, Langnas AN, Stratta RJ, et al: Optimal therapy for patients with biliary atresia: Portoenterostomy ("Kasai" procedures) versus primary transplantation. J Pediatr Surg *25*:153, 1990.
85. Paradis KJG, Freese DK, Sharp HL: A pediatric perspective on liver transplantation. Pediatr Clin North Am *35*:409, 1988.
86. Davis PJ, Cook DR: Anesthetic problems in pediatric liver transplantation. Transplantation Proc *21*:3493, 1989.
87. Lichtor JL, Emond J, Chung MR et al: Pediatric orthotopic liver transplantation: Multifactorial predictions of blood loss. Anesthesiology *68*:607, 1988.
88. Gordon R, Iwatsuki S, Esquival C, et al: Liver transplantation across ABO groups. Surgery *100*:342, 1986.
89. O'Kelly B, Jayais P, Veroli P, et al: Dose requirements of vecuronium, pancuronium, and atracurium during orthotopic liver transplantation. Anesth Analg *73*:794, 1991.
90. Lawless S, Ellis D, Thompson A, et al: Mechanisms of hypertension during and after orthotopic liver transplantation in children. J Pediatr *115*:372, 1989.
91. Swygert TH, Roberts LC, Valek TR, et al: Effect of intraoperative low-dose dopamine on renal function in liver transplant recipients. Anesthesiology *75*:571, 1991.
92. Todani T, Watanabe Y, Narusue M, et al: Congenital bile duct cysts. Am J Surg *134*:263, 1977.
93. Martin LW, Torres AM: Hirschsprung's disease. Surg Clin North Am *65*:1171, 1985.
94. deVries PA, Cox KL: Anorectal anomalies. Surg Clin North Am *65*:1139, 1985.
95. deVries PA, Pena A: Posterior sagittal anorectoplasty. J Pediatr Surg *17*:638, 1982.
96. Vaughan VC, McKay RJ, Behrman RE (Eds.): Nelson Textbook of Pediatrics. 14th edition. Philadelphia, WB Saunders, 1992, pp 195–211.
97. McGowin M: Clinical Management of Electrolyte Disorders. Boston, Martinus Nijhoff, 1983, p 90.
98. Santosham M, Daum RS, Diuman L, et al: Oral rehydration therapy of infantile diarrhea. A controlled study of well-nourished children hospitalized in the United States and Panama. N Engl J Med *306*:1070, 1982.
99. Hamilton JR: Treatment of acute diarrhea. Pediatr Clin North Am *32*:419, 1985.
100. Collins RD: Illustrated Manual of Fluid and Electrolytes. 2nd edition. Philadelphia, JB Lippincott, 1983, p 107.
101. Wilmore DW: Factors correlating with successful outcome following extensive intestinal resection in infants. J Pediatr *80*:88, 1972.
102. Klish WJ, Putman TC: The short gut. Am J Dis Child *135*:1056, 1981.
103. Heird WC, Winters RW: Total parenteral nutrition: The state of the art. J Pediatr *86*:2, 1975.
104. Zlotkin SH, Stallings VA, Pencharz PB: Total parenteral nutrition in children. Pediatr Clin North Am *32*:381, 1985.
105. Miller RC, Grogan JB: Incidence and source of contamination of intravenous nutritional infusion systems. J Pediatr Surg *8*:195, 1973.

106. Farago S: Compatibility of antibiotics and other drugs in total parenteral nutrition solutions. Can J Hosp Pharm *36*:43, 1983.
107. Salem MR, Wong AY, Mani M, et al: Premedicant drugs and gastric juice pH and volume in pediatric patients. Anesthesiology *44*:216, 1976.
108. Goudsouzian NG, Cote CJ, Liu LMP, et al: The dose response effect of oral cimetidine on gastric pH and volume in children. Anesthesiology *55*:533, 1981.
109. Albibi R, McCallum RW: Metoclopramide: Pharmacology and clinical application. Ann Intern Med *98*:86, 1983.
110. Stanciu C, Bennett JR: Metoclopramide in gastroesophageal reflux. Gut *14*:275, 1973.
111. Lou HC, Lassen NA, Friis-Hansen B: Impaired autoregulation of cerebral blood flow in the distressed newborn infant. J Pediatr *94*:118, 1979.
112. Salem MR, Wong AY, Fizzotti GF: Efficacy of cricoid pressure in preventing aspiration of gastric contents in paediatric patients. Br J Anaesth *44*:401, 1972.
113. Salem MR, Wong AY, Lin YH: The effect of suxamethonium on intra-gastric pressure in infants and children. Br J Anaesth *44*:166, 1972.
114. Roy WL: Intraoperative aspiration in a paediatric patient. Can Anaesth Soc J *32*:639, 1985.
115. Tolia V, Fleming SL, Kauffman RE: Randomised, double-blind study of midazolam and diazepam for endoscopic sedation of children. Dev Pharmacol Ther *14*:141, 1990.
116. Nahata MC, Murray RD, Zingarelli J, et al: Efficacy and safety of a diazepam and meperidine combination for pediatric gastrointestinal procedures. J Pediatr Gastroenterol Nutr *10*:335, 1990.
117. Lee MG, Hanna W, Harding H: Sedation for upper gastrointestinal endoscopy: A comparative study of midazolam and diazepam. Gastrointest Endosc *35*:82, 1989.
118. Tolia V, Brennan S, Aravind MK, Kauffman RE: Pharmacokinetic and pharmacodynamic study of midazolam in children during esophagogastroduodenoscopy. J Pediatr *119*:467, 1991.
119. Rimmer KP, Graham K, Whitelaw WA, Field SK: Mechanism of hypoxia during panendoscopy. J Clin Gastroenterol *11*:17, 1989.
120. Casteel HB, Fiedorek SC, Kiel EA: Arterial blood desaturation in infants and children during upper gastrointestinal endoscopy. Gastrointest Endosc *36*:489, 1990.
121. Bendig DW: Pulse oximetry and upper intestinal endoscopy in infants and children. J Pediatr Gastroenterol Nutr *12*:39, 1991.
122. Andrus CH, Dean PA, Ponsky JL: Evaluation of safe, effective intravenous sedation for utilisation in endoscopic procedures. Surg Endosc *4*:179, 1990.
123. Ellet ML: General anesthesia: An alternative to sedation for pediatric endoscopic procedures. Gastroenterol Nurs *13*:166, 1991.
124. American Academy of Pediatrics, Committee on Drugs and Section on Anesthesiology: Guidelines for the elective use of conscious sedation, deep sedation, and general anesthesia in pediatric patients. Pediatrics *76*:317, 1985.
125. American Academy of Pediatrics, Committee on Drugs and Section on Anesthesiology: Guidelines for monitoring and management of pediatric patients during and following sedation for diagnostic, dental, and therapeutic procedures. Pediatrics *89*:1110, 1992.

CHAPTER

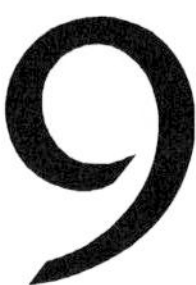

Pediatric Head and Neck Syndromes

C. F. WARD, M.D.

Several decades have passed since the discovery of the vaccine and the conquest of polio. The organization that once devoted itself to polio alone now largely concerns itself with birth defects and has recruited a medical ally, the dysmorphologist, who possesses special knowledge concerning anatomical associations and the probabilities of recurrence of malformations. These specialists and the organization both have tremendously expanded the understanding of human malformation, as well as presenting another etiological concept of abnormal anatomy, that of in utero growth restraint leading to deformation. Much of what follows is based on this foundation, which has been provided over the past 30 years.

This chapter is the first of three constrained by anatomy and morphology. Where possible, I have attempted to remain within the assigned boundaries; however, it is important to realize that numerous other diseases and syndromes have craniofacial presentation that may be of anesthetic significance and will not be so easily restricted. For example, Table 9–1 presents a compilation of the many syndromes associated with micrognathia. By no means will all such issues be dealt with here, and investigation of other publications may well be necessary to understand thoroughly some pathology, especially that resulting from chromosome abnormalities or trauma.

The question of nomenclature is prominent in any discussion of birth defects. Descriptions applied in this chapter are those found in Bergsma's *Birth Defects Compendium,* with additional titles or descriptions added as thought appropriate to assist in historical correlation.

EMBRYOLOGY

Typically, those engaged in the practice of anesthesia possess a dominant interest in physiology and pharmacology, with a near aversion to anatomy, except as it pertains directly to the clinical situation. This aversion usually becomes withdrawal when embryology is mentioned; however, tracing the origin of head and neck anatomy is worthwhile because of the understanding such pursuit lends to what *may be.* Many an operating room visit planned for the child with unusual craniofacial appearance is an aggressive examination with the child under anesthesia, occasionally followed by removal or rearrangement of malpositioned or malproportioned parts. Those who schedule such visits

References are grouped by topic at the end of the chapter.

Table 9–1. SYNDROMES ASSOCIATED WITH MICROGNATHIA

Abnormality, Primary Name	Associated Names, Descriptions
Syndromes Caused by Known Chromosome Abnormality	
4 p−	Wolf's
5 p−	Cri du chat
13 trisomy	
14 q proximal partial trisomy	
11 q−	
11 q partial trisomy	
18 q−	
18 p−	
18 trisomy	Edwards'
21 monosomy	
Syndromes Caused by Other Than Known Chromosome Abnormality	
Acrocephalopolysyndactyly	
Acrocephalosyndactyly	
Arthro-ophthalmopathy	Stickler's
Auditory canal arresia	
C syndrome	
Campomelic dysphasia	
Cerebrocostomandibular	
Cerebrohepatorenal	Bowen's or Zellweger's
Cerebro-oculofacioskeletal	COFS
Chondrodystrophic myotonia	
Cleft palate	
Craniofacial dysostosis with diaphyseal hyperplasia	
Craniofacial dyssynostosis	
Deafness and ear pits	
Dubowitz'	
Ear, absent tragus	
Fetal trimethadione	
Frontometaphyseal dysplasia	
G syndrome	Opitz-Frias
Gingival fibromatosis, Cowden's type	
Hanhart's	
Hemifacial microsomia	
Laryngomalacia	
Lissencephaly	
Mandibulofacial dysostosis	
Marden-Walker	
Meckel's	
Megalocornea–mental retardation	
Mesomelic dysplasia, Langer's type	
Noonan's	
Nose, posterior atresia	Choanal atresia
Oculoauriculovertebral dysplasia	Goldenhar's
Oculomandibulofacial dysplasia	Hallermann-Streiff
Opitz-Kaveggia PG	
Osteodysplasty	Melnick-Needles
Pierre Robin	
Progeria	Hutchinson-Gilford
Pyle's disease	
Seckel's	
Smith-Lemli-Opitz	
Thrombocytopenia with absent radius	TAR
Thymic agenesis	DiGeorge's
Trichorhinophalangeal, type II	Langer-Giedion
Turner's	
Williams'	

p− Nomenclature indicates partial or total absence of chromosome short arm.

q− Nomenclature indicates partial or total absence of chromosome long arm.

usually know well the anatomical possibilities. As the surface area in question encompasses the brain and the airway, both of which are of interest to anesthetists, it seems prudent to review development briefly as an aid to foreseeing what these possibilities may be.

THE SKULL

The upper portion of the cranial vault develops from mesenchyma that undergoes membranous ossification. This part of the skull consists of flat bones that join edge-to-edge to form sutures, or to form fontanelles where more than two bones meet. The two frontal bones oppose at the mid-forehead, forming the metopic suture. The frontal bones oppose the parietal bones bilaterally, creating the coronal suture, and the anterior fontanelle results from both matched bone pairs joining in the midline. The two parietal bones oppose to form the sagittal suture and posteriorly contact the occipital bone to form the lambdoid suture. At the junction of these three bones, the posterior fontanelle is formed.

The base of the skull is formed from separate cartilage that creates the base of the occipital bone, the sphenoid, the ethmoid, and the petrous bone, along with portions of the temporal bone. Where the base of the skull, consisting primarily of the squamous temporal bone, opposes the parietal bone, the squamous suture is created; where these two bones meet the frontal bone and occipital bone, the anterolateral and posterolateral fontanelles, respectively, are formed.

The face develops from two origins. Upper midline structures develop primarily from the frontal prominence, whereas lateral and middle facial anatomy traces its origin to the branchial or pharyngeal arches. The arches are originally bars of mesenchymal tissue, separated from one another by the branchial or pharyngeal clefts. Both these structures develop coincidentally with the foregut, or pharyngeal, pouches. Each of these three structures will be described in turn. It is well worthwhile remembering the various arch components, especially the first, for developmental abnormalities involving a visible portion of an arch may also affect other, less prominent, anatomy.

The first branchial arch gives origin to the maxilla, the mandible, the zygoma, and a portion of the temporal bone. A small portion of this arch also contributes the incus and malleus. The muscles of mastication, the mylohyoid, the tensor tympani, tensor palatini, and anterior belly of the digastric, also originate here. Each arch has its own cranial nerve component, in this case the trigeminal nerve.

The second arch gives rise to the stapes, the styloid process of the temporal bone, the stylohyoid ligament and the lesser horn, and a portion of the body of the hyoid bone. The muscles are the stapedius, stylohyoid, posterior belly of the digastric, the auricular, and all the facial expression muscles. The nerve supply is from the facial nerve.

The third arch gives rise to the remainder of the hyoid, while the lone muscle derived from this structure is the stylopharyngeal, with innervation from the glossopharyngeal nerve.

The fourth arch provides the laryngeal cartilage, along with the pharyngeal constrictors, the levator palatini, and the cricothyroid muscles, with innervation from the fourth arch nerve, the superior laryngeal branch of the vagus. The sixth arch provides the intrinsic laryngeal muscles with nerve supply from the recurrent branch of the vagus.

The first pharyngeal pouch creates the eustachian tube and middle ear, the second pouch forms the tonsillar fossa, and the third pouch creates the thymus and a portion of the parathyroid. The fourth pouch contributes the rest of the parathyroids, while the fifth pouch develops into the portion of the thyroid gland that secretes calcitonin.

Of the clefts, only the first, between the first and second arches, forms a definitive structure—the external ear. However, if the second arch does not grow caudally over the third and fourth arches, as it normally should, the second, third, and fourth clefts can remain in contact with skin surface, forming branchial fistulas anywhere between the inferior border of the mandible and the clavicle, anterior to the sternocleidomastoid muscle. The tongue surface, although originating primarily from first arch structures, also receives major contributions from the second, third, and fourth arches, as evidenced by its changing sensory nerve supply. To complicate matters still further, the bulk of the tongue probably originates from occipital somites, thus accounting for the hypoglossal nerve innervation of the tongue musculature.

The thyroid gland originates as a cell proliferation at the foramen cecum in the tongue, then migrates, anterior to the gut, caudad to its eventual location anterior to the larynx. During this transition, the gland remains connected to the tongue via the thyroglossal duct, which eventually disappears. Should this not occur, it is worth recalling the migration, for although 75 percent of thyroglossal cysts are near the hyoid, they may be found anywhere along the track from the foramen cecum.

The midface is created by a very complex lateral-to-medial transition of first arch structures, along with evolution of the frontal prominence. The first arch contributions begin as maxillary, medial nasal, and lateral nasal swellings. During their midline fusion process, these structures create the intermaxillary segment. If one considers the upper jaw as an arch, this segment is the keystone. It comprises the philtrum of the lip, a jaw segment with the four incisor teeth, and a triangular component, called the primary palate, the vertex of which is the incisive foramen. This foramen marks the demarcation point between a cleft lip and a cleft (secondary) palate. The majority of the definitive palate arises from the maxillary swellings and grows medially to a midline fusion, also giving rise to the uvula. Returning to the arch analogy, it becomes easier to comprehend the location of the usual cleft lip, along the off-midline border of the "keystone" intermaxillary segment, and equally well, the midline location of the isolated cleft palate.

GENERAL ASSESSMENT

Prior to discussion of specific pathology, and immediately after discussion of embryology, I draw to the reader's attention that there is a separate chapter (Chapter 4) that concerns itself with central nervous system disease. This is quite appropriate, and it is equally so to note that despite the close proximity of the face, skull, and brain, they are not subject to a uniform pathological discussion. That lovely children may develop debilitating brain disease seems intellectually acceptable. Slightly more awkward, however, is the fact that an infant with near-monstrous appearance may, for the moment at least, be intellectually normal and quite able to survive. One must overlook the overall appearance of the package and instead consider the contents. A physician's initial expression of dismay when first viewing a child with a cloverleaf skull or facial burn may be witnessed by the parents and accidentally destroy all chance to establish confidence with them. The goal, then, must be to evaluate such children strictly as a physician without contamination from personal aesthetic values. To do otherwise does all concerned a terrible disservice.

CONGENITAL CRANIOFACIAL DEFORMITIES

The *Birth Defects Compendium* of Bergsma provides an encyclopedic approach to development gone awry and provides descriptions of over 1000 birth defects. Numerous tables in the volume list anatomical areas involved by these defects; the face alone receives nearly 300 such citations, with mention of the facial segments and skull proper receiving about an equal number. Obviously, many of these tables involve duplicate listings of the same syndrome. Nevertheless, a discussion of congenital craniofacial deformities must cover a panoply of anatomy, roughly divided into three areas: (1) chromosome defects; (2) syndromes named for the original author(s) involved; and (3) syndromes named to describe the anatomical defect. A failure to recognize members of category 1 or 2 has always seemed somewhat understandable to me, for many are exceedingly rare and complex; furthermore, disease descriptions involving proper names are somewhat passé. The third category is rather more embarrassing, for specific anatomical information is available in the names; unfortunately, the words are alien to the rest of medicine and seem altogether more appropriate to a description of long-deceased reptiles. Therefore, the following is a guide to the terms involved in this subject.

A *synostosis* is a union between adjacent bones. A *dysostosis* refers to a defect in ossification. A cranial suture dysostosis refers in a nonspecific way to a primary defect in suture formation. *Craniosynostosis* refers to a premature closure of a skull suture. Harken back to the description of embryology and it becomes apparent that the resultant anatomy will be highly dependent on which suture is involved. Keep clearly in mind that brain growth is the driving force behind cranial expansion; if one dimension is eliminated, growth may well be diverted to the others.

Closure of the sagittal suture prevents lateral skull growth. This results in an elongated skull, referred to as *scaphocephaly (scapho*, boat-shaped) or *dolichoscaphocephaly (dolicho*, long, narrow). Closure of the coronal suture prevents anteroposterior skull growth. This results in a widened skull, referred to as *brachycephaly (brachy*, broadened) or *acrobrachycephaly (acro*, extreme). If both the sagittal and coronal sutures close, skull growth is impeded in two dimensions, resulting in vertical growth. The result is *turricephaly (turri*, tower), *oxycephaly (oxy*, pointed), or *oxyturricephaly*. An unusual variant of multiple suture closure results in vertical and inferolateral expansion, referred to as *Kleeblattschädel* or more simply as a *cloverleaf* dysostosis. Premature closure of the metopic suture creates the very visible *trigonocephaly* (*trigono,* triangular), characterized by a midforehead "keel." Finally, an asymmetrical suture closure may create a tilted cranium, referred to as *plagiocephaly* (*plagio,* slanting). Reduced symmetrical cranial size is *microcephaly*, usually due to deficient brain growth, whereas nonspecific symmetrical skull enlargement is *macrocephaly*, which may be due to causes other than hydrocephalus, to which it is often reflexly attributed.

CRANIOSYNOSTOSES

Given the foregoing terms, logic would dictate a unified classification scheme, probably based primarily on suture involvement and resultant cranial vault shape. However, even if the specific pathology of each defect were known (they are not), this classification model would be valid only if syndrome anatomy proved relatively constant (it does not). Each leading text rearranges some or all of these defects, based on the particular author's viewpoint. This sort of internecine activity is useful in an evolutionary sense, but it makes the occasional reader's task a good bit more difficult. To those interested in a previously diagnosed specific syndrome, much of this is superfluous. Consequently, what follows is a consensus compilation of craniosynostosis syndromes, listed in alphabetical order, with an inclusion of anatomy that either generally occurs with the syndrome or has special relevance to anesthesia.

Particular note should be taken of what is *not* included here—anesthesia for craniofacial reconstructive surgery. The strides made by Gilles, Obwegeser, Converse, Munro, and especially Tessier in remodelling the entire cephalad portion of a deformed human being are absolutely astounding. In these aggressive techniques, only the brain and attendant cranial nerve–supplied organs are sacrosanct; everything else is movable or removable. However, the most liberal estimate of centers required to perform this surgery is 1 per 20 million population. Assuming, then, that I am in one such hospital, a discussion of anesthesia for this radical surgical therapy would be directed to 11 other centers in the United States, in turn

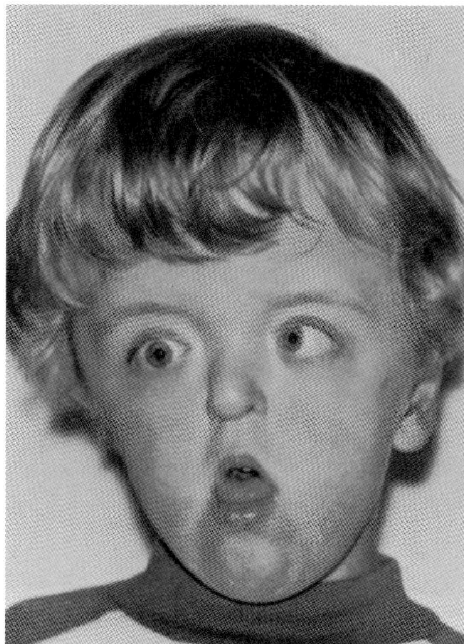
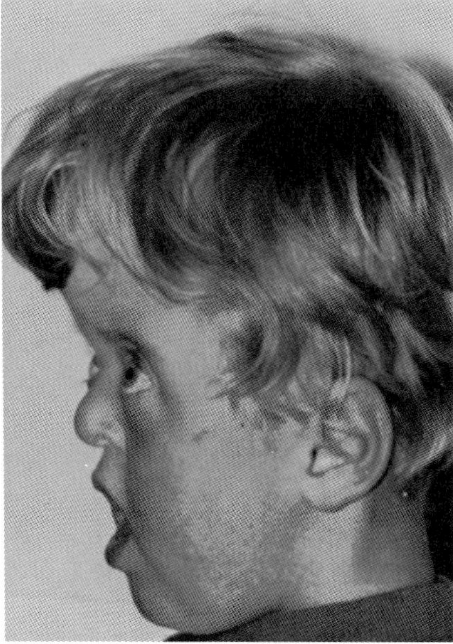

FIGURE 9–1. Apert's syndrome (Reproduced by permission from Cohen MM Jr: Dysmorphic syndromes with craniofacial manifestations. *In* Stewart RE, Prescott GH [eds]: Oral Facial Genetics. St. Louis, CV Mosby, 1976.)

attending to about 1200 to 1500 patients per year requiring plastic repair.

Therefore, rather than simply being presented with a rearrangement of published phrases, the interested reader is directed to obtain and read original articles thoroughly. In such reading it should be noted particularly that major postoperative neurological sequelae, blood loss of 25 to 400 percent, and intraoperative demise are almost invariably mentioned, usually of groups consisting of only 15 to 20 patients. (For an exception to small numbers, note the Toronto experience of Crysdale and associates from Ian Munro's group.) In this context, the fact that the trachea can be extubated because the entire midface advances 3 cm seems almost insignificant. It is, therefore, my opinion that operation *on* a patient with a craniosynostosis is reasonable when and wherever indicated. However, *for* the craniosynostosis is a much different matter and literally requires a cast of thousands, of which the anesthesiologist is but one. Following a perusal of the literature, patient referral for definitive repair will usually appear eminently reasonable.

ACROCEPHALO(POLY)SYNDACTYLIES

This group of deformities includes Apert's syndrome, Carpenter's syndrome, Pfeiffer's syndrome, and Saethre-Chotzen syndrome. In addition to these, the following syndromes are listed for the sake of completeness, although often only one report of each is present in the literature: Hermann-Opitz type, Sakati's syndrome, Summitt's type, and Waardenburg's type (not Waardenburg syndrome). Because of their extraordinary rarity, these will not be discussed further.

Apert's Syndrome (Fig. 9–1)

In 1906, Apert first noted a syndrome of acrobrachycephaly with syndactyly or webbing between the fingers and toes (usually second to fifth). This particular combination is in general referred to as acrocephalopolysyndactyly; Apert described but one variation. This syndrome is thought to occur in about 1 in 160,000 live births, is transmitted as autosomal dominant with a male:female ratio of 1:1, and is rarely linked with advanced paternal age. Mental retardation is common, and life span should be normal.

Clinical Features. Craniosynostosis is of a variable degree, primarily affecting the coronal suture, associated with sphenoethmoidomaxillary hypoplasia. The characteristic appearance is of turribrachycephaly with a wide, high forehead, marked in infancy by a supraorbital ridge. As the midface is hypoplastic, the mandible is relatively prominent. There is hypertelorism, proptosis, downward slanting palpebral fissures, and generally a small nasal bridge. Hydrocephalus, with several presentations, has been variably reported. The symmetrical limb defect creates a fusiform mass that generally contains the second, third, and fourth digits at a minimum. Slightly less than one third of these patients will also have a cleft palate. Later in life, there is progressive skeletal involvement, which has been reported to involve the cervical spine.

Pfeiffer's Syndrome (Fig. 9–2)

A recent addition to the category of acrocephalopolysyndactyly was made in 1964 when Pfeiffer described eight members of one family with what is now "his" syndrome. Owing to the recentness of the report, statements concerning incidence are unwarranted. The male:female ratio is probably 1:1, and transmission is autosomal dominant with complete penetrance and variable expressivity. Intelligence is usually unaffected, and life span should be normal, although the latter statement has only 2 decades of support at this writing.

Clinical Features. The skull is towering and wide, with "syndactyly" usually presenting in the form of unusually broad thumbs and great toes. The maxilla is hypoplastic, as is the nasal bridge, leading to relative prognathism. There may also be hypertelorism, downward slanting palpebral fissures, proptosis, and strabismus.

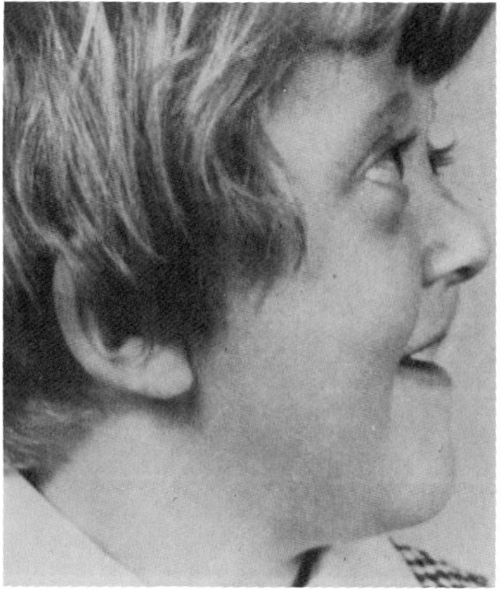

FIGURE 9–2. Pfeiffer's syndrome. (Reproduced by permission from Goodman RM, Gorlin RJ: Atlas of the Face in Genetic Disorders. 2nd edition. St. Louis, CV Mosby, 1977.)

Malocclusion and submucous cleft palate, along with low set ears, have been associated also.

Saethre-Chotzen Syndrome (Fig. 9–3)

Saethre, in a 1931 report of three patients, followed in 1932 by Chotzen with a further three patients, described another variant of acrocephalopolysyndactyly. The incidence of this syndrome is uncertain, with the male:female ratio probably 1:1. Transmission is autosomal dominant, with a high degree of penetrance and variable expressivity. Intelligence is frequently normal, and life span is presumedly unaffected. Some experts content this is a frequently misdiagnosed syndrome, either being labelled as a mild normal variant or as another of the acrocephalopolysyndactylies.

Clinical Features. The skull is usually wide and towering, with a flat forehead and low anterior hairline. Frequently the involvement is asymmetrical, causing plagiocephaly. The nasal bridge is small, while the mandible is prominent. Hypertelorism, strabismus, lacrimal duct defects, high-arched palate, and low-set ears have also been associated. Mild conductive hearing loss is common. The limb malformations are generally minimal, presenting as webbing between the second and third fingers and/or clinodactyly (medially or laterally "bent" fingers).

Carpenter's Syndrome (Fig. 9–4)

In this case, history has been kind, for Carpenter's description of this syndrome in 1909 was not placed into perspective until Temtamy's observations in 1966, yet the original name remained somehow associated. This is a variant of acrocephalopolysyndactyly, of rare but uncertain incidence, transmitted in an autosomal recessive manner. The male:female ratio is probably 1:1. Mental retardation is severe. Life span is adversely affected by the occurrence of congenital heart disease; as of 1978, the oldest known patient was 25 years old.

Clinical Features. The skull is widened and towering, often to an extreme degree. This is thought to be due to premature closure of all cranial sutures, with the coronal being last to fuse. Occasionally, this produces a cloverleaf skull. The eyes are wide-spread and "downthrust." The nasal bridge is flat, and the mandible hypoplastic. The patient is often short, with a particularly short neck; weight is commonly above average. Omphalocele and atrial ventricular septal defect, pulmonary stenosis, and tetralogy of Fallot have been associated.

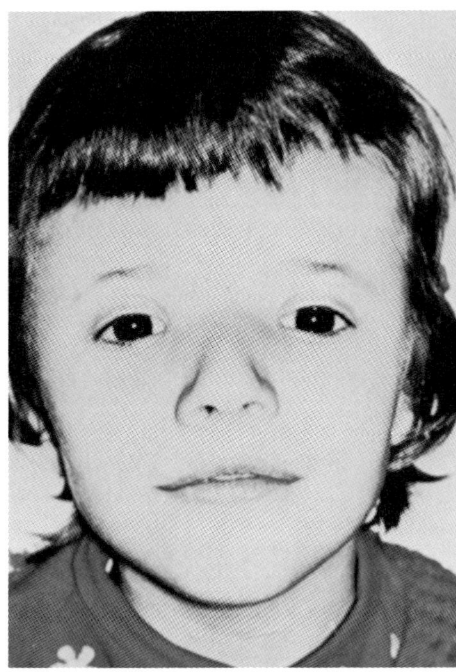
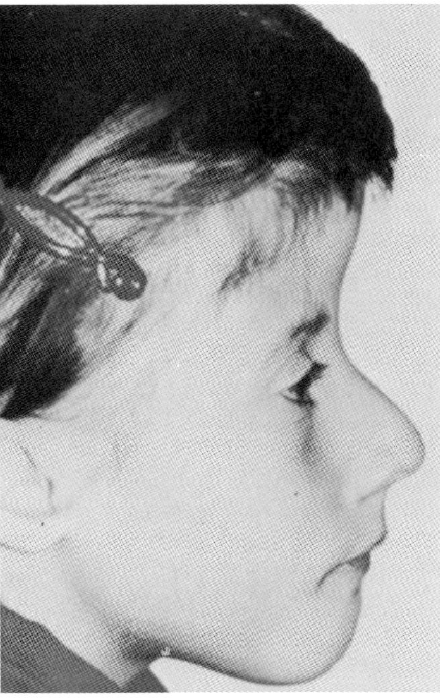

FIGURE 9–3. Saethre-Chotzen syndrome. (From Cohen MM Jr: An etiologic and nosologic overview of craniosynostosis syndromes. *In* Bergsma D [ed]: Malformation Syndromes. New York, American Elsevier Publishing Co., for the National Foundation—March of Dimes, BD: OAS X(2):137–189, 1975.)

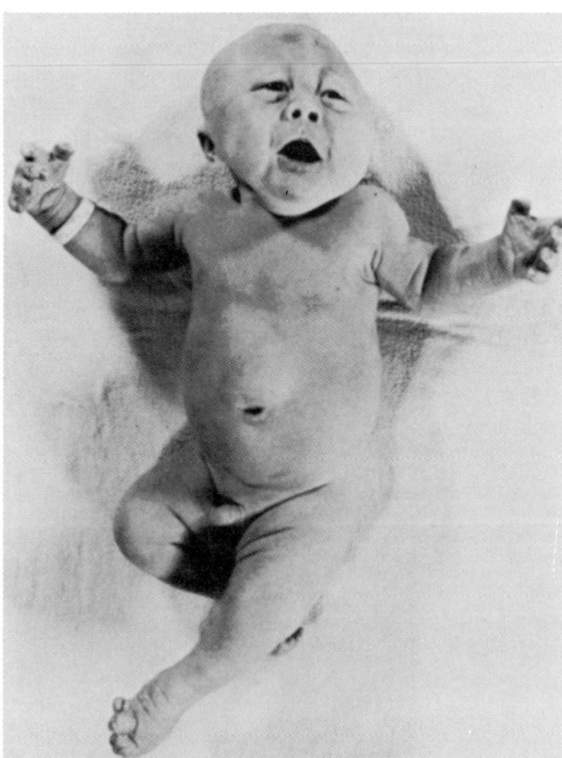

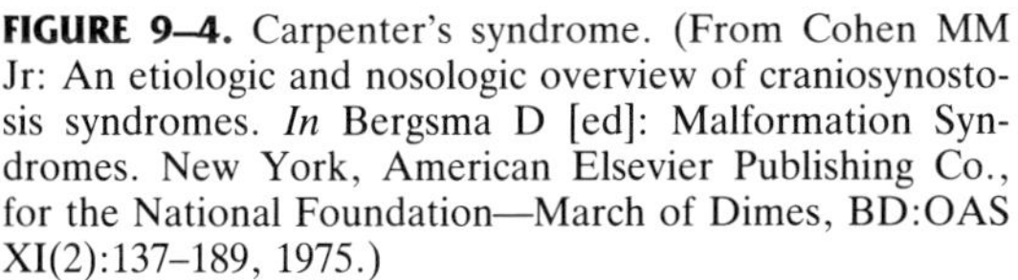

FIGURE 9–4. Carpenter's syndrome. (From Cohen MM Jr: An etiologic and nosologic overview of craniosynostosis syndromes. *In* Bergsma D [ed]: Malformation Syndromes. New York, American Elsevier Publishing Co., for the National Foundation—March of Dimes, BD:OAS XI(2):137–189, 1975.)

The upper limbs are often short, with webbing between the third and fourth digits. There may be associated minor lower extremity defects as well.

CROUZON'S SYNDROME (Fig. 9–5)

Crouzon reported, in 1912, the association of a widened, towering skull with proptosis, maxillary hypoplasia, and a beaked nose. This initial report, in both a mother and her son, is the first description of craniofacial dysostosis; subsequent descriptions have variously added and subtracted features, largely owing to the variability of the syndrome. Transmission is autosomal dominant, with complete penetrance and highly variable expressivity. This latter characteristic makes statements concerning incidence somewhat suspect; additionally, about 25 percent of reported cases seem to represent fresh mutations. Life span should be normal, while mental capacity may be highly dependent on the interaction between suture closure and brain growth. Generally, intelligence is normal. The male:female ratio is 1:1.

In 1963, Stanesco reported a syndrome, found in seven members of one family, that may be a variant of Crouzon's syndrome. The seven patients all had the craniofacial features found in Crouzon's syndrome, plus diaphyseal hyperplasia and small stature. Referred to as Stanesco's dysostosis, or craniofacial dysostosis with diaphyseal hyperplasia, this syndrome is transmitted as autosomal dominant with nearly complete expression. The incidence is unknown.

Clinical Features. In distinction from many other forms of craniosynostosis, suture closure generally begins well after birth in Crouzon's syndrome, usually becoming complete by age 2 years or so. The involved sutures commonly include the lambdoidal as well. Because of this variability, no characteristic cranial shape can be described. Brachycephaly, scaphocephaly, trigonocephaly, and even the cloverleaf skull have been reported. Hypertelorism and exophthalmos are fairly constant features, as are strabismus and nystagmus. The maxillae are hypoplastic, creating the appearance of prognathism. The palate is often high-arched, short, and occasionally cleft, and malocclusion is common. Increased intracranial pressure may be associated with Crouzon's syndrome, although this is not the norm.

CRANIOFACIAL DYSSYNOSTOSIS

This syndrome was reported by Neuhauser in 1976. It is transmitted as autosomal recessive,

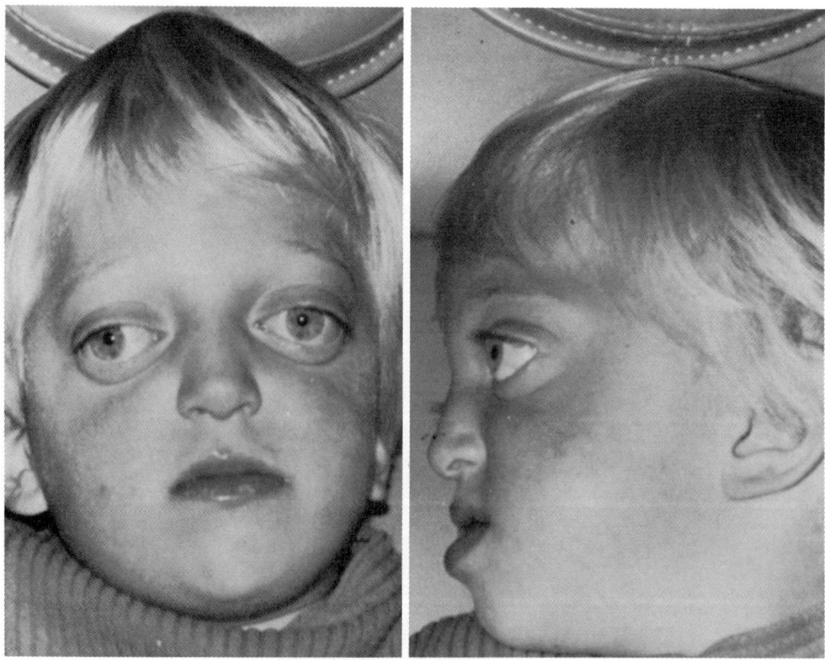

FIGURE 9–5. Crouzon's syndrome. (Reproduced by permission from Cohen MM Jr: Dysmorphic syndromes with craniofacial manifestations. *In* Stewart RE, Prescott GH [eds]: Oral Facial Genetics. St. Louis, CV Mosby, 1976.)

although there is some thought that this syndrome has several different possible etiologies. The male:female ratio is 1:1, and the incidence is unknown. The majority of children are mentally retarded, perhaps secondary to elevated intracranial pressure.

Clinical Features. The skull may be long or wide and towering with occipital prominence, usually secondary to lambdoid and posterior sagittal suture closure. There may also be facial or cranial asymmetry or both. Macrocephaly and microcephaly have both been reported. The face is characterized by hypoplastic supraorbital ridges, short maxillae, and micrognathia. Ocular signs include strabismus and nystagmus. EEG recordings are often abnormal, and seizures may be associated. Hydrocephalus is common, and almost all patients are of short stature. Associated congenital heart disease has been reported as well.

CRANIOCARPOTARSAL DYSPLASIA (WHISTLING FACE OR FREEMAN-SHELDON SYNDROME) (Fig. 9–6)

This extraordinarily rare disorder was first reported by Freeman and Sheldon in 1938. Burian applied the description by which most patients are now identified in 1962. The hallmarks of the syndrome are microstomia with pursed lips, camptodactyly with ulnar deviation, and talipes equinovarus. Frequent associations are coloboma alae, strabismus, high arched palate, flattened midface, kyphoscoliosis, and short stature. At the moment, the syndrome is thought to be due to a slowly progressive myopathy that primarily affects the facial, limb, and respiratory muscles. It is transmitted as an autosomal dominant, is of unknown incidence, and presents a male:female ratio of 1:1. Intelligence should be normal, while life span will be a function of the progression of the myopathy of respiratory muscles.

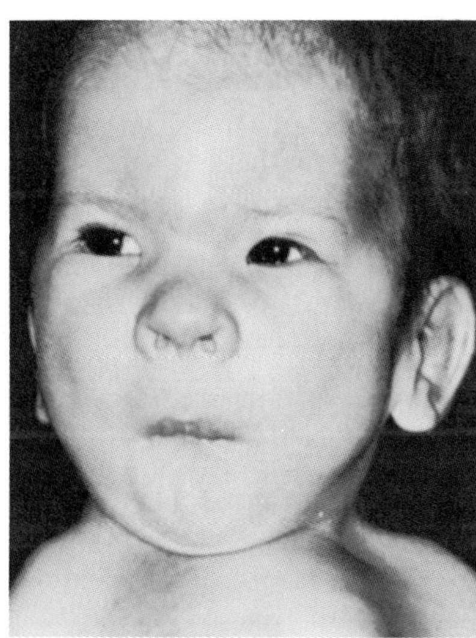

FIGURE 9–6. Freeman-Sheldon syndrome. (Reproduced by permission from Goodman RM, Gorlin RJ: Atlas of the Face in Genetic Disorders. 2nd edition. St. Louis, CV Mosby, 1977.)

Clinical Features. The face is flat, stiff, and masklike. The eyes are sunken; hypertelorism, strabismus, and blepharophimosis are common. The central segment of the cheeks bulge as though the patient were whistling, apparently secondary to a facial muscle defect. The mouth is frequently strikingly small and the lips pursed, often with a V-shaped fibrous tissue band at the midchin. Bilateral talipes equinovarus is associated, causing delay in ambulation.

Three reports of anesthetic experiences are in the literature, the most recent by Duggar and associates in 1989. They pointed out that many previous reports from outside the surgical arena noted severe respiratory morbidity, due, in some cases, to a near-total immobility of the thoracic cage. Duggar and associates employed regional analgesia in their patient, specifically because of their concern with respiratory inadequacy postoperatively. They also emphasized that the peculiar appearance of the mouth in these patients is due to diffuse fibrosis within the orbicularis oris, which does *not* relax after the induction of anesthesia or the use of relaxant drugs. As a consequence, they intubated their 7 month old patient awake.

ANESTHETIC CONSIDERATIONS

The unusual appearance of many children with congenital craniofacial abnormalities, in conjunction with an impressive syndrome title, can at times become the definitive statement about the patient's health. Unfortunately, when this occurs, the anesthesiologist is left with numerous unanswered questions about the current status of the life-support system for this strange craniofacial complex. Not only is it necessary temporarily to overlook the obvious, it is also necessary to question the usual—children with Crouzon's disease still get upper respiratory infections, for example. Only after the questions about associated defects and other diseases have been answered can the more obvious anesthetic problems of these children be addressed.

The mental and neurological status of the child must be assessed early in the planning of anesthetic treatment, based on how well the patient has met developmental milestones and current evaluations. The more severe the deformity, the more thoroughly the chart should be reviewed, if for no other reason than to facilitate the rapid development of the parents' confidence during the interview. As well, this information allows for a thoughtful approach to premedication and induction plans. For the infant, general activity and muscle tone are primary, with lesser attention paid to intellectual progression, as it little affects initial drug selection. The older child should be premedicated based on physical status and developmental age. As a general rule, all children, and perhaps these especially, look with disfavor on injection; this suggests use of oral premedicants, given 60 to 90 minutes prior to transport to the operating room.

Intracranial pressure (ICP) obviously influences the premedication and induction sequence significantly. In this group of patients, only about one third will have normal ICP. It is probably safest to depend only on "certain" statements and discard usual assumptions. "Certain" statements are those that clearly note the presence or absence of raised ICP based on examination, whereas much less "certain" is the child with an unusual cranium about whom nothing has been said regarding ICP. Furthermore, beyond documented elevated ICP is the consideration of intracranial compliance. The safe administration of drugs that cause rises in Pa_{CO_2} or cerebral blood volume depends in large measure on the assumption that the cranial vault is not only fairly accommodative, but uniformly so. A child with turricephaly may have marginally sufficient total intracranial volume to tolerate 1.3 MAC N_2O/O_2/halothane with spontaneous ventilation, yet lack the necessary room in one or more dimensions. In essence, although blood and cerebrospinal fluid can follow the path of least resistance, the brain may not.

In one series of patients with craniosynostosis, 14 percent of children with single suture involvement were found to have elevated ICP. Given this uncertainty, the most reasonable course seems to be to select premedication associated with lesser degrees of respiratory depression—for example, chloral hydrate or midazolam instead of morphine—and administer more potent drugs only under personal control at induction. Finally, if drugs known to raise Pa_{CO_2} and/or cerebral blood volume are selected, thought must be given to emergence and the postoperative period; no matter how efficacious, hyperventilation eventually must cease, and spontaneous ventilation must resume.

Although, as stated earlier, many strange-appearing children are intellectually normal, the complete picture is that many are not. As a part of this, the ability of one mentally retarded child to defeat the efforts of a half dozen supposedly bright adults concerning elimination of preoperative oral intake is living testimony to the motivational power of hunger. In my experience, the probability of a full stomach rises in the environmental progression: concerned, bright parents → hospital → unconcerned, less intelligent parents → custodial nursing facility. This situation is magnified by the number of hours the patient is awake and starved, which strongly suggests a rapid transition from A.M. awakening to the operating room.

Laboratory assessment should include hematocrit at the minimum, along with liver function tests for patients received from chronic institutional care. Chest radiograph and ECG are usually not needed unless indicated by the history or physical examination.

Adding up the features noted thus far, we find a variably retarded child with a potential for an unusual airway, a full stomach, and a raised ICP. As with most such complex situations, there is no "right" answer. However, one approach is oral midazolam premedication, rectal barbiturates (if needed), N_2O/O_2 with controlled mask hyperventilation (with cricoid pressure) as indicated, and then volatile vapor, until the patient is intubated and IV access is established. At this point, the stomach should be decompressed and relaxants or narcotic or both employed as desired. If the stomach proves relatively empty, the patient can be extubated at operation's end, airway permitting, while still anesthetized, switching to mask ventilation to decrease anesthetic depth. If the stomach proves full, ventilation must continue via the endotracheal tube until drug effects are eliminated, dissipated, or reversed, at which time the patient is extubated awake. The use of H_2-blockers remains controversial in children, with many experts of the opinion that they are little indicated in view of the very low incidence of aspiration. I take the somewhat different view that "low" is not "zero" and recommend that serious consideration be given to pharmacologic reduction of acid secretion. Admittedly, this will have no impact on the intraoperative course, but it does add a measure of protection after extubation.

The problem of pain control in a patient with a potentially raised ICP requires caution in the use of narcotics; preferably, small incremental doses should be given IV rather than a larger dose IM. When applicable, the use of regional analgesia may also provide a reasonable alternative in these patients, although narcotics may still be required for the child with defects of mentation, hearing, or vision. The recent introduction of a potent nonsteroidal anti-inflammatory drug, ketorolac tromethamine, with the potency of morphine suggests an option for pain control. However, at this writing, this drug is not approved for use in pediatrics (in the United States), does have a recognized incidence of somnolence after administration, and is a potent inhibitor of cyclooxygenase with a subsequent mild prolongation of the bleeding time. None of these facts preclude use, but at the very least the impact on coagulation suggests that communication with the surgeon should take place prior to ketorolac injection. Acetaminophen, on the other hand, can be administered rectally 1 hour before emergence with little such concern.

In conjunction with these considerations of analgesia, those responsible for care of this strange-appearing child must be given a very clear understanding of the patient's preoperative neurological status, developmental age, and any defects in sensory reception or speech. Parental visitation in the recovery room, or, for that matter, the induction room, is very much a matter of local policy, but in many cases a visit by the child's mother may be more helpful, as well as safer, than morphine.

ACQUIRED CRANIOFACIAL DEFORMITIES

TRAUMA

Infants and children are highly exposed to head and neck trauma, suffering damage from falls and motor vehicle accidents like their parents while at risk for birth injury, dog bites, and child abuse in a way their elders are not. The injuries are adversely affected by derangement of suture lines, osseous development, and tooth eruption, along with an increased ease of airway obstruction from hemorrhage or aspiration. All this is without consideration of the devastating psychological impact on a child of suddenly becoming unattractive or blind and then perhaps facing several attempts at surgical reconstruction.

Any attempt to consider pediatric trauma restricted along anatomical boundaries immediately runs afoul of a child's construction and the forces of physics. Children have relatively larger heads, weaker necks, and thinner and more flexible bones; the patient's smaller size makes it likely that more than the skull will be injured and that mass-velocity relationships will transfer tremendous amounts of kinetic energy to the patient. As a consequence, blunt thoracoabdominal injuries and head injuries are more likely to be coincident in children than in adults. The evaluation of this combination is very difficult and must be performed in a logical manner, without any regard to the initial training and orientation of the physician responsible. For those working in trauma centers, this is already accomplished. For those anesthesiologists working elsewhere, a frequently discovered principle is that each specialist perceives a human being to be a mobile life support system for an organ system of interest. Neurosurgery excepted, adherence to this concept has the potential for great misadventure.

Any child who presents with upper body trauma must first have established the basics of cardiopulmonary resuscitation. An airway must be assured or established (while accounting for deciduous teeth), respiration and oxygenation assured, and circulation confirmed. Any bleeding must be stopped, followed by a rapid evaluation of the central nervous system (CNS), skull, and cervical spine. In this process, it must be remembered that actually immobilizing the cervical spine is nearly impossible, and attempts to do so create a situation seemingly guaranteed to maximize aspiration opportunities. Fortunately, the actual incidence of spinal cord injury, with or without fracture, is low in children below age 13 years. Clinical evaluation is made more difficult because the majority of cases of pediatric cord trauma do *not* have associated fractures. In fact, evaluation of the upper cervical spine in young children may not be possible from plain radiographs and may require a computed tomographic scan for completeness. Therefore, any history of paresthesia or weakness should be considered very seriously, despite a "normal spine film."

Next, cardiothoracic and abdominal evaluation should proceed in conjunction with a bladder catheter, and, if indicated, an intravenous pyelogram. Moving peripherally, long bone and other fractures are evaluated and soft tissue injuries dealt with. In this sequence, the head and neck are at the periphery if the CNS is considered independently. The patient who is cardiovascularly stable should be nursed head up (semisitting, not reverse Trendelenburg), with the chin midline to decrease ICP and swelling. Conversely, the unstable patient should be cared for with the lower extremities elevated, not in Trendelenburg position. Lowering a child's skull below the heart provides a large reservoir for blood pooling while accomplishing absolutely nothing positive for critical cerebral perfusion pressure. The only significance afforded to the head and neck during the first critical moments should be because: (1) blood loss from scalp and facial lacerations, even though now no longer active, may have been substantial; and (2) any evidence of a major midface fracture, although not found commonly in children, is a relative contraindication to the blind nasal passage of anything, nasogastric tubes included, lest the skull be entered.

Following this evaluation, there is often pressure to operate on the child to close lacerations and stabilize facial fractures. This is usually motivated by a desire to obtain a quick return to normal appearance, coupled with the knowledge that the face will rapidly swell and fractures become "sticky," making subsequent work difficult. However, before this occurs the anesthesiologist must ensure that the patient is stable from a neurological and cardiopulmonary standpoint. If a major cerebral concussion was sustained, the neurosurgeon must be made aware that no neurological examination will be possible for several hours during the operation. On occasion, this may prompt the insertion of a device to monitor ICP as, and while, the patient is anesthetized. Any evidence of blunt trauma to the body absolutely demands a recent postresuscitation hematocrit measurement and chest radiograph—hours-old data are insufficient. Additionally, if anterior thoracic trauma is suspected, an ECG should be obtained. The anesthesiologist should ensure that blood and blood products are available as needed. Finally, intravenous access must be well established (while avoiding surgical access) and hydration accomplished, not only to ensure hemodynamic stability but to allow for rapid drug administration when required.

The patient should be brought to the operating room with analgesic premedication as tolerated by CNS status. The induction process is often a matter of selecting the drugs less contraindicated by the injuries; for example, ketamine offers hemodynamic stability and analgesia, but adversely affects ICP. Despite concerns about adrenal suppression and myoclonic movement, etomidate may have special merit in this situation. Whatever sequence is selected, several points are worth mentioning.

1. Suction capability must be redundant and assured—the stomach is full.
2. Mask oxygenation preinduction should be complete, timed by clock, and verified by oximetry, not by guess.
3. Oral intubation is generally best, at least initially. Any hint that the airway has been disrupted, i.e., crepitus, strongly suggests that laryngoscopy be done awake. Strangely, tracheal continuity can be disrupted without profound respiratory distress—while awake. Terrifying pictures in the surgical literature attest to the fact that respiration can occur via a serpentine path that will not easily allow for intubation from above. In such a situation, spontaneous respiration is absolutely lifesaving.
4. Cricoid pressure, gently before and firmly following induction, is absolutely required. Contrary to common practice, this is best accomplished bimanually.
5. The incidence of cervical cord injuries in children is low, but not zero. Current restraint devices, tongs excepted, do not immobilize the cervical spine. There are definite occasions when the trachea must be intubated, under direct vision, in the face of uncertain spine status. In such a situation, an assistant should apply very gentle traction during laryngoscopy to immobilize, *not distract*, the cervical spine.
6. Laryngoscopy must be visually analyzed from start to finish and near to far, as loose teeth, aspiration, hemorrhage, or airway disruption may be so diagnosed. In rapid sequence inductions, this is easier said than done, as target fixation on the vocal cords tends to eliminate visual depth of field.
7. One method of tube fixation in the burn or trauma patient is illustrated in Figure 9–7.
8. The incidence of oxygenation defects after major trauma, from aspiration, pulmonary contusion, pneumothorax or hemothorax, and so forth, is so high as to suggest use of more than 90 percent oxygen until blood gases are sampled.

A fair amount of information will be presented after induction, which requires interpretation. The response to positive-pressure ventilation often unmasks occult hypovolemia; crystalloid infusion to correct this will lower a marginal hematocrit level yet further. Obviously, if the induction commenced with a hematocrit that met personal transfusion criteria, the blood should be on the way before the drugs are. As well, this same ventilation may

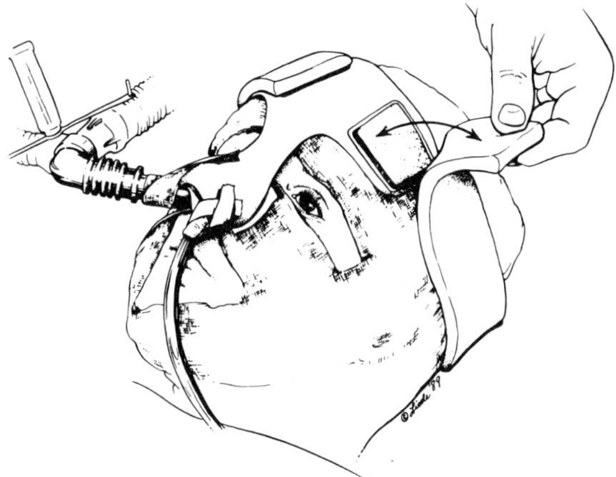

FIGURE 9–7. Tube fixation in the burn or trauma patient. (Reprinted with permission from Ward CG, Gorhan K, Hammond J, Varas R: Securing endotracheal tubes in patients with facial burns or trauma. Am J Surg *159*:339, 1990.)

rapidly enlarge an undiagnosed pneumothorax, requiring constant reassessment of symmetrical chest movement for at least 10 to 15 minutes after intubation. Abrupt collapse with the onset of positive pressure ventilation suggests pulmonary venous gas embolism, resuscitation from which may require transition to a head-down position and immediate thoracotomy.

For the patient brought very suddenly to operation, hypothermia is a major concern. Rapid infusion of cold blood and crystalloid can compound this situation; a blood warmer should be used from the outset. Beyond the usual issues that are part of hypothermia, body temperature can fall so low following transport as to adversely affect clotting. The other side of this issue is the good news that a cold brain requires less perfusion and may therefore protect a hypotensive patient. Although usually difficult to accomplish, body temperature should not be returned to normal before perfusion pressure. Later in the hospital course, patients with maxillofacial trauma often develop fever, frequently intraoperatively.

During the major portion of the operation, the anesthesiologist should add to his or her usual duties the continuing reevaluation of the acute patient. Despite the heroic image associated with liver and spleen trauma or pelvic factures, slow blood loss can occur from these injuries, and this can be diagnosed intraoperatively by increased fluid requirements, falling hematocrit, and enlarging abdomen. If some aspects of a case do not make sense, questions should be verbalized, as the pattern may be recognizable to others.

Finally, special vigilance is reserved for the airway itself. Tube malfunction, circuit disconnections, and surgical transgression of the airway all can occur, occasionally presenting as unusual one-way partial obstructions to gas exchange that are difficult to diagnose.

At the end of the operation, a full stomach and a generally swollen face are indications for leaving the patient intubated. The frequent use of intermaxillary fixation usually requires an intraoperative transition to a nasal tube, or, when the nasal complex or meninges are involved, even a tracheostomy. The latter, fortunately, eliminates the temptation to remove the tube prematurely; no matter how easy nasal intubation was initially, it will not be so straightforward to reinsert the tube in an awake patient who now has a nearly perfectly spherical skull. When the time seems eventually appropriate for extubation, any question concerning airway status should be assessed via direct visualization of the upper airway with a fiberoptic device. My experience with such endoscopy, following massive fluid resuscitation, has revealed examples of supraglottic edema suggestive of supraglottitis. Certainly, one direct view is worth 1000 rules of thumb, based on past experience. Any mechanical difficulty in actual tube removal requires AP and lateral skull x-ray films to rule out transfixation by wires or pins.

The patient should be nursed semi-sitting in the recovery room and supplied with humidified air/oxygen. Pain should be very carefully controlled with small incremental doses of narcotics (morphine, 0.025 mg/kg), neurological status permitting. Often the patients will have one nostril filled with nasogastric tube, while the mouth may be wired shut and completely filled with a swollen tongue. One somewhat edematous nostril leaves little margin for error in gas exchange; if respiratory difficulty ensues, a nasal airway should be gently inserted, midfacial or skull factures notwithstanding, before the oral wires are hurriedly cut. This airway can be in the form of a shortened endotracheal tube that can be easily connected to an oxygen source and used to buy time to reevaluate the situation.

BURNS

Burn injuries account for over 3000 deaths per year in children below age 15 years, with three times this number being disabled. Thermal and electrical burns are the second most common cause of death from age 1 to 4 years. The majority of childhood burns, fortunately, are not serious and do not require inpatient therapy. Such burns are due to scalds from a bathtub, usually affecting the lower body, or from spilled liquids, affecting the upper body. The child is otherwise subjected to burns for the same reason as the parent, substituting curiosity for stupidity where matches and flammable liquids are concerned. As with other forms of trauma, there is also the disturbing possibility that a child has been burned in abuse by another.

The general tendency in the care of these patients has been to refer patients with burns over a large surface area, those with more complicated burn injuries, or younger burned children to centers specializing in their care. This is appropriate management in intellectual isolation, but reality is the chance that any combination of child plus uncontrolled heat can create a critical mass demanding initial, or very late stage, anesthetic care wherever the child happens to be. This can be for anything from life-saving intubation and establishment of vascular access, to anesthesia for scar revision. The elaborate detail required to describe this full spectrum requires, and has received, a chapter unto itself (Ward, 1984). The following is a consolidation of pertinent facts that represents the *minimum* data base for caring for a child with damage to a portion of his or her largest organ, where the center of the injury area is occupied by multiple special senses and access to the respiratory tract.

Anesthetic Management

The preanesthetic assessment of a burned child is truly an emotionally difficult task. Even with substantial experience in an adult burn population, everyone who in any way cares for children must steel themselves for the sight of an infant or small child suffering the pain and disfigurement of a head and neck burn. As a part of this, the anesthesiologist must also prepare for a preanesthetic interview with parents, who often seem to possess a terribly short attention span and who oscillate between twin pillars of rage and guilt. In general, the majority of these children will have been healthy prior to the thermal insult, thus easing the interview, but the incidence of associated diseases is still high enough to deserve the usual questions. Additionally, there is a significant probability of other associated trauma compounding the burn, for which major allowances must be made in management.

Beyond the medical history of the child who *was*, obtained from the parents, there is the medical history of the child who *is*, obtained from the current chart. Preeminent in this review must be the evaluation of pulmonary function, for facial burns are often associated with significant airway damage. The awareness of everyone caring for burn patients that the upper airway may be injured is very high, and although criteria may vary from unit to unit, a request by an experienced burn surgeon to intubate a child, on admission or preoperatively, should be very seriously considered—nearly taken as mandatory, in fact. While true lung burn, steam inhalation excepted, is rare, upper airway burns are common; furthermore, the rate of edema formation after a major burn can be absolutely astounding. A straightforward, apparently unnecessary intubation can become critical and impossible in 4 hours as normally mobile anatomy becomes swollen and woodlike. The last topic in this chapter is management of the difficult airway, yet an extra concern for the burn patient is tube fixation. When the face is freshly burned, adhesive tape is not useful. Later, during reconstruction, such tape may injure new grafts. The useful approach of Ward and associates (1990) utilizes a nasotracheal tube support splint that is held in place by a circumferential strip of Velfoam and Velcro (see Figure 9–7). This can be used in children with extensive facial burns. The swelling that ensues after resuscitation will actually enlarge the head, so any form of circumcranial tube restraint may need to be acutely readjusted to remain nonconstrictive.

Another interesting technique to stabilize a nasal tube, reported by Galvis and Mestad (1981), is to split the tube longitudinally down to the nostril and tie umbilical tape to the resultant ends. One other method is a back-and-forth suture in the nasal membranous septum, tied around the tube. Although this is not the place to discuss the issue, a nasal tube seems more secure than an oral tube in these patients and is recommended as the final airway. However, their use requires an index of suspicion for otitis media and sinus infection whenever an unexplained fever occurs. Lastly, whatever tube is selected must have an airway leak, if uncuffed; if cuffed, it must be minimally inflated. Previously damaged tracheal cartilage cannot tolerate further insult.

There is a reasonable possibility that a child with burns of the head and neck, oral electrical injury excepted, will also have burns of the remainder of the upper body. These, in turn, may require escharotomy, and if anesthesia is requested for this, the anesthesiologist must remember to inquire about inhalation injury and carbon monoxide poisoning. The former demands anesthetic gas heat and humidification, along with arterial gas sampling; the latter suggests greater than 90 percent oxygen if more than 10 percent carboxyhemoglobin is measured.

During the preoperative visit to these patients, obtaining excessive detail about ongoing care is nearly impossible. The airway and ventilation data must include (1) tube size, depth of insertion (external and internal measure), leak/cuff pressure, and ease of suctioning; (2) ventilator settings with matched blood gases; and (3) chest radiograph and endoscopic evaluation of airway insult. The intake and output data must also include not just quantity but how administered, as venous access can be very difficult. Although NPO orders usually deal adequately with feeding by nasogastric tube, it is best to be certain and specifically discontinue such feedings at a desired time. Monitoring must be noted; usually easy questions such as "where to place ECG electrodes" often evolve innovative answers. Drug therapy must be recorded and then reflected upon. The chronic pain and analgesic therapy these patients receive requires a readjustment in thinking, lest the anesthesiologist discover that the selected preoperative intravenous dose of opiate is 50 percent *less* than the patient's usual increment. My preference is to order analgesic premedication alone, with little else, for patients in the acute phase of a burn, unless ventilation is mechanically controlled. When the patient is under the anesthesiologist's direct and continuous care, intravenous benzodiazepines can be useful to provide amnesia. Once the chronic phase begins, the usual individual premedication practice for patients subjected to multiple painful procedures should be followed. Beware the perfectly calm child; an emotional decompensation in the operating room can be expected if he or she is treated as if the inside matched the outside.

Burned children resemble premature babies in their vulnerability to cold. The operating room should be warm and draft-free when these patients arrive. A heating blanket should be on the bed, with an initial temperature set at 37°C, to be then decreased to 30 to 32°C for any situation in which the patient essentially sits semi-upright on the blanket. Although difficult to quantify exactly, the time-related potential for thermal injury to weight-bearing surfaces only requires consideration of how well the anesthesiologist would enjoy sitting absolutely immobile on a 37°C surface for several hours to prompt moderation in temperature settings. A heated gas humidifier is strongly recommended for all but short, late-stage reconstruction. Prolonged ventilation with cool, dry gas is not appropriate therapy for an already insulted airway. The drugs selected for the anesthetic are usual in name, but not in quantity. Narcotics, thiopental, and nondepolarizing relaxants should all be at least available in larger quantities; the patient with burns is likely to be resistant to the effects of each of these. Succinylcholine should be eliminated from use in all but chronic, fully covered burns—and probably even from those, as it is potentially harmful and rarely essential. For larger surface area burns, calcium chloride is very useful to have readily at hand, in a dilution such that 5 mg/kg is easy to administer as treatment for unexplained cardiovascular depression.

Monitoring again needs consideration, with an automatic blood pressure cuff or Doppler monitor nearby if the legs alone are available and an arterial catheter is not desired. Fluids should be passed through a warmer, most especially if the venous catheter tip is central. Additionally, if this is the case, flow must be evaluated early—fluid in a 6-inch, 18-gauge central catheter may flow less than half as well as in the usual 18-gauge peripheral catheter.

During induction and maintenance, the anesthesiologist must attend to the airway problems (see last section) while striving to keep up with fluid and thermal caloric losses. Keep very clearly in mind just how stressed these patients already are and that the skin preparation is noxious and actually begins the operation. The anesthetic should require large quantities of busy preparation, but should be designed to run on automatic pilot during the case. I favor moderate muscle paralysis, 50 percent N_2O/O_2, low-dose volatile vapor, and morphine, or perhaps methadone, 0.2 to 0.5 mg/kg, all with controlled ventilation. For prolonged operations, the presence of bowel dysfunction or distention may suggest the elimination of N_2O from the inspired gas mixture. The task then becomes vernier adjustment of anesthesia, monitoring, and intake and output control—the latter to maintain perfusion and urine output at 0.5 to 1 ml/kg/h.

Deliberate induction of hypotension may have a place in head and neck burn surgery, provided the patient, anesthetist, monitoring, and vascular access all coincide. The entire subject is much too broad to deal with here, except for three caveats: (1) induced hypotension should never be a last-minute addition to the anesthetic; (2) hypovolemia and high MAC-multiple inhalation anesthesia is a terrible combination that devastates the cardiac index, and it should not be employed; and (3) positioning and anesthesia should be flawless before hypotensive pharmacology is employed.

Once the débridement has finished and grafts have been placed, the wound must be covered and the patient awakened. If the wound extends onto the chest and circumferential dressings are to be applied, it becomes easy to impede thoracic wall and upper abdominal respiratory movement during this process. Five to ten centimeters of positive end-expiratory pressure at this stage, carried through until the patient is awake and breathing well, will assist in maintaining functional residual capacity and oxygenation. Extubation, if indicated, usually should be a thoughtful process in a comfortable patient, perhaps an hour or so postoperatively, unless the operation was minor. Striving for rapid extubation without analgesia has no place in the care of such chronically tormented children. Postextubation stridor is particularly common in the patient with facial burns, especially if there is no detectable air leak prior to extubation. Hence, the greatest caution should be exercised in planning any extubation. Those who require continued intubation should receive therapy to minimize airway damage, and a slight air leak should be ensured. In the recovery room, the anesthetic record should be reviewed thoroughly for detail. Whether the immediately preceding anesthetic was perfect or not, it represents a significant data point in the child's history and can be invaluable to those care providers who follow. The paradigm of senseless morbidity is the same error on the same patient—occasionally by the same anesthesiologist. These children are much too ill for repetitive first-order approximations at optimum anesthesia.

DEFORMITIES OF THE EXTERNAL EAR

The auricle serves as a gathering device. By design, it is a gathering device for sound energy, but when deformed it becomes, by default, a gathering device for attention. Many of the adjectives applied to the deformed external ear, excepting complete agenesis, are subjective and involve terms descriptive of size and location. As such, barring interference with hearing, such defects would appear to be of concern to the patient and his or her surgeon solely because of cosmetic considerations. However, review briefly the embryology, and the possibilities for associated defects loom large. The external ear originates from the first pharyngeal, or branchial, cleft; the first pharyngeal pouch opposes the cleft and creates the eustachian tube and middle ear. The ossicles develop from the first and second branchial arch, and the entire apparatus rests along the base of the skull near the temporal bone. Potentially, then, an event affecting the external ear could equally well disrupt development in the near vicinity.

In addition to malformations related by embryological continuity, external ear defects may also serve as a marker for more significant generalized abnormalities. There are therefore two general categories in which external ear defects may be placed. The first, primary ear defects, is presented in Table 9–2, along with a listing of associations, genetics, incidence, intelligence and life span predictions, and appropriate clinical features. The second category, in Table 9–3, is that of external ear abnormalities generally found in specific syndromes, although the described abnormality is by no means the primary diagnosis. Some, such as skin tags associated with Goldenhar's syndrome, are visually obvious. Others, such as the association of peripheral pulmonary stenosis with large ears, are far from apparent but nonetheless significant.

The preoperative assessment may find significant systemic disease, but this is not usually the case. What may be discovered instead is a 6-year-old who knows he or she is going to have an operation because he or she looks funny. For those unable to relate to this, the Walt Disney movie "Dumbo" is recommended. Premedication should be ordered accordingly. Otherwise, these diagnoses rarely demand special measures.

ANESTHETIC MANAGEMENT

Access to both ears is generally crucial during reparative operation, not only for the obvious reasons that defects may be bilateral, but because symmetry is so important to appearance. As a consequence, the surgeon may well request that both ears be visible and that 270° access to the head be afforded. If the former alone is desired, an endotracheal tube in line with the patient's longitudinal axis will suffice. This can be either an oral precurved tube (see next

Table 9–2. PRIMARY EXTERNAL EAR DEFECTS AND ASSOCIATIONS

Defect	Associated	Genetics	Incidence	Intelligence/ Life Span	Clinical Features
Absent tragus	Agnathia	?	?	Normal/normal	Absent tragus
AV fistula	—	?	?	Normal/normal	Enlarged pink or blue pulsatile auricle
Cupped ear	Pierre Robin	Autosomal dominant	?	Normal/normal	Pinna cupped forward, ear projects laterally, usually bilateral
Ectopic pinna	Middle ear malformation	?	?	Normal/normal	Pinna located without relation to ear canal
Echondrosis	—	Autosomal dominant	?	Normal/normal	Cartilaginous lump on posteromedial pinna
Absent lobe	Bird-headed dwarfism	?	?	Normal/normal	Absent ear lobe
Lobe pit	—	Autosomal dominant	?	Normal/normal	Incomplete pit, or hole, in ear lobe
Attached lobes	—	?	High in Germany	Normal/normal	Lower portion of ear attached to skull without free-hanging lobes
Hypertrophic lobes	Malformed incus	Autosomal dominant	?	Normal/normal	Fibrotic large ear lobes, conductive hearing loss
Long, narrow, posteriorly rotated ears	Rubinstein-Taybi syndrome, osteogenesis imperfecta	?	?	Normal/normal	Elongated ear, rotated backwards on skull more than 10%
Lop ear	Trisomy 21, conductive hearing loss	Autosomal dominant	1:5000	Normal/normal	Large concha, protruding ear, floppy helix
Low-set ears	Multiple syndromes	?	?	Retardation/normal or reduced	Helix below line from outer canthus to occipital protuberance
Mozart's ear	—	?	?	Normal/normal	Bulging superior aspect of pinna
Ear pits	Branchial fistulas, cleft palate, spina bifida, imperforate anus, renal defects	Autosomal dominant	2:1000	Normal/normal	Frequently draining tracts on/near helix
Prominent anthelix	Multiple syndromes and chromosome defects	?	?	Variable/variable	Prominent anthelix, poorly formed helix
Small ear with folded-down helix	Trisomy 21, conductive hearing loss	?	?	Normal/normal	Small ear; poorly developed, folded helix

section on Cleft Lip and Palate) or a nasal tube, again precurved if possible. If free 270° availability is needed, then the oral tube is best, leading to an anesthesia circuit that also follows the longitudinal axis. Generally, the operating table is eventually turned 90° to 180° from the traditional orientation, influenced by preference and the possible intent to take a skin graft for the ear repair.

The patient should be placed slightly head up (20°) to prevent bleeding, with little fear of air emboli unless bone is to be entered. Lidocaine with epinephrine is often injected along the incision line for hemostasis, markedly decreasing the anesthetic requirements—until the surgeon moves to an unanesthetized area or turns the head (for epinephrine dose limits with halothane, see page 339). This situation, except for a more favorable position for ventilation, is akin to that found in a cleft palate repair. The anesthesiologist must watch the airway move 4 feet away and then disappear beneath drapes, all the while maintaining the patient's spontaneous ventilation prompted by minimal stimulus. Muscle paralysis is one answer to this quandary, while another is controlled ventilation alone. In either case, the troublesome period is the start of the operation, when anesthetic concentration is rising; I generally employ controlled ventilation early on, changing to spontaneous ventilation, if possible, as the case progresses. Whatever the solution arrived at, a probably unacceptable combination is high inspired concentrations of volatile anesthetic, spontaneous ventilation, and minimal or absent surgical stimulation. The hypoventilation and myocardial depression associated with this combination can be literally deadly.

A prominent exception to this low anesthetic requirement is the harvesting of costal cartilage, usually from the eighth, ninth, and tenth ribs. Not only does this necessitate a second incision,

Table 9–3. SECONDARY EXTERNAL EAR DEFECTS AND ASSOCIATIONS

Defect	Association
Cauliflower ear	Diastrophic dwarfism
Crumpled ear	Contractural arachnodactyly
	Microtia-atresia
Cup ear	Syndrome with conductive deafness
	Fetal trimethadione
Folded ear	Cranio-oculodental syndrome
	Syndrome with conductive deafness
Lop ears	Anus-hand-ear syndrome
	Chromosome 18 p− syndrome
	Deafness and ear pits
Preauricular fistula	Deafness and ear pits
	Mandibulofacial dysostosis
	Oculoauriculovertebral dysplasia (Goldenhar's)
Preauricular pit	Chromosome 4 p− syndrome
	Deafness and ear pits
	Lip pits
Preauricular tag	Chromosome 5 p− syndrome
	Deafness and ear pits
	Lateral facial clefts
	Hemifacial microsomia
	Iris coloboma and anal atresia syndrome
	Limbal dermoid
	Mandibulofacial dysostosis
	Marden-Walker syndrome
	Microtia-atresia
	Oculoauriculovertebral dysplasia (Goldenhar's)
Large ears(s)	Auditory canal atresia
	Cerebro-oculofacial syndrome (COPS)
	Chromosome 8 trisomy syndrome
	Chromosome 18 p− syndrome
	Chromosome 13 q− syndrome
	Chromosome 21 monosomy syndrome
	Deafness, peripheral pulmonary stenosis, and brachytelephalangy
	Ear AV fistula
Large ear(s) *Continued*	Leprechaunism
	Macrotia
	Osteodysplasty
	Bilateral renal agenesis
	Trichorhinophalangeal syndrome, type II
	Small ear(s)
	Auditory canal atresia
	Auriculo-osteodysplasia
	C syndrome
	Chromosome 13 trisomy syndrome
	Chromosome 21 trisomy syndrome
	Cranio-oculodental syndrome
	Craniosynostosis-radial aplasia syndrome
	Deafness and ear pits
	Hemifacial microsomia
	Hypertelorism, microtia, facial clefting, and conductive deafness
	Microtia-atresia
	Renal, genital, and middle ear anomalies
Dysplastic ear(s)	Acrocephalopolysyndactyly(ies)
	C syndrome
	Cervico-oculoacoustic syndrome
	Chromosome 18 trisomy syndrome
	Chromosome 4 p− trisomy syndrome
	Pierre Robin syndrome
	Craniofacial dysostosis
	Craniosynostosis–radial aplasia syndrome
	Lateral facial cleft
	Fetal warfarin syndrome
	Limb-oto-cardiac syndrome
	Lissencephaly syndrome
	Mandibulofacial dysostosis
	Median clefts of lip, mandible, and tongue
	Prader-Willi syndrome
	Short rib–polydactyly syndrome, Majewski's type
	Thymic agenesis

but the area in question can never be fully immobilized to decrease pain. Additionally, this raises the possibility of pneumothorax, with the attendant concerns of N_2O use thereafter. Regional anesthesia, in the form of intercostal block, may be very useful in this situation.

Strangely, given the preceding warnings about diminished anesthetic requirements, small doses of narcotics (morphine, 0.025 mg/kg) may be required in the recovery room for children who have undergone bilateral repairs, as they awaken functionally deaf from surgical dressings. Obviously, the requirement for analgesia will be substantially greater for the child from whom costal cartilage was harvested for the auricular repair, unless regional anesthesia is utilized prior to emergence to provide postoperative pain relief. A chest x-ray examination in the recovery room is probably worthwhile to ensure the absence of pneumothorax.

CLEFT LIP AND PALATE

This topic would seem relatively straightforward, requiring brief mention of several combinations and variations on two central themes. The realization that this anatomy has an entire medical journal devoted to it, and that the abnormality occurs in association with over 150 syndromes (accounting, however, for less than 10 percent of clefts), exclusive of the Pierre Robin anomalad, points out the spectrum of the malformations. A good bit of this interest is due to a combination of two features: (1) surgically reparable defects in appearance and speech, and (2) frequency. Cleft lip and palate occur at a rate of about 1.5 per 1000 live births, with isolated cleft lip, or cleft palate, occurring about one third as often. Complicating these statements, however, is the realization that while cleft lip is almost invariably reported by birth certificate, cleft palate often is not; indeed, estimates of under-reporting are as high as 60 percent. The left:right:bilateral relationship is about 6:3:1. There is a male excess in cleft lip and palate, with female excess in isolated cleft palate. Intelligence and life span should both be normal, although an estimated 10 to 20 percent of infants do not survive the first year of life, usually owing to associated other defects, especially congenital heart disease.

CLINICAL FEATURES

Much of the distinction between cleft lip and cleft palate is based on an arcane landmark, the incisive foramen, and a missing word—secondary. Cleft *lip* usually refers to a pre–incisive foramen defect that may be anything from a minor incomplete skin cleft to a complete interruption of skin, gum, alveolar ridge, and primary palate. Cleft *palate* actually refers to cleft secondary post–incisive foramen palate. Bilateral cleft lip usually involves both primary and secondary palates, but may involve only the primary. As a consequence of all this, the diagnosis of cleft lip may refer to a highly variable spectrum of defects, whereas cleft palate may not be apparent in any way until the patient's mouth is opened. Indeed, some forms of palate defects may not be obvious even then. In addition to the cosmetic defects, however, cleft lip may present major impediments to the development of normal dentition, whereas cleft palate may cause velopharyngeal incompetence with resultant hypernasality of speech. Cleft palate may also present feeding problems in infancy, as the normal separation between food and air is absent, creating a nonphysiological mixing chamber in the nasopharynx. This often is associated with chronic rhinorrhea that must be distinguished preoperatively from infection.

Beyond the familiar clefts of the lip and palate, there is also a range of much rarer midline, median, and lateral facial clefts. These occur in an incidence of 1 to 4 percent of all clefts. Several classification schemes have been proposed to make sense of these unusual defects, with none being totally satisfactory. Their rarity and variability defy general statements, although in all such cases a thorough search should be made for other associated abnormalities. A number of these rarer defects seem to pose significant difficulties to airway management by mask; intubation does not appear so formidable, as almost all these malformations affect only the midface.

Although clefts of the lip and palate appear to be in anatomical continuity, it seems fairly clear that isolated cleft palate is somewhat unique. Although the incidence of simultaneously occurring additional abnormalities varies from series to series, isolated cleft palate almost invariably has twice the percentage of such associations when compared with isolated cleft lip or cleft lip with cleft palate. The most common nonsyndrome-related abnormalities found in association with any of these clefts are umbilical hernia, clubfoot, and limb and ear deformities; the most common syndromes are Klippel-Feil syndrome and the Pierre Robin anomalad. The incidence of congenital heart disease is fairly low in surgical series; however, this is because a large number of infants younger than 6 months with severe cardiac malformations are too ill, or have not survived, to enter such series. Among such infants, 66 percent have severe heart disease, whereas less than 2 percent of infants older than 6 months have heart disease. There is also an increased incidence of cervical spine abnormalities in cleft palate patients, although these generally do not become symptomatic in children.

ANESTHETIC MANAGEMENT

Repair of an isolated cleft lip usually will take place between the ages of 3 months and 6 months; repair of cleft secondary palate is delayed until age 12 months or more, so that growth can occur and ease the technical problems of the procedure. Preoperative assessment is typical for a child of this age, modified by the presence of additional defects. Intraoperative blood transfusion can be anticipated very rarely for lip repairs, uncommonly for palate repairs, and occasionally for pharyngoplasty. For any of these procedures, the patient should be brought to the operating room unpremedicated, excepting atropine, 0.01 to 0.02 mg/kg, given 30 minutes or less prior to, or coincident with, induction. The operating room should be warm (25°C) and draft-free, with a heating blanket (37°C) placed on the table. Induction is usually uneventful, utilizing N_2O/O_2/halothane and spontaneous ventilation, although a large palate defect may require placement of an oral airway fairly early. Laryngoscopy in a patient with a cleft lip is generally straightforward, but a cleft palate has the capability to trap and immobilize a straight blade, occasionally in a subtle fashion that befuddles an endoscopist unaware of the possibility. Should this occur, the anesthesiologist must first recognize the lateral immobility of the laryngoscope for what it is (this requires some thought, for the problem area is not always in direct view) and then consider inserting a gauze pack or dental roll in the cleft prior to the next attempt to visualize the vocal cords. Some anesthesiologists feel that specific laryngoscope blades such as the Robertshaw's or Oxford infant blades (Fig. 9–8), are especially useful in this setting.

The endotracheal tube itself is chosen for internal diameter (ID), according to age; in children older than 12 months, this can be determined by using the formula:

$$\frac{16 + \text{age in years}}{4} = \text{ID in mm}$$

Although some prefer a straight tube with a curved 15-mm connector, most anesthesiologists now select a precurved (RAE) tube for lip and/or palate surgery. Insertion of such a precurved tube may be somewhat easier with a stylet, and use of a stylet should be considered. It is worth noting at this point that tubes with manufactured conformation force the acceptance of a length/internal diameter relationship. For most patients, in most positions, this is acceptable, but not always. For the unusual combination, a tube with a soda-straw flexible extension (Flex-Bend) may prove useful. To achieve a cosmetic repair, symmetry is essential, so the tube should exit from the mouth in the midline without facial distortion from either the tube itself or the securing tape. As this tape will disappear beneath the surgical drapes, the use of a cutaneous adhesive, such as benzoin, is recommended to ensure adherence. It may be necessary to suture the tube to the lower gum in some circumstances.

The type of operation dictates the need for tube restraint. If a tongue blade is part of the surgical retractor, then the tube will be immobilized by the gag. If not, adhesive tape for precurved tube stabilization should be applied in two layers. The first layer crosses the straight external tube extension parallel to the lower lip and fixes the tube laterally. However, if narrow tape is used for this purpose (as is most often the case), the tube can still pivot or rotate. Consequently, a second piece of tape should be placed farther distal on the tube extension, with divided ends extending to the face over the right and left mandibular rami. This layer effectively restricts longitudinal and axial motion. Following tube fixation, stomach decompression with an in-and-out orogastric tube is recommended. After this step, bilateral chest ventilation should

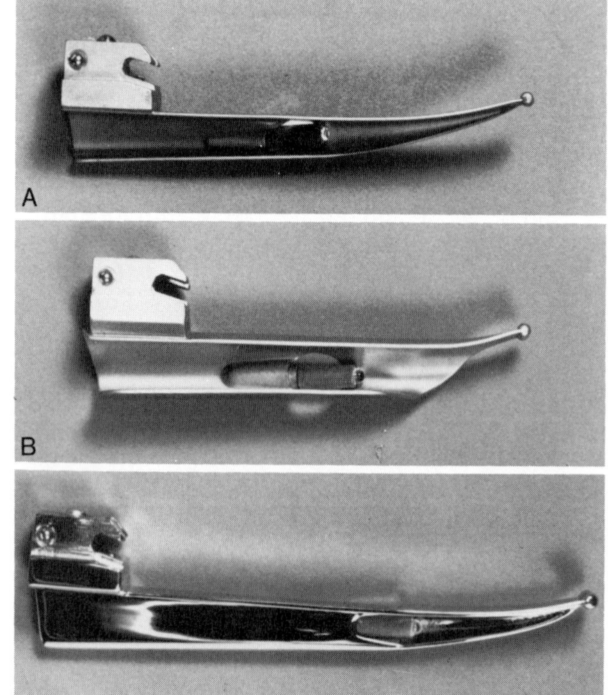

FIGURE 9–8. Blades for laryngoscopy. *A*, Robertshaw blade. *B*, Oxford infant blade. *C*, Seward blade. (Courtesy of Penlon USA, Division of Bear Medical Systems, Inc., Riverside, Cal.)

be assured with the patient in essentially the position required for the operation. For a cleft lip, this is fairly neutral, but for a cleft palate, moderately extreme cervical extension is required. Next, a pharyngeal pack of moistened ribbon gauze is inserted for cleft lip repairs; cleft palate surgery requires a tongue gag, and this cannot be placed correctly if the pack is in place. Once the gag has been inserted into a cleft palate patient, the surgeon can insert a pharyngeal pack, if it does not interfere with the surgical anatomy. Following gag and pack insertion, ventilation should be reassessed, as tube compression may have occurred. If a pack is used, consider writing the word "pack" on a piece of tape applied to the anesthesia machine or the patient's forehead, as a reminder at the end of the operation. Sterile ointment should be placed in both eyes; the application of tape to close the eyelids is according to surgical preference. If not already placed, secondary monitors (temperature, ECG, BP) should be applied and intravenous access established. The latter should be selected for cleft palate patients with the distinct possibility that blood transfusion might be required, especially if a pharyngeal flap is planned. If thought desirable, rectal acetaminophen can be administered at this point for procedures planned for less than 2 hours in length.

The patient can now be positioned for operation. The top of the infant's skull should be as near the head of the table as possible. For the cleft lip patient, this is generally sufficient, but the cleft palate patient frequently requires exaggerated neck hyperextension with a 15° Trendelenburg tilt that, following 90 to 180° table rotation, nearly places the patient's head in the surgeon's lap. In either situation, a low metal screen can sometimes be mounted on the table, with the horizontal bar a few centimeters over the patient's abdomen, serving to support the surgical drapes free of the infant's thorax.

Following positioning and surgical preparation, the drapes are applied. If the patient's temperature has not fallen below 36°C, external heating devices should be turned off at this point, as hyperthermia is easily achieved when all but 5 percent or so of the patient's surface area is covered. If the temperature has fallen substantially, warming should continue until 36°C is reached. In any case, the room can now be cooled, as the patient is environmentally isolated.

Occasionally in cleft lip repair, and always in cleft palate repair, lidocaine with epinephrine is injected early. The volume is small, to prevent anatomical distortion, but nevertheless raises the recurrent question of "How much epinephrine is allowed?" In general, children seem less susceptible to dysrhythmias than adults, although the reasons for this are not clear. The most specific and aggressive recommendations are those of Karl and associates (1983), who suggest a maximum epinephrine dose of 10 μg/kg through a wide range of end-tidal halothane concentrations—in *normocapnic children*. This should be placed in the context of a 1-year-old infant, covered in layers of surgical drapes, positioned head down and breathing through a convoluted, long, high-resistance tube.

The decision to utilize a spontaneous or controlled ventilation technique involves a number of considerations, but the obstacles to adequate spontaneous alveolar ventilation, for the cleft palate patient to a major degree and the cleft lip patient somewhat less, are substantial. Clearly, if a dysrhythmia does occur following epinephrine injection, one available option is to assure normocapnia via controlled ventilation; a second option is to change the volatile agent from halothane to another one with less arrhythmogenic potential. A further consideration following this injection of local anesthesia is the elimination of some, or all, of the surgical stimulus to the patient. The failure to adjust the inspired anesthetic concentration in response to this can lead to a relative overdose.

At the conclusion of the procedure, extubation should occur only when the patient is fully awake. Any other decision raises the specter of postextubation airway problems in which oral and nasal airways, and perhaps even masks, threaten the surgical repair. Many anesthesiologists make it a practice to remove any pharyngeal packs under direct vision while the patient is still anesthetized, to ensure an airway free of blood at the time of tube removal. Massive macroglossia causing airway obstruction, presumed to be a result of intraoperative pressure from the tongue blade, has been described to occur following cleft palate repair. The tongue should be examined prior to intubation; if there is any swelling, the patient is left intubated until this resolves.

To prevent the infant from disrupting the repair, patient arm restraints are utilized; these may interfere with the function of upper extremity intravenous infusions as well as requiring blood pressure to be measured in the legs rather than the arms. Before the patient is taken to the recovery room, the anesthesiologist must ensure that the flow of intravenous infusions can be maintained and the blood pressure can be monitored.

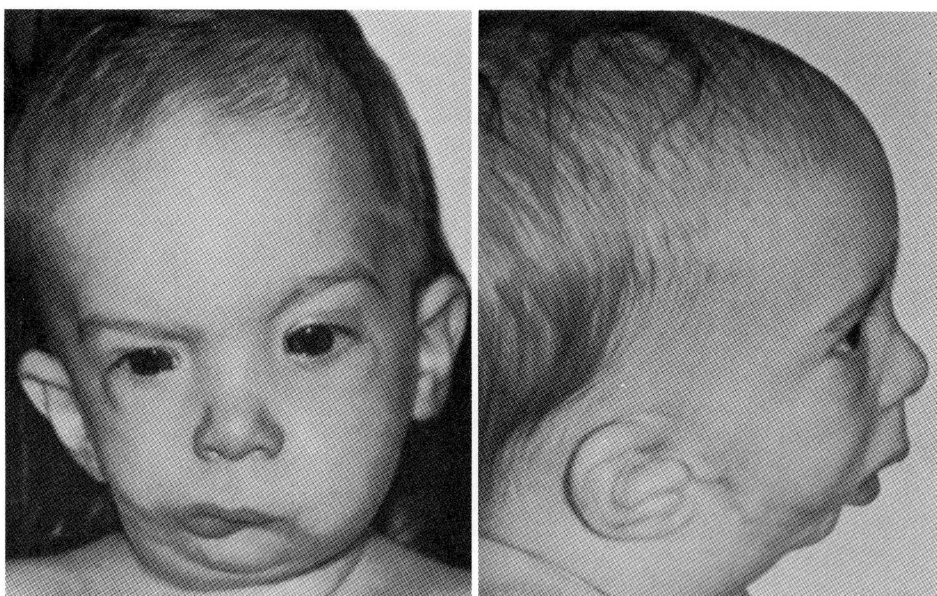

FIGURE 9–9. Hemifacial microsomia. (Reproduced by permission from Cohen MM Jr: Dysmorphic syndromes with craniofacial manifestations. *In* Stewart RE, Prescott GH [eds]: Oral Facial Genetics. St. Louis, CV Mosby, 1976.)

Pain therapy in the infant is a matter of some discussion. Options available vary from mother's comfort and oral intake to small doses of narcotics. If the parents are prepared for the postoperative appearance of their infant, their presence may be quite beneficial. If narcotics are felt needed, a suggested increment is morphine, 0.025 mg/kg intravenously, repeated no more frequently than every 10 minutes, to a total dose not to exceed 0.1 mg/kg. My habit is to write no repeat orders for any patient after pharyngoplasty but instead to reevaluate them personally from time to time, as these patients are at risk postoperatively from airway obstruction. Many institutions require that, following pharyngoplasty, children be retained in the recovery room for 24 hours and have close nursing observation. The possibility of later obstructive sleep apnea in such patients also must be considered.

If possible, these infants should be nursed slightly head up in the postoperative period to decrease edema formation. A variety of so-called infant seats can be employed to accomplish this.

BRANCHIAL ARCH DEFECTS

The clarity of this embryologically based title belies the facts, or at least the facts as different specialists perceive them. For example, one dysmorphology text presents a syndrome of high-arched palate, beak nose, micrognathia, zygomatic hypoplasia, antimongoloid palpebral fissures, broad thumbs, and broad great toes—the Rubinstein-Taybi syndrome—as one of the most important first arch syndromes. Another similar text places this syndrome in a separate classification, while a plastic surgery text doesn't mention the syndrome at all. At the outset, then, there appears to be not only confusion about what belongs in this classification but also whether, indeed, more than one syndrome "qualifies." The *Birth Defects Compendium* applies this primary title of first (and second) branchial arch syndrome to hemi(cranio)facial microsomia. The ensuing discussion follows this convention.

HEMIFACIAL MICROSOMIA
(Fig. 9–9)

Also known as otomandibular dysostosis, this syndrome was apparently described as early as 2000 B.C. By 1845, it was recognized that the structures involved were primarily derived from the first and second branchial arches, including the intervening first cleft. Providing a reasonable estimate of incidence is made difficult by yet another disagreement over terminology—in this case, whether or not this syndrome can cause *bilateral* deformity. However, as the supposed incidence of bilateral disease is only about 10 to 12 percent, it has little impact on an estimated incidence of 1 in 4000 to 6000 live births. As will be apparent from the description of the unilateral version, a bilateral presentation seems barely distinguishable from the Treacher Collins syndrome, except possibly by genetics. The male:female ratio has been variably reported at 1:1 or 2:1. The etiology is unknown. The patient's intelligence and life span generally should not be affected.

Clinical Features. The minimal diagnostic criteria are unilateral ear abnormalities and unilateral hypoplasia of the mandibular condyle and ramus. The ear abnormalities may vary from absence of the external ear to mild prominence of the auricle. Mandibular hypoplasia may virtually eliminate the ramus, causing the body of the mandible to curve up and join the condyle. The chin is generally deviated toward the affected side. Malocclusion and late tooth eruption occur frequently. The muscles of mastication, especially the lateral pterygoid, are impaired in some of these patients. This can limit the patient's ability to move the mandible, either forward or laterally, and when the mandible is externally depressed, the unaffected side may nearly dislocate downward and laterally while the affected condyle barely moves. Abnormalities of the eye and eyelid have been reported, including deviated palpebral fissure and choroid coloboma, along with strabismus. Pulmonary hypoplasia on the affected side has been noted as well. Agenesis of a portion of the facial nerve is the most common CNS defect noted, but any cranial nerve can be affected. Hearing loss on the affected side obviously may be associated; usually, this is of a conductive type and is due to the canal abnormalities.

OCULOAURICULOVERTEBRAL DYSPLASIA (GOLDENHAR'S SYNDROME) (Fig. 9–10)

In 1952, Goldenhar described in detail a syndrome of preauricular appendages and fistulae, associated with mandibulofacial dysostosis. Since that time, slightly more than 110 cases have been reported, extending the clinical presentation widely. The incidence is uncertain, as are the genetics. The male:female ratio is 1:1; life span and intelligence are both usually normal. This syndrome is currently thought to be a variation of the first (and second) branchial arch syndrome.

Clinical Features. There is no universally accepted constellation of features. Eye abnormalities include epibulbar dermoids, extraocular muscle defects, and coloboma. Auricular defects include external ear abnormalities, skin tags, and hearing loss. Rather more interesting from the anesthesiologist's view is micrognathia, unilateral mandibular hypoplasia, and cleft palate, in association with a 40 percent incidence of vertebral abnormalities and a 35 percent incidence of congenital heart disease. The former association frequently involves the upper neck, with vertebral fusion and odontoid elongation being noteworthy. The cardiac defects include septal defects and tetralogy of Fallot.

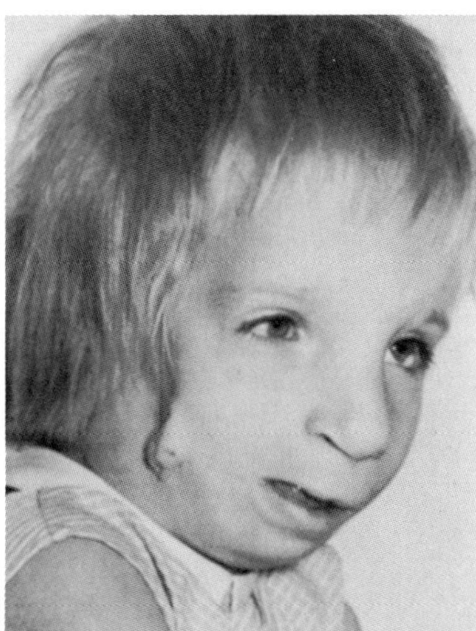

FIGURE 9–10. Goldenhar's syndrome. (Reproduced by permission from Goodman RM, Gorlin RJ: Atlas of the Face in Genetic Disorders. 2nd edition. St. Louis, CV Mosby, 1977.)

Increasingly, the term *facioauriculovertebral anomalad* has been applied to both this and hemifacial microsomia, owing to increasing clinical experience that suggests a continuum rather than a separation.

MANDIBULOFACIAL DYSOSTOSIS (BERRY'S SYNDROME; TREACHER COLLINS SYNDROME; FRANCESCHETTI-ZWAHLEN-KLEIN SYNDROME)

Simply based on the number of names involved, the struggle involved in classifying this constellation of defects can be easily surmised. Berry, an ophthalmologist, reported several family members with lower lid coloboma, and Treacher Collins subsequently reported an 8-year-old child who also had malar hypoplasia.

Finally, Franceschetti and colleagues pointed out the associated ear and mandibular deformities and emphasized that the minimal manifestation of the syndrome may be simply downward-slanting palpebral fissures and lid coloboma. As well, these latter investigators subdivided the syndrome into five categories: complete, incomplete, unilateral, abortive, and atypical. The so-called unilateral form is probably actually hemi(cranio)facial microsomia and will not be further considered here. The incidence is approximately 1 in 8000 to 10,000 live births, and over 200 cases have been reported. The syndrome is transmitted as autosomal dominant, with high penetrance and highly variable expressivity.

Patients with this syndrome generally do not suffer intellectual impairment, except as a function of hearing loss. However, those patients with pronounced facial maldevelopment in conjunction with such hearing loss may suffer enormously from being perceived as retarded. The prognosis for a normal life span is excellent, provided the patient survives infancy. Unfortunately, a number of children suffer fatal respiratory complications during the first few months of life.

Clinical Features. The complete form includes downward-slanting palpebral fissures, notching or coloboma of the lower eyelid, hypoplasia of facial bones (especially the zygoma and mandible), malformation of the ear (external, middle, and occasionally inner), macrostomia with high palate and abnormal dentition, blind fistulae between the ear and the angle of the mouth, and patchy projections of hair from the sideburns onto the cheeks. Very commonly, the palate may be cleft, as well. As a matter of interest, Tessier, in presenting a new classification of craniofacial clefts in 1973, felt that the entire syndrome could be explained by a combination of three different clefts (numbers 6, 7, and 8 in his system). Although a decade is insufficient time to establish this concept, it may provide an attractive unification of the syndrome presentations.

The incomplete form usually presents with a lesser degree of deformity, frequently with associated deafness. This presentation is probably the original Treacher Collins syndrome. The abortive form involves only the eyes, whereas the atypical type consists of defects, partly typical and partly quite unusual, such as microphthalmos and temporomandibular joint dysfunction. The inclusion of cases into this category is often subject to debate.

The incomplete form, or Treacher Collins syndrome (Fig. 9–11), has received a rather large amount of attention considering its rarity. Externally, many children with Treacher Collins syndrome somewhat resemble those with Pierre Robin anomalad, suggesting upper airway obstruction from similar causes—glossoptosis and micrognathia. However, several investigators have examined children with Treacher Collins syndrome in some detail and have discovered a slightly more complex situation. Utilizing multiview video-fluoroscopy and fiberoptic nasopharyngoscopy, patients with Treacher Collins syndrome were compared with normal controls and with a group of patients with isolated cleft palate. It was clearly demonstrated that every patient with Treacher Collins syndrome had pronounced narrowing of the pharynx in the lateral dimension, usually at the tongue base. This was associated with some anteroposterior narrowing as well, markedly reducing the cross-sectional area of the airway at a point well above the larynx. To put this finding into perspective, the mean pharyngeal width reported for controls was 32 mm, whereas patients with the Treacher Collins syndrome were reported to have a mean width of 14 mm—including one 11-year-old child with a lateral measurement of only 5 mm. To worsen the situation, the correlation between the visible penetrance of the syndrome and pharyngeal hypoplasia was adjudged poor, so that predicting an excessively

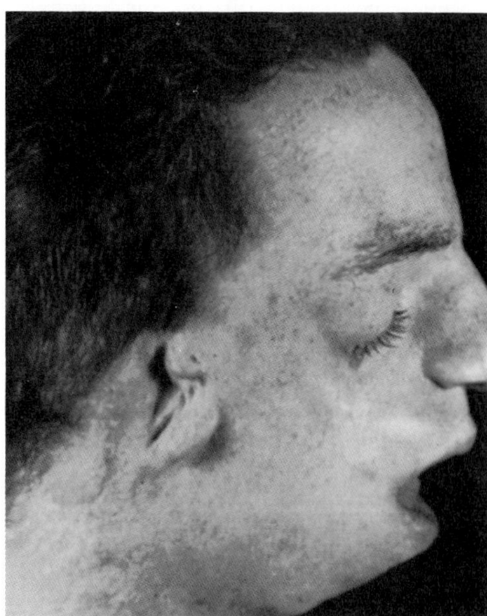

FIGURE 9–11. Treacher Collins syndrome. (Reproduced by permission from Goodman RM, Gorlin RJ: Atlas of the face in Genetic Disorders. 2nd edition. St. Louis, CV Mosby, 1977.)

narrow airway from the patient's appearance was improbable.

It is interesting that despite the fact that 80 percent of the patients in this report with Treacher Collins syndrome also had cleft palates, those patients with isolated cleft palate possessed increased lateral pharyngeal dimensions—mean width 36 mm—emphasizing that similar features do not create identical situations. However, it is worth considering the implications of cleft palate and Treacher Collins syndrome, for if such a patient speaks with a nasal quality, the traditional approach might be to correct velopharyngeal incompetence with a pharyngoplasty. In at least one reported Treacher Collins patient, this produced a subsequent sleep apnea syndrome; this demonstrates that despite the multifactorial requirements currently thought necessary to develop sleep apnea, a major contribution from any one sector can precipitate the syndrome. (For further considerations, see the following discussion of Pierre Robin anomalad and the latter section on chronic airway obstruction.)

Two questions are immediately generated from this progression. First, does this pharyngeal hypoplasia occur in the other forms of mandibulofacial dysostosis? Second, how many other syndromes primarily manifested in maldevelopment of the first and second branchial arch might involve airway constriction? At the moment, both questions await further data.

PIERRE ROBIN ANOMALAD

(Fig. 9–12)

Micrognathia and glossoptosis (tongue falling backward), often in association with cleft palate, compose this assemblage, which is more correctly called an anomalad, or group of anomalies. It was undoubtedly known prior to Pierre Robin's 1923 paper, but he does deserve credit for drawing attention to the clinical significance of the association. (In further writings, Robin developed the significance of this combination to the point he felt that it was present in 60 percent of children and caused, among other things, flat feet.) The anomalad may occur in isolation in about 1 in 30,000 live births or as a part of other syndromes, especially the campomelic syndrome, the cerebrocostomandibular syndrome, the persistent left superior vena cava syndrome, and Stickler's sequence. The etiology is uncertain, although intrauterine malposition and pressure are frequently mentioned. While this initially seems a simplistic explanation, al-

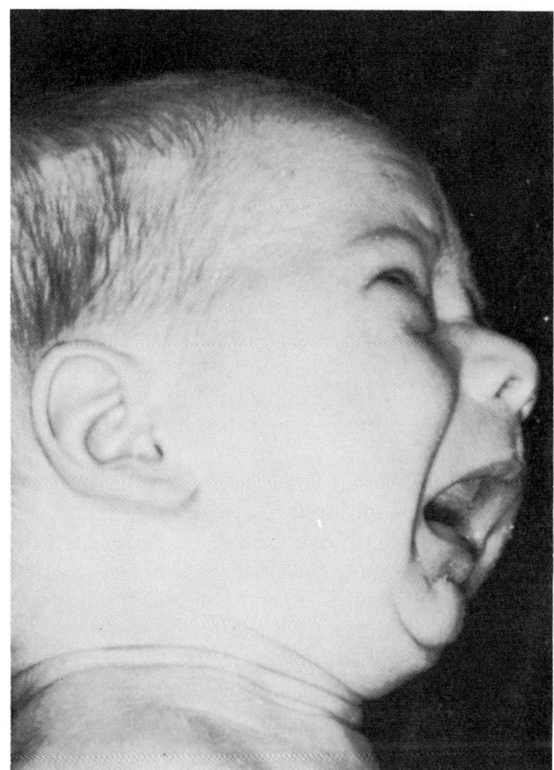

FIGURE 9–12. Pierre Robin anomalad. (Reproduced by permission from Goodman RM, Gorlin RJ: Atlas of the Face in Genetic Disorders. 2nd edition. St. Louis, CV Mosby, 1977.)

ternatives are not clearly available, as the structures involved develop at different times and from different sources. The male:female distribution is 1:1. The patient's intelligence and life span are normal, except in cases involving significant airway compromise and associated other defects. Unfortunately, 60 percent of patients have such other defects, largely accounting for the associated mortality of 20 to 25 percent.

Clinical Features. The essential features of the anomalad are micrognathia and glossoptosis. Cleft palate is almost an invariable addition; the defect is usually U-shaped, thought secondary to tongue interference with palatal fusion. Twenty-five percent of cases are associated with known syndromes; 36 percent of patients have other defects, most frequently cardiac, not associated with identified syndromes.

These infants can present major problems almost immediately after delivery, although a more typical history is of development of airway obstruction over the first 4 weeks of life. It is fascinating that premature infants may not develop problems until reaching the same gestational age. It is actually difficult to imagine upper airway anatomy more vexing than in this anomalad. In pronounced cases, the nasopharynx will fill with tongue (via the cleft palate) whenever the baby is supine, causing total airway occlusion, with the generation of negative respiratory pressures of up to 60 mm Hg serving only to aggravate the posterior tongue displacement. The baby frequently may try to maintain its airway by constant struggling and crying, only to suffer obstruction very abruptly when exhausted. Prodigious amounts of nursing attention, prone positioning, and extraordinary care in feeding may buy time during which the tongue-mandible relationship may improve or, alternatively, time in which the infant improves tongue musculature control.

When traditional medical means have been inadequate, traditional surgical measures usually have been employed. Such measures include suturing the tongue anteriorly in one of several methods (including permanent glossopexy) or passing a Kirschner's wire anterior to the mandibular angles and transfixing the tongue.

Two unusual management techniques recently have been employed with these babies. One is to nurse the baby prone, with the skull suspended by a traction cap. The other concept, very comfortable to anesthesiologists, is to use an 8- to 9-cm long, 3- to 3.5-mm internal diameter endotracheal tube as a nasopharyngeal airway. This latter technique has been evaluated in some detail, and with appropriate nursing care it appears to have substantial merit. However, this is very dynamic anatomy, and the margin for error in naso-pharyngeal tube placement is minuscule.

Chronic upper airway obstruction represents a constant threat to these unfortunate infants in two ways. First, prolonged hypoventilation and marginal oxygenation may cause pulmonary artery hypertension and cor pulmonale. This clinical situation has been associated with an increased incidence of pulmonary edema, which was originally thought to be due to changes in central blood volume and intrapleural pressure but, in view of current research on right-left ventricular interaction, may also be partly due to interventricular septal shift secondary to chronic right ventricular overload. Associated with this cardiopulmonary dysfunction may well be failure to thrive subsequent to feeding difficulties and to a two- to threefold increase in the work of breathing. The second threat is abrupt respiratory failure, superimposed on chronic disease, due to exhaustion, aspiration, or infection, all of which are common.

With time, usually a few months, infants with this anomalad generally, but not always, "improve" so that the airway is less perilous. However, cleft palate repair involving the use of a pharyngeal flap may recreate the neonatal situation of airway compromise. This particular sequence has been implicated in the postoperative demise of a child.

The preceding discussion sets the basis for considerations of elective tracheostomy in these children, with full recognition that decannulation may require months. While this may be viewed as somewhat archaic in this advanced age of oral and nasal plastics, note well the duration and severity of the pathology before rejecting a permanent artificial airway. As will be discussed on page 352, supraglottic intubation of a child with a severe form of this syndrome may simply prove nearly impossible, leaving no other option.

Until recently, the evaluation of these children depended on the experience level of the physicians involved and a history of cyanosis or severe feeding difficulties. The tremendous interest in sleep disorders during the past decade has created a unique modality to quantify airway obstruction in these patients—polysomnography. In conjunction with oximetry, it has now become possible to measure frequency, duration, and severity of airway obstruction, with subsequent specific recommendations for therapy. A recent series of 21 patients so evaluated reported a mortality of zero, with surgical intervention required for 50 percent of patients. Not surprisingly to anesthesiologists, it was noted that desaturation frequently occurred without obvious cyanosis. It was also noted that obstruction without desaturation also occurred on occasion. Furthermore, by utilizing a pharyngeal pH probe, it was determined that a subset of these patients, during periods of obstruction, also had significant evidence of acid aspiration and went on to antireflux surgical therapy.

OCULOMANDIBULOFACIAL (HALLERMANN-STREIFF) SYNDROME (Fig. 9–13)

As is often the case, history has been unkind, for this syndrome was probably first described by C. Audry in 1893. Hallermann and Streiff, independently, further clarified the components of the syndrome and pointed out the ophthalmological aspects, thus gaining lasting recognition. Although this syndrome has constant manifestations that extend well beyond the head and

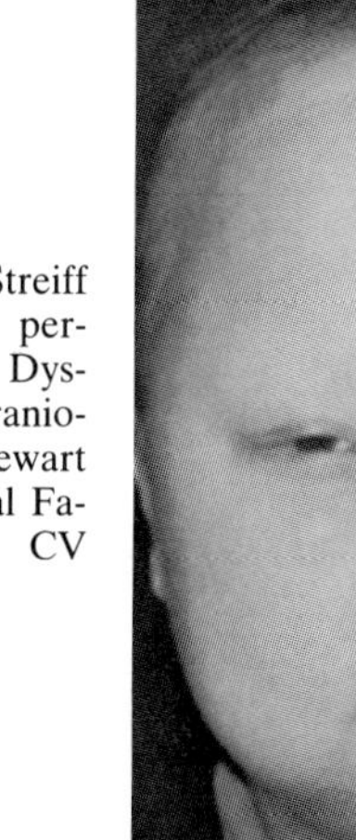
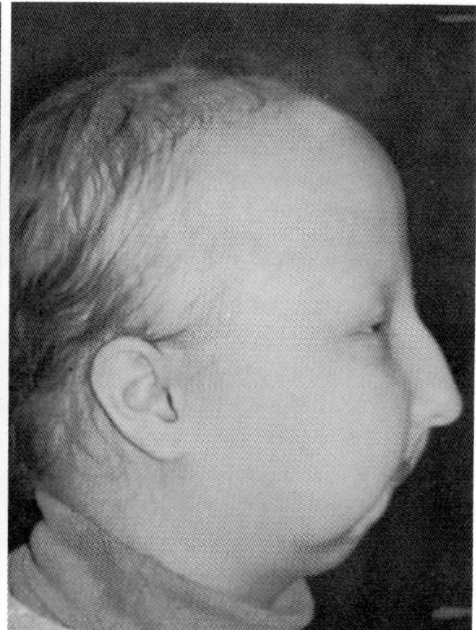

FIGURE 9–13. Hallermann-Streiff syndrome. (Reproduced by permission from Cohen MM Jr: Dysmorphic syndromes with craniofacial manifestations. *In* Stewart RE, Prescott GH [eds]: Oral Facial Genetics. St. Louis, CV Mosby, 1976.)

neck, it is included in discussion here because the anatomical description seems to warrant it.

This syndrome is very rare, with somewhat more than 50 cases in the literature. The male:female ratio is 1:1, with the mode of genetic transmission unknown. In theory, life span should be normal, but the impact of lower facial malformation has led to death in childhood, usually directly linked to recurrent respiratory infections and feeding problems. Intelligence should be normal, although the effect on development of strange facies, possibly diminished hearing, and probably decreased vision may be profound.

Clinical Features. Proportionate dwarfism is almost invariably present, along with diminished scalp and body hair. The skull is often wide, occasionally with macrocephaly and lambdoid suture dehiscence, although microcephaly also has been reported. Ophthalmological defects include microphthalmia, downward slanting palpebral fissures, blue sclerae, congenital cataracts (which, strangely, may spontaneously resorb), nystagmus, strabismus, and decreased visual acuity. The face usually appears small, with a narrow beaked nose that generates an impression of a "birdlike" face. Malar bone hypoplasia may be present; micrognathia and mandibular hypoplasia are almost invariably so. It is interesting that the entire temporomandibular joint may be displaced up to 2 cm forward. The palate has a high arch, and dentition is disturbed, allowing for severe malocclusion, absent teeth, extra teeth, and persistent deciduous teeth. Deafness is occasionally noted, as are general skeletal problems such as lordosis, scoliosis, and spina bifida. The scalp veins are often noted to be prominent, generally secondary to cutaneous atrophy, not to hydrocephalus.

ANESTHETIC MANAGEMENT

In general, hemifacial microsomia, oculoauriculovertebral dysplasia, mandibulofacial dysostosis, Pierre Robin anomalad, and oculomandibulofacial syndrome all present to the anesthesiologist the dual challenge of the difficult airway and difficult intubation, compounded by other assorted systemic defects. The airway constraints are very real and, despite the progression described in the last section on Management of the Difficult Pediatric Airway and Intubation, can defeat a very skilled anesthesiologist on any given day.

Hemifacial microsomia, strictly speaking, is unilateral, and the unaffected side may represent a point of attack, especially for lateral laryngoscope insertion. The three-dimensional asymmetry can be expected to make fitting a mask very difficult.

Oculoauriculovertebral dysplasia poses the very tough combination of cervical spine abnormalities, including odontoid elongation, with micrognathia. Not only can this serve to make mask fit and intubation difficult, but also the possibility of actual cord trauma exists. Compounded with congenital heart disease, especially a tetralogy, this can set the stage for disaster. Airway management is often extremely difficult in affected children, and the capability to add tracheostomy rapidly to the scheduled procedure is a must. The concept of a continuum of facioauriculovertebral anomalad suggests that the anesthetic considerations applying to the entire continuum should be kept in mind in managing patients with oculoauriculovertebral dysplasia or hemifacial microsomia.

Mandibulofacial dysostosis is highly variable in appearance and difficulty. The detailed description of Treacher Collins syndrome should probably be assumed to apply to all variations until proved otherwise. The very narrow posterior upper airway should be kept in mind during laryngoscopy, as distortion of this plane, at this location, could adversely affect blade mobility and tube passage.

Pierre Robin anomalad is the best known of these very difficult airways. The difficulty here is related to a large palate defect, other systemic abnormalities, and micrognathia. These infants, too, may require tracheostomy because intubation cannot be accomplished by the outlined measures. However, with Pierre Robin anomalad and all these syndromes, it is worth considering a request for help from the best pediatric fiberoptic endoscopist available if personal expertise is not up to the task.

Oculomandibulofacial syndrome presents a risk for obstructive sleep apnea and a difficult airway with difficult intubation. The occasional displacement of the temporomandibular joint is difficult to assess, as it might possibly diminish problems. By no means, however, should this be counted on, as clinical experience is minimal. The isolated case report of anesthesia for a patient with this syndrome commented on micrognathia, fragile teeth, and temporomandibular joint restrictions, along with diminished nostril size, as potential problems. In point of fact, the actual management of this case involved awake direct laryngoscopy and oral intubation without much difficulty. The patient, however, was an adult; management would probably have been more difficult for a child.

All the children should be carefully assessed postoperatively and extubated awake. Experience seems to be greatest with Pierre Robin patients, and the tendency seems to be a longer period (3 to 5 days) following any form of airway operation before extubation. Near-prone positioning may help the patient sustain a natural airway, and humidified oxygen should be supplied after extubation. Serious thought should be given to staffing patterns in the recovery room. If continuous one-on-one coverage with an experienced nurse who is comfortable with children is not the plan, then the plan must be rearranged, the anesthesiologist must stay close at hand or, perhaps best, the patient should be extubated following resolution of surgical edema in the intensive care unit. To have one of these patients slip into difficulty in the immediate postoperative period, after all the anxiety and effort in the operating room, is truly to snatch defeat from the jaws of victory.

BRANCHIAL CYSTS AND FISTULAE

Despite the brief and seemingly straightforward opening discussion of branchial cleft embryology, uniform agreement about the true origin of these cysts and fistulae has yet to be achieved. The most generally accepted theory is that presented in the initial review of embryology, and, for discussion purposes, this will be accepted here. From the management standpoint, however, it is worthwhile to note that some investigators feel the cysts are of a different origin than the fistulae and will therefore refer to these lesions as cervical cysts instead. By themselves, neither cysts nor fistulae generally have an impact on the patient's life span, intelligence, or well being. A rare exception to this is a case of malignant degeneration in a cyst or fistula late in life.

Clinical Features. These lesions may present at any age, are more common in males, and are generally unilateral. Cysts outnumber fistulae about three to one. A confusing entity in this area is the very common preauricular sinus, which may be associated with other defects but generally exists independently. This type of sinus presents as a dimple anterior to the tragus and usually ends in a blind pouch against the superior conchal fossa. Unless inflamed, such a sinus usually requires little medical attention.

A first branchial cleft cyst or fistula is found entirely above the hyoid bone, communicates with the external auditory canal, and can be easily confused with a parotid tumor. The primary significance of these lesions, as with parotid tumors, is their proximity to the facial nerve. A more common sinus or fistula originates from the second branchial cleft. They may appear externally anywhere along the anterior border of the lower two thirds of the sternocleidomastoid muscle, generally most often at the junction of the lower and middle third. About 50 percent of these particular cleft defects will have a fistula with origins in the tonsillar fossa, traversing between the internal and external carotid arteries and presenting at the skin. The third branchial cleft opens externally at about the same location as the second, but presents internally at the pyriform sinus after travelling down the sheath of the common carotid, deep to the internal carotid artery. Cysts or fistulae of the fourth cleft are theoretically possible but are reported rarely; they should pass from upper esophagus to mediastinum.

ANESTHETIC MANAGEMENT

The symptoms presented by these cysts or fistulae are generally only cosmetic, although the possibility of infection and prior attempts at removal may certainly be part of the patient's history. Preoperative assessment and preparation are unremarkable for this diagnosis.

The patient will eventually be positioned with the neck extended and the head rotated away from the lesion. There exists some possibility that intraoral manipulation will be required, suggesting a contralateral nasal tube as a final airway. If a nasal tube is chosen, the precurved variety provides for a low profile as well as minimizing dead space. Recommendations for passing a nasal tube are found in the section on the difficult Pediatric Airway (see pages 352 to 358). During the actual procedure, the patient should be positioned slightly (20°) head up (not, however, in the reverse Trendelenburg position) to decrease bleeding. Overaggressiveness in elevating the head also raises the possibility of air emboli; this should be avoided unless the position is felt to be so beneficial that all the measures associated with a sitting craniotomy are also taken. For procedures on first cleft defects, the proximity of the facial nerve suggests minimal use of long-acting relaxants, particularly if a nerve stimulator is included on the sterile field. Defects of the lower clefts involve dissection around the carotid artery with the attendant problem of bradycardia; after hypoxia has been eliminated as a cause, such heart rate changes may require atropine therapy.

Following an excision of a first cleft lesion, extubation can usually be performed immediately. Procedures for second and third cleft defects may involve substantially more paratracheal dissection, with the possibility of attendant cervical swelling, and this suggests awake extubation. In either case, the patient should be nursed semi-sitting in the postoperative period to minimize swelling.

CYSTIC HYGROMA

Adolph Wernher published a monograph in 1843 concerning one variety of what is today called a lymphangioma. Wernher described the gross pathology of these lesions; pointed out that while they are common in the neck, they may occur elsewhere (as in the abdomen); and applied the clinically established but nonspecific term *cystic hygroma*. It remained for a number of pathologists to establish the lymphatic origin of these lesions, and even today there is controversy concerning their true nature. The current leading hypothesis is that cystic hygromas are the result of congenital dysplasia of lymphatics, although the possibility still exists that hamartoma or true neoplasm may be a more applicable classification.

Lymphangioma may be classified into one of three general categories: (1) simplex, made up of small lymphatics, usually confined to skin or mucous membranes; (2) cavernous, made up of larger lymphatics, with deep diffuse extension; and (3) cystic, or cystic hygroma, involving multilobular, multilocular collections of small cysts filled with clear, yellow-tinged, or bloody fluid. None of these presentations are considered common.

Clinical Features. Cystic hygroma most often occurs in the neck (60 to 70 percent), generally in the posterior triangle, although occasionally a cyst will communicate beneath the clavicle with a hygroma in the axilla, the next most common location (20 percent). Less frequently, a hygroma will appear in the anterior triangle, generally high up, and will then be associated with intraoral lymphangiomas. This presentation is the one most often associated with airway compromise, occasionally compounded by mediastinal extension of the hygroma. This latter possibility strongly suggests radiological evaluation of the chest in all infants with a diagnosis of cystic hygroma.

The usual history of these lesions is presentation at birth or shortly thereafter, often with subsequent alarmingly rapid enlargement. Infection is certainly possible; spontaneous regression is doubtful. Simple incision and drainage lead to chronic fluid loss, while decompression of the cyst or cysts, pre- or intraoperatively, has been described as a major impediment to complete cure—being then, in turn, partly responsible for the 10 to 25 percent recurrence rate of hygromas. The word *recurrence* requires some elaboration, for on occasion these cysts have refilled, with either clear fluid or blood, in periods of only a few days.

ANESTHETIC MANAGEMENT

First and foremost, it is necessary for the anesthesiologist to have a clear picture of the limits of the disease. In general, these lesions are tolerated amazingly well by the infants, but any history vaguely suggestive of respiratory problems, feeding difficulties, or even cough should be pursued to discover possible intraoral or mediastinal disease. The presence of cysts in the visible oral cavity may warn of extension into the supraglottic area, while mediastinal compression may require endotracheal tube insertion to, or perhaps beyond, the carina. Although such preoperative assessment must be thorough, it should not be tardy, for the possibility that the cysts will enlarge is quite real, thus making a known difficult situation into an unknown worse one.

The patient should be brought to the operating room unpremedicated except for atropine, given 30 minutes or less prior to, or coincident with, induction. For a neonate, an awake intubation with continuous oxygen insufflation may be preferred. For the older infant, a spontaneous ventilation halothane mask induction, with or without N_2O, allows for gradual assumption of the airway. Upon demonstration of bilateral chest expansion without gastric distention during a positive-pressure breath, the anesthesiologist has total airway control—as yet, however, without assurance of intubation. Even at this stage, it is best to maintain spontaneous ventilation until the trachea has been intubated, since, despite preoperative assessment, the supraglottic airway may possess unsuspected abnormalities, such as epiglottic cysts. In general, these structures can be avoided under direct vision, given the time available with adequate oxygenation and anesthesia. If the intubation is prolonged, it may be worthwhile to insufflate the anesthetic mixture via a nasopharyngeal catheter or airway, provided it does not also serve to anesthetize the endoscopist. (See also the concluding section on the difficult airway and intubation.)

After the trachea has been intubated orally, some thought may be given to substituting a nasal tube, especially if the lesion extends into the mouth. To change the tube is very much the decision of the anesthesiologist, and no further steps should be taken if the maneuver is thought excessively difficult. In either case, bilateral ventilation must be reconfirmed once the baby is finally positioned for operation.

Taking advantage of halothane-induced cutaneous vein prominence, it is highly desirable to insert at least one, preferably two, substantial intravenous catheter(s) early, not only to offset the dehydration/inhalation combination, but also in anticipation of the occasionally substantial blood and fluid losses that occur in the resection of these cysts. An intra-arterial catheter is suggested if the cyst is large, and *strongly* suggested if the lesion extends into the mediastinum. Central venous pressure monitoring is desirable; unfortunately, the most direct access to the right atrium, via the jugular veins, may be impossible. For all but the most limited lesions, an indwelling bladder catheter connected to calibrated drainage is indicated.

Following tracheal intubation, spontaneous or controlled ventilation techniques may be employed, as indicated. The anesthesiologist's task then becomes fluid and thermal energy replacement in the face of steady substantial losses of both. Clearly identifying what type of fluid is being lost may be rather difficult, emphasizing the value of intermittent blood sampling.

The possibility of surgically induced bradycardia should be considered whenever the dissection nears branches of the vagus nerve or the carotid sinus. However, bradycardia remains foremost a warning of hypoxia in infants, despite the anatomy. Only after this cause is eliminated should atropine be employed.

Postoperative airway management is largely dictated by the procedure. For removal of an isolated small cyst, extubation is straightforward. In general, however, the possibility of oropharyngeal edema suggests a cautious delay in extubation. Indeed, if the situation so warrants, elective tracheostomy may even be indicated at the time of the excision, rather than delaying 2 weeks and performing the operation under less optimal conditions.

The patient should spend a short stay in an intensive care unit following most such operations. If the nasal or oral endotracheal tube is left in place, its position should be confirmed by chest radiograph. Provisions for humidified air/oxygen should be made, and all those responsible for postoperative care should be informed of fluid therapy, the potential for swelling, and possible nerve dysfunction (such as vocal cord weakness) from the operation. As well, the connection between massive swelling and hypovolemia should be gently emphasized lest intravascular volume slowly translocate, without replacement, into the neck.

THYROGLOSSAL DUCT CYST

This is the most common case of a midline neck mass in a child. The two other fairly common causes are dermoid cysts and midline cervical clefts, both of which are simply and easily locally excised. As was reviewed in the discussion of embryology, thyroglossal duct cyst represents a somewhat more complex situation.

Clinical Features. The thyroid gland originates as a cellular rest at the foramen cecum in the tongue and migrates in the anterior midline of the neck to its permanent location by the eighth week of development. In the usual situation, the thyroglossal duct is obliterated by the tenth week, but should this not occur, a neck mass may present anywhere along the path followed by the gland. In fact, over 75 percent of these cysts present in close proximity to the hyoid bone. Early excision is recommended before infection or occasional malignant degeneration occurs. The majority of these cysts appear after the child's second birthday, with 50 percent being identified by age 10 years.

The removal of the cyst requires dissection of the tract to the foramen cecum. Rather than widely opening the anterior neck, the surgeon should employ a series of stepladder-style incisions until digital pressure, applied intraorally over the foramen cecum, brings the tongue nearer the skin incision, so that the entire tract can be removed flush with the tongue epithelium.

ANESTHETIC MANAGEMENT

The symptoms presented by these cysts are generally only cosmetic, occasionally compounded by external drainage and rarely by infection. Thyroid function is not involved. Preoperative assessment and preparation are unremarkable for this diagnosis. Very rarely, fluid can be expressed from the cyst into the mouth, but neither the frequency nor the quantity recommends special airway precautions.

The patient eventually will be placed in a position essentially like that for tracheostomy. The surgical field can be expected to include the mouth, as intraoral digital pressure assists the dissection. The patient can be intubated orally, although it seems more reasonable to progress from an oral tube, the insertion of which confirms correct tracheal fit, to a nasal tube, thus removing the airway from the surgical field. If a nasal tube is chosen, the precurved variety provides for a low profile as well as minimizing dead space. A pharyngeal pack is rarely indicated, as the operation never truly enters the oral cavity. During the actual procedure, the patient should be positioned slightly (20°) head up to decrease bleeding. Overaggressiveness in elevating the head raises the possibility of air embolism; this should be avoided unless the position is felt to be so beneficial that all the measures associated with a sitting craniotomy are also taken.

Following a straightforward excision in an older child, the tube can be removed and the patient then awakened. A more difficult procedure, or operation on a smaller infant, suggests awake extubation. In either case, the patient should be nursed semi-sitting in the postoperative period to minimize swelling.

SALIVARY GLAND TUMORS

This topic generally brings to mind tumors of the parotid gland, or radical extirpative surgery for oropharyngeal cancer—all in adults. Salivary gland tumors constitute about 3 percent of all tumors, with only about 0.3 to 1.3 percent of this 3 percent found below a patient age of 16 years. Unfortunately, when such tumors are found in children, the majority are malignant. The anatomical possibilities include the paired glands—parotid, submandibular, and sublingual—or any of the 400 to 800 individual glands found in the oropharynx; however, 75 percent will be located in the parotid gland. In those circumstances in which the other paired glands are involved, the incidence of malignancy may be as high as 70 percent. As with most cases of malignant disease, the etiology is unknown, although a history of head and neck radiation has been estimated to increase the incidence ninefold. The majority of patients should be cured by surgical therapy.

Clinical Features. The usual clinical presentation is of a 1- to 2-cm, firm, slowly enlarging mass, often in the parotid gland, brought to a physician's attention when the patient is about 1 year of age. The facial nerve is rarely involved, and the child does not otherwise appear to have cancer. Airway compromise is extraordinarily uncommon in the usual case; occasionally a ranula, a cyst of the sublingual gland duct, may present some minor difficulty.

The surgical approach to the parotid is via an incision anterior to the auricle, to the submandibular gland via an incision parallel to the horizontal ramus of the mandible beneath the floor of the mouth, and to the sublingual gland intraorally. In general, the largest element of concern is preserving vital structures while removing the entire tumor, as recurrences can be more aggressive. The most prominent vital structure is the facial nerve as it divides and weaves its way through the parotid gland, in one of multiple patterns. On occasion, despite the importance of the facial nerve, it or one of its branches must be sacrificed; in such a situation, immediate repair, either by direct anastomosis or free nerve grafting, is recommended. The nerve is rather sensitive to trauma, and facial muscle weakness after nerve manipulation is not uncommon.

ANESTHETIC MANAGEMENT

The symptoms presented by these lesions are usually cosmetic, although terribly magnified by the fear of malignancy. The airway is rarely involved. Therefore, preoperative assessment and preparation for these tumors are unremarkable.

The patient will be placed in moderate cervical extension, with the head possibly rotated away from the lesion. An oral tube will usually suffice, although a nasal tube certainly can be used. A pharyngeal pack is not indicated. A lesion in the parotid suggests that long-acting neuromuscular block be avoided.

Following operation, the tube usually can be removed in a straightforward manner, although dissection in the floor of the mouth may favor extubation awake. In either case, the patient should be nursed semi-sitting in the postoperative period to minimize swelling.

CHRONIC UPPER AIRWAY OBSTRUCTION AND SLEEP APNEA

Examination of one of any number of anesthesia textbooks could lead to the assumption that the trachea is separated from the environment by an uninteresting and amorphous area simply referred to as "the upper airway." This construct is not unique to anesthesiology, for until recently, this anatomy was also largely ignored by respiratory physiologists and clinicians in other specialties. In the mid-1960s, the key feature of the pickwickian syndrome was recognized to be oropharyngeal occlusion that occurred only during sleep. In 1978, Remmers and colleagues presented a concept of airway occlusion during sleep that emphasized the role of oropharyngeal inspiratory muscle activity. Following these prominent advances, a number of studies have increased general knowledge of this unknown territory between the teeth and trachea. Some of these studies, in attempting to answer why the airway closes during sleep in some patients, have posed an even more fundamental question: Why does the airway stay open in anyone during sleep? Initially, this research was directed toward a seemingly small adult population, but as has proved true in other newly described entities, the actual scope and size of the population affected by upper airway obstruction was soon found to be substantially greater than expected.

The current understanding of sleep apnea generally includes two categories: central, or arrhythmic, apnea characterized by absent gas flow and lack of respiratory effort, and obstructive apnea, characterized by absent gas flow despite respiratory effort. Given that most patients with this problem do not have obstruction when awake, the majority of obstructive types must have some defect in central drive to airway musculature, leading to a third group aptly called mixed apnea. Perfectly normal people may experience short (10- to 20-second) episodes of apnea during sleep, usually on a nonrecurring basis. It has been suggested that those with sleep apnea syndromes demonstrate repetitive (20 per hour) episodes, each greater than 10 seconds in duration. The exact pathology responsible for these syndromes—there may be multiple causes—is unclear, but theories include the following:

1. A small airway that requires greater inspiratory pressure than a normal-sized airway, and that passively closes as tone is reduced in sleep.
2. A small airway that requires active dilator muscle activity to remain patent—inspiratory pressure is normal.
3. A normal airway with excessive loss of muscle tone (predominantly the genioglossus).
4. A normal airway, including muscle tone, with abnormal respiratory control/feedback.

A number of syndromes also are associated with sleep apnea, related to abnormalities of the cranial base. Apparently, children with Crouzon's, Apert's, Pfeiffer's, Stickler's, and Treacher Collins syndromes all have a shorter anterior, and abnormally angled posterior, cranial base. This has the effect of decreasing the anteroposterior diameter of the pharynx and causing the syndrome.

The usual symptoms are snoring, enuresis, sleepwalking, daytime sleepiness, morning headaches, personality changes, dyspnea with exercise intolerance, and insomnia. However, failure to thrive in infants and diminished stature have also been attributed to this syndrome.

The pediatric literature initially approached chronic obstruction from the perspective of mechanical high-grade occlusion from "visible" sources, such as hypertrophied adenoids and tonsils or severe micrognathia. This situation was often the source for case reports of chronic hypercapnia and hypoxemia with subsequent right ventricular dysfunction from pulmonary artery hypertension. Beyond this presentation, there was a suggested possible association with sudden infant death syndrome that is still unclear. However, the parallel adult and pediatric approaches to upper airway disorders have become more nearly coincident recently, and a number of investigators have suggested a continuum in age and presentation, extending from infants with Pierre Robin anomalad to sixth-decade males (it is a male-preponderant population) with severe snoring.

Evaluation of patients thought to have the syndrome first begins by obtaining a history of snoring or interrupted breathing or both during sleep. Obviously, this infers that either the parents volunteer the information or a physician asks pointed questions. There may also be a history of chronic night cough, thought secondary to recurrent aspiration of pharyngeal secretions. This, in turn, can markedly aggravate prior respiratory disease, such as asthma. Children with sleep apnea often suffer from daytime somnolence and behavior disorders. Polysomnography is the definitive method of diagnosis, but this multichannel system, although the gold standard, is complex and expensive. As an alternative, the parents can obtain a tape recording of their child's respiration during sleep, which can be analyzed via computer to present a graphic display of respiration.

Although the emphasis in pediatric patients was originally on airway obstruction with subsequent right heart disease, a connection to adult sleep apnea research was made in a report of postoperative sleep obstruction in a patient with Treacher Collins syndrome. Admittedly, the pharyngeal hypoplasia associated with Treacher Collins syndrome would seem to present an unusual mechanical restriction in the airway, but even so, there must be some additional component responsible for sleep obstruction, since few of these patients are in distress while awake. Studies of nonsyndrome-related sleep apnea patients have also suggested combinations of reduced airway cross-sectional area in conjunction with some deficiency in respiratory drive during natural sleep. In general, this deficiency is best described as a respiratory dysrhythmia, or failure of rhythm control, but there is also an element of decreased responsiveness to carbon dioxide (CO_2). Furthermore, during sleep, the breathing of increased oxygen concentration will improve saturation at the cost of prolongation of apnea duration. Clearly, a patient with a natural unresponsiveness to CO_2, failure of respiratory rhythm control, reduced cross-sectional area of the airway, and a tendency to retain CO_2 when administered oxygen requires strict attention to airway management and respiratory monitoring in the postanesthetic recovery period.

Unfortunately, the only visible clue available to identify these patients, other than morbid obesity, comes from the work of Coccagna and associates (1976, 1978), who noted that a bird-like facies with micrognathia was highly suggestive of sleep apnea. For the moment, the anesthesiologist must remain aware of the syndrome, in its several presentations, and be advised to question the patient, or parents, about sleeping problems or snoring whenever obesity or facial anatomy suggests the syndrome. If responses to this line of questioning support the diagnosis, premedication should be ordered cautiously. (As an example of the risks involved, consider the case of a 4-year-old child with sleep apnea who succumbed following ingestion of a usual dose of cough syrup containing promethazine and codeine, ostensibly due to the effect of these two drugs on deficient respiratory drive.)

Analgesia after surgery presents a major concern, and no best method has been clearly indentified. However, regional anesthesia and nonsteroidal anti-inflammatory drugs may have merit in this situation, while patient-controlled analgesia could have increased risk of exacerbating the syndrome. In theory, mixed agonist-anatogonists, such as dezocine, potentially have increased safety in sleep apnea, but this has *not* been evaluated.

The postoperative management of sleep apnea patients may be benefited by the application of nasal continuous positive airway pressure (CPAP), which seems to offer great promise for amelioration of symptoms during normal unmedicated sleep. For those fortunate enough to work in close proximity to a sleep study laboratory, nasal CPAP capability is close by and very useful in the recovery room. However, as of this writing, it is not a modality that can be requested on the spur of the moment. Rather, it requires fine tuning to define correct pressure settings—and can cost up to $500 for initial equipment setup. It is most useful for those patients who come to operation with a preoperative diagnosis of the syndrome and already have an ongoing program of therapy.

PULMONARY EDEMA ASSOCIATED WITH UPPER AIRWAY OBSTRUCTION

Beginning with the report by Travis and associates in 1977, attention has been drawn to the abrupt appearance of florid pulmonary edema in otherwise healthy patients following relief of upper airway obstruction. On occasion, these episodes were attributed to drugs that were used during the event, adding more confusion to an already uncertain physiology. The simplest explanation of the appearance of lung fluid was that vigorous inspiratory effort against a closed glottis "pulled" fluid from within vessels into the alveoli. The actual physiology responsible for the appearance of alveolar fluid remains, 15 years later, still uncertain.

The complexity of monitoring the heart and great vessels within the thorax raises very confusing issues as to just what constitutes negative pressure between chambers or cavities. Laboratory work has thus far seemed to dispel the simple notion that negative pressure alone can cause this situation. Instead, it now seems that the negative pressure must also be associated with hypoxia and, possibly, with acute transient left ventricular dysfunction in otherwise normal patients. In general, most case reports note quick resolution, but by no means is this absolute enough to be depended on. Should this situation occur in a patient with no prior history of cardiac dysfunction, it generally can be assumed that this qualifies as non-cardiac pulmonary edema, and as such, can be managed with endotracheal intubation, PEEP, oxygen, and mild diuresis. Invasive monitoring of central pressures, postedema formation, is usually not helpful, as values are normal. Resolution often occurs in hours, but a delay of up to a day or so is not unusual. What seems most effective in foreshortening recovery is quick intervention, which, in turn, is based on awareness that edema can occur in a matter of minutes postobstruction.

MANAGEMENT OF THE DIFFICULT PEDIATRIC AIRWAY AND INTUBATION

Achieving control of a patient's airway is the anesthesiologist's forte and primary task. Without expertise in this area, the rendering of a person unconscious with respiratory depressant drugs becomes unacceptably hazardous. A first consideration of this crucial subject might therefore place "intubation" into the larger category of "airway" management; on further thought and clinical experience, it is clear that difficulty with management of the nonintubated airway is not always associated with difficulty in intubation. Laryngotracheomalacia is one example of such a situation. Furthermore, given reasonable assurance that the airway is manageable, most anesthesiologists face the difficult elective intubation as a challenge, armed with numerous techniques, publications, and mechanical devices. The difficult airway, on the other hand, is an altogether undesirable addition to any anesthetic, for which the publications and devices have much less to offer. Indeed, many investigators seem to feel that their principal task, and a major contribution, is to forewarn the anesthetist of a difficult airway and trust to experience thereafter. The following is an approach to the recognition and management of the difficult airway, and then to its less threatening associate, the difficult intubation. This is necessitated by the fact that a number of head and neck syndromes present both problems in rapid succession.

Preoperative assessment begins the management of the difficult airway and difficult intubation, for first the problem must be recognized. Every anesthesiologist has memories of dealing with such challenges, but the clearest recall is always of the unsuspected difficulty or the uncertain situation in which someone thought all would be well and pressed on, only to be completely defeated in a few short minutes. It is interesting to reflect for a moment on the concept of a "difficult airway," as perceived by an anesthesiologist, for often at the time this description is applied, the patient appears completely unperturbed by this problem. (However, it is worth noting that many patients with Pierre Robin anomalad also appear unperturbed and are intermittently hypoxic.) Significant trouble, therefore, is that resulting from the combination of anesthetic-induced muscle relaxation, respiratory depression, preexisting anatomy, and the supine position.

Consider an extreme example of a difficult airway, the Pierre Robin anomalad. Micrognathia is a hallmark here, along with a tongue that "falls backward." White and Kander (1975) examined the difficult intubation in adults and found that the most significant anatomical measurement associated with difficulty in laryngeal visualization was the depth (or vertical height) of the mandible as measured from the alveolar ridge at the third molar to the lower border of the mandible. They felt that this anatomy, especially if it was combined with a relatively short mandible, placed soft tissue more posteriorly into the oropharynx and hindered intubation. When this line of reasoning is applied to the aforementioned child with Pierre Robin anomalad, the similarity is striking. Practically every illustration drawn to describe a child with micrognathia and glossoptosis portrays a condensed mass of soft tissue, including the tongue, in the posterior oropharynx. In essence, the compression of soft tissue into a space defined by a mandible relatively deficient in length seems to pose a spectrum of problems, varying in severity from functional intrusion into the airway, patient awake, to functional intrusion, patient anesthetized, to the least threatening situation, that of interference only with laryngeal visualization.

This continuum was also recently suggested, somewhat obliquely, in a study of airway stability in micrognathic infants. In general, the transition through the panoply appears to be part of normal growth, which allows for relative airway enlargement beyond critical lower limits, perhaps in conjunction with improvement in oropharyngeal muscle tone and control. That this airway improvement should occur is probably due to the impact of fluid flow being inversely proportional to the fourth or fifth power of the length of the radius, and is analogous to the enormous declines in flow resistance associated with the smallest endotracheal tubes as they increase internal diameter by 0.5-mm increments.

Another approach to the difficult airway was offered by Nichol and Zuck (1983), who looked at a frequent preanesthetic exercise, that of asking a patient to tip the head back as far as possible, from the view of determining what actually restricts the movement. They noted that the atlanto-occipital distance largely defines these limits, and attempts forcefully to continue extension after atlanto-occipital contact apply leverage to the cervical spine posteriorly, producing an anterior bowing of the vertebral column, thereby lifting the larynx farther anteriorly out of view. This relationship was examined in adults and children only, but, despite the anatomical differences in infants, it is interesting in view of the strong clinical dictum not to extend an infant's head beyond neutral for laryngoscopy.

It is certainly easy to suspect that the very prominent occiput of an infant may restrict this axis of motion. Unfortunately, although this is intriguing, the clinical recommendation must remain simply to continue the current practice of evaluating head extension preoperatively, as cervical spine radiographs on every patient are impractical. Furthermore, functional demonstration is probably more valuable than static measurement. However, a limited number of congenital abnormalities of the cervical spine may adversely affect ease of laryngoscopy, or spinal cord function, during neck hyperextension. These may require further radiological evaluation; they are listed in Table 9–4.

Consequent to this and previous evaluations, the patient's appearance and the range of mo-

Table 9–4. CONGENITAL ABNORMALITIES OF THE CERVICAL SPINE AND ASSOCIATIONS

Abnormalities	Association	Symptom Onset
Basilar impression (for platybasia)	Atlanto-occipital fusion, atlas hypoplasia, abnormal odontoid, Klippel-Feil syndrome, skeletal dysplasia, bifid postatlas arch	Uncommon until 2nd, 3rd decade
Congenital atlantoaxial instability	Congenital scoliosis, Down's syndrome, bone dysplasia, spondyloepiphyseal dysplasia, osteogenesis imperfecta, neurofibromatosis	Usually by 2nd decade; childhood presentation; generalized weakness
Atlanto-occipital fusion	Jaw anomalies, cleft palate, ear deformities, cervical rib, urinary tract anomalies	Usually in 3rd, 4th decade
Odontoid hypoplasia/aplasia or os odontoideum	Down's syndrome, Klippel-Feil syndrome, skeletal dysplasias, spondyloepiphyseal dysplasia	Variable; frequently diagnosed after episode of significant trauma
Congenital laxity of transverse atlantal ligament	Down's syndrome (20%)	Variable; recommend C1–C2 articulation be evaluated in all Down's patients prior to general anesthesia
Klippel-Feil syndrome (congenital synostosis of cervical vertebrae)	Scoliosis, renal abnormalities, Sprengel's deformity, deafness, synkinesia, congenital heart disease	Symptoms uncommon

tion at the temporomandibular and atlanto-occipital joints must be examined in detail. The child's face must be seen in three dimensions, so a full lateral view must be obtained. This will reveal defects in proportion, such as small jaw or malar hypoplasia. The former's significance should now be clear; the latter may create an almost flat face that cannot be well matched to a traditional semi-rigid Rendell-Baker mask but instead requires a more adult-style small mask with a moldable pneumatic cushion. The anterior gliding movement of the temporomandibular joint can be evaluated by asking the child to oppose the upper and lower incisors, while a request to open the mouth wide is the best test of that axis of movement. For the infant, it may be possible to test mandible movement manually.

From the perspective of the endoscopist, the atlanto-occipital and temporomandibular joints seem to represent the only available sites of motion that can possibly assist in the task of "straightening" the upper airway into alignment with the trachea. However, the larynx is one end of a movable conduit and, as such, can itself be repositioned to assist in visualization. In circumstances when full displacement of both skeletal sites is inadequate to visualize the larynx, manual pressure posteriorly, laterally, and/or cephalad over the thyroid cartilage will often bring at least some recognizable anatomy into view. As intubation under direct vision requires both of the endoscopist's hands to be occupied, an assistant can stand to the patient's right and provide this extra degree of movement on command from the anesthesiologist. As well, the assistant can insert one of any number of atraumatic surgical retractors (Green's loop, vein, Army-Navy, small Richardson's) into the right corner of the mouth, laterally and superiorly displacing the entire orifice so that substantially more working room is available for intubation. Decreasing the soft tissue obstruction caused by the ipsilateral cheek often can ease actual tube passage to a striking degree. Yet another role for the assistant can be to "elevate" the larynx into view by tongue withdrawal with forceps, as described by Miyabe and colleagues (1985).

In dealing with a subject as vexing as this, any absolute statement is suspect. However, a strong recommendation to preserve spontaneous ventilation comes reasonably close to being such an absolute. Even following a successful induction, maintaining the option offered by a breathing patient will occasionally rescue the situation from an unanticipated last-moment obstacle, as well as serving to prevent the reduction in the anesthesiologist's coronary artery flow associated with the sudden appreciation of the obstacle. Many a pediatric airway has been rescued by the passage of an endotracheal tube through a small air bubble perched on the glottis.

Accepting this concept, premedication should be selected to assist, rather than impair, the induction process. Consequently, drugs such as barbiturates, benzodiazepines, or chloral hydrate are suggested as examples of suitable choices instead of narcotics, which are more prone to decrease minute ventilation. Although atropine is usually given primarily to block the cardiac response to vagal stimulation, in this situation atropine can also be given by mouth, primarily to decrease secretions. As all of these sedating compounds, except the newer benzodiazepines, are long-acting in effective doses, their use must be based on both the preoperative and postoperative situations—chloral hydrate, 50 mg/kg, is not well suited to early same-day discharge. Another consideration for the difficult airway is that of gastric contents. Although it is far from universal practice, I administer ranitidine, 2 to 3 mg/kg BID in pill or syrup form, beginning the night prior to operation, to selected patients anticipated to have problems with a difficult airway.

Finally, the method of anesthetic induction seems crucial to success, as spontaneous ventilation and oxygenation both must be preserved. Undoubtedly, a "proper" dose of ketamine or barbiturate can be selected so that apnea does not occur, but the consequences of misjudgment must be recognized. My preference is to administer oxygen alone for several minutes, followed by halothane, increased by 0.25 percent every three breaths, until 4 to 5 percent inspired concentration is reached. On occasion this may have to be accomplished with the patient semi-sitting, at least initially, to prevent abrupt obstruction while the patient is still awake. A useful adjunct to this sequence is an intravenous infusion, established several hours preoperatively so the child does not develop a fluid deficit. A full right atrium assists the smooth, leisurely establishment of inhalation anesthesia remarkably well, especially if the patient must be positioned head up during the induction.

Having clearly stated a preference for inhalation anesthesia, to be thorough it is worth noting that I first used subanesthetic ketamine in 1979 to provide improved conditions for bronchoscopic intubation. The combination of analgesia, amnesia, minimal respiratory depression, and adequate airway muscle tone remains difficult to achieve with any other single drug in current use. In combination with topical anesthesia and prior antisialogogue treatment, ketamine deserves reconsideration for this purpose.

Initial operating room management of the airway usually centers on the interface between the anesthesia mask and the patient's face. All anesthesia masks roughly create a funnel with a small peripheral invagination for the chin and a larger one for the nose. A lateral facial view of a child with Pierre Robin anomalad, as an example, shows that the usual plane created by the maxilla and mandible does not exist, thereby creating a break in the mask-to-face seal over the mandible. One answer to this might be a custom mask; another and more practical answer might be to build up the mandible artificially with gauze until contact is obtained. While either may help achieve a mask fit that ensures oxygen and anesthetic delivery to the face, the basic pathology remains unaffected and the airway may still be obstructed.

Therefore, in contradistinction to usual practice, the airway must first be established prior to general anesthesia. Consequently, assuming mask positive pressure alone appears insufficient, the nasopharynx or oropharynx should be topically anesthetized (lidocaine, maximum 4 mg/kg, tetracaine, maximum 1 mg/kg) and the appropriate device inserted. When a nasal airway is used, the lubricant should be only that, not a concentrated anesthetic preparation, as drug administration will be neither recognized nor controlled. Furthermore, some topical anesthetic preparations use a methylcellulose base that dries into stalactites and potentially can cause airway obstruction. If a shortened endotracheal tube is used as a nasal airway, ready connection with an anesthetic apparatus will be facilitated via the 15-mm connector.

Complications to the foregoing are epistaxis, emesis, and failure to establish an airway. Epistaxis is rarely a problem with infants; for the older child, topical application of 0.125 percent phenylephrine or 0.025 percent oxymetazoline will effectively vasoconstrict the mucosa. When applied before drug instillation, this step also should theoretically decrease absorption of local anesthetic. This is especially effective when the vaosconstrictor is sprayed into the nostrils prior to patient arrival in the operating room. The older child also is at risk of having a cylindrical biopsy of hypertrophied adenoids taken during nasal tube insertion. This can be avoided by first passing a small, soft catheter through the tube, then (through the nostril) into and (via the mouth) back out of the oropharynx. A heat-softened tube is then passed into the oropharynx via the nose while gentle tension is maintained on the catheter, thus directing the tube anteriorly away from the adenoids; once the tip passes these tissues, the catheter is removed and the tube is placed in final position in a conventional manner. Obviously, this step generally requires an anesthetized patient.

Emesis, like epistaxis, does not seem to be a major problem with infants. For the older child, topical anesthesia to the oropharynx will usually limit this. Failure to establish an airway is generally due to the variation of Murphy's Law that predicts the device selected will be too large or too small. An excessively large oral airway has the potential to aggravate the obstruction by occluding or compressing the larynx, whereas an airway that is too small simply fails to displace the tongue from the posterior pharyngeal wall. An oversized nasal tube either will not pass the nostril or, after insertion, extends into the esophagus and worsens the entire situation. To avoid this, an external estimate of length should be made before the nasal airway is inserted. In any case, if the situation does not improve following airway insertion, the tube should be removed immediately and the approach to intubation should be reassessed.

All the preceding serves to establish a passage for gas exchange and possibly even for mask positive-pressure ventilation. This may prove adequate for some operations, but more likely what it serves to do is provide a calm, well-oxygenated patient for intubation attempts or possibly tracheostomy. However, one exception to this progression to endotracheal intubation is provided by the use of a supraglottic nasal endotracheal tube, or nasal airway with an added 15-mm connector, as a final method to administer anesthesia. With sufficient patience to achieve adequate depth, even assisted ventilation can be provided in this way. Obviously, this situation is not as desirable as a properly fitting translaryngeal endotracheal tube, but it is superior to a tracheostomy for a revision of a syndactyly repair. If this method is eventually selected, a high degree of vigilance is required to detect gastric distention; if that is suspected, a 10- to 14-gauge catheter must be quickly passed via the mouth into the stomach. As this is such a distinct possibility, the presence of any form of esophageal pathology that makes gastric intubation hazardous poses a relative contraindication to this nasopharyngeal technique, at least if positive airway pressure is to be employed.

If endotracheal intubation is indicated, the tube generally will be inserted via the mouth, at least initially. For the overwhelming majority of patients, this is a straightforward task. The variety of laryngoscope blades commercially available stands in mute testimony to the exceptions. The occasional pediatric anesthetist may be acquainted with numerous adult blades, but perhaps only one, frequently the Miller's, for children. (It is enlightening to compare the currently available Miller's blade with the original; from this, one can speculate that the first version may well have been the best.) Often other blades are useful for the difficult intubation, and it is worthwhile having a selection at hand for this situation. In the United States, the following are generally available: Miller's, Wisconsin, Wis-Foregger, Wis-Hipple, Alberts', Michaels', Flagg's, Guedel's, Bennet's, Seward's, Robertshaw's, and Oxford Infant. When the patient's anatomy allows the usual right-sided oral laryngoscope insertion, followed by lateral movement to the midline, I have found the Seward's or Robertshaw's blade (see Figure 9–7) useful. For those situations in which the blade must be passed via, and remain in, the far right lateral aspect of the mouth, the smaller cross-sectional area of the Miller's blade seems best. The limited view of the glottis afforded by this lateral approach may require removal of the 15-mm connector from the tube to prevent loss of view of the larynx during intubation.

A very interesting variation of this technique utilizes a pediatric Jackson's anterior commissure laryngoscope to visualize the larynx, followed by tube insertion over an optical stylet through the laryngoscope. The tube is then fixed in position with long alligator forceps while the stylet and laryngoscope are withdrawn and the 15-mm connector is inserted into the tube. In this, or any situation in which the connector has been left off during insertion, the tube must be left long enough to grasp, and the connector must be initially firmly preinserted to facilitate subsequent reinsertion after intubation. Often during these maneuvers the tube becomes slippery; the silent struggle to control 1 cm of lubricated plastic of 4-mm ID tube well enough to insert a connector without extubating the child is amusing only to the uninitiated. Vanishing adult tubes can be tethered by the pilot balloon; pediatric tubes have no such safety line. A suture can be passed through the tube side wall to provide restraint and control when deemed necessary.

In any of the techniques involving difficult laryngoscopy, two additional general measures must be attended to: someone must observe and care for the patient, and oxygen, usually with anesthetic, must be provided. The answer to the former is to obtain assistance. The latter is satisfied by insufflation, intermittently via the laryngoscope, or preferably continuously via a nasopharyngeal catheter or airway. Finally, the child's fragile teeth must be protected, either by a commercial dental guard or by cotton gauze.

A recent combination of features from the conventional laryngoscope and fiberoptic bronchoscope created the Bullard's laryngoscope. The device has a three-dimensional cross-sectional area not much greater than an endotracheal tube and seems to have a wide field of view when inserted. The terminal portion of the device describes a narrow-radius 90° turn that can be used in the form of either a Miller's or MacIntosh's blade. The general design of the device seems to be of most benefit to patients in whom skull movement is undesirable, or in whom mouth opening is quite restricted. Experience in infants or children is minimal, experience in the abnormal pediatric airway is even less, and the limiting factor in gathering such experience is a cost (more than $3000) near to that of a bronchoscope, with much less versatility in the Bullard's laryngoscope.

An alternative to conventional laryngoscopy is the use of a fiberoptic bronchoscope, as a flexible stylet, as a visualization device when the bronchoscope is too large to pass through the tube, or as the first step of a guide wire–cardiac catheter-endotracheal tube sequence. Expertise with the device comes with practice, most easily acquired in adult patients first. The difficult small airway is most certainly not the place to launch a new skill. Recently, the technique of retrograde-assisted intubation (described later) has been modified by passing the transtracheal guide through the suction channel of a 2.8-mm bronchoscope. This allows the novice endoscopist the luxury of a guaranteed passive guide through the larynx without concern for scope control, passing anatomy, or depth of field through this unusual lens. This technique allows for intubation with tube-over-scope down to a 4.0-mm internal diameter. Bronchoscopes are now available with an outer diameter as small as 1.8 mm, but, as can be imagined, without a suction channel, thus precluding this technique with the smallest instruments. For those with some skill in fiberoptic endoscopy in adults, it is worth emphasizing that even an ultra-thin scope fills a substantial portion of a small endotracheal tube. Therefore, while it is quite reasonable to pass a tube over a bronchoscope and linger in the adult airway, to do so in a very small child may well create another citation in the airway obstruction–pulmonary edema literature.

The Hopkins telescope can be used as a rigid optical stylet in certain cases, either as previously described or as part of a more conventional laryngoscopy-bronchoscopy technique. Although it has been some time since this technique was first described, it seems to have taken a definite secondary position to flexible fiberoptics, despite the fact that the rod-lens has infinitely superior optics.

A large number of devices have been used as nonoptical guides to direct tube passage into the larynx in instances when only the most posterior aspect of the larynx could be visualized. Any malleable object thin enough to pass through a tube and long enough to be manageable while intubating can be, and probably has been, used. An interesting commercially produced variation allows for variable flexion of the guide tip; this device has recently become available in a size that will accommodate tubes as small as 4.5 mm ID, at a cost of about that of a laryngoscope blade.

If laryngoscopy and oral intubation prove impossible, blind nasal intubation is usually the next option. The endotracheal tube is passed with the same consideration as when used as an airway, except it is cut somewhat longer. This method is much less hurried in a patient spontaneously breathing an anesthetic mixture via an airway in the other nostril, although occasionally the airway may need to be withdrawn slightly to prevent interference with the advancing tube. Alternatively, the anesthesia circuit may be connected directly to the endotracheal tube being passed, although this removes the audible cues to intubation. Atraumatic insertion can be facilitated by heating the tube, in a warmer or in fluids, to a temperature of 40 to 50°C. Berry recently reported an impressive 96 percent success rate for blind nasal intubation aided by an 8- or 14-gauge pliable stylet, formed to desired shape and inserted into the endotracheal tube *after* the tube tip was in the oropharynx. Interested readers should consult the original, very specific, reference. Great care must be taken with these blind techniques in children, as the larynx may be easily traumatized by intubation attempts. A recent report of arytenoid dislocation in a child, caused by vigorous coughing, emphasizes the fragility of these periglottic structures.

During a difficult nasal intubation, it is possible to tunnel the tube submucosally, generally via a tear near the sphenoid prominence. Once this tissue plane has been entered, it is surprisingly easy to advance the tube, although obviously never successfully into the airway. Consequently, whenever a tube appears to have passed from the nasopharynx into the oropharynx, without accompanying audible evidence of respiration emanating from the tube, it is worthwhile to inspect the oropharynx visually and confirm the proper plane of advance.

On occasion, following a successful oral intubation, a transition to a nasal tube is planned. One device that facilitates this exchange under direct vision is an Aillon's tube forcep, which can nicely redirect an anterior tube tip down the tracheal axis, thereby eliminating the "hang-up" so often encountered with a nasal tube.

An interesting technique, now largely forgotten, may prove useful when visual and traditional blind methods fail. Well described by Hudon, this method is perhaps more appropriately titled tactile intubation. This technique involves guiding the tube through the glottis with fingers inserted into the oral cavity, after ensuring adequate anesthesia and with the mouth held open with a gag. The initial route of intubation, oral or nasal, appears immaterial in this technique; Hudon actually seemed to feel this represented a preferred means of intubation. This approach can be useful in difficult situations, provided some prior practice is obtained in straightforward cases. The original article should be read in some detail by those interested, as it is extremely thorough.

A useful addition to a stylet is a light source at the tip, creating a device referred to as a "lightwand." This provides optical assistance to an otherwise blind technique, by allowing visualization of light source entry into the cervical trachea via transillumination of the thyroid cartilage. This adaptation is most often described as an adjunct to Hudon's technique but recently was suggested as a means to confirm endotracheal tube tip location in the cervical trachea. However, as always, there must be some negative component to this addition; in this case, it was the loss of the light bulb into a bronchus from the earliest version of the device. The most familiar version of this device, commercially available for limited re-use, will pass through a tube no smaller than 5.0-mm ID. A permanent alternative for smaller tubes can also be purchased at about three times the price, but still less than $100.

If intubation from above proves initially impossible, a reasonable next step would be to establish a reliable mechanical path into the airway from below. This technique was initially made popular with a large-bore needle–epidural catheter–retrograde oral tube sequence across the cricothyroid membrane, but has recently been reported as a modified Seldinger's technique, utilizing a 20-gauge needle and a 0.021-inch guide wire. When this technique is employed, the wire should be passed into the endotracheal tube via the Murphy's side hole rather than the larger end hole, to allow insertion of an additional 1 cm or so of tube into the larynx before wire withdrawal. Obviously, this technique also demands a fairly still patient during needle insertion to prevent internal laryngeal injury.

Should none of these techniques prove effective, three options remain: tracheostomy, the laryngeal mask, and other. Tracheostomy seems quite attractive at first but often proves less so when the entire picture of small child, movement, possible supine airway obstruction, and unfavorable anatomy becomes clearer. In essence, the very problems initially confronting the anesthesiologist are still there, compounded by surgical access requirements. It is important to remember that tracheostomy is still surgery, and there are good reasons why an operation without general anesthesia is rarely scheduled for children. This is most especially true if the child is mentally retarded or has a hearing or vision defect.

The laryngeal mask (LM) was introduced in the United Kingdom in 1983 by Dr. Brain, whose name was quickly associated with the device. This was much to the confusion of American readers, who spent the next eight years sorting out how an airway into the CNS could possibly function, even in Great Britain. It is amazing that, despite skeptics and the United States tort system, the device entered the U.S. in 1991. This has relevance, because a pediatric version has been employed for cleft palate repair in a Robin syndrome patient. From even a brief reading of the literature about the Brain's airway, one becomes certain that a quite anesthetized airway is required for its employment. It clearly might be thought to have the greatest application in patients with manageable airways for whom intubation has proved very difficult to impossible by conventional methods, but caution has been advised not to consider this a substitute for tracheal intubation. It is difficult to advance the LM into the pharynx of some patients without extending the neck, hence caution is required in those with cervical spine pathology. It is generally unsuitable for those with a pathological lesion within the pharynx. Finally, it does *not* protect the trachea and bronchial tree from aspiration.

"Other" refers to the innovation required when all else fails. For example, although most extremity procedures are performed while patients are supine, it may be possible to obtain reasonable operating conditions with the patient in a lateral or semi-prone position that more favors the natural airway. Perhaps the most extreme example of how useful position may be is a report of blind nasal intubation in the prone position, employed in an infant with Pierre Robin anomalad, for whom all other techniques had failed. Additionally, local or regional anesthesia may play a role, providing *very* strict attention to protection from overdose is maintained, as convulsion or cardiac depression without airway control seems a highly undesirable situation. Finally, alternative methods of analgesia or relative immobility, such as a continuous ketamine infusion, alone or in conjunction with the previous variations, may allow successful surgery. This infusion technique has often been useful for the burned child with severe cervical flexion contractures, for whom other techniques would have been quite difficult.

For any of these approaches, it is critical that the team members be made aware of the anesthesiologist's concerns and management plan, because proceeding with an operation without any reasonable possibility of providing general endotracheal anesthesia, even if required, is a major departure from usual practice. A hasty discussion about the situation after a request for muscle paralysis is untimely and seems poorly designed for good future working relations.

REFERENCES

EMBRYOLOGY

Wilson DB: Embryonic development of the head and neck. Part 2. The branchial region. Head Neck Surg *2*:59, 1979.

Wilson DB: Embryonic development of the head and neck. Part 3. The face. Head Neck Surg *2*:1435, 1979.

CONGENITAL CRANIOFACIAL DEFORMITIES

Apert E: De l'acrocephalosyndactylie. Bull Soc Med *23*:1310, 1906.

Bergsma D: Birth Defects Compendium. New York, Alan R. Liss, 1979.

Broennle AM, Teller L: Anesthesia for craniofacial procedures. Clin Plast Surg *14*:17, 1987.

Burian F: Sign of "whistling face" in polyvalent syndrome. Acta Chir Orthop Traumatol Cech *29*:481, 1962.

Carpenter G: Two sisters showing malformations of the skull and other congenital abnormalities. Rep Soc Study Dis Child Lond *1*:100, 1901.

Chotzen F: Eine eigenartige familiare Entwicklungsstorung.

(Akrocephalosyndaktylie, Dysostosis craniofacialis und Hypertelorismus.) Monatsschr Kinderheilkd *55*:97, 1932.

Cohen MM: Dysmorphic syndromes with craniofacial manifestations. *In* Steward R, Prescott G (eds): Oral Facial Genetics. St. Louis, CV Mosby, 1976.

Converse JQ, Wood-Smith D, McCarthy JG: Report of a series of 50 craniofacial operations. Plast Reconstr Surg *55*:283, 1975.

Crouzon O: Dysostose cranio-faciale hereditaire. Bull Mem Soc Med Hop (Paris) *33*:545, 1912.

Crysdale WS, Kohli-Dang N, Mullins GC, et al: Airway management in craniofacial surgery. J Otol *16*:207, 1987.

Davies DW, Munro IR: The anesthetic management and intraoperative care of patients undergoing major facial osteotomies. Plast Reconstr Surg *55*:50, 1975.

Duggar RG, DeMars PD, Bolton VE: Whistling face syndrome: General anesthesia and early postoperative caudal anesthesia. Anesthesiology *70*:545, 1989.

Dyken P, Miller M: Facial Features of Neurologic Syndromes. St. Louis, CV Mosby, 1980.

Freeman EA, Sheldon JH: Cranio-carpo-tarsal dystrophy. Arch Dis Child *13*:277, 1938.

Golabi M, Edwards MS, Ousterhout DK: Craniosynostosis and hydrocephalus. Neurosurgery *21*:63, 1987.

Gorlin RJ: Developmental anomalies of the face and oral structures. *In* Gorlin RJ, Goldman HM (eds): Thoma's Oral Pathology. 6th edition St. Louis, CV Mosby, 1970.

Handler SD, Beaugard ME, Whitaker LA, et al.: Airway management in the repair of craniofacial defects. Cleft Palate J *16*:16, 1978.

Laishley RS, Roy WL: Freeman-Sheldon syndrome. Can Anaesth Soc J *33*:388, 1986.

Marchac D: Discussion: Early surgery for craniofacial synostosis: An 8-year experience. Plast Reconstr Surg *73*:531, 1984.

McCarthy JG, Epstein F, Sandove M, et al: Early surgery for craniofacial synostosis: An 8-year experience. Plast Reconstr Surg *73*:521, 1984.

Pfeiffer RA: Dominant erbliche Akrocephalosyndactylie. Z Kinderheilkd *90*:301, 1964.

Powazek M, Billmeier GJ: Assessment of intellectual development after surgery for craniofacial dysostosis. Am J Dis Child *133*:151, 1979.

Renier D, Sainte-Rose C, Marchac D, et al: Intracranial pressure in craniostenosis. J Neurosurg *57*:370, 1982.

Saethre H: Ein Beitrag zum Turmschadelproblem. (Pathogenese, Erblichkeit und Symptomatologie.) Dtsch Z Nervenheilkd *117*:533, 1931.

Shillito J, Matson DD: Craniosynostosis: A review of 519 surgical patients. Pediatrics *41*:829, 1968.

Smith DW: Recognizable Patterns of Human Malformation. 2nd edition. Philadelphia, WB Saunders, 1976.

Stanesco V, Maximilian C, Poenaru S, et al: Syndrome hereditaire dominant reunissant une dysostose craniofaciale de type particulier, une insuffisance de croissance d'aspect chondrodystrophique et un epaississement massif de la corticale des os longs. Rev Fr Endocrinol *4*:219, 1963.

Tateishi M, Imaizumi H, Namiki A: Anesthetic management of a patient with Freeman-Sheldon syndrome. Masui *35*:1114, 1986.

Temtamy SA: Carpenter's syndrome: Acrocephalopolysyndactyly, an autosomal recessive syndrome. J Pediatr *69*:111, 1966.

Tessier P: Anatomical classification of facial, cranio-facial and latero-facial clefts. J Maxillofac Surg *4*:69, 1976.

ACQUIRED CRANIOFACIAL DEFORMITIES: TRAUMA

Converse JM: Facial injuries in children. *In* Mustarde JC (ed): Plastic Surgery in Infancy and Childhood. Edinburgh, Churchill Livingstone, 1979.

Karlson TA: The incidence of facial injuries from dog bites. JAMA *251*:3265, 1984.

Kissoon N, Dreyer J, Walia M: Pediatric trauma: Differences in pathophysiology, injury patterns and treatment compared with adult trauma. Can Med Assoc J *142*:27, 1990.

Luce EA, Tubb T, Moore A: Review of 1,000 major facial fractures and associated injuries. Plast Reconstr Surg *63*:26, 1979.

Palmer J, Rees M: Dog bites of the face: A 15-year review. Br J Plast Surg *36*:315, 1983.

Sayers M: Craniocerebral trauma. *In* Touloubian R (ed): Pediatric Trauma. New York, John Wiley, 1978.

Venes J, Collins W: Spinal cord injury. *In* Touloubian R (ed): Pediatric Trauma. New York, John Wiley, 1978.

Wiseman NE, Chochinov H, Fraser V: Major dog attack injuries in children. J Pediatr Surg *18*:533, 1983.

ACQUIRED CRANIOFACIAL DEFORMITIES: BURNS

Galvis AG, Mestad PH: Modified endotracheal tube for airway management of children with facial burns. Anesth Analg *60*:116, 1981.

Kemper KJ, Benson MS, Bishop MJ. Predictors of postextubation stridor in pediatric trauma patients. Crit Care Med *19*:352, 1991.

Molinaro JR: The social fate of children disfigured by burns. Am J Psychiatry *135*:979, 1978.

Ward CF: Anesthesia for head and neck burn surgery. *In* Wachtel T, Frank D (eds): Burns of the Head and Neck. Philadelphia, WB Saunders, 1984, pp 34–55.

Ward CF, Alfery DD, Saidman LJ, et al: Deliberate hypotension in head and neck surgery. Head Neck Surg *2*:185, 1980.

Ward CF, Gorhan K, Hammond J, Varas R: Securing endotracheal tubes in patients with facial burns or trauma. Am J Surg. *159*:339, 1990.

DEFORMITIES OF THE EXTERNAL EAR

Bergsma D: Birth Defects Compendium. New York, Alan R. Liss, 1979.

Edgerton M: Auricular deformities. *In* Ravitch M, Welch K, Benson C, et al (eds): Pediatric Surgery. 3rd edition. Chicago, Year Book Medical Publishers, 1979.

Posivillo D: The pathogenesis of the first and second branchial arch syndromes. Oral Surg *35*:302, 1973.

Tanzer R, Bellucci R, Converse J, et al: Deformities of the auricle. *In* Converse JM (ed): Reconstructive Plastic Surgery. Vol 3, 2nd edition. Philadelphia, WB Saunders, 1977.

CLEFT LIP AND PALATE

Bell C, Oh TH, Loeffler JR. Massive macroglossia and airway obstruction after cleft palate repair. Anesth Analg *67*:71, 1988.

Bethmann W, Hockstein H: Anesthesiological experiences in 4,000 operations on infants and children for cleft lip and palate. Plast Reconstr Surg *41*:129, 1968.

Cohen MM: Syndromes with cleft lip and cleft palate. Cleft Palate J *15*:306, 1978.

Conway H, Bromberg B, Hochn R, et al: Causes of mortality in patients with cleft lip and cleft palate. Plast Reconstr Surg *37*:51, 1966.

Fraser GR, Cahran JS: Cleft lip and palate: Seasonal incidence of birth weight, birth rank, sex, and site, associated malformations and parental age. Arch Dis Child *36*:420, 1961.

Furnas DW, Allison GR: Circummandibular or nasomaxillary suture with pullout loop for secure placement of endotracheal tube. Am J Surg *139*:887, 1980.

Gorlin RJ, Cervenba J, Pruzansky S: Facial clefting and its syndromes. Birth Defects 7:3, 1971.

Halpern L, Roy L. Anaesthetic morbidity associated with surgical correction of velopharyngeal insufficiency in children. Can J Anaesth *38*:A91, 1991.

Karl HW, Swedlow DB, Lee KW, et al: Epinephrine-halothane interactions in children. Anesthesiology *58*:142, 1983.

Kravath RE, Pollack CP, Borowiecki B, Weitzman ED: Obstructive sleep apnea and death associated with surgical correction of velopharyngeal incompetence. J Pediatr *96*:645, 1980.

Maue-Dickson W, Dickson DR: Anatomy and physiology related to cleft palate: Current research and clinical implications. Plast Reconstr Surg *65*:83, 1980.

McClelland RM, Patterson TJ: The preoperative, anesthetic and postoperative management of cleft lip and palate. Plast Reconstr Surg *29*:642, 1962.

Morgan GA, Steward DJ: A preformed paediatric orotracheal tube design based on anatomical measurements. Can Anaesth Soc J *29*:9, 1982.

Morgan GA, Steward DJ: Linear airway dimensions in children: including those with cleft palate. Can Anaesth Soc J *29*:1, 1982.

Salanitre E, Rackow H: Changing trends in the anesthetic management of the child with cleft lip-palate malformation. Anesthesiology *23*:610, 1962.

Shah CV, Pruzansky S, Morris W: Cardiac malformations with facial clefts. Am J Dis Child *119*:238, 1970.

Wall MA: Infant endotracheal tube resistance: Effects of changing length, diameter, and gas density. Crit Care Med *8*:38, 1980.

Whalen JS, Conn AW: Improved technics in anesthetic management for repair of cleft lips and palates. Anesth Analg *56*:355, 1978.

Zook EG, Salmon JH: Anomalies of the cervical spine in the cleft palate patient. Plast Reconstr Surg *60*:96, 1977.

BRANCHIAL ARCH DEFECTS

Abadir AR, Cottrell J: Anesthesia for craniofacial surgery. *In* Abadir AR, Humayun SG (eds): Anesthesia for Plastic and Reconstructive Surgery. St Louis, Mosby Year Book, 1991.

Audry C: Variete d'alopecie congenitale; Alopecie suturale. Ann Dermatol Syph (Ser 3) *4*:899, 1983.

Augarten A, Sagy M, Yahav J, et al: Management of upper airway obstruction in the Pierre Robin syndrome. Br J Oral Maxillofac Surg *28*:105, 1990.

Berry GA: Note on a congenital defect (coloboma) of the lower lid. Ophthal Hosp Rep *12*:255, 1888.

Braver RD: Congenital cysts and tumors of the neck. *In* Converse JM (ed): Reconstructive Plastic Surgery. Vol 5, 2nd edition. Philadelphia, WB Saunders, 1977.

Bull MJ, Givan DC, Sadove AM, et al: Improved outcome in Pierre Robin sequence. Pediatrics *86*:294, 1990.

Burge D, Middleton A: Persistent pharyngeal pouch in the neonate. J Pediatr Surg *18*:230, 1983.

Cafiero T, Gargiulo G, Carideo P, et al: Anesthetic problems in the surgery of craniofacial dysostosis. Min Anesthesiol *53*:351, 1987.

Carey J, Fineman R, Ziter F: The Robin sequence as a consequence of malformation, dysplasia and neuromuscular syndromes. J Pediatr *101*:858, 1982.

Collins S: The pathogenesis of the Treacher Collins syndrome. Br J Oral Surg *13*:1, 1975.

Crysdale WS, Kohli-Dang N, Mullins GC, et al: Airway management in craniofacial surgery: Experience in 542 patients. J Otol *16*:207, 1987.

Deane SA, Telander R: Surgery for thyroglossal duct and branchial cleft anomalies. Am J Surg *136*:348, 1978.

Dennison WM: The Pierre Robin syndrome. Pediatrics *36*:336, 1965.

Feingold M, Baum J: Goldenhar's syndrome. Am J Dis Child *132*:136, 1978.

Fletcher M, Blum S, Blanchard C: Pierre Robin syndrome: Pathophysiology of obstructive episodes. Laryngoscope *79*:547, 1969.

Franceschetti A, Klein D: Mandibulo-faciale dysostosis; A new hereditary syndrome. Acta Ophthalmol *27*:143, 1949.

Franceschetti A, Zwahlen P: Un syndrome nouveau, la dysostose mandibulofaciale. Bull Schweiz Akad Med Wissensch *1*:60, 1944.

Freed G, Pearlman MA, Brown AS, et al: Polysomnographic indications for surgical intervention in Pierrre Robin sequence. Cleft Palate J *25*:151, 1988.

Freeman MK, Manners JM: Cor pulmonale and the Pierre Robin anomaly. Anaesthesia *35*:282, 1980.

Goldenhar M: Associations malformatives de l'oeil et de l'orielle, en particular le syndrome et dermoide epibulbaire-appendices, auriculaires-fistula, auris congenita et ses relations avec le dysostose mandibulo-faciale. J Genet Humaine *1*:253, 1952.

Grabb WC: The first and second branchial arch syndrome. Plast Reconstr Surg *36*:485, 1965.

Hallerman W: Vogelgesicht und Cataracta congenita. Klin Monatsbl Augenheilkd *113*:315, 1948.

Hanson JW, Smith DW: U-shaped palatal defect in the Robin anomalad: Developmental and clinical relevance. Pediatrics *87*:30, 1975.

Heaf DP, Helms PJ, Dinwiddie R, et al: Nasopharyngeal airways in Pierre Robin syndrome. J Pediatr *100*:698, 1982.

Henzel J, Pories W, DeWeese M: Etiology of lateral cervical cysts. Surg Gynecol Obstet *125*:87, 1967.

Jackson P, Whitaker LA, Randall P: Airway hazards associated with pharyngeal flaps in patients who have the Pierre Robin syndrome. Plast Reconstr Surg *58*:184, 1976.

Jeresaty RM, Huszar RJ, Basu S: Pierre Robin syndrome. Cause of respiratory obstruction, cor pulmonale, and pulmonary edema. Am J Dis Child *117*:710, 1969.

Johnson G, Todd D: Cor pulmonale in severe Pierre Robin syndrome. Pediatrics *65*:152, 1980.

Luke MJ, Mehrizi A, Folger GM, et al: Chronic nasopharyngeal obstruction as a cause of cardiomegaly, cor pulmonale, and pulmonary edema. Pediatrics *37*:762, 1966.

Madan R, Trikha A, Venkataraman RK, et al: Goldenhar's syndrome, an analysis of anaesthetic management; A retrospective study of seventeen cases. Anaesthesia *45*:424, 1990.

Mallory SB, Paradise JL: Glossoptosis revisited: On the development and resolution of airway obstruction in the Pierre Robin syndrome. Pediatrics *64*:946, 1979.

Olsen KD, Maragos N, Weiland L: First branchial cleft anomalies. Laryngoscope *90*:423, 1980.

Pearl W: Congenital heart disease in the Pierre Robin syndrome. Pediatr Cardiol *2*:307, 1982.

Posivillo D: The pathogenesis of the first and second branchial arch syndromes. Oral Surg *35*:302, 1973.

Rasch DK, Browder F, Barr M, et al: Anaesthesia for Treacher Collins and Pierre Robin syndromes. Can Anaesth Soc J *33*:364, 1986.

Ravidson R, Stoops CM: Anesthetic management of a patient with Hallermann-Streiff syndrome. Anesth Analg *53*:254, 1979.

Roa NL, Moss KS: Treacher-Collins syndrome with sleep apnea: Anesthetic considerations. Anesthesiology *60*:71, 1984.

Robin P: Backward lowering of the root of the tongue causing respiratory disturbances. Bull Acad Nat Med *89*:37, 1923.
Robin P: De la physiologique de la tetee au sein et de la forme que doit avoit tetine dur bibeion. Bull Soc Pediat Paris *27*:55, 1929.
Ross ED: Treacher Collins syndrome. Anaesthesia *18*:350, 1963.
Shprintzen RJ, Croft C, Berkman MD, et al: Pharyngeal hypoplasia in Treacher Collins syndrome. Arch Otolaryngol *105*:127, 1979.
Sklar GS, King BD: Endotracheal intubation and Treacher Collins syndrome. Anesthesiology *44*:247, 1976.
Stehling L: Goldenhar syndrome and airway management. Am J Dis Child *132*:818, 1978.
Stern LM, Fonkalsrud EW, Hassakis P, et al: Management of Pierre Robin syndrome in infancy by prolonged naso-esophageal intubation. Am J Dis Child *124*:78, 1972.
Streiff EB: Dysmorphie mandibulofaciale et alterations oculaire. Ophthalmologica *120*:79, 1950.
Thomson A: A description of congenital malformation of the auricle and external meatus of both sides in three persons. Proc R Soc Edinburgh *1*:443, 1845.
Treacher Collins E: Case with symmetrical congenital notches in the outer part of each lower lid and defective development of the malar bones. Trans Ophthal Soc UK *20*:190, 1900.
Weissman C, Damask MC, Yang J: Noncardiogenic pulmonary edema following laryngeal obstruction. Anesthesiology *60*:163, 1984.
Williams AJ, Williams MA, Walker CA, et al.: The Robin anomalad (Pierre Robin syndrome)—a follow up study. Arch Dis Child *56*:663, 1981.

CYSTIC HYGROMA

Barrand KG, Freeman NV: Massive infiltrating cystic hygroma of the neck in infancy. Arch Dis Child *48*:523, 1973.
Bill AH, Sumner DS: A unified concept of lymphangioma and cystic hygroma. Surg Gynecol Obstet *120*:79, 1965.
Braver RD: Congenital cysts and tumors of the neck. *In* Converse JM (ed): Reconstructive Plastic Surgery. Vol 5, 2nd edition. Philadelphia, WB Saunders, 1977.
Evans P: Intubation problem in a case of cystic hygroma complicated by a laryngotracheal haemangioma. Anaesthesia *36*:696, 1981.
Grosfeld J, Weber T, Vane D: One-stage resection for massive cervicomediastinal hygroma. Surgery *92*:693, 1982.
Lindsay WK: The neck. *In* Mustarde JC (ed): Plastic Surgery in Infancy and Childhood. 2nd edition. New York, Churchill Livingstone, 1979.
Ninh TN, Ninh TA: Cystic hygroma: A report of 126 cases. J Pediatr Surg *9*:191, 1974.
Pounds L: Neck masses of congenital origin. Pediatr Clin North Am *28*:841, 1981.
Weller RM: Anaesthesia for cystic hygroma in a neonate. Anaesthesia *29*:588, 1974.
Wernher A: Die angeborenen Zysten-Hygrome und die ihnen verwandten Geschwulste in anatomischer, diagnostischer und therapeutischer Beziehung. Giessen, G.F. Heyer, 1843, p 76.
Wilson RD, Putnam L, Phillips MT, et al: Anesthetic problems in surgery for varying levels of respiratory obstruction in infants and children. Anesth Analg *53*:878, 1974.
Zitelli B: Neck masses in children. Pediatr Clin North Am *28*:813, 1981.

THYROGLOSSAL DUCT CYST

Braver RD: Congenital cysts and tumors of the neck. *In* Converse JM (ed): Reconstructive Plastic Surgery. Vol 5, 2nd edition. Philadelphia, WB Saunders, 1977.
Brereton RJ, Symonds R: Thyroglossal cysts in children. Br J Surg *65*:507, 1978.
Deane SA, Telander R: Surgery for thyroglossal duct and branchial cleft anomalies. Am J Surg *136*:348, 1978.
Pounds L: Neck masses of congenital origin. Pediatr Clin North Am *28*:841, 1981.
Zitelli B: Neck masses in children. Pediatr Clin North Am *28*:813, 1981.

SALIVARY GLAND TUMORS

Attie JN: Tumors of major and minor salivary glands: Clinical and pathologic features. Curr Probl Surg *18*:65, 1981.
Bianchi A, Cudmore RE: Salivary gland tumors in children. J Pediatr Surg *13*:519, 1978.
Krolls SD, Tradahl JN, Boyers RC: Salivary gland lesions in children. Cancer *40*:459, 1972.
Schuller DE, McCabe BF: The firm salivary mass in children. Laryngoscopy *87*:1891, 1977.
Tipton JB: Carcinoma of a minor salivary gland in an 18 month old child: case report. Plast Reconstr Surg *62*:790, 1978.

CHRONIC UPPER AIRWAY OBSTRUCTION AND SLEEP APNEA

Brouilette RT, Fernbach SK, Hunt CE: Obstructive sleep apnea in infants and children. J Pediatr *100*:31, 1982.
Cherniak NS: Sleep apnea and its causes. J Clin Invest *73*:1501, 1984.
Coccagna G, Cirignotta F, Lugaresi E: Sleep Apnea Syndromes. New York, Alan R. Liss, 1978.
Coccagna G, di Donatta G, Verucchi P, et al: Hypersomnia with periodic apnea in acquired micrognathia. Arch Neurol *33*:769, 1976.
Conway WA, Bower GC, Barnes ME: Hypersomnolence and intermittent upper airway obstruction. JAMA *237*:2740, 1977.
Felman A, Loughlin G, Leftridge C: Upper airway obstruction during sleep in children. Am J Roentgenol *133*:213, 1979.
Gastaut H, Tassinari CA, Duron B: Polygraphic study of the episodic diurnal and nocturnal (hypnic and respiratory) manifestations of the Pickwick syndrome. Brain Res *2*:167, 1966.
Kravath RE, Pollak CP, Borowiecki B, et al: Obstructive sleep apnea and death associated with surgical correction of velopharyngeal incompetence. J Pediatr *96*:645, 1980.
Littner M, Young E, McGinty D, et al: Awake abnormalities of control of breathing and of the upper airway. Chest *86*:573, 1984.
Mealer WR, Fisher JC: Cor pulmonale and facio-auriculovertebral sequence. Cleft Palate J *21*:100, 1984.
Potsic WP: Obstructive sleep apnea. Pediatr Clin North Am *36*:1435, 1989.
Remmers JE, de Groot WJ, Sauerland EK, et al: Pathogenesis of airway occlusion during sleep. J Appl Physiol *44*:931, 1978.
Remmers JE, Sterling JA, Thoratinsson B, et al: Nasal airway positive pressure in patients with occlusive sleep apnea. Methods and feasibility. Am Rev Respir Dis *130*:1152, 1984.
Roberts JL, Reed WR, Mathew OP, et al: Assessment of

pharyngeal airway stability in normal and micrognathic infants. J Appl Physiol *58*:290, 1985.

Rowland TW, Norstrom LG, Bean MS, et al: Chronic upper airway obstruction and pulmonary hypertension in Down's syndrome. Am J Dis Child *135*:1050, 1981.

Singer LP, Saenger P: Complications of pediatric obstructive sleep apnea. Otol Clin North Am *23*:665, 1990.

Sullivan CE, Berthon-Jones M, Issa FG, et al: Reversal of obstructive sleep apnoea by continuous positive airway pressure applied through the nares. Lancet *1*:862, 1981.

VanDercar DH, Martinez AP, De Lisser EA: Sleep apnea syndrome: A potential contraindication for patient-controlled analgesia. Anesthesiology *74*:623, 1991.

Weinberg S, Kravath R, Phillips L, et al: Episodic complete airway obstruction in children with undiagnosed obstructive sleep apnea. Anesthesiology *60*:356, 1984.

PULMONARY EDEMA SECONDARY TO AIRWAY OBSTRUCTION

Barin ES, Stevenson IF, Donnelly GL: Pulmonary edema following acute upper airway obstruction. Anaesth Intensive Care *14*:54, 1986.

Brown RE. Negative pressure pulmonary edema. *In* Berry FA (ed): Anesthetic Management of Difficult and Routine Pediatric Patients. New York, Churchill Livingstone, 1986.

Hansen TN, Gest AL, Landers S: Inspiratory airway obstruction does not affect lung fluid balance in lambs. J Appl Physiol *58*:1314, 1985.

Kanter RK, Watchko JF: Pulmonary edema associated with upper airway obstruction. Am J Dis Child *138*:356, 1984.

Lee KWT, Downes JJ: Pulmonary edema secondary to laryngospasm in children. Anesthesiology *59*:347, 1983.

Lorch DG, Sahn SA: Post-extubation pulmonary edema following anesthesia induced by upper airway obstruction. Chest *90*:802, 1986.

Loyd JE, Nolop KB, Parker RE, et al. Effects of inspiratory resistance loading on lung fluid balance in awake sheep. J Appl Physiol *60*:198, 1986.

Tami TA, Chu F, Wildes TO, et al: Pulmonary edema and acute upper airway obstruction. Laryngoscope *96*:506, 1986.

Travis KW, Todres ID, Shannon DC. Pulmonary edema associated with croup and epiglottis. Pediatrics *59*:695, 1977.

Warner LO, Beach TP, et al: Negative pressure edema secondary to airway obstruction in an intubated infant. Can J Anaesth *35*:507, 1988.

Wilder RT, Belani KG: Fiberoptic intubation complicated by pulmonary edema in a 12-year-old child with Hurler syndrome. Anesthesiology *72*:205, 1990.

MANAGEMENT OF THE DIFFICULT PEDIATRIC AIRWAY AND INTUBATION

Alfrey DD, Ward CF, Harwood IR, et al: Airway management for a neonate with congenital fusion of the jaws. Anesthesiology *51*:340, 1979.

Asai T, Fujise K, Uchida M: Use of the laryngeal mask in a child with tracheal stenosis. Anesthesiology *75*:903, 1991.

Audenaert SM, Montgomery CL, Stone B, et al: Retrograde-assisted fiberoptic tracheal intubation in children with difficult airways. Anesth Analg *73*:660, 1991.

Berry FA: The use of a stylet in blind nasotracheal intubation. Anesthesiology *61*:469, 1984.

Beveridge ME: Laryngeal mask anaesthesia for repair of cleft palate. Anaesthesia *44*:656, 1989.

Borland LM, Swan DM, Leff S: Difficult pediatric endotracheal intubation: A new approach to the retrograde technique. Anesthesiology *55*:577, 1981.

Bourke D, Levesque PR: Modification of retrograde guide for endotracheal intubation. Anesth Analg *53*:1013, 1974.

Brain A: Proper technique for insertion of the laryngeal mask. Anesthesiology *73*:1053, 1990.

Brown AC, Sataloff T: Special anesthetic techniques in head and neck surgery. Otolaryngol Clin North Am *14*:587, 1981.

Burtner DD, Goodman M: Anesthetic and operative management of potential upper airway obstruction: Arch Otolaryngol *104*:657, 1978.

Chatterji S, Gupta NR, Mishra TR: Valvular glottic obstruction following extubation. Anaesthesia *39*:246, 1984.

Crowley DS, Giesecke AH: Bimanual cricoid pressure. Anaesthesia *45*:588, 1990.

Fan LL, Flynn JW: Laryngoscopy in neonates and infants: Experience with the flexible fiberoptic bronchoscope. Laryngoscope *91*:451, 1981.

Fisher JA, Ananthanarayan C, Edelist G: Role of the laryngeal mask in airway management. Can J Anaesth *39*:1, 1992.

Grebenik CR, Ferguson C, White A: The laryngeal mask airway in pediatric radiotherapy. Anesthesiology *72*:474, 1990.

Handler SD, Keon TP.: Difficult laryngoscopy/intubation: The child with mandibular hypoplasia. Ann Otol Rhinol Laryngol *92*:401, 1983.

Hemmer D, Lee T, Wright BD: Intubation of a child with a cervical spine injury with the aid of a fiberoptic bronchoscope. Anaesth Intens Care *10*:163, 1982.

Hensinger RN, MacEwen GD: Congenital anomalies of the spine. *In* Rothman RH, Simeon FA (eds): The Spine. Philadelphia, WB Saunders, 1982.

Howardy-Hansen P, Berthelsen P: Fiberoptic bronchoscopic nasotracheal intubation of a neonate with Pierre Robin syndrome. Anaesthesia *43*:121, 1988.

Hudon F: Intubation without laryngoscopy. Anesthesiology *6*:476, 1945.

Katz RL, Berci G: The optical stylet—a new intubation technique for adults and children, with specific reference to teaching. Anesthesiology *51*:251, 1979.

Knuth TE, Richards JR: Mainstem bronchial obstruction secondary to nasotracheal intubation. Anesth Analg *73*:487, 1991.

Mikawa K, Maekawa N, Goto R, et al: Transparent dressing is useful for the secure fixation of the endotracheal tube. Anesthesiology *75*:1123, 1991.

Miller RA: A new laryngoscope. Anesthesiology *2*:317, 1941.

Miyabe M, Dohi S, Homma E: Tracheal intubation in an infant with Treacher Collins syndrome—pulling out the tongue by a forceps. Anesthesiology *62*:213, 1985.

Muzzi DA, Losasso TJ, Cucchiara RF: Complication from a nasopharyngeal airway in a patient with a basilar skull fracture. Anesthesiology *74*:366, 1991.

Nichol HC, Zuch D: Difficult laryngoscopy—the "anterior" larynx and the atlanto-occipital gap. Br J Anaesth *55*:141, 1983.

Peterson MD: Making oral midazolam palatable for children. Anesthesiology *73*:1053, 1990.

Populaire C, Lundi JN, Pinaud M: Elective tracheal intubation in the prone position for a neonate with Pierre Robin syndrome. Anesthesiology *62*:214, 1985.

Salem MR, Mathrubhutham M, Bennett EJ: Difficult intubation. N Engl J Med *295*:879, 1976.

Seraj MA, Yousif M, Channa AB: Anaesthetic management of congenital fusion of the jaws in a neonate. Anaesthesia *39*:695, 1984.

Stiles CM: A flexible fiberoptic bronchoscope for endotracheal intubation of infants. Anesth Analg *53*:1017, 1974.

Stone DJ, Stirt JA, Kaplan MJ, et al: A complication of lightwand-guided nasotracheal intubation. Anesthesiology *61*:780, 1984.

Stool SE: Intubation techniques in difficult airways. Pediatr Infect Dis J *7*:S154, 1988.

Ward CF, Salvatierra CA: Special intubation techniques for the adult patient. *In* Benumof J (ed): Clinical Procedures in Anesthesia and Intensive Care. Philadelphia, JB Lippincott, 1991.

Watson CB, Clapham M: Transillumination for correct tube positioning: Use of a new fiberoptic endotracheal tube. Anesthesiology *60*:253, 1984.

White A, Kander PL: Anatomical factors in difficult direct laryngoscopy. Br J Anaesth *47*:468, 1975.

CHAPTER

10 Ophthalmological Diseases

NANCY KNUTSEN FRANCE, M.D.

Anesthetic considerations specific to pediatric eye surgery are the same for both normal children and those with syndromes of congenital abnormalities. For example, maintaining stable intraocular pressure (see the sections on Congenital Cataracts, Penetrating Trauma, and Glaucoma later in this chapter) and an awareness of the potential for eliciting the oculocardiac reflex (see the section on Retinoblastoma) are important concerns for the anesthesiologist with *all* pediatric patients.

However, children with uncommon diseases and congenital abnormalities have a disproportionate number of ophthalmic lesions requiring surgery. In formulating a preoperative anesthetic plan for such children, the anesthesiologist must be aware of any associated systemic abnormalities apart from the eye lesion. Table 10–1, designed to provide a handy reference for the anesthesiologist, outlines ocular lesions associated with pediatric syndromes and the manifestations of these syndromes, including associated systemic disorders, and highlights the major anesthesia concerns. It is beyond the scope of this table to elaborate on details of anesthesia for multisystem anomalies, although a few are listed. One frequent problem is upper airway deformity leading to a difficult or impossible intubation, especially in cases of craniofacial anomalies. In such cases, topical anesthesia followed by an awake intubation, either blind or with the aid of a small-diameter fiberoptic bronchoscope, is often required.

The purpose of this chapter is to inform the anesthesiologist of the surgical approach and anesthetic concerns related to the relatively uncommon pediatric ocular lesions. The more common lesions such as strabismus or lacrimal duct probe are amply described elsewhere.

CONGENITAL CATARACTS

Clouding of the crystalline lens of the eye is termed a cataract. Congenital cataracts of sufficient size or density severely limit retinal stimulation and restrict development of vision. Cataracts never regress; therefore, early identification and treatment are necessary.[1]

The most effective treatment of bilateral complete congenital cataracts is surgical removal as early in life as possible. This operation may be performed on both eyes simultaneously to reduce anesthesia time or avoid a second anesthetic.[2] A unilateral complete congenital cataract also should be removed in the neonatal period to prevent severe deprivation amblyopia and a poor visual outcome. These conditions are likely to develop when surgery is delayed beyond 6 months of age.[1, 3]

Approximately 50 percent of congenital cataracts are idiopathic. The remainder are associated with various pediatric syndromes, including inborn errors of metabolism, chromosomal disorders, intrauterine infections, trauma that ruptures the lens capsule, or drugs (for example, corticosteroids)[1, 3, 4] (see Table 10–1). At least 30 percent of children with congenital cataracts have an associated nonocular anomaly of another organ system;[1] cardiac anomalies, as commonly occur in the congenital rubella syndrome and Down's syndrome, are of particular concern to the anesthesiologist.

Lenses that become malpositioned owing to dislocation or subluxation, as seen in Marfan's syndrome and homocystinuria (80 percent and 100 percent of patients, respectively) require similar surgical removal[5] (Table 10–2).

Anterior chamber aspiration of the lens is

performed using an operating microscope and a mechanical suction–cutting instrument. An optimal surgical field requires an immobile, maximally dilated pupil for observation of the red reflex to assure complete removal of lens material.[3]

A gravity infusion of 1:200,000 epinephrine in saline via a small needle inserted into the anterior chamber will immediately induce dilation of the iris and intense vasoconstriction, which presumably also delays absorption of intraocular epinephrine. Simultaneous with the epinephrine infusion, a second motorized cutting needle is placed in the anterior chamber for aspiration of its contents along with a considerable volume of the epinephrine-saline solution.[3] The total volume of epinephrine infusion required varies considerably from patient to patient and depends on the duration of the procedure and on fluid losses from needle sites in the anterior chamber.

The arrhythmogenic potential of systemically absorbed epinephrine in the child receiving a potent inhalation anesthetic is a very real concern to the anesthesiologist. Compared with adults, children appear to have a higher threshold to and lower incidence of dysrhythmias induced by exogenous epinephrine during halothane anesthesia.[6–10] However, studies determining the upper limit of subcutaneously injected epinephrine compatible with halothane cannot necessarily be applied to the absorption of intraocular epinephrine. Measurements of systemic epinephrine levels in children have not been reported during this infusion technique, and there are no reports of adverse dysrhythmias with intraocular epinephrine infusion in adults under anesthesia.[11, 12] Nevertheless, caution is warranted, and halothane may be avoided in favor of less arrhythmogenic agents, such as isoflurane, enflurane, or a narcotic-relaxant combination.[6]

EFFECTS OF ANESTHETIC DRUGS AND TECHNIQUES ON INTRAOCULAR PRESSURE

Maintaining a near-normal intraocular pressure (IOP) throughout the operation is essential to prevent loss of vitreous or intraocular contents associated with elevated IOP in the surgically opened eye. IOP is determined by the balance between aqueous humor formation and drainage in the anterior segment of the eye. The most important determinant of IOP is the systemic central venous pressure; it is reflected in the periocular venous system, which receives both blood and aqueous humor drainage from the eye. A sudden explosive Valsalva maneuver or cough immediately raises the central venous pressure, retards drainage of aqueous humor into the venous plexus, increases the intraocular blood volume, and markedly elevates the intraocular pressure.[13] An adequate depth of anesthesia until the last suture has closed the open wound is the best protection against such an unfortunate occurrence. If necessary, a nondepolarizing muscle relaxant can be used to immobilize the patient. If the child unexpectedly moves in response to surgical stimulation, immediate and rapid administration of thiopental will quiet the patient. In this instance, succinylcholine should be avoided as it may acutely raise the IOP owing to its unique effect of tonic contracture of the extraocular muscles.[14]

All the central nervous system depressants in the anesthesiologist's armamentarium tend to decrease intraocular pressure and are, therefore, all acceptable agents in intraocular surgery.[15–20] Similarly, the nondepolarizing muscle relaxants, atropine premedication, alteration in arterial blood pressure, and modest variations in P_{CO_2} have minimal or no effect on IOP.[14, 19, 21–24] Studies of ketamine effects on the normal eye have shown conflicting results of either elevated or unchanged IOP; it should be used cautiously if at all in the open eye.[25–28]

Succinylcholine has been considered to be contraindicated when the eye is surgically open but may be used during the early induction and intubation period. The transiently increased IOP returns to baseline within 5 minutes of intravenous succinylcholine, presumably by autoregulation with increased outflow of aqueous humor; however, the tonic contracture of the extraocular muscles persists for up to 15 to 20 minutes.[14] In theory, the continued contracture and pull of the extraocular muscles on the sclera may cause the ocular contents to be expelled upon incision into the globe. In practice, however, succinylcholine has been widely used to facilitate laryngoscopy without documented increased hazard during cataract surgery.

Many of the patients presenting for congenital cataract aspiration are infants—term or premature—in the first few days of life. An effective and safe anesthetic technique for the neonate includes fentanyl (5 μg/kg) and pancuronium (0.06 mg/kg) or atracurium (0.4 mg/kg), titrated and reversed with the aid of ulnar nerve stimulation. The potential for hyperoxia-induced retinopathy of prematurity dictates maintenance of an arterial oxygen saturation of less than 100

Text continued on page 375

Table 10–1. OCULAR SURGICAL LESIONS IN PEDIATRIC SYNDROMES

Disorder	Inheritance	Defect	Surgical Lesions	Manifestations	Anesthesia Concerns
Chromosomal Aberrations					
Numerical Abnormalities					
Trisomy 13 (Patau's syndrome)	Sporadic; rarely inherited as translocation	Trisomy of chromosome 13	Cataracts, glaucoma, retinal detachment	Cleft lip/palate; digital abnormalities; CHD; arhinencephaly; MR; hypotonia; low-set ears; deafness; high infant mortality (18% survive first year); surgical therapy probably not indicated	
Trisomy 18 (Edwards' syndrome)	Sporadic; rarely inherited as translocation	Trisomy of chromosome 18	Cataracts, glaucoma, ptosis	MR; microcephaly; digital, central venous, and renal abnormalities; rocker-bottom feet; apneic spells; micrognathia; majority die before 1 year	Difficult intubation; CHD precautions; caution with renally excreted drugs
Trisomy 21 (Down's syndrome)	Sporadic; 5% familial translocation	Trisomy of chromosome 21	Cataracts, strabismus	Mental and physical retardation; hypotonia; chronic infections; partial upper airway obstruction during sleep; characteristic facies; atlanto-occipital instability or dislocation; CHD: endocardial cushion defect, ventricular septal defect, PDA, tetralogy of Fallot, ± pulmonary vascular disease	Standard doses of atropine; heavy sedation pre- or postop likely to accentuate airway obstruction and hypoventilation; cannulation may be difficult owing to hypoplastic peripheral vessels; small subglottic area—choose endotracheal tube that allows air leak with ventilation; gentle manipulation of cervical spine during laryngoscopy; blood pressure significantly lower than normal; ketamine, inhalation agents satisfactory; CHD precautions
"Cat eye" syndrome		Extra acrocentric chromosome	Cataracts	Imperforate anus; variable renal, central venous, and digital anomalies; micrognathia; MR; iris resembles the cat's vertical pupil	Difficult intubation
Cornelia de Lange's syndrome	Unknown	Small % chromosomal aberrations	Ptosis, strabismus	Short stature; MR; microcephaly; hirsutism and bushy eyebrows; weak cry; malformed hands and feet	
Fanconi's syndrome with pancytopenia	Autosomal recessive	High % of chromated breaks and unusual chromosomal alignments	Strabismus, ptosis	Microcephaly and short stature; MR; pigmentation of skin; absence of radii and thumbs; pancytopenia; leukemia frequently occurs	Severe anemia, leukopenia—Rx with blood transfusions and androgenic steroids
Prader-Willi syndrome	Unknown	Occasional chromosome 15 abnormalities	Strabismus	Uncontrollable hyperphagia; small, obese stature; MR; hypotonia; cryptorchidism; ± diabetes	Monitor for hypoglycemia—Rx glucose infusion; extreme obesity may impair ventilation postop

Structural Abnormalities					
Deletion 4p− (Wolf-Hirschhorn syndrome)	Sporadic or may be familial	Deletion (4p−)	Strabismus, cataracts	MR; seizures; cleft lip/palate; deformed nose; hydrocephalus	
Deletion 5p− (Cri-du-chat)	Sporadic, may be familial	Deletion (5p−)	Cataracts, strabismus	Catlike cry secondary to abnormal larynx; cleft lip/palate; microcephaly; micrognathia; ± CHD; hypotonia; MR	Airway stridor due to laryngomalacia; difficult intubation; CHD precautions
Deletion 11p−	Sporadic or familial translocation	Deletion (11p−)	Glaucoma, cataracts	Aniridia; MR; genitourinary anomalies; associated with Wilms' tumor	± Hypertension—Rx with hydralazine and propranolol; avoid ketamine
Deletion 13q−	Sporadic or familial translocation	Deletion (13q−)	Cataract, retinoblastoma, strabismus, ptosis	Microcephaly; micrognathia; MR; hypospadias	Avoid ketamine
Deletion 18p−	Sporadic, occasional familial translocation	Deletion (18p−)	Ptosis, strabismus	Microcephaly; MR; webbed neck; immunoglobulin abnormalities; diabetes; thyroiditis; severe form has cyclopia	
Deletion 18q−	Sporadic, occasional familial translocation	Deletion (18q−)	Cataracts	Microcephaly; midface hypoplasia; carplike mouth; deafness; abnormalities of hands and feet	
Sex Chromosomes					
Turner's syndrome (monosomy X)	Sporadic	XO (80% have 45 chromosomes, a single X, no sex chromatin) XO/XX mosaics	Strabismus, ptosis, cataracts	Sexual infantilism; short stature; webbed neck; small mandible; cubitus valgus; coarctation of aorta; dissecting aneurysm of aorta; autoimmune disease (diabetes and thyroiditis); recurrent ear infections	± Hypertension secondary to coarctation of aorta; avoid ketamine
Klinefelter's syndrome	Sporadic	XXY XXXY XXXXY XXYY XYY (for chromatin positive)	Strabismus, retinal detachment, dislocation of lens	± MR; scoliosis; microcephaly; CHD; gynecomastia; prognathism; tall stature; aggressive or bizarre behavior; hypogenitalism; increasing X chromosomes associated with mental and physical impairment	
Defects of Lipid Metabolism					
Familial Hypolipoproteinemia					
Bassen-Kornzweig syndrome (abetalipoproteinemia)	Autosomal recessive	Absent betalipoprotein	Retinal abnormalities, strabismus, ptosis	Spinocerebellar degeneration with ataxia; steatorrhea; acanthocytes; vitamin A deficiency	
Tangier disease (analphalipoproteinemia)	Autosomal recessive	Deficiency of high-density lipoprotein	Corneal haziness	Accumulation of cholesterol esters in RE system (large orange tonsils, hepatosplenomegaly); peripheral neuropathy and muscle wasting; anemia and thrombocytopenia; premature coronary disease; decreased plasma cholesterol and phospholipids	Check hemoglobin and platelets

Table continued on following page

Table 10–1. OCULAR SURGICAL LESIONS IN PEDIATRIC SYNDROMES *Continued*

Disorder	Inheritance	Defect	Surgical Lesions	Manifestations	Anesthesia Concerns
Lipoidoses					
Gaucher's disease I, II, III	Autosomal recessive	Defect in glucocerebrosidase; ceramide glucosidase accumulates	Corneal opacities, strabismus	Hepatosplenomegaly; hypersplenism and abnormal bruising; elevated serum acid phosphatase; bone pain, joint swelling, and fractures; chronic lung disease secondary to aspiration; spasticity; tremors; failure to thrive; progressive dementia	Anemia and coagulation disorders second to platelet deficiency
Fabry's disease (angiokeratoma corporis diffusum)	X-linked recessive	Deficiency of ceramide trihexosidase	Corneal dystrophy, cataracts	Lipid deposition in blood causes painful extremities and dark purple maculopapular eruption; edema of legs and face; hypertension; progressive renal failure; myocardial ischemia and premature death in adulthood	Cardiac and renal function compromised
Gangliosidoses					
Tay-Sachs disease (GM2 type I) (infantile cerebromacular degeneration)	Autosomal recessive	Deficiency of hexosaminidase A	Optic atrophy, blindness	Begins 6–12 mos—death by 3 yr; dementia; hypotonia; hyperacusis; visceromegaly; spastic paralysis; seizures	Neurological deficit leads to respiratory disability
Refsum's syndrome (heredopathia atactica polyneuritiformis)	Autosomal recessive	Deficiency of phytanic acid alpha-hydroxylase	Optic nerve atrophy, cataracts, glaucoma	Peripheral polyneuropathy; ichthyosis; limb weakness; nerve deafness; cerebellar ataxia; ECG changes and premature death in adulthood	
Familial cerebrotendinous xanthomatosis	Autosomal recessive	Increased serum cholestanol	Cataracts	Cerebellar ataxia; enlargement of tendons	
Defects of Amino Acid Metabolism					
Albinism 1. Oculocutaneous 2. Ocular	1. Autosomal recessive 2. X-linked	Defect in converting tyrosine to melanin	Strabismus	Hypopigmentation; increased susceptibility to skin neoplasia	
Cystinosis (Fanconi's syndrome with renal tubular defects)	Autosomal recessive	Enzyme defect unknown	Corneal transplant (benign or adult form)	Deposition of cystine in RE system, renal tubular cells, and cornea; small stature; aminoaciduria; renal tubular acidosis; hypophosphatemic rickets; nephrotic syndrome and renal failure (benign form, kidneys spared)	Monitor acid-base and electrolytes Caution when using renally excreted drugs
Homocystinuria	Autosomal recessive	Deficiency of cystathionine B synthase	Dislocated lens, secondary glaucoma, strabismus, retinal detachment	MR; seizures; marfanoid habitus; osteoporosis; thromboembolic episodes secondary to platelet adhesiveness	Preop correction of platelet function; maintain hydration and peripheral perfusion

Alkaptonuria and ochronosis	Autosomal recessive	Deficiency of homogentisic acid oxidase	Scleral pigmentation	Renal calculi; osteoarthritis; valvular heart disease and atherosclerosis; black urine on standing secondary to homogentisic acid	Cardiac and renal precautions
Hyperlysinemia	Autosomal recessive	Deficiency of lysine ketoglutarate reductase	Subluxation of lens, strabismus	Lax ligaments; hypotonic muscles; seizures; hyperlysinemia and lysinuria	
Defects of Carbohydrate Metabolism					
Galactosemia	Autosomal recessive	1. Deficiency of galactose-1-phosphate uridyl transferase	Cataracts	Galactosemia and galactosuria; hepatosplenomegaly; hepatic failure and jaundice; MR; vomiting and failure to thrive; Rx eliminate galactose from diet	
		2. Deficiency of galactokinase	Cataracts	More benign; galactosuria and galactosemia; Rx eliminate galactose from diet	
Mucopolysaccharidoses (Types I–VII)	All autosomal recessive except Hunter's syndrome, which is X-linked recessive	Defects in lysosomal acid hydrolases	Cloudy cornea, retinal changes, glaucoma	Variable changes depending on type—coarse facies, short neck, hepatosplenomegaly, dwarfism, stiff joints, cardiac involvement, respiratory disability	Upper airway obstruction Difficult intubation
Hurler's syndrome (gargoylism)	Autosomal recessive	Deficiency of L-iduronidase	Cloudy cornea, ptosis, strabismus, glaucoma	Deposition of acid mucopolysaccharide in every system of body; MR; large head; short neck; coarse features; dwarfism; kyphoscoliosis; hepatosplenomegaly; myocardial and valvular infiltration cause angina, myocardial infarction, CHF; respiratory difficulties; infections, abnormal tracheobronchial cartilages, large tongue, infiltration of lymphoid tissue of larynx and lungs; most die by 10 years of age	Upper airway obstruction; difficult intubation; CHF; arrhythmias, postop respiratory difficulties
Glycogen storage disease (Von Gierke's disease) unknown (hepatorenal glycogenosis type I)		Deficiency of glucose-6-phosphatase	Macular lesions	Hepatosplenomegaly; renal hyperplasia; poor muscular development; macroglossia; hypoglycemia; lactic acidosis; hyperlipemia; dwarfism; bleeding diathesis with thrombocytosis	Dehydration and acidosis—monitor acid base; fasting blood glucose very low—maintain at physiological levels
Glucose-6-phosphate dehydrogenase deficiency (favism)	X-linked recessive	Deficiency of glucose-6-phosphate dehydrogenase	Cataracts, vitreous hemorrhage	Fava beans, sulfonamides, antimalarials, and phenacetin induce an acute hemolytic anemia	
Defects of Metal Metabolism					
Wilson's disease (hepatolenticular degeneration)	Autosomal recessive	Deficiency of serum ceruloplasmin	Kayser-Fleischer rings of cornea; "sunflower" cataracts	Copper accumulation in liver, brain, kidney, and cornea; degeneration of lenticular nucleus and basal ganglia; hepatic cirrhosis and jaundice; malabsorption syndrome; renal tubular damage and aminoaciduria	Treatment with penicillamine (copper chelator that lowers body content of copper); anemia; anesthetic compatible with hepatic and renal failure

Table continued on following page

Table 10–1. OCULAR SURGICAL LESIONS IN PEDIATRIC SYNDROMES *Continued*

Disorder	Inheritance	Defect	Surgical Lesions	Manifestations	Anesthesia Concerns
CNS Disorders					
Marinesco-Sjögren syndrome	Autosomal recessive		Cataracts, strabismus	Oligophrenia and spinocerebellar ataxia; MR	
Sjögren's syndrome	Autosomal recessive		Cataracts	Oligophrenia	
Meckel's syndrome	Autosomal recessive		Cataracts	Occipital encephalocele; polycystic kidneys; polydactyly; CHD; abnormal genitalia	
Musculoskeletal Disease					
Chondrodysplasia punctata	Autosomal recessive and autosomal dominant	Bone dysplasia	Cataracts	Bone dysplasia; joint contractures; calcification of tracheal cartilages; recessive form lethal in 1st year of life	
Myotonic dystrophy (Steinert's disease)	Autosomal dominant	Muscle defect	Ptosis, cataracts, strabismus	Myotonia with muscle atrophy and weakness; conduction defects and arrhythmias; impaired ventilation, frequent aspiration and pneumonia; hypogonadism	Can induce myotonia with succinylcholine, neostigmine, halothane; jaw easily dislocated; sensitive to respiratory depressants—anticipate postop pulmonary problems; regional or local anesthesia preferred
Albright's hereditary osteodystrophy	Autosomal dominant	Skeletal dysplasia	Cataracts	Skeletal dysplasia; obesity; MR; intracranial and subcutaneous calcifications; neuromuscular problems and seizures	
1. Pseudohypoparathyroidism (PH)				1. Hypocalcemic	Hypocalcemia with possible cardiac conduction defects, neuromuscular problems; avoid relaxants
2. Pseudo-pseudohypoparathyroidism (PPH)				2. Normocalcemic	
Stickler's syndrome (progressive arthro-ophthalmomyopathy)	Autosomal dominant		Cataracts, retinal detachment, glaucoma	Tall; joint laxity with arthritis; cleft palate; kyphoscoliosis; deafness; micrognathia; flat facies	Difficult intubation
Robert's syndrome	Autosomal recessive		Cataracts	Tetraphocomelia; cleft lip/palate	
Marfan's syndrome	Autosomal dominant	Connective tissue degeneration of the elastic lamellae	Subluxation of lens, glaucoma, retinal detachment, strabismus	Arachnodactyly; hyperextensibility; hypotonia; scoliosis; hernias; aortic aneurysm; aortic valve insufficiency; mitral valve prolapse	± Propranolol therapy
Weill-Marchesani syndrome	Autosomal recessive	Connective tissue disorder	Dislocation of lens, secondary to glaucoma	Brachydactyly; short stature; stiff immobile joints; ± cardiac anomalies	
Ehlers-Danlos syndrome (7 forms)	Autosomal dominant Also recessive Also X-linked	Connective tissue disorder; deficiency of protocollagen lysyl hydroxylase	Subluxation of lens, keratoconus, glaucoma, retinal detachment	Hyperextensibility of joints and skin; easy bruisability; wide nasal bridge; gastrointestinal bleeding; kyphoscoliosis; dissecting aortic aneurysm; mitral valve prolapse; conduction defects; hernias	Avoid trauma to skin, eyes, joints; difficult to maintain IV routes; adequate vascular access; risk of excessive bleeding; potential for spontaneous pneumothorax

Bird-headed dwarfism (Seckel's syndrome)	Autosomal recessive		Strabismus	Microcephaly; prominent nose; intrauterine growth retardation; short stature; MR	
Klippel-Feil syndrome	Autosomal dominant, ? autosomal recessive		Strabismus	Congenital fusion of cervical vertebrae, especially synostosis of atlas and axis; short neck, immobile, often torticollis; spastic paraplegia; deafness; ± MR	Difficult intubation
Mieten's syndrome	Autosomal recessive		Strabismus	MR; small stature; short forearms, dislocation of radius with flexion contracture elbow	
Spondyloepiphyseal dysplasia, congenital (pseudoachondroplasia)	Autosomal dominant		Retinal detachment, cataracts	Short trunk and limbs; deformity of sternum, hands, and feet; skeletal abnormalities of vertebral column and hips; deafness	
Thrombocytopenia—absent radius syndrome	Autosomal recessive		Strabismus	Thrombocytopenia, ± eosinophilia; absence or hypoplasia of radius; ± CHD; 35% die in 1st year of life of intracranial hemorrhage	Platelet transfusion pre- and intraop
Renal Diseases					
Lowe's syndrome (oculocerebrorenal syndrome)	X-linked recessive		Cataracts, glaucoma, strabismus	MR; hypotonia; renal tubular dysfunction with hyperchloremic acidosis; aminoaciduria; osteoporosis; renal rickets; seizures	Rx large doses vitamin D, Ca, Na supplements; monitor acid base, electrolytes, calcium; caution with renally excreted drugs
Alport's syndrome (hereditary nephritis with deafness and ocular abnormalities)	X-linked recessive or ? Autosomal dominant		Cataracts, retinal detachment	Sensorineural deafness; glomerulopathy and chronic renal failure	Caution with renally excreted drugs
Cerebrohepatorenal syndrome (Zellweger's syndrome)	Autosomal recessive		Glaucoma, cataracts	Mental and growth retardation; flat facies; hepatomegaly; polycystic kidneys and albuminuria; hypotonia; PDA; hypospadias; calcific deposits in long bones; death in early infancy	Rx hypoprothrombinemia; caution with renally excreted drugs
Hartnup's disease	Autosomal recessive	Defect in transport of tryptophan by intestinal mucosa and renal tubules	Strabismus	Aminoaciduria; photosensitive skin and pellagra-like skin rash; ataxia; mental deterioration; excess urinary indole excretion; Rx with nicotinamide and high-protein diets	
Dermatological Disorders					
Cockayne's syndrome	Autosomal recessive		Cataracts	Dwarfism with prognathism; MR; deafness; thick skull bones; hepatosplenomegaly; photosensitive dermatitis; premature senility	
Rothmund-Thomson syndrome (poikiloderma atrophicans vasculare)	Autosomal recessive		Cataracts	Atrophic telangiectatic dermatosis; sparse hair; defective dentition; congenital bone defects; hypogenitalism	

Table continued on following page

Table 10–1. OCULAR SURGICAL LESIONS IN PEDIATRIC SYNDROMES *Continued*

Disorder	Inheritance	Defect	Surgical Lesions	Manifestations	Anesthesia Concerns
Bloch-Sulzberger syndrome (incontinentia pigmenti)	X-linked dominant (lethal in male)	Mesenchymal and ectodermal defect	Cataracts, strabismus	Generalized ectodermal dysplasia; bullous eruptions; hyperpigmentation; hypoplasia of dentition; MR; skeletal abnormalities; microcephaly; ± cardiac abnormalities	
Goltz's syndrome (focal dermal hypoplasia)	Unknown	Mesenchymal and ectodermal defect	Strabismus	Areas of hypoplasia and altered pigmentation of skin; dystrophic nails; enamel hypoplasia; syndactyly; multiple papillomas of mucous membranes and skin; occurs mainly in females	Airway may contain papillomas
Histiocytic dermatoarthritis	Autosomal dominant		Glaucoma, cataracts	Histiocytic nodules on face, hands, feet; seronegative arthritis; bony resorption of hands, wrists	
Ataxia-telangiectasia (Louis-Bar syndrome)	Autosomal recessive	Probable thymus dysfunction	Strabismus	Cutaneous telangiectasia of ears, cheeks, antecubital space; cerebellar ataxia; deficiency of IgA; lymphoreticular malignancy; recurrent sinopulmonary infections (bronchiectasis); anemia; MR	Correct anemia; anesthesia for chronic lung disease; reverse isolation techniques
Ichthyosis					
Ichthyosis vulgaris	Autosomal dominant	Abnormal stratum corneum	Cataracts	Skin changes appear after 3 mon. of life (mildest form); dryness; keratosis pilaris, increased markings on palmar and plantar skin	
Congenital ichthyosis (harlequin fetus)	Autosomal recessive	Abnormal stratum corneum	Cataracts	Hyperkeratosis with thick scaly skin and hyperhidrosis (lethal in neonatal period)	
Ichthyosis and cataracts	Autosomal recessive	Abnormal stratum corneum	Cataracts	Same as congenital ichthyosis	
Oculocerebral syndrome with keratosis follicularis and aminoaciduria	X-linked		Cataracts, glaucoma	Keratosis follicularis; aminoaciduria; alopecia; MR	
Hamartoses (Abnormal Mixtures of Normal Tissues)					
Sturge-Weber syndrome (encephalotrigeminal angiomatosis)	Unknown		Glaucoma when hemangioma involves lid or conjunctiva	Flat facial hemangioma (usually unilateral), 5th cranial nerve distribution; meningeal hemangiomas; seizures; paresis; mental deficiency, cerebral calcifications	Angioma may involve airway
Klippel-Trenaunay-Weber syndrome (giant hemangioma with localized hypertrophy or gigantism)	Unknown		Glaucoma when hemangioma involves lid or conjunctiva	Similar to Sturge-Weber syndrome, except hemangioma also affects body and limbs with hypertrophy of one or more limbs; varicose veins	

Von Recklinghausen's syndrome (neurofibromatosis)	Autosomal dominant		Glaucoma	Multiple neurofibromas in skin and meninges; café-au-lait spots; skeletal defects; scoliosis; neurological symptoms with involvement of cranial or spinal nerve roots	Hypertension may indicate pheochromocytoma
Oculodermal melanocytosis (nevus of Ota)	Sporadic		Glaucoma	Unilateral ocular melanocytosis; increased pigmentation of lids and periorbital skin	
Basal cell nevus (carcinoma) syndrome	Autosomal dominant		Glaucoma, strabismus, cataracts	Multiple cutaneous nevoid basal cell carcinomas; cysts of mandible; scoliosis; intracranial calcifications; mental deficiency	
Craniofacial Malformations					
Hallermann-Streiff syndrome (oculomandibulo) or Françqis' syndrome	Autosomal dominant or sporadic		Cataracts, strabismus	Dyscephaly; mandibular and malar hypoplasia; small mouth; faulty dentition; atrophy of skin and hypotrichosis; dwarf stature; limitation of mouth opening secondary to maldevelopment of temporomandibular joint	
Rubinstein-Taybi syndrome	Unknown, ? recessive	Unknown, ? small Chromosomal abnormality	Cataracts, glaucoma, ptosis, strabismus	Broad thumbs and toes; beaked nose; MR; antimongoloid slant of eyelids; very short stature; may have vertebral, cardiac, renal abnormalities	Cardiac (pulmonary stenosis) and renal compromise
Smith-Lemli-Opitz syndrome	Autosomal recessive		Ptosis, cataracts, strabismus	Microcephaly; micrognathia; hypotonia; pyloric stenosis; MR; hypospadias and cryptorchidism; syndactyly	Difficult intubation
Marshall's syndrome (? synonymous with Stickler's syndrome)	Autosomal dominant		Cataracts	Saddle nose; sensorineural deafness	
Cerebro-oculofacial–skeletal (COFS) syndrome	Autosomal recessive	Degenerative disorder	Cataracts, blepharophimosis	Hypotonia; microcephaly; micrognathia; flexion contractures; death common in first few years of life	
Möbius' syndrome	Autosomal dominant	Cranial nerve palsy VI and VII, bilateral	Strabismus, ptosis	Deafness; muscular weakness of tongue, neck, and chest; immobility (palsy) of face; difficulty chewing and swallowing	
Crouzon's disease (craniofacial dysostosis) (Apert's syndrome is a manifestation of greater expressivity and penetrance)	Autosomal dominant	Defect unknown	Cataracts, strabismus, tarsorrhaphy	Craniofacial dysostosis; deafness; beaked nose; hypoplastic maxilla; hypertelorism and proptosis; soft palate against posterior pharyngeal wall, mouth breathing necessary; syndactyly associated with Apert's syndrome	Difficult intubation; upper airway obstruction
Pierre Robin syndrome	? Autosomal dominant	1st and 2nd arch syndrome	Cataracts, glaucoma, retinal detachment, strabismus	Micrognathia with glossoptosis and cleft palate; upper airway obstruction and swallowing difficulties	Upper airway obstruction; difficult intubation

Table continued on following page

Table 10–1. OCULAR SURGICAL LESIONS IN PEDIATRIC SYNDROMES *Continued*

Disorder	Inheritance	Defect	Surgical Lesions	Manifestations	Anesthesia Concerns
Goldenhar's syndrome (oculoauriculovertebral syndrome)	Sporadic	Anomalies of development of 1st and 2nd branchial arches	Glaucoma, cataracts, strabismus	Bulbar dermoids or lipodermoids; ± cleft lip/palate; ± CHD; deafness; malar and mandibular hypoplasia; malformed, low-set ear; hypoplasia of cervical vertebrae; condition usually unilateral	Difficult intubation
Oculodentodigital syndrome	Unknown		Glaucoma	Hypoplastic tooth enamel; abnormal digits; ± cleft lip/palate; deafness; hip dislocation	
Rieger's syndrome	Autosomal dominant		Glaucoma	Hypodontia; malar hypoplasia; myotonic dystrophy; MR; hypertelorism	
Axenfeld's syndrome and Peter's anomaly			Glaucoma	Similar to Rieger's syndrome, probably represents a different manifestation of same dysgenetic defect	
Miscellaneous Disorders					
Kartagener's syndrome	Autosomal recessive		Cataracts	Dextrocardia; bronchiectasis and sinusitis; dysfunctional cilia; heart block; male sterility	Anesthesia for chronic pulmonary disease
Laurence-Moon syndrome	Autosomal recessive		Strabismus	Hypogenitalism; MR; spastic paraplegia; ± CHD and renal abnormalities; retinitis pigmentosa	Precautions if cardiac or renal abnormalities present
Werner's syndrome	Autosomal recessive		Cataracts	Retinitis pigmentosa; arrest of growth at puberty; ± MR, scleroderma-like changes; premature graying, alopecia; arteriosclerosis; hypogonadism; diabetes	Manage as for atherosclerotic heart disease and diabetes
Hypercalcemia (Williams' syndrome)	Unknown		Strabismus	Elfin facies; supravalvular aortic stenosis; hypercalcemia in infancy, dental abnormalities	Monitor serum calcium; avoid cardiac depressants if fixed cardiac output, left ventricular failure, and myocardial ischemia, cardiac surgery; correction must precede eye surgery

CHD = congenital heart disease; MR = mental retardation; PDA = patent ductus arteriosus; RE = reticuloendothelial; CHF = congestive heart failure.
Data from references 105 to 112.

Table 10–2. ECTOPIA LENTIS REQUIRING SURGICAL REMOVAL

	Abnormalities of Eye	Abnormalities of Skeleton	Abnormalities of Cardiovascular System	Therapy
Marfan's syndrome	Lens subluxated or dislocated (also glaucoma, retinal detachment, strabismus)	Arachnodactyly; tall, slender build; kyphosis; scoliosis; chest deformities; muscles flaccid with joint hyperextensibility; caution with positioning and neck movement	Aneurysm of ascending aorta; aortic or mitral regurgitation; mitral valve prolapse	Propranolol (? retard aortic dilation) Antibiotic prophylaxis (not necessary for eye surgery, for intubation)
Homocystinuria	Lens dislocated (also glaucoma, retinal detachment, strabismus)	Marfanoid habitus; osteoporosis	Thromboembolic lesions	Pyridoxine (vitamin B_6)
			Deficiency of cystathionine-beta-synthase Homocystine irritates vascular endothelium and induces platelet consumption and thrombosis	Dipyridamole (antiplatelet utilization) Operation when platelet function within normal limits Anesthesia: adequate hydration and peripheral blood flow; hypoglycemia second to hyperinsulinemia requires monitoring serum glucose

Data from references 36 to 42.

percent in the premature infant; monitoring saturation by pulse oximetry is very helpful in determining safe concentrations of nitrous oxide and oxygen to be administered.[29–34] The SPO_2 should be maintained at ± 95 percent.

Avoiding prolonged periods of high inspired oxygen in the full-term neonate is recommended because of variations in retinal maturation until 44 weeks postconceptional age.[35]

Postoperatively, it is desirable to have a quiet, drowsy patient and again to minimize large swings in venous pressure and IOP. The very young infant who has received a narcotic-balanced combination of anesthetics will continue to have residual sedation in the recovery room, but the older infant or child who received inhalation anesthetics may require additional postoperative sedation with diazepam (0.1 to 0.2 mg/kg) or droperidol (0.075 to 0.1 mg/kg).

PENETRATING TRAUMA OF THE GLOBE

Perforating wounds of the eye are common in children and vary from small punctures to extensive lacerations complicated by prolapse of intraocular contents. Apart from mechanical damage at the time of injury, the subsequent risk of intraocular infection and the potential for development of sympathetic ophthalmia involving the contralateral eye are very real hazards.[43]

The need for early wound closure and removal of any foreign body presents the anesthesiologist with the dual challenge of maintaining a stable IOP to prevent further ocular damage and inducing anesthesia in the small child with a full stomach.

IOP can best be maintained within a normal range by preventing elevated central venous pressure due to breath-holding, crying, struggling, and vomiting, and by avoiding drug-induced IOP changes.

The use of succinylcholine to permit rapid sequence induction in patients with open eye injury, previously condemned, is now accepted by many anesthesiologists. Reports of two large series of patients who were anesthetized in referral eye centers and given succinylcholine at induction suggest that none of them demonstrated any deterioration in the condition of the injured eye following induction.[44, 45] Furthermore, studies of uninjured eyes during a rapid sequence induction using thiopental and succinylcholine indicate that under these conditions IOP did not rise above baseline awake levels.[46] Similar findings were reported in patients given lidocaine 1 minute prior to induction with thiopental and succinylcholine, in whom no increase in IOP above baseline occurred during rapid sequence induction and intubation.[47] Lidocaine does not, however, prevent a rise in intraocular pressure if succinylcholine is given during halothane/nitrous oxide anesthesia.[48]

These reports suggest that when succinylcholine is considered to be the drug of choice in the management of a patient with a full stomach, the presence of an open eye injury may not compromise this decision, provided a rapid sequence induction with lidocaine and thiopental is used. The conditions for intubation are usually better following succinylcholine than after a nondepolarizing drug, and a more rapid, gentle intubation is possible.

There are, however, some possible alternatives in the anesthesia management of the child with an open eye injury. A safe, rapid induction technique designed to minimize IOP elevation includes preoxygenation of a well-sedated child and gentle mask placement to prevent extrinsic pressure on the globe; thiopental, 5 to 7 mg/kg intravenously; a nondepolarizing muscle relaxant of intermediate-acting duration such as pancuronium,* 0.15 mg/kg, or atracurium, 0.4 mg/kg; cricoid pressure, which will allow gentle positive-pressure ventilation, minimizing gastric inflation and passive regurgitation; intravenous lidocaine, 1 mg/kg, to blunt the stimulation of intubation and its adverse effect on IOP; and laryngoscopy as soon as the child is fully paralyzed as indicated by a peripheral nerve stimulator.[48–50]

However, the small, frightened, uncooperative child may do considerable additional damage to the open eye injury by excessive crying or struggling during attempts to place an intravenous catheter. Flexibility and an alternative induction technique are necessary for this situation. A rectal barbiturate in the presence of the parents or a gentle mask induction followed by cricoid pressure and intravenous catheter placement as soon as the child is asleep is acceptable; the remainder of induction is as previously described.[51, 52]

*In practice, the relaxant drug can be given immediately *before* the thiopental to further hasten good intubating conditions.

Finally, if the risk of aspiration during induction is considered very high, the use of a rapid sequence induction with succinylcholine is justified. This will permit rapid control of the airway with optimal conditions for intubation. After a suitable period of gentle preoxygenation, lidocaine (1.5 mg/kg) should be administered intravenously, followed in 3 minutes by the rapid injection of a sleep dose of thiopental and succinylcholine (1 to 2 mg/kg).

At the conclusion of wound closure, the stomach should be aspirated and the trachea extubated when the child is awake, with full return of airway reflexes. Again, intravenous lidocaine, 1 to 2 mg/kg, will diminish vigorous coughing on the endotracheal tube while the child is awaiting an awake extubation.[53]

GLAUCOMA

In infants and children, glaucoma, which is an elevated IOP that produces damage to ocular structures or function, is caused either by maldevelopment of the eye (developmental glaucoma) or, secondarily, by other ocular diseases such as neoplasm or trauma.[54] In addition, many syndromes and anomalies may have associated glaucoma (see Table 10–1).

Congenital glaucoma occurs at or shortly after birth; 75 percent of the cases are bilateral. A history of prematurity is common. The cardinal signs in the infant are enlarged and cloudy cornea due to edema, tearing, photophobia, and blepharospasm. Under 3 years of age the eye is quite elastic and will enlarge as a result of increased IOP; this is termed buphthalmos or ox eye.[54, 55] Glaucomatous cupping of the optic disc appears early in infants with increased IOP and may also disappear rapidly after the IOP is controlled.[55]

Congenital glaucoma occurs because of impaired outflow; surgical therapies such as goniotomy, trabeculotomy, and trabeculectomy are designed to open a route for aqueous flow into Schlemm's canal, normalizing IOP. Cases that fail to respond to such operation may require cyclocryotherapy, which reduces the formation of aqueous humor. This technique involves freezing (to −60 to −80°C) the aqueous-producing portion of the ciliary body; the lesions are extremely painful postoperatively, and patients require generous narcotic analgesia.

Early diagnosis is essential if treatment is to be successful. The infant suspected of having congenital glaucoma requires a general anesthetic for an examination and IOP measurement. Preparations should be made to follow the examination with a surgical procedure if the diagnosis is confirmed. A sleep dose of rectal methohexital plus a topical ocular anesthetic is often sufficient for the initial examination.[52]

All general anesthetics and central nervous system depressants tend to lower IOP (with the exception of ketamine) and are also acceptable. One simply needs to be aware of the modest lowering or slight elevation (ketamine) of IOP from the baseline levels in the unanesthetized eye when evaluating the measured pressure.[56, 57] Optimally, IOP should be measured during the first 10 minutes after induction with nitrous oxide and halothane, but before intubation.[57] Fortunately, the diagnosis of congenital glaucoma is not based solely on the numerical IOP reading, but also on the unmistakable ocular signs of glaucoma (corneal edema, tears in Descemet's membrane, cupping of the optic nerve).[55]

Succinylcholine and intubation, which may alter IOP, should be avoided before the IOP reading but may be used in preparation for the subsequent operative procedure.[58]

The operation of goniotomy or trabeculectomy for glaucoma is a delicate intraocular procedure that requires the optimal surgical conditions, which can be provided only by very careful general endotracheal anesthesia. Adequate levels of anesthesia, together with neuromuscular block and controlled ventilation, should be employed to ensure absolute immobility and optimal control of IOP.[59]

Smooth emergence and extubation without coughing or straining are essential. Lidocaine, 1.5 mg/kg IV, followed by careful suctioning of the pharynx, should precede removal of the endotracheal tube.[53]

Infants with glaucoma should be examined periodically with repeat IOP measurements under general anesthesia. In order to evaluate the success of therapy, the drugs must be continued up to the time of anesthesia and consideration given to the potential systemic side effects (Table 10–3).

RETINOBLASTOMA

Retinoblastoma is an intraocular tumor that occurs in 1 per 20,000 live births and accounts for 1 percent of all cancer-related deaths in children.[76] The tumor is either inherited in an autosomal dominant gene, as a chromosomal abnormality with a partial deletion of the long arm of chromosome 13 (13 q), or as a sporadic mutation.[77, 78] One third of retinoblastoma cases are bilateral. The tumor is very aggressive and may extend along the optic nerve to the brain and metastasize to skull, long bones, lung, and lymph nodes. The affected child may present clinically with a white pupil, strabismus, a red painful eye, glaucoma, or poor vision.[76] An urgent examination with the patient under anesthesia is required to determine the extent of the disease. Enucleation and irradiation are the primary modes of therapy and, depending on the tumor staging, secondary treatment may also include chemotherapy, photocoagulation, and cryotherapy. The remaining eye should be examined periodically for tumor and treatment as necessary.

The potential to elicit the oculocardiac reflex (a trigeminovagal arc) is fairly high during the manipulation of enucleation through traction on the extraocular muscles and during digital pressure deep within the empty orbit. Occasionally persistent bleeding from the central retinal artery requires prolonged digital compression. Vigorous (as opposed to gentle) surgical handling of the extraocular muscles will increase the frequency and severity of the oculocardiac reflex, as will hypercapnia.[79] The incidence of the oculocardiac reflex can be minimized by atropine (0.04 mg/kg PO; 0.02 to 0.03 mg/kg IM; 0.01 to 0.02 mg/kg IV) either preoperatively or during the induction period.[80–85]

The most common manifestation of the oculocardiac reflex is a sinus bradycardia, but multiple varieties of dysrhythmias may occur, including junctional rhythm, periods of sinus arrest, and extrasystoles. No treatment is necessary for modest decreases in heart rate; however, the anesthesiologist should observe the electrocardiogram and blood pressure closely and wait for vagal escape or fatigue of the reflex.[79, 85]

Should the oculocardiac reflex decrease the heart rate to less than 100 beats per minute in small infants, less than 80 beats per minute in young children, or less than 60 beats per minute in older children, the surgeon should promptly discontinue traction or stimulation of the globe. The rate can be expected to return to baseline, and (particularly when hypotension has accompanied the relative bradycardia) small intravenous increments of atropine (0.01 mg/kg) should be given before resumption of surgical traction.[80]

On the rarer occurrence of ventricular dysrhythmias, increments of lidocaine, 1 to 2 mg/kg IV, may return the rhythm to a normal sinus pattern. These dysrhythmias are more difficult

Table 10–3. SIDE EFFECTS AND INTERACTIONS OF OPHTHALMIC DRUGS

Drug	Indications and Suggested Dose	Side Effects	Contraindications and Possible Interactions
Topical Drugs			
Parasympatholytic Agents			
Atropine	To produce mydriasis, 1 drop 1% solution	Flushing, thirst, tachycardia, dry skin, pyrexia, agitation	Contraindicated in closed-angle glaucoma or shallow anterior chamber
Scopolamine	To produce mydriasis and cycloplegia, 1 drop 0.25% solution	Excitation, disorientation; treat with physostigmine, 0.01 mg/kg IV	Contraindicated in closed angle glaucoma or shallow anterior chamber
Cyclopentolate (Cyclogyl)[60, 61]	To produce mydriasis, 0.5% solution (infants); 1% solution (children)	Disorientation, ataxia, dysarthria, convulsions, psychosis (especially with 2% solutions)	Contraindicated in closed angle glaucoma or shallow anterior chamber. May interact and interfere with other antiglaucoma drugs (carbachol and pilocarpine and anticholinesterases)
Tropicamide (Mydriacil)[62]	To produce mydriasis and cycloplegia, 1 drop 0.5–1% solution	Behavior disturbances, psychotic reactions, vasomotor collapse (rare)	Contraindicated in closed angle glaucoma or shallow anterior chamber
Sympathomimetic Agents			
Phenylephrine (Neosynephrine)[63, 64]	To produce mydriasis and vasoconstriction, 1 drop 2.5% solution	Severe hypertension, tachycardia, headache (especially likely with > 2.5% solution or in patients with inflamed conjunctivae)	Contraindicated in closed angle glaucoma or shallow anterior chamber. Serious interactions with MAO inhibitors or tricyclic antidepressant drugs
Epinephrine[64]	To decrease aqueous outflow and IOP, 1 drop 0.5% solution	Hypertension, tachycardia, pallor and fainting	Contraindicated in patients with tetralogy of Fallot or history of arrhythmia. May interact with halothane to cause arrhythmias
Cholinergic Agents			
Pilocarpine (Pilocar)	To produce miosis and decrease IOP, 1 drop 0.5% solution	Hypertension, tachycardia, bronchospasm, nausea, vomiting, and diarrhea	
Anticholinesterase Agents			
Echothiophate (Phospholine)[65–69]	To produce miosis and reduce IOP, 0.03–0.25% solution	Bronchospasm, vomiting, hypotension, abdominal pain, exacerbation of asthma	Contraindicated in patients with asthma or epilepsy. Contraindicated in closed-angle glaucoma. Duration of action is prolonged for weeks after withdrawal of therapy. Prolonged apnea may occur after succinylcholine. Delayed metabolism of ester-type local anesthetics.
Nonselective β-Blocking Drug			
Timolol (Timoptic)[70–73]	To reduce IOP, 1 drop 0.25–0.5%	Fatigue, disorientation, CNS depression, severe exacerbation of asthma. Postoperative apnea in infants[74]	Contraindicated in asthma, congestive heart failure, and heart block. May interact with digitalis and calcium channel blockers. May exacerbate myasthenia gravis. Caution in infants: may cause postoperative apnea
Intraocular Drugs			
Acetylcholine	To produce miosis after lens extraction	Increased secretions, salivation, bronchospasm, bradycardia	May interact with halothane to produce brachycardia. Contraindicated in patients with a history of asthma
Sulfur hexafluride[75]	Injected to assist in retinal reattachment	Rapid increase in IOP if nitrous oxide in use. May result in retinal ischemia	Discontinue nitrous oxide 20 minutes before sulfur hexafluride or air is injected into eye
Systemic Drugs			
Carbonic Anhydrase Inhibitor			
Acetazolamide (Diamox)	To decrease aqueous humor and reduce IOP	Metabolic acidosis and loss of sodium, potassium, water. Anaphylaxis, Stevens-Johnson syndrome, bone marrow depression	Contraindicated in patients with hepatic or renal impairment. Serious arrhythmias may occur during anesthesia secondary to electrolyte disturbance

to treat and frequently are abolished only at the conclusion of the operation and ocular traction.

ANESTHESIA FOR RADIOTHERAPY

Frequently, infants and children with retinoblastoma require daily radiation therapy for many weeks. The children need to be motionless for a short time (about 10 minutes) during radiotherapy and ideally should return to normal activity and eating within a few hours. Satisfactory anesthetic agents and techniques include rectal (25 mg/kg) or intramuscular (10 mg/kg) methohexital, intravenous or intramuscular ketamine combined with atropine, or a brief period of an inhalational agent.[86–89] Ketamine is usually quite satisfactory as long as the anesthesiologist is mindful of its potential to produce tachyphylaxis and the need for increasing dosage over time.[90] Atropine should be given to prevent excessive salivation following ketamine. An indwelling catheter may be placed (with the patient under intramuscular ketamine) and securely taped, and patency can be maintained by flushing with heparinized (50 μg/ml) saline solution four times a day.[91] This can simplify daily intravenous administration of the anesthesiologist's drug of choice without the trauma of multiple injections or the unpredictability of rectal absorption. Recommendations for care of the indwelling cannula include a 5-day (Monday through Friday) period of use, removal during the weekend, and reinsertion each Monday for the following week of treatment.[91]

If the treatment required is short, IV propofol (2.5 to 3.5 mg/kg) will permit a brief period of immobility, which is followed by a very rapid awakening. For slightly longer treatments an infusion of propofol may be appropriate.

Improved radiotherapy techniques for the treatment of retinoblastoma may require modifications to the anesthesia technique used. A lens-sparing technique of radiotherapy may be used which requires that the child's head be firmly immobilized, and this may compromise the airway. In such cases the use of a general inhalation anesthetic administered via the laryngeal mask airway has proved very satisfactory.[92] The laryngeal mask is inserted blindly into the pharynx to surround and seal the larynx, thus avoiding the necessity to instrument the larynx repeatedly.[93]

Photoradiation therapy using a hematoporphyrin derivative (HpD) and the argon laser has also been used to treat retinoblastoma. HpD is administered intravenously and persists longer in the tumor cells than in adjacent normal cells. When treated with light of specific wavelength, the HpD-containing tumor cells are destroyed, sparing adjacent normal tissue. The administration of HpD requires that the patient be kept in total darkness to avoid skin pigmentation and burns. Thus anesthesia in almost total darkness is required. Fortunately, pulse oximetry is safe and reliable in the presence of HpD, and intubation and other procedures can be carried out using a night vision scope.[94]

RETINOPATHY OF PREMATURITY

The continuing problem of retinopathy of prematurity (ROP) has long been a concern of neonatologists and ophthalmologists. Increasingly, anesthesiologists too are sharing this concern, as the very young premature infant requires a general anesthetic and oxygen administration for cardiovascular, gastrointestinal, or central nervous system surgery.[29–32]

ROP acutely presents as a vascular retinopathy at the developing edge of the eye and evolves to a cicatricial form in which scar tissue places the retina under traction, causing detachment and loss of vision.

Each year in the United States, about 2000 neonates incur some degree of permanent ROP, and a quarter of these are affected by blindness. It is well known that the incidence of ROP is inversely related to birth weight, although one third of healthy premature infants who received high concentrations of oxygen (for example, FIO_2 0.5 for 28 days) developed cicatricial ROP, according to data from the 1950's. However, we do not know the incidence of ROP in the tiny sick premature population receiving only moderate concentrations of oxygen for short periods of time, such as during the course of a general anesthetic.[32]

Logistical risk analysis considering surgery (requiring use of anesthetic gases) as a risk variable demonstrated that surgery does not contribute to the risk of ROP in small prematures as compared with those who did not require surgery.[32]

Arbitrarily, anesthesiologists regulate the FIO_2 of oxygen-nitrous oxide or oxygen-air mixtures to maintain PaO_2 at less than 100 torr, as monitored by intra-arterial blood sampling or by a transcutaneous sensor, both of which must sample the oxygen tension above the level of the ductus arteriosus. Any condition, such as systemic hypotension or the pulmonary hypertension syndrome, that places the infant's circulation in the fetal pattern of right-to-left shunting at the ductus level requires assessment of the oxygen tension in the ascending aorta as an indication of oxygen concentration perfusing the eye.[29, 33, 34]

But the old dogma that stresses oxygen as the sole culprit responsible for inducing ROP is being challenged by the recognition that it is a multifactorial disease.[31, 95] The continued high incidence of ROP among very low birth weight infants in spite of frequent monitoring of oxygen use, the reports of ROP in premature infants who have received little or no oxygen, the occurrence of ROP in premature infants with cyanotic congenital heart disease, and its rare occurrence in full-term neonates all suggest causes other than oxygen-induced vasoconstriction.

In infants smaller than 1250 g there is a significant correlation of ROP with apnea, requiring mask and bag ventilation without an increase in oxygen concentration, prolonged parenteral nutrition, a greater number of blood transfusions, and episodes of hypoxemia (PaO_2 less than 40 torr), hypercapnia, and hypocapnia.[96] Specifically, episodes of hypocapnia with $PaCO_2$ less than 25 torr and an arterial pH above 7.55 were often associated with ROP. It appears that the retinal vasculature may also be responsive to this deficit, and the anesthetic plan should include monitoring to avoid severe hyperventilation.[96]

Thirty years after the initial observation that vitamin E supplements were associated with a reduced incidence of ROP, therapy with prophylactic intramuscular and oral vitamin E is again showing promise in protecting the preterm infant against severe ROP. Vitamin E is an andogenous antioxidant that protects against free radical damage (plasma levels are severely depressed in the premature), and supplementation to adult physiological levels is nontoxic.[97, 98] The drug must be initiated on the first day of life and maintained continuously until the retinal vasculature matures.

The maturation of the retinal vasculature shows considerable variation until 44 weeks postconception, suggesting that excessively long periods of high oxygen concentration should be minimized throughout the neonatal period.[35]

Caution is necessary when an infant who was born prematurely requires eye or nonocular operation early in life. Those younger than 41 to 46 weeks' conceptual age with a history of idiopathic apnea are predisposed to postoperative life-threatening apneic episodes.[99] Nonessential surgery in preterm infants should be delayed until 44 weeks' conceptual age or later. When surgical therapy is necessary, these infants must be monitored for apnea for 18 hours postoperatively, and the means to ventilate the infant mechanically should be kept at hand.[100]

RETINAL DETACHMENT

A retinal detachment occurs when subretinal fluid causes a separation of the outer layers of the sensory retina away from the retinal pigment epithelial layer.[101, 102] Retinal detachments in the pediatric age group are classified as rhegmatogenous, traction, or exudative.

Rhegmatogenous retinal detachments in children are most frequently a sequela of trauma, usually contusion of the globe, and to a lesser extent of myopia, aphakia, and retinopathy of prematurity. Breaks through all of the inner areas of the retina allow vitreous fluid to enter the subretinal space, dissecting it off the retina. Classic scleral buckling procedures are successful in reattaching this type of detachment in most cases.[101]

The traction detachment is a complication seen with retinopathy of prematurity, diabetes, and sickle retinopathy and occurs when vitreoretinal traction separates the retinal pigment epithelium from the retina. Scleral buckling, scleral resection, or vitrectomy may be indicated in cases of traction detachment that extend into the macular or foveal area.[101]

Exudative retinal detachments follow accumulation of subretinal fluid without evidence of retinal break and can be seen with retinoblastoma, choroidal hemangioma or melanoma, angiomatosis retinae, and severe renal disease.[101]

Reattachment of the retina to the pigment epithelium is managed with scleral buckling surgical therapy consisting of a combination of techniques.[102] First, cryotherapy or laser therapy may be used to produce a chorioretinal scar, sealing the retinal break. The second part of the surgical procedure consists of physical indentation of the sclera by a variety of buckling materials to bring the retinal tear closer to the pigment epithelium. Third, reattachment may be facilitated by external drainage of the subretinal fluid. In more complicated cases, vitrectomy surgery using a suction–cutting instrument may be combined with scleral buckling.

In addition, an intraoperative technique of internal tamponade by air injected into the vitreous may help hold the retina in place; the air remains in the eye for 6 to 10 days until resorbed.[102] Use of this technique is of special concern regarding the concurrent use of nitrous oxide. Because nitrous oxide rapidly diffuses into the air-containing space, the volume of gas increases two- to threefold and is responsible for an associated significant increase in intraocular pressure.[103, 104] Compromised retinal circulation poses a potential risk to the eye as a consequence of elevated intraocular pressure.[75, 103] Conversely, when nitrous oxide is discontinued at the conclusion of the operation, the sudden washout of nitrous oxide and shrinkage of the gas bubble (causing a lower than original IOP) may also be detrimental to the surgical outcome.[103, 104]

This potential problem can be avoided by discontinuing nitrous oxide 20 minutes before the air is injected into the vitreous so that there will be little change in bubble size. An inhalation agent and 100 percent oxygen can be used for the balance of the procedure without affecting intravitreal gas dynamics.[104]

Any combination of induction and inhalation anesthetic agents is acceptable for retinal detachment procedures, applying the basic principles of anesthetic care for pediatric ophthalmic surgical therapy as previously discussed. Regard for the potential to elicit the oculocardiac reflex with traction on the globe, especially during placement of the scleral buckle, is also an important consideration.

REFERENCES

1. O'Neill JF, Bateman JB: The lens and pediatric cataracts. *In* Metz HS, Rosenbaum AL (eds): Pediatric Ophthalmology. New York, Medical Examination Publishing Company, 1982, pp 235–261.
2. Guo S, Nelson LB, Calhoun J, Levin A: Simultaneous surgery for bilateral congenital cataracts. J Pediatr Ophthalmol Strabismus *27*:23, 1990.
3. France TD, Baker JD, Rogers GL, et al: Diagnosis and treatment of cataracts in children. American Academy of Ophthalmology, 1980, Instruction Section, Course 58.
4. Kohn BA: The differential diagnosis of cataracts in infancy and childhood. Am J Dis Child *130*:184, 1976.
5. Cross HE, Jensen AD: Ocular manifestations in the Marfan syndrome and homocystinuria. Am J Ophthalmol *75*:405, 1973.
6. Johnston RR, Eger EI, Wilson C: A comparative interaction of epinephrine with enflurane, isoflurane, and halothane in man. Anesth Analg *55*:709, 1976.
7. Rao CC, Dierdorf SF, Wolfe TM, et al: Effect of age on epinephrine-induced arrhythmias during halothane anaesthesia in pigs. Can Anaesth Soc J *31*:20, 1984.
8. Karl HW, Swedlow DB, Lee KW, et al: Epinephrine-halothane interactions in children. Anesthesiology *58*:142, 1983.
9. Ueda W, Hirakawa M, Mae O: Appraisal of epinephrine administration to patients under halothane anesthesia for closure of cleft palate. Anesthesiology *58*:574, 1983.
10. Pepple J: Epinephrine-halothane interaction in children versus adults. Anesthesiology *60*:76, 1984.
11. Smith RB: Intra-ocular adrenaline and halothane anaesthesia. Br J Anaesth *43*:1200, 1971.
12. Smith RB, Douglas H, Petruscak J, et al: Safety of intraocular adrenaline with halothane anaesthesia. Br J Anaesth *44*:1314, 1972.
13. MacDiarmid IR, Holloway KB: Factors affecting intraocular pressure. Proc R Soc Med *69*:601, 1976.
14. France NK, France TD, Woodburn JD, et al: Succinylcholine alteration of the forced duction test. Ophthalmology *87*:1282, 1980.
15. Kornblueth W, Aladjemoff L, Magora F, et al: Influence of general anesthesia on intraocular pressure in man. Arch Ophthalmol *61*:84, 1959.
16. Joshi C, Bruce DL: Thiopental and succinylcholine: Action on intraocular pressure. Anesth Analg *54*:471, 1975.
17. Famewo CE, Odugbesan CO, Osuntokun OO: Effect of etomidate on intra-ocular pressure. Can Anaesth Soc J *24*:712, 1977.
18. Runciman JC, Bowen-Wright RM, Welsh NH, et al: Intraocular pressure changes during halothane and enflurane anaesthesia. Br J Anaesth *50*:371, 1978.
19. Ausinsch B, Graves SA, Munson ES, et al: Intraocular pressures in children during isoflurane and halothane anesthesia. Anesthesiology *42*:167, 1975.
20. Presbitero JV, Ruiz RS, Rigor B, et al: Intraocular pressure during enflurane and neurolept anesthesia in adult patients undergoing ophthalmic surgery. Anesth Analg *59*:50, 1980.
21. Litwiller RW, DiFazio CA, Rushia EL: Pancuronium and intraocular pressure. Anesthesiology *42*:750, 1975.
22. Cunningham AJ, Kelly CP, Farmer J, et al: The effect of metocurine and metocurine-pancuronium combination on intraocular pressure. Can Anaesth Soc J *29*:617, 1982.
23. Balamoutsos NG, Tsakona H, Kanakoudes PS, et al: Alcuronium and intraocular pressure. Anesth Analg *62*:521, 1983.
24. Schwartz H, de Roetth A, Papper EM: Preanesthetic use of atropine and scopolamine in patients with glaucoma. JAMA *165*:144, 1957.
25. Corssen G, Joy JE: A new parenteral anesthetic—CI-581: Its effect on intraocular pressure. J Pediatr Ophthalmol *4*:20, 1967.
26. Yoshikawa K, Murai Y: The effect of ketamine on intraocular pressure in children. Anesth Analg *50*:199, 1971.
27. Peuler M, Glass DD, Arens JF: Ketamine and intraocular pressure. Anesthesiology *43*:575, 1975.
28. Ausinsch B, Rayburn RL, Munson ES, et al: Ketamine and intraocular pressure in children. Anesth Analg *55*:773, 1976.
29. Phibbs RH: Oxygen therapy: A continuing hazard of the premature infant. Anesthesiology *47*:486, 1977.
30. Betts EK, Downes JJ, Schaffer DB, et al: Retrolental fibroplasia and oxygen administration during general anesthesia. Anesthesiology *47*:518, 1977.
31. Merritt JC, Sprague DH, Merritt WE, et al: Retrolental fibroplasia: A multifactorial disease. Anesth Analg *60*:109, 1981.
32. Flynn JT: Oxygen and retrolental fibroplasia: Update and challenge. Anesthesiology *60*:397, 1984.
33. Horbar JD, Clark JT, Lucey JF: The newborn oxygram: Automated processing of transcutaneous oxygen data. Pediatrics *66*:848, 1980.
34. Lucey JF: Transcutaneous diagnosis in the high-risk neonate. Hosp Pract *16*:108, 1981.

35. Quinn GE, Betts EK, Diamond GR, et al: Neonatal age (human) at retinal maturation. ASA Abstracts, Anesthesiology *55*:A326, 1981.
36. Pyeritz RE, McKusick VA: The Marfan syndrome: Diagnosis and management. N Engl J Med *300*:772, 1979.
37. Boucek RJ, Noble NL, Gunja-Smith Z, et al: The Marfan syndrome: A deficiency in chemically stable collagen cross-links. N Engl J Med *305*:988, 1981.
38. Harker LA, Slichter SJ, Scott CR, et al: Homocystinemia: Vascular injury and arterial thrombosis. N Engl J Med *291*:537, 1974.
39. Brown BR, Walson PD, Taussig LM: Congenital metabolic diseases of pediatric patients: Anesthetic implications. Anesthesiology *43*:197, 1975.
40. Crooke JW, Towers JF, Taylor WH: Management of patients with homocystinuria requiring surgery under general anaesthesia. Br J Anaesth *43*:96, 1971.
41. McGoldrick KE: Anesthetic management of homocystinuria. Anes Rev *8*:42, 1981.
42. Parris WC, Quimby CW: Anesthetic considerations for the patient with homocystinuria. Anesth Analg *61*:708, 1982.
43. Hicks E: Ocular trauma. *In* Metz HS, Rosenbaum AL (eds): Pediatric Ophthalmology. New York, Medical Examination Publishing Company, 1982, pp 25–47.
44. Libonati MM, Leahy JJ, Ellison N: The use of succinylcholine in open eye surgery. Anesthesiology *62*:637, 1985.
45. Donlon JV: Succinylcholine and open eye injury. Part II. Anesthesiology *64*:524, 1986.
46. Edmondson I, Lindsay SL, Lanigan LP, et al: Intraocular pressure changes during rapid sequence induction of anesthesia. Anaesthesia *43*:1005, 1988.
47. Grover VK, Lata K, Sharma S, et al: Efficacy of lignocaine in the suppression of the intraocular pressure response to suxamethonium and tracheal intubation. Anaesthesia *44*:22, 1989.
48. Warner LO, Bremer DL, Davidson PJ, et al: Effects of lidocaine, succinylcholine, and tracheal intubation on intraocular pressure in children anesthetized with halothane–nitrous oxide. Anesth Analg *69*:687, 1989.
49. Salem MR, Wong AY, Mani M, et al: Efficacy of cricoid pressure in preventing gastric inflation during bag-mask ventilation in pediatric patients. Anesthesiology *40*:96, 1971.
50. Brown EM, Krishnaprasad D, Smiler BG: Pancuronium for rapid induction technique for tracheal intubation. Can Anaesth Soc J *26*:489, 1979.
51. Smith RM: Choice of inhalation agents. *In* Anesthesia for Infants and Children. St. Louis, CV Mosby, 1980, pp 109–127.
52. Goresky GV, Steward DJ: Rectal methohexitone for induction of anaesthesia in children. Can Anaesth Soc J *26*:213, 1979.
53. Baraka A: Intravenous lidocaine controls extubation laryngospasm in children. Anesth Analg *57*:506, 1978.
54. Hoskins HD: Pediatric glaucomas. *In* Metz HS, Rosenbaum AL (eds): Pediatric Ophthalmology. New York, Medical Examination Publishing Company, 1982, pp 262–302.
55. Kolker AE, Hetherington J: Congenital glaucoma. *In* Kolker AE, Hetherington J (eds): Diagnosis and Therapy of the Glaucomas. St. Louis, CV Mosby, 1976, pp 276–321.
56. Adams AK: Ketamine in paediatric ophthalmic practice (letter). Anaesthesia *28*:212, 1973.
57. Watcha MF, Chu FC, Stevens JL, Forestner JE: Effects of halothane on intraocular pressure in anesthetised children. Anesth Analg *71*:181, 1990.
58. Donlon JV: Anesthesia factors affecting intraocular pressure: Succinylcholine and endotracheal intubation. Anesth Rev *8*:13, 1981.
59. McGoldrick KE: Considerations for pediatric eye surgery. Int Anesthesiol Clin *28*:78, 1990.
60. Kennerdall JS, Wucher FP: Cyclopentolate associated with two cases of grand mal seizure. Arch Ophthalmol *87*:634, 1972.
61. Binkhorst RD, Weinstein GW, Baretz RM, et al: Psychotic reaction induced by pentolate: Results of pilot study and a double blind study. Am J Ophthalmol *55*:1243, 1963.
62. McGoldrick KE: Ocular drugs and anesthesia. Int Anesthesiol Clin *28*:72, 1990.
63. Wellwood M, Goresky GV: Systemic hypertension associated with topical administration of 2.5% phenylephrine HCl. Am J Ophthalmol *93*:369, 1982.
64. Lansche RK: Systemic reactions to topical epinephrine and phenylephrine. Am J Ophthalmol *61*:95, 1966.
65. Eilderton TE, Farmati O, Zsigmond EK: Reduction in plasma cholinesterase levels after prolonged administration of echothiophate iodide eyedrops. Can Anaesth Soc J *15*:291, 1968.
66. Ellis PP, Esterdahl M: Echothiophate iodide therapy in children. Arch Ophthalmol *77*:598, 1967.
67. Pantuck EJ: Echothiophate iodide eye drops and prolonged response to suxamethonium. Br J Anaesth *38*:406, 1966.
68. Donati F, Bevan DR: Controlled succinylcholine infusion in a patient receiving echothiophate eye drops. Can Anaesth Soc J *28*:488, 1981.
69. Brodsky JB, Campos FA: Chloroprocaine analgesia in a patient receiving echothiophate iodide eye drops. Anesthesiology *48*:288, 1978.
70. Kim JW, Smith PH: Timolol-induced bradycardia. Anesth Analg *59*:301, 1980.
71. Schoene RB, Martin TR, Charan NB, et al: Timolol-induced bronchospasm in asthmatic bronchitis. JAMA *245*:1460, 1981.
72. Samuels SI, Maze M: Beta-receptor blockade following the use of eye drops. Anesthesiology *52*:369, 1980.
73. Williams T, Ginther WH: Hazard of ophthalmic timolol (letter). N Engl J Med *306*:1485, 1982.
74. Bailey PL: Timolol and postoperative apnea in neonates and young infants. Anesthesiology *61*:622, 1984.
75. Wolf GL, Capuano C, Hartnung J: Nitrous oxide increases intraocular pressure after intravitreal sulfur hexafluride injection. Anesthesiology *59*:547, 1983.
76. Rosenbaum AL, Bremer DL: Ocular tumors in children. *In* Metz HS, Rosenbaum AL: Pediatric Ophthalmology. New York, Medical Examination Publishing Company, 1982, pp 391–403.
77. Bensinger RE, Mills M: Retinoblastoma: Diagnosis and treatment. Res Staff Phys 46–49, 1982.
78. Weichselbaum RR, Zakov ZN, Albert DM, et al: New findings in the chromosome 13 long-arm deletion syndrome and retinoblastoma. Ophthalmology *86*:1191, 1979.
79. Blanc VF, Hardy JF, Milot J, et al: The oculocardiac reflex: A graphic and statistical analysis in infants and children. Can Anaesth Soc J *30*:360, 1983.
80. Meyers EF, Tomeldan SA: Glycopyrrolate compared with atropine in prevention of the oculocardiac reflex during eye-muscle surgery. Anesthesiology *51*:350, 1979.
81. Steward DJ: Anticholinergic premedication for infants and children. Can Anaesth Soc J *30*:325, 1983.
82. Mayhew JF: Are anticholinergics needed in strabismus surgery? Anesth Rev *11*:24, 1984.
83. Joseph MC, Vale RJ: Premedication with atropine by mouth. Lancet *2*:1060, 1960.

84. Brzustowicz RM, Nelson DA, Betts EK, et al: Efficacy of oral premedication for pediatric outpatient surgery. Anesthesiology *60*:475, 1984.
85. Moonie GT, Rees DL, Elton D: The oculocardiac reflex during strabismus surgery. Can Anaesth Soc J *11*:621, 1964.
86. Amberg HL, Gordon G: Low-dose intramuscular ketamine for pediatric radiotherapy: A case report. Anesth Analg *55*:92, 1976.
87. Cronin MM, Bousfield JD, Hewett EB, et al: Ketamine anaesthesia for radiotherapy in small children. Anaesthesia *27*:135, 1972.
88. Samuels SI, Lim F, Maze A: Failure to produce satisfactory operating conditions following large doses of ketamine hydrochloride. Anesth Rev *5*:23, 1978.
89. Smith HS: Anaesthesia for radiotherapy (letter). Can Anaesth Soc J *31*:236, 1984.
90. Byer DE, Gould AB: Development of tolerance to ketamine in an infant undergoing repeated anesthesia. Anesthesiology *54*:255, 1981.
91. Rodarte A: Heparin-lock for repeated anesthesia in pediatric radiation therapy. Anesthesiology *56*:316, 1982.
92. Grebenik CR, Ferguson C, White A: The laryngeal mask in pediatric radiotherapy. Anesthesiology *72*:474, 1990.
93. Taylor DH, Child CS: The laryngeal mask for radiotherapy in children. Anaesthesia *45*:690, 1990.
94. Uchida U, Kinouchi K, Tashiro C: A new photoradiation therapy and anesthesia. Anesth Analg *70*:222, 1990.
95. McGoldrick KE: Factors influencing development of retrolental fibroplasia (letter). Anesth Analg *60*:539, 1981.
96. Shohat M, Reisner SH, Krikler R, et al: Retinopathy of prematurity: Incidence and risk factors. Pediatrics *72*:159, 1983.
97. Hittner HM, Speer ME, Rudolph AJ, et al: Retrolental fibroplasia and vitamin E in the preterm infant—comparison of oral versus intramuscular:oral administration. Pediatrics *73*:238, 1984.
98. Hittner HM, Kretzer FL, Rudolph AJ: Prevention and management of retrolental fibroplasia. Hosp Pract *19*:85, 1984.
99. Liu LM, Cote CJ, Goudsouzian NG, et al: Life-threatening apnea in infants recovering from anesthesia. Anesthesiology *59*:506, 1983.
100. Gregory GA, Steward DJ: Life-threatening perioperative apnea in the ex-"premie" (editorial). Anesthesiology *59*:495, 1983.
101. Hammer ME: Pediatric diseases of the retina. *In* Metz HS, Rosenbaum AL (eds): Pediatric Ophthalmology. New York, Medical Examination Publishing Company, 1982, pp 331–373.
102. Marcus DF, Bovino JA: Retinal detachment. JAMA *247*:873, 1982.
103. Smith B, Carl B, Linn JG, et al: Effect of nitrous oxide on air in vitreous. Am J Ophthalmol *78*:314, 1974.
104. Stinson TW, Donlon JV: Interaction of intraocular SF_6 and air with nitrous oxide. ASA Abstracts, Anesthesiology, *51*:S16, 1978.

GENERAL REFERENCES FOR TABLE 10–1

105. Harley RD (ed): Pediatric Ophthalmology. 2nd edition. Philadelphia, WB Saunders, 1983.
106. Metz HS, Rosenbaum AL (eds): Pediatric Ophthalmology. New York, Medical Examination Publishing Company, 1982.
107. Behrman RE, Vaughan VC III (eds): Nelson Textbook of Pediatrics. 12th edition. Philadelphia, WB Saunders, 1983.
108. Gregory GA: Pediatric Anesthesia. New York, Churchill Livingstone, 1983.
109. Steward DJ: Manual of Pediatric Anesthesia. New York, Churchill Livingstone, 1979.
110. Stehling LC: Common Problems in Pediatric Anesthesia. Chicago, Year Book Medical Publishers, 1982.
111. Stehling LC, Zauder HL (eds): Anesthetic Implications of Congenital Anomalies in Children. New York, Appleton-Century-Crofts, 1980.
112. Kobel M, Creighton RE, Steward DJ: Anaesthetic considerations in Down's syndrome: Experience with 100 patients and a review of the literature. Can Anaesth Soc J *29*:593, 1982.

CHAPTER

11 Otolaryngological Diseases

JAMES D. MORRISON, M.D.

Diseases and operations that directly involve the airway present an enormous challenge to all those involved in the care of the patient. No other field of surgical therapy demands closer cooperation between anesthesiologist and surgeon than does that of the upper airway. By the same token, no other area of operative procedures offers the special professional satisfactions and rewards that come from the mutual cooperation, understanding, and respect generated when colleagues are so closely involved in each other's endeavor. However, such a cooperative ideal will be achieved only by the anesthesiologist and surgeon who each undertake to have a complete understanding of the diseases, lesions, and procedures with which they are dealing. The anesthesiologist in the role of resuscitator also requires the ability to recognize and appropriately treat respiratory obstruction, especially in neonates and infants. Not only is it important to know when tracheostomy is required, it is also necessary to know when it, and its associated morbidity, can safely be avoided. An informed anesthesiologist also can perform a valuable diagnostic role, in that he or she is often the first physician to examine the larynx in the case of acute respiratory obstruction.

The diseases discussed in this chapter are uncommon, and perhaps for most practitioners will remain textbook descriptions of lesions that they will never see at first hand. A few are trivial, but most are serious and life threatening, some devastatingly so. Almost all, by their intimate involvement with the airway, have the potential for rapid progression to ventilatory problems of frightening proportions. These problems can be greatly compounded by medical, especially anesthetic, mismanagement.

Throughout this chapter, discussion is limited to those conditions that occur within the boundaries of traditional otolaryngological practice. The reader may find closely related material in Chapter 9, Pediatric Head and Neck Syndromes, and Chapter 4, Central Nervous System Diseases.

NOSE AND NASOPHARYNX

CHOANAL ATRESIA

Lack of continuity of the air passages between the nasal cavity and the nasopharynx is a rare congenital defect and varies from partial unilateral obstruction to complete bilateral atresia. The defect is usually due to obstruction by a bony plate, but in 10 percent of patients the obstruction lies more posteriorly and is membranous rather than bony. Unilateral choanal atresia is of much lesser importance, as significant respiratory obstruction is unlikely; patients with such atresia may go undetected for many years, eventually presenting with symptoms of unilateral nasal obstruction, such as chronic discharge or reduced olfactory sensation.

Congenital Bilateral Choanal Atresia. This condition presents as respiratory distress in the newborn infant. Because the neonate may not rapidly convert to mouth breathing if the nose is obstructed, bilateral choanal atresia is life threatening and demands urgent treatment. Choanal atresia is usually due to a bony plate occluding the posterior nares; in about 10 percent of cases the obstruction is more posterior and is membranous rather than bony. As many as 70 percent of these infants have other concurrent major congenital defects, including in about one third the CHARGE association* of multisystem defects.[1] Unilateral atresia is seen but is of much lesser significance as total respiratory obstruction does not occur; nonetheless, most of these patients will be seen before the age of 2 years with symptoms of persistent, unilateral nasal discharge, often associated with feeding difficulties. Rarely such patients may remain undiagnosed until much later in life. Indeed there are also rare incidents of patients with bilateral choanal atresia surviving undiagnosed to adulthood.[2]

DIAGNOSIS

The presence of bilateral choanal atresia should be suspected in any newborn infant who displays signs of respiratory obstruction, especially if this obstruction appears to improve spontaneously during crying (this is because the seal between the tongue and the palate is broken during crying, thus allowing mouth breathing).

The diagnosis is confirmed by failure to pass a soft catheter through the nose into the pharynx. Later evaluation should include computed tomography (although the possibility of misleading appearances due to accumulation of mucus in the nasal cavities must be borne in mind),[3] rhinoscopy, and possibly contrast radiological studies. It is also important to examine the infant carefully for evidence of other anomalies.

FIRST AID

Immediate relief of respiratory obstruction is simple: a tongue depressor or oropharyngeal airway inserted into the mouth enables mouth breathing. Such measures are only temporary, however, and do not permit feeding of the infant. Although immediate puncture of the atretic area at the time of diagnosis was suggested as long ago as the middle of the 19th century, this is ineffective because of invariable rapid restenosis. Instead, conservative management during the first year of life, followed by definitive repair in the older infant, has been a more or less universally adopted treatment.

Effective conservative treatment followed the demonstration by Hough that placement of an orogastric tube would not only maintain the oral airway and hence effective mouth breathing, but also would provide a route by which the infant could be fed a normal diet.[4] Although effective, this treatment is not easy, demanding prolonged close supervision in hospital, since infants are often slow to learn spontaneous mouth breathing, and until this skill has been acquired the orogastric tube must remain in place. Formerly more or less universally used, this conservative treatment now is reserved for those patients in whom accompanying defects indicate a poor prognosis or present a higher priority for treatment.

Tracheostomy is also a possible conservative treatment but is rarely used because of its own associated morbidity and possible mortality in this age group. It is reserved for those patients in whom associated anomalies affect the airway, such as Crouzon's syndrome, or other defect in which intubation might be impossible.

DEFINITIVE SURGICAL CORRECTION

Recently attention has returned to early definitive surgical correction, and significant progress toward this ideal has been made. It is now quite common to attempt repair of choanal atresia in the neonate. There are three possible anatomical approaches, none of which is clearly superior and each of which has its own particular disadvantages:

Transpalatal. Operation through the palate has been the traditional approach in older infants, allowing good access. However, the operations are long, involve significant blood loss, and require lengthy convalescence.[5] There also may be secondary effects on normal facial bone growth and function that necessitate later reconstructive surgery and orthodontic treatment.

Transseptal. This approach has been used mainly in unilateral atresia and is similar in most respects to the transpalatal route.

Transnasal. The transnasal route avoids the growth disturbance produced by transseptal and transpalatal approaches but provides poorer access to the atretic area. Formerly, operations done by this route had a very high rate of recurrence, but recent improvements in technique, including the use of nasal endoscopes and drilling rather than curettage, along with postoperative stenting, have greatly improved the outcome. This approach is now emerging as

---

*Coloboma, congenital **h**eart defect, choanal **a**tresia, growth and mental **r**etardation, **g**enitourinary anomalies, **e**ar anomalies, genital hypoplasia.

the preferred method of neonatal repair,[1, 6, 7] offering a fairly simple operation with good initial results. The procedure allows the infant to feed and breathe normally and often obviates the need for later additional surgery. This technique is particularly effective in the case of membranous atresia, for which the initial success rate approaches 100 percent. In bony atresia, the long-term success is rather less (80 percent), and a proportion of these recurrences will necessitate future transpalatal repair. Complications of the transnasal approach include recurrence in spite of stenting, palatal fistula, and ulceration of the columella or alae or both because of pressure necrosis from the stents.

Osteotomy. In much older patients presenting for correction of unilateral choanal atresia, access by LeFort I maxillary osteotomy has been utilized.[8]

OPERATION

The infant is anesthetized and orally intubated. With the mouth held open by a cleft palate gag, a nasopharyngoscope is inserted through the mouth into the pharynx. Under direct vision, a metal bougie is passed through the nose to puncture the atretic plate or membrane. In the neonate, unlike the older infant, there is usually no difficulty in perforating the atresia. The choanae are then enlarged, if necessary, by drilling away the excess bone, inserting the drill through a speculum placed in the nose to protect the anterior nasal structures. The procedure is repeated on the other side, and a double-barreled stent is inserted. The stent is made from a soft plastic tracheal tube folded and partially cut through to give patency to each side. It is inserted into the nostrils from the nasopharynx and secured in place by suturing the two ends together in front of the nasal columella. Various differences in stenting technique have been suggested to reduce the incidence of columella ulceration, including shortening of the stents without columella fixation[9] and a reduced period of stenting.[6] In all cases, however, it is important that the tube fit loosely to avoid pressure against the posterior nasal septum and possible interference with growth.

The stent is left in place for 6 to 12 weeks. After its removal, weekly dilatation of the choanae may be required to prevent constriction by scar tissue. If, despite all, stenosis recurs, a second operation and a further period of stenting will be required.

Postoperatively, the infant usually establishes normal feeding and breathing patterns within a few days and does not require prolonged hospitalization. In older children, operation is technically much more difficult because of growth of the atresia into a substantial bony obstruction that requires destructive surgical dissection; in such cases, the transpalatal approach is used most often.

Neonates. Endonasal puncture of the atresia in the neonate presents several problems for the anesthesiologist: the general problems of neonatal anesthesia related to immaturity and size, thermoregulation, and fluid and electrolyte balance, and the additional problems of operating within the airway. Access to the patient is limited, especially if the operating microscope is used. Postoperatively, the presence of foreign bodies within the nose may cause problems.

If induction of anesthesia before intubation is desired, care must be taken to ensure that a good oral airway can be maintained until successful intubation is achieved. If there is any doubt about the ability to maintain the airway after induction of anesthesia, then intubation is probably better performed with the patient awake. An oral RAE or similar tube should be used, brought down over the chin, and secured so as neither to impede operation nor risk accidental displacement or disconnection by the operator. After intubation, the chest should be auscultated to confirm bilateral aeration, and anesthesia may be continued using assisted or controlled ventilation with halothane, or halothane and a muscle relaxant. Other agents may be substituted, but narcotic-based techniques should be used with caution to avoid postoperative respiratory depression. A reliable intravenous cannula should be placed, and minimal monitoring should include precordial stethoscope, pulse oximetry, capnography, blood pressure, electrocardiograph, and body temperature. Blood loss is not usually significant during endonasal puncture in the neonatal period. Before extubation at the end of operation, the anesthesiologist must ensure that the new nasal airway is clear and that the stents are secure and will not themselves be liable to cause obstruction. Postoperatively, the nasal stents must be kept clear by frequent suctioning, using small, soft catheters.

Older Infants. For the reasons mentioned earlier, definitive operation in older infants is a much greater undertaking than neonatal endonasal puncture. The operation is usually performed through the palate and is usually prolonged, involving substantial blood loss that often will require replacement. Anesthetic management is similar to that just outlined for the neonate. Limited access to the patient while the microscope is in use necessitates particular care in securing the tracheal tube and monitors, and particular attention must be given to accurate measurement of blood loss and careful maintenance of intravascular volume.

NASOPHARYNGEAL TUMORS

The majority of tumors of the nose in children are benign. Nonetheless, some can be life threatening owing to respiratory obstruction, the potential for serious bleeding, or aggressive local expansion. They also may cause considerable interference with normal growth of the face.

ANGIOFIBROMA

Juvenile nasal angiofibroma is a rare, benign tumor with an aggressive local growth pattern that renders it a dangerous disease for the patient.[10] It occurs predominantly in males, usually at about the age of adolescence, but may also be found in older and younger patients.[11, 12] These tumors are deep seated, arising from the vault of the posterior wall of the nasopharynx, and they have a tendency to grow and extend through the tissues surrounding the nasopharynx. Although they are not usually invasive, extensive pressure erosion of bone may occur. Their growth is accompanied by considerable destruction of surrounding tissues, and the tumor may extend into the cranium through the base of the skull or orbit.

The usual presenting symptoms are those of nasal obstruction and episodic epistaxis, and the presence of a tumor is confirmed by x-ray, rhinoscopy, computed tomography, and carotid angiography. These tumors are very vascular, and because of their inaccessibility bleeding can be difficult to control. For this reason it is usual to avoid diagnostic biopsy; diagnosis depends rather on definition of the extent of the tumor by computed tomography, and determination of its major vascular components (which are usually derived from the internal maxillary artery) by selective carotid angiography.

Surgical removal of these tumors usually involves a staged procedure. The first requirement is to reduce vascularity, and this may be done by selective embolization of the feeder vessels under radiological control at the time of carotid angiography or by ligation of the feeders, if accessible. Although it has never been convincingly demonstrated that these tumors are endocrine dependent,[13] some surgeons believe that preoperative estrogen therapy helps reduce vascularity.[11]

Following successful devascularization, a variety of possible surgical approaches is available, including the infratemporal, transmaxillary, and lateral rhinotomy routes, but by far the commonest approach is through the palate.[11, 14, 15] Dissection is often difficult, and bleeding may still be troublesome in spite of the devascularization. Incomplete removal may necessitate repeated operation. However, recent reports suggest that with modern techniques the recurrence rate may be less than 30 percent.[11, 12, 16] Those tumors that extend into the cranium or orbit are particularly difficult to treat surgically and are more often treated by radiotherapy.[17] In a very small proportion of cases, the tumor may undergo change to sarcoma.[18]

The special problems of anesthetic management and operation of nasal angiofibromas are the preexisting nasal airway obstruction, possible preexisting anemia due to recurrent epistaxis, and the possibility of considerable, sometimes massive, bleeding during dissection. Postoperatively, nasal obstruction will continue to present a problem. Because of the staged nature of surgical management, the patient is likely to have a series of investigations or operations requiring repeated general anesthetics in a relatively short time. Preoperative assessment pays particular attention to the degree of nasal obstruction and the possible need for preoperative blood transfusion.

During induction of anesthesia, early insertion of an oral airway is indicated to bypass nasal obstruction. The trachea should be intubated orally using a cuffed RAE or similar tube and a pharyngeal pack inserted. The endotracheal tube must be secured very carefully as it will be inaccessible once the operation is underway. A reliable large-bore intravenous cannula and blood-warming equipment are essential in case rapid blood infusion becomes necessary. Maintenance of anesthesia can be by any suitable method, but generally a relaxant technique with controlled ventilation is preferred, particularly when controlled hypotension is to be used. The value of hypotensive anesthesia is controversial, but some surgeons believe that it contributes to simplifying the dissection and therefore ensuring a better result. If sodium nitroprusside is used to induce hypotension, monitoring should include means to assess blood volume, including central venous pressure and direct arterial blood pressure measurement.

Postoperatively there may be residual nasal

obstruction and continuous oozing from the operation site. The tracheal tube, therefore, should be left in place until the patient is fully awake.

Nasopharyngeal Mucocele

Nasal polyps are comparatively rare in children but do occur in association with cystic fibrosis.[19] A high percentage of nasal polyps in children extend into the sinuses, and antrochoanal polyps may account for a quarter or more of all nasal polyps.[20] This has clinical importance, since such polyps may mimic the appearance of more serious pathology—for example, meningoencephalocele or nasopharyngeal malignancy. Nasal polyps inevitably lead to obstruction of the nasal airway and chronic nasal infection, hence surgical removal is necessary.

The treatment of uncomplicated nasal polyps is simple avulsion: for antrochoanal polyp, the antral portion may be removed through a Caldwell-Luc or similar antrostomy. However, recent advances in nasal endoscopic surgical therapy now allow complete removal of such polyps through the middle meatus,[21] making the operation a much simpler and less traumatic event for the patient. In more severe cases in which there is persisting involvement of the ethmoid or sphenoid, radical operation may still be required.

Anesthetic management is complicated not only by local obstruction from the polyps but also in many patients by the presence of a chronic respiratory disease. Such patients may have severely reduced pulmonary function, chronic hypoxia, and copious purulent sputum. They must be carefully prepared for operation, with every effort made to reduce the volume of retained secretions by physiotherapy, postural drainage, and bronchodilators, along with antibiotics to control the infection. Anesthetic management should take into account the local obstruction caused by the lesion and its propensity to bleed during removal, in addition to the special requirements of the chronic respiratory disease.

Preoperatively, it is usual to avoid all sedative and anticholinergic drugs because of effects on ventilation and on the viscosity of secretions, respectively. Careful preoxygenation, intravenous induction, and oral intubation, followed by oxygen and halothane anesthesia with controlled ventilation, is a suitable technique that ensures control of the airway and allows optimal ventilation with reduced airway reactivity. Humidified gases should be used for ventilation. Throughout the operation, the tracheal tube should be aspirated frequently but gently, using a soft catheter. Profuse bleeding may occur during polypectomy in these circumstances, and blood transfusion occasionally may be required.

At the end of the operation, the tracheal tube must remain in place until the patient is fully awake. It is important to recommence active chest treatment as soon as possible in the postoperative period, preferably in the recovery room. The preoperative regimen of physiotherapy, postural drainage, bronchodilators, and antibiotics should be continued.

Other Nasal Tumors in Children

Teratomas,[22] dermoids, meningiomas,[23] paragangliomas, nasal encephaloceles, and gliomas all may occur as abnormal embryological intrusions of intracranial contents into the nose and may present as congenital nasal masses which, if large, may cause airway obstruction.[24, 25] In neonates, nasal airway obstruction is tantamount to complete respiratory obstruction because of the obligatory nasal breathing, but a patent airway may be restored readily by insertion of an oropharyngeal airway. Regardless of the particular pathological nature of the tumor, the principles of treatment are the same: careful surgical dissection, preserving as far as possible the normal anatomical structures. Proper treatment thus depends on accurate diagnosis and delineation of the extent of the tumor by radiology, including computed tomography. A special search must be made for any intracranial extension of the tumor.

Operation should not be undertaken until these investigations have been completed, as these lesions are often more extensive than first anticipated. Tumors that do extend into the cranium must be approached by frontal craniotomy rather than through the nose. Purely intranasal tumors may be approached through a midline or lateral rhinotomy. Anesthetic management is similar to that for nasal angiofibroma, except that bleeding is less likely to be a major problem, and deliberate hypotension rarely will be required.

Malignant tumors of the nose and nasopharynx, although common in older patients, are exceedingly rare in childhood. When such a lesion does occur, radiotherapy is usually the treatment of choice.[26]

MOUTH AND PHARYNX

ORAL TUMORS

Numerous congenital solid and cystic lesions occasionally occur in the soft tissues of the mouth and pharynx, which are amenable to surgical correction. Small, benign tumors lend themselves to simple excision and present few problems to the surgeon or anesthetist. Ranulas, for example, are simple, thin-walled cysts with a characteristic bluish appearance. They occur in the floor of the mouth and are formed by myxomatous degeneration of the salivary glands. Ranulas occur in all age groups, including infants and older children. They may burst and drain spontaneously but invariably recur. Although uncomfortable, they rarely, if ever, cause obstruction. The only reliable way of avoiding recurrence is total excision of the cyst, but this is often technically difficult because of the very thin wall. Marsupialization, with high probability of recurrence, may be the best that can be offered. Dissection is made easier by partial removal of the contents of the cyst, but unfortunately these contents are usually too viscid to allow easy aspiration. Ranulas, therefore, are frustrating for surgeon and patient alike but cause little morbidity and are of no danger to the patient except insofar as multiple operations are likely to be required for eventual elimination. Rarely the ranula may extend below the mylohyoid, in which case it will present as a swelling in the neck.[27] General endotracheal anesthesia via a nasal tube, with packing-off of the pharynx as for any other straightforward intraoral operation, will give satisfactory operating conditions. Blood loss is usually minimal.

Large tumors, and those that have eroded bone,[28] present more serious problems in terms of delineation and dissection but also may cause preoperative respiratory obstruction or difficulty during intubation. Teratomas of the head and neck may occur as respiratory obstruction in the neonate,[25] and indeed may even be diagnosed prenatally, allowing a planned approach to management to be made in advance of the event. In the initial care of such patients, the primary objective is to secure the airway, usually by intubation.[29] Acquired tumors of the mouth present similar problems; malignant tumors arising from the salivary glands do occur occasionally in childhood and are best treated by resection followed by radiotherapy.[30] Other sources of childhood malignancy in the pharynx include the tonsil and other lymphoid tissue, bone, and embryological rests of abnormally placed tissue—for example, thyroid and brain.

Surgical management of such tumors is by careful preoperative delineation of the extent of the tumor by computed tomography and magnetic resonance imaging, possibly aided by angiography, so that an appropriate surgical approach may be planned.[31] Anesthetic management places emphasis on securing the airway, replacement of intraoperative fluid losses, and maintenance of a secure and clear airway in the postoperative period. Nasal intubation is usually preferred to improve surgical access. Temporary tracheostomy may have to be considered in those patients expected to have continued postoperative respiratory obstruction.

PHARYNGEAL INFECTIONS OF SURGICAL IMPORTANCE

Although it is generally accepted that serious infective complications of tonsillitis are less common than a generation or two ago, and that the severity of such abscesses has been reduced following the availability of specific antibiotic therapy, this may not be entirely true. There is some evidence that the incidence of extratonsillar abscess is rising again, and that this increase may be related to a generally decreased rate of tonsillectomy.[32] Nonetheless, early antibiotic treatment of pyogenic extratonsillar pharyngeal infection usually prevents progression to frank abscess formation and the necessity for surgical drainage. This is fortunate, because a large pharyngeal abscess is a life-threatening condition. Not only does the airway become obstructed by the pharyngeal swelling, but also there is the added risk of sudden aggravation of this obstruction by rupture of the abscess, flooding the pharynx with pus and possibly allowing aspiration of infected material into the trachea and lungs. Rupture occurring during induction of anesthesia, when the patient's protective reflexes are obtunded and before the airway has been secured and adequately sealed off from the pharynx, is particularly dangerous. General anesthesia in these circumstances can be hazardous in the extreme.[33]

PERITONSILLAR ABSCESS (QUINSY)

Peritonsillar abscess forms by the spread of infection beyond the tonsillar capsule, most usually into the soft palate in the region of the superior pole of the tonsil, although abscesses around the middle and lower poles may also occur. In most cases, peritonsillar abscess affects one side only, but in a few patients, fewer than 10 percent, bilateral abscesses may occur. Older children and young adults account for most cases, and rather more males are affected than females.[34] Bacteriological examination usually shows a mixed infection of aerobes and anaerobes, with only about one quarter of all cases showing aerobes alone. The most commonly cultured organisms are streptococci, including beta-hemolytic streptococci, but pneumococci, enterococci, and occasionally *Haemophilus* species are also seen. Common anaerobes include peptostreptococci, peptococci, and bacteroides. Since many of the patients have been treated with antibiotics, a proportion of the abscesses prove to be sterile on culture.[35]

The usual presentation is of a patient who complains of severe sore throat, with trismus and difficulty in swallowing, along with signs of systemic toxicity. There is usually dysphonia, with speech becoming difficult and muffled. If there is marked swelling of the pharynx, there may also be signs of respiratory obstruction. Most patients with signs of early peritonsillar infection may be managed successfully by conservative treatment with antibiotics and do not proceed to abscess formation.[34, 36] The choice of antibiotic traditionally has relied heavily on penicillin alone. However, the probable presence of anaerobic pathogens makes addition of an antibiotic such as clindamycin or metronidazole more appropriate. Such patients are usually offered elective tonsillectomy as soon as possible after the infective episode, because it is thought that the incidence of recurrence is very high.[37, 38] The evidence for this is quite variable, and rather lower recurrence rates have, in fact, been reported in children;[39] hence the need for tonsillectomy in such patients has again been questioned.[34]

If frank abscess formation has already occurred and there is an apparent urgent need for surgical drainage in addition to antibiotic therapy, this can be accomplished in one of three ways:

1. *Needle aspiration of the abscess;* this has the advantage of being easily accomplished without general anesthesia in the cooperative patient (but thus may not therefore be a practical proposition in the younger child). It is easily repeated, gives an excellent sample for bacteriological evaluation, and does not in itself require admission to hospital so that many patients may be successfully treated as outpatients.[40, 41]
2. *Incision and drainage;* this does require general anesthesia and admission to hospital and often fails to drain the abscess adequately. It is associated with a recurrence rate of up 60 percent[34] and an unavoidable risk of pulmonary aspiration of infected material.
3. *Tonsillectomy à chaud* (immediate, or quinsy, tonsillectomy); immediate tonsillectomy is a practical option, and bleeding, although increased, has not proved to be an unmanageable problem. At operation, the tonsil on the unaffected side is removed first, and under no circumstances is adenoidectomy carried out at the same time. Bleeding on the affected side is usually greater than in most tonsillectomies but is readily controlled by the usual means. The results of immediate tonsillectomy are encouraging, as judged by duration of hospitalization. They are as good as if not better than those of conservative treatment alone, and there is the added benefit for the patient of not requiring later interval tonsillectomy.[32]

Patients with obviously pointing large abscesses are not suitable for tonsillectomy à chaud and require incision and drainage into the pharynx. Because of the hazard of aspiration this should be done, if at all possible, in the fully awake patient, with neither general anesthesia nor deep sedation.[42] Unfortunately this is not usually possible in children, and general anesthesia will be required.

Management of General Anesthesia in Patients with Peritonsillar Abscess

The special problems of anesthesia in these circumstances are as follows:

1. The likelihood of aggravating preexisting respiratory obstruction during induction and loss of consciousness.
2. Trismus may not resolve even with muscle relaxation, thus making laryngoscopy and intubation difficult or impossible.
3. Pharyngeal swelling and distortion of normal anatomy add to the difficulty of intubation.
4. The abscess may rupture at any time during induction or laryngoscopy and flood the pharynx with pus. This causes immediate respiratory obstruction with aspiration of infected material into the lungs, also adding greatly to the immediate difficulty of intubation.
5. Patients with large abscesses may be severely ill, pyrexial, toxic, and dehydrated.

A seriously toxic and dehydrated patient must be prepared for operation by rehydration with intravenous fluids, antibiotic therapy, and measures to lower the temperature. The most difficult problem for the anesthesiologist then remains management of the airway. If, after examination of the patient's mouth and pharynx, the anesthesiologist has any doubt that the patient can be intubated successfully, the safer course is to perform a preliminary tracheostomy under local anesthesia. General anesthesia can then be induced after the airway has been secured. However, most instances of peritonsillar infection are not so florid, and it is reasonable to proceed to induction of general anesthesia in those patients in whom it has been possible to inspect the throat preoperatively, in whom there is no significant respiratory obstruction, and when the abscess is still intact. In these circumstances, preoxygenation, followed by a rapid sequence intravenous induction and intubation (avoiding positive-pressure ventilation of the patient before intubation if at all possible), is a suitable technique.

If, on the other hand, preoperative examination of the patient shows a degree of trismus sufficient to make opening of the mouth difficult, or if there has been any suggestion of respiratory obstruction due to the pharyngeal swelling, then it becomes imperative to maintain spontaneous ventilation until absolutely sure that intubation can be achieved. Anesthesia should be induced in these circumstances with oxygen and halothane, and the patient should be allowed to become sufficiently deeply anesthetized, provided adequate ventilation can be maintained, to allow laryngoscopy. The administration of lidocaine, 1 mg/kg intravenously 3 minutes prior to laryngoscopy, reduces the incidence of coughing or breathholding. If the glottis can be easily seen and there is no apparent hindrance to intubation, the trachea may be intubated directly. Alternatively, to avoid coughing and straining and possible abscess rupture, an assistant can give succinylcholine intravenously while the anesthesiologist maintains direct vision of the glottis and proceeds to intubate when the cords are fully relaxed. The prolonged period of oxygen breathing during induction usually allows 1 or 2 minutes of apnea without leading to hypoxia, and most often it is unnecessary to ventilate the patient artificially before intubation. Once the airway has been secured by intubation, the hazards are greatly reduced and anesthesia can be continued in any appropriate way. The area of incision is hyperemic, and considerable bleeding that may be difficult to control is common. Particular attention must be paid to adequate fluid replacement. At the end of operation, the patient should be turned onto the side and allowed to regain consciousness before extubation.

Occasionally a similar clinical picture is seen in infectious mononucleosis, in which marked involvement of the lymphoid tissue of the nasopharynx can cause gross enlargement of the tonsils and respiratory obstruction, sometimes severe enough to be fatal.[43] If there is no response to conservative treatment, tonsillectomy will become urgently required. However, because of the friability and hyperemia of the tonsillar and other lymphoid tissue in the nose and pharynx, along with the possibility of secondary pyogenic bacterial infection, the problems and hazards of attempting induction of general anesthesia are the same as those in peritonsillar abscess. Whenever there is any doubt about the ease of intubation, preinduction tracheostomy offers much greater safety for the patient.[44]

RETROPHARYNGEAL ABSCESS

There are two distinct types of retropharyngeal abscess. The first, which is related to acute pyogenic infection and abscess formation in the lymphatic tissue that lies between the prevertebral fascia and the posterior pharyngeal wall in children, occurs as a direct extension of infection from the tonsil, nose, or middle ear. The clinical features are severe sore throat, respiratory obstruction due to forward dislocation of the posterior pharyngeal wall, and marked general toxicity. Retropharyngeal abscess of this type presents the same threat to the patient's airway as does quinsy, for if it ruptures it does so into the pharynx itself. The treatment is similar to that described for peritonsillar abscess. Drainage, if required, has of necessity to be into the pharynx because of the abscess's position relative to the prevertebral fascia.

The other form of retropharyngeal abscess occurs behind the prevertebral fascia, usually by extension from osteomyelitis of a vertebral body, and is more usually chronic than acute. Because of the barrier presented by the prevertebral fascia, these abscesses do not tend to point into the pharynx, and the appropriate drainage route is to the exterior of the neck. This may be readily accomplished through a skin incision made behind the sternomastoid. Induction of general anesthesia in these circumstances is much safer and simpler than in other forms of pharyngeal abscess, because of the lesser degree of obstruction of the pharynx by swelling and the prevention of pharyngeal soiling by the intact prevertebral fascia.

LUDWIG'S ANGINA

This is a severe pyogenic (usually streptococcal or staphylococcal) cellulitis of the submandibular and sublingual region associated with inflammatory edema of the mouth and tongue. Edema develops rapidly, and the tongue swells and is pushed forward through the opened mouth and upward against the palate. Cellulitis spreads into the neck below the deep cervical fascia, and respiratory obstruction may occur with great rapidity. Intubation of the trachea is usually impossible and should respiratory obstruction become severe, there is no option but to perform emergency tracheostomy with local anesthesia alone. Attempts at blind nasal intubation or nasal intubation using a flexible bronchoscope in the face of severe respiratory obstruction are likely to lead to disaster. General anesthesia is fraught with the danger of provoking complete respiratory obstruction and must be avoided. If an abscess forms, which is unusual, it should be incised and drained externally through a submental cervical incision. Indeed, even in the absence of a defined abscess, if edema and swelling of the neck do not subside rapidly following institution of antibiotic therapy, a similar incision may still be indicated to decompress the closed fascial space beneath the mylohyoid muscle and reduce the potential for airway obstruction. This incision should be made with local anesthesia alone and is left open until the swelling subsides.

TONGUE

By its occupancy of the pharynx, disturbances of function or form of the tongue can have profound effects on the vital functions of breathing, swallowing, and speech as well as possibly influencing the growth of surrounding tissues, notably the dentition and associated bony structures.

ANKYLOGLOSSIA (TONGUE-TIE)

Primary tethering of the tongue in infants and children is caused by shortening of the lingual frenulum. Secondary ankyloglossia, such as that which occurs in carcinoma of the tongue or following damage to the glossopharyngeal nerve, is exceedingly rare in childhood.

Tongue-tie is difficult to evaluate in terms of functional impairment of speech, and it is doubtful whether there is ever serious interference with sucking in infancy. Difficulty in clearing the buccal sulcus with the tongue is the main indication for operation. For these reasons, there is no particular urgency to perform release of tongue-tie. If release is thought to be indicated, it can safely be postponed until the child is about a year old without affecting the normal development of speech.

Although lingual frenulectomy is a simple operation, there is a danger of bleeding, and such bleeding may be difficult for the surgeon to control in less than ideal operating conditions. For this reason, the patients should be treated as for any intraoral operation—that is, given general anesthesia with nasotracheal intubation and pharyngeal packing. Postoperative analgesia can be provided by applying lidocaine gel to the surgical site at the end of the operation.

MACROGLOSSIA

Macroglossia is a term which is often very loosely applied to pediatric patients. The tongue may be truly enlarged, owing, for example, to hypertrophy of its own tissues or to invasion by tumor, or there may be merely apparent enlargement secondary to a relative diminution in the size of the oral cavity, such as occurs in Down's syndrome (Table 11–1).

The definition of macroglossia has been extended by some to include all cases in which the tongue is incapable of being withdrawn behind the anterior teeth (or gums). Others have limited its application only to those instances in which obstructive symptoms occur. Because of this problem of definition, estimates of the incidence of macroglossia in the population are equally confusing. Primary macroglossia has thus been described as being common,[45] uncommon,[46] and rare.[47]

Symptoms associated with an enlarged tongue are proportional to the degree of enlargement relative to the size of the mouth and vary from minor effects on development of speech and dentition to profound obstruction of both respiration and swallowing. Of course, speech cannot be evaluated in infancy, but in older children secondary macroglossia causes interference with speech. This is related not only to the overall

Table 11–1. CLASSIFICATION OF MACROGLOSSIA IN CHILDHOOD

Category	Examples
Apparent	Down's syndrome
(Pseudoenlargement)	Cerebral palsy
Acute	
Inflammatory edema	Trauma
	Infection
	Allergy
	Hereditary angioedema
	Postoperative
Actual Enlargement	
Chronic	
Diffuse	
Congenital	Idiopathic macroglossia
	Hypothyroidism
	Beckwith's syndrome
	Glycogen storage diseases
Acquired	Hypothyroidism
	Amyloidosis
Nodular	
Congenital	Hemangioma
	Lymphangioma
	Lingual thyroid
Acquired	Trauma
	Infection
	Simple tumors
	Carcinoma

degree of enlargement of the tongue but also to the exact site of the swelling, particularly with smaller lesions. Minor degrees of obstruction cause little noticeable effect apart from excess salivation, but more pronounced obstruction causes dysphagia. Almost all patients with primary or secondary macroglossia of any significant degree have difficulty in swallowing, often being able to manage only liquids. When enlargement is marked, the anterior part of the tongue is permanently exteriorized, hence the surface becomes dry and fissured, and ulceration is common. Respiratory obstruction is also a feature of these grosser forms of macroglossia and occurs particularly when the pathology involves not only the tongue but also the floor of the mouth and tissues of the neck (for example, lymphangioma).

Some specific causes of enlarged tongue are discussed next.

Acute Glossitis. Rapidly developing, diffuse swelling of the tongue, usually caused by inflammatory edema and associated with trauma or allergy, may require an artificial airway. It might be possible to do this by oral intubation before the swelling becomes too great. If the swelling is limited to the anterior part of the tongue, a nasal airway or nasal intubation (possibly aided by flexible endoscopy) may be possible. However, in some cases of rapidly increasing size, particularly when the enlargement involves the posterior part of the tongue, the degree of obstruction may make intubation entirely impossible, with no alternative but to proceed to tracheostomy.

A particular form of this acute glossitis has been described following cleft palate repair,[48] and it is suggested that the mouth and tongue should always be examined prior to extubation in such patients. If there is swelling of the tongue, the endotracheal tube should not be removed. Macroglossia has also been described following posterior fossa craniotomy; this may be due at least partially to venous obstruction, but a primary neurogenic component also has been suggested.[49] Whatever the precise cause, this kind of acute enlargement of the tongue usually will persist for days or even weeks rather than hours, and need for an artificial airway will be prolonged.

Chronic Macroglossia. A chronically enlarged tongue in children may be more apparent than real. Some conditions, for example Down's syndrome, are associated with a rather small oropharynx in which a normal-sized tongue gives the appearance of being too large. Problems of neuromuscular coordination, such as cerebral palsy, also may give the appearance of a large tongue when in fact no such enlargement exists. True macroglossia may be due to intrinsic hyperplasia of the tongue tissue or to the development of discrete lesions within the tongue. Bleeding into a small chronic lesion can cause rapid expansion with sudden onset, or worsening, of obstructive symptoms. Regardless of the cause of the enlargement, a reduction in the size of the tongue may become necessary to relieve the oral obstruction.

In lesser degrees of enlargement, the normal growth of the oral cavity (which enlarges more rapidly than the tongue) will allow relatively better accommodation of the enlarged tongue as the child's age increases. There may also be a primary indication for reduction glossoplasty in order to prevent later dental malocclusion, speech problems, and disordered facial growth. Thus the indications for surgery in any individual case of macroglossia are far from being clear-cut.[47]

Surgical Lesions of Special Interest

Lymphangioma. Cystic hygroma usually occurs in infancy: most cases are seen soon after birth and almost all are seen before the age of 2 years.[50, 51] It most commonly occurs in the posterior triangle of the neck but rarely may arise in the anterior triangle close to the mandible. In this latter group the tumor usually extends into the floor of the mouth at the base of the tongue. Cystic hygroma involving the tongue is much rarer than other forms of cervical lymphangioma but is more urgent because it may cause severe pharyngeal obstruction; such patients are usually seen with acute respiratory obstruction at birth. The histological appearance of cystic hygroma is that of a multilocular, endothelium-lined, thin-walled tumor arising from lymphatic vessels but often containing areas of more solid lymphoid tissue with a large number of thin-walled blood vessels. It is not malignant but infiltrates widely, making dissection difficult and often necessitating multiple operations for its eradication.[52] The tumor is prone to sudden enlargement, sometimes due to hemorrhage or infection, but frequently for no apparent reason.

Lingual Thyroid. Incomplete descent of the thyroid gland during development from the thyroglossal duct may cause the only functioning thyroid tissue to be in the tongue rather than in its usual anatomical location. In other instances, when there is indeed a normally located thyroid, a thyroid nodule in the tongue probably represents an ectopic rest of thyroid tissue occurring along the track of the duct. Lingual thyroid is a rare entity, more common in females than in males, and it is usually found as a mass in the posterior third of the tongue, between the foramen cecum and the epiglottis.[53] Thyroid tissue thus located is nonetheless subject to all the potential pathology of thyroid tissue generally, although the incidence of malignancy may be lower than formerly suggested.[54] Lingual thyroid dysfunction seems to be more often associated with hypothyroidism than with thyrotoxicosis. Lingual thyroid may remain asymptomatic and be detected only incidentally. In symptomatic cases, the common presentation is of dysphagia or a choking sensation, often provoked by sudden enlargement of the nodule due to bleeding. Once suspected, the diagnosis can be confirmed by radionuclide scanning.

Treatment largely depends on the degree of symptoms: if the patient is asymptomatic there may be no need for any treatment at all. If the patient is symptomatic, thyroid supplementation therapy usually results in reduction in the size of the gland, often to the point of rendering the patient asymptomatic. Alternatively, the ectopic thyroid tissue may be excised, in which case the patient often will require thyroid replacement therapy. To avoid the need for lifelong replacement therapy, the excised thyroid tissue may be implanted elsewhere in the body.[55]

Cysts of the Tongue. Solitary cysts of a variety of pathological types, including salivary, dermoid, and epidermoid growths, occur in the tongue. Symptoms depend on the size and site, and most cysts will require operation. Simple salivary cysts usually can be effectively cured by marsupialization, but most others will require definitive removal.[56]

Other Tumors of the Tongue. Apart from lymphangioma, other diffuse neoplastic tumors, including hemangioma, fibroma, and fibrolipomatous dysplasia, are also rare causes of macroglossia. Smaller, discrete simple tumors of the tongue also have been reported occasionally.[57] Malignant tumors of the tongue are exceedingly rare in childhood, but lingual carcinoma and rhabdomyosarcoma have been known to occur.[58, 59] Treatment of malignant tumors of the tongue in children is similar to that in adults, including radiation and aggressive surgical therapy, possibly with hemimandibulectomy and radical cervical node dissection.

Surgical Therapy for Macroglossia

When any operation of the tongue is contemplated, it is imperative that it be designed not only to remove the bulk of the tumor or cyst but also to preserve as far as possible the function and appearance of the tongue. This means that attention must be given to the final shape and mobility of the tongue as well as to the overall size, and that preservation of speech and taste should be ensured if at all possible. Various operations have been devised to meet these goals,[45] and among the least damaging partial glossectomies are those that are limited to the anterior and superficial two thirds of the tongue, avoiding the lingual and hypoglossal nerves. Operations necessarily involving the posterior part of the tongue are more mutilating and may damage not only the lingual and hypoglossal nerves but also the glossopharyngeal nerve.

Anesthesia for Glossectomy

The special problems that may be encountered by the anesthesiologist during operations on the tongue are related to the following:

1. *The degree of pharyngeal obstruction.* Severe macroglossia will cause marked obstruction of the airway, although if the enlargement is confined to the anterior part of the tongue obstruction in the oropharynx may be bypassed by the nasal airway. Thus, even in the absence

of obvious respiratory obstruction in the preoperative period, there may be sufficient intraoral obstruction to make laryngoscopy and intubation difficult. Lesions involving the floor of the mouth as well as the tongue are particularly likely to cause difficulty during laryngoscopy and intubation.

2. *The need to secure the airway* and isolate it from the surgical field.

3. *Intraoperative bleeding,* which may be considerable and require aggressive volume replacement.

4. *Acute postoperative edema and swelling,* which may cause severe, albeit temporary, pharyngeal and respiratory obstruction. This is particularly likely if the operation involves the posterior part of the tongue. Swelling of the anterior two thirds is usually well tolerated by patients who have unobstructed nasal airways. In the preoperative assessment of patients requiring glossectomy, particular attention, therefore, should be paid to signs and symptoms of respiratory obstruction, and even in patients without clinical evidence of significant obstruction a careful examination of the pharynx and neck should be made for the degree of soft tissue enlargement. The nasal airways also should be checked for patency.

Intraoperative Management

Patients Without Respiratory Obstruction. Laryngoscopy and intubation in this group, although occasionally difficult, is rarely impossible. Nevertheless, if there are any doubts after preoperative examination that intubation will be other than straightforward, it is wise to avoid intravenous agents or muscle relaxants until the airway has been secured. Awake laryngoscopy and intubation may be possible in some patients, particularly infants: otherwise a gentle inhalation induction to a deep plane of anesthesia sufficient to allow intubation is the technique of choice (as described earlier for peritonsillar abscess). If the tongue lesion is placed anteriorly and there are no indications of potential difficulty in intubation, any technique of induction that might otherwise be used will be suitable.

Nasotracheal intubation is the route of choice. It offers the advantage of removing the tube as far as possible from the surgical field, allows better fixation, and is more suitable for continuing care into the immediate postoperative period. Pharyngeal packing to protect against tracheobronchial soiling is necessary. Monitoring and maintenance of anesthesia are as for any other common pharyngeal operation, but with particular attention to accurate estimation and appropriate replacement of blood losses.

At the end of the operation, it is important to assess the possible degree of postoperative respiratory obstruction that may occur secondary to edema and swelling. This is particularly likely to cause trouble if the operation has involved the posterior part of the tongue or the patient has preexisting nasal obstruction. If there is any indication that there may be some postoperative obstruction of this nature, then the airway must be secured and maintained by artificial means until postoperative edema and swelling have subsided. This may be achieved either by maintaining nasotracheal intubation for 1 or 2 days postoperatively, or by elective tracheostomy. It is much easier to anticipate problems and provide for them than to cope with an acute episode of severe respiratory obstruction occurring perhaps hours after operation.

Patients with Preexisting Respiratory Obstruction. These are usually infants with a cystic hygroma involving the anterior tongue, and the usual presentation is with acute respiratory distress at birth. It is emphasized that only a very small proportion of infants with cystic hygromas fall into this group.[60] The primary objective is to achieve and maintain an adequate airway. Although intubation may be difficult, there is little alternative as these tumors often infiltrate the floor of the mouth and the neck, making tracheostomy technically very difficult (and unlikely to be successful if required to be done urgently for resuscitation). Every effort, therefore, should be directed to intubating the trachea as the initial resuscitative measure. A selection of laryngoscope blades, endotracheal tubes, and stylets should be prepared, and skilled assistants should be available.

In some instances it may be possible to establish the airway only by using a bronchoscope, and in this case a tracheostomy may be performed with the bronchoscope in place. Once the airway is secured by intubation, the immediate emergency is over and time can be taken to complete resuscitation and assessment of the child. Because of the difficult dissection of these tumors and their unpredictable behavior in terms of acute size changes, long-term tracheostomy is usually required for airway management. Other patients may require tracheostomy for the immediate perioperative period. As just emphasized, tracheostomy should be carried out as a planned procedure in an already intubated patient. Once a satisfactory airway has been secured, further management is as described for nonobstructed patients, except that in this group it is absolutely mandatory to maintain the artificial airway well into the postoperative period.

Patients with lesser degrees of respiratory obstruction will not require immediate respiratory resuscitation but must be considered to be in danger of complete respiratory obstruction during induction of anaesthesia and treated accordingly. The techniques that may be most safely used are awake intubation; intubation following gentle inhalation induction alone; or, for those patients whose lesions do not involve the neck, primary tracheostomy using infiltration anesthesia alone.

ACUTE OBSTRUCTIVE INFECTIONS OF THE UPPER AIRWAY

Any lesion producing partial obstruction of the larynx or trachea causes characteristic noisy breathing (stridor). In previously healthy children, stridor of acute onset is almost always due to laryngotracheobronchitis, epiglottitis, or a foreign body. Rarer causes include trauma, smoke inhalation, and external compression of the trachea.

Acute infectious diseases that commonly cause respiratory obstruction and stridor in children can be classified into two main categories. Laryngotracheobronchitis, commonly simply called croup, is of rather slow onset and usually runs a benign course over a few days. Epiglottitis, on the other hand, is characterized by sudden onset and very rapid progression to potentially lethal respiratory obstruction within a few hours. Although there is characteristically a completely different clinical picture in typical cases of laryngotracheobronchitis and acute epiglottitis, in many patients the initial differential diagnosis may be difficult. Sometimes it may be quite impossible to distinguish one from the other.[61–63] Even within the laryngotracheobronchitis group, a small proportion of patients will go on to develop respiratory obstruction of sufficient severity to require airway intervention of the same sort as that described next for the management of acute epiglottitis—indeed, every instance of sudden onset of stridor in a child must be considered to herald a potentially lethal condition and be treated accordingly. The system of initial airway management described for epiglottitis can be followed usefully in any such circumstance, regardless of the precise cause, and will allow the airway to be secured, after which definitive diagnostic steps can proceed in an orderly fashion.

ACUTE EPIGLOTTITIS (SUPRAGLOTTITIS)

This potentially fatal, fulminant inflammation of the epiglottis and other supraglottic structures has a notably rapid onset, characterized by progressive respiratory obstruction. The infection predominantly involves the supraglottic structures, that is, the epiglottis, aryepiglottic folds, arytenoid cartilages, and surrounding tissues. Inflammatory swelling and edema of the involved tissues not only produces the characteristic swollen, cherry red epiglottis but also, by encroaching on the airway, progressively decreases the cross-sectional area of the lumen until severe and even complete obstruction occurs.

Acute epiglottitis occurs in all age groups; most cases occur either in young children (18 months to 8 years of age) or young adults (15 to 30 years),[64] although it has also been reported in infants less than 2 years old[65, 66] and in older adults.[67, 68] Incidence rates reported from North America,[69] Europe,[64, 70] and Australasia[71] do not vary greatly and suggest an annual rate of about 1 in 10,000 to 15,000 for children and 1 in 50,000 for adults. The course of the disease in adults is generally more benign than that in children.[72] In children, more boys are affected than girls. These incidence rates refer to conditions in which widespread immunization had not been available and are likely to be modified significantly when public health programs of immunization against *Haemophilus influenzae* group b are introduced. The mortality, which was formerly high, is now lower, reflecting better awareness of the potential for respiratory obstruction and the need to secure the airway as the primary event in management.

Complications of epiglottitis are almost entirely attributable to the hypoxic sequelae of respiratory obstruction, but other rare complications include acute onset of pulmonary edema following relief of obstruction,[73] and effects of the infection in other tissues and organs, including meninges,[74] joints, and pericardium, and pneumonia and septic shock.[75] Provided an adequate airway is maintained, most cases respond quickly to antibiotic treatment, and the patient recovers fully and rapidly.

BACTERIOLOGY

In most cases of acute epiglottitis in children the causative organism is *Haemophilus influenzae* group b.[76] This strain is also the commonest cause of bacterial meningitis in North America.

It is widely distributed, with nasopharyngeal carrier rates of up to 5 percent. Its virulence in young children is attributed to deficiency of antibody, with infection usually becoming established in the upper respiratory tract from where it may extend by direct spread though tissues (sinusitis; epiglottitis) or by blood-borne dispersal (meningitis). In epiglottitis, the organism often may be recovered from both blood cultures and throat swabs, and diagnosis may be confirmed rapidly by countercurrent immunoelectophoresis of serum or cerebral spinal fluid.

H. influenzae b is generally sensitive to ampicillin, but more recently there is apparently an increasing incidence of β-lactamase-producing strains resistant to ampicillin. For this reason it has been recommended to start treatment with both ampicillin and chloramphenicol, later modifying the antibiotic regime according to the results of sensitivity tests from the blood cultures. Chloramphenicol-resistant strains[77] do occur, however, and the cephalosporin cefuroxime is now preferred, as it has a high margin of safety and penetrates into the cerebrospinal fluid.[78] The recommended dose is 100 to 200 mg/kg/day intravenously in divided doses.

Very young infants have a reduced immune response to *H. influenzae,*[74] but universal immunization of children at 18 months of age with *H. influenzae* b polysaccharide vaccine would be expected to reduce the incidence of *H. influenzae* meningitis and epiglottitis, and significant strides in this direction have already been reported.[79] In a minority of cases other causative organisms have been identified, including group A β-hemolytic streptococci, in which circumstances the illness usually runs a more protracted course.[80] On occasion other, more exotic organisms have been implicated,[81] especially in immunocompromised hosts,[82] and a similar syndrome of necrotizing epiglottitis has been described in infectious mononucleosis.[83]

Clinical Picture

The classic presentation of acute epiglottitis is sudden onset of sore throat in a previously well child. Increasing dysphagia, shortness of breath, and inspiratory stridor follow. The total time span from the onset of symptoms to severe respiratory distress is usually only 6 to 12 hours. On examination the child is obviously toxic, with pyrexia, tachycardia, and tachypnea, and prefers to sit upright, leaning forward with the chin pushed out and the neck hyperextended. There is no cough, and the child usually makes little effort to speak or cry. Drooling often occurs because of the pain on attempted swallowing. The symptoms are exacerbated by lying down. As respiratory obstruction worsens, hypercapnia and hypoxia cause further distress, and the onset of cyanosis or obvious air hunger signals impending respiratory arrest. Even when dyspnea does not appear to be particularly severe, sudden complete respiratory obstruction and arrest may be caused at any time by laryngospasm. Stress, anxiety, and crying all can contribute to an increased oxygen requirement and exacerbation of symptoms.[84]

In some patients, notably younger infants, the clinical features may be atypical and suggest a diagnosis of croup or pharyngitis[85–87] or may be masked by other clinical conditions—for example, suspected foreign body aspiration.[88] It would seem wise, therefore, to include acute epiglottitis in the differential diagnosis of any child who presents with fever and respiratory distress.

Diagnosis

Acute epiglottitis in children remains a clinical diagnosis made on the basis of history and examination rather than on the results of laboratory tests or special investigations. The important differential diagnoses in acute epiglottitis are viral laryngotracheobronchitis and laryngotracheal foreign body. The characteristic clinical features are summarized in Table 11–2. Although it may appear from this table that laryngotracheobronchitis and acute epiglottitis can readily be distinguished on clinical grounds, occasionally this may be very difficult.[61, 62] It is not unknown for severe cases of laryngotracheobronchitis to develop profound respiratory distress similar to that seen in acute epiglottitis, usually attributable to laryngeal edema, secondary bacterial laryngitis, or retention of tenacious secretions.

Precise diagnosis at this stage is of secondary importance; the urgent need is obvious: to secure a clear airway and improve the patient's ventilatory status. It is essential to proceed with active airway management rather than to delay intervention to allow more diagnostic effort while the patient's condition rapidly deteriorates. The diagnosis of laryngeal foreign body usually causes fewer difficulties, being characterized by the onset of stridor after choking, eating, or playing with small objects, and a lack of signs of any systemic toxicity. Nonetheless even here there are potential pitfalls for the diagnostician, and the finding of acute epiglot-

Table 11–2. ACUTE EPIGLOTTITIS AND LARYNGOTRACHEOBRONCHITIS

	Acute Epiglottitis	Laryngo-tracheobronchitis
Incidence	Rare (<5%)*	Common (>80%)*
Age	Mostly 2–6 yr	6–36 mon
Onset	Sudden: <24 h	Gradual: 2–3 days
Clinical Features		
1. Stridor	Yes Lessens as respiratory obstruction increases	Yes
2. Cough	No	Yes
3. Voice	Hoarse	Does not speak
4. Posture	Sits upright, head forward	
5. Drooling	Yes	No
X-ray Results	Swollen epiglottis	Narrow subglottis
Laryngoscopy	Erythema and edema of epiglottis and periglottic tissues	Normal glottis
Etiology	Bacterial: *H. influenzae* b	Viral: parainfluenzal, influenzal
Treatment	Intubation Antibiotics Rehydration	Humidification Racemic epinephrine Steroids Intubation (rarely)
Course	24–48 h	3–6 days

*Proportion of all hospital admissions for stridor.

titis in a child with a classic history of inhaled foreign body has been reported.[88]

The diagnosis of acute epiglottitis can best be confirmed by direct examination of the throat, but the extent of the examination compatible with safety remains controversial. In general, pediatric anesthesiologists are agreed that, in respiratory distress, attempts at awake laryngoscopy inevitably will lead to increasing agitation and struggling in the child. This will increase the degree of respiratory obstruction while simultaneously increasing the patient's oxygen demand and may precipitate total airway obstruction. It is generally advised to avoid examination of the larynx until definitive airway management is immediately available (that is, in an operating room or intensive care unit and usually after induction of anesthesia). Others suggest that direct examination of the larynx is perhaps not so fraught with danger, particularly if carried out by a skilled physician well accustomed to the technique;[89] however, advocates of this approach still advise that such examination take place only when the apparatus and expertise to secure an artificial airway immediately are present.[90]

The usefulness of lateral neck radiographs is well attested,[91] particularly in patients first seen at an early stage of the disease, before significant respiratory distress has developed. Typical radiographic appearances of acute epiglottitis include swelling and rounding of the epiglottitis and distention of the hypopharynx. Attention to precise interpretation of the radiological appearances of soft tissue images and comparison of ratios such as epiglottic width to third cervical body width will allow a very high degree of correlation with subsequent definitive diagnosis[92] and are of great help in differentiating laryngotracheobronchitis from acute epiglottitis. Of course such x-ray films will also be useful in revealing or excluding radiopaque laryngotracheal foreign bodies.

Blood tests are of absolutely no immediate useful diagnostic value and indeed may be positively dangerous if they lead to crying and laryngospasm in the patient or temporizing by the medical staff. Such tests as are required for whatever purpose are best left undone until after the airway has been secured. In particular, arterial blood gas determinations are of no value in assessing the need for airway intervention. Laboratory studies that are useful (but that can also be postponed until the airway has been, or is being, secured) include blood samples for culture along with direct swabs from the throat so that retrospective precise bacteriological diagnosis may be made.

TREATMENT

The preferred management of children with severe stridor is immediate admission to a pediatric intensive care unit or, when this is not possible, to the best-equipped emergency area in the hospital that has the necessary airway support resources. As soon as possible thereafter laryngoscopy should be performed, with the patient anesthetized and the airway secured by tracheal intubation. Blood is drawn for culture, and surface swabs are taken for specific diagnosis, after which expectant antibiotic therapy is continued until specific bacteriological sensitivities are reported, and attention is given to ensuring rehydration of the patient.

Most pediatric hospitals have established protocols to be followed in cases of suspected acute epiglottitis, and the following scheme for management of these patients is that which is followed in my hospital.

Upon notification that a patient with suspected or possible acute epiglottitis is being sent to the hospital, the anesthesia and intensive care unit staffs are alerted to ensure the presence of an anesthesiologist in the emergency room when the patient arrives and to allow arrangements to be made for probable admission to the intensive care unit and immediate availability of an operating room. (In some institutions, primary care of these cases is undertaken by the otolaryngology service, in which case an otolaryngologist would be called in addition to the anesthesiologist). On arrival, the patient is subjected to the very minimum of examination or interference and can generally be immediately classified into one of three categories by simple inspection:

Category 1. The patient is unconscious, in gross respiratory distress, cyanotic, and moribund. Immediate resuscitation must be attempted, hence the need for skilled airway management to be available from the moment of arrival. Oral intubation should be attempted but, if not immediately successful, an attempt should be made to ventilate the patient with a bag, face mask, and positive pressure:[93] if these measures do not suffice to overcome the respiratory obstruction at least to the degree of allowing adequate oxygenation of the patient, immediate cricothyroidotomy is performed. Following successful resuscitation and securing of the airway, the patient is transferred to the intensive care unit for specific treatment of the epiglottitis, along with all necessary measures to minimize the effects of tissue hypoperfusion and hypoxia that will have occurred during the period of respiratory (and possibly cardiac) arrest. Particular attention is paid to instituting specific measures to ensure optimal cerebral recovery.

Category 2. If the patient is conscious but has obvious stridor and air hunger (evidenced by use of accessory respiratory muscles and flaring of nostrils) he or she is not examined or x-rayed but allowed to remain sitting up and, accompanied by the parents if present, is transferred at once to the intensive care unit or operating room for immediate laryngoscopy and intubation under anesthesia. Time should not be wasted in applying monitoring devices other than a pulse oximeter—it is apparent that immediate first aid is required and monitoring in this circumstance will not provide any additional security for the patient. The only therapeutic endeavor allowed during transport is oxygen (preferably humidified) by face mask: in particular, examination of the throat is forbidden for fear of provoking laryngospasm and acute respiratory obstruction. No therapeutically useful knowledge will be gained by such examination at that time, as any patient in this degree of respiratory distress will require an artificial airway regardless of the findings on examination. Nor, in the face of established respiratory distress, is there any indication for delaying treatment to obtain lateral cervical radiographs. Routine blood work is postponed until after the airway is secure, not only because it is noncontributory at this stage but also to avoid increasing the patient's distress.

Category 3. In these patients there is less urgency: although there is obvious stridor, there are no signs of air hunger. The patient is conscious and alert, not in a state of respiratory distress. The chief diagnostic problem here is to distinguish those patients in the early stage of epiglottitis who will require active airway intervention from those with laryngotracheobronchitis who would probably not require any airway treatment beyond humidification and possibly racemic epinephrine. The value of a lateral cervical radiograph is well proved in this group.[92, 94]

Nonetheless, the potential for rapid deterioration in ventilatory status is ever present, so the patient should be accompanied at all times during this process by a physician with the capability and necessary equipment to establish an emergency artificial airway should this become necessary. Following the x-ray film, the patient is admitted to the intensive care unit as before: those with a radiological diagnosis of epiglottitis will proceed to the operating room for laryngoscopy and probable intubation; those with no radiological changes but in whom stridor persists will be treated for laryngotracheobronchitis, with frequent reassessment of their respiratory status. Should this worsen to the point of producing respiratory distress, then this patient will also be taken to the operating room for laryngoscopy. On the other hand, if stridor lessens, then the patient will be assumed to have resolving laryngotracheobronchitis and will be transferred out of the intensive care unit to a general pediatric ward.

LARYNGOSCOPY AND INTUBATION

All necessary airway equipment, including a range of tracheal tubes, laryngoscopes, rigid bronchoscopes, and an emergency tracheostomy set, should be assembled and checked before the patient arrives in the operating room. On arrival, the child, preferably accompanied by a parent or other familiar person, should be disturbed as little as possible. On transfer to the operating room, the child should be allowed to sit up rather than be forced to lie down, as this may induce sudden, complete respiratory obstruction. A gentle inhalation induction of anesthesia, using halothane in oxygen, should be initiated. As induction proceeds and the mask is more firmly applied to the patient's face, a little positive pressure should be given via the reservoir bag, as this often improves ventilation significantly. So long as the patient does not become desaturated, anesthesia should be continued in this way until the patient is in a fairly deep plane of surgical anesthesia. The time required to achieve this will be quite long, probably in excess of 15 minutes, but while the patient's status remains reasonably stable there is no need to hurry.

Opportunity may be taken, after consciousness is lost, to apply the customary monitors (particularly pulse oximeter, electrocardiographic leads, and blood pressure cuff), establish an intravenous infusion, administer atropine, and draw blood for culture and any other test that may be required. These procedures should be avoided while the patient is still responsive for fear of disturbing the smooth induction. Lidocaine, 1 to 1.5 mg/kg intravenously, may be administered at this stage to reduce further the likelihood of coughing or breathholding during laryngoscopy.

When adequate anesthesia has been achieved, laryngoscopy is performed, note taken of the appearance of the glottis and surrounding tissues, and an oral tracheal tube passed without the aid of muscle relaxants. Generally this is fairly easy, although a smaller than usual tube may be required. If the entrance to the glottis is obscured because of swelling and edema, external pressure on the chest usually will reveal the position of the glottis by the expulsion of air bubbles into the pharynx. If an endotracheal tube cannot be inserted into the glottis, then a small-diameter rigid bronchoscope should be substituted. If in spite of this it is still impossible to intubate the trachea and total respiratory obstruction occurs, an attempt to ventilate the patient by face mask and positive pressure should be made but, if there is not almost immediate relief of obstruction, cricothyroidotomy should be performed without further delay.

Once the airway has been established, anesthesia is continued with assisted ventilation. Blood for cultures, if not already obtained, is taken at this stage, along with surface glottic bacteriology swabs; when this has been achieved, intravenous antibiotic therapy is started. To increase the patient's comfort and decrease nursing difficulties, the orotracheal tube should be changed for a nasotracheal tube while the patient is still anesthetized. Generally this presents no particular difficulty, provided the patient has been kept at a reasonable depth of anesthesia. Because of the period of stenting by the oral tube, the glottic edema has already to some degree been "pushed back," and the glottic opening is more easily defined. In these new circumstances, it is quite reasonable to change the tube with the aid of a muscle relaxant. After careful securing of the nasotracheal tube, the patient is returned to the intensive care unit and allowed to awaken. A restraint jacket with rigid arms that do not allow the patient to raise the hands to the endotracheal tube is useful.

Treatment is continued with antibiotics and intravenous fluids; the tracheal tube is usually well tolerated, but all patients require close supervision during emergence to guard against self-extubation. Some patients will require continued sedation so long as the tube remains in place. Spontaneous ventilation using humidified air or oxygen-enriched air is usually all that is required. Accidental displacement of the tube at this stage is not usually followed by immediate total airway obstruction, and reintubation can be undertaken in a measured and controlled fashion. All patients with epiglottitis must be kept in an intensive care unit and all routine care for an intubated patient given.

Pulmonary edema following relief of profound respiratory obstruction has been reported.[95] This occurrence is treated in the usual way, with continuous positive-pressure ventilation and diuretics. The mechanism of this pulmonary edema may include the physical effects of sudden change in the pressure environment within the chest and lungs, and the cell membrane effects of the bacteremia. A similar syndrome is seen in other forms of upper airway obstruction.[96] The concept of a physical etiology as the primary cause is supported by the short duration and relatively benign course of this pulmonary edema.

Alternative protocols have been described from other institutions. One relies upon nasotracheal intubation, using intravenous induction and muscle relaxants in an intensive care unit by pediatric intensive care specialists. All patients are paralyzed and intubated to avoid accidental extubation, to decrease laryngeal trauma caused by movement of the tube, and to facilitate repeated laryngoscopy. This has been associated with no serious complications, although the average duration of intubation is rather longer than usual.[97] Another protocol describes management of clinically mild cases without intubation, relying instead on close observation in a pediatric intensive care unit with constant availability of physicians skilled in intubation.[98] This plan should be followed only in a unit with 24-hour immediate expert physician attendance.

Haemophilus influenzae epiglottitis usually resolves very quickly, within 24 to 48 hours, although infection by other bacterial pathogens, notably streptococci, may persist for much longer; durations for up to 3 weeks have been reported.[80] There is no precise guide to the timing of removal of the tracheal tube. Evidences of improvement in the patient include resolution of the pyrexia and toxemia and the development of an air leak around the tube. These events are usually a better guide to the patient's ability to do without the artificial airway than relying on repeated laryngoscopic examinations under general anesthesia. Not only does this avoid the need for repeated anesthesia, but also it has been shown that the appearance of the larynx in these circumstances does not necessarily correlate well with the patient's ability to maintain an adequate airway.[84] The safety and freedom from complications of relatively short-term nasotracheal intubation in acute epiglottitis have been well established.[94, 97] This may not be equally true for the longer-term intubation occasionally required in the treatment of laryngotracheobronchitis or in those rare instances of streptococcal epiglottitis, particularly in children less than 1 year of age in whom the incidence of postintubation subglottic stenosis remains high.[99] The average duration of nasotracheal intubation in *H. influenzae* epiglottitis is about 36 hours, although there is considerable individual variation.[100]

The use of expectant corticosteroid therapy to reduce inflammation and edema is becoming more common; although doubt remains whether this has any specific effect on the rate of resolution of the disease,[84] it may have a useful role in reducing postintubation sequelae. A more controversial aspect of steroid therapy in acute epiglottitis is reliance on this to reduce the edema to avoid the necessity for intubation or tracheostomy.[93, 98] This approach has received little support and, indeed, has been specifically condemned for management of childhood epiglottitis.[101] Undoubtedly, the safest option at this time is to provide an artificial airway for every child in whom a diagnosis of acute epiglottitis is made.

It must always be remembered that acute epiglottitis is an infectious disease and that contacts of the patient are at risk of developing *H. influenzae* infections, including meningitis. Accordingly, the immediate family and other intimate contacts of the patients, particularly children, should be offered rifampicin prophylaxis.[90]

In recently published series, there has been almost no mortality or serious complication reported from acute epiglottitis in children admitted directly to pediatric centers that follow this or a similar protocol. Patients transferred from other hospitals, especially those in whom an artificial airway had not been established prior to transfer, remain at risk of significant morbidity and mortality.[94]

DIPHTHERIA

This is an acute and deadly infectious disease that occurs primarily in children and is caused by *Corynebacterium diphtheriae.* Although the infection is limited to the nose, throat, larynx, and, occasionally, skin, profound systemic disturbances are caused by release of bacterial exotoxin. Fortunately, diphtheria has largely disappeared from the developed world since the adoption of universal active immunization, but it has not been wholly eradicated, as evidenced by continuing sporadic outbreaks,[102, 103] and it remains an endemic disease in some parts of the world.[104] In recent years, outbreaks in industrialized countries have generally occurred in subjects who were debilitated or immune deficient.[105] These events serve to remind us that epidemics of diphtheria may occur once again if universal active immunization lapses. Indeed, there is already some evidence that immunization programs are no longer applied as effectively as in the past.[106, 107] Diphtheria can be spread by asymptomatic carriers and can also be brought into a country by travelers or immigrants arriving from regions in which diphtheria is endemic.[108] Thus, the community is constantly at risk for reintroduction of infection. For these reasons, diphtheria cannot be disregarded, and it is important to maintain public health measures to ensure widespread immunity.[109, 110] It is equally necessary for physicians to maintain a degree of clinical awareness of this disease and its treatment.

Diphtheria occurs predominantly in temperate zones and, prior to universal immunization, was characterized by epidemics that occurred in all seasons but were more common in winter.

Children accounted for almost all the victims; it was uncommon before the age of 6 months due to transplacental transfer of maternal antibody, but the incidence thereafter increased to peak at about 6 years of age, with only a few cases occurring in children older than 10 years old. Although a greater number of cases occurred in girls, there was usually a higher mortality in boys, explained in part by a higher incidence of laryngeal involvement in boys.

While these epidemiological features would probably still hold true for an epidemic of diphtheria occurring in a nonimmunized community, even partial programs of immunization may have a significant effect on the population at risk. Thus, in one recent instance, the proportion of patients younger than 5 years old was shown to be dramatically decreased.[104] Recent outbreaks in Western communities have predominantly involved older patients and largely reflect individual immune deficiency (owing, for example, to the avoidance of active immunization for religious reasons) or have involved patients with generalized debility, alcoholism, and poor hygiene.[111, 112] In this latter group, almost all cases occurred as cutaneous diphtheria.

There are three morphological variants of *C. diphtheriae* (*mitis, intermedius,* and *gravis*), but the severity of the disease is entirely related to the degree to which the organism produces exotoxin, and there is no consistent relationship between morphological differences and toxigenicity. *C. diphtheriae* is usually transmitted by droplet, and the infection remains largely localized to the site of initial invasion, with the severity of the resulting illness depending on the systemic effects of the exotoxin. Nontoxigenic strains cause symptomatic diphtheria, but the clinical course is milder, shorter, and free from complications. The incubation period is short, 1 to 4 days. The prodromal period likewise is short: the patient initially complains of feeling unwell, perhaps with a sore throat and mild fever, but little is found on physical examination apart from mild infection of the pharynx. Within 12 to 24 hours, whitish spots appear on the tonsils, rapidly enlarging and coalescing so that by the second day the typical leathery pseudomembrane has appeared. This pseudomembrane consists of necrotic tissue, debris, and blood, and varies in color from dirty white to nearly black, with sharply defined margins. It is very adherent, and attempts to remove it will leave a raw and bleeding surface. At the same time, the systemic effects of the exotoxin may become obvious: organs particularly at risk are the heart and the peripheral nervous system.

Clinical evidence of myocardial involvement is seen in about 50 percent of all patients with diphtheria, and histological evidence of myocarditis can be demonstrated in almost all patients dying of this disease. Heart failure is a common mode of death. Peripheral nerve palsies occur in about one fifth of patients. Both local and systemic symptoms begin to subside by about the fifth day, but even after apparent complete resolution late cardiac and neurological complications may occur, although there are usually no permanent neurological or cardiac sequelae. Mortality rates of up to 30 percent were not uncommon before immunization. Death may occur at any time and is most commonly caused by respiratory obstruction or myocardial failure.

Variations of Diphtheria

1. *Malignant or "bull neck" diphtheria* is a particularly severe manifestation in which the disease follows an accelerated course, progressing to involve the entire pharynx, with swelling, necrosis, cervical lymphadenitis, and cellulitis. Toxemia is marked and mortality is high.
2. *Nasal diphtheria.* The infection is limited to the anterior nares and does not produce constitutional symptoms. The patient, however, is a carrier and as such is a great danger to the community and therefore must be sought out and treated to eradicate the infection.
3. *Laryngeal diphtheria.* In most patients, involvement of the larynx is by direct spread from the pharynx, but in a few the larynx is the primary site of infection and the patient's presenting complaints are of hoarseness and loss of voice. Patients with laryngeal diphtheria are at particular risk of respiratory obstruction, and the mortality is high.
4. *Cutaneous diphtheria* is more common in tropical than in temperate zones and occurs when otherwise insignificant skin wounds are invaded by *C. diphtheriae,* leading to chronic ulceration, membrane formation, and secondary toxic complications.

Treatment

The treatment of diphtheria, if it is to be effective in healing the patient and preventing spread of the disease, involves use of specific antitoxins, antibiotics, relief of respiratory obstruction, prolonged bed rest, isolation, and public health measures, including reimmunization of contacts and follow-up surveillance to detect carriers. When diphtheria is suspected, efforts must be made to confirm the diagnosis bacteriologically. Swabs should be taken from the pharynx before antibiotics are given. Definitive diagnosis will depend on the result of culture testing and therefore takes some time—if the diagnosis is made clinically, treatment with antitoxin (following all precautions for serum sensitivity) should begin as soon as possible, since the antitoxin will not neutralize toxin already bound to cells. Penicillin and erythromycin are effective in controlling the growth of *C. diphtheriae* and should be given along with the antitoxin. Bed rest is important and should continue for 2 to 3 weeks after local manifestations have resolved—that is, until the usual period has passed during which toxic myocarditis may occur.

Respiratory Obstruction in Diphtheria

The risk of respiratory obstruction is always present when there is pharyngeal membrane formation of moderate degree, and the risk increases if the membrane spreads to the glottis, larynx, and trachea. Even in the recovery period, sudden death may still occur by laryngeal obstruction owing to loosened membrane being aspirated from the pharynx or coughed up from the trachea.

Formerly, tracheostomy was reserved for severe diphtheritic respiratory obstruction and was frequently performed in circumstances of great urgency. With modern facilities, elective tracheostomy should be performed early in patients with any form of membranous pharyngitis, even before the onset of respiratory symptoms.[109] Indications for tracheostomy in these circumstances might include stridor, membrane extending beyond the tonsils to encroach on the periglottic tissues, and any other evidence of laryngeal involvement. If tracheostomy is delayed until evidence of respiratory obstruction or failure becomes apparent, it may be too late.[111] Emergency intubation of such patients is likely to be difficult due to involvement of the periglottic tissues and difficulty in clearing away the obstructing membrane. Should complete respiratory obstruction occur in patients with diphtheria, it will probably be better to proceed directly to cricothyroidotomy rather than to attempt intubation. Because of the high incidence of toxic myocarditis, general anesthesia is probably best avoided in these patients, and tracheostomy should be carried out using local infiltration anesthesia without prior intubation.

Prognosis

The outcome in diphtheria not only depends on the toxigenicity of the particular strain of *C. diphtheriae* involved and the degree of immunity possessed by the patient but also is related to the age of the patient, the location and extent of the membrane, the promptness of diagnosis, and specific antitoxin and antibiotic treatment. Older patients tend to do better than younger, probably because older persons have larger laryngeal airways and are therefore relatively more tolerant of partial obstruction. The spread of the membrane from the pharynx into the larynx and trachea is associated with a higher mortality. Mortality overall, however, is greatly reduced if the antitoxin is given early.

Other Conditions Causing Membranous Pharyngitis. Membranous pharyngitis is not pathognomonic of diphtheria, and similar pseudomembranes may be found in association with infection due to other members of the *Corynebacterium* family, for example *C. haemolyticum,* and in infectious mononucleosis, streptococcal pharyngitis, candidiasis, and Vincent's infection. However, in all these conditions, the membrane is much less adherent and does not leave a bleeding surface. Nonetheless, the potential for respiratory obstruction, although slight, is still present, and active airway management similar to that for diphtheria may be required. A similar but nonbacterial pharyngitis can be caused by oral ingestion of the herbicide paraquat.[113]

LARYNX AND TRACHEA

The immediate threat to the child with deformity or disease of the larynx is respiratory obstruction. Although the individual anatomical lesions may each be quite rare, laryngeal diseases are responsible for a great deal of morbidity and mortality in infancy and childhood. Improved endoscopy equipment, better understanding of etiological factors, more aggressive and refined surgical procedures, and much better postoperative care all have combined to improve this situation dramatically. Particularly in the treatment of acquired stenotic lesions of the larynx, laryngotracheal reconstructive surgical therapy using a variety of techniques is finding greater acceptance and offers better functional and cosmetic results than does the alternative of long-term tracheostomy.[114, 115]

Nonetheless, laryngeal obstructive problems remain a major challenge for pediatrician, laryngologist, anesthesiologist, and intensive care specialist. Congenital malformations and lesions involving the larynx are rare and usually cause respiratory symptoms at birth or shortly thereafter: acquired laryngeal diseases commonly occur in older children and are responsible for the general syndrome of croup. Some of the causes of laryngotracheal obstruction in children are shown in Table 11–3.

CONGENITAL LARYNGEAL ANOMALIES

Stridor, or noisy breathing, is the cardinal symptom of laryngeal obstruction but is not a diagnosis in itself and may have many different causes.[91, 115, 116] High-pitched inspiratory stridor suggests obstruction at the glottic or supraglottic level; addition of an expiratory component indicates a level below that of the glottis. Expiratory wheeze alone is associated with bronchial rather than laryngeal obstruction. The quality of the child's cry may give further evidence of the site of obstruction, in that the cry is usually weak or absent in laryngeal lesions (even when there is little respiratory obstruction). Hoarseness indicates a lesion at the level of the glottis.

The presence of stridor does not necessarily mean that respiratory distress will follow inevitably, but stridor along with signs of respiratory distress indicates that airway support probably will be necessary and adds urgency to the need for a definitive diagnosis. Signs of increasing respiratory distress in infants are a rising respiratory rate, flaring of the alae nasi, sternal indrawing, decreased breath sounds, head retraction, tachycardia, restlessness, and cyanosis. Overflow of saliva and aspiration pneumonia will also occur when there is interference with normal laryngeal protective functions.

The assessment of an infant with stridor requires considerable care because of the myriad causes of respiratory problems in this age group. In particular, the occurrence of stridor in an infant with respiratory distress cannot be assumed to indicate that the distress is due to a laryngeal lesion (although it could be). Nor should the absence of respiratory distress in the infant with stridor be assumed to mean that there is no danger, for in such patients otherwise trivial events such as a minor upper respiratory infection can provoke profound respiratory obstruction. For these reasons, it is necessary to make every effort to obtain a correct anatomical diagnosis and to assess the degree of respiratory obstruction accurately. A careful history and physical examination will help exclude other common causes of respiratory distress, notably congenital heart disease. When a laryngeal lesion is suspected, diagnostic clues may be gleaned from the degree of stridor, quality of the cry, presence or absence of palpable cervical masses, and diagnostic imaging. Definitive diagnosis usually requires laryngoscopy, and when respiratory distress exists this may have to be undertaken urgently.

Table 11–3. SOME CAUSES OF LARYNGOTRACHEAL OBSTRUCTION IN CHILDREN

Category	Example
Congenital (intralaryngeal)	Laryngomalacia
	Congenital subglottic stenosis
	Laryngeal web
	Laryngotracheal cleft
	Congenital laryngeal paralysis
	Congenital tumors
	Hemangioma
	Lymphangioma
	Saccular cyst
	Laryngocele
Congenital (extralaryngeal)	Macroglossia
	Cervical lymphangioma
Infection	Laryngotracheobronchitis
	Acute epiglottitis
	Diphtheria
	Infectious mononucleosis
	Pharyngeal abscess
Trauma	Inhaled foreign body
	Laryngeal edema
	Postintubation
	Chemical
	Thermal
	Acquired subglottic stenosis
	Cervical trauma
	Open
	Closed
Neoplasms	Laryngeal papillomatosis
	Extrinsic tumors of tongue and neck

LARYNGOMALACIA

This is the most common form of congenital laryngeal obstruction in infants, found in about 75 percent of all infants with stridor.[117] The laryngeal cartilages are abnormally soft and flexible, the epiglottis is long and narrow, and the aryepiglottic folds are short and floppy. In these patients, during inspiration, the supraglottic tissues tend to fold in toward the glottis, causing partial obstruction and the characteristic inspiratory noise. Thus, the supraglottic tissues act rather like a one-way valve. The etiology of this condition is unknown, and it is perhaps best considered a relative immaturity of the cartilages, representing no more than a slowing of normal development. Babies born with this condition usually have stridor from birth, or within a few days of birth, although it may be intermittent and tends to disappear during periods of rest and to be exaggerated during crying. The stridor is usually most marked when the infant lies on the back,[116] decreasing when the child lies prone with the neck extended. Respiratory distress is rare in laryngomalacia. Although a lateral neck radiograph will usually show a characteristic anterior and downward displacement of the aryepiglottic folds, definitive diagnosis is made by laryngoscopy in the awake patient. The characteristic appearances on endoscopy have prompted the alternative name of *inspiratory laryngeal collapse* for this condition.

Laryngomalacia almost always runs a benign course, and symptoms tend to disappear with growth, usually by about 18 months of age. Treatment is rarely required, and there are no long-term sequelae. However, in a very small proportion of cases, severe respiratory obstruction does occur, and in these patients airway support is necessary, which in the past has invariably meant long-term tracheostomy. Epiglottoplasty,[118] or suture of the epiglottis to the base of the tongue,[119] in those in whom the laryngomalacia is secondary to excessive tissue in the posterior aryepiglottic region, or laser division of the aryepiglottic folds for those in whom these are shortened, may enable tracheostomy to be avoided.

Another, much rarer form of congenital laryngeal cartilage dystrophy is the complete absence of the epiglottis. This does not cause respiratory obstruction, but inadequate protection of the glottis during swallowing causes choking and persistent aspiration pneumonia.

Tracheomalacia is a similar condition of decreased cartilaginous rigidity affecting the trachea, producing the same sort of obstructive symptoms as does laryngomalacia. It may be associated with tracheoesophageal fistula or vascular ring or may be seen as an isolated defect. The treatment of choice is aortopexy to reduce the degree of tracheal collapse.

Congenital Laryngeal Web

Obstruction of the larynx by membranous webs or partial fusion of the cords is a very rare cause of stridor in infants.[120] Commonly the web occurs at the level of the cords and may consist of a thin membrane lying across the cords, a thick web, or a partial fusion in which the cords are firmly joined together. The supraglottic web, the most common form of this defect, is a partial fusion of the false cords. In extreme cases there is total obstruction by a web, which is incompatible with life unless immediately recognized and treated at birth. A few cases have been reported in which immediate tracheostomy or forceful bronchoscopy has been successful in resuscitation of infants with this anomaly. It is likely that laryngeal atresia is the cause of occasional stillbirths in which the respiratory obstruction has gone unrecognized, and this may be true even after routine autopsy in which the larynx is often only superficially examined.[121] Laryngeal webs produce symptoms of respiratory obstruction proportional to the degree of narrowing, and definitive diagnosis is made by laryngoscopy.

Treatment depends on the severity of obstruction. Thin, membranous anterior webs may be divided by simple surgical incision or by use of the carbon dioxide laser,[122] possibly followed by repeated laryngeal dilatation. Thicker, stronger webs will usually require temporary stenting to prevent recurrence; the most severe forms are probably best repaired by open laryngofissure and insertion of a glottic keel. The risk of recurrence is high, and, unless meticulous technique is followed, including mucosal grafting of all raw areas created by dissection of the web, there is also a high probability of permanent voice impairment. Such operations are probably better left until considerable growth of the larynx has taken place, although this also increases the possibility of acquired subglottic stenosis secondary to the prolonged tracheostomy.[123]

Congenital Subglottic Stenosis

Soft tissue thickening of the larynx, usually most marked 2 to 3 mm below the level of the true cords, and possibly accompanied by a narrowed cricoid diameter, may produce biphasic stridor and other symptoms of respiratory obstruction shortly after birth, depending on the severity. In some patients the onset of symptoms of subglottic stenosis may be delayed for 6 months or longer.[99] Indeed, mild cases may remain asymptomatic but are at risk of developing laryngeal obstruction secondary to upper airway infection or edema. Such cases may present first because of recurrent episodes of laryngotracheobronchitis or are noted to require a smaller than usual endotracheal tube at the time of operation for an unrelated condition. This anomaly may be associated with other congenital anomalies, particularly Down's syndrome[124] and congenital heart disease.

Diagnosis is confirmed by endoscopy, and treatment depends on the severity of the obstruction. Mild cases require no active treatment, whereas more severe forms may be treated by repeated endoscopic dilatation,[125] although the efficacy of this has been questioned.[99] Infants with persisting severe respiratory obstruction will require either tracheostomy[115] or open laryngeal reconstruction (which is discussed later with acquired laryngeal stenosis). In general, the prognosis is good, with gradual lessening of stenosis with growth, and eventual achievement of normal laryngeal patency without serious sequelae.[126] However, patients who require tracheostomy are less fortunate, having the added risk of developing a secondary, and often intractable, acquired subglottic stenosis.

Congenital Tracheal Stenosis

Congenital tracheal stenosis is a rare and usually lethal condition, often found in association with other gross anomalies, in which the trachea is narrow, rigid, and inelastic. Infants so affected present with symptoms of respiratory obstruction at birth or shortly thereafter, and diagnosis is confirmed by bronchoscopy. Although temporary improvement may be obtained from endoscopic dilatation, respiratory failure inevitably occurs. The only prospect for lasting improvement is permanent enlargement of the stenotic segment by tracheoplasty. Anesthesia is particularly hazardous for these patients because tracheostomy will be of no help (unless the distal trachea is not involved in the stenosis) should control and patency of the airway be lost, and efforts to overcome obstruction by endotracheal intubation are prone to produce complete respiratory obstruction unless the greatest care is taken in sizing and placement of the tube. For this reason, if this diagnosis is suspected every effort must be made to minimize trauma to the trachea by endoscope or tube lest subsequent edema cause complete ventilatory obstruction.

Management of ventilation during tracheoplasty will present considerable problems and will require careful planning and total cooperation between surgeon and anesthesiologist: in some cases it may be better to avoid these problems entirely by electing to perform the operation with cardiopulmonary bypass, which will also give the advantage of better surgical access.[127]

Laryngotracheoesophageal Cleft

This is a very rare family of congenital anomalies in which there is incomplete separation of the larynx from the esophagus. The degree of malformation varies from simple absence of the interarytenoid muscle, producing only mild symptoms, to complete fusion of the larynx, trachea, and esophagus into one tube in the most severe form,[128] with extension of the defect into a bronchus also being possible.[129] Between these extremes, intermediate degrees of cleft are represented by failure of posterior fusion of the cricoid and possibly the first one or two tracheal cartilages.

The infant presents with a clinical picture similar to that of tracheoesophageal fistula (which may coexist in about 20 percent of these patients). The most prominent features are respiratory distress aggravated by feeding, profuse pharyngeal secretions, choking, and aspiration pneumonia; stridor may or may not be present. A wide variety of other congenital anomalies occur in association with laryngotracheoesophageal cleft. The endoscopic appearances are confusing and difficult to interpret and frequently fail to provide the diagnosis.[128] A diagnosis is best made by probing the posterior wall of the larynx during rigid endoscopy, when parting of the mucosal folds may not only reveal the cleft but also allow its extent to be determined.[129, 129a, 130]

Tracheostomy to secure the airway is comparatively ineffective except in very minor degrees of cleft, because of the propensity for the tracheostomy tube to find its way through the cleft and into the esophagus. The same problem may well be encountered with endotracheal intubation, and extreme care must be taken in placing, securing, and maintaining the airway.

In all but the mildest cases, there is little alternative to early reconstructive surgery. In some cases the cleft can be repaired intraluminally, using the suspension laryngoscope and simply suturing the mucosal defect, but if this is not possible, or if such repair persistently breaks down, then correction by an open operation will be required, in which case a lateral pharyngotomy is made and the larynx reconstructed over a tracheal tube that remains in place postoperatively as a stent. A gastrostomy is maintained throughout the period of healing. Anesthetic management largely revolves around airway maintenance[131] and may involve various changes in approach during operation—for example, insertion of a sterile tracheal tube through the wound directly into the distal trachea may offer better surgical access to the larynx during the early stages of repair. As far as possible the details of the operation and the options and procedures for airway management must be planned in advance by surgeon and anesthesiologist together. Theoretically, cardiopulmonary bypass might be used to secure good operating conditions without the need for ventilation, but the very long duration of these operations, along with the additional morbidity due to cardiopulmonary bypass itself, would have to be weighed carefully against the potential advantage.

Such reconstructions are technically very difficult, and the relative avascularity of the tissues involved makes the repair prone to necrosis and breakdown. Nonetheless, an increasing number of successful neonatal reconstructions have been reported.[129, 129a, 131]

LARYNGOCELES AND CONGENITAL LARYNGEAL CYSTS

Epithelium lined simple cystic tumors of the larynx are rare causes of respiratory obstruction in children and may occur in one of two forms: laryngocele or congenital laryngeal cyst.[132] A laryngocele is an abnormal development of the saccular appendage of the laryngeal ventricle and communicates freely with the lumen of the larynx. This free communication accounts for the most remarkable feature of the laryngocele, that is, the great variation in size that can take place rapidly with changes in intralaryngeal pressure. On the other hand, congenital laryngeal cysts, or saccular cysts, although also arising from the saccular appendage, do not communicate with the laryngeal cavity and are fluid filled.

Laryngeal symptoms are proportional to the degree of respiratory obstruction, and investigation is largely by radiology and endoscopy, but definitive diagnosis is frequently evasive and may require repeated examination. Laryngoscopy may occasionally provoke a sudden increase in size (due to bleeding or edema) and cause severe respiratory obstruction. Such obstruction, however, can usually be relieved by endoscopic aspiration of the cyst, although relief is likely to be temporary as recurrence after aspiration is almost invariable. A better approach is endoscopic unroofing of the cyst with removal of the lining epithelium,[133] and the carbon dioxide laser may offer advantages for this.[134] Occasionally extralaryngeal operation through the neck may be necessary.[116]

Other congenital cystic swellings in the neck, for example cystic hygroma, also may cause laryngeal obstruction either by external compression or by extension into it.

CONGENITAL LARYNGEAL PARALYSIS

Neurogenic paralysis of the vocal cords is the second most common cause of congenital laryngeal obstruction:[116] it may arise from a variety of primary causes and is often associated with gross anomalies in other systems. The respiratory obstruction may be apparent at birth or, when resulting from expanding lesions elsewhere, there may be a considerable delay in onset of symptoms. Among central causes of laryngeal paralysis are intracerebral hemorrhage, cerebral agenesis, myelomeningocele with Arnold-Chiari malformation, and hydrocephalus, and in these cases spontaneous resolution of the paralysis may follow reduction of intracranial pressure.[135] Peripheral motor nerves may be damaged by birth trauma or by involvement in congenital lesions in the mediastinum and neck[136] or may be damaged during operations to relieve other congenital problems, for example during thoracotomy for repair of heart and esophageal malformations. In many cases a definite cause cannot be identified, and the paralysis is often temporary. Half of all patients with unilateral congenital cord paralysis eventually recover fully, as does a rather smaller proportion, about a third, of those with bilateral paralysis. As a general rule, the longer the duration of paralysis the poorer the prognosis. Symptoms are proportional to the severity of the obstruction and the degree of laryngeal incompetence, the infant presenting with varying degrees of stridor, respiratory distress, dysphagia, and aspiration pneumonia. Dysphonia is uncommon. Diagnosis is best made by awake laryngoscopy with careful observation of cord motility, while a definitive neurological origin may be confirmed by electrodiagnostic studies.[115]

Unilateral paralysis, which is usually caused by a peripheral lesion, is more common than bilateral paralysis, and the left side is more commonly affected than the right, presumably because the longer course of the recurrent laryngeal nerve on the left exposes it to greater risk of damage. Unilateral lesions are often associated with quite severe feeding problems, marked by coughing and choking. Accompanying stridor may be dependent on position—lessening or even disappearing when the infant lies on the affected side. Bilateral paralysis usually indicates a central nervous system cause: respiratory obstructive symptoms are more obvious and of greater degree than in unilateral paralysis.

The need for treatment is determined by the degrees of respiratory obstruction and laryngeal incompetence. In some cases of isolated unilateral paralysis, no treatment is required, and good phonation can develop by compensation by the normal cord, even without recovery on the affected side. Teflon injection of the paralyzed cord will bring it to a more medial position, improving laryngeal competence in unilateral paralysis. However, tracheostomy inevitably will be required if there are persisting problems of respiratory obstruction or continuing aspiration. Arytenoidectomy to remove the obstructive component should be delayed for several years to allow for spontaneous recovery. Alternatively, the use of innervated muscle pedicle grafts to restore function is possible.[137]

Congenital Hemangioma

Laryngeal and subglottic hemangiomas commonly occur in association with similar cutaneous lesions[138] and should be suspected in any child with a strawberry nevus in the head region who also develops stridor. Girls are affected twice as frequently as boys. Obstructive symptoms generally appear before 6 months of age and are first noticed as stridor during crying; these tend to worsen as the tumor grows. Phonation is not affected as the hemangioma lies below, and does not involve, the cords, so this diagnosis should be suspected in any baby with a history of intermittent respiratory obstruction but a normal cry. Diagnosis is confirmed by radiography of the airway, possibly helped by contrast radiography of the esophagus, and by endoscopy. However endoscopic diagnosis is not always easy, because the overlying mucosa is normal and the angioma empties as pressure is applied so that inspection with a laryngoscope may show only an apparently normal larynx.

The growth of the tumor is usually limited, and most laryngeal hemangiomas tend to regress, many patients becoming asymptomatic by the age of 2 years. However, it is difficult to predict the behavior of any individual hemangioma, and repeated endoscopy is required to follow the progression of the disease. Spontaneous bleeding from these tumors is not a problem, nor does bleeding usually occur during diagnostic laryngoscopy or tracheal intubation.[139] The combination of the natural history of the disease tending to spontaneous regression, along with the often unsatisfactory results of operation, indicates that treatment should be conservative and limited to those patients in whom the degree of respiratory obstruction makes relief imperative. Endoscopic resection, using the carbon dioxide laser in preference to sharp dissection so that bleeding is minimized, may completely obliterate the lesion, particularly if it is relatively small and well localized,[140] although attempted removal of larger tumors by this means may be complicated by postoperative subglottic stenosis.[141, 142] Other forms of treatment that have been advocated include radiotherapy,[143] although there remains considerable apprehension about the long-term neoplastic complications of laryngeal radiation,[144] and intralesional injection of steroids.[145]

LARYNGEAL TUMORS

Simple squamous papillomas, although rare, are the most common laryngeal tumors in children and may be seen as multiple or discrete lesions.

Juvenile Papillomatosis

Multiple papillomas (juvenile laryngeal papillomatosis) may occur at any age but are most often seen in children between the ages of 5 and 15 years and usually present initially with hoarseness. These tumors, although benign, are aggressive in growth and local spread.[146] They tend to recur frequently and rapidly and may spread through the larynx, pharynx, and trachea and occasionally into lung tissue itself. Their presence within the laryngotracheal tract presents a constant and serious threat of respiratory obstruction, and overall mortality may be in excess of 10 percent. The natural history of these tumors is that of variable and unpredictable growth. Long periods of quiescence may be ended by a sudden outburst of activity, and apparently good initial results from local therapy may not be maintained, making evaluation of different treatment modalities particularly difficult and necessitating long-term follow-up even after apparent complete regression. Although it is widely believed that in most cases the disease tends to regress and disappear around the time of puberty, this may not always be true.[147]

These tumors are now known to be of viral etiology. The human papilloma virus has been shown to be associated with a wide variety of epithelial lesions, including invasive carcinomas,[148] and virus-containing respiratory cancers have been identified in patients who have had laryngeal papillomatosis,[149] although malignant change in papillomatosis is rare. The identification of a viral cause for laryngeal papillomas has provoked interest in augmenting surgical treatment by modification of the patient's immune response[150] or by antiviral therapy, but the effectiveness of these approaches remains unproved.[151]

The mainstay of treatment is repeated endoscopic removal, using the microscope, and removing the tumors either by sharp dissection using forceps or, preferably, the carbon dioxide laser, which is more accurate and therefore causes less damage to the surrounding tissues. Even after apparent complete removal, recurrence is likely, and if the papillomatous mass becomes very big, respiratory obstruction may dictate the need for tracheostomy. Unfortunately, this brings the added danger of papillomas seeding to the tracheostomy site itself,[152] and so tracheostomy should be avoided if at all possible. In spite of the undoubted advances in endoscopic microsurgery, the treatment of juvenile laryngeal papillomatosis remains frustrating and achieves little more than control of the growth of the tumors until, in most cases, spontaneous regression occurs. The prognosis appears to be less favorable when the disease first occurs in infancy.[153] Anesthesia management for resection will be discussed later.

Vocal Cord Nodules

Vocal cord nodules, which are fairly common in adults as "singer's nodes," are less common in childhood, in which they are possibly better described as "screamer's nodes." The usual presentation is of hoarseness in a child with a history of voice abuse.[119] These nodules are harmless and are treated conservatively in the first instance by voice rest and speech therapy. Very occasionally persistent nodules require surgical removal. Postintubation granulomas are similar in most respects to singers' nodes but tend to not resolve spontaneously and generally require surgical removal.

Malignant Tumors of the Larynx

Malignancy arising in the larynx in childhood is exceedingly rare but not unknown[154] as is involvement of the airway in malignancy arising in other tissues of the neck.[155]

ACQUIRED STRUCTURAL DEFECTS OF THE LARYNX

Acquired Subglottic Stenosis

The commonest cause of acquired subglottic stenosis, which is usually more severe than the congenital form,[115] is prolonged tracheal intubation. The premature infant with respiratory distress syndrome is particularly at risk, and better survival rates for such infants have been paralleled by an increased incidence of postintubation subglottic stenosis. This may affect up to one tenth of all neonates requiring ventilator support. Much less frequently subglottic stenosis occurs as a complication of tracheostomy, particularly when it is performed at a high level; direct laryngeal trauma; aspiration of caustic liquids; and respiratory burns.[156, 157]

Most acquired stenoses are at the level of the cricoid cartilage. Initially, mucosal ulceration and necrosis occur where the tracheal tube lies against the glottis posteriorly or in the region of the cricoid ring: such ulceration may take place very quickly, within 1 or 2 days of initial intubation, and may be aggravated by mechanical trauma and infection. Later, healing with fibrosis and consequent narrowing of the larynx occurs.[99] Subglottic stenosis is more likely after prolonged intubation but may occur even after a period of a week or less.[158] Careful attention to correct size, design, and material of the tracheal tube, along with adequate fixation so that there is the least possible movement of the tube in relation to the larynx, will greatly reduce the incidence, but not eliminate the risk, of stenosis, regardless of whether the oral or nasal route is used.[159] The stenosis may be apparent at the time of attempted extubation, but more usually there is a variable interval between extubation and onset of symptoms of respiratory obstruction.

In contrast to congenital subglottic stenosis, the acquired form does not tend to resolve and is much more difficult to manage. The need for treatment is likely to span years rather than months. Almost all patients with acquired subglottic stenosis will require tracheostomy (unless treated by immediate reconstructive surgical therapy), compared with fewer than 50 percent of those with congenital subglottic stenosis. Thus there is an inevitably higher degree of associated morbidity and mortality, and mortality rates in infants with acquired stenosis and long-term tracheostomy have been reported as high as 24 percent.[160]

The treatment of acquired subglottic stenosis is difficult, and many differing methods have been explored. In general, the initial approach is a conservative one, similar to the management of congenital subglottic stenosis: tracheostomy to maintain the airway while the patient undergoes repeated endoscopic dilatations. The aim each time is to achieve sufficient stretching to increase the airway diameter while simultaneously avoiding any degree of trauma sufficient to cause more scarring and hence the possibility of increased stenosis. If the airway grows satisfactorily, the patient may be decannulated without any other treatment, but failure of the airway to enlarge will indicate a need for surgical intervention, which may involve anything from repeated scar excision by sharp dissection, cautery, or laser, to laryngotracheoplasty.[161] Successful treatment following this plan requires considerable judgment, because overenthusiastic dilatation may simply cause further scarring and eventual worsening of the degree of stenosis.

With conservative treatment it may be difficult to know when decannulation of the trachea will be tolerated, and indeed restoration of the tracheostomy may be required weeks, or even months, after apparently successful decannulation.[126] If the stenosis persists in spite of repeated dilatation, surgical reconstruction of the larynx offers the only hope of avoiding permanent tracheostomy. A wide variety of techniques has been used, but recent reports suggest that ultimate successful decannulation can be expected in 80 to 90 percent of laryngeal reconstructions.[114, 162]

Possible operations include laryngofissure with grafting, open laryngotracheoplasty, and vertical incision of the cricoid cartilage with insertion of a cartilage graft to maintain a wider lumen.[163] These operations do not remove the need for prolonged postoperative tracheostomy and are burdened by all the complications thereof. This fact, along with the relatively poor results of conservative treatment of acquired subglottic stenosis, has encouraged attempts at immediate surgical correction of acquired stenoses with avoidance of tracheostomy. This is possible by the anterior cricoid split operation,[164, 165] in which the cricoid cartilage and upper trachea are exposed in the neck and a vertical midline incision made through the cricoid cartilage and mucosa down onto the tracheal tube, and extended downward through the first two tracheal rings. No effort is made to close the incision by grafting or other means. The tracheal tube is left in place as a stent, and every effort is made to minimize further laryngeal trauma, including in some instances keeping the patient paralyzed and artificially ventilated. The endotracheal tube can usually be removed after 7 to 10 days.

Post-traumatic laryngeal stenosis that occurs in association with blunt cervical trauma can be among the most difficult of all to treat, particularly in small children. Excision of the scarred area and medium to long-term use of a prosthetic stent may be required.[166]

Anesthetic management of laryngeal reconstruction of this type is usually straightforward, as a secure airway in the form of the tracheostomy is already available. Some anesthesiologists prefer to pass an endotracheal tube through the tracheostomy to facilitate positive-pressure ventilation, but particular care in positioning and securing the tube must be taken lest it become displaced during operation, and provision for easy intraoperative suctioning must be made. A suitable-sized reinforced endotracheal tube that is sutured to the skin adjacent to the tracheostomy is often very satisfactory. This can be isolated from the surgical site by means of a sterile plastic adhesive dressing. Access to the patient will be limited during operation, so all monitors and intravascular lines must be well tested and secured before starting.

ACQUIRED LARYNGEAL PARALYSIS

The distinction between congenital and acquired is of little importance, for the results of acquired laryngeal paralysis are in all respects similar to those of congenital laryngeal paralysis. The investigation and treatment are the same. Causes of acquired vocal cord paralysis in children include surgical trauma (particularly associated with mediastinal operations and thyroid surgery), blunt trauma to the neck, and compression by cervical tumors. Laryngeal paralysis is usually unilateral and may be asymptomatic or present as hoarseness. The diagnosis is confirmed by awake indirect endoscopic examination, which reveals an immobile cord fixed in an intermediate position.

ANESTHETIC CONSIDERATIONS IN LARYNGOSCOPY

Of all therapeutic interventions requiring general anesthesia in infants and children, few have greater potential than laryngoscopy for producing danger for the patient, urgent problems for the anesthesiologist, and considerable difficulty for the operator. Disaster can strike with great rapidity if respiratory obstruction occurs, and when this happens, tragedy can be averted only by rapid action. The appropriate action demands a clear understanding of what is happening and immediate implementation of predetermined plans to deal with complications.

The particular problems associated with laryngoscopy include the following:

1. The airway has to be shared between operator and anesthesiologist, but the anesthesiologist must ensure constant control of the airway lest the patient's safety be compromised.
2. Adequate alveolar ventilation must be maintained despite the upper airway pathology and the additional obstruction due to surgical instruments and manipulations.
3. During the operation, blood and debris must be removed to prevent its aspiration into the lower respiratory tract.
4. Laryngoscopy and the operation are compromised if there is any movement. Reflex coughing, bucking, laryngospasm, or indeed any movement must be suppressed.
5. Sophisticated instruments and operative techniques (for example, the carbon dioxide laser) demand special considerations and add further constraints to anesthetic management.
6. Speedy recovery of protective reflexes at the end of operation is essential, unless an artificial airway is to remain in place.
7. Severe respiratory obstruction may arise in the postoperative period because of laryngeal edema.
8. Finally, it is usually essential to view the structures as the patient is breathing spontaneously. Dynamic airway obstruction (e.g., due to laryngomalacia or tracheomalacia) will not be detected during controlled or assisted ventilation.

These sometimes apparently conflicting requirements can be met only by cooperation and understanding between anesthesiologist and surgeon and require that each be fully aware of the other's problems, plans, and actions. Many different anesthetic techniques have been described for laryngoscopy, and none is ideal in all respects. The choice of technique of anesthetic management will depend on the nature of the disease and the planned operative procedure. Precise details will have to be matched to the individual patient. However, certain general principles apply and are discussed in the following paragraphs.

DIAGNOSTIC LARYNGOSCOPY IN NEONATES

The usual indication for laryngoscopy is the presence of stridor, and a proper endoscopic examination requires evaluation of vocal cord movements as well as inspection of laryngeal anatomy. This requires observation of the glottis during normal inspiration and expiration and during phonation or crying. For these reasons, and because newborn infants often tolerate awake laryngoscopy surprisingly well, general anesthesia is not used. However, because there is always danger of provoking respiratory arrest or obstruction, the examination should take place in a fully equipped operating room, with the assistance of an anesthesiologist to monitor the baby. The anesthesiologist should be prepared to intubate and ventilate the patient should respiratory problems arise, or to induce anesthesia should tracheostomy or other operation become indicated.

Although general anesthesia is not often required, these patients should be given atropine prior to the examination. Reflex bradycardia commonly occurs from stimulation of the larynx, and reduction of secretions contributes to the ease of endoscopy. During neonatal laryngoscopy, the tip of the blade should be placed in the vallecula; if the blade is inserted under the epiglottis it not infrequently fixes the right cord, and this could be misinterpreted as right-sided vocal paralysis.

If a more complete examination of the respiratory tract is planned, sometimes it is appropriate to anesthetize the patient for this examination and then to view the movement of the vocal cords as the patient emerges from anesthesia.

DIAGNOSTIC DIRECT LARYNGOSCOPY IN OLDER INFANTS AND CHILDREN

Older infants and children will not readily tolerate awake laryngoscopy, and general anesthesia is required. In order to allow the endoscopist an unimpeded view of the glottis, it is preferable to avoid intubation, and this is most readily accommodated using volatile anesthesia agents and having the patient maintain spontaneous ventilation throughout the examination. Sedative premedications should be avoided in patients with obstructive respiratory symptoms, but atropine should be given for the reasons outlined earlier. Anesthesia is induced with oxygen and halothane, with or without the addition of nitrous oxide. When the patient is deeply anesthetized, the anesthetic is continued with halothane and oxygen alone and the glottic area sprayed with lidocaine (maximum dose, 4 mg/kg). After a further few minutes of oxygen and halothane, the face mask is removed and endoscopy can take place. With the face mask removed, the level of anesthesia begins to lighten but usually there is sufficient time to allow adequate examination of the laryngeal anatomy. Maintaining the endoscope in place as the level of anesthesia lightens also allows movements of the cords to be observed. During laryngoscopy, oxygen and halothane can be delivered to the pharynx by catheter.

Throughout the procedure the patient must be monitored fully and carefully. At any sign of respiratory inadequacy the laryngoscope should be removed and the child ventilated, using face mask and bag if possible, or if not possible then the airway should be secured by intubation or by rigid bronchoscope and the patient ventilated. Again, if the endoscopy shows the need for immediate tracheostomy or other operative intervention, the patient should be intubated and anesthesia continued according to the requirements of the particular operation.

Most pediatric laryngologists prefer rigid endoscopes for diagnostic investigation of the upper airway in infants and children. However, some find the transnasal use of small flexible fiberoptic bronchoscopes to be efficient even in infants and claim excellent visualization of the supraglottic and subglottic structures.[167]

Anesthesia for Suspension Microlaryngoscopy

The combination of suspension laryngoscopy and a microscope is commonly used for both diagnostic and operative purposes. Preoperative sedative drugs should be avoided in patients with preexisting respiratory obstruction, who should be given atropine alone. Endotracheal tubes and a rigid bronchoscope of appropriate size should be available, and the patient must be fully monitored to allow immediate detection of ventilatory inadequacy. Good conditions for general diagnostic and operative laryngoscopy are obtained by maintenance of spontaneous ventilation using inhalation agents.[168] This technique allows the minimum of competition between surgeon and anesthesiologist for access to the airway, along with retention of normal laryngeal function, which greatly eases the interpretation of any apparently abnormal appearances and movements of the airway structures. Other advantages claimed for this method include excellent surgical access, a quiet and unreactive glottis, reduced postoperative coughing and edema, and a history of safety in use.

Following induction with nitrous oxide, oxygen, and halothane, the glottis is sprayed with lidocaine in an appropriate dosage, and a small endotracheal tube or catheter[169] is passed through the cords. Anesthesia is continued by insufflation of oxygen and halothane, with a constant check being made to ensure that the tube does not become obstructed by surgical manipulation. An alternative method of insufflation is to use a side channel incorporated in the laryngoscope blade. If the trachea is intubated, it is important that the size of the tube be such that it does not impede the surgeon's access to the particular area of the larynx in which she or he is interested. Anesthetic gases emerging from the mouth can be scavenged by means of a suction apparatus.

Following operative interventions in the larynx, edema is likely and may cause significantly increased obstruction. Postoperative laryngeal edema may not be entirely avoidable, but it can be reduced by maintaining a meticulous and gentle approach to laryngeal manipulations and dissection. Its effects can be minimized in the immediate postoperative period by routine administration of humidified gases by mask or tent.

Many alternative techniques for ventilation of the lungs during operative laryngoscopy have been described, and the relative merits of each remain a matter of some controversy. Among these are the jet ventilation system, which has the advantages of offering an unobstructed view of the larynx and enabling good alveolar ventilation in a paralyzed but unintubated patient. Its disadvantage, particularly in the presence of laryngeal obstruction or if the tip of the injector is in the trachea rather than in the laryngoscope,[170, 171] is the potential for producing very high airway pressures, with the risk of mediastinal emphysema, tension pneumothorax, and death. The risk of barotrauma is increased in the smaller-diameter airways of children, and for this reason jet ventilation is generally considered unsuitable for use in children,[172] although, because of the absolute immobility of the cords ensured in the paralyzed patient, some advocate it as the technique of choice for laser surgery even in smaller children.[173]

High-frequency ventilation using a small-bore catheter within the trachea has been suggested as a safer technique than jet ventilation,[174, 175] providing the same advantages of good surgical access and reliable alveolar ventilation without the risk of barotrauma, although its usefulness in children remains largely unexplored. Intubation of the trachea using a relatively small-bore cuffed tube to allow controlled ventilation and muscle paralysis during laryngoscopy has been used in adults but is not a suitable technique for small children because of the relative sizes of tube and trachea.

LASER SURGERY

Lasers, particularly the carbon dioxide laser, offer several potential advantages to the surgeon that have made this instrument particularly useful in operations of the airway. Among these qualities are an intrinsic hemostatic effect, precision of dissection, and reduced tissue reactivity and scarring. At the same time it is acknowledged that the laser has the potential to produce great harm if used inappropriately or in unskilled hands.[134, 176] The advantages offered are of particular benefit in laryngotracheal surgery and the CO_2 laser is now a well-established tool for the pediatric laryngologist, particularly in the treatment of choanal atresia, laryngotracheal and nasal papillomas, laryngeal webs and stenoses, and subglottic hemangiomas. Laser technology is constantly expanding, and other forms—for example argon and KTP lasers—are also being used for specific applications in surgical therapy of the head and neck.

Energy from the laser is concentrated into a very narrow beam, which is invisible but otherwise acts like light, that is, it will be reflected from metallic and other surfaces until it reaches a material that will absorb its energy, converting it to heat. It is this heat that produces the destructive tissue effect. These properties produce several problems for the anesthesiologist, chief of which is the danger of fire in the airway, especially in the presence of high local concentrations of oxygen.[177] Rubber or plastic tracheal tubes are liable to ignite if struck directly by the laser beam. Plastic tubes are best avoided entirely: foil wrapped red rubber tubes are theoretically more acceptable but technically difficult to assemble and use in small sizes, and a preferred solution is to use one of the metallic tubes now available[178] or to avoid the use of a tracheal tube entirely. This may be achieved by employing the technique of spontaneous ventilation and topical anesthesia described earlier, or by using high-frequency jet ventilation by a metal catheter.[173] The latter method may direct smoke and debris down into the tracheobronchial tree but in practice this hazard seems more theoretical than real. Precise focusing enables laser dissection also to be very precise, but accuracy is possible only if the patient is absolutely immobile: deep anesthesia or anesthesia with muscle paralysis is required.[179] The concentration of oxygen in the inspired gases should be reduced and nitrous oxide discontinued while the laser is in use.

In addition to these specific airway considerations, general precautions to ensure the safety of all personnel in the operating room are required, and these include occlusive protection for the patient's eyes and the wearing of filtering goggles by all others present. The risk of random reflection can be greatly reduced by ensuring that all metal surfaces near the operation site are matte black. The occurrence of fire in the airway demands immediate action: the tube must be removed at once and all gases discontinued until the fire is extinguished.

LARYNGOTRACHEAL TRAUMA

Injuries to the neck may involve the larynx or cervical trachea, or both. Unfortunately, children are not immune to such accidents, although serious injury to the laryngotracheal airway in the neck is uncommon. Open injuries of the neck are usually the result of automobile accidents and are most commonly caused by laceration by broken glass; they almost always involve injuries to other systems and organs, so that evaluation of the degree of airway involvement may present considerable diagnostic difficulty.[180] Other forms of open wounds of the neck, such as the suicidal cut throat or gunshot wounds, are mostly met in older patients but are not unknown in children.[181] The larynx is less at risk in this type of injury than is the cervical trachea, being relatively well protected by the laryngeal cartilages. The larynx also can be severely damaged by compression against the cervical spine, even in the absence of any external evidence of injury to the neck. In many ways this is more dangerous than an open neck injury, for it is easy to overlook closed injury since the symptoms and signs may be confusing and often do not correspond well with the degree of disruption of the airway.[182] Such laryngeal fractures may be caused by sharp blows on the front of the neck, such as might be sustained by running against a taut rope or wire or falling against the edge of a table or across the handlebar of a bicycle.

Although tracheal damage in these circumstances usually takes the form of longitudinal tears, laryngeal damage may involve complete anatomical disruption, with dislocation of the arytenoid cartilages and disruption of the cricoarytenoid joints, so that the arytenoid itself may obstruct the glottis. Respiratory obstruction by such injuries will be further aggravated by the associated bleeding, swelling, and edema formation.

In large open wounds, involvement of the larynx or trachea may be obvious on inspection, but subcutaneous emphysema, dyspnea, hoarseness, coughing, and hemoptysis are all signs of airway involvement, and the onset of respiratory distress with stridor or cyanosis is evidence of critical respiratory obstruction. Voice change after a blow on the neck almost always signifies laryngeal damage. Anterior cervical emphysema can quickly produce a dangerous vicious circle in which increasing respiratory obstruction causes increased respiratory effort and further increases the air leak, which in turn increases the emphysema. Positive-pressure ventilation, struggling, and coughing also will increase the degree of emphysema. There is no constant relationship between the degree of injury and the degree of emphysema.

Isolated damage to the airway is unlikely in cervical injuries, owing to the concentration of vital structures within the neck. Associated injuries that may add to the difficulties of managing these patients include gross hemorrhage, arterial or venous or both, with the possibility of cerebral ischemia if the carotid vessels are involved or compressed;[183] air embolization through torn cervical veins; pneumothorax where penetrating neck wounds involve the dome of the pleura; and cervical spine injury.

Surgical Management

Injuries to the larynx and trachea are usually fairly simple to repair. Tracheal injuries require little more than suturing. Even quite complex laryngeal fractures are reconstructed by wiring: a good potential for recovery of function exists if they are treated early.[184] In general, a tracheostomy is performed below the level of the injury and the air leak closed with reconstruction of the airway. If possible, the use of a stent is avoided. The tracheostomy is maintained until healing is complete. However, the operation in cervical trauma is rarely limited to the airway. There are likely to be associated injuries to the blood vessels, pharynx, and esophagus, and such injuries must be sought and treated at the same time the airway is repaired. Esophageal tears, in particular, cause a marked increase in morbidity and mortality if overlooked.

Initial Airway Management

Emergency resuscitation of patients with cervical wounds who develop respiratory distress presents an urgent problem of restoration of the airway. Unfortunately, it also presents the danger that therapy will further aggravate the degree of injury and respiratory obstruction.[185] In rare cases, a transsected cervical trachea may be seen in the wound, and the distal segment can then be intubated directly. In other circumstances in which there is suspicion of laryngotracheal injury, attempts at intubation may produce further disruption of anatomy, or the tube, apparently passed safely through the glottis, may in fact leave the airway through the tear, creating a false passage and total respiratory obstruction. For this reason it is better to secure the airway by bronchoscopy if this is possible, or, in those cases with gross disruption of anatomy, to proceed to immediate tracheostomy or cricothyroidotomy.

Anesthetic Management

Most patients with cervical injury who survive and arrive at the hospital do not develop respiratory distress so quickly as to require resuscitation as described earlier, but most will require early surgical exploration. The particular problems facing the anesthesiologist in these circumstances include the following:

1. The general problems of induction of anesthesia in the injured patient, especially those of hypovolemia and full stomach.
2. The risk of laryngotracheal damage causing sudden respiratory obstruction during induction, and the danger that positive-pressure ventilation may increase emphysema.
3. Difficulty in laryngoscopy and intubation because of distortion of the normal anatomy by injury and swelling.
4. The presence of blood and debris (including foreign bodies) in the pharynx, adding further difficulty in laryngoscopy along with the risk of aspiration.
5. Associated injuries, particularly of the cervical spine.
6. The risk of venous air embolism in open cervical wounds.
7. Distant injuries (for example, ruptured spleen) resulting from the same accident.

In older patients, awake intubation is preferable in these circumstances if at all possible, but this is unlikely to be a viable approach with most children. The alternatives are to perform tracheostomy with local anesthesia, or to postpone intubation until after induction of anesthesia. Although the patient must be assumed to have a full stomach, it is probably unwise to attempt to aspirate stomach contents through a gastric tube for fear that the tube will aggravate the injury. Similarly, cricoid pressure must not be used over a damaged larynx; quite apart from aggravating the damage, this maneuver is likely to cause complete respiratory obstruction if the structural integrity of the larynx has been lost.

Use of intravenous induction agents or muscle relaxants before the airway has been secured is contraindicated in all patients in whom there is a risk of total respiratory obstruction and in those with traumatic emphysema. The preferred technique is gentle inhalation induction with halothane and oxygen (nitrous oxide should be avoided in the presence of emphysema) and maintenance of spontaneous ventilation until the patient will tolerate laryngoscopy and intubation. Intravenous lidocaine prior to laryngoscopy can be used to help prevent coughing.

A rigid bronchoscope must be available in case there is difficulty in passing or positioning the tracheal tube. If ventilation is adequate, it may be advantageous to postpone intubation until after the larynx and trachea have been exposed and the extent of the damage has been assessed. The trachea can then be intubated with certainty that the tube has been properly placed in relation to the damaged airway. Once the airway is secure, anesthesia can be continued in any appropriate way, but positive-pressure ventilation should not be used so long as there is any doubt about the extent of the laryngotracheal damage. Positive-pressure ventilation is safe only when the damaged region has been isolated by the use of a cuffed endotracheal or endobronchial tube.

REFERENCES

1. Morgan DW, Bailey CM: Current management of choanal atresia. Int J Pediatr Otorhinolaryngol *19*(1):1, 1990.
2. Rizzo KA, Kelly MF, Lowry LD: Diagnosis and treatment of congenital choanal atresia. Trans Pa Acad Ophthalmol Otolaryngol *41*:842, 1989.
3. Kearns D, Wickstead M, Choa D, et al: Computed tomography in choanal atresia. J Laryngol Otol *102*:414, 1988.
4. Hough JVD: The mechanism of asphyxia in bilateral choanal atresia. South Med J *48*:588, 1955.
5. Pirsig W: Surgery of choanal atresia in infants and children: Historical notes and updated review. Int J Pediatr Otorhinolaryngol *11*(2):153, 1986.
6. Singh B: Bilateral choanal atresia: Key to success with the transnasal approach. J Laryngol Otol *104*(6):482, 1990.
7. Stankiewicz JA: The endoscopic repair of choanal atresia. Otolaryngol Head Neck Surg *103*(6):931, 1990.
8. Resouly A, Barnard JD, Purnell AN: Access by LeFort 1 osteotomy for correction of unilateral choanal atresia. Clin Otolaryngol *15*(3):281, 1990.
9. Grundfast KM, Thomsen JR, Barber CS: An improved stent method for choanal atresia repair. Laryngoscope *100*(10 Pt 1):1132, 1990.
10. Bremner JW, Neel HB, DeSanto LW, Jones GC: Angiofibroma: Treatment trends in 150 patients during 40 years. Laryngoscope *96*(12):1321, 1986.
11. Maharaj D, Fernandes CMC: Surgical experience with juvenile nasopharyngeal angiofibroma. Ann Otol Rhinol Laryngol *98*(4):269, 1989.
12. Roberts JK, Korones GK, Levine HL, et al: Results of surgical management of nasopharyngeal angiofibroma. The Cleveland Clinic experience, 1977–86. Cleve Clin J Med *56*(5):529, 1989.
13. Lee DA, Roa BR, Meyer JS, et al: Hormonal receptor determination in juvenile nasopharyngeal angiofibromas. Cancer *46*(4):547, 1980.
14. Andrews JC, Fisch U, Valvavanis A, et al: The surgical management of extensive nasopharyngeal angiofibromas with the infratemporal fossa approach. Laryngoscope *99*(4):429, 1989.
15. Wood GD, Stell PM: Osteotomy at the LeFort 1 level. A versatile procedure. Br J Oral Maxillofac Surg *27*(1):33, 1989.
16. McCombe A, Lund VJ, Howard DJ: Recurrence in juvenile angiofibroma. Rhinology *28*(2):97, 1990.
17. Cummings BJ, Blend R, Keane T, et al: Primary radiation therapy for juvenile nasopharyngeal angiofibroma. Laryngoscope *94*(12):1599, 1984.
18. Witt TR, Shah JP, Sternberg SS: Juvenile nasopharyngeal angiofibroma. A 30 year clinical review. Am J Surg *146*(4):521, 1983.
19. Drake-Lee AB, Morgan DW: Nasal polyps and sinusitis in children with cystic fibrosis. J Laryngol Otol *103*(8):753, 1989.
20. Chen JM, Schloss MD, Azouz ME: Antro-choanal polyp: A 10 year retrospective study in the pediatric population with a review of the literature. J Otolaryngol *18*(4):168, 1989.
21. Kamel R: Endoscopic transnasal surgery in antrochoanal polyp. Arch Otolaryngol Head Neck Surg *116*(7):841, 1990.
22. Ward RF, April M: Teratomas of the head and neck. Otolaryngol Clin North Am *22*(3):621, 1989.
23. Costantino PD, Friedman CD, Pelzer HJ: Neurofibromatosis type II of the head and neck. Arch Otolaryngol Head Neck Surg *115*(3):380, 1989.
24. Bradley PJ, Singh SD: Congenital nasal masses: Diagnosis and treatment. Clin Otolaryngol *7*(2):87, 1982.
25. Zerella JT, Finberg FJ: Obstruction of the neonatal airway from teratomas. Surg Gynecol Obstet *170*(2):126, 1990.
26. Sumitsawan Y, Lorvidhaya V, Martin M: Carcinoma of the nasopharynx in Chiang Mai University Hospital: A review of 205 cases. J Med Assoc Thai *73*(8):450, 1990.
27. de Visscher JG, van der Wal KG, de Vogel PL: The plunging ranula. Pathogenesis, diagnosis and management. J Craniomaxillofac Surg *17*(4):182, 1989.
28. Vally IM, Altini M: Fibromatoses of the oral and paraoral soft tissues and jaws. Review of the literature and report of 12 new cases. Oral Surg Oral Med Oral Pathol *69*(2):191, 1990.
29. Sauter ER, Diaz JH, Arensman RM, et al: The perioperative management of neonates with congenital oropharyngeal teratomas. J Pediatr Surg *25*(9):925, 1990.
30. Tran L, Sidrys J, Horton D, et al: Malignant salivary gland tumors of the paranasal sinuses and nasal cavity. The UCLA experience. Am J Clin Oncol *12*(5):387, 1989.
31. Carrau RL, Myers EN, Johnson JT: Management of tumors arising in the parapharyngeal space. Laryngoscope *100*(6):583, 1990.

32. Richardson KA, Birck H: Peritonsillar abscess in the pediatric population. Otolaryngol Head Neck Surg *89*(6):907, 1981.
33. Majumdar B, Stevens RW, Obara LG: Retropharyngeal abscess following tracheal intubation. Anaesthesia *37*(1):67, 1982.
34. Hall SF: Peritonsillar abscess: The treatment options. J Otolaryngol *19*(3):226, 1990.
35. Jokinen K, Sipila P, Jokipii AMM, Sorri M: Peritonsillar abscess: Bacteriological evaluation. Clin Otolaryngol *10*(1):27, 1985.
36. Brodsky L, Sobie SR, Korwin D, Stanievich JF: A clinical prospective study of peritonsillar abscess in children. Laryngoscope *98*:780, 1988.
37. Herbild O, Bonding P: Peritonsillar abscess. Arch Otolaryngol *107*(9):540, 1981.
38. Neilson VM, Greison O: Peritonsillar abscess. J Laryngol Otol *95*(8):801, 1981.
39. Holt GR, Tinsley PP: Peritonsillar abscesses in children. Laryngoscope *91*(6):1226, 1981.
40. Herzon FS: Permucosal needle drainage of peritonsillar abscess. Arch Otolaryngol *110*(2):104, 1984.
41. Richardson GS: Peritonsillar abscess (letter). Arch Otolaryngol *111*(2):135, 1985.
42. Tucker R: Peritonsillar abscess—a retrospective study of medical treatment. J Laryngol Otol *96*(7):639, 1982.
43. Wolfe JA, Rowe LD: Upper airway obstruction in infectious mononucleosis. Ann Otol Rhinol Laryngol *89*(5):430, 1980.
44. Catling SJ, Asbury AJ, Latif M: Airway obstruction in infectious mononucleosis. A case report. Anaesthesia *39*(7):699, 1984.
45. Velcek FT, Klotz DH, Hill CH, et al: Tongue lesions in children. J Pediatr Surg *14*(3):238, 1979.
46. Gupta OP: Congenital macroglossia. Arch Otolaryngol *93*(4):378, 1971.
47. Schafer AD: Primary macroglossia. Clin Pediatr *7*(6):357, 1968.
48. Bell C, Oh TH, Loeffler JR: Massive macroglossia and airway obstruction after cleft palate repair. Anesth Analg *67*:71, 1988.
49. Moore JK, Chaudhri S, Moore AP, Easton J: Macroglossia and posterior fossa disease. Anaesthesia *43*(5):394, 1988.
50. Ricciardelli EJ, Richardson MA: Cervicofacial cystic hygroma. Patterns of recurrence and management of the difficult case. Arch Otolaryngol Head Neck Surg 117(5):546, 1991.
51. Kennedy TL: Cystic hygroma-lymphangioma: A rare and still unclear entity. Laryngoscope 99(10 Pt 2; Suppl 49):1, 1989.
52. al-Samarrai AY, Jawad AJ, al-Rabeeah A, et al: Cystic hygroma in Saudi Arabian children. J R Coll Surg Edinb *35*(3):178, 1990.
53. Katz AD, Zager WJ: The lingual thyroid. Arch Surg *102*(6):582, 1971.
54. Harvey HK: Diagnosis and management of the thyroid nodule. Otolaryngol Clin North Am *23*(2):303, 1990.
55. Wertz ML: Management of undescended lingual and sublingual thyroid glands. Laryngoscope *84*(4):507, 1974.
56. Flom GS, Donovan TJ, Landgraf JR: Congenital dermoid cyst of the anterior tongue. Otolaryngol Head Neck Surg *100*(6):602, 1989.
57. Grime PD: Giant enterocystoma within an infant's tongue. J Laryngol Otol *104*(10):814, 1990.
58. Simmons WB, Haggerty HS, Ngan B, Anonsen CK: Alveolar soft part sarcoma of the head and neck. A disease of children and young adults. Int J Pediatr Otorhinolaryngol *17*(2):139, 1989.
59. Solomon MP, Tolete-Velcek F: Lingual rhabdomyoma (adult variant) in a child. J Pediatr Surg *14*(1):91, 1979.
60. Ninh TN, Ninh TX: Cystic hygroma in children: A report of 126 cases. J Pediatr Surg *9*(2):191, 1974.
61. Valman HB: Stridor. BMJ *283*(6286):294, 1981.
62. Rowlandson P: Stridor (letter). BMJ *283*(6295):863, 1981.
63. Couriel J: Acute stridor in preschool child (letter). BMJ *288*(6424):1162, 1984.
64. Carenfelt C, Sobin A: Acute infectious epiglottitis in children and adults: Annual incidence and mortality. Clin Otolaryngol *14*(6):489, 1989.
65. Brilli RJ, Benzing G, Cotcamp DH: Epiglottitis in infants less than two years of age. Pediatr Emerg Care *5*(1):16, 1989.
66. Losek JD, Dewitz-Zink BA, Melzer-Lange M, Havens PL: Epiglottitis: Comparison of signs and symptoms in children less than two years old and older. Ann Emerg Med *19*(1):55, 1990.
67. Stanley RE, Liang TS: Acute epiglottitis in adults (the Singapore experience). J Laryngol Otol *102*(11):1017, 1988.
68. Mayosmith MF, Hirsch PJ, Wodzinski SF, Schiffman FJ: Acute epiglottitis in adults. An eight-year experience in the state of Rhode Island. N Engl J Med *314*(18):1133, 1986.
69. Wurtele P: Acute epiglottitis in children and adults: A large scale incidence study. Otolaryngol Head Neck Surg *103*(6):902, 1990.
70. Trollfors B, Nylen O, Strangert K: Acute epiglottitis in children and adults in Sweden 1981–3. Arch Dis Child *65*(5):491, 1990.
71. Gilbert GL, Clements DA, Broughton SJ: *Haemophilus influenzae* type b infections in Victoria, Australia, 1985 to 1987. Pediatr Infect Dis J *9*(4):252, 1990.
72. Fontanarosa PB, Polsky SS, Goldman GE: Adult epiglottitis. J Emerg Med *7*(3):223, 1989.
73. Bonadio WA, Losek JD: The characteristics of children with epiglottitis who develop the complication of pulmonary edema. Arch Otolaryngol Head Neck Surg *117*(2):205, 1991.
74. Foweraker JE, Millar MR, Smith I: Meningitis caused by *Haemophilus influenzae* type b infection after epiglottitis. BMJ *298*(6679):1003, 1989.
75. Gonzales C, Gartner JC, Casselbrant ML, Kenna MA: Complication of acute epiglottitis. Int J Pediatr Otorhinolaryngol *11*(1):67, 1986.
76. Briggs WH, Althenau MM: Acute epiglottitis in children. Otolaryngol Head Neck Surg *88*(6):665, 1980.
77. Smith MD, Kelsey MC, Scott GM, Rom S: Acute epiglottitis due to a chloramphenicol-inactivating strain of *Haemophilus influenzae* type b (letter). J Infect *13*(1):93, 1986.
78. Sendi K, Crysdale WS: Acute epiglottitis: Decade of change—a 10 year experience with 242 children. J Otolaryngol *16*:196, 1987.
79. Granoff DM, Sheetz K, Pandey JP, et al: Host and bacterial factors associated with *Haemophilus influenzae* type b disease in Minnesota children vaccinated with type b polysaccharide vaccine. J Infect Dis *159*(5):908, 1989.
80. Lacroix J, Ahronheim G, Arcand P, et al: Group A streptococcal supraglottitis. J Pediatr *109*(1):20, 1986.
81. Mehtar S, Bangham L, Kalmanovitch D, Wren M: Adult epiglottitis due to *Vibrio vulnificus*. BMJ (Clin Res) *296*(6625):827, 1988.
82. Parment PA, Hagberg L: Fatal *Serratia marcescens* epiglottitis in a patient with leukaemia (letter). J Infect *14*(3):280, 1987.

83. Biem J, Roy L, Halik J, Hoffstein V: Infectious mononucleosis complicated by necrotizing epiglottitis, dysphagia, and pneumonia. Chest *96*(1):204, 1989.
84. Welch DB, Price DG: Acute epiglottitis and severe croup. Experience in two English regions. Anaesthesia *38*(8):754, 1983.
85. Blackstock MB, Adderley RJ, Steward DJ: Epiglottitis in young infants. Anesthesiology *67*(1):97, 1987.
86. Goldhagen JL: Supraglottitis in three young infants. Pediatr Emerg Care *5*(3):175, 1989.
87. Schuh S, Huang A, Fallis JC: Atypical epiglottitis. Ann Emerg Med *17*(2):168, 1988.
88. Howell PR: Acute epiglottitis (letter). Anaesthesia *43*(5):425, 1988.
89. Fried MP: Controversies in the management of supraglottitis and croup. Pediatr Clin North Am *26*(4):931, 1979.
90. Diaz JH: Croup and epiglottitis in children: The anesthesiologist as diagnostician. Anesth Analg *64*(6):621, 1985.
91. Maze A, Bloch E: Stridor in pediatric patients. Anesthesiology *50*(2):132, 1979.
92. Rothrock SG, Pignatiello GA, Howard RM: Radiologic diagnosis of epiglottitis: Objective criteria for all ages. Ann Emerg Med *19*(9):978, 1990.
93. Glicklich M, Cohen RD, Jona JZ: Steroids and bag and mask ventilation in the treatment of acute epiglottitis. J Pediatr Surg *14*(3):247, 1979.
94. Vernon DD, Sarnaik AP: Acute epiglottitis in children: A conservative approach to diagnosis and management. Crit Care Med *14*(1):23, 1986.
95. Soliman MG, Richer P: Epiglottitis and pulmonary oedema in children. Can Anaesth Soc J *25*(4):270, 1978.
96. Lynch M, Underwood S: Pulmonary oedema following relief of upper airway obstruction in the Pierre-Robin syndrome: A consequence of early palatal repair? Br J Anaesth *66*(3):391, 1991.
97. Kimmons HC Jr, Peterson BM: Management of acute epiglottitis in pediatric patients. Crit Care Med *14*(4):278, 1986.
98. Butt W, Shann F, Walker C, et al: Acute epiglottitis: A different approach to management. Crit Care Med *16*(1):43, 1988.
99. Healy GB: Subglottic stenosis. Otolaryngol Clin North Am *22*(3):599, 1989.
100. Rothstein P, Lister G: Epiglottitis—duration of intubation and fever. Anesth Analg *62*(9):785, 1983.
101. Hawkins DB: Corticosteroids in the management of laryngotracheobronchitis. Otolaryngol Head Neck Surg *88*(3):207, 1980.
102. Hodes HL: Diphtheria. Pediatr Clin North Am *26*(2):445, 1979.
103. Coyle MB, Groman NB, Russell JQ, et al: The molecular epidemiology of three biotypes of *Corynebacterium diphtheriae* in the Seattle outbreak, 1972–82. J Infect Dis *159*(4):670, 1989.
104. Loevinsohn BP: The changing age structure of diphtheria patients: Evidence for the effectiveness of EPI in the Sudan. Bull WHO *68*(3):353, 1990.
105. Christenson B, Hellstrom L, Aust-Kettis A: Diphtheria in Stockholm, with a theory concerning transmission. J Infect *19*(2):177, 1989.
106. Masterton RG, Tettmar RE, Pile RLC, et al: Immunity to diphtheria in young British adults. J Infect *15*:27, 1987.
107. Bjorkholm B, Wahl M, Granstrom M, Hagberg L: Immune status and booster effect of low doses of diphtheria toxoid in Swedish medical personnel. Scand J Infect Dis *21*(4):429, 1989.
108. Hatton P: A report of the investigation and control measures instituted after the isolation of toxin-producing *Corynebacterium diphtheriae mitis* from a child in Leeds. Community Med *11*(4):316, 1989.
109. Bowler ICJ, Mandal BK, Schlecht B, Riordan T: Diphtheria—the continuing hazard. Arch Dis Child *63*(2):194, 1988.
110. Karzon DT, Edwards KM: Diphtheria outbreaks in immunized populations. N Engl J Med *318*(1):41, 1988.
111. Dobie RA, Tobey TN: Clinical features of diphtheria in the respiratory tract. JAMA *242*(20):2197, 1979.
112. Harnisch JP, Tronca E, Nolan CM, et al: Diphtheria among alcoholic urban adults. A decade of experience in Seattle. Ann Intern Med *111*(1):71, 1989.
113. Stevens DS, Walker DH, Schaffner W, et al: Pseudodiphtheria: Prominent pharyngeal membrane associated with fatal paraquat ingestion. Ann Intern Med *94*(1):202, 1981.
114. Cotton RT, Gray SD, Miller RP: Update of the Cincinnati experience in pediatric laryngotracheal reconstruction. Laryngoscope *99*(11):1111, 1989.
115. Zalzal GH: Stridor and airway compromise. Pediatr Clin North Am *36*(6):1389, 1989.
116. Cotton RT, Richardson MA: Congenital laryngeal anomalies. Otolaryngol Clin North Am *14*(1):203, 1981.
117. Holinger LD: Etiology of stridor in the neonate, infant and child. Ann Otol Rhinol Laryngol *89*(5):397, 1980.
118. Zalzal GH, Anon JB, Cotton RT: Epiglottoplasty for the treatment of laryngomalacia. Ann Otol Rhinol Laryngol *96*(1):72, 1987.
119. Fearon B: Laryngeal surgery in the pediatric patient. Ann Otol Rhinol Laryngol (Suppl) *89*(5, Pt 2):146, 1980.
120. Holinger PH, Brown WT: Congenital webs, cysts, laryngoceles and other anomalies of the larynx. Ann Otol Rhinol Laryngol *76*(4):744, 1967.
121. Cundy RL, Bergstrom LB: Congenital subglottic stenosis. J Pediatr *82*(2):282, 1973.
122. McGill T, Friedman EM, Healy GB: Laser surgery in the pediatric airway. Otolaryngol Clin North Am *16*(4):805, 1983.
123. Isshiki N, Taira T, Nose K, Kojima H: Surgical treatment of laryngeal web with mucosa graft. Ann Otol Rhinol Laryngol *100*(2):95, 1991.
124. Miller R, Gray SD, Cotton RT, et al: Subglottic stenosis and Down syndrome. Am J Otolaryngol *11*(4):274, 1990.
125. Kotton B: The treatment of subglottic stenosis in children by prolonged dilatation. Laryngoscope *89*(12):1983, 1979.
126. Fearon B, Crysdale WS, Bird R: Subglottic stenosis of the larynx in the infant and child. Ann Otol Rhinol Laryngol *87*(5):645, 1978.
127. Murphy PM, Lloyd-Thomas A: The anaesthetic management of congenital tracheal stenosis. Anaesthesia *46*(2):106, 1991.
128. Zaw-Tun HI: Development of congenital laryngeal atresias and clefts. Ann Otol Rhinol Laryngol *97*(4):353, 1988.
129. Armitage EN: Laryngotracheo-oesophageal cleft. A report of three cases. Anaesthesia *39*(7):706, 1984.
129a. Ogawa T, Yamataka A, Miyano T, et al: Treatment of laryngotracheoesophageal cleft. J Pediatr Surg *24*(4):341, 1989.
130. Benjamin B, Inglis A: Minor congenital laryngeal clefts: Diagnosis and classification. Ann Otol Rhinol Laryngol *98*(6):417, 1989.
131. Chitwood WR, Bost WS, Pories WJ, et al: Laryngotracheoesophageal cleft: Endoscopic diagnosis and surgical repair. Ann Thorac Surg *48*(2):292, 1989.

132. Donegan JO, Strife JL, Seid AB, et al: Internal laryngocele and saccular cysts in children. Ann Otol Rhinol Laryngol *89*(5):409, 1980.
133. Holinger LD, Barnes DR, Smid LJ, Holinger PH: Laryngocele and saccular cysts. Ann Otol Rhinol Laryngol *87*(5):675, 1978.
134. Crockett DM, Reynolds BN: Laryngeal laser surgery. Otolaryngol Clin North Am *23*(1):49, 1990.
135. Holinger PC, Holinger LD, Reichert TJ, Holinger PH: Respiratory obstruction and apnea in infants with bilateral abductor vocal cord paralysis, meningomyelocele, hydrocephalus, and Arnold-Chiari malformation. J Pediatr *92*(3):368, 1978.
136. Cohen SR, Geller KA, Birns JW, Thompson JW: Laryngeal paralysis in children. A long-term retrospective study. Ann Otol Rhinol Laryngol *91*(4):417, 1982.
137. Tucker HM: Human laryngeal reinnervation: Long-term experience with the nerve-muscle pedicle technique. Laryngoscope *88*(4):598, 1978.
138. Enjolras O, Riche MC, Merland JJ, Escande JP: Management of alarming hemangiomas in infancy: A review of 25 cases. Pediatrics *85*(4):491, 1990.
139. Lee MH, Ramanathan S, Chalon J, Turndorf H: Subglottic hemangioma. Anesthesiology *45*(4):459, 1976.
140. Healy GB, McGill T, Friedman EM: Carbon dioxide laser in subglottic hemangioma. Ann Otol Rhinol Laryngol *93*(4):370, 1984.
141. Cotton RT, Tewfik TL: Laryngeal stenosis following carbon dioxide laser in subglottic hemangioma. Report of 3 cases. Ann Otol Rhinol Laryngol *94*(5):494, 1985.
142. McCaffrey TV, Cortese DA: Neodymium:YAG laser treatment of subglottic hemangioma. Otolaryngol Head Neck Surg *94*(3):382, 1986.
143. Dutton SC, Plowman PN: Paediatric haemangiomas: The role of radiotherapy. Br J Radiol *64*(759):261, 1991.
144. Lindeberg H, Elbrnd O: Malignant tumours in patients with a history of multiple laryngeal papillomas: The significance of irradiation. Clin Otolaryngol *16*(2):149, 1991.
145. Meeuwis J, Bos CE, Hoeve LJ, van der Voort E: Subglottic hemangiomas in infants: Treatment with intralesional corticosteroid injection and intubation. Int J Pediatr Otorhinolaryngol *19*(2):145, 1990.
146. Cohen S, Geller KA, Seltzer S, Thompson JW: Papilloma of the larynx and tracheobronchial tree in children. Ann Otol Rhinol Laryngol *89*(6):497, 1980.
147. Lindeberg H, Elbrnd O: Laryngeal papillomas: Clinical aspects in a series of 231 patients. Clin Otolaryngol *14*(4):333, 1989.
148. Cripe TP: Human papilloma viruses: Pediatric perspectives on a family of multifaceted tumorigenic pathogens. Pediatr Infect Dis J *9*(11):836, 1990.
149. Lindeberg H, Syrjanen S, Karja J, Syrjanen K: Human papilloma virus type II DNA in squamous cell carcinomas and pre-existing multiple laryngeal papillomas. Acta Otolaryngol (Stockh) *107*(1–2);141, 1989.
150. Perrick D, Wray BB, Leffell MS, et al: Evaluation of immunocompetency in juvenile laryngeal papillomatosis. Ann Allergy *65*(1):69, 1990.
151. Healy GB, Gelber RD, Trowbridge AL, et al: Treatment of recurrent papillomatosis with human leukocyte interferon: Results of a multicenter randomized clinical trial. N Engl J Med *319*(7):401, 1988.
152. Cole RR, Myer CM 3rd, Cotton RT: Tracheotomy in children with recurrent respiratory papillomatosis. Head Neck *11*(3):226, 1989.
153. Chipps BE, McClurg FL Jr, Friedman EM, Adams GL: Respiratory papillomas: Presentation before six months. Pediatr Pulmonol *9*(2):125, 1990.
154. Schwartz DA, Katin L, Lesser RD, et al: Juvenile laryngeal carcinoma: Correlation of computed tomography and magnetic resonance imaging with pathology. Ann Clin Lab Sci *20*(3):225, 1990.
155. Snow JB: Neoplasms of the head and neck in children. Adv Otorhinolaryngol *23*:115, 1978.
156. Weber TR, Connors RH, Tracy TF: Acquired tracheal stenosis in infants and children. J Thorac Cardiovasc Surg *102*(1):29, 1991.
157. Flexon PB, Cheney ML, Montgomery WW, Turner PA: Management of patients with glottic and subglottic stenosis resulting from thermal burns. Ann Otol Rhinol Laryngol *98*(1):27, 1989.
158. Holinger PH, Kutnik SL, Schild JA, Holinger LD: Subglottic stenosis in infants and children. Ann Otol Rhinol Laryngol *85*(5):591, 1976.
159. Laing IA, Cowan DL, Hume R: Prevention of subglottic stenosis. J Laryngol Otol (Suppl) *17*:11, 1988.
160. Fearon B, Cotton R: Surgical correction of subglottic stenosis of the larynx in infants and children. Ann Otol Rhinol Laryngol *83*(4):428, 1974.
161. Bailey CM: Surgical management of acquired subglottic stenosis. J Laryngol Otol (Suppl) *17*:45, 1988.
162. Luft JD, Wetmore RF, Tom LW, et al: Laryngotracheoplasty in the management of subglottic stenosis. Int J Pediatr Otorhinolaryngol *17*(3):297, 1989.
163. Cotton R: Management of subglottic stenosis in infancy and childhood: A review of a consecutive series of cases managed by surgical reconstruction. Ann Otol Rhinol Laryngol *87*(5):649, 1978.
164. Cotton RT, Seid AB: Management of the extubation problem in the premature child. Anterior cricoid split as an alternative to tracheotomy. Ann Otol Rhinol Laryngol *89*(6):508, 1980.
165. Frankel LR, Anas NG, Perkin RM, et al: Use of anterior cricoid split operation in infants with acquired subglottic stenosis. Crit Care Med *12*(4):395, 1984.
166. Schuller DE: Long-term stenting for laryngotracheal stenosis. Ann Otol Rhinol Laryngol *89*(6):515, 1980.
167. Vauthy P, Reddy R: Acute upper airway obstruction in infants and children. Evaluation by the fiberoptic bronchoscope. Ann Otol Rhinol Laryngol *89*(5):417, 1980.
168. Kennedy MG, Chinyanga HM, Steward DJ: Anaesthetic experience using a standard technique for laryngeal surgery in infants and children. Can Anaesth Soc J *28*(6):561, 1981.
169. Young PN, Robinson JM: Anaesthesia for microsurgery of the larynx (letter). Ann R Coll Surg *65*:135, 1983.
170. Vivori E: Anaesthesia for laryngoscopy (letter). Br J Anaesth *52*(6):638, 1980.
171. Craft TM, Chambers PH, Ward ME, Goat VA: Two cases of barotrauma associated with transtracheal jet ventilation. Br J Anaesth *64*(4):524, 1990.
172. Steward DJ, Fearon B: Anaesthesia for laryngoscopy (letter). Br J Anaesth *53*(3):320, 1981.
173. Tsui SL, Woo DCS, Lo JR: Anaesthetic management of a 2-month-old infant for laser resection of vocal cord granuloma. Br J Anaesth *66*(1):134, 1991.
174. Borg U, Eriksson I, Sjostrand U: High frequency positive pressure ventilation: A review based upon its use during bronchoscopy and for laryngoscopy and microlaryngeal surgery under general anesthesia. Anesth Analg *59*(8):594, 1980.
175. Smith RB: Ventilation at high respiratory frequencies. High frequency positive pressure ventilation, high frequency jet ventilation and high frequency oscillation. Anaesthesia *37*(10):1011, 1982.

176. Crockett DM, Strasnick B: Lasers in pediatric otolaryngology. Otolaryngol Clin North Am *22*(3):607, 1989.
177. Cozine K, Rosenbaum LM, Askanazi J, et al: Laser-induced endotracheal tube fire. Anesthesiology *55*(5):583, 1981.
178. Hunton J, Oswal VH: Anaesthesia for carbon dioxide laser surgery in infants. Anaesthesia *43*(5):394, 1988.
179. Paes ML: General anaesthesia for carbon dioxide laser surgery within the airway: A review. Br J Anaesth *59*(12):1610, 1987.
180. Brierley JK, Oates J, Bogod DG: Diagnostic and management dilemmas in a patient with tracheal trauma. Br J Anaesth *66*(6):724, 1991.
181. Hamilton-Farrell MR, Edmondson L, Cantrell WDJ: Penetrating tracheal injury in a child. Anaesthesia *43*(2):123, 1988.
182. Fuhrman GM, Steig FH, Buerk CA: Blunt laryngeal trauma: Classification and management protocol. J Trauma *30*(1):87, 1990.
183. Oxorn D, Clark K: Crico-tracheal disruption and common carotid artery occlusion: A case of blunt trauma. Can J Anaesth *37*(8):913, 1990.
184. Schaefer SD: Primary management of laryngeal trauma. Ann Otol Rhinol Laryngol *91*(4):399, 1982.
185. Sirkir D, Clarke MM: Rupture of the cervical trachea following a road traffic accident. Br J Anaesth *45*(8):909, 1973.

CHAPTER

12 Diseases of the Endocrine System

THOMAS P. KEON, M.D., and
JOSEPHINE J. TEMPLETON, M.D.

Abnormalities of endocrine function may be the primary indication for a surgical procedure or may be present in patients who require an operation for unrelated diseases. An understanding of the pathophysiology of diseases of the endocrine glands is essential for optimal anesthetic management of these patients. This chapter reviews normal endocrine physiology and diagnostic studies, pathology, and current management of endocrine diseases in the pediatric patient. Anesthetic considerations including preoperative assessment, operative management, and postoperative care will be discussed with emphasis on the infant, child, or adolescent. Inevitably, for some disorders, the majority of the data that are available have been taken from studies in adult patients.

PITUITARY GLAND

The pituitary, a complex endocrine gland located in the sella turcica at the base of the brain, is connected to the hypothalamus by the pituitary stalk, which is composed of glandular, vascular, and neural elements. The anterior pituitary (adenohypophysis) develops from an outgrowth of the buccal mucosa called Rathke's pouch and is connected to the hypothalamus by a complex portal vascular system that provides hypothalamic control of pituitary function. The posterior pituitary (neurohypophysis) is composed of the terminal endings of neurons that originate in the hypothalamus.

NORMAL PITUITARY FUNCTION

Anterior Pituitary (Adenohypophysis)

Hormones secreted by the anterior pituitary gland include adrenocorticotropic hormone (ACTH), thyroid-stimulating hormone (TSH), growth hormone (GH), prolactin (PRL), luteinizing hormone (LH), follicle-stimulating hormone (FSH), and melanocyte-stimulating hormone (MSH). The regulation of hormone secretion from the anterior pituitary is controlled by hypothalamic neurohormonal substances (releasing and inhibiting hormones) produced in the neurons of the tuber cinereum, particularly within the median eminence.[1] These hypothalamic hormones are secreted intermittently in response to decreasing levels of circulating end-organ hormones or to neural stimuli, and they are transported by the venous system of the pituitary stalk to the sinusoidal capillaries of the anterior lobe of the pituitary gland.

The median eminence, which forms the base of the hypothalamus and third ventricle, appears to be the common pathway for humoral and neural control of the anterior pituitary. The identification in the median eminence of nerve endings containing dopamine, norepinephrine, and serotonin that arise from neurons in the hypothalamus suggests that the secretion of hypothalamic-releasing hormones and consequently pituitary hormones is controlled by secretion of biogenic aminergic neurons. In addition, target organ products such as estrogen, testosterone, thyroid, and adrenal hormones can exert feedback at either the hypothalamic or the pituitary level (Fig. 12–1).

Posterior Pituitary (Neurohypophysis)

The supraoptic and paraventricular nuclei of the hypothalamus synthesize the posterior pituitary hormones vasopressin (antidiuretic hormone; ADH) and oxytocin. These hormones are attached to specific carrier proteins, neurophysins, and are transported along the pituitary stalk in secretory granules. The stimulus for the release of these hormones arises in the hypothalamus.

The primary functions of antidiuretic hormone are regulation of plasma osmolality and maintenance of extracellular fluid volume. ADH secretion, hence extracellular fluid osmolality, is regulated by osmoreceptors in the region of the supraoptic nuclei and blood volume receptors located in the left atrium and pulmonary veins. The most potent stimulus to ADH secretion is hypotension due to blood loss. The release of ADH produces peripheral vasoconstriction in addition to conservation of water by the kidneys. ADH acts on the distal tubules, collecting tubules, and a portion of the loops of Henle to make them permeable to water such that most of the water in the urine is reabsorbed. In the absence of ADH these structures are almost impermeable to water.[2] Conservation of free water as a result of the release of antidiuretic hormone also results in a decrease in urinary output. Painful stimulation due to trauma or surgery and positive airway pressure are additional factors that result in the release of antidiuretic hormone and conservation of free water.[3] Disorders of posterior pituitary function are manifested as either diabetes insipidus (inadequate ADH secretion) or inappropriate (excessive) antidiuretic hormone secretion. The physiological role of oxytocin is to stimulate contraction of the uterus and to promote milk secretion by the mammary glands.

The endocrine disorders associated with tumors in the pituitary hypothalamic area result from disruption of pituitary function by the tumor. The clinical manifestations of endocrine abnormalities vary with the age of the patient as well as the type of lesion. Tumors involving the pituitary-hypothalamic area usually result in deficiency of pituitary trophic hormones and less commonly in excessive secretion. In children, the tumors most frequently associated with endocrine dysfunction are craniopharyngiomas, gliomas of the optic nerve and optic chiasm, hypothalamic gliomas, hamartomas, and pineal tumors. Pituitary adenomas, more common in adults, are rarely encountered in the first two decades of life.

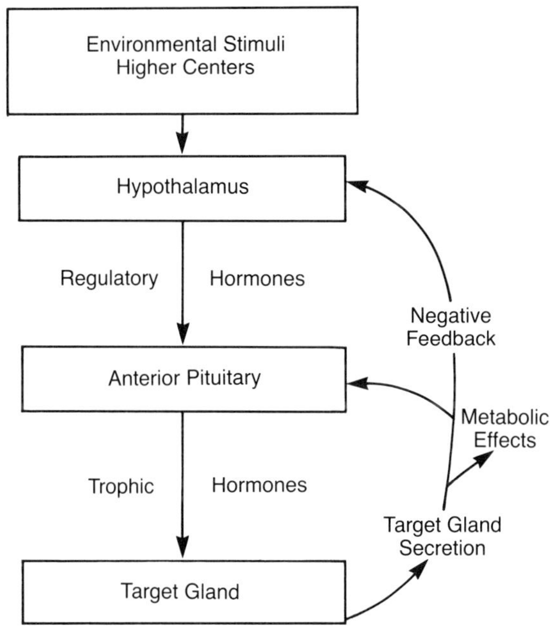

FIGURE 12–1. The endocrine system. Hormonal control by feedback mechanisms.

HYPOPITUITARISM

The most common demonstrable cause of panhypopituitarism in children is compression of the pituitary gland by a craniopharyngioma. Hypothalamic tumors, tuberculosis, sarcoidosis, toxoplasmosis, and aneurysms are less common causes. In more than half of children with hypopituitarism the cause is not known,[4] and there is no demonstrable lesion of the pituitary or hypothalamus. Panhypopituitarism may also follow head injury, radiation therapy, or surgical hypophysectomy and is manifested as multiple endocrine gland dysfunction. Deficiency of growth hormone in childhood results in dwarfism, but when it occurs in adults it does not produce symptoms. Treatment of panhypopituitarism is with specific hormone replacement, which may include gonadotropins, cortisol, and thyroxine. The administration of a mineralocorticoid is usually unnecessary because aldosterone release continues in the usual fashion.[5]

CRANIOPHARYNGIOMA

This tumor accounts for approximately 10 percent of all intracranial tumors in patients under 14 years of age.[6] Peak incidence occurs at age 7 years, with boys more frequently affected than girls. The lesion is benign and usually well encapsulated, and its size may vary from that of an olive to that of an orange. In the majority of cases it extends above the sella, indenting the hypothalamus and stretching the optic chiasm.

The characteristic triad of clinical features includes growth failure, increased intracranial pressure, and visual loss. Tumors presenting in childhood frequently produce hydrocephalus and symptoms of increased intracranial pressure, which may obscure the endocrine abnormalities. However, multiple endocrine abnormalities may be manifested by short stature, hypothyroidism, diabetes insipidus, lack or arrest of sexual development, obesity, and less commonly hypoadrenalism. Skull radiographs may reveal suprasellar calcifications, and a computed tomography scan revealing a calcified suprasellar tumor is virtually pathognomonic.

Surgical removal of the tumor is the treatment of choice. Radiation therapy is prescribed for tumors that cannot be removed completely.[7] Deficiencies of adrenocorticotropic hormone and antidiuretic hormone may exist prior to operation or develop following extirpation of the tumor.

HYPOTHALAMIC TUMORS

Tumors growing in the region of the hypothalamus, optic nerves, and optic chiasm may be associated with specific endocrine and metabolic abnormalities. The diencephalic syndrome, with a peak incidence in the first 6 months of age, is manifested by extreme emaciation, hyperkinesis, vomiting, inappropriate euphoria, nystagmus, and pallor without anemia.[8] Endocrine abnormalities include growth hormone deficiency and lack of diurnal variation in plasma cortisol levels.

Precocious puberty may be associated with tumors in the floor of the third ventricle, the posterior hypothalamus, and the tuber cinereum, often in the median eminence. Boys are more commonly affected, and clinical features include all the signs of puberty associated with gonadal maturation. The mechanism by which these tumors produce sexual precocity is unclear. Pressure from the tumor may result in increased secretion of gonadotropin-releasing hormone by interference with inhibitory neural stimuli.

PITUITARY TUMORS

Pituitary adenomas are uncommon in children and represent only 1 percent of all intracranial tumors. The endocrine abnormalities associated with pituitary tumors result from lack of secretion due to compression of the normal gland, impairment by the tumor of the hypophyseal-portal circulation, or excessive production of pituitary hormones. The diagnosis is suggested by the presence of endocrine abnormalities and visual field defects and confirmed by abnormalities of the sella turcica seen on radiography. In prepubertal children the earliest clinical findings are decreased linear growth and delayed development of secondary sex characteristics. Hypothyroidism and hypoadrenalism may occur later.

DIABETES INSIPIDUS

Diabetes insipidus is a syndrome characterized by hypotonic polyuria and normal or elevated plasma osmolality. Central diabetes insipidus occurs when insufficient ADH is released from the posterior pituitary. Nephrogenic diabetes insipidus results from relative insensitivity of the renal tubules to antidiuretic hormone. Central diabetes insipidus, if not present before pituitary surgical therapy, usually becomes manifest 6 to 12 hours after operation, as a result of direct hypothalamic injury or ischemia, stalk edema, or high pituitary stalk transection. In some patients diabetes insipidus lasts only 24 to 36 hours, after which urine output decreases and urine specific gravity increases, suggesting normal ADH activity. However, in the majority, this recovery lasts for only 3 to 5 days, following which permanent diabetes insipidus develops. Transient recovery of ADH function is thought to result from lysis of surgically damaged cells containing ADH.

Urine volume and specific gravity and serum electrolytes should be monitored in the intraoperative and postoperative periods. The urine volume may be as high as 10 to 20 ml/kg/h, with urine osmolality usually between 50 and 150 mOsm/L. Urine specific gravity will be between 1.001 and 1.005, and a urine-to-serum osmolality ratio of less than 1.1 indicates a negative water balance. The differential diagnosis includes diuresis from mannitol, glucose, or excessive crystalloid fluid administration.[9]

Perioperative management will frequently include the administration of vasopressin (Pitressin) or desmopressin (1-deamino-8-D-arginine vasopressin, DDAVP). Vasopressin administered as continuous infusion or subcutaneously at 6- to 8-hour intervals will control the symptoms of ADH deficiency. A wide variation in the dose of desmopressin exists and does not seem to relate to the age or size of the child. A reasonable starting dose is 2.5 μg administered by nasal insufflation or subcutaneous injection. The effect may last for 8 to 20 hours and therefore dosing needs to be individualized carefully for each patient.[10]

HYPERPITUITARISM

GIGANTISM

Gigantism is rare in early childhood but is usually recognized during adolescence when clinical features of both acromegaly and gigantism are present.[11] It is due to excessive secretion of growth hormone associated with an eosinophilic or chromophobic pituitary adenoma. Clinical features in children include increased growth velocity, excessive height, and enlargement of hands and feet without associated virilization. The diagnosis is confirmed by measuring an increased basal growth hormone concentration and the presence of sellar abnormalities. Lack of suppression or a paradoxical increase in growth hormone levels during hyperglycemia is characteristic. Glucose intolerance and hyperinsulinemia are commonly found.[12]

ACROMEGALY

Excessive growth hormone secretion following puberty results in acromegaly. Clinical manifestations result from a general overgrowth of skeletal, soft, and connective tissues. Facial features are coarse, and the mandible increases in thickness and length. Excessive enlargement of the tongue and epiglottis may contribute to upper airway obstruction, and intubation may be difficult.[13] Stridor or a history of dyspnea suggests involvement of the larynx, and subglottic narrowing of the trachea may be present.[14] Peripheral neuropathies occur because of trapping of nerves by skeletal, connective, and soft tissue overgrowth.

CUSHING'S DISEASE

This condition is the result of excessive secretion of adrenocorticotropic hormone (ACTH). The characteristic clinical features in children consist of obesity, stunted growth, retarded bone age, and osteoporosis. Bilateral hyperplasia of the adrenal glands is found, although a pituitary adenoma may not be evident. A high incidence of pituitary microadenomas has been documented at operation in patients with Cushing's disease even when sellar changes were not detected on routine skull films.[15] The diagnosis is confirmed by demonstrating elevated plasma ACTH and cortisol levels, absence of diurnal variation, and failure of dexamethasone to suppress serum cortisol and urinary 17-hydroxycorticosteroids. Cushing's disease and syndrome are thoroughly discussed in the section on adrenal diseases later in this chapter.

SYNDROME OF INAPPROPRIATE ANTIDIURETIC HORMONE (SIADH) SECRETION

This condition exists in patients when excessive quantities of ADH are produced in the absence of a physiological stimulus. It is found in association with a variety of illnesses, including brain diseases of inflammatory, neoplastic, vascular, and traumatic origin, pulmonary disease, and malignancies of the larynx, duodenum, and pancreas. Clinical features include hyponatremia, decreased serum osmolality, reduced urine output, and urine with a high osmolality. Acute reductions in serum sodium can lead to seizures. Diagnosis is based on evidence that the urine osmolality is unusually high when related to the markedly decreased osmolality of the plasma. Patients with SIADH usually do not show signs of impaired renal, adrenal, or hepatic function. Peripheral edema and arterial hypertension are not present. Hyponatremia occurs because of decreased free water clearance as well as excessive natriuresis, which even in conjunction with a high sodium input generally leads to a negative sodium balance. Treatment is initiated by restriction of fluid intake, which may be sufficient for asymptomatic patients. Demeclocycline (DMC), lithium, furosemide, and hypertonic saline may be necessary in selected patients unresponsive to fluid restriction.[16]

OTHER PITUITARY HORMONE–SECRETING TUMORS

Pituitary tumors that secrete thyrotropin (TSH), prolactin (PRL), and the gonadotropins luteinizing hormone (LH) and follicle-stimulating hormone (FSH) have not been reported in children. However, pituitary adenoma may result from long-standing hypothyroidism and hypogonadism, suggesting that early diagnosis and treatment of hormonal deficiencies with continuous replacement therapy may be important in the prevention of some pituitary tumors.[17]

ANESTHETIC MANAGEMENT

PREOPERATIVE ASSESSMENT

Preoperative evaluation of patients with pituitary dysfunction requires a familiarity with normal anterior and posterior pituitary physiology. Panhypopituitarism is more common with nonfunctioning tumors than with hormone-producing tumors. In the former, diagnosis is usually delayed until the growth of the tumor disrupts normal pituitary function. The important anesthetic considerations are assessment and management of the endocrine dysfunctions as well as management of intracranial hypertension or reduced intracranial compliance. Adrenocortical, thyroid, and antidiuretic hormone dysfunction are the three principal endocrine problems that must be evaluated. Accurate radioimmunoassay methods are presently available for all hormones, but traditional laboratory tests are still frequently utilized.

Adrenocortical hormone activity must be maintained when pituitary-adrenocortical function has been or will be disrupted. The normal secretory rate of cortisol in children is 12 mg/m^2/day, and a maximal adrenal cortisol production rate of 270 mg/1.73 m^2/day has been reported.[18] Cortisol measurements in adults under conditions of major stress have revealed maximal cortisol production of 250 to 300 mg/day. Intramuscular hydrocortisone hemisuccinate in a dosage of 100 mg every 6 hours in adults produces plasma corticosteroid values that compare favorably with levels observed in normal adult patients undergoing operation.[19] Commercial steroid preparations have variable absorption rates. The hemisuccinate and phosphate ester conjugates are water soluble and readily absorbed parenterally, hence are useful for infusions during surgical procedures. The acetate and diacetate forms are relatively insoluble in water and are absorbed slowly over days to weeks when given intramuscularly. Different coverage protocols have been recommended, but the administration of 2 mg/kg of hydrocortisone every 6 hours should exceed the maximal cortisol production of a normal adrenal gland and hence is appropriate for major surgical procedures.

Thyroid function, as measured by blood levels of TSH, triiodothyronine (T_3), and thyroxine (T_4) as well as clinical signs, should be determined. Hypothyroidism must be corrected with appropriate amounts of thyroxine. The patient may require up to 2 weeks to achieve a euthyroid state. Patients with normal preoperative thyroid function who undergo hypophysectomy usually will not need thyroid replacement therapy for a few weeks following operation (see the section on the Thyroid Gland later in this chapter).

Diabetes insipidus is rarely present preoperatively but commonly occurs in the immediate postoperative period. Urine output, serum sodium, serum osmolality, and urine osmolality are necessary for diagnosis and must be monitored frequently. Therapy has been discussed previously.

Hypophysectomy causes minimal alterations in carbohydrate metabolism in nondiabetic patients. However, in patients with diabetes mellitus the postoperative requirements for insulin are markedly reduced. Usually about one third of the preoperative dose of insulin will be required postoperatively. Sex hormone and mineralocorticoid hormone replacement are not necessary in the immediate postoperative period but may be required on a long-term basis.[20]

Signs of raised intracranial pressure must be sought in children with brain tumors. Headache, vomiting, papilledema, tense fontanelle in infants, and alteration of consciousness are indicative of increased intracranial pressure. Preoperative treatment with corticosteroids, fluid restriction, and diuretics usually results in temporary improvement.

Premedication with central nervous system depressants should not be given to patients with reduced intracranial compliance or signs of increased intracranial pressure. Preoperative anticholinergics are useful to reduce oral secretions and permit secure fixation of the endotracheal tube. Corticosteroid coverage should begin in the preoperative period.

OPERATIVE MANAGEMENT

The three surgical approaches that have been utilized are stereotactic, transsphenoidal, and frontal craniotomy. The transsphenoidal operation involves incision through the nasal septum and vomer to the sphenoid or through an incision in the maxilla. A frontal craniotomy necessitates retraction and elevation of the frontal lobe. When evidence exists of extension of the tumor into the cavernous sinuses, an increased risk of air embolism and excessive blood loss must be anticipated.[21, 22]

A neuroanesthesia induction sequence that minimizes changes in vital signs and intracranial pressure is desired. Intravenous thiopental, 4 to 6 mg/kg, and vecuronium, 0.15 mg/kg, are administered, and hyperventilation through cricoid pressure is initiated. Fentanyl, 6 to 8 μg/kg, and lidocaine, 1.5 mg/kg, are administered prior to tracheal intubation to attenuate cardiovascular and intracranial pressure changes associated with laryngoscopy and insertion of the endotracheal tube. The tip of the endotracheal tube should be placed at midtrachea and the tube securely taped. The eyes are protected by instillation of sterile lubricant and taped closed.

Intraoperative monitors include an esophageal stethoscope, noninvasive blood pressure apparatus, electrocardiogram, temperature probe, pulse oximetry, capnography, and nerve stimulator. An intra-arterial catheter is inserted for continuous monitoring of arterial pressure as well as being a sampling port for intermittent measurement of hematocrit, electrolytes, osmolality, glucose, and blood gases. Continuous end-tidal CO_2 monitoring permits control of arterial carbon dioxide tension, reduces the number of arterial gas samples, and is a sensitive monitor for air embolism. If the patient is in the sitting position or there is an increased risk of air embolism, a central venous catheter should be placed through the internal jugular, brachial, or femoral vein. Additional monitoring for venous air embolism should include the ultrasonic precordial Doppler device. A urinary catheter is inserted for accurate measurement of urine output.

Maintenance of anesthesia is continued with oxygen (30 percent), nitrous oxide (70 percent), isoflurane (0.5 to 1.2 percent) and fentanyl (1 to 2 μg/kg/h). Neuromuscular blockade should be continued and a peripheral nerve stimulator used to ensure paralysis. The arterial carbon dioxide tension is usually maintained at 25 to 30 torr. Clinical swelling of the brain is treated with hyperventilation, mannitol, 0.5 g/kg, thiopental, 2 to 3 mg/kg, and elevation of the head.

Intraoperative fluid management must consider preoperative volume status, intraoperative blood loss, urine output, and the need to minimize cerebral edema. Five percent dextrose and lactated Ringer's solution is used as the maintenance solution for children under 6 years of age and plain lactated Ringer's solution for older children. An intraoperative serum glucose determination will permit changes in the administered glucose concentration to assure a normal serum glucose concentration. The hourly maintenance rate should be administered and the fasting deficit not replaced unless it is required to maintain cardiovascular stability.

Patients operated upon in the sitting position are prone to venous air embolism. Management of this complication includes lowering the head, flooding the operative field with saline, discontinuation of nitrous oxide, application of bilateral jugular venous pressure, and aspiration of air through a previously placed right atrial catheter.[23]

Nasogastric tubes should not be inserted in patients with pituitary tumors. Large tumors may erode the sella and the sphenoid sinus and permit direct intracranial penetration of tubes or catheters, with potentially serious complications.

At the end of intracranial operation, most children can be extubated in the operating room. Intravenous lidocaine, 1.5 mg/kg, may be given to prevent coughing on the tracheal tube. The neuromuscular blockade is reversed with atropine, 0.02 mg/kg, and neostigmine, 0.07 mg/kg. Criteria for extubation include a regular respiratory pattern, normal neuromuscular function, and spontaneous eye opening. The patient is transferred to the intensive care unit with the same vigilant monitoring that was used during the surgical procedure.

Postoperative Management

Vigilant, comprehensive monitoring must be continued in the postoperative period. The following complications or problems should be anticipated:

Diabetes Insipidus. The most significant complication is diabetes insipidus. Urine output, serum sodium and osmolality, and urine osmolality must be measured frequently. If the urine output exceeds 3 ml/kg/h, hypernatremia is present, urine osmolality is decreased, and the urine-to-serum osmolality ratio is less than 1:1, vasopressin should be administered. Diabetes insipidus occurs in approximately 20 percent of patients and may subside in a few days.[24] Therapy includes replacement of urine losses with a hypotonic solution, replacement of potassium, and subcutaneous vasopressin tannate or nasal insufflation of DDAVP. Administration of glucose solutions must be carefully monitored because hyperglycemia may contribute to the diuresis. Preoperative prophylactic therapy with vasopressin is not advised because excessive fluid retention with volume overload could result and diabetes insipidus may occur in a minority of patients. Diabetes insipidus occurs with greater frequency following a transfrontal craniotomy than with the transsphenoidal approach.

Hormone Deficiency. Adrenocortical hormone therapy at maximum stress dosage (8 mg/kg/day) should be continued for 48 hours before reduction to maintenance levels is begun. Unless thyroxine was required preoperatively, this hormone can be started in 1 to 2 weeks. Testosterone (in males), estrogen and progesterone (in females), and mineralocorticoid are usually begun a few weeks following operation.

Reduced Insulin Requirement. Insulin-dependent diabetics develop a drastically reduced insulin requirement. Urine and blood sugar determinations must be done frequently, and the daily insulin dose is often only one third of the preoperative dose.

Hyperthermia. Hypothalamic temperature-regulating mechanisms may be disrupted, and temperature should be monitored continuously. Symptomatic therapy is indicated to maintain normothermia.

Seizures. Postoperative seizures may occur, and phenytoin medication may be given as a prophylactic measure.

Cerebrospinal Fluid Leak. Following transsphenoidal hypophysectomy, cerebrospinal fluid leak is an infrequent complication. Therapy includes antibiotic administration to prevent meningitis and may require surgical reexploration.

THYROID GLAND

Thyroid hormones influence many physiological processes but are particularly important in the maintenance of body temperature, cardiovascular activity, gastrointestinal motility, and reflex neurological function. During fetal life and in the first 2 years they are essential for normal growth and development of the central nervous system and the skeletal system. Thyroid hormones play a role in the biological processes of essentially every organ system.

NORMAL THYROID FUNCTION

Thyroxine (tetraiodothyronine, T_4) and triiodothyronine (T_3) are the active thyroid gland hormones that influence cells to alter the rate of biochemical reactions. Approximately one third of T_3 comes from thyroid gland secretion, whereas two thirds is the result of peripheral tissue deiodination of T_4.[25] T_3 is approximately four to five times as active as T_4 in bioassays. Circulating T_4 and T_3 are more than 99 percent bound to serum proteins, especially thyroxine-binding globulin and prealbumin.[26] Only the free thyroid hormone is biologically active, and therefore the ratio of free hormone to bound hormone, rather than the total serum concentration, will determine the level of metabolic activity.

The major regulator of thyroid hormone production is thyroid-stimulating hormone (TSH), which is secreted from the anterior pituitary. A closed feedback loop functions to control the production of thyroid hormones (Fig. 12–2). The negative feedback produced by circulating T_4 or T_3 on the production of TSH has the dominant effect. TSH release is also affected by thyrotropin-releasing hormone (TRH), which is produced in the hypothalamus and transported to the anterior pituitary by the hypophyseal portal venous system. Hence, thyroid gland dysfunction can reflect disease processes involving the hypothalamus, the anterior pituitary, or the thyroid gland itself.

The biosynthesis of thyroid hormone can be

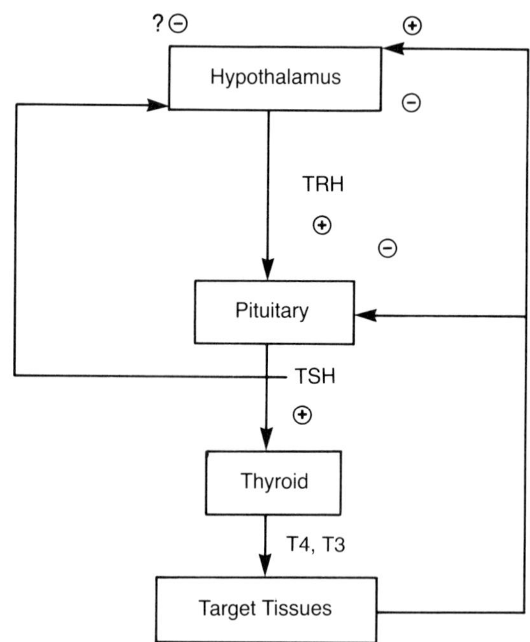

FIGURE 12–2. Concept of the hypothalamic-pituitary-thyroid axis. The closed feedback loop controls the production of thyroid hormones. ⊕, stimulation of gland; ⊖, inhibition of gland.

divided into four steps: (1) iodide trapping by the gland, (2) oxidation and iodination of tyrosine, (3) coupling of iodotyrosines and hormone storage as part of thyroglobulin, and (4) proteolysis with release of T_3 and T_4. Various drugs are administered to alter thyroid function and may act at different stages of thyroid hormone production. Thiocyanate and perchlorate both inhibit iodine trapping by the gland. Propylthiouracil and methimazole inhibit the oxidation of inorganic iodide and formation of monoiodotyrosine and diiodotyrosine. The proteolytic step necessary for the release of active hormone is stimulated by thyroid-releasing hormone and inhibited by the administration of iodides or lithium.[27]

The mechanism of action of thyroid hormone at the cellular level is complex, with multiple mechanisms rather than a solitary mode of action. Effects occur on the plasma membrane and the mitochondrial inner membrane with activation of mitochondrial energy metabolism. The activation of mitochondrial energy metabolism probably accounts for the increased oxygen consumption seen within a few hours of injection of T_3.[28]

Development of Thyroid Function

The embryonic thyroid gland is evident in the first month of fetal life as an invagination of the endoderm of the foregut. The first evidence of thyroid activity is the synthesis of thyroglobulin as early as the eighth fetal week.[29] By the twelfth week, colloid formation is apparent histologically, and fetal pituitary TSH secretion occurs. The fetal hypothalamic-pituitary-thyroid axis is functional by 20 weeks and develops free from maternal influence. Neither thyroid-stimulating hormone (TSH), thyroxine (T_4), nor triiodothyronine (T_3) crosses the placental barrier to any significant degree.[30] Thus, the fetal pituitary-thyroid axis functions independently of the maternal axis, and maternal thyroid hormones do not protect against congenital hypothyroidism.

Premature infants delivered prior to maturation of the hypothalamic-pituitary-thyroid system respond to extrauterine life with qualitatively similar but quantitatively decreased changes in serum TSH and iodothyronine concentrations. The TSH response to birth is reduced and, although a subsequent increase in T_4 concentration occurs, T_4 levels remain below those seen in full-term infants throughout the first few weeks of life.[31] Thyroid hormone levels are highest in infancy, gradually decline throughout childhood, and reach adult levels at about the age of 15 years.

THYROID FUNCTION TESTS

Tests of thyroid function include (1) quantitation of thyroid hormone levels in blood, (2) measurement of iodine turnover in the thyroid gland, (3) assessment of peripheral effects of thyroid hormone, and (4) tests of the hypothalamic-pituitary-thyroid axis.

Serum Thyroxine and Triiodothyronine

Most of the T_4 and T_3 circulating in the blood is bound to various thyroid-binding proteins. The bound forms of the hormone are inactive, and only the small proportion of circulating free hormone is active at the tissue level. Radioimmunoassay levels of T_4 and T_3 measure both the bound and free moieties. Drugs or conditions that alter the level of thyroid-binding proteins can cause major changes in the levels of total serum T_4 or T_3 and therefore do not reflect a thyroid abnormality or an excess of free hormones at the tissue level. A list of the more common conditions and medications altering total T_4 and T_3 appears in Table 12–1. Correction of the total T_4 or T_3 levels for thyroid-binding protein abnormalities has been achieved by combining them with the direct measurement of thyroid-binding protein levels or, more commonly, with the T_3 resin uptake test.

Triiodothyronine Resin Uptake

This test measures the unsaturated binding sites available to bind radioactive T_3. When the

Table 12–1. FACTORS AFFECTING THYROID BINDING PROTEINS

Increase
High total T_4 + low T_3RU
Estrogens
Pregnancy
Methadone
Liver disease
Porphyria
Decrease
Low total T_4 + high T_3RU
Androgens
Anabolic steroids
Asparaginase
Steroids
Phenytoin—competes with T_4 for binding
Salicylates—compete with T_4 for binding
Severe liver disease
Severe illness

level of binding proteins is normal but the patient's serum T_4 or T_3 levels are high (hyperthyroidism) or low (hypothyroidism), the T_3 resin uptake (T_3RU) is similarly raised or lowered. However, elevation or lowering of blood levels of thyroid-binding proteins alters the T_3RU inversely to serum T_4 or T_3. Thus, in most cases, multiplying the T_4 or T_3 with the T_3RU corrects for thyroid-binding protein abnormalities. This is the basis of the free thyroxine index (FTI) test reported by some laboratories.

FREE THYROXINE

New techniques have been developed to measure free T_4 and free T_3 in the serum, and these tests will soon replace the combination of measurements of the total serum T_4 or T_3 level with the T_3RU or measurement of thyroid-binding proteins.

RADIOACTIVE IODINE UPTAKE (RAIU)

This test measures the uptake of radioactive iodine by the thyroid gland in a given period of time. The uptake of isotopes by the thyroid gland is influenced by the iodine content of the body. Although elevations of iodine-131 uptake usually indicate hyperthyroidism and decreases usually indicate hypothyroidism, iodine deficiency or excess can give similar results. An alternative test measures uptake of radioactive technetium.

THYROID-STIMULATING HORMONE

The measurement of serum TSH has become an essential tool in the diagnosis of primary and secondary hypothyroidism. Primary hypothyroidism will result in a low level of serum T_4 and an elevated serum TSH.

THYROID SCANNING

Various isotopes of iodine can be used, but the most common scanning material is technetium-99, which gives off lower doses of radiation than the standard iodine-131. Isotope scanning gives an outline picture of the thyroid tissue, including its size, shape, and location. In addition, scanning can outline areas of decreased function (cold) or increased function (hot) in a gland. It cannot distinguish the malignant from the nonmalignant or, in the case of a cold area, whether it is solid or cystic.

ADDITIONAL TESTS

Ultrasonography of the thyroid gland permits reliable discrimination between cystic and solid nodules. Computed tomography (CT) may be used to complement the other structural investigations of the thyroid gland. Xerography is an x-ray technique that is useful in determining the degree of tracheal or esophageal compression from a large goiter or nodule. The detection of thyroid antibodies (antithyroglobulin and antimicrosomal) is important in the diagnosis of Hashimoto's thyroiditis.

HYPOTHYROIDISM

Hypothyroidism results from deficient production of thyroid hormone and is among the most common of the endocrine disorders of childhood. Hypothyroidism in children may be congenital or acquired; however, when symptoms appear after a period of apparently normal thyroid function, a disorder may appear "acquired" but result from a congenital defect in which the manifestation of the deficiency is delayed. In the pediatric age group, approximately one third of patients with hypothyroidism present in infancy (less than 1 year of age), and two thirds during childhood.

GOITER

A goiter is an enlargement of the thyroid gland. Goiter may be congenital, acquired, endemic, or sporadic. A patient with an enlarged thyroid gland may have normal function of the gland (euthyroidism), thyroid deficiency (hypothyroidism), or overproduction of hormones (hyperthyroidism). A large goiter may be seen rarely in an infant born to a mother who has received thionamide medication or iodide for hyperthyroidism. Both these goitrogens cross the placenta to the fetal side and inhibit fetal thyroid hormone production. The resultant fetal TSH secretion and thyroid gland hypertrophy may produce life-threatening airway obstruction.

CONGENITAL HYPOTHYROIDISM

The estimated frequency of congenital hypothyroidism is between 1 in 4000 and 1 in 7000 live births.[29] An unexplained 2:1 ratio of affected girls to affected boys exists with this disorder. Developmental defects of the thyroid gland are the most common causes of congenital hypothyroidism and are referred to as thyroid dysgenesis. Other causes include maternal goitrogen ingestion or radioactive iodine treatment, iodine deficiency (endemic goiter), autoimmune thyroiditis, and hypopituitarism.

The term *cretinism* is often used synonymously with congenital hypothyroidism but is best applied to infants with neurological sequelae of congenital hypothyroidism.

ACQUIRED HYPOTHYROIDISM

The incidence of acquired hypothyroidism is difficult to estimate, but it is approximately twice as common as congenital hypothyroidism. Causes include chronic lymphocytic thyroiditis, previous thyroidectomy or iodine-131 treatment, infiltrative diseases (cystinosis, histiocytosis X), sick euthyroid syndrome, and hypopituitarism.

MANIFESTATIONS OF HYPOTHYROIDISM

At birth, signs of hypothyroidism are usually absent or so nonspecific that the diagnosis is missed. Because irreversible damage to the central nervous system may take place before clinical manifestations suggest the diagnosis, screening programs have been developed to detect the disorder in newborn infants by laboratory testing before signs become clinically manifest.

It is uncommon for infants to present with a palpable goiter. Classical features of congenital hypothyroidism include a puffy face; wide fontanelles and sutures; flattened nasal bridge with pseudohypertelorism; a large, protruding tongue with an open mouth; a hoarse cry; a protuberant abdomen with an umbilical hernia; cold, mottled, or jaundiced skin; and sluggish reflexes. The risk of mental retardation appears to exist when hypothyroidism is present in a child under 2 years of age.

Hypothyroidism in childhood or adolescence may be insidious in onset, and the most common sign is a decrease in growth velocity. Clinical features include lethargy, cold intolerance, bradycardia, low pulse pressure, myxedema, delayed dentition, goiter, precocious sexual development, and a dull, placid expression. Myxedema coma is rare in children and is characterized by extreme lethargy, severe hypothermia, respiratory depression, hyponatremia, and congestive heart failure.

LABORATORY DIAGNOSIS

The biochemical hallmarks of primary hypothyroidism are a low serum T_4, normal or low serum T_3 resin uptake, and an elevated TSH. The elevated TSH is the most sensitive test for primary hypothyroidism. Serum cholesterol is elevated in hypothyroidism in childhood (not in infants), but this is not a diagnostic finding. The development of programs for screening neonates is an important advance in the diagnosis of congenital hypothyroidism. Most of the programs perform an initial T_4 on a filter paper blood sample obtained at a few days of life; if this is low, a TSH assay is performed on the same filter paper specimen.

TREATMENT

Untreated congenital hypothyroidism will have devastating effects on the growth and development of a child. Synthetic sodium levothyroxine is administered in a dose of 5 to 6 μg/kg in the first year of life, then 4 μg/kg after age 2 years and 3 to 4 μg/kg in late childhood and adolescence.[32]

In the infant one will observe an increase in activity, an improvement in skin color and temperature, reversal of other signs of hypothyroidism, plus normal growth and skeletal advancement. Serum T_4, T_3 resin uptake, and TSH should be monitored. Serum TSH that is in the normal range appears to be the best biochemical indicator of adequate therapy. If hypothyroidism develops after age 2 years, there does not appear to be a risk of permanent intellectual impairment, and all changes should be reversible with treatment.

ANESTHETIC MANAGEMENT

Preoperative Assessment. The degree of dysfunction in hypothyroidism may range from subclinical to overt with myxedema coma. Hypothyroidism should be corrected prior to a planned surgical procedure. At least 2 weeks are usually necessary to render a patient euthyroid. Treatment must begin slowly in patients with underlying myxedematous heart disease because of rare reports of sudden deaths in infants after 2 to 3 weeks of treatment.[29] Both serum T_4 and TSH will be normal in adequately treated patients.

Depending on the degree of physiological derangement, any or all of the following problems should be anticipated.

Sensitivity to Depressant Drugs. Cardiovascular and respiratory depression occurs more readily with sedative, narcotic, or anesthetic agents.[33] Narcotics, including fentanyl and morphine, may be associated with prolonged recovery from anesthesia.[34] The increased sensitivity of hypothyroid patients to morphine may in part be related to decreased hepatic metabolism.[35]

Hypodynamic Cardiovascular Function. Cardiac output may decrease as much as 40 percent owing to reductions in both stroke volume and heart rate. Peripheral vascular resistance is increased with narrowing of the pulse pressure. Myocardial depression may be partly due to myxedematous infiltration but also reflects impaired cellular metabolism resulting from deficient thyroid hormone activity.[36] Baroreceptor dysfunction has been demonstrated and may contribute to the hypotension that occurs with anesthetic agents.[37]

Impaired Respiratory Function. The normal ventilatory response to hypoxia and hypercapnia is impaired in overt hypothyroidism.[38] Depressant anesthetic drugs and hypothermia may further impair this function, necessitating postoperative ventilation.

Decreased Intravascular Volume. Intravascular volume may be reduced 10 to 24 percent below normal values. Chronic peripheral vasoconstriction is present. Use of drugs or anesthetic agents that cause vasodilation will lead to marked hypotension.[36]

Hypothermia. The basal metabolic rate may be reduced to 55 percent of normal because of a decrease in the activity of mitochondrial enzymes and a general slowing of substrate oxidation. This results in an inability to increase core temperature, which renders these patients susceptible to intraoperative and postoperative hypothermia. In infants such hypothermia is associated with apnea, bradycardia, and hypotension.

Adrenal Insufficiency. There is an increased incidence of adrenocortical insufficiency in patients with hypothyroidism, and the adrenocorticotropic hormone (ACTH) response to stress is impaired. Patients with severe hypothyroidism should receive daily steroid coverage during any acute stress.[39]

Hyponatremia. Inappropriate secretion of ADH as well as changes in renal function may also be of consequence in drug elimination.

Anemia. Anemia is often present and is refractory to treatment with hematinics.

Hypoglycemia. Intravenous dextrose solutions are necessary to prevent hypoglycemia from prolonged fasting.

Delayed Gastric Emptying Time. Emptying of the stomach is delayed and precautions to prevent gastric regurgitation and pulmonary aspiration are necessary.

Reduced Response to Peripheral Nerve Stimulation. Acute severe hypothyroidism may interfere with both proper intraoperative monitoring of neuromuscular excitability and estimation of neuromuscular blockade. A unique case is reported of a completely absent response to peripheral nerve stimulation prior to and after the administration of neuromuscular blocking drugs in a normothermic, severely hypothyroid patient.[40]

Premedication. Sedative premedication should be avoided in hypothyroid patients who are symptomatic. Anticholinergics can be administered intravenously prior to the induction of anesthesia. Patients taking thyroid replacement therapy should continue the usual dose regimen in the perioperative period. Full stress response doses of hydrocortisone (2 mg/kg every 6 hours) should be given if concomitant pituitary disease exists or if associated adrenal insufficiency is suspected.

Operative Management. Regional nerve blocks offer a major advantage for some procedures but frequently are not accepted and may be unsatisfactory in the pediatric patient. The dose of any local anesthetic agent used should be minimal to avoid toxicity secondary to impaired rates of metabolism of these drugs.

Induction. Because of increased sensitivity to all anesthetic agents, the induction agent must be administered in small increments with continuous monitoring of the cardiovascular system. Excessive peripheral vasodilation or myocardial depression may precipitate cardiovascular collapse. Inhalation agents must be titrated slowly. Ketamine may offer advantages in these functionally hypovolemic patients by stimulating increased sympathetic activity. Thiopental must be used cautiously in small doses to avoid excessive myocardial depression.[41] Endotracheal intubation is recommended both for airway protection and for controlled ventilation. Respiratory dysfunction should be expected.

Maintenance. Balanced anesthesia with nitrous oxide in oxygen and small amounts of fentanyl and diazepam with a muscle relaxant have been used successfully.[34] Muscle relaxation utilizing pancuronium is advantageous because of the drug's sympathomimetic effects. Curare may induce vasodilatation and hypotension. Potent inhalational agents must be used cautiously because of the known reduced myocardial reserve of these patients.

Animal studies indicate that the level of thyroid activity has minimal effect on anesthetic requirements or MAC.[42] The increased sensitivity of hypothyroid patients to anesthetic agents may represent secondary effects. Decreases in cardiac output shorten induction time with inhalation agents. This, combined with a decreased intravascular volume and altered baroreceptor function, may readily produce hypotension in the hypothyroid patient. In addition, reduced hepatic drug metabolism and renal drug excretion can prolong elimination of drugs and delay recovery from anesthesia.[36]

Patients undergoing major surgical procedures with significant blood loss require continuous arterial monitoring of blood pressure. Central venous pressure also should be measured because of a contracted blood volume and the need to maintain an adequate but not excessive intravascular volume. Intraoperative fluids must contain dextrose to prevent hypoglycemia. Administration of sodium-containing solutions and monitoring of serum electrolyte levels will prevent serious hyponatremia.

Aggressive practices must be used to prevent hypothermia. The temperature of the operating suite should be maintained at 25°C or above. An overhead radiant heater, warming mattress, heated humidified inspired gases, warmed irrigation solutions, and a blood warmer have proved effective. Reduction of the patient's temperature reduces anesthetic requirements for volatile drugs and slows the hepatic biotransformation and renal elimination of injected drugs.

Postoperative Management. The vigilance of the operative period must be continued postoperatively. Emergence from anesthesia may be delayed, with a prolonged obtunded period. Continued respiratory and cardiovascular monitoring is essential until the effects of the anesthetic drugs have dissipated. Normal body temperature should be restored and maintained. Hypothermia will contribute to incomplete reversal of neuromuscular blockers, respiratory depression, and bradycardia. Corticosteroid therapy must continue and thyroid maintenance is reinstituted.

HYPERTHYROIDISM

Hyperthyroidism results from excessive secretion of thyroid hormone. The most common causes in children are congenital (transient neonatal) hyperthyroidism and Graves' disease. Rare causes of hyperthyroidism observed in children include toxic uninodular goiter (Plummer's disease), hyperfunctioning thyroid carcinoma, thyrotoxicosis factitia, and acute suppurative thyroiditis. Hyperthyroidism is a frequent concomitant of McCune-Albright syndrome (precocious puberty with polyostotic fibrous dysplasia and abnormal pigmentation).[43] Graves' disease is often associated with other autoimmune disorders such as pernicious anemia, idiopathic adrenal insufficiency, myasthenia gravis, and disseminated lupus erythematosus.

Congenital Hyperthyroidism

Transient neonatal hyperthyroidism is considered to result from the transplacental transfer of thyroid-stimulating immunoglobulins from the mother, but the thyroid function status of the mother does not seem to play a role in the transmission of the disease. The hyperthyroid state is short-lived because of the half-life of maternal immunoglobulins (up to 3 months). Frequently, long-acting thyroid stimulator (LATS) can be demonstrated in both infant and mother when the mother has a history of active or recently active Graves' disease.[44]

Affected infants are frequently premature, and the majority will have a goiter. Sex predominance is not found. Hypermetabolic signs may be severe, with tachycardia, respiratory distress, and congestive heart failure. Accelerated bone maturation with premature craniosynostosis may be present. When the mother has been taking antithyroid medication, all symptoms in the infant may be suppressed until a week after birth owing to the effect of maternal antithyroid medication.

Graves' Disease

This is the most common cause of juvenile thyrotoxicosis, with the peak incidence occurring during adolescence. The disease is four to five times more common in girls than in boys.[45] There is substantial evidence that immune factors are important in the pathogenesis, and immunoglobulins, such as long-acting thyroid stimulator, can be identified.[46] In general, the disease is less debilitating and not as fulminant in children as in adults. Thyroid storm and apathetic hyperthyroidism rarely occur in children.[44]

Manifestations of Hyperthyroidism

The onset of the disease is usually gradual, with nervousness, increased sweating, heat intolerance, increased appetite, and palpitations. Physical findings include thyroid enlargement (goiter), eye prominence and exophthalmos, tremor, tachycardia, hypertension, and a wide pulse pressure. Skeletal muscle weakness is frequently present.

The hyperdynamic cardiovascular system is characterized by tachycardia, increased cardiac output, and low peripheral resistance. Though this is a sympathetic-type response, serum catecholamines are not elevated, suggesting that adrenergic receptors may be sensitized by thyroid hormone. Nevertheless, there is no direct evidence that cardiovascular responsiveness to exogenous catecholamines is altered by increased or decreased activity of the thyroid gland. Persistent excessive release of thyroid gland hormones may produce an increase in the number of beta-adrenergic receptors.[5]

LABORATORY DIAGNOSIS

Serum T_4 and T_3 levels are usually elevated. Elevation of T_3 with normal T_4 (T_3 toxicosis) is frequently described in adults but is rare in children. However, at the time of presentation of the disease the T_3 level is usually markedly elevated, making it the best single screening test for hyperthyroidism. Levels of thyroid hormone are higher in children, and an erroneous diagnosis of hyperthyroidism can be made if age-adjusted normal values are not used.[47] T_3 resin uptake will help distinguish abnormally elevated values associated with excess thyroid-binding globulin. Radioactive iodide uptake testing may be utilized, and the detection of immunoglobulins is useful in confirming the diagnosis.

TREATMENT

Initial treatment of congenital hyperthyroidism attempts to control the excessive cardiovascular stimulation. A beta-adrenergic antagonist, such as propranolol, 1 to 2 mg/kg/day divided into three doses, is administered. In addition, hypersecretion of the thyroid gland is suppressed using propylthiouracil, 5 to 10 mg/kg/day, and saturated solution of potassium iodide, one drop every 8 hours. Symptomatic improvement occurs in 1 or 2 weeks, whereas laboratory abnormalities may not return to normal until 4 to 6 weeks after initiation of therapy.

Radioactive iodide therapy in children may be associated with genetic damage, thyroid cancer induced by the radiation, and development of hypothyroidism. Surgical treatment necessitates that the patient be well controlled with medical therapy prior to the operation. Generally, the indications for treatment by radioactive iodides or operation are a drug reaction or noncompliance. Medical therapy is the treatment of choice for children, and remission occurs in one third of patients in 2 to 3 years.[47]

THYROID STORM

Thyroid storm, or acute, uncompensated thyrotoxicosis, is extremely rare in children. In adults, it most commonly occurs 6 to 18 hours postoperatively and is manifested by hyperthermia, tachyarrhythmias, hypotension, and coma. Thyrotoxic storm is a clinical diagnosis and may mimic malignant hyperthermia.[48]

Treatment of thyroid storm must be aggressive, with both specific and supportive therapy. Hyperthermia may require ice packs, a cooling blanket, and cold crystalloid solutions. Glucose-containing solutions and balanced salt solutions are necessary to maintain intravascular volume. Propranolol intravenously is titrated to reduce the peripheral effects of thyroid gland hormones on the cardiovascular system. Propylthiouracil, 5 to 10 mg/kg, inhibits the synthesis of thyroid gland hormone. Sodium iodide can be administered following the thiouracil; the iodide will inhibit the release of active hormone from the gland. Hydrocortisone, 2 mg/kg every 6 hours, has been reported to increase survival, although documented adrenal insufficiency among patients in thyroid storm is rare.[49]

ANESTHETIC MANAGEMENT

Preoperative Assessment. Patients should be pharmacologically euthyroid prior to a planned surgical procedure. Six to eight weeks of thiouracil therapy is usually necessary, and Lugol's iodine solution is started 1 week prior to surgery to decrease vascularity and hyperplasia of the overactive gland. Propranolol is administered to reduce the heart rate to a normal range and should be continued on the day of operation. The euthyroid state is substantiated by improvement of clinical symptoms, a normal resting pulse, and normal laboratory findings. A large goiter should be evaluated with lateral neck radiographs, xeroradiography, or computed tomography scans to determine the length and extent of tracheal compression.

Premedication. A calm, sedated patient is the goal. Pentobarbital, 4 mg/kg, provides effective sedation with the advantage that barbiturates suppress thyroid gland function. Anticholinergics have been avoided because they interfere with the sweating mechanism and normal heat regulation. Chronically administered antithyroid drugs and beta-adrenergic blockers should be administered on the morning of the operating day.

Operative Management. Patients with large goiters or signs of upper airway obstruction should be managed with techniques appropriate for children with upper airway obstruction. The airway must be secured awake, or an inhalation induction is used with the maintenance of spontaneous ventilation until a satisfactory airway has been established. A firm, armored endotracheal tube should be placed beyond the area of obstruction if tracheal compression has been demonstrated.

Induction. Thiopental is preferred because the thiourea structure lends antithyroid activity to this agent. Inhalational inductions are prolonged in patients with an increased cardiac output because additional time is required to increase the alveolar concentration of inhaled agent. In contrast to a common clinical impression, an increased anesthetic requirement has not been demonstrated in well-controlled animal studies.[42] Airway instrumentation and stimulation should be avoided until a deep level of anesthesia has been achieved. Prominent eyes will demand meticulous care with the instillation of lubricant and careful protective covering.

Muscle relaxants with the least cardiovascular effect (atracurium and vecuronium) are recommended. Continuous monitoring of neuromuscular blockade will permit assessment of the degree of coexisting muscle weakness that may be present.

Maintenance. Anesthetic agents that stimulate the sympathoadrenal axis or have sympathomimetic effects should be avoided (ether, cycloproprane, ketamine, pancuronium). Because of accelerated drug biotransformation in hyperthyroidism, drugs exhibiting a significant degree of biotransformation to toxic products are potentially more hazardous. An animal model made hyperthyroid by pretreatment with triiodothyronine resulted in hepatotoxicity associated with halothane anesthesia, which did not occur with enflurane anesthesia.[50] Isoflurane, which does not undergo significant biotransformation and does not sensitize the myocardium to catecholamines, appears to be a good choice for the maintenance of anesthesia. Nevertheless, there are no controlled studies in humans that have demonstrated differences in outcome depending on the choice of anesthetic agents.[51]

Controlled mechanical ventilation will prevent hypercapnia with consequent sympathetic activity. Carotid sinus stimulation resulting from surgical manipulations can produce profound bradycardia. Continuous electrocardiographic and esophageal stethoscope monitoring will permit immediate detection. Treatment consists of stopping the stimulation as well as administering atropine intravenously. Venous air embolism is rare but is possible because of head elevation and large neck veins.

Continuous intraoperative and postoperative monitoring is essential to detect increased thyroid activity and thyroid storm. Temperature elevation, tachycardia, and cardiovascular instability are indications for invasive monitoring and institution of the steps outlined previously to treat thyroid storm.

Postoperative Management. A number of postoperative complications may occur and therefore continuous postoperative monitoring is essential. Problems include airway obstruction, hypoparathyroidism, thyroid storm, and thoracic air dissection.[52]

Upper airway obstruction may occur owing to mucosal edema (postintubation croup), tracheomalacia, vocal cord paralysis, or compression by hematoma. Postintubation croup can be managed with humidified air and/or oxygen and racemic epinephrine inhalation. Bilateral recurrent laryngeal nerve injury secondary to surgical trauma results in obstruction due to unopposed adduction of the vocal cords and closure of the glottic aperture. This unusual complication necessitates reintubation followed by tracheotomy. Unilateral recurrent nerve injury often is not noticed because of compensatory overadduction of the uninvolved cord. Tracheal collapse due to preexisting chondromalacia of the tracheal rings may necessitate intubation for a period of time postoperatively. Postoperative hematoma in the neck may obstruct the trachea and requires the prompt removal of the dressing and opening of the surgical incision.

Hypoparathyroidism may occur because of inadvertent surgical removal of the parathyroid glands. Signs of hypocalcemia commonly do not develop for 24 to 72 hours but may become manifest immediately in the recovery room. Below-normal serum ionized calcium is diagnostic. Signs of tetany, including spasm of the laryngeal muscles, will diminish with the intravenous administration of calcium.

Thyroid storm is rare in children but in adults occurs most commonly 6 to 18 hours postoperatively. Supportive and specific therapy for thyroid storm was discussed earlier.

Subcutaneous emphysema, pneumothorax, and pneumomediastinum may occur with the surgical dissection of extensive thyroid tumors. A postoperative chest film should be reviewed for these complications.

THYROIDITIS

Chronic Lymphocytic Thyroiditis

Also known as Hashimoto's thyroiditis, this disease is the most common thyroid disorder in children and adolescents. The overall incidence in children is 1 percent, with a 4:1 to 8:1 female predominance. It is the most common cause of nontoxic goiter, and thyroid enlargement occurs in 90 percent of cases.[53]

Clinical features may include signs of hypothyroidism or hyperthyroidism. The usual course is either uneventful recovery or slow progression to hypothyroidism. Thyroid hormone supplementation in replacement doses is indicated when laboratory tests confirm hypothyroidism.

The disease is caused by an autoimmune process, and antibodies to thyroglobulin or thyroid microsomes can be demonstrated. It is commonly seen in Down's syndrome (trisomy 21) and in sex chromosome abnormalities, such as Turner's and Klinefelter's syndromes, and is associated with diabetes mellitus, Addison's disease, congenital rubella, and toxoplasmosis.[54] Corticosteroids in pharmacological doses may have some temporary effect in reducing goiter size and increasing the serum T_4 level but do not change the long-term outlook.

Anesthetic considerations will be determined by the functional status of the thyroid gland and have been outlined previously.

THYROID TUMORS

Thyroid tumors in children are uncommon. The important benign lesions are thyroiditis, thyroid adenoma, thyroid cysts, and ectopic thyroids. A solitary and nonfunctioning ("cold") nodule in the thyroid gland will be malignant in 10 to 30 percent of patients, with the greatest incidence occurring in patients less than 20 years of age. Common features of thyroid carcinoma in children include abnormal cervical lymph nodes, metastatic lesions, abnormal hardness of the nodule, and a history of radiation to the head and neck.[55]

Medullary thyroid gland carcinoma characteristically produces large amounts of calcitonin, but hypocalcemia does not occur despite an excess of calcitonin in the circulation. Multiple endocrine adenomatosis (MEA) comprises a group of endocrine disorders that can occur by autosomal dominant genetic transmission. Sipple's syndrome (MEA II) consists of medullary carcinoma of the thyroid, pheochromocytoma, and parathyroid hyperplasia. The important anesthetic considerations for medullary carcinoma of the thyroid are the presence or absence of these syndromes.

ADRENAL GLAND

The adrenal gland consists of two distinct endocrine systems: The cortical system responsible for the synthesis of glucocorticoid, mineralocorticoid, and androgenic hormones, and the medullary system, which synthesizes the endogenous catecholamines dopamine, norepinephrine, and epinephrine.

ADRENAL CORTEX

The cortex is divided into three functional zones, each responsible for the synthesis of a specific group of hormones. The zona glomerulosa, located beneath the capsule, is responsible for the synthesis of mineralocorticoids, important in salt and water balance. The glucocorticoids, so called for their ability to conserve glucose at the expense of other substrates, are synthesized in the zona fasciculata. The zona reticularis, which forms a network around the medulla, is responsible for the synthesis of androgens.

Cortisol, the major glucocorticoid synthesized by the adrenal cortex, affects the metabolism of most tissues (Fig. 12–3). Cortisol exerts a catabolic effect, resulting in a degradation of protein into amino acids with subsequent formation of glucose. In addition, cortisol inhibits utilization of glucose by the cells, an effect that is in direct opposition to the action of insulin. Hyperglycemia, present in syndromes of hypercorticism, is in part a reflection of both gluconeogenesis and decreased peripheral utilization of glucose. In the liver, cortisol has a prominent anabolic effect, which results in an increase of protein and glycogen synthesis.

In the medulla, cortisol must be present for the conversion of norepinephrine to epinephrine. As a result hypertension is a common feature in syndromes of hypercorticism. Another important property of cortisol is its ability to stabilize cell membranes and decrease the inflammatory response. Such a feature is used to advantage in treating conditions of hypersensitivity. The mean cortisol production rate has been reported to be 12 mg/m^2/day, although more recent information seems to indicate that

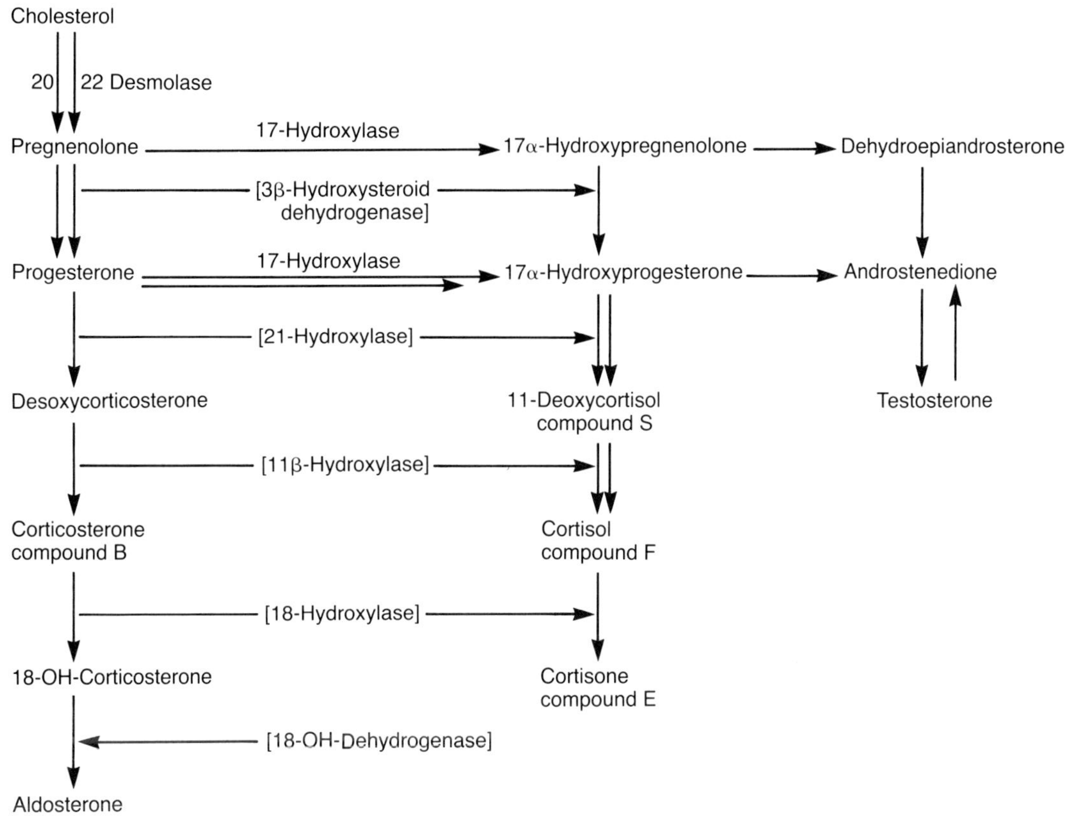

FIGURE 12–3. Synthesis of hydrocortisone. Double arrows indicate principal pathway of steroid synthesis. Single arrows indicate alternate pathways. Brackets denote enzymatic defects leading to virilizing adrenal hyperplasia.

cortisol production in children is 7 mg/m²/day.[56] Plasma levels range from 7 to 18 μg/dl in the early morning hours, with lower plasma concentrations of 2 to 9 μg/dl occurring at midnight, thereby establishing a diurnal variation. The diurnal variation in the secretion of ACTH is used to advantage during steroid therapy. To minimize suppression of the hypothalamic-pituitary-adrenal axis, exogenous steroids are best administered in the early morning hours when cortisol levels are at their peak and ACTH secretion is low.

Aldosterone is the principal mineralocorticoid. Desoxycortisone and corticosterone also have mineralocorticoid activity, but are secreted in small quantities. The synthesis and secretion of aldosterone is regulated by the renin-angiotensin system and the serum concentration of potassium (see Fig. 12–3). Renin is a proteolytic enzyme released from the juxtaglomerular cells of the kidney in response to hypovolemia, hypotension, or hyponatremia. In the presence of the angiotensin-converting enzyme secreted by the lung, angiotensin I is converted to angiotensin II, which acts primarily on the adrenal cortex to secrete aldosterone. The kidney responds to aldosterone by increasing sodium reabsorption and increasing potassium excretion.

Dehydroepiandrosterone, androstenedione, and testosterone are androgenic hormones synthesized in the adrenal cortex (see Fig. 12–3). These hormones are metabolized in the liver and are excreted by the kidney in the form of 17-ketosteroids. In the female, urinary measurement of 17-ketosteroids can be accepted as an index of their production, whereas in the male, only two thirds of the urinary 17-ketosteroids are of adrenal cortical origin. The remaining one third are produced by the testicle. Prior to 8 to 10 years of age, the urinary excretion of these hormones is small, but there is a constant increase throughout adolescence until adult levels are reached. The androgenic properties of these hormones are most conspicuous under pathological conditions, such as congenital adrenal hyperplasia.

Laboratory Tests of Adrenal Function

Maintenance of the hypothalamic-pituitary-adrenal (HPA) axis is vital to the normal response of the patient to anesthetic and surgical stress. The relationship between plasma cortisol level and ACTH forms the HPA axis. A decrease in plasma cortisol stimulates the hypothalamus to secrete corticotropin-stimulating factor, which is transported by way of the hypophyseoportal vessels to the anterior pituitary, resulting in ACTH secretion. Several laboratory methods are available to test the integrity of the HPA axis.

Metapyrone Test. Metapyrone inhibits the conversion of 11-deoxycortisol to cortisol. 11-Deoxycortisol, or compound S, is physiologically inert and therefore cannot suppress ACTH output by the pituitary. The absence of cortisol causes the pituitary to increase the secretion of ACTH. Thus the adrenal gland is stimulated to increase production of 11-deoxycortisol. A normal pituitary ACTH secretion and a normal adrenal responsiveness are indicated by a sharp increase in compound S or 11-deoxycortisol following the administration of metapyrone. If the measured level of 11-deoxycortisol in plasma, after metapyrone is injected, is greater than 7 μg/dl, it can be concluded that the subject has a normal pituitary-adrenal axis. The metapyrone test remains the best method for demonstrating cortisol deficiency with a normal adrenal responsiveness.

ACTH or Cortrosyn Stimulation Test. The ACTH or cosyntropin (Cortrosyn) stimulation test is used to establish whether the abnormality of the pituitary-adrenal axis is located in the pituitary, hypothalamus, or adrenal glands. The test is carried out by administering 250 μg of Cortrosyn intravenously. Serum cortisol levels are then measured 1 hour after injection. A normal test is one in which there is a baseline cortisol level of at least 5 μg/dl, an increment between baseline and stimulated level greater than 7 μg/dl, and a stimulated cortisol level of greater than 18 μg/dl.

Dexamethasone Suppression Test. The dexamethasone suppression test is the most useful method for screening hypercorticism. This test is carried out by administering 1 mg of dexamethasone in older children (10 years and older) and 0.5 mg in younger children at 11:00 P.M. and then measuring the plasma cortisol levels the next day at 8:00 A.M. prior to ingestion of food. In the normal individual the cortisol level should be below 5 μg/dl. It is also useful to determine whether a diurnal variation of cortisol levels is present. A serum cortisol level at 6:00 P.M. that measures 75 percent or less of the 8:00 A.M. level is considered normal and establishes a diurnal variation.

ADRENAL INSUFFICIENCY

The syndrome of adrenal insufficiency as originally described by Addison was the result of destruction of the adrenal gland by tuberculosis. We now recognize two distinct forms of hypoadrenalism with different clinical manifestations. Primary adrenal insufficiency is now considered to be due to an autoimmune mechanism and may be associated with other autoimmune diseases, such as chronic lymphocytic thyroiditis, hyperthyroidism, and diabetes mellitus.[57, 58] Tuberculosis, fungal infections, adrenogenital hyperplasia, and cytotoxic factors are responsible for the syndrome. A fulminant form of adrenal insufficiency is caused by meningococcemia and is known as Waterhouse-Friderichsen syndrome.

Clinical Manifestations. The clinical manifestations of adrenal insufficiency depend on the type of hypoadrenalism. Primary adrenal insufficiency is associated with both glucocorticoid and mineralocorticoid deficiency. Progressive weakness, anemia, and hyperpigmentation are the salient features. The pigmentation, which is characteristic for its distribution on the flexor surfaces of the body giving a dirty skin appearance, is caused by increased levels of ACTH and β-lipoprotein, which stimulate melanocyte receptors. Hypoglycemia without electrolyte imbalance is present in hypoadrenalism from pituitary or hypothalamic failure. Hyponatremia, if present, is thought to be due to increased vasopressin activity. If adrenal insufficiency is not recognized, an adrenal crisis may supervene in which the patient suddenly becomes cyanotic and dyspneic, with a weak, rapid pulse and cold extremities. Unless treatment is immediate and aggressive, death ensues. In patients with inadequately treated adrenal insufficiency, adrenal crises can be precipitated by trauma, infection, excessive fatigue, or drugs such as morphine, barbiturates, thyroid hormone, laxatives, or insulin.

Laboratory findings depend on the type of hypoadrenalism. Hyponatremia, hyperkalemia, and anemia with increased eosinophils are present in primary adrenal insufficiency. Hypoglycemia without electrolyte imbalance is present in secondary hypoadrenalism. Urinary electrolytes mirror serum findings, with increased excretion of sodium and chloride and a decrease in urinary potassium. Roentgenographic examination of the chest will reveal a small, narrow heart.

Treatment. Administration of glucocorticoids and mineralocorticoids forms the basis for the treatment of adrenal insufficiency. Daily administration of cortisol, 12 to 15 mg/m^2, is considered adequate replacement. Lower amounts may be sufficient. In times of illness or stress, the dosage is increased by 50 to 100 percent. Fludrocortisone (Florinef), an oral mineralocorticoid, is administered in a dosage of 0.05 to 0.1 mg irrespective of age or weight. This dose is adjusted to maintain normal serum levels of sodium and potassium without producing hypertension. An intramuscular preparation of mineralocorticoid is used when the patient is unable to ingest oral medications.

Acute adrenal insufficiency is initially treated with 5 to 10 percent glucose in isotonic saline, at a rate of 100 to 120 ml/kg for the first 24 hours. Twenty to 25 percent of the total replacement is administered in the first 2 hours. Fluid therapy after the initial 24 hours will depend on the status of the child and assessment of continuing losses. A water-soluble form of hydrocortisone such as hydrocortisone hemisuccinate, initial dose of 2 mg/kg, is administered and followed by an infusion at 0.6 mg/kg/h until symptoms subside. In this manner high levels of cortisol can be achieved instantaneously. Invasive monitoring with an arterial cannula, central venous pressure line, and urinary catheter is instituted early and continued until cardiovascular stability is attained.

Intramuscular injections of cortisone acetate, 2 mg/kg, are given daily for a few days to provide a sustained and prolonged cortisol level. These doses can then be reduced progressively over 24 hours if progress is satisfactory. A salt-retaining hormone in the form of intramuscular deoxycorticosterone (DOCA) in doses of 1 to 3 mg is added daily to maintain electrolyte balance. This therapy is administered for 48 hours. If oral intake is satisfactory, the intravenous fluids are discontinued and cortisol can be given orally at 0.5 mg/kg in three divided doses. DOCA is administered daily and continued throughout the period of treatment.

Once the acute episode is under control, the patient will require chronic replacement therapy with cortisol and mineralocorticoid. The intramuscular administration of DOCA is replaced by the oral administration of fluorohydrocortisone in doses of 0.05 mg to 0.1 mg daily regardless of age. Appropriate dosage of fluorohydrocortisone is regarded as that at which electrolyte balance can be maintained without signs of hypertension.[59]

Anesthetic Management. The anesthetic management of the child with documented adrenal insufficiency must include the provision for exogenous corticosteroids. Preoperative assessment should focus particularly on the adequacy of corticosteroid supplementation (refer to the section on The Steroid-Treated Patient later in this chapter). However, the selection of anesthetic agents is not influenced by the presence of treated hypocorticism. Plasma cortisol concentrations predictably increase during operation, but the rise is in response to surgical stimulus rather than the anesthetic agent.[60] In the literature there are frequent suggestions that unexplained intraoperative hypotension and even death reflect undiagnosed adrenal insufficiency, but there is no supportive evidence for this etiology.[61]

Should emergency operation become necessary in a situation of untreated or partially treated hypoadrenocorticism, the patient is regarded as one with impending acute adrenal insufficiency and is therefore treated aggressively with fluids, glucocorticoids, and a mineralocorticoid.

Corticosteroids are administered well above the physiological dose of 12 mg/m^2/day. The preparation of choice is cortisone succinate, which provides an immediate serum level. The administration of 2 mg/kg of hydrocortisone every 6 hours is appropriate for most surgical procedures. Anesthetic agents are carefully titrated since patients with adrenal insufficiency are sensitive to the myocardial depression induced by potent anesthetic agents. Muscle relaxants are administered in response to peripheral muscle stimulation in view of the skeletal muscle weakness present in patients with adrenal insufficiency. Continuous monitoring of arterial and cardiac filling pressures is indicated for major procedures. Serum concentrations of electrolytes and blood glucose are evaluated frequently in the perioperative period. Glucocorticoid and mineralocorticoid supplemenation is continued in the postoperative period.

Congenital Adrenal Hyperplasia

Congenital adrenal hyperplasia is an autosomal recessive disorder characterized by ambiguous genitalia, virilization, severe salt-losing crises, and in rare cases hypertension. Clinical manifestations are the result of decreased cortisol production, which leads to unsuppressed ACTH secretion. ACTH acts upon the zona reticularis of the adrenal cortex to increase production of androgenic hormones with subsequent virilization.

There are several forms of congenital adrenal hyperplasia, the most common of which is 21-

hydroxylase deficiency (Table 12–2) with failure of conversion of 17-hydroxyprogesterone. In females, virilization is manifested by ambiguous external genitalia, which if untreated will lead to premature growth of pubic and axillary hair and enlargement of the clitoris. Muscles are well developed and ossification is well advanced for chronological age, with early epiphyseal closure and short stature in the untreated patient.

Salt-losing crises occur in about half of all patients with 21-hydroxylase deficiency as a result of a concomitant aldosterone deficiency. In those patients who do not have salt-wasting crises in times of stress, there is actually an increase in aldosterone production. Salt loss is aggravated by the presence of two metabolic intermediates, 17-hydroxyprogesterone and progesterone, both of which antagonize the action of aldosterone on the renal tubule. Adrenal hyperplasia is to be suspected in an infant with ambiguous genitalia, poor feeding, vomiting, lethargy, and shock. Low serum sodium concentration and abnormally high serum potassium lend support to the diagnosis. The electrocardiogram may show sharply peaked T waves and shortening of the S-T segment, consistent with hyperkalemia. Urea nitrogen and creatinine are increased secondary to prerenal diversion of the circulation. Evidence of increased plasma concentration of 17-hydroxyprogesterone establishes the diagnosis. Serum concentrations of 200 ng/dl are considered normal in the first month of life, after which there is a gradual decrease to 100 ng/dl until puberty.

Treatment. There are three essential components to treating salt-losing crises: intravenous fluids containing sodium, mineralocorticoids (deoxycorticosterone), and cortisol. If the infant is moribund, initial treatment is begun with the intravenous infusion of normal saline at 20 ml/kg administered over a short period of time. With improvement of the circulatory status, treatment is then continued as for acute adrenal insufficiency crises.

In the patient receiving fludrocortisone (Florinef), blood pressure is measured frequently, since hypertension is an early sign of overdosage. Fludrocortisone is administered in a dosage of 0.05 to 1 mg orally; the requirements do not seem to increase with age, although the reasons for this are unclear. The dosage of cortisol to maintain adequate bone maturation, growth, and steroid levels is normally two and one half to three times the normal secretory rate of cortisol. The average dose of cortisol for patients with congenital adrenal hyperplasia is in the range of 30 to 36 mg/m^2/day or 3 to 3.5 mg/kg/day.[62] Two thirds of the dose is administered in the evening hours, when the major surge of ACTH occurs, and one third in the morning hours.

In salt losers, discontinuation of mineralocorticoids at any time carries the risk of acute adrenal insufficiency. These children will need close observation should infection develop and in preparation for surgery. In these situations their requirements for corticosteroids and mineralocorticoids will be increased.

Table 12–2. CONGENITAL ADRENAL HYPERPLASIA

Enzymatic Defect	Urine	Plasma	Electrolyte Abnormality	Symptoms	Treatment
21-Hydroxylase, salt-losing	↑ Pregnanetriol ↑ 17-Ketosteroids ↓ Aldosterone	↑ 17-Hydroxyprogesterone ↑ Dehydroepiandrosterone ↑ Renin ↓ Aldosterone	↓ Na ↑ K	Virilization Muscle weakness Dehydration	DOCA + cortisol for acute crisis Fluorohydrocortisone + cortisone for maintenance therapy
21-Hydroxylase, non–salt-losing	↑ Pregnanetriol ↑ 17-Ketosteroids	↑ 17-Hydroxyprogesterone ↑ Dehydroepiandrosterone ↑ Renin ↑ Aldosterone	Normal	Virilization	Cortisone
11-Hydroxylase	↑ Tetrahydro-S → Pregnanetriol	↑ Compound S →↓ Renin →↓ Aldosterone	↑ NA ↓ K	Incomplete virilization Hypertension	Cortisone
17-Hydroxylase	↓ 17-Ketosteroids	↑ Progesterone ↑ Corticosterone ↑ 11-Deoxycorticosterone	Normal		
3-β-Dehydrogenase, salt-losing	↑ 17-Ketosteroids	↑ Pregnenolone	↓ Na ↑ K	Dehydration	DOCA + cortisol for acute crisis Fluorohydrocortisone + cortisone for maintenance therapy

Table 12–3. DIFFERENCES IN STEROID PREPARATIONS

	Biological Half-Life (h)	Plasma Half-Life (min)	Glucocorticoid Potency	Equivalent Glucocorticoid (mg)	Mineralocorticoid Activity
Short-Acting					
Cortisol	8–12	90	1	20	2+
Cortisone	24–36	30	0.8	25	2+
Prednisone	24–36	30	4	5	1+
Prednisolone	12–36	200	4	4	1+
Methylprednisolone	12–36	200	5	4	0
Intermediate-Acting					
Triamcinolone	12–36	200	5	4	0
Long-Acting					
Betamethasone	36–54	300	25	0.60	0
Dexamethasone	36–54	300	30	0.75	0

Anesthetic Management. The preoperative assessment of patients must include evaluation of the state of hydration, serum electrolytes, urea nitrogen, blood glucose, and acid-base status. Glucocorticoids and mineralocorticoids are continued in the usual doses up to the time of surgery. Serial preoperative blood pressure measurement is important to evaluate the adequacy of mineralocorticoid replacement. On the day of operation, the usual therapeutic cortisone dose is increased by 50 to 100 percent. Thus a child receiving a daily morning dose of 8 mg of cortisone should have the dose increased to 12 mg, administered by intravenous injection. The initial dose should be followed by a continuous infusion of 0.4 mg/kg/h throughout the period of surgery or given as individual doses of 1.5 to 2 mg/kg at 6-hour intervals. Intramuscular DOCA should be administered in dosages of 1 to 3 mg daily and continued until the patient is able to resume oral medication. The use of invasive monitoring is dictated by the severity of the surgical procedure and physical status of the patient. Electrolytes, blood glucose, and acid-base status are evaluated frequently during the surgical procedure. Any anesthetic agent, whether volatile or intravenous, may be used; one agent does not seem to have any advantage over another. Postoperatively, these patients must be observed closely for signs of adrenal insufficiency.

The Steroid-treated Patient

Cortisone, when administered, must be converted to cortisol to become biologically active. This conversion occurs even in the absence of adrenals.[5] Similarly, prednisolone, a synthetic steroid, must be converted to prednisone to become biologically active. In managing patients on corticosteroid therapy it is important to distinguish between plasma and biological half-life of the steroid preparations (Table 12–3). The biological half-life appears to be manifested well after the glucocorticoid has left the circulation and is reflected in the duration of the hypothalamic-pituitary-adrenal (HPA) suppression. It is also known that the duration of the HPA suppression approximates the duration of the anti-inflammatory activity of the glucocorticoid when this is given orally. By examining the HPA suppression, it has been possible to estimate the duration of the therapeutic effects of cortisol and its analogues.

Important factors in determining the degree of HPA suppression are not only the potency and the tissue half-life of the glucocorticoid but also the dosage, the time of day, and the total duration of steroid therapy. The peak activity of the pituitary-adrenal interaction occurs in the early morning hours, with high levels of plasma cortisol being measured at approximately 8:00 A.M. The resultant feedback maximally suppresses further ACTH release. If exogenous steroids are administered at this time, there will be minimal suppressive effect on the pituitary-adrenal axis.[63]

It is generally accepted that significant HPA suppression occurs after 10 days of high-dose corticosteroid therapy and may be detected as early as 5 days. The recovery time from HPA suppression is not as definite and can be as long as 12 months after only 2 weeks of supraphysiological doses of steroids (Table 12–4).

In the recovery phase, ACTH levels increase before the adrenal cortex is capable of responding to ACTH. However, without evaluation of the axis, it is difficult to draw conclusions regarding recovery of the HPA axis. Preoperative evaluation of the pituitary-adrenal axis, as suggested by Symreng and colleagues, would pro-

Table 12–4. RECOVERY OF HYPOTHALAMIC-PITUITARY-ADRENAL FUNCTION AFTER WITHDRAWAL OF STEROIDS

Recovery Time (mon)	Plasma 17-Hydroxycorticoid Values	Plasma ACTH Values	Adrenal Response to Exogenous ACTH	Response to Metyrapone
1	Low	Low	Low	Low
2–5	Low	High	Low	Low
6–9	Normal	Normal	Low	Low
> 9	Normal	Normal	Normal	Normal

vide a more intelligent approach to coverage of the corticosteroid-treated patient.[64] However, since evaluation of the HPA axis is often difficult and impractical, it is wise to administer steroid supplementation to patients who will experience medical or surgical stress within 1 year of cessation of corticosteroid therapy.

Knowledge of the absorption rates of commercial steroid preparations is important in preparing these patients for operation. For example, the hemisuccinates and phosphate are water soluble preparations and readily absorbed when administered by a parenteral route. They are useful in acute situations as well as for prolonged infusions. The acetate and diacetate forms are insoluble in water and when given intramuscularly are absorbed slowly over a period of days or weeks and can be used parenterally for short-term continuous therapy in place of oral steroids. The pivalates and hexacetonide are long-acting and are absorbed over weeks or months.

The preoperative coverage of the corticosteroid-treated pediatric patient is based on adult protocols. We know that the adrenal cortex of the normal adult under perioperative conditions is able to secrete 116 to 185 mg of cortisol daily.[65] During periods of maximum stress, the adult is able to secrete 200 to 500 mg daily. Good correlation also seems to exist between the response of the adrenal gland and the severity and duration of surgical stress. In one study, the mean maximal plasma cortisol level during the major surgical procedure was 47 μg/dl (range, 22 to 75 μg/dl), and values remained above 26 μg/dl for a maximum of 72 hours. The mean maximal cortisol level during minor surgery was 28 μg/dl (range, 10 to 44 μg/dl).[19]

In the child, hydrocortisone hemisuccinate, 2 mg/kg, is administered every 6 hours on the day of operation. For major surgery, this therapy is continued for the next 3 days and either discontinued abruptly or tapered over the next 5 days. For minor operations, such as a herniorrhaphy, 24-hour coverage with 2 mg/kg of hydrocortisone hemisuccinate every 6 hours is sufficient protection, whereas for short procedures like esophagoscopy a single injection of 2 mg/kg of hydrocortisone hemisuccinate on the day of operation is sufficient.[66]

Hypercorticism

Cushing's syndrome is characterized by chronic excessive production of glucocorticoid hormones. In 1932, Harvey Cushing described bilateral adrenal hyperplasia secondary to basophilic adenomas. This form of the syndrome, bilateral adrenal hyperplasia caused by excessive production of ACTH, became known as Cushing's disease and is distinguished from other forms of the syndrome. Cushing's disease was formerly thought rare but is now being detected with increasing frequency. The initiating factor appears to be a hypothalamic disturbance giving rise to pituitary tumors. However, enlargement of the sella turcica in children is extremely rare. Characteristic of the syndrome is increased secretion of corticotropin, with loss of the circadian rhythm and resistance to suppression by the dexamethasone test.

Excessive production of biologically active ACTH by nonendocrine tumors such as thymoma, bronchogenic carcinoma, islet tumor of the pancreas, neuroblastoma, and ganglioneuroblastoma will give rise to a symptom complex known as ectopic Cushing's syndrome. More commonly in children, a clinical pattern identical to Cushing's syndrome results from prolonged exogenous administration of glucocorticoids.

In infants with adrenal involvement, the lesion is usually a functioning tumor, frequently a malignant cortical carcinoma. These patients present with increased production of androgens, estrogens, and aldosterone, giving a mixed picture of hypercorticism.

Clinical Features. A moon facies and centripetal fat distribution with thin extremities and truncal obesity are the most outstanding features. Growth retardation is a useful sign to distinguish this syndrome from exogenous obesity, which is usually characterized by excessive growth. Osteoporosis is present, with delayed epiphyseal maturation due to decreased matrix formation and impaired calcium reabsorption. Hypertension occurs as a result of increased catecholamine secretion with salt and fluid retention. Hyperglycemia or frank diabetes mellitus results from inhibition of peripheral utilization of glucose and concomitant gluconeogenesis. Hypokalemic alkalosis may be present, although this is more commonly seen in the ectopic ACTH syndrome. The lympholytic and immunosuppressive effects of glucocorticoids make these patients more susceptible to infections. Glucocorticoids also have a negative effect on wound healing, which is only in part reversed by vitamin A.[67]

Diagnosis. Demonstration of increased plasma and urine concentrations of cortisol forms the basis of the diagnosis of hypercorticism. Dexamethasone will suppress production of cortisol in the normal patient but not in the patient with hypercorticism; testing for cortisol production after administration of dexamethasone is the most useful method for screening patients for hypercorticism. An elevated plasma level of adrenocorticotropic hormone suggests the presence of a pituitary gland tumor or an ectopic hormone-producing tumor. A very high level of ACTH is highly suggestive of an ectopic tumor. Carcinoma of the adrenal cortex, which produces an excess of glucocorticoids, is likely to cause secretion of an excess of androgens, leading to increased urinary excretion of 17-ketosteroids and sometimes to signs of virilization.

Preoperative Evaluation. Special preoperative considerations in children with hypercorticism are directed toward the establishment of the diagnosis, the indication for surgery, and the specific hormonal abnormalities present. In cases of glucocorticoid excess, emphasis is placed on regulating hyperglycemia and hypertension, ensuring that the intravascular volume is adequate and that electrolyte concentrations are normal. Evaluation of acid-base disturbances is particularly important in cases of ectopic ACTH production, in which hypokalemic alkalosis may be marked. Radiographs of the skeletal system should be reviewed for evidence of osteoporosis and the presence of subclinical pathological fractures. This is important in terms of subsequent positioning of the patient.

In addition to the evaluation of the specific medical conditions of the patient, specific considerations are directed to the particular operation contemplated.

There is no reason to alter the preoperative medication schedule, since hypercorticism does not influence drug metabolism. Holaday and associates report decreased morphine metabolism in patients following bilateral adrenalectomy.[68]

Anesthetic Management. Surgical stress will predictably increase the release of cortisol from the adrenal cortex. It does not seem likely, however, that these patients would be affected differently from normal patients. Halothane, ethrane, isoflurane, or a nitrous oxide-narcotic relaxant technique can be chosen according to the personal preference of the anesthesiologist. Mechanical ventilation of the lungs is suggested in view of the muscle weakness that frequently accompanies hypercorticism. Muscle relaxant doses may need to be reduced, especially if hypokalemia coexists. The need for invasive monitoring is dependent on the type of operation and the physical status of the patient. For adrenalectomy, the size, vascularity, and location of the tumor must be considered. Once the secreting tumor is removed the patient should receive supplemental exogenous intravenous glucocorticoids (as discussed previously in the section on Adrenal Insufficiency). Supplementation is required by patients undergoing unilateral as well as bilateral adrenalectomy, since the contralateral adrenal may be quiescent as a result of low levels of ACTH. Postoperatively, the glucocorticoid may be tapered to a maintenance therapy level.

PRIMARY ALDOSTERONISM

Primary aldosteronism usually occurs in the third decade of life and is rare in children. It is generally attributable to a functional adrenal tumor. In children, hyperaldosteronism has been associated more commonly with adrenal hyperplasia. However, demonstration of a low renin serum level should suggest a primary adrenal defect.

Clinical Manifestations. The clinical symptoms are due to excess production of mineralocorticoids, which results in hypertension. Other symptoms include polydipsia, polyuria, nocturia, paresthesias, visual disturbance, intermittent paralysis, tetany, fatigue, muscle weakness, and discomfort. The severe growth retardation and muscle weakness that may occur are probably a result of potassium depletion. The urine is alkaline or neutral, and the kidneys lose their ability to concentrate urine. The serum pH, carbon dioxide content, and sodium concentration are all elevated, and serum potassium and chloride levels are decreased. Tetany may occur in spite of a normal serum calcium. Urinary excretion of 17-ketosteroids and 17-hydroxycorticosteroids is within normal limits, but urinary excretion of aldosterone is increased.

Primary aldosteronism must be differentiated from secondary hyperaldosteronism, in which there is an increased secretion of aldosterone secondary to low body sodium and excessive accumulation of potassium and/or dehydration. Secondary hyperaldosteronism is present in congestive cardiac failure, cirrhosis of the liver, and the nephrotic syndrome. The most important diagnostic clue is the level of serum renin, which is high in secondary hyperaldosteronism but low in primary aldosteronism, in which the renin-angiotensin system is suppressed.

Diagnosis. A serum potassium level of less than 3.5 mEq/L in a patient with hypertension suggests hyperaldosteronism. The diagnosis is confirmed by the demonstration of an increased plasma concentration of aldosterone and elevated urinary potassium. Measurement of plasma renin activity allows differentiation between primary hyperaldosteronism with low activity and secondary hyperaldosteronism with increased secretion. The patient's drug history should be considered in interpreting laboratory values (Table 12–5).

Anesthetic Management. The preoperative evaluation of the patient with hyperaldosteronism is directed toward assessment of the electrolyte status and correction of hypertension and hypokalemia. The anesthetic management is simplified if hypokalemia is corrected preoperatively, since hyperventilation can further decrease the serum concentration of potassium.

Either intravenous or inhaled anesthetic agents are acceptable choices; however, the choice of ethrane may be questionable if a nephropathy exists preoperatively. Invasive monitoring of arterial blood pressure and central venous pressure is suggested for adequate evaluation of intravascular volume as well as of the response to intravenous fluids. Unexpected hypotension in response to vasodilating anesthetic agents and positive-pressure ventilation may be the result of aggressive preoperative preparation to reduce the excess intravascular volume. Acid-base status and serum electrolytes must be monitored frequently during the perioperative period. Supplementation with exogenous cortisol is not indicated in the case of a solitary adenoma. However, when multiple adenomas are to be excised with bilateral mobilization of the adrenal gland, transient hypocorticism may develop, and the need for exogenous cortisol exists. In this situation a continuous infusion of cortisone hemisuccinate should be administered to attain immediate high serum levels.

Table 12–5. DRUGS THAT ALTER PLASMA RENIN ACTIVITY

Increased Activity	Decreased Activity
Thiazide diuretics	Propranolol
Nitroprusside	Alpha-methyldopa
Hydralazine	Clonidine
Chlorpromazine	
Thyroxine	

ADRENAL MEDULLA

The adrenal medulla is composed of chromaffin tissue derived from the neural crest. By its capability to synthesize epinephrine and norepinephrine, the medulla becomes an integral part of the sympathetic nervous system (Fig. 12–4). Norepinephrine forms the neurotransmitter for the postganglionic fibers of the sympathetic nervous system, with the exception of the sweat glands and the pilomotor nerves. Epinephrine is produced entirely in the medulla from methylation of norepinephrine by the action of the enzyme phenylethanolamine transferase. The presence of cortisol is essential for this reaction to take place. This synergistic action of cortisol partly explains the hypertension that occurs in syndromes of hypercorticism.

The half-life of catecholamines is short because deactivation occurs rapidly by means of enzymatic degradation (catechol-*O*-methyltransferase) or conjugation (with sulfate or glucuronide). The secretion of catecholamines is under the direct control of the nervous system. Factors such as mental stress, hypoxia, and acidemia favor the release of epinephrine. In addition, histamine can stimulate the release of epinephrine from the adrenal medulla. This explains why the administration of D-tubocurarine, which releases histamine, can produce a rise in blood pressure when used in a patient with pheochromocytoma.

Knowledge of the pharmacology of catecholamines is important in understanding the clinical and anesthetic implications of catecholamine-secreting tumors. Alquist's classification of catecholamines as possessing alpha- or beta-adrenergic activity was artificially based on chemical and pharmacological differences.[69] Under this

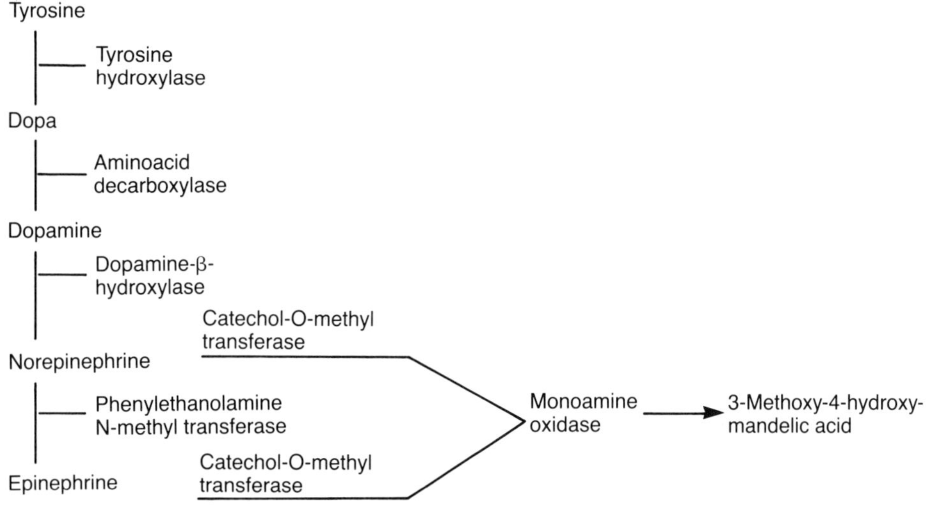

FIGURE 12–4. Biosynthesis of catecholamines.

classification, norepinephrine was described as possessing alpha-adrenergic activity and producing systemic vasoconstriction with reflex bradycardia. However, as a neurotransmitter of the sympathetic nervous system, norepinephrine has direct cardiac effects or beta activity. The beta activity of norepinephrine will become evident in the presence of an agent such as phentolamine, which will block the alpha-receptors.

Epinephrine is considered to possess both alpha and beta activity. The peripheral vascular effects of epinephrine vary in different vascular beds and with different drug concentrations. In the arterioles of skeletal muscle where both alpha- and beta-receptors are present, vasodilatation occurs at a low concentration of epinephrine. By contrast, in the presence of a high concentration of epinephrine, the alpha effects predominate and vasoconstriction occurs. The vessels of the skin and mucous membranes will respond almost always with vasoconstriction. The effect of epinephrine on the heart is similar to that of norepinephrine. The major difference between norepinephrine and epinephrine is the effect on body metabolism. Epinephrine is associated with a sharp increase in oxygen consumption. Insulin secretion is inhibited by epinephrine, resulting in increased levels of glucose, lactate, and glycerol.

Dopamine is now generally accepted as a neurotransmitter with specific receptors in certain organs such as the kidney.[70] At low concentrations the beta-adrenergic activity of dopamine is evident, whereas at higher concentrations the alpha effects predominate. Dopamine is often the major catecholamine secreted by a neuroblastoma.

NEUROBLASTOMA

Neuroblastoma is a malignant solid tumor of childhood that arises from the adrenal medulla or paravertebral ganglia. As a tumor derived from the neural crest, a neuroblastoma may occur in the mediastinum or abdomen or invade the spinal canal, where it can cause compression of the spinal cord. A neuroblastoma generally will reach a large size before clinical symptoms become evident. Common sites of metastases include bone marrow, liver, and brain. Radiological studies, including intravenous urograms, computed tomography, and radionuclide scans, are used together with bone marrow and spinal taps to establish the diagnosis. If there is evidence of cord compression, myelography is performed in preparation for emergency decompression.

The diagnosis of neuroblastoma is established by measurement of urinary catecholamines and their metabolites. Abnormally high levels of dopamine, homovanillic acid, norepinephrine, normetanephrine, vanillylmandelic acid, and other metabolites are found in the urine of most patients with neuroblastoma. Radioisotope studies and tumor analysis show that there is increased catabolism of catecholamines, with release of metabolically inactive compounds. As a result, hypertension secondary to catecholamine secretion is not always present.

Anesthetic Management. The size and location of the tumor, extent of the disease, biological effects of the tumor, symptoms related to the presence of the tumor, and the extent of chemotherapy are important factors for the anesthetic management of the child with neuroblastoma.

In a large number of children, metastases may be present at the time of diagnosis. Since neuroblastomas frequently metastasize to the liver, lymph nodes, bone marrow, and skeleton, the preoperative evaluation should include x-ray views of the abdomen and chest, intravenous pyelography, and a skeletal survey. Serum electrolytes and urea nitrogen are measured in addition to hemoglobin/hematocrit. Vomiting and diarrhea may result from vasoactive peptide secreted by some neuroblastomas.

Blood loss equal to the patient's blood volume during the resection of a neuroblastoma is not uncommon. Third space fluid sequestration secondary to the generous exposure needed for the resection should be replaced by lactated Ringer's solution at 8 to 10 ml/kg/h.

In the young child the size of the tumor may cause symptoms of intestinal obstruction, and, particularly in the infant, respiratory failure may be present. Where spinal compression is suspected and an emergency myelogram required, the induction of anesthesia may be further complicated by the presence of a full stomach.

Intravenous catheters must be placed in the upper extremities so that infusion of fluids occurs independently of the status of the inferior vena cava. Urine output is measured by means of a urinary catheter. In thoracic tumors as in large abdominal tumors, a pulse oximeter in addition to measurement of arterial blood gas levels is useful to detect sudden changes in arterial oxygenation. Invasive arterial monitoring is necessary to measure changes in blood pressure. A central vein catheter is used to measure cardiac filling pressure and to administer added volume and resuscitation drugs. Heat losses are common in these patients, and precautions to avoid hypothermia are taken.

Anesthesia may be induced with thiopental or by the use of an inhalation agent, preferably enflurane or isoflurane. If signs of intestinal obstruction are present, a rapid sequence induction is preferred. Isoflurane and enflurane, with their ability to protect the myocardium from catecholamine stimulation and control blood pressure, remain the anesthetic agents of choice. Atracurium and vecuronium are similarly chosen for their minimal cardiovascular effects, and pancuronium has been used in the past without difficulty. Hypertension may be present, and alpha-adrenergic blocking agents such as nitroprusside and phentolamine should be available.

Since most children with neuroblastoma have normal pulmonary function, extubation of the trachea is usually possible at the completion of the surgical procedure. The postoperative care of these patients requires close monitoring of the fluid status as measured by arterial and central venous pressure and urine output. If the cardiovascular or respiratory system is not stable, or losses of blood and fluid have been substantial, these patients should be admitted to the intensive care unit for more attentive supervision.

PHEOCHROMOCYTOMA

Pheochromocytoma is a catecholamine-secreting tumor that originates from chromaffin cells. It is most commonly found in the adrenal medulla but may be found wherever chromaffin tissue is present. Extra-adrenal tumors are usually located in the abdomen along the sympathetic chain, although they have been described in the neck and in the mediastinum. In the bladder they may arise from sympathetic ganglia present in the wall. Pheochromocytoma is a rare tumor in the pediatric population and occurs more commonly at puberty. Over 95 percent of the tumors arise in the abdominal cavity, including approximately 90 percent in the adrenal medulla, with a predilection for the right side. A malignant pheochromocytoma is rare in children. Bilateral or multiple tumors may occur. A pheochromocytoma may occur as part of multiple endocrine adenomatosis (Table 12–6) in association with pituitary and/or parathyroid gland adenoma.[71]

Clinical Manifestations. The symptoms of pheochromocytoma are the result of the physiological and pharmacological effects of an increased plasma concentration of norepinephrine and epinephrine. Headache, nausea, and vomiting are common findings in the child with hypertension due to a pheochromocytoma. Arterial blood pressure may reach levels of over 250 mm Hg systolic with concomitant elevated diastolic pressure. The child often appears pale,

Table 12–6. MULTIPLE ENDOCRINE ADENOMATOSIS

	Organ	Disorder
Werner's syndrome (Type I)	Pituitary	Hypoglycemia
	Parathyroid	Hypercalcemia
	Pancreas	Peptic ulcer
Sipple's syndrome (Type II)	Thyroid	Medullary carcinoma
	Parathyroid	Hyperplasia
	Adrenal medulla	Pheochromocytoma
(Type III)	Nervous system	Multiple neuromas
	Thyroid	Medullary carcinoma
	Adrenal medulla	Pheochromocytoma

weak, and anxious and has cool extremities. Abdominal pain, polydipsia, and polyuria are also common findings.[72] Hypertensive encephalopathy may occur and may be confused with intracranial neoplasm.

Diagnosis. The importance of diagnosing a pheochromocytoma before anesthesia and operation cannot be overemphasized. Pheochromocytoma can be totally quiescent when the tumor is not actively secreting catecholamines but suddenly cause a stormy hypertensive crisis as catecholamines are rapidly secreted into the circulation. Cardiomyopathy is rare in children but more common in the adult patient. Small tumors are more likely to produce the classic intermittent type of hypertension with normotension between crises. Apparently small tumors release active metabolites, including normetanephrine and metanephrine. Sustained hypertension is more common in children and is a feature of large tumors, which predominantly secrete norepinephrine.[73] The catecholamine composition of the tumor will regulate the type and severity of hypertensive crises even to the extent that a hypotensive crisis may occur in dopamine-epinephrine mixed tumors. Measurement of urinary catecholamines or their metabolites provides a useful screening method, but diagnosis is difficult owing to the high percentage of false positives. Measurement of plasma catecholamines reliably establishes the presence of a pheochromocytoma even in those cases in which normotension exists.[74]

Preoperative Preparation. The child should be admitted several days before operation, at which time any additional laboratory tests and preparation may be conducted. Although not common in the pediatric age group, active myocarditis was found in 15 of 26 patients with pheochromocytoma in a study reported by the Mayo Clinic.[75] James reported that the coronary arteries of one patient with pheochromocytoma had platelet aggregates, supporting the role of catecholamines in platelet aggregation.[76]

The preoperative preparation of the patient with pheochromocytoma should include measurement of serum electrolytes, creatinine, and fasting blood glucose levels and, if indicated, a glucose tolerance test. Cardiac evaluation with an electrocardiogram and an echocardiogram is performed to exclude cardiomyopathy. The blood volume in patients with pheochromocytoma is contracted. A falling hematocrit in response to alpha-adrenergic blocking drugs is generally an indication of restoration of blood volume. The function of other endocrine glands is reviewed by history and laboratory evaluation.

Preoperative localization of the tumor can be achieved by the use of computed tomography. Arteriography will establish the vascular connections of the tumor, which are important for surgical resection. General anesthesia for arteriography should be conducted with the same precautions as are taken for anesthesia for resection of the tumor. Radiocontrast materials may cause histamine release when injected during the vascular study, and this may cause the tumor to secrete catecholamines. Provocative tests with agents such as histamine, glucagon, and phentolamine are rarely used because of their associated risks. Venous samples from different locations in the vena cava often can supplement radiological evaluation.[77]

Phenoxybenzamine given orally in increasing doses several days to weeks prior to operation is the drug of choice for the preoperative preparation of the patient with pheochromocytoma. Phenoxybenzamine, a long-acting alpha-blocking drug, acts by strongly binding with the receptor so that it cannot be displaced by circulating catecholamines. Thus, excessive vasoconstriction is prevented in spite of variable surges of catecholamines that can occur during manipulation of the tumor,[78] and the preoperative intravascular volume is partly restored.

Cardiac arrhythmias and tachycardia are very rare in the pediatric patient with pheochromocytoma. If supraventricular arrhythmias should occur, control can be attained by the use of a beta-blocker such as propranolol. Beta-blockade should not be instituted in the absence of alpha-adrenergic block.[79] There is at least a theoretical concern that a heart depressed by beta-blockade could not maintain an adequate cardiac output in the face of unopposed alpha-mediated vasoconstriction. Beta-blockade is not generally required in children with pheochromocytoma.

An additional approach to the preparation of the child with pheochromocytoma is the use of alpha-methyltyrosine, which interferes with the hydroxylation of tyrosine and thereby inhibits the further production of catecholamines. This mode of therapy has been used with some success in children.[79]

Anesthetic Management. Patients with pheochromocytoma require adequate preoperative medication to minimize anxiety-induced catecholamine release. Oral diazepam, 0.1 mg/kg approximately 90 minutes before induction of anesthesia, followed by morphine sulfate, 0.1 mg/kg, and glycopyrrolate, 0.01 mg/kg, 1 hour before produces reliable sedation. Glycopyrrolate is the preferred anticholinergic agent because of its minimal effects on heart rate, whereas scopolamine may produce behavioral dysfunction in some children. The use of morphine with the release of histamine has been questioned in patients with pheochromocytoma, but hypertensive crises have not been reported in well-blocked patients.

Anesthesia is induced by the intravenous administration of thiopental or diazepam or by inhalation of isoflurane or enflurane. Thiopental releases histamine and might cause a hypertensive response, although this has never been reported in children. Enflurane and isoflurane are selected because they do not sensitize the myocardium to the dysrhythmic effects of catecholamines, and they are able to reduce the activity of the sympathetic nervous system. In contrast, halothane increases myocardial sensitivity to catecholamines. Intubation is facilitated by the use of a nondepolarizing muscle relaxant, such as atracurium, metacurine, or vecuronium, that produces minimal cardiovascular effects.[80] The histamine release produced by D-tubocurarine and the vagolytic effects of pancuronium and gallamine make these drugs unattractive in the patient with pheochromocytoma.[81] Succinylcholine has been used in patients with pheochromocytoma without adverse effects, but there is concern that fasciculations may cause release of catecholamines. Clinical experience, however, has not supported this theory.

Intubation of the trachea should be performed only after establishment of an adequate depth of anesthesia and muscle relaxation as determined by a nerve stimulator. To further minimize increases in blood pressure, the administration of intravenous lidocaine, 1 to 2 mg/kg 3 minutes before intubation, is quite effective.[82] Nitroprusside, 1 to 4 μg/kg/min, or phentolamine, 30 to 60 μg/kg, is effective for treating acute rises in blood pressure.

Maintenance of anesthesia can be accomplished with enflurane or isoflurane and nitrous oxide.[83-85] The delivered concentration of these agents is adjusted in response to blood pressure changes. Nitrous oxide narcotic combinations do not suppress sympathetic activity; in addition, should hypotension occur, the reduction in depth of anesthesia is not as easily attainable when intravenous agents are used. Droperidol may provoke hypertension by interfering with the uptake of norepinephrine into the postganglionic sympathetic nerve endings or may stimulate the release of catecholamines directly into the tumor.[86]

Continuous infusions of nitroprusside or phentolamine are necessary if hypertension should occur in the presence of adequate anesthesia.[87] Trimetaphan is not recommended because of histamine release and frequent occurrence of tachyphylaxis. The potential rapidity and magnitude of blood pressure changes require continuous intra-arterial pressure measurements. An intra-arterial catheter is introduced after the induction of anesthesia. During induction of anesthesia arterial blood pressure can be measured reliably by means of a Doppler flowmeter. The use of a pulmonary artery catheter, which permits determination of cardiac output, left heart function, and vascular resistance, generally has been limited to patients in whom there is evidence of myocardial dysfunction. In children, a central venous pressure catheter is used as an alternative, with the understanding that left ventricular dysfunction may not be appreciated by this method.

Serial measurement of arterial blood gases, electrolytes, blood glucose concentration, urine output, and body temperature is required to follow rapid changes in these parameters. The blood glucose level is followed closely, since hypoglycemia may occur when catecholamine secretion decreases following the removal of the tumor.[88] Serial electrocardiograms also should be taken. Also with tumor removal, rapid blood and fluid infusions are usually required to combat hypotension, even if apparently full alpha-blockade was established preoperatively.

Reversal of the neuromuscular blockade at the completion of the procedure is accomplished by the use of anticholinesterase and anticholinergic agents. There is no evidence to suggest that this combination should be avoided.

Postoperatively, invasive monitoring should be continued until cardiovascular stability has been established. Generally, the arterial blood pressure will return to normal within 24 to 48 hours after operation; failure to do so is an indication that residual catecholamine tumor is still present. While the blood pressure will return to normal levels, the plasma concentration of catecholamines will not for at least 7 to 10 days after excision of the pheochromocytoma.

PARATHYROID GLANDS

The parathyroid glands, located behind the upper and lower poles of the thyroid, synthesize a polypeptide known as parathyroid hormone (PTH). Secretion of PTH into the circulation depends on the serum calcium concentration and indirectly on the serum concentration of phosphorus and magnesium. Thus an increased concentration of calcium will inhibit the secretion of PTH, whereas a decreased concentration of calcium will stimulate secretion of parathyroid hormone. An increase in serum concentration of phosphorus will cause a decrease in serum concentration of calcium to maintain the calcium-times-phosphorus product constant. The resulting decrease in calcium concentration will further stimulate the parathyroids to secrete PTH. Magnesium impairs secretion of PTH as well as decreasing the peripheral response to PTH.

The function of PTH is to maintain a normal serum concentration of calcium by promoting the absorption of calcium from three main sites: the kidney, the intestinal tract, and the skeletal system. In the kidney, PTH promotes the conversion of 25-hydroxycalciferol (vitamin D_3) to 1,25-dihydroxycalciferol, the active metabolite. Vitamin D increases tubular reabsorption of calcium while it enhances renal excretion of phosphorus. In renal disease in which phosphorus clearance is decreased, accumulation of phosphate in the circulation will result in a decrease in the serum concentration of calcium and stimulation of the parathyroid gland to secrete PTH.

Similarly, the effect of PTH on the gastrointestinal tract is to induce the synthesis of vitamin D, which in turn enhances calcium absorption. In the skeletal system, PTH releases calcium by its activity on the osteoclastic cells. Evidence of this activity is seen in cystic areas in bone, which may be the cause of pathological fractures.

Calcium exists in the body in two main forms: an inactive protein-bound fraction and an active ionized fraction. Several factors will alter the distribution between these two fractions and must be considered in interpreting serum calcium levels (Table 12–7). A fall in total protein concentration of 0.8 mg will decrease serum calcium by 1 mg/dl. Unless other conditions such as alkalosis exist, this decrease may not be accompanied by symptoms of hypocalcemia since it occurs only in the protein-bound fraction and not in the ionized fraction. Similarly, an increase in total protein may increase the total serum calcium but not the ionized fraction, and symptoms of hypocalcemia may exist.[89]

The ionized calcium fraction regulates the permeability of cell membranes to sodium and potassium. Thus, calcium becomes important in the excitation of skeletal and cardiac muscle. As the serum concentration of ionized calcium increases, the permeability of the cell membrane to sodium and potassium decreases. The effect will be a spontaneous slowing of the cardiac rhythm with an increase in the ventricular arrhythmogenicity, decreases in muscular excitability, and disturbances in mentation. In contrast, when the ionized calcium level is decreased, membrane permeability to sodium and potassium increases, thereby increasing muscle and nervous tissue excitability.

Finally, calcitonin produced by the C cells of the thyroid and thymus glands is important in maintaining serum calcium equilibrium by directly opposing the actions of PTH. Secretion of calcitonin decreases the serum calcium concentration.

Table 12–7. SERUM CALCIUM CONCENTRATION IN VARIOUS CONDITIONS

Increased	Decreased
Milk alkali syndrome	Malabsorption syndrome
Hyperparathyroidism	Hypoparathyroidism
Vitamin A and D excess	Subtotal parathyroidectomy
Idiopathic hypercalcemia of infants	Neonatal tetany
Adrenocortical deficiency	Excessive fluoride intake
PTH-like neoplasms	
Acidosis increases ionized fraction	Alkalosis increases protein fraction
Sarcoidosis	
Immobilization	
Thiazide diuretics	
Acute renal failure	

From Nimmagadda U, Salem MR, Ivankovich AD: Anesthesia and parathyroid disease. Semin Anesth *3*:175, 1984.

HYPERPARATHYROIDISM

The recognition of hyperparathyroidism has increased in recent years for several reasons: routine evaluation of serum calcium levels, increased survival of patients undergoing renal dialysis who may need a parathyroidectomy to control bone and metastatic calcification; increased awareness of hyperparathyroidism as a cause of renal stones; fluoridation of drinking water, which decreases calcium and magnesium content with subsequent stimulation of the parathyroid glands; and iatrogenic factors such as the use of steroids and diuretics.

Hyperparathyroidism can be classified into a primary or idiopathic form, a secondary form, and pseudohyperparathyroidism.

PRIMARY HYPERPARATHYROIDISM

Primary hyperparathyroidism is the result of malregulated hypersecretion of the parathyroid gland. Although considered more common in the adult, hyperparathyroidism is now recognized increasingly frequently in children as a result of improved methods of diagnosis. Hyperparathyroidism may be the result of generalized hyperplasia, a benign adenoma, or carcinoma of the parathyroid gland. It also may exist in association with other endocrine disorders as in multiple endocrine adenomatosis. In childhood, a parathyroid adenoma is the more common etiology.

The clinical manifestations of hyperparathyroidism are secondary to hypercalcemia and can be grouped according to the major bodily systems they affect (Table 12–8). In the newborn infant, primary hyperparathyroidism presents with hypotonia, poor feeding, weight loss, dehydration, anemia, and respiratory distress from a poorly developed rib cage.

Diagnosis. The presence of an elevated ionized serum calcium concentration is diagnostic of primary hyperparathyroidism. The serum chloride is also elevated. This reflects increased renal excretion of bicarbonate, producing a mild metabolic acidosis. Serum concentration of phosphate is decreased with increased urinary excretion of phosphate. As the disease progresses, renal dysfunction is reflected by elevation of serum creatinine. The finding of an increased serum concentration of parathyroid hormone establishes the diagnosis of hyperparathyroidism.

Secondary Hyperparathyroidism

Secondary hyperparathyroidism results from a compensatory increase in the secretion of parathyroid hormone in response to hypocalcemia, hyperphosphatemia, or hypomagnesemia produced by other disease processes. A common cause is renal disease, which impairs the elimination of phosphorus and the synthesis of vitamin D. Gastrointestinal diseases that impair calcium absorption will result in hypocalcemia. After renal transplantation, transient hypercalcemia may exist as a result of the inability of a hyperactive parathyroid to adapt to the normal renal handling of calcium, phosphorus, and vitamin D. In time the parathyroid function will generally return to normal.

Table 12–8. CLINICAL MANIFESTATIONS OF HYPERCALCEMIA

Nervous system	Psychosis Somnolence Hypesthesia
Cardiac	Hypertension Short Q-T interval Prolonged P-R interval
Gastrointestinal	Abdominal pain Peptic ulcer Pancreatitis Vomiting
Renal	Polyuria Lithiasis Decreased GFR
Neuromuscular	Muscle weakness
Articular	Calcifications
Ocular	Band keratopathy Conjunctivitis
Hematopoietic	Anemia

Pseudohyperparathyroidism

Sometimes called ectopic hyperparathyroidism, pseudohyperparathyroidism results from the increased secretion of parathyroid hormone or of a substance with similar endocrine properties from tissues other than the parathyroid glands. More commonly this is caused by carcinoma of the lung, breast, pancreas, kidney, or lymphoid tissues.

Secondary Hypercalcemia

Hypercalcemia may be present in association with conditions not related to the parathyroid gland. Certain tumors can be the cause of hypercalcemia, as occurs with carcinoma of the lung, hepatoma, fibrosarcoma, renal cancer, leukemia, pheochromocytoma, and bone metastases.[90, 91–93] Ectopic parathyroid tissue may also produce hypercalcemia. Hypercalcemia in these conditions is related to the secretion of PTH, similar hormone production of prostaglandin (PGE_2) with osteoclastic activity, or tumor-produced osteoclast-stimulating factor.

Hypercalcemia can result from vitamin D intoxication when doses above 400 units are ingested daily or from vitamin A overdosage as a result of food faddism or treatment for acne.

Thiazide therapy potentiates the hypercalcemic effect of PTH.[94] Milk alkali syndrome similarly can be an important cause of hypercalcemia in patients using large quantities of milk and alkali for peptic ulcer disease.

Immobilization for fractures, burns, or other causes can lead to a rise in serum calcium, which is seen beginning on the fourth day and reaches a peak in 6 days.[95] Total calcium levels may reach 18 mg/dl. Nephrocalcinosis, hypertension, and hypertensive encephalopathy occur in addition to other more typical signs. Thyrotoxicosis and decreased glucocorticoid secretion have been associated with elevated calcium levels as well.[96]

Benign familial hypercalcemia is inherited as an autosomal dominant trait and presents as mild hypercalcemia with serum calcium levels generally under 12 mg/dl and without apparent ill effects.

In infants fat necrosis can lead to calcium levels as high as 19 mg/dl. Fat necrosis occurs in traumatic vaginal deliveries, especially of large infants. Areas subjected to greatest pressure, including shoulders, upper arms, back, and outer thighs, can form necrotic lesions. Hypercalcemia develops after a week or several weeks, suggesting gradual mobilization of calcium to extracellular space from the existing necrotic areas.

Idiopathic hypercalcemia of infancy is thought to be part of a syndrome consisting of mental retardation, elfin facies, and supravalvular aortic stenosis. Clinically, failure to thrive, vomiting, constipation, hypotonia, and nephrocalcinosis may be present.

TREATMENT

The treatment of hyperparathyroidism is directed toward the lowering of the serum concentration of calcium by decreasing bone resorption and increasing urinary calcium excretion. The intravenous infusion of normal saline alone can decrease calcium levels by 2 to 3 mg/dl. Loop diuretics such as furosemide are used to promote urinary calcium loss. This mode of therapy results in the loss of large quantities of electrolytes in the urine; therefore, close monitoring of the cardiovascular and electrolyte status is necessary. Electrocardiography is important to monitor changes in Q-T intervals and occurrence of arrhythmias.[97]

Mithramycin as an inhibitor of RNA synthesis when administered in a dose of 25 μg/kg will block osteoclastic activity induced by parathyroid hormone. A rapid reduction in the serum concentration of calcium occurs within 12 to 36 hours.[98, 99] Mithramycin has a tendency to produce rebound hypercalcemia after an initial decrease, thereby decreasing its effectiveness.

Calcitonin causes no toxicity and can be administered intravenously and intramuscularly in doses of 8 units per kg every 6 hours. Dialysis is used when renal failure is present. By the use of a low-calcium dialysate, approximately 300 mg/h can be removed. Ethylene-diaminetetraacetic acid is a chelating agent that binds calcium but has a substantial nephrotoxicity. Phosphate is administered orally to avoid causing symptoms of hyperphosphatemia.

Specific therapy of hypercalcemia is aimed at treating the cause of hyperparathyroidism. In patients with diffuse hyperplasia, familial hyperplasia, multiple endocrine adenomatosis syndrome, or several adenomas, a subtotal parathyroidectomy is performed to lessen the incidence of postoperative hypocalcemia.

A particular group of patients are the hyperparathyroid patients with a serum calcium level above 15 mg/dl. These patients are seriously ill with a condition referred to as hypercalcemic crisis, which if not treated promptly can lead to coma and even death. If scheduled for emergency operation, these patients are lethargic and are dehydrated, with electrolyte imbalance from vomiting and polyuria. Hypertension is a common finding.

Preoperative Evaluation. The preoperative evaluation of the hyperparathyroid patient includes a careful history and physical examination, with particular emphasis on the cardiovascular, renal, and gastrointestinal systems. Blood pressure and electrolytes should be carefully noted. Several investigators have described electrocardiographic changes in hyperparathyroidism. These include a prolonged P-R interval and a rate-corrected, Q-T interval that is inversely proportional to the serum calcium level up to 16 mg/dl. Above this level T waves are prolonged and rounded and the Q-T interval becomes disproportionately long. Although tachycardia is often mentioned, Bronsky and associates found no change in cardiac heart rate in 35 patients with hypercalcemia.[100]

The patient should be well hydrated, the serum calcium should be decreased to an acceptable level, and other electrolyte abnormalities should be corrected before parathyroidectomy is attempted. The bones are very fragile in these patients, who must be handled very gently to avoid pathological fractures.

Anesthetic Management. Anesthesia can be induced by means of intravenous thiopental or the use of an inhalational agent. Before or soon after the induction of anesthesia a large-bore intravenous catheter should be inserted. Alterations in heart rate with severe bradycardia may occur if the carotid sinus is stimulated during mobilization of the parathyroid glands. A precordial stethoscope is used to monitor cardiac rhythm and ventilation. The use of an esophageal stethoscope is felt by some surgeons to interfere with neck dissection and to cause laryngeal edema.[101] There is experimental and clinical evidence that nasogastric tubes left in place for prolonged periods of time give rise to laryngeal edema,[102] but there is as yet no definite evidence that the same occurs with short-term placement of the esophageal stethoscope.

Urine output should be monitored by means of a Foley catheter. This is particularly important in cases of acute hypercalcemic crises to diagnose renal shutdown. Temperature monitoring is necessary, especially in the young child, in whom heat loss may be a cause of acidosis and increased serum calcium concentration. Lidocaine, 1 to 2 mg/kg, intravenously or by spray 1 minute before intubation, is useful to suppress laryngeal reflexes. The airway may then be secured by a well-positioned endotracheal tube, allowing for air leak below 30 cm of H_2O as suggested by Lee and associates.[103] A supine position with slight elevation of the head and moderate extension of the neck will provide good surgical conditions, increase venous drainage, and decrease bleeding.

In patients with hypercalcemic crises, ketamine may be useful in avoiding precipitous falls in blood pressure. Arterial and venous hypertension are to be avoided, and slight hypotension may be useful in providing a bloodless surgical field. Mild respiratory alkalosis will reduce ionized calcium levels in the blood. Hyperventilation must be used carefully in the patient with hypercalcemic crises, in whom alkalosis may cause calcium to precipitate with further damage to the kidney. The action of calcium on the cell membrane may alter the effect of muscle relaxants; in general, this is a problem only in hypercalcemic crises, and in this case the dose of muscle relaxants should be decreased.

Blood loss generally is not significant. Possible exploration of the mediastinum must be considered whenever operation on the parathyroid glands is undertaken. At the end of the surgical procedure when vital signs are stable, intravenous lidocaine, 1 to 2 mg/kg, is administered to suppress laryngeal reflexes, and the trachea is extubated.

Postoperative Management. During the early postoperative period the patient must be observed in a high-surveillance area. The patient's head is maintained in a 30° elevation, and humidified oxygen is administered. The immediate postoperative complications may lead to airway obstruction. These include hematoma with airway obstruction, bilateral recurrent laryngeal nerve injury, and laryngeal edema.

Bilateral vocal cord paralysis in the postoperative period is a result of bilateral recurrent laryngeal nerve injury.[104] The vocal cords appear flaccid and paralyzed in an intermediate position; the airway may or may not be compromised. Bilateral vocal cord paralysis is suspected in patients with stridor and cyanosis shortly after extubation. If the stridor is mild and laryngeal edema is suspected, treatment with humidified oxygen is warranted. Racemic epinephrine in normal saline administered by nebulizer is useful for airway edema causing obstruction.

Muscular hyperexcitability, with muscle cramps, paresthesias, and cardiac irregularities with prolongation of the Q-T interval, may be present in milder forms of hypocalcemia. The more serious forms are manifested by tetany. Symptoms may appear 3 or 4 days after operation and may persist for 3 to 6 months until the remaining parathyroid tissue is able to produce an adequate amount of parathyroid hormone. Treatment for symptomatic hypocalcemia is administration of calcium gluconate, 30 mg/kg, or calcium chloride, 10 mg/kg, through a central catheter. Calcium should be administered with ECG monitoring.

A rare complication is injury to the cervical sympathetic trunk leading to a Horner's syndrome. Other complications may involve damage to the phrenic nerve, transection of the spinal accessory nerve, and damage to the right lymphatic duct.

HYPOPARATHYROIDISM

In the pediatric age group there are two classic forms of hypoparathyroidism: primary or idiopathic, in which there is decreased production of parathyroid hormone, and pseudohypoparathyroidism, in which there is an increase of parathyroid hormone production with deficient end-organ responsiveness.

Pseudohypoparathyroidism is an inherited disorder in which the release of parathyroid hormone is intact. The children are typically short in stature, with round faces; short, thick necks; and short metacarpals. Mental retardation is a prominent feature. Pseudopseudoparathyroidism is characterized by similar findings, but there is an inadequate secretion of parathyroid hormone.

More commonly, hypoparathyroidism results from the inadvertent removal of parathyroid glands during thyroid operation or during subtotal parathyroidectomy, when the function of the residual parathyroid is decreased.[104]

Deficiency of parathyroid hormone decreases serum and urinary phosphorus excretion, resulting in an elevated serum phosphorus level with a decreased calcium level.

Clinical Manifestations

Signs and symptoms of hypoparathyroidism are a reflection of the serum concentration of calcium. The severity of the symptoms depends on the rapidity of the reduction in serum calcium concentration. Acute hypocalcemia, such as that which occurs when parathyroids are inadvertently removed, manifests itself with perioral paresthesias, restlessness, and neuromuscular irritability. A positive Chvostek's or Trousseau's sign is confirmatory of neuromuscular irritability. In the nonverbal child, inspiratory stridor may be the first sign of hypocalcemia.

A chronic reduction in serum concentration of calcium is associated with fatigue and skeletal muscle cramps. The common cause of chronic hypocalcemia is chronic renal failure. A prolonged P-R interval with unchanged QRS complex frequently provides electrocardiographic evidence of hypocalcemia. Cardiac rhythm remains normal.

Diagnosis

The diagnosis of hypoparathyroidism is based on a reduced serum calcium concentration. Urinary excretion of calcium and phosphorus is decreased. A decrease in urinary excretion of cyclic adenosine monophosphate is an indication of low serum concentration of parathyroid hormone. Diagnosis of pseudohypoparathyroidism is made on the basis of the presence of hyperphosphatemia.

Treatment

Treatment of acute hypocalcemia is with intravenous infusion doses of calcium gluconate 10 percent (0.45 mEq/ml), 30 mg/kg, or calcium chloride 10 percent (1.36 mEq/ml), 10 mg/kg, until signs of neuromuscular irritability, particularly cardiac irritability, disappear. Calcium is administered with the use of electrocardiography to monitor cardiac rhythm until a serum level of 4 mEq/dl is reached.

Hypocalcemia from chronic hypoparathyroidism is treated by the administration of oral calcium and vitamin D. Thiazide diuretics cause sodium depletion without calcium excretion. This tends to increase serum calcium concentration and can be used as an alternative mode of therapy.

Anesthetic Management. Elective surgical procedures in patients with hypoparathyroidism should be postponed until appropriate therapy to raise the serum concentration of calcium can be administered. If the procedure cannot be postponed, intravenous calcium therapy is administered with continuous ECG monitoring.

If emergency operation is to be performed, the anesthetic management is designed to prevent further decreases in the serum concentration of calcium. Respiratory or metabolic alkalosis, which can occur with hyperventilation or after the infusion of bicarbonate for the treatment of a metabolic acidosis, can cause a decrease in the serum ionized calcium concentration. Administration of whole blood with a citrate preservative does not reduce serum calcium concentrations appreciably since the body can mobilize calcium rapidly from its stores. However, the rapid administration of citrated whole blood (1 ml/kg/min) or plasma may cause hypocalcemia, particularly in patients with cirrhosis, in whom a decreased metabolism of citrate may occur.

Arterial blood gases must be monitored frequently during anesthesia with particular regard to pH, serum protein level, and ionized calcium concentration. Muscle relaxants should be administered with the use of a nerve stimulator, but the choice of anesthetic agents should be dictated by the needs of the particular patient and the preference of the anesthesiologist.

Hypocalcemia in the Newborn Infant

The anesthetic management of the newborn infant during the first week of life can be further complicated by the presence of hypocalcemia and hyperphosphatemia. Three groups of infants are particularly prone to neonatal hypocalcemia: premature infants, infants of diabetic mothers, and infants with birth asphyxia.

Hypocalcemia in the neonate is thought to be related to several factors: renal immaturity, direct action of phosphate on calcium deposition and/or resorption, and a relative hypoparathyroidism. The newborn kidney excretes phosphate less efficiently as a result of its low glomerular filtration rate. To increase urinary phosphate excretion the neonate must increase the serum concentration of phosphate. The high serum phosphorus concentration inhibits calcium resorption in order to maintain a normal calcium-times-phosphorus product. In addition, the newborn kidney is relatively refractory to parathyroid hormone, with the result that phosphate excretion is further decreased. Connelly and Crawford found that the newborn infant responded to exogenous parathyroid hormone on the first day of life with an increase in serum phosphate concentration, but the renal phosphaturic response was minimal.[105] By the third day, the renal response was adequate to lower the serum phosphorus level. An increase in urinary cyclic AMP excretion during the first 3 days of life is associated with an increase in phosphate excretion and phosphate clearance. At the end of the second week of life, the renal response to parathyroid hormone is similar to that of the adult.[106, 107] Thus, the hypoparathyroidism that exists in the neonate is transient, lasting a few days, and calcium serum concentration should return to normal after the first week of life. The term newborn infant is capable of maintaining a normal serum calcium concentration, probably by parathyroid bone calcium mobilization.[108]

The decrease in parathyroid function is a prominent factor in premature infants and infants of diabetic mothers,[109, 110] whereas increased production of calcitonin may play a role in the hypocalcemia seen in the infant with birth asphyxia.

GONADS

TESTIS

In the male, testosterone is the principal hormone secreted by the testis. Testosterone is responsible for the development of secondary sex characteristics and spermatogenesis in the adult. Dysfunction of the testis is reflected by Klinefelter syndrome, which is characterized by the presence of two X chromosomes and one Y chromosome. Plasma concentration of testosterone is reduced and the testes are small. Diagnosis is made by the demonstration of clumps of Barr's bodies in mucosal cells. The syndrome does not pose anesthetic problems.

OVARY

The principal hormones produced by the ovary are estrogen and progesterone. Dysfunction of hormonal secretion includes gonadal dysgenesis and polycystic ovary.

Gonadal Dysgenesis

Gonadal dysgenesis, or Turner's syndrome, is due to absence of the second X chromosome, giving a chromosome pattern of XO. These patients generally are of short stature, are mildly obese, and have a webbed neck that may present problems at intubation. Their anesthetic management may be further complicated by the presence of coarctation of the aorta and pectus excavatum.

Polycystic Ovary

Polycystic ovary syndrome (Stein-Leventhal syndrome) is characterized by an increased production of androgens with associated findings of primary amenorrhea, hirsutism, and muscularity. Height is usually normal, and congenital anomalies are unlikely. The patients do not present particular anesthetic problems.

PANCREAS

The pancreas contains two types of secreting glands: acinar tissue responsible for exocrine secretion, and islet cells (islands of Langerhans) responsible for endocrine secretion. This section is not concerned with disorders of the exocrine pancreas. Islet cells secrete insulin (beta-cells) and glucagon (alpha-cells). Hypofunction of these cells results in diabetes mellitus, and hyperactivity results in hypoglycemia.

DIABETES MELLITUS

Diabetes mellitus is the most common endocrine disease in childhood. It results from an absolute or functional deficiency of insulin, which leads to an impairment of glucose transport, a decrease in the storage and synthesis of lipid, and a decrease in the synthesis of protein. These metabolic abnormalities produce long-term effects through changes in small and large vessels resulting in retinopathy, nephropathy, neuropathy, ischemic heart disease, and large vessel obstruction. The accumulated clinical, experimental, and biochemical evidence links the development of complications from diabetes to the degree of control of the metabolic disturbances found in diabetes. Hence, the pediatrician's aim is to maintain as near normal metabolism as is compatible with the well-being of each individual child.

Diabetes mellitus has an overall prevalence of 1.89 per 1000 school-age children and affects some 100,000 persons under the age of 20 in the United States.[111] Males and females appear to be equally affected, and there is no correlation to socioeconomic status. Prevalence rates in the United States are similar to those reported in England and Sweden.[112]

The Diabetes Branch of the National Institutes of Health (NIH) recommends dividing patients with diabetes mellitus into two principal types: type I, the insulin-dependent group (IDDM) and type II, the non-insulin-dependent group (NIDDM). Diabetes in children is of the insulin-dependent variety previously called juvenile diabetes mellitus. However, insulin-dependent diabetes may present in adulthood, and hence the term juvenile diabetes mellitus should be abandoned. Type I diabetes is characterized by insulin deficiency, intermittent ketoacidosis, and association with other autoimmune diseases. Type II diabetes is characterized by normal or high plasma insulin levels, absence of ketoacidosis, a strong hereditary pattern, and onset in the third or fourth decade of life or later.[113]

Pathogenesis

The cause of pancreatic beta-cell failure in IDDM may be an autoimmune destruction of pancreatic islets in predisposed individuals. Type I diabetes is known to be associated with disorders such as Addison's disease and Hashimoto's thyroiditis, in which autoimmune disturbances are known to be pathogenic.[114]

Circulating antibodies directed against the surface components of islet cells have been demonstrated and are not the insulin antibodies found universally in insulin-treated diabetic patients. Environmental triggering factors such as a viral infection may initiate the immune response in susceptible individuals. A diabetes-producing variant of Coxsackie B4 virus has been isolated from the pancreas of a child who died of diabetic ketoacidosis.[115]

Although insulin deficiency is the primary defect, secondary hormonal changes also contribute to metabolic abnormalities. Levels of growth hormone, catecholamines, and cortisol are elevated in decompensated diabetes and are restored to normal with adequate insulin therapy.[111] The important metabolic effects of insulin include the transfer of glucose across the cell membrane into the cell, the formation of glycogen, the conversion and storage of glucose as fatty acids in adipose tissue, and the passage of potassium into cells with glucose. Insulin deficiency results in hyperglycemia secondary to glycogenolysis; gluconeogenesis and decreased peripheral glucose utilization; and lipolysis in fat tissue, which increases free fatty acids and conversion of free fatty acids to ketone bodies (acetoacetic acid and betahydroxybutyric acid). Acetone formed from acetoacetic acid is responsible for the characteristic fruity odor of the breath.

Epinephrine produces hyperglycemia by stimulating liver glycogenolysis, decreasing glucose uptake by muscle, and directly inhibiting pancreatic insulin release. The glucocorticoids exert their diabetogenic action by increasing hepatic gluconeogenesis from proteins, decreasing glucose uptake by adipose tissue, and stimulating the formation of an ill-defined circulating insulin antagonist.

Clinical Features

Initially, children usually present with a history of polyuria, polydipsia, polyphagia, and weight loss. An insidious onset with lethargy, weakness, and weight loss is also quite common. A minority of children (10 to 20 percent) present with frank diabetic ketoacidosis manifested by hyperglycemia, ketonemia, vomiting, dehydration, obtundation, air hunger, acetone breath, glucosuria, and ketonuria.

Abdominal pain with a leukocytosis that mimics appendicitis is common in children with ketoacidosis and may be associated with an elevated serum amylase level that does not necessarily indicate the existence of pancreatitis.[116] Hyperglycemia with blood glucose exceeding 300 mg/dl must be demonstrated for this diagnosis to be made. With the administration of fluid and electrolyte therapy and insulin replacement, the abdominal pain resolves after several hours.

Renal glycosuria, either as an isolated finding or as part of the Fanconi's syndrome in a child with vomiting and starvation ketosis, may mimic the urinary findings of ketoacidosis (glycosuria and ketonuria). Blood glucose levels are normal, however, and insulin therapy is not indicated.

The average total daily dose of insulin in children when replacement is necessary is on the order of 0.5 to 1.0 units per kg. With a single daily-dose regimen, two thirds of the total dose is intermediate-acting insulin (NPH, lente), and the remainder is fast-acting regular insulin, given 30 minutes before breakfast. Adjustments in the dose are made depending on the pattern of blood glucose or urine glucose. Each increase should be approximately 10 percent, and subsequent changes should be made at 2- to 3-day intervals, depending on response. Twice daily injections may also be utilized, with two thirds given before breakfast and one third before the evening meal; each injection consists of intermediate- and short-acting insulin in the proportion of 2:1 or 3:1. For infants and children less than 5 years old, twice daily injections result in smoother control of blood glucose and fewer episodes of hypoglycemia.

Nearly all patients can be demonstrated to

have antibodies to insulin after several months of insulin therapy. Rarely, children with antibodies develop true insulin resistance characterized by an insulin requirement in excess of 2 units/kg/day. A change to a preparation of pure beef or pure pork insulin usually resolves the problem; if it does not, a course of steroids may be necessary.[111]

Following initial stabilization when insulin requirements are quite high, there is in many children a progressive reduction in insulin requirements to daily doses of 0.3 unit per kg or less. The duration of this honeymoon phase is variable, lasting a few months or as long as 1 to 2 years.

Hypoglycemic reactions occur in all diabetic children at some time during the course of their disease. The signs of hypoglycemia develop suddenly over a few minutes, whereas signs of diabetic ketoacidosis develop over hours or days. Symptoms and signs of hypoglycemia include trembling, shaking, sweating, apprehension, tachycardia, mood changes, mental confusion, seizures, and coma. When the child is cooperative, a drink with sugar or candy should be taken. Glucagon, 0.5 to 1 mg intramuscularly, is useful when the patient is losing consciousness or vomiting. When intravenous access is available, 1 ml/kg of 50 percent dextrose, diluted to 10 percent before injection, should by given until symptoms improve.

Hypoglycemic episodes that alternate with hyperglycemia, ketosis, glycosuria, and ketonuria should suggest the diagnosis of Somogyi's phenomenon.[117] This syndrome has been described as "hypoglycemia begetting hyperglycemia," and is believed to be caused by excessive insulin and the counterregulation of its hypoglycemic effects by hyperglycemic hormones. The occurrence of "brittle" diabetes with daily insulin doses of more than 2 units per kg suggests that the phenomenon is present and the insulin dose should be reduced. Somogyi's phenomenon is the most common cause of instability or brittleness.

Diabetic Ketoacidosis

The criteria for diagnosis include hyperglycemia (glucose greater than 300 mg/dl), ketonemia (ketones strongly positive at greater than 1:2 dilution of serum), acidosis (pH less than 7.30), glycosuria, and ketonuria. Clinical findings include dehydration, hyperventilation, obtundation, and a strong odor of acetone on the breath. A few other conditions with ketoacidosis, such as starvation, organic acidemias, and ingestion of ethanol or salicylates, have to be considered and excluded. Precipitating factors include stress, such as trauma, infections, vomiting, and psychological disturbances.

Insulin deficiency results in a pattern of starvation and catabolism with gluconeogenesis, ketogenesis, and enhanced lipolysis. Overproduction of ketones and glucose results in their accumulation in the blood and urine. Hyperglycemia increases serum osmolality, with a shift of water from the intracellular space producing intracellular dehydration. Excessive diuresis results in a net loss of water greater than that of electrolytes and a decrease in the intravascular fluid volume. In the presence of acidosis, potassium leaves the cells and, although serum potassium may be high, total body stores are depleted. Metabolic acidosis occurs mainly because of the buildup of organic acids. Dehydration and impairment in renal acidification also contribute to acidosis. Severe systemic acidosis may cause hypotension and impair myocardial function. Hyperosmolality and brain cell dehydration are the main causes of obtundation. In the treated patient, further obtundation may occur, with a rapid lowering of blood glucose to 250 mg/dl and below. A shift of water from the extracellular fluid to the relatively hyperosmolar brain cells causes cerebral edema.[118]

The treatment of diabetic ketoacidosis consists of fluid and electrolyte replacement, insulin administration, and frequent laboratory and clinical monitoring. The child differs little from the adult in basic pathophysiological disturbances and clinical features. However, in children there is a greater need for precision in the quantity, composition, and rate of fluid and electrolyte therapy, as well as in insulin dosage. A flow chart should include fluid intake and output, weight, vital signs, blood glucose, electrolytes, bicarbonate, and pH. These parameters should be monitored at intervals of 2 to 4 hours. Hourly blood glucose readings should be made during the first 6 to 10 hours.

A fluid and electrolyte deficit of 10 percent or more is present in moderate-to-severe diabetic ketoacidosis. This deficit of 1 dl/kg of fluid should be replaced over 24 hours in addition to the normal maintenance requirements. Normal saline solution (20 ml/kg) should be given in the first hour. Half the deficit should be replaced in the first 8 hours. When the serum glucose declines below 300 mg/dl, 5 percent glucose and 0.45 normal saline solution should replace the normal saline solution. Potassium should be added to the solution in the absence of hyperkalemia, provided renal function is intact. Therapy results in a shift of potassium back to the intracellular compartment and may result in hypokalemia if potassium supplementation is inadequate. The administration of potassium phosphate will also replace phosphate, which can be significantly depleted in acidosis. Provision of phosphate promotes the formation of 2,3-diphosphoglycerate (2,3-DPG), which shifts the oxygen dissociation curve to the right, releasing oxygen to tissues and resulting in correction of acidosis.[119]

Metabolic acidosis usually corrects spontaneously with the administration of fluids, electrolytes, and insulin owing to the interruption of ketogenesis, the metabolism of ketones to bicarbonate, and the generation of bicarbonate by the distal renal tubule. Bicarbonate administration may be deleterious because alkalosis shifts the oxygen dissociation curve to the left, accelerates entry of potassium into the intracellular space, and may lead to worsening in cerebral acidosis. Hence bicarbonate is not administered unless the pH is below 7.0. Bicarbonate should be infused at a rate of 1 mEq/kg/h to raise the pH to 7.15.[120]

A regimen of constant infusion of small doses of insulin is simple to follow and permits close monitoring of the relationship of dose to effect.[121] Initially, 0.1 unit per kg of regular insulin is administered by bolus intravenously. This is followed by the administration of 0.1 unit/kg/h intravenously by constant infusion. Fifty units of regular insulin in 250 ml of isotonic saline yields 0.2 unit of insulin per milliliter of solution. A few milliliters are run through the tubing and discarded, to saturate the insulin-binding sites in the tubing. The rate of insulin infusion can be modified to produce a decrease of 75 to 100 mg/dl/h in blood glucose concentration. When the blood glucose concentration reaches 250 to 300 mg/dl, 5 percent glucose should be added to the intravenous solutions. The infusion is discontinued when control has been achieved, and regular insulin can be given subcutaneously every 6 to 8 hours. Intermediate-acting insulin is usually begun within 24 to 36 hours after commencing therapy, but 3 to 5 days is the usual time required to stabilize the insulin dose.

PREOPERATIVE ASSESSMENT

General Principles. The majority (85 to 90 percent) of adult patients with diabetes in the United States have type II, non-insulin-dependent diabetes and are treated with diet and the oral hypoglycemic agents (tolbutamide, tolazamide, chlorpropamide, acetohexamide). Some of these agents have hypoglycemic effects for 24 to 36 hours, which may result in hypoglycemic episodes in fasting patients. A review of the perioperative management of adult diabetics has recently been published.[122]

Diabetic patients in the pediatric age group virtually all have type I, insulin-dependent diabetes. In children, a careful history must be obtained with respect to age of onset, types and dose of insulin, dietary habits, and frequency of hypoglycemic or ketotic episodes. The perioperative management of children is best accomplished with the help of the patient's pediatrician or endocrinologist. Their familiarity and knowledge of the patient will be useful in formulating a mutually acceptable management plan. There are advantages to "same day" operation for patients with stable, well-controlled diabetes undergoing relatively minor surgical procedures. However, those with unstable or brittle diabetes may need hospitalization for a few days prior to operation for stabilization and optimal preparation.

Associated Conditions. The complications of diabetes, including microangiopathy of the kidneys, coronary artery disease, hypertension, retinopathy, and peripheral neuropathies, are rarely observed in children. The "functional age" of a diabetic is estimated to equal the sum of the patient's chronological age and the number of years following onset of the disease. Hence a prematurely senile vascular system may be present in youthful-appearing patients. Autonomic neuropathy affects cardiovascular reflexes and may impair the catecholamine response to hypoglycemia.[123] Gastric emptying may be delayed on the same basis. In children, delayed puberty and a reduction of height are the major sequelae. The designation *Schmidt's syndrome* is applied to the association of insulin-dependent diabetes, chronic lymphocytic thyroiditis, pernicious anemia, and vitiligo.[115]

Laboratory Studies. Frequent preoperative determinations of blood glucose and ketones will be necessary for unstable patients. Urinary sugar and ketone levels are optimally recorded before each meal and at bedtime. Monitoring of serum electrolytes, creatinine, and blood urea nitrogen values may also be indicated. Associated physiological disturbances that require surgical intervention demand more extensive investigation in some patients.

PREMEDICATION

Anxiety, trauma, and stress associated with illness and surgery result in sympathetic discharge and neuroendocrine changes termed the *stress response.* Reduction of anxiety and the establishment of rapport with the diabetic child during the preoperative visit will prove beneficial. Premedication with barbiturates, diazepam, narcotics, and anticholinergics does not have a significant effect on glucose metabolism and these agents should be administered in the usual doses. Solid food is withheld for 12 hours, and clear fluids are permitted 3 hours prior to induction of anesthesia.[124] The surgical procedure should be scheduled for the early morning to avoid a prolonged period of fasting. The plan for insulin administration and glucose infusion should be individualized for each patient after consultation with the child's pediatrician or endocrinologist.

Operative Management

The primary goals of management are the avoidance of hypoglycemia and excessive hyperglycemia with ketosis. Ketosis and protein breakdown can be prevented by the administration of dextrose and insulin. Many plans have been described for the management of diabetic patients undergoing operation, but no particular perioperative regimen has been shown to be superior to others.[125, 126] An infusion of 5 percent dextrose and 0.45 normal saline solution should be started prior to 8 A.M. on the day of operation and continued at a calculated maintenance rate until oral intake is reinstituted. The method of insulin administration will depend on the individual patient's needs and the preference of the anesthesiologist and pediatrician.

One method is to give one half the usual intermediate-acting insulin dose in the morning following the initiation of the dextrose infusion. Blood glucose determinations prior to induction and at 2-hour intervals permit further therapy to maintain plasma glucose between 100 and 250 mg/dl. Regular insulin, 0.1 mg/kg, can be given intravenously when the plasma level approaches 250 mg/dl. However, the administration of the partial dose of insulin in the morning has been associated with hypoglycemia, and an intravenous bolus of regular insulin may not reach the peak effect for 3 hours.[125, 127] Another alternative to the preoperative administration of a portion of the normal daily dose of insulin is the continuous intravenous infusion of a low dose of regular insulin during the procedure. A constant infusion of 5 percent dextrose is maintained, and the rate of insulin infusion is adjusted to maintain blood glucose levels between 100 and 200 mg/dl.[126] New electronic techniques for monitoring and infusing insulin and glucose are being tested, and these automated devices may someday improve on current practices.

The effects of anesthetic drugs on blood glucose concentration and insulin release are clinically insignificant to the total management of anesthesia in the diabetic patient. Hyperglycemia occurs with surgery and is probably due to increases in cortisol, growth hormone, and sympathetic stimulation.[127, 128] No particular anesthetic agents are specifically beneficial for diabetes, nor are any of the agents contraindicated. Fluid and electrolyte administration should follow the usual guidelines for operation, which should include a continuous infusion of dextrose at the appropriate maintenance rate for the patient's weight.

Postoperative Management

A blood glucose determination should be done in the recovery room and a plan formulated in conjunction with the surgeon and pediatrician for subsequent management. Walts and associates were impressed at finding a large number of adult patients who had postoperative plasma glucose values of greater than 400 mg/dl.[123] They attributed the hyperglycemia to poorly monitored dextrose infusion rates and infrequently monitored plasma glucose values. Children will need monitoring every 4 to 6 hours until they are able to resume their normal oral intake.

HYPERINSULINISM

Hyperinsulinism is the most common cause of persistent hypoglycemia in the first year of life. At this age, hypoglycemia is often severe and intractable; if it is not treated effectively, irreversible brain damage is likely to result. Hyperinsulinism may result from a number of pancreatic abnormalities termed *islet cell dysmaturation syndrome.* The pathology of islet cell dysmaturation syndrome ranges from microadenomas and islet cell adenomas to islet cell dysplasia and nesidioblastosis. At the present time no way has been found to predict the nature of the lesion responsible for hyperinsulinism in infants and children preoperatively. In infants under 1 year of age, diffuse pancreatic involvement appears to be as likely as a localized resectable lesion.[129] In the older child, an islet cell adenoma is likely and operation is indicated. A trial of medical therapy with diazoxide (10 to 20 mg/kg/day) is indicated in infants because diffuse lesions are frequently present and subtotal pancreatectomy has not necessarily been curative.

Anesthetic Management

During the preoperative evaluation a plan is formulated that will continue the current medical therapy on the day of operation. The patient must be transported to the surgical suite without disruption of the glucose infusion. An infusion rate of 12 mg/kg/h may be necessary to maintain adequate blood glucose levels during the operation.[130]

Patients receiving diazoxide, which inhibits release of insulin from the pancreas, may be susceptible to profound hypotension if thiopental is administered. Thiopental may displace diazoxide from plasma protein binding sites, thereby releasing pharmacologically active diazoxide that can produce peripheral vascular dilatation.[131] Ketamine has been used as an induction agent in patients receiving oral diazoxide and hypotension did not occur.[130] An arterial catheter or central venous line should be inserted to permit frequent monitoring of serum glucose concentration. Glucose determinations should be made every 15 minutes with Dextrostix and laboratory samples sent every 30 minutes for confirmation. Transient decreases in blood glucose may occur with surgical manipulation of the tumor. Complete removal of an insulinoma may produce a rise in blood sugar within 30 minutes; nevertheless, this is not reliable evidence that an adenoma has been removed.

The anesthetic technique and selection of agents will have minimal influence on intraoperative blood glucose levels. The concentration of potent inhalational agents and dose of narcotics should be sufficient to suppress the stress response associated with light anesthesia.

Postoperatively, frequent monitoring of blood glucose should continue for early detection of persistent hypoglycemia or hyperglycemia. Diabetes mellitus can develop when only minimal pancreatic tissue is left behind. Some children will continue to exhibit hypoglycemia and must undergo exploration with an extended subtotal pancreatectomy.

REFERENCES

1. Blackwell RE, Guillemin R: Hypothalamic control of adenohypophysial secretions. Annu Rev Physiol *35*:357, 1973.
2. Hays RM: Antidiuretic hormone. N Engl J Med *295*:659, 1976.
3. Philbin DM, Coggins CH: Plasma antidiuretic hormone levels in cardiac surgical patients during morphine and halothane anesthesia. Anesthesiology *49*:95, 1978.
4. Behrman RE, Vaughan VC III (eds): Nelson Textbook of Pediatrics. Philadelphia, W.B. Saunders, 1983, p 1435.
5. Tasch MD: Endocrine diseases. *In* Stoelting RK, Dierdorf SF (eds): Anesthesia and Co-Existing Disease. New York, Churchill Livingstone, 1983.
6. Banna M, Hoare RD, Stanley P, et al: Craniopharyngioma in children. J Pediatr *83*:781, 1973.
7. Hoffman HJ, Hendrick EB, Humphreys RP, et al: Management of craniopharyngioma in children. J Neurosurg *47*:218, 1977.
8. Burr IM, Slonim AE, Danish RK, et al: Diencephalic syndrome revisited. J Pediatr *88*:439, 1976.
9. Robertson GL: Differential diagnosis of polyuria. Annu Rev Med *39*:425, 1988.
10. Gregor NG, Kirkland RT, Clayton GW, et al: Central diabetes insipidus; 22 years' experience. Am J Dis Child *140*:551, 1986.
11. Costin G, Fefferman RA, Kogut MD: Hypothalamic gigantism. J Pediatr *83*:419, 1973.
12. Nelson JC, Kollar DJ, Lewis JE: Growth hormone secretion in pituitary disease. Arch Intern Med *133*:459, 1974.
13. Southwick JP, Katz J: Unusual airway difficulty in the acromegalic patient—indication for tracheotomy. Anesthesiology *51*:72, 1979.
14. Hassan SZ, Matz G, Lawrence AM, et al: Laryngeal stenosis in acromegaly. Anesth Analg *55*:57, 1978.
15. Tyrell JB, Brooks RM, Fitzgerald PA, et al: Cushing's disease—selective transsphenoidal resection of pituitary microadenomas. N Engl J Med *298*:753, 1978.
16. Finsterer U, Beyer A, Jensen R, et al: The syndrome of inappropriate secretion of antidiuretic hormone (SIADH)—treatment with lithium. Intens Care Med *8*:223, 1982.
17. Samaan NA, Osborne BM, MacKay G, et al: Endocrine and morphologic studies of pituitary adenomas secondary to primary hypothyroidism. J Clin Endocrinol Metab *45*:903, 1977.
18. Kenny FM, Preeyasombat C, Migeon CJ: Cortisol production rate in normal infants, children and adults. J Pediatr *37*:34, 1966.
19. Plumpton FS, Besser GM, Cole PV: Corticosteroid treatment and surgery. I. Investigation of the indications for steroid cover. II. The management of steroid cover. Anaesthesia *24*:3, 1969.
20. Raven MB, Feinberg G: Anesthetic management of hypophysectomy. NY State J Med *24*:776, 1968.
21. Newfield P, Albin M, Chestnut JS, et al: Air embolism during transsphenoidal pituitary operations. Neurosurgery *2*:39, 1978.
22. Messick JM, Laws ER, Abboud CV: Anesthesia for transsphenoidal surgery of the hypophyseal region. Anesth Analg *57*:206, 1978.
23. Munson ES: Effect of nitrous oxide on the pulmonary circulation during venous air embolism. Anesth Analg *50*:785, 1971.
24. Shucart WA, Jackson I: Management of diabetes insipidus in neurosurgical patients. J Neurosurg *44*:65, 1976.
25. Surks MI, Schadlow AR, Stock JM: Determination of iodothyronine absorption and conversion of L-thyroxine (T_4) to L-triiodothyronine (T_3) using turnover rate techniques. J Clin Invest *52*:805, 1973.

26. Inglar SH, Woebar KA: The thyroid gland. *In* Williams RH (ed): Textbook of Endocrinology. Philadelphia, W.B. Saunders, 1981, pp 117–247.
27. Gilman AG, Murad F: Thyroid and antithyroid drugs. *In* Goodman LS, Gilman A (eds): The Pharmacological Basis of Therapeutics. New York, Macmillan, 1980, pp 1397–1419.
28. Dillman WH: Mechanism of action of thyroid hormones Med Clin North Am *69*:849, 1985.
29. La Franchi SH: Hypothyroidism. Pediatr Clin North Am *26*:33, 1979.
30. Fisher DA, Drissault JH, Sach J, et al: Ontogenesis of hypothalamic-pituitary-thyroid function and metabolism in man, sheep and rat. Recent Prog Hormone Res *33*:59, 1977.
31. Fisher DA, Klein AH: Thyroid development and disorders of thyroid function in the newborn. N Engl J Med *304*:702, 1981.
32. Rezvani I, DiGeorge AM: Reassessment of the daily dose of oral thyroxine for replacement therapy in hypothyroid children. J Pediatr *90*:291, 1977.
33. White VA, Kumagai LF: Preoperative endocrine and metabolic considerations. Med Clin North Am *63*:1321, 1979.
34. Kim JM, Hackman L: Anesthesia for untreated hypothyroidism: Report of three cases. Anesth Analg *56*:299, 1977.
35. Kato R, Takanaka A, Takahashi A: Effect of thyroid hormone on the substrate interaction with P-450 in the oxidation of drugs by liver microsomes. J Biochem *68*:613, 1970.
36. Murkin JM: Anesthesia and hypothyroidism: A review of thyroxine physiology, pharmacology and anesthetic implications. Anesth Analg *61*:371, 1982.
37. McBrien DJ, Hindle W: Myxoedema and heart failure. Lancet *1*:1066, 1963.
38. Zwillich CW, Pierson DJ, Hofeldt FD, et al: Ventilatory control in myxedema and hypothyroidism. N Engl J Med *292*:662, 1975.
39. James ML: Endocrine disease and anaesthesia. Anaesthesia *25*:232, 1970.
40. Miller LR, Benumof JL, Alexander L, et al: Completely absent response to peripheral nerve stimulation in acutely hypothyroid patient. Anesthesiology *71*:779, 1989.
41. Abbott TR: Anaesthesia in untreated myxoedema: Report of two cases. Br J Anaesth *39*:510, 1967.
42. Badad AA, Eger EI: The effects of hyperthyroidism and hypothyroidism on halothane and oxygen requirements in dogs. Anesthesiology *29*:1087, 1968.
43. Jones KL: Smith's Recognizable Patterns of Human Malformation. 4th edition. Philadelphia, WB Saunders, 1988, p 454.
44. Lee WN: Thyroiditis, hyperthyroidism, and tumors. Pediatr Clin North Am *26*:53, 1979.
45. Barnes HV, Blizzard RM: Antithyroid drug therapy for toxic diffuse goiter (Graves' disease): Thirty years experience in children and adolescents. J Pediatr *91*:313, 1977.
46. Brown J, Solomon DH, Beall GN, et al: Autoimmune thyroid diseases, Graves' and Hashimoto's. Ann Intern Med *88*:379, 1978.
47. Fisher DA, Sack J, Oddie TH, et al: Serum T_4, TBG, T_3 uptake, T_3, reverse T_3, and TSH concentrations in children 1 to 15 years of age. J Clin Endocrinol Metab *45*:191, 1977.
48. Peters KR, Nance P, Wingard DW: Malignant hyperthyroidism or malignant hyperthermia? Anesth Analg *60*:613, 1981.
49. Mackin JF, Canary JJ, Pittman CS: Thyroid storm and its management. N Engl J Med *291*:1396, 1974.
50. Wood M, Berman ML, Harbeson RD, et al: Halothane-induced hepatic necrosis in triiodothyronine pretreated rats. Anesthesiology *52*:470, 1980.
51. Roizen MF, Hansel P, Lichtor JL, Schreider BD: Patients with disorders of thyroid function. Anesthesiol Clin North Am *5*:277, 1987.
52. Caldarelli DD, Holinger LD: Complications and sequelae of thyroid surgery. Otolaryngol Clin North Am *13*:85, 1980.
53. Rallison ML, Dobyns BM, Kealing FR, et al: Occurrence and natural history of chronic lymphocytic thyroiditis in childhood. J Pediatr *86*:675, 1975.
54. Fisher DA, Oddie TH, Johnson DE, et al: The diagnosis of Hashimoto's thyroiditis. J Clin Endocrinol Metab *40*:795, 1975.
55. Fisher, DA: Thyroid nodules in childhood and their management. J Pediatr *89*:866, 1976.
56. Linder LB, Esteban NV, Yergev AL, et al: Cortisol production in childhood and adolescence. J Pediatr *17*:892, 1990.
57. Knowlton AI: Addison's disease: A review of its clinical course and management. *In* Christy NR (ed): The Human Adrenal Cortex. New York, Harper and Row, 1971, pp 329–358.
58. Blizzard RN, Solomon IL: Autoimmune disorders of endocrine glands. J Pediatr *63*:1021, 1963.
59. Kaplan SA: Disorders of the adrenal cortex. Pediatr Clin North Am *26*:70, 1979.
60. Oyama T: Endocrine response to general anesthesia and surgery. *In* Endocrinology and the Anesthetist. Monographs in Anesthesiology. Vol 11. Amsterdam, Elsevier, 1983.
61. Knudsen L, Christiansen LA, Lorentzen JE: Hypotension during and after operation in glucocorticoid patients. Br J Anaesth *53*:295, 1981.
62. Kaplan S: Diseases of the adrenal cortex. II. Pediatr Clin North Am *26*:77, 1979.
63. Axelrod L: Glucocorticoid therapy. Medicine *55*:39, 1976.
64. Symreng T, Karlberg BE, Kagedal B, et al: Physiological cortisol substitution of long-term steroid-treated patients undergoing major surgery. Br J Anaesth *53*:949, 1981.
65. Roizen MF, Lampe GH: Adrenal cortex malfunction: Implications for the anesthetist. Semin Anesth *3*:186, 1984.
66. Keheler H: A rational approach to dosage and preparation of parenteral glucocorticoid substitution therapy during surgical procedures. Acta Anaesth Scand *19*:260, 1975.
67. Ehrlich HP, Hunt TP: Effects of cortisone and vitamin A on wound healing. Ann Surg *167*:324, 1968.
68. Holaday JW, Law P-Y, Loh HH, et al: Adrenal steroids indirectly modulate morphine and beta-endorphin effects. J Pharmacol Exp Ther *208*:176, 1979.
69. Alquist RP: Studies on the adrenotropic receptors. Am J Physiol *153*:586, 1948.
70. Goldberg LI: Cardiovascular and renal actions of dopamine: Potential clinical applications. Pharmacol Rev *24*:1, 1972.
71. Voorhees ML: Disorders of the adrenal medulla and multiple endocrine adenomatoses. Pediatr Clin North Am *26*:209, 1979.
72. Melicow NM: One hundred cases of pheochromocytoma at the Columbia Medical Center. Cancer *40*:1987, 1977.
73. Iversen LL: Uptake of circulating catecholamines into tissues. *In* Blasko H, Sayers G, Smith AD (eds): Handbook of Physiology, Section 7: Endocrinology. Vol 6: Adrenal. Washington, DC, American Physiological Society, 1975, pp 713–722.

74. Bravo EL, Tarazi RC, Ray WG, et al: Circulatory and urinary catecholamines in pheochromocytoma. N Engl J Med *301*:682, 1978.
75. Van Vliet PD, Burchell HB, Titus JL: Focal myocarditis associated with pheochromocytoma. N Engl J Med *274*:1102, 1966.
76. James TN: On the cause of sudden death in pheochromocytoma. Circulation *54*:348, 1976.
77. Davies RA, Patt NL, Sole MJ: Localization of pheochromocytoma by selective venous catheterization and assay of plasma catecholamines. Can Med Assoc J *120*:539, 1979.
78. Maddern PJ, McGrew I, Oh T: Pheochromocytoma: Aspects and management. Anaesth Intens Care *4*:156, 1976.
79. Robinson RG, DeQualtro V, Grushkin CM, et al: Childhood pheochromocytoma: Treatment with alphamethyl tyrosine for resistant hypertension. J Pediatr *91*:143, 1977.
80. Amaramath L: Atracurium and pheochromocytoma. Anesth Analg *67*:1127, 1988.
81. Jones RB, Hill AB: Severe hypertension associated with pancuronium in a patient with pheochromocytoma. Can Anaesth Soc J *28*:394, 1981.
82. Stanley T, Chung F, et al: Intravenous lidocaine: Optional time of injection before intubation. Anesth Analg *66*:1036, 1987.
83. Desmonts JM, le Houelleur J, Remond P, et al: Anaesthetic management of patients with phaeochromocytoma. A review of 102 cases. Br J Anaesth *49*:991, 1977.
84. Suzukawa M, Michaels IAL, Ruzbarsky J, et al: Use of isoflurane during resection of pheochromocytoma. Anesth Analg *62*:100, 1983.
85. Janeczko GF, Ivankovich AD, Glisson SN, et al: Enflurane anesthesia for surgical removal for pheochromocytoma. Anesth Analg *56*:61, 1977.
86. Bittar DA: Innovar-induced hypertensive crises in patients with pheochromocytoma. Anesthesiology *50*:366, 1979.
87. Csanky-Treels JC, Lawick van Pabst WP, Brands JW, et al: Effects of sodium nitroprusside during the excision of pheochromocytoma. Anaesthesia *31*:60, 1976.
88. Martin R, St. Pierre B, Molinar OR, et al: Pheochromocytoma and postoperative hypoglycemia. Can Anaesth Soc J *26*:260, 1979.
89. Melian FC, Hastings AB: Clinical estimation and significance of calcium ion concentration in blood. Am J Med Sci *189*:601, 1935.
90. Knill-Jonens RP, Buckle RM, Parson V, et al: Hypercalcemia and increased parathyroid hormone activity in primary hepatoma. N Engl J Med *282*:704, 1970.
91. Stein RC: Hypercalcemia in leukemia. J Pediatr *89*:1029, 1976.
92. Swinton NW: Hypercalcemia and familial pheochromocytoma correction after adrenalectomy. Ann Intern Med *76*:455, 1972.
93. Stapleton FB, Lukert BP, Linshaw MA: Treatment of hypercalcemia associated with osseous metastases. J Pediatr *89*:1029, 1976.
94. Porter RH, Cox BG: Treatment of hypoparathyroid patients with chlorothiazide. N Engl J Med *198*:577, 1978.
95. Heath H III, Earle JM: Serum ionized calcium during bed rest in fracture patients in normal man. Metabolism *21*:633, 1972.
96. Rude RK, Oldham SB, Singer FR, et al: Treatment of thyrotoxic hypercalcemia with propranolol. N Engl J Med *294*:431, 1976.
97. Heath DA: Emergency management of disorders of calcium and magnesium. Clin Endocrinol Metab *9*:487, 1980.
98. Nimmagadda U, Salem MR, Ivankovich AD: Anesthesia and parathyroid disease. Semin Anesth *3*:175, 1984.
99. Schweitzer VG, Thompson NW, Harness JK, et al: Management of severe hypercalcemia caused by primary hyperparathyroidism. Arch Surg *113*:373, 1978.
100. Bronsky D, Dubin A, et al: Calcium and the electrocardiogram. Electrocardiographic manifestation of hyperparathyroidism and of marked hypercalcemia from various etiologies. Am J Cardiol *7*:833, 1961.
101. Paloyan E, Lawrence AM: Hyperparathyroidism. New York, Grune and Stratton, 1973, p 180.
102. Friedman H, Baun H: Laryngeal injuries secondary to nasogastric tubes. Ann Otol Rhinol Laryngol *90*:469, 1981.
103. Lee KW, Dougal RM, Templeton JJ, et al: Tracheal gas leak and intraoperative tracheal aspiration in children. Anesth Analg *64*:185, 1985.
104. Waldster SS: Medical complications of thyroid surgery. Otolaryngol Clin North Am *13*:99, 1980.
105. Connelly JP, Crawford JD: Studies of neonatal hyperphosphatemia. Pediatrics *30*:425, 1962.
106. McCrory WW, Forman CW, McNamara H, et al: Renal excretion of inorganic phosphate in newborn infants. J Clin Invest *31*:357, 1952.
107. Linarelli LG: Newborn urinary cyclic AMP and developmental renal responsiveness to parathyroid hormone. Pediatrics *50*:14, 1972.
108. David L, Anast C: Calcium metabolism in newborn infants. J Clin Invest *54*:187, 1974.
109. Tsang RC, Chen IW, Friedman MA, et al: Neonatal parathyroid function: Role of gestational age and postnatal age. J Pediatr *83*:728, 1973.
110. Tsang RC, Chen IW, Friedman MA, et al: Parathyroid function in infants of diabetic mothers. J Pediatr *86*:399, 1975.
111. Sperling MA: Diabetes mellitus. Pediatr Clin North Am *26*:149, 1979.
112. Calnan M, Peckham CS: Incidence of insulin dependent diabetes in the first 16 years of life. Lancet *1*:589, 1977.
113. Cahill GF Jr, McDevitt HO: Insulin dependent diabetes mellitus: The initial lesion. N Engl J Med *304*:1454, 1981.
114. MacCuish AC, Irvine WJ: Autoimmunological aspects of diabetes mellitus. Clin Endocrinol Metab *4*:435, 1975.
115. Yoon JW, Austin M, Onodera T, et al: Virus-induced diabetes mellitus. Isolation of virus from a pancreas of a child with diabetic ketoacidosis. N Engl J Med: *300*:1173, 1979.
116. Valerio D: Acute diabetic abdomen in childhood. Lancet *1*:66, 1976.
117. Bloom ME, Mintz DH, Field JB: Insulin-induced posthypoglycemic hyperglycemia as a cause of "brittle" diabetes: Clinical clues and therapeutic implications. Am J Med *47*:891, 1969.
118. Krane EJ, Rockoff MA, Wollman JK, Wolfsdorf JI: Subclinical brain swelling in children during treatment of diabetic ketoacidosis: N Engl J Med *312*:1147, 1985.
119. Alberti KG, Hockaday TD: Diabetic coma: A reappraisal after five years. Clin Endocrinol Metab *6*:421, 1977.
120. Sanson TH, Levine SN: Management of diabetic ketoacidosis. Drugs *38*:289, 1989.
121. Edwards GA, Kohaut EC, Wehring B: Effectiveness of low-dose continuous intravenous insulin infusion in diabetic ketoacidosis. A prospective comparative study. J Pediatr *91*:701, 1977.

122. Stevens A, Roizen MF: Patients with diabetes mellitus and disorders of glucose metabolism. Anesthesiol Clin North Am *5*:339, 1987.
123. Loughran PG, Giesecke AH: Diabetes mellitus: Anesthetic considerations. Semin Anesth *3*:207, 1984.
124. Schreiner M, Triebwasser A, Keon T: Ingestion of liquids compared with preoperative fasting in pediatric patients. Anesthesiology *72*:593, 1990.
125. Walts LF, Miller J, Davidson MB, et al: Perioperative management of diabetes mellitus. Anesthesiology *55*:104, 1981.
126. Meyer EJ, Lorenzi M, Bohannon WV, et al: Diabetic management by insulin infusion during major surgery. Am J Surg *137*:323, 1979.
127. Fletcher J, Langman MJS, Kellock TD: Effect of surgery on blood sugar levels in diabetes mellitus. Lancet *2*:52, 1965.
128. Clarke RSJ.: Anaesthesia and carbohydrate metabolism. Br J Anaesth *45*:237, 1973.
129. Gauderer M, Stanley CA, Baker L, et al: Pancreatic adenomas in infants and children: Current surgical management. J Pediatr Surg *13*:591, 1978.
130. Yamashita M, Tsuneto S: Anesthesia for an infant with severe hyperinsulinism treated by pancreatectomy. Anesthesiology *67*:985, 1987.
131. Burch PG, McLeskey CH: Anesthesia for patients with insulinoma, treated with oral diazoxide. Anesthesiology *55*:472, 1981.

CHAPTER

13 Genetic Metabolic Diseases

LINDA C. STEHLING, M.D.

The history of human biochemical genetics began when Sir Archibald Garrod initiated studies of patients with alkaptonuria at the turn of the century. He developed the concept that certain diseases are due to deficiencies of enzymes that regulate specific metabolic steps.[1] The first enzyme defect in a human genetic disease was identified in 1948.[2] The following year, Pauling and his associates presented evidence that human mutations produce alterations in the primary structure of proteins.[3] By the 1970's it was possible to identify individual chromosomes. Advances in molecular biology have led to characterization of the human genome and identification of the chromosomal location of genes responsible for hundreds of diseases. It is known, for example, that mutations involving chromosome 1 cause Gaucher's disease, whereas chromosome 15 is involved with Tay-Sachs disease. Mutations of chromosomes 3, 5, 7, and 22 are associated with different types of mucopolysaccharidoses.[4]

Children with genetic metabolic diseases may require anesthesia for procedures, such as organ transplantation, that are intended to prevent or treat complications of the underlying disease state. More frequently, the anesthesiologist is called upon to care for children with one of these disorders who are undergoing common surgical procedures, such as myringotomy or hernia repair. Few clinicians are conversant with the pathophysiology of even the more common genetic metabolic disorders. Eponyms, acronyms, biochemical defects, physical features, and the names of patients are used singly or in combination to describe the disorders, complicating access to the literature. Relatively few articles have been published dealing with the anesthetic implications of specific genetic metabolic diseases. Indeed, many of them have no features that alter anesthetic management or predispose the children to untoward events.

The anesthesiologist can usually rely upon a combination of common sense, experience, and basic anesthesia knowledge when caring for children with these disorders. However, some children with genetic metabolic diseases, most notably the mucopolysaccharidoses, can present significant challenges. In some circumstances, such as liver transplantation, the implications of the surgical procedure outweigh most features of the metabolic derangement. This review will consider primarily diseases with specific implications for anesthetic management. Procedures such as liver and bone marrow transplantation are dealt with elsewhere.

DETECTION OF METABOLIC DISEASES

Detection of the carrier state for some of the genetic metabolic diseases facilitates reproductive counseling for couples at risk of having affected children. Prenatal diagnosis is possible for many of the disorders, and newborn screening programs identify children with several of the diseases at a stage when medical intervention can prevent or ameliorate symptoms. Unless otherwise specified, the mode of inheritance of the disorders discussed is presumed to be autosomal recessive.

POPULATION-BASED SCREENING PROGRAMS

Population-based genetic screening programs are employed to detect disorders with high prevalence in defined groups. For example, the carrier frequency of Tay-Sachs disease is 1 in 30 to 1 in 40 in the Jewish population of Central and Eastern European ancestry—approximately tenfold higher than in the general population.[5] Not only is antenatal detection possible, there is also a reliable test for identification of the carrier state. Large-scale screening programs were initiated in Jewish communities in North America in the 1970's and are now conducted in many areas of the world.

ANTENATAL DIAGNOSIS

Transabdominal amniocentesis, which came into widespread use during the 1960's, is usually required for the antenatal diagnosis of genetic diseases. More recently, transcervical or transabdominal chorionic villus sampling has been introduced for obtaining tissue of fetal origin. The major advantage of this technique is that it can be performed earlier in pregnancy. Although direct examination of amniotic fluid is useful in detecting abnormalities such as neural tube defects, in vitro culture of the fetal cells for biochemical studies is usually required for diagnosing the metabolic diseases. Enzyme assays have traditionally been employed. However, molecular diagnosis using deoxyribonucleic acid (DNA) obtained from the cultured cells is becoming a useful alternative.

NEONATAL SCREENING

Neonatal screening programs were initiated with testing for phenylketonuria (PKU). It is estimated that approximately 10 million newborn infants worldwide are screened annually for hyperphenylalaninemia.[6] Although liquid blood samples can be used, the most common technique involves collection of a capillary blood specimen on filter paper. The filter paper is then sent to a central facility for testing. The most widely used technique, Guthrie's test, employs a microbiological inhibition assay for phenylalanine content. More sophisticated quantitative methods are also available.

Although PKU screening has proved extremely successful over the last quarter of a century, changes in medical practice in the last decade have made modification of testing procedures necessary. More neonates are being discharged from the hospital within 24 hours or less of birth. The potential for false-negative test results when a blood specimen is obtained on the first day of life necessitates lowering cutoff levels or obtaining a second specimen when the infant is approximately 2 weeks of age. Despite the expense, the latter procedure is still recommended.[7] Screening is also available for several other inborn errors of metabolism.

SCREENING IN LATER LIFE

The primary purpose of screening procedures performed in older children and adults is detection of diseases for which medical intervention is possible. A secondary benefit is identification of patients with disorders for which genetic counseling is beneficial. Some inborn errors of metabolism are identified by accumulated or missing metabolites in urine. Diagnosis of enzymatic defects can be made by direct assay of blood or tissue. When tissue diagnosis is necessary, general anesthesia may be required. For example, local anesthesia is suitable for percutaneous liver biopsy in adults but is not appropriate for children. Patients of all ages require general or regional anesthesia when open liver biopsies are performed. It may be anticipated that screening programs will proliferate as new diagnostic techniques are introduced and more treatment options become available.

TREATMENT OF METABOLIC DISEASES

Conventional therapeutic approaches are often nutritional or pharmacological. Dietary restriction of a particular substrate is effective in some disorders involving accumulation of toxic precursors. For example, diets restricted in phenylalanine or the branched-chain amino acids are effective in preventing mental retardation associated with phenylketonuria and maple syrup urine disease, respectively. Replacement of deficient products is another therapeutic alternative. Frequent intake of glucose or glucose polymers is employed in patients with some types of glycogen storage disease.

In some neonates, irreversible tissue damage, particularly injury to the central nervous system, is inevitable if urgent measures are not taken to reduce the levels of circulating toxic metabolites. Exchange transfusion, peritoneal dialysis, hemodialysis, and forced diuresis can be employed. More recently, continuous venovenous hemofiltration has been used. The primary advantage of this technique is that only venous access is required, making the technique more available to infants with a wide range of inborn errors of intermediary metabolism.[8]

Research efforts are being directed toward protein replacement therapy for several of the disorders. Although more success has been achieved in the area of hormone replacement, recombinant DNA technology may offer a means of producing deficient enzymes for patients with metabolic diseases. The newest area of research, however, is somatic gene replacement. Among the disorders considered possible candidates for this type of therapy are Lesch-Nyhan syndrome, phenylketonuria, Tay-Sachs disease, and the lysosomal storage diseases.

Organ transplantation lies on the borderline between therapy at the level of the dysfunctional protein and gene therapy. The transplanted organ supplies the deficient protein but also brings new genetic information to the recipient. Kidney, liver,[9] and bone marrow (Table 13–1) transplants are being employed with increasing frequency. In one series of childhood liver transplantations, 29 percent were performed for metabolic disorders.[10] For some children, transplantation is performed to supply tissue that can provide missing proteins. Examples include bone marrow transplantation for lysosomal storage diseases and liver transplantation for type I glycogen storage disease. In other circumstances, such as renal transplantation for cystinosis, the transplanted organ replaces the damaged, native organ.

Table 13–1. METABOLIC DISORDERS FOR WHICH BONE MARROW TRANSPLANTATION MAY BE AN ALTERNATIVE THERAPY

Wolman's disease
Sanfilippo's syndrome
Farber's disease
Hunter's syndrome
Hurler's syndrome
Fabry's disease
Gaucher's disease
Metachromatic leukodystrophy
Niemann-Pick disease
Krabbe's disease

From The Hematologist's/Oncologist's Guide to Unrelated Donor Marrow Transplantation, published by the National Heart, Lung, and Blood Institute, 1991.

DISORDERS OF CARBOHYDRATE METABOLISM

The glycogen storage diseases, of which there are at least ten types, are the most significant of the disorders of carbohydrate metabolism and will be discussed in some detail. Clinical manifestations of the diseases and their anesthetic implications are listed in Table 13–2.

GLYCOGEN STORAGE DISEASES (Table 13–3)

TYPE I (VON GIERKE'S DISEASE)

Children with type I glycogen storage disease are deficient in glucose-6-phosphatase, the enzyme that causes release of glucose from glucose-6-phosphate. However, the glucose-6-phosphate does not accumulate. Some enters the Embden-Meyerhof pathway, resulting in lactic acid accumulation; it is also shunted into the pentose phosphate pathway, leading to elevated uric acid levels. Pyruvate, triglyceride, phosphate, and cholesterol levels are also higher than normal. Glycogen accumulation in the liver results in massive hepatomegaly, usually evident at birth. The large liver may preclude palpation of the kidneys, which are also enlarged. Splenomegaly is rare. The patients are of short stature with poorly developed musculature.

Severe hypoglycemia and acidosis are characteristic of the disorder. Although convulsions may occur because of hypoglycemia, profound hypoglycemia often occurs without clinical

Table 13–2. DISORDERS OF CARBOHYDRATE METABOLISM

Disorder	Prevalence	Clinical Features	Anesthetic Implications
Galactosemia	1:30,000 to 1:60,000	Cataracts, vomiting, jaundice, hepatomegaly, cirrhosis, hypoglycemia, failure to thrive, mental retardation	Hypoglycemia
Galactokinase deficiency	1:40,000 to 1:100,000	Cataracts (severe form may resemble galactosemia)	None
Benign fructosuria	1:130,000	1+ test for reducing substances in urine, negative for glucose	Confusion with diabetes
Hereditary fructose intolerance	1:20,000 Swiss	Hypoglycemia, vomiting, jaundice, hepatosplenomegaly, failure to thrive	Dehydration, hypoglycemia, acidosis, hypokalemia
Fructose-1,6-diphosphatase deficiency	Rare	Hypoglycemia, hypotonia, acidosis, hepatomegaly	Dehydration, acidosis, hypoglycemia
Glycogen storage diseases—see Table 13–3			

symptoms. This is thought to be due to high lactate levels, which substitute for glucose as an energy source in the brain.[11] Ketosis is unusual. The respiratory compensation for the chronic metabolic acidosis is usually adequate to maintain the pH in the normal range. A Fanconi-like syndrome characterized by aminoaciduria, glycosuria, and phosphaturia is seen in some patients. A bleeding diathesis characterized by epistaxis and easy bruising is not uncommon. Clotting studies are normal, but the bleeding time is prolonged. The platelet count is normal, indicating that platelet dysfunction is the underlying pathology. Patients with type Ib von Gierke's disease exhibit a predisposition to infection, particularly recurrent otitis media and pneumonia. In addition to a neutropenia, impaired neutrophil function may be a feature of this variant of the disease.

The diagnosis of von Gierke's disease is made by assaying glucose-6-phosphatase in liver tissue, usually obtained by open liver biopsy. Despite the severe metabolic derangements and multisystem disease, many patients live to adulthood. Dietary treatment has significantly improved the prognosis. Portacaval diversion has been performed in some patients with variable results. Early experience with orthotopic liver transplantation is encouraging.[12]

The primary perioperative problem is avoid-

Table 13–3. GLYCOGEN STORAGE DISEASES

Disorder		Prevalence	Clinical Features	Anesthetic Implications
Type I	von Gierke's disease	1:100,000 to 1:200,000	Hypoglycemia, hepatomegaly, short stature, lactic acidosis, hyperlipidemia, bleeding diathesis, nephropathy, hyperuricemia	Increased intra-abdominal pressure, hypoglycemia, bleeding, acidosis
Type II	Pompe's disease	1:100,000 to 1:200,000	Hypotonia, hepatomegaly, cardiomegaly, macroglossia, recurrent pneumonia	Airway difficulties, congestive heart failure, pulmonary disease
Type III	Cori's disease	1:100,000 to 1:150,000	Hepatomegaly, splenomegaly, cardiomegaly, hypoglycemia, seizures, muscle wasting, growth retardation	Hypoglycemia, myopathy
Type IV	Andersen's disease	1:500,000 to 1:1,000,000	Hepatosplenomegaly, failure to thrive, cirrhosis	Muscle weakness, hypoglycemia
Type V	McArdle's disease	1:500,000 to 1:1,000,000	Muscle cramps, myoglobinuria	Muscle damage secondary to tourniquet, myoglobinuria or hyperkalemia with depolarizing relaxants, confusion with malignant hyperthermia
Type VI	Hers' disease	1:200,000	Hepatomegaly	Hypoglycemia
Type VII	Tarui's disease	1:500,000 to 1:1,000,000	Muscle cramps, myoglobinuria	Confusion with malignant hyperthermia

ance of hypoglycemia. The child should receive a glucose-containing solution intravenously, and the blood sugar should be measured frequently. A rapid sequence induction is indicated because of the increased intragastric pressure caused by the enlarged liver. None of the halogenated anesthetic agents currently in use are contraindicated. Renal function is not ordinarily impaired to a degree that warrants omission of muscle relaxants that depend upon renal excretion. Monitoring of arterial blood gases to detect metabolic acidosis is recommended during long procedures.[13] If the history suggests easy bruising or other evidence of coagulopathy, a bleeding time should be determined prior to operation. Consultation with a hematologist may be required. Prophylactic platelet administration is not recommended.

Type II (Pompe's Disease)

Deficiency of lysosomal acid alpha-glucosidase results in the accumulation of glycogen in virtually all cells of the body. However, skeletal and cardiac muscle are the most profoundly affected. Hypotonia and muscle weakness are evident, although the muscle mass appears normal. Macroglossia occurs in some children. Cardiomegaly is often severe. The electrocardiogram usually shows marked left axis deviation, a short P-R interval, large QRS amplitude, and T wave inversion. Mental retardation is not a feature of the disease.

In the most common variant, the infantile form of the disease, symptoms appear before 6 months of age, and death usually occurs within the first year from cardiorespiratory failure. The liver is normal in size or only moderately enlarged, and liver function is normal. There are no abnormalities of glucose metabolism, and lactate, uric acid, and lipid levels are normal. The diagnosis is made on the basis of determination of acid alpha-glucosidase activity in muscle, liver, or leukocytes. There is no therapy for the disorder, although bone marrow transplantation has been suggested.

In the juvenile form of the disease, symptoms occur in early childhood and progress more slowly. Muscle weakness and hypotonia are pronounced, but cardiac disease is not a feature. Death due to respiratory failure usually occurs by the mid to late teens. In a few reported cases, onset of the disease occurred in adulthood and was characterized by a girdle myopathy but no hepatic or cardiac signs.

Children with Pompe's disease may require anesthesia for muscle or liver biopsy. Cardiac arrest[14] and ventricular fibrillation[15] have been described with induction of anesthesia in patients with this disorder. The primary concerns are the cardiomyopathy, macroglossia that can lead to airway obstruction and difficulty with intubation, and the frequent occurrence of atelectasis and pneumonia secondary to inability to clear secretions, as well as compression of major bronchi by the enlarged heart. A chest radiograph and an electrocardiogram should be obtained preoperatively. Echocardiography may also be indicated.

The anesthetic technique employed is determined primarily by the degree of cardiomyopathy; myocardial depressants should be avoided. Nondepolarizing muscle relaxants of short duration are recommended unless postoperative mechanical ventilation is planned. Theoretically, one might want to avoid the use of succinylcholine in patients with Pompe's disease because of concerns regarding hyperkalemia following its administration. If macroglossia is evident, awake intubation or the use of specialized techniques of intubation such as the Bullard's intubating laryngoscope may be required. Following all but the most minor procedures, children should be observed in a special care unit. Mechanical ventilation may be required. Narcotics should be administered with caution because of their respiratory depressant effects.

Type III (Cori's Disease)

It may be difficult to differentiate this disorder clinically from von Gierke's disease, though the clinical course may be milder. The hyperglycemic response to galactose is normal or exaggerated, and lactate and uric acid levels are lower. Biochemical analysis can be performed on erythrocytes, although muscle or liver biopsy may be required for confirmation. Hepatomegaly is not severe and may resolve at puberty. Symptomatic hypoglycemia may occur. Myopathy may be evident only in adult life and is slowly progressive. Although cardiomegaly may occur, signs and symptoms of heart disease are not prominent features of the disease. Bleeding tendencies may occur; check history and order coagulation studies.

Anesthetic management is influenced by the severity of the disease. The principles outlined for types I and II disease apply.

Type IV (Andersen's Disease, Branching Enzyme Deficiency)

Type IV glycogenosis, also known as amylopectinosis, is very rare. The children usually appear normal for the first several months. Progressive hepatosplenomegaly, muscle weakness, and failure to thrive become evident within a few months, and death due to cirrhosis usually occurs before 5 years of age. Mild fasting hypoglycemia is common. The diagnosis is confirmed by assay of branching enzyme in leukocytes, cultured fibroblasts, or muscle. Although the abnormal glycogen is deposited in muscle as well as liver, cardiomyopathy does not occur. A recent report of liver transplantation in several patients with this disorder indicated that growth and development were normal almost 4 years following transplantation.[16]

Type V (McArdle's Disease)

Children with deficiency of muscle phosphorylase are usually asymptomatic. Adolescents and adults complain of easy fatigability, severe muscle cramps, and inability to perform vigorous exercise. Muscle wasting is evident in older patients. Exercise tolerance is limited because rapid glycogenolysis cannot occur because of the myophosphorylase deficiency. Liver phosphorylase is normal. Cardiac disease is not a feature of the disorder. A few cases of acute renal failure secondary to myoglobinuria associated with excessive exercise have been reported.[17] A venous blood sample drawn from an extremity that has been vigorously exercised will not have an elevated lactate level. Biochemical analysis of muscle tissue reveals absence of phosphorylase activity. The only therapy is avoidance of strenuous exercise.

The history of severe muscle cramping and myoglobinuria in at least half these patients is suggestive of malignant hyperthermia. However, there is no association between the two disorders. Theoretically, malignant hyperthermia is unlikely because of the patient's limited ability to generate a hypermetabolic state.[14]

A glucose-containing solution should be infused in the perioperative period to serve as an energy source. Succinylcholine should be avoided in older patients because of the risk of myoglobinuria and potential renal failure. In addition, succinylcholine theoretically could induce hyperkalemia, particularly in patients with muscle wasting. The successful use of atracurium during a modified rapid sequence induction has been reported.[18] Should myoglobinuria occur, forced diuresis with mannitol and furosemide might be beneficial. The absence of acidosis could readily differentiate myoglobinuria associated with McArdle's disease from that occurring during a malignant hyperthermic episode.

Intravenous regional (Bier block) anesthesia may be contraindicated because muscle ischemia is thought to lead to atrophy.[14] However, if the success of a surgical procedure on the extremity depends upon provision of a bloodless field, use of a tourniquet is justified.

Type VI (Hers' Disease)

Children with hepatic phosphorylase complex deficiency usually have only mild hepatomegaly secondary to glycogen accumulation. Mild fasting hypoglycemia occurs in some patients and should be considered when NPO orders are written. Acidosis is not a feature of the disease. Anesthesiologists should be aware that life-threatening hypoglycemia can be precipitated by severe illness in these patients. The disease improves with increasing age.

Type VII (Tarui's Disease)

The conversion of glucose to pyruvate does not proceed normally when there is a deficiency of muscle phosphofructokinase. The muscles are unable to utilize glucose for energy, and lactate does not accumulate during exercise. Children are usually asymptomatic; however, vigorous exercise produces muscle cramping and myoglobinuria in some adults. Although the disease is much less severe than McArdle's disease, the same anesthetic considerations apply.

Types VIII, IX, and X

Progressive brain degeneration and hepatomegaly are the clinical features of the few patients with type VIII disease. Types IX and X are even less well described. However, there has been a case report of hyperthermia and ketoacidosis during anesthesia in a child thought to have type IX disease.[19] This was thought to be due to a hypermetabolic state not related to malignant hyperpyrexia.

DISORDERS OF GALACTOSE METABOLISM

Disorders caused by deficiency of the enzymes that metabolize galactose result in cataract formation. It is estimated that inborn errors of galactose metabolism are responsible for approximately 4 percent of cataracts occurring in children under 1 year of age. As galactose accumulates, it diffuses into the lens and is converted to galactitol, which cannot diffuse out of the lens. Osmotic overhydration and swelling occur, and the lens fibers are eventually destroyed. The only consistent pathology in children with galactosemia due to galactokinase deficiency is cataracts. "Classic" galactosemia, which is due to deficiency of galactose-1-phosphate uridyl transferase, is often initially manifest by failure to thrive. Vomiting, dehydration, hypoglycemia, jaundice, hepatomegaly, and cirrhosis ensue. Diagnosis is made by enzyme assay of liver tissue, erythrocytes or leukocytes, or cultured fibroblasts. Elimination of galactose from the diet is essential and is accomplished by avoiding milk products. Cataracts and cirrhosis regress if not advanced at the time of diagnosis and initiation of dietary restriction. There are no known special anesthesia considerations for these patients.

DISORDERS OF FRUCTOSE METABOLISM

Fructokinase deficiency does not produce any pathology beyond the inability to metabolize ingested fructose and is referred to as benign fructosuria. Infants who lack hepatic fructose-1-phosphate aldolase are asymptomatic until they ingest fructose or the disaccharide sucrose. Symptoms include hypoglycemia, vomiting, and failure to thrive. Hepatosplenomegaly, coagulopathy, and renal tubular defects may also occur. Albuminuria and excessive loss of potassium result in hypoproteinemia and hypokalemia. Acidosis is the result of excessive renal bicarbonate excretion and enhanced conversion of fructose to lactate. Exchange transfusion has been employed in critically ill children; however, omission of fructose, sucrose, and sorbitol from the diet is all that is required for remission of symptoms and normal growth in most patients.

Symptoms of fructose-1,6-diphosphatase deficiency are initiated with introduction of fructose-containing foods in the diet. Children are free of symptoms as long as they ingest only human milk. Hypoglycemia is the usual presentation, and hyperventilation is the most common sign in the newborn infant. Hypotonia, hepatomegaly, and metabolic acidosis may also occur. Manifestations of the disease are exacerbated by infection or prolonged fasting.

Since hypoglycemia occurs with prolonged fasting, especially during febrile episodes, it is important to minimize the amount of time children with these disorders are kept NPO prior to operation. The anesthesiologist must also remember not to order fruit juice or other foods containing fructose for oral hydration. Intravenous solutions containing glucose can be administered liberally. Intermittent sampling of blood for glucose and pH determinations is indicated during major operation to ensure that hypoglycemia and acidosis do not occur.[20] All surgical procedures except those for life-threatening conditions must be deferred in children who are severely acidotic or hypokalemic.

DISORDERS OF AMINO ACID METABOLISM

Disorders of amino acid metabolism played an important role in the evolution of diagnostic techniques for children with inborn errors of metabolism. The current approach to phenylketonuria exemplifies the merits of both screening procedures and dietary restrictions.

PHENYLKETONURIA (PKU)

Hyperphenylalaninemia can be either benign (non-PKU hyperphenylalaninemia) or associated with severely impaired cognitive development. Both disorders are the result of deficiency of phenylalanine hydroxylase. The overall incidence is approximately 100 per million births. There is significant geographic and ethnic variation in PKU, with the reported incidence being 5 to 190 cases per million births.[6]

The most significant consequence of hyperphenylalaninemia is mental retardation, which first becomes manifest in midinfancy. Less than 2 percent of untreated children have an IQ above 70; in most it is less than 20. However, with scrupulous dietary management, mental development should proceed normally. Affected children are usually hyperactive and aggressive. Occasionally the disorder is confused with autism. At least one fourth of the patients have seizures. Untreated children have hypopigmentation of the skin, hair, and irises. A mousey or musty odor, due to accumulation of phenylacetic acid, is characteristic. Eczema is common. It is of interest that an increased incidence of pyloric stenosis has been reported in association with the disorder.

There are no unique anesthetic considerations for children with PKU. In fact, it should not be seen in countries with neonatal screening programs. Affected children with seizures should be maintained on anticonvulsant medication in the perioperative period. If eczema is present, careful handling and positioning are indicated to prevent further damage to the skin. Although it has been stated that children with PKU are very sensitive to narcotics and central nervous system depressants,[21] no documentation for this statement is provided, and it does not seem intuitively obvious that such should be the case.

TYROSINEMIA

Transient Neonatal Tyrosinemia

Hypertyrosinemia occurs in many newborn infants, especially premature babies. Although the levels of tyrosine may be very high, the liver and kidneys are not affected. Aside from transient lethargy, there are no clinical findings. Most cases are controlled by reducing protein intake or by breast-feeding. The tyrosine levels decrease to normal within a few weeks.

Tyrosinemia Type I

This is due, at least in part, to a deficiency of para-hydroxyphenyl pyruvic acid oxidase. Tyrosinemia I occurs in two forms: as an acute infantile disease or as a more chronic disorder of later onset. With the acute infantile form, vomiting, diarrhea, failure to thrive, hepatosplenomegaly, and jaundice occur within the first few months. A renal tubular defect causes acidosis, aminoaciduria, and polyuria. Rickets may result from phosphaturia. Glucosuria can lead to hypoglycemia. Rapid deterioration of liver function occurs, and most children with this form of the disorder die before 1 year of age.

The chronic form of the disease has a later onset with similar but milder manifestations. However, the majority of children with this variant die within the first decade of life. Abdominal crises and polyneuropathy are related to acute, intermittent, porphyria-like chemical abnormalities. Hypertension is not unusual. Hepatoma occurs in a significant percentage of patients. Normocytic anemia and leukocytosis are usually present, and coagulation defects are common. Dietary restriction is the mainstay of therapy, but liver transplantation has been employed in a few children.

Modifications of anesthetic techniques for these children may be required, depending upon the degree of hepatic and renal disease. Chronic anemia is common, but transfusion is not indicated unless the hematocrit is very low or acute blood loss occurs. Hypoglycemia must be prevented by limiting the NPO interval and infusing a glucose solution. The presence of liver or renal disease does not preclude the use of a volatile anesthetic agent. Renal excretion of muscle relaxants is not affected unless renal disease is severe; in such cases atracurium, which does not depend upon renal excretion, is preferable.

Tyrosinemia Type II

Tyrosinemia II (Richner-Hanhart syndrome) is a rare oculocutaneous syndrome characterized by keratosis of the soles and palms and corneal lesions. The severity of the skin and ocular lesions is related to the degree of tyrosine deposition. Mental retardation is an inconsistent feature of the disorder. There are no hepatic or renal abnormalities.

MAPLE SYRUP URINE DISEASE

There are several clinical phenotypes of maple syrup urine disease (MSUD). Increased concentrations of the branched-chain amino and alpha-keto acids are found in body cells and fluids. The incidence of the disorder depends upon the population screened, ranging from 1 in 290,000 in a heterogeneous population to 1 in 760 in an inbred Mennonite group.[22]

Poor feeding, vomiting, and a high-pitched cry are noted within the first week or two of life. The typical maple syrup or burnt sugar odor of the urine may be the first clue to the diagnosis. Hypotonicity or hypertonicity may occur, and these conditions may alternate initially. In untreated babies, severe hypoglycemia, ketoacidosis, coma, seizures, and death occur within weeks to months. Treatment must be initiated within the first week to 10 days to prevent central nervous system damage and physical and mental retardation. The primary approach to therapy is dietary. However, exchange transfusion, hemodialysis, peritoneal dialysis, or venovenous hemofiltration[8] can be employed to reduce the toxic metabolites rapidly. Administration of branched-chain amino acid–free parenteral nutrition is also useful in treating acute metabolic decompensation in these patients.[23]

The primary anesthetic consideration in children who are well controlled and require elective surgery is prevention of hypoglycemia and acidosis.[24] The period of dietary restriction should be minimized and glucose administered intravenously. If the surgical procedure is prolonged, blood sugar and arterial blood gas determinations should be performed intermittently. The child who is in a catabolic state as a result of an infectious process or trauma may require dialysis prior to operation.

HOMOCYSTINURIA

Cystathionine beta-synthase deficiency is the most frequent cause of homocystinuria. Clinical manifestations include optic lens dislocation, mental retardation, and thromboembolism affecting large and small arteries as well as the venous system. Although osteoporosis is common, several other skeletal disorders also occur, including pectus excavatum or carinatum, kyphosis, scoliosis, and arachnodactyly. Some patients have a Marfan-like habitus. Growth retardation has also been reported. Many of the children have a "Charlie Chaplin" type of gait. Afflicted children usually have fair skin and light-colored, brittle hair. Mental retardation is common.

By far the most serious manifestation of the disease is arterial and venous thrombosis. Although the exact mechanism of the thrombotic diathesis is not defined, both abnormalities of the arterial walls and hypercoagulability appear to contribute. The latter is probably due to increased platelet adhesiveness. Vascular occlusion may occur as early as the first decade and is common in older children. Death results from vascular thrombosis by the midtwenties in half the patients.

Administration of pyridoxine (vitamin B_6) is beneficial in some patients. Dietary restriction is practiced in those unresponsive to pyridoxine. More recently, therapy with the methyl donor betaine has proved successful in some patients nonresponsive to pyridoxine.[25]

Although spontaneous thrombosis of the cerebral, pulmonary, renal, mesenteric, and coronary arteries occurs, it is more likely in the perioperative period. Any preexisting neurological deficit must be carefully documented. A preoperative electrocardiogram should be obtained in all patients. Dehydration and vascular stasis should be avoided. Perioperative administration of dextran 40 has been suggested to decrease platelet aggregation and possibly reduce the incidence of thrombosis.[26] Acute normovolemic hemodilution, by decreasing viscosity, might be a useful adjunct in patients having major surgical procedures. Dextrose solutions also should be administered intraoperatively, as patients with homocystinuria are prone to develop hyperinsulinemia and hypoglycemia. During lengthy operative procedures it is critical that the patient be positioned in a manner to minimize venous stasis. Wrapping the legs with Ace bandages and elevating the foot of the operating room table is recommended. The goals of anesthetic management are to maintain peripheral perfusion, avoid dehydration or stasis, and promote early recovery and ambulation. Hypothermia should be avoided as it increases viscosity and predisposes to thrombosis.

Invasive radiographic studies requiring intravenous administration of contrast media are especially hazardous because the dye produces an osmotic diuresis, which may lead to dehydration and increased blood viscosity. It is imperative that intravenous fluid administration equal or exceed urinary losses.

DISORDERS OF ORGANIC ACID METABOLISM

ALCAPTONURIA

Alcaptonuria is the disorder that led to elucidation of the concept of inborn errors of metabolism by Garrod in 1902. It is a rare disease in which homogentisic acid, an intermediary product in the metabolism of phenylalanine and tyrosine, cannot be further metabolized, leading to pigmentation of connective tissue (ochronosis). Progressive degenerative arthropathy and spondylitis occur in adults, but symptoms are not present in children. The relationship between the metabolic defect and the clinical syndrome has not been explained. Dietary restrictions and various pharmacological agents have been utilized, but at this time there is no specific treatment. There are no special anesthetic considerations for children with this disorder.

LACTIC ACIDEMIA

Several inborn errors of metabolism present with metabolic acidosis in which lactic acidosis is prominent. In others, not characterized by acidosis, the blood lactate level is also elevated chronically or intermittently. The high lactic acid levels are usually associated with unusual organic acids in the urine, distinguishing the disorders from nongenetic conditions in which lactic acidosis is a manifestation of various types of severe organ damage.

The differential diagnosis of lactic acidemia is based on biochemical and pathological information as well as the child's signs and symptoms. Blood lactate and pyruvate levels are assayed, serum amino acids are quantified, urine organic acids are analyzed by gas chromatography/mass spectrometry, and a glucose determination is performed. Muscle biopsy also may be necessary for diagnosis. Most of the disorders are rare, and the clinical presentations vary from hypoglycemia and coma to myopathy, cardiomyopathy, and psychomotor retardation. The most common of the disorders, resulting from deficiency of the pyruvate dehydrogenase complex, is characterized by a spectrum of presentations varying from overwhelming lactic acidemia in the neonatal period to mild acidemia accompanied by psychomotor retardation.[27]

Modifications of anesthetic technique depend upon the type of disorder and metabolic derangement. Adequate hydration and avoidance of hypoglycemia are essential. Monitoring of arterial blood gases is indicated during major procedures; however, attempts should not be made to achieve a normal pH in children who are chronically acidotic.

DISORDERS OF LIPID METABOLISM

CARNITINE DEFICIENCY SYNDROMES

Fatty acids are the predominant substrate for energy production during periods of fasting. Oxidation of fatty acids also accounts for up to 60 percent of muscle oxygen consumption during prolonged aerobic exercise. The fatty acids are taken up by the liver and other tissues by concentration-dependent mechanisms that are not fully elucidated. Once inside cells, the fatty acids are activated to form coenzyme A (CoA) esters that can serve as substrates for triglyceride, phospholipid, and cholesteryl ester synthesis. However, during periods of fasting, they are directed primarily toward mitochondrial beta-oxidation. Long-chain acyl-CoA esters must first be transesterified to carnitine by the outer mitochondrial membrane enzyme carnitine palmityltransferase I (CPT I) before they can cross mitochondrial membranes. Transmembrane transfer of acylcarnitines is mediated by carnitine translocase. Carnitine palmityltransferase II (CPT II) is required for re-esterification of acylcarnitines to form CoA esters.

There are a number of carnitine deficiency syndromes. Fasting can induce episodes of vomiting and lethargy as well as hypoglycemic coma. A presentation difficult to differentiate from Reye's syndrome, usually preceded by a viral infection, has also been desribed.[28] In the myopathic form of the disorder, rhabdomyolysis can occur with prolonged fasting or exercise since the muscle tissue cannot utilize fatty acid as an alternative energy source. Patients may also experience episodes of pain and muscle rigidity in association with exercise. There is a case report of severe rhabdomyolysis and acute renal failure following anesthesia in a patient who, after the event, was determined to be CPT-deficient.[29] There is also a case report of massive rhabdomyolysis and cardiac arrest associated with general anesthesia in a child with CPT deficiency.[30]

Avoidance of prolonged fasting in the perioperative period is essential. Since the patients are primarily dependent upon glucose for energy production, glucose should be administered intravenously. Administration of succinylcholine is contraindicated as it, too, has been reported to induce rhabdomyolysis.[31] Although it has been stated that the disorder may be associated with malignant hyperthermia,[29] it is more likely to be confused with malignant hyperthermia rather than associated with it.

DISORDERS OF LIPOPROTEIN METABOLISM

Much has been learned in recent years about the process of lipid transport in the blood. In three genetic diseases of lipoprotein metabolism associated with hypercholesterolemia the molecular defect has been defined.[32] The disorders are classified on the basis of total cholesterol and triglycerides in the plasma as well as the concentration of total cholesterol in major lipoprotein classes. At least two types of familial hyperlipoproteinemia during childhood are associated with significant morbidity and mortality.

FAMILIAL LIPOPROTEIN LIPASE DEFICIENCY

Children with lipoprotein lipase deficiency have episodes of severe abdominal pain because of recurrent acute pancreatitis. The children may be subjected to laparotomy if pancreatitis is confused with other intra-abdominal pathology such as appendicitis. The disease may present in infancy with colicky pain and failure to thrive. Cutaneous xanthomatosis occurs in about half the patients, and hepatomegaly is very common. Serum levels of chylomicrons, cholesterol, and triglycerides are high, and the severity of symptoms correlates with the degree of chylomicronemia. Premature atherosclerosis is not a feature of the disease.[33] Dietary restriction and avoidance of unnecessary laparotomies are the cornerstones of therapy.

FAMILIAL COMBINED HYPERLIPIDEMIA

Familial combined hyperlipidemia is transmitted through a single autosomal dominant gene. Although the incidence of homozygosity is only about 1 in a million, the heterozygous state may be as frequent as 1 in 500. Homozygotes have severe disease that is manifest early in childhood. Generalized atherosclerosis with severe coronary artery disease often leads to death before the age of 20 years. Xanthomas are evident by 4 years of age and may even be present at birth. Arcus corneae usually develops within the first decade. Neither dietary nor medical therapy is very effective in patients with the homozygous form of the disease. In contrast, dietary restriction and therapy with cholestyramine or colestipol exchange resins are beneficial in heterozygotes.

The anesthetic considerations for children with the homozygous form of the disorder are those applicable to any patient with coronary artery disease. Extensive invasive monitoring may be indicated in children undergoing major surgical procedures.

DISORDERS OF LYSOSOMAL ENZYMES

Lysosomal enzyme deficiencies result in accumulation of mucopolysaccharides, glycoproteins, and sphingolipids, singly or in combination (Table 13–4). The skeleton, central nervous system, and viscera are affected. Although deposition of the stored material begins prior to birth, the onset of clinical manifestations can be delayed for several years. The mucopolysaccharidoses constitute the largest subgroup of disorders and are associated with the most significant anesthetic problems.

Table 13–4. DISORDERS OF LYSOSOMAL ENZYMES

Disorder	Prevalence
Mucopolysaccharidosis, type I	
Hurler's syndrome	1:100,000
Scheie's syndrome	1:600,000
Hurler-Scheie syndrome	1:100,000
Mucopolysaccharidosis, type II (Hunter's syndrome)	1:70,000 in Israel
Mucopolysaccharidosis, type III (Sanfilippo's syndrome)	1:24,000 in Netherlands
Mucopolysaccharidosis, type IV (Morquio's syndrome)	1:300,000
Mucopolysaccharidosis, type VI (Maroteaux-Lamy syndrome)	Rare
Mucopolysaccharidosis, type VII (Sly's syndrome)	Rare
Acid lipase deficiency (Wolman's disease)	Rare
Ceramidase deficiency (Farber's disease)	Rare
Niemann-Pick disease	Rare
Gaucher's disease, type I	1:600 Ashkenazi Jews
type II, type III	Rare
Galactosylceramide lipidosis (Krabbe's disease)	1:50,000 Swedes
Metachromatic leukodystrophy	1:100,000
Alpha-galactosidase A deficiency (Fabry's disease)	1:40,000
Tay-Sachs disease	1:3000 US Jews

Modified from Scriver CR, Beaudet AL, Sly WS, Valle D (Eds.): The Metabolic Basis of Inherited Disease. 6th ed. New York, McGraw-Hill, 1989, pp 137–140; with permission.

MUCOPOLYSACCHARIDOSES

Deficiency of the lysosomal enzymes involved in the degradation of dermatan sulfate, heparan sulfate, and keratan sulfate leads to accumulation and increased urinary excretion of partially degraded mucopolysaccharides. There is clinical similarity between the different enzyme deficiencies but a wide spectrum of severity within each type of deficiency. Diagnosis and prognosis are based on enzymatic and clinical evaluation. Simple enzyme assays utilizing fibroblasts, leukocytes, or serum are available. Prenatal diagnosis is also possible. Except for Hunter's syndrome, which is X-linked, the pattern of inheritance is autosomal recessive. Enzyme replacement therapy may prove to be an effective treatment. Bone marrow transplantation has been successfully employed in children with several of the disorders. In some, there was dramatic improvement in the clinical course of the disease.

TYPE I (HURLER'S, SCHEIE'S, AND HURLER-SCHEIE SYNDROMES)

Alpha-L-iduronidase deficiency has three different forms that can be distinguished on the basis of age of onset and clinical course. The first, Hurler's syndrome, is the prototype for all the mucopolysaccharidoses. The children appear normal in infancy, but toward the end of the first year they are noted to be unusually large with proportionately large heads. Dwarfing and increased head size become evident by 2 or 3 years. Coarse facies are a prominent characteristic of the disorder. Macroglossia and patulous lips are accentuated, since the children are usually mouth breathers because the nose is obstructed by secretions and the adenoids and tonsils are large. The gums are hyperplastic and the teeth abnormally shaped and widely spaced. The neck is short and thick. Narrowing of the laryngeal inlet and tracheobronchial tree may occur as a result of deposition of mucopolysaccharides.[34] Progressive clouding of the cornea occurs, and some children also develop glaucoma. Hydrocephalus may occur secondary to thickening of the meninges. The skin is thickened, and there is generalized hirsutism. The abdomen is protuberant and the liver and spleen are enlarged. Umbilical and inguinal hernias are frequent. Joint mobility is decreased, flexion contractures and thoracolumbar kyphosis usually occur, and the hands are often said to be clawlike. Sensorineural deafness is frequent. Coronary artery and valvular disease occur in young children.[35, 36] Cardiomyopathy also results from deposition of mucopolysaccharides in the myocardium. Severe mental retardation is a consistent feature of the disorder. Death from cardiac failure usually occurs in the first decade. Restrictive lung disease due to thoracic cage abnormality is compounded by recurrent pulmonary infections.

Children with Scheie's syndrome generally are less severely affected than those with Hurler's syndrome. Coarse facial features, corneal clouding, glaucoma, retinal degeneration, deafness, and aortic valvular disease are common. Sleep apnea severe enough to require tracheostomy has been reported.[37] Intelligence and life span are usually normal. The more common procedures for which these patients are seen are carpal tunnel release, aortic valve replacement, and ophthalmological procedures.

Hurler-Scheie disease is an intermediate phenotype. Patients are short, have joint involvement, and are usually of moderate intelligence. Valvular lesions are more severe than in children with Scheie's disease. Micrognathia is a consistent feature. Death usually occurs by the second decade.

Type II (Hunter's Syndrome)

The Hunter syndrome occurs in severe and mild forms. The facies are coarse and mild, and moderate dwarfism is characteristic. Corneal clouding does not occur, but retinitis pigmentosa may. Vision and hearing deteriorate progressively. Virtually all patients become deaf. Nodular, ivory-colored skin lesions are characteristic. Mental retardation and joint disease are less pronounced than in Hurler's syndrome. Hydrocephalus may be severe and lead to premature death. Valvular and ischemic heart disease are frequent, although patients with mild forms of the disease survive into adulthood. Although usually less severe, the same airway difficulties may occur as with Hurler's syndrome, and tracheostomy may be required.[38]

Type III (Sanfilippo's Syndrome)

The four biochemically distinct forms of the Sanfilippo syndrome are not clinically distinguishable. Severe, progressive mental retardation is the primary feature of the disorder. The somatic manifestations are relatively mild. Facial features are less coarse than in types I and II disease, joint stiffness is not as severe, and corneal clouding does not occur. Patients rarely survive into the second decade.

Type IV (Morquio's Syndrome)

These children are usually of normal intelligence. The degree of facial coarseness is mild to moderate; the maxilla is usually prominent, the nose short, and the teeth widely spaced. Partial deafness is the rule. Skeletal abnormalities are severe. The neck and trunk are short, and progressive pectus carinatum develops. Genu varum, joint laxity, and severe dwarfism are present. Absence or marked hypoplasia of the odontoid process of the second vertebra and resulting atlantoaxial instability may lead to spinal cord compression.[39] Progressive neurological degeneration, acute quadriparesis,[40] and death from respiratory arrest have been reported. Upper airway obstruction due to collapse of the trachea during head flexion has also been reported.[41] Chronic pulmonary disease secondary to thoracic deformity and repeated pulmonary infections is common.[42] Aortic regurgitation may accompany the disorder. Most patients live to adulthood. Prophylactic posterior cervical fusion has been performed in some patients and may lead to longer survival.

Type VI (Maroteaux-Lamy Syndrome)

This disorder is characterized by short stature, joint stiffness, coarse facial features, and corneal clouding. There is a spectrum of disease severity. Less consistent features are hydrocephalus, valvular disease, hypoplasia of the odontoid, lumbar kyphosis, and genu valgum. Patients usually die by the second decade.

Type VII (Sly's Syndrome)

Extremely rare and of variable severity, this type of mucopolysaccharidosis is characterized by coarse facies, corneal clouding, hepatosplenomegaly, umbilical and inguinal hernias, pectus carinatum, joint deformities, and aortic disease.

The primary anesthetic consideration for children with all these disorders is airway management. Several reviews have been published that emphasize this aspect of the mucopolysaccharidoses.[43–45] In the latest, the overall incidence of airway problems was 26 percent, but it was 53 percent in those with Hurler's or Hunter's syndromes.[45] It is often difficult to determine the optimal time for elective surgical procedures because most of the children have chronic otitis media and nasal stuffiness that can be difficult to differentiate from acute infectious processes.

Because of the frequency of ischemic and valvular disease, an electrocardiogram should be obtained preoperatively, and an echocardiogram may be indicated. Radiographs of the cervical spine are advisable to check for odontoid hypoplasia and atlantoaxial subluxation. If there is reason to suspect tracheal compression, a CT scan or tomography can be considered. However, the risks of sedating or anesthetizing the child for radiographic studies may very well outweigh the benefits of the tests.

An antisialogogue should be administered preoperatively. Sedatives should be used in small doses or avoided completely because of the risks of airway obstruction. If sedation is indicated, it is probably best to administer it rectally or intravenously in a holding area where the patient can be continuously observed rather than on the ward. Intravenous access is often difficult due to the child's thick skin and abnormal anatomy secondary to joint contractures.

It should be assumed that airway maintenance and endotracheal intubation will be difficult. The large tongue often leads to obstruction with induction of anesthesia. Intubation may be complicated by micrognathia as well as macroglossia. A plan should be formulated prior to induction of anesthesia for management of the airway if conventional measures fail. Specialized techniques of intubation such as fiberoptic endoscopy or use of the Bullard laryngoscope should be considered. Nasotracheal intubation should not be attempted unless mandated by the nature of the surgical procedure because of the danger of bleeding and the potential for hyperplastic adenoid tissue being dislodged and possibly impacted in the endotracheal tube. The size of tube that can be passed is often smaller than predicted, mandating the ready availability of several sizes of tubes. The child should be extubated only when fully awake.

METACHROMATIC LEUKODYSTROPHY

Metachromatic leukodystrophy, of which there are at least seven variants, is an inherited disorder of myelin metabolism. The initial signs appear at any time from birth to old age, but the most common ages of onset are between 1 and 2 years for the late infantile variant, 4 and 6 years for the juvenile type, and 16 and 26 years for the adult form. Signs in children with the infantile type are developmental delay, weakness, optic atrophy, ataxia, and progressive spastic quadriparesis. Older children usually have mental confusion, postural abnormalities, and pyramidal and extrapyramidal signs. In one variant the children have the habitus of children with mucopolysaccharidoses. The principles of anesthetic management previously described for children with mucopolysaccharidoses apply to children with this variant. Neither dietary nor pharmacological therapy is useful. Bone marrow transplantation has been employed in a few children with varying degrees of success.

ACID LIPASE DEFICIENCY (WOLMAN'S DISEASE)

Deficiency of lysosomal acid lipase leads to massive accumulation of cholesteryl esters and triglycerides in most tissues. The onset of symptoms is within the first few weeks of life. Vomiting, diarrhea, hepatosplenomegaly, abdominal distention, and anemia are progressive, and death usually occurs before the age of 1 year. Calcification of the adrenal glands is consistently demonstrated. Should these childen require an operation, the primary considerations are increased intragastric pressure secondary to the large liver, anemia, and the potential for adrenal insufficiency. Liver and bone marrow transplantations have been performed in a limited number of children with the disorder.

CERAMIDASE DEFICIENCY (FARBER'S DISEASE)

Deficiency of a lysosomal acid ceramidase results in tissue accumulation of ceramide in patients with Farber's disease. The classic signs, which are usually evident between 2 weeks and 4 months of age, are subcutaneous nodules, arthritis, and hoarseness. The nodules are most prominent around involved joints, which are swollen and painful. Hoarseness usually progresses to aphonia. Dysphagia and respiratory difficulty are due to granuloma formation in the epiglottis and larynx. The laryngeal inlet may be markedly reduced in diameter, and tracheostomy may be required. Macroglossia may compromise the airway. Hepatomegaly, cardiomyopathy, and mental deterioration are less common. Diagnosis usually can be made clinically but is confirmed by histological examination of a biopsied nodule, assay of enzyme activity in cultured skin fibroblasts or leukocytes, or chromatographic analysis of ceramide in tissue or body fluid. There is no specific therapy, and the children usually die by 2 years of age. Bone marrow transplantation may offer some hope.

Anesthetic experience with these children is extremely limited. It seems prudent to avoid endotracheal intubation if the operative procedure can be safely performed with inhalation anesthesia by mask. Perhaps a laryngeal mask airway could be employed. When endotracheal intubation is indicated, the tube should be smaller than that usually used for a child of the same age in order to minimize trauma to the vocal cords. Measures normally employed in children with postextubation croup can be utilized if necessary.

SPHINGOMYELIN-CHOLESTEROL LIPIDOSES (NIEMANN-PICK DISEASE)

Niemann-Pick disease is characterized by tissue accumulation of sphingomyelin owing to deficiency of sphingomyelinase. There are six variants of the disorder. Hepatosplenomegaly is a constant feature, and foam cells are found in the bone marrow of affected children. Involvement of the nervous system and lung is common. Often, a cherry-red spot is evident in the retina. The acute form of the disease is characterized by massive visceromegaly, rapid progression, and death prior to 5 years of age. Occasionally, splenectomy is performed if the organ is extremely large. Such children should have a rapid sequence induction because the enlarged spleen and liver render the patient susceptible to regurgitation and aspiration.

GLUCOSYLCERAMIDE LIPIDOSES (GAUCHER'S DISEASE)

Gaucher's disease is the most prevalent lysosomal storage disorder. The subtypes are clinically very different, although all are related biochemically in that patients are deficient in glucocerebrosidase. The diagnosis should be considered in any patient with unexplained splenomegaly and is confirmed by assay of glucocerebrosidase in white cells or fibroblasts. The highest incidence (1 in 2500) is found in the Ashkenazi Jewish population.

The age of onset and severity of symptoms in type I or chronic non-neuronopathic Gaucher's disease are quite variable. Painless splenomegaly, thrombocytopenia, anemia, and leukopenia are the usual initial manifestations. Hepatomegaly is not pronounced, and hepatic function usually remains normal. Degenerative bone changes are the leading cause of disability in these patients. Bone scans reveal decreased bone density in the long bones, hip joints, and vertebrae. Aseptic necrosis of the femoral head and vertebral fractures are common. Severe episodes of bone pain—"bone crises," often accompanied by fever, may be mistaken for osteomyelitis. Pulmonary involvement is common and can lead to pulmonary hypertension and cor pulmonale. The disease usually progresses slowly. In April, 1991, the Food and Drug Administration approved Ceredase, the first agent available to treat type I Gaucher's disease. The enzyme replacement therapy decreases splenic enlargement and reverses the anemia characteristic of the disease.

Severe deficiency of enzymatic activity causes accumulation of large amounts of glucocerebroside in patients with type II disease. Hepatosplenomegaly is the usual presenting sign. Neurological signs are usually evident within 6 months of birth. Dysphagia, difficulty in handling secretions, and recurrent aspiration pneumonitis occur, and most children die within the year from pulmonary infection. Progressive spasticity, hyperreflexia, and pathological reflexes are present. The triad of trismus, strabismus, and retroflexion of the head is classic.

Type III Gaucher's disease has a more heterogeneous presentation, with onset in childhood or adolescence. Hepatosplenomegaly and skeletal and neurological involvement usually become evident in adolescence. The course of the disease is variable.

A hematological profile should be obtained for any child with Gaucher's disease who is scheduled for operation. Mild anemia is common. Patients may have platelet counts below 50,000/μL without a bleeding diathesis. Conversely, some with normal bleeding and clotting studies bleed excessively during operation. Prophylactic platelet administration is not indicated, but the availability of platelets should be assured prior to operation. Therapy should be administered only if warranted by the clinical situation. A hematology consultation is recommended. As many as one third of patients have significant pulmonary pathology, and pulmonary hypertension is not uncommon.[46] Difficult endotracheal intubation must be anticipated in patients with type II disease, because of the trismus and the abnormal head position.

Although liver transplantation does not cure Gaucher's disease, it may prolong life in selected children.[47] Allogeneic bone marrow transplantation has resulted in partial clinical improvement of visceral symptoms in several patients.[48]

GALACTOSYLCERAMIDE LIPIDOSIS (KRABBE'S DISEASE)

This is a rapidly progressive disease, usually manifest at 3 to 6 months of age by irritability, hypertonicity, vomiting, and failure to thrive. Progressive mental and motor deterioration, spastic quadriparesis, blindness, and deafness ensue, and most children die by age 2 years. Bone marrow transplantation may have a place in treatment of affected patients, but currently no other therapy is available.

ALPHA-GALACTOSIDASE A DEFICIENCY (FABRY'S DISEASE)

Fabry's disease is an X-linked disorder that is usually manifest in children although the onset can be delayed until adulthood. The most common presenting symptoms are severe, intermittent pain and paresthesias in the extremities that are triggered by exercise, stress, climatic changes, or hyperpyrexia. Vessel ectasia (angiokeratoma) occurs in skin and mucous membranes, and hypohidrosis, diarrhea, nausea, and vomiting are common. Cardiac conduction defects, cerebrovascular occlusion, and renal disease are also features of the disease. Many patients live to adulthood, with death resulting from vascular or renal complications.

Diphenylhydantoin often provides relief from the excruciating pain. Dialysis and renal transplantation are employed for severe renal disease. The first renal transplantation for this disorder was performed in 1967. Although there are approximately 50 documented renal transplants in patients with Fabry's disease, reports of long-term survival are rare.[49] Bone marrow transplantation may have a role in therapy of children with Fabry's disease.

The disease must not be confused with malignant hyperthermia in which vigorous exercise may induce muscle cramping. Patients controlled on diphenylhydantoin should continue to receive the drug in the perioperative period. No contraindications to specific anesthetic agents or techniques are known.

GANGLIOSIDOSES (TAY-SACHS DISEASE)

At least three subtypes of gangliosidoses are recognized. Neonates may present with a rapidly progressive neurological deterioration that results in death in infancy. Facial features in these children often resemble those of children with the Hurler's syndrome. At the other end of the spectrum are patients with normal intelligence who survive to adulthood.

Tay-Sachs disease is the most common ganglioside storage disease and the most severe form of the disorder. Testing for the carrier state is recommended in Ashkenazi Jewish populations, since the carrier state is prevalent in that population. An exaggerated startle response is usually noted early. Motor weakness is evident by 6 months of age, and psychomotor deterioration progresses rapidly. Deafness, blindness, convulsions, and cherry-red spots in the macula are characteristic. Most children die by age 3 or 4 years. There is no therapy.

Most of the children have severe pulmonary disease as a result of recurrent aspiration. A feeding gastrostomy may be required as swallowing becomes progressively ineffective. Patients should be considered at risk for aspiration of gastric contents and either intubated awake or with a rapid sequence induction. Preoperative administration of metoclopramide and cimetidine may be helpful.

DISORDERS OF PURINE METABOLISM

LESCH-NYHAN SYNDROME

This devastating disease is due to a virtual absence of hypoxanthine-guanine phosphoribosyl transferase, which is essential for normal purine metabolism. Uric acid accumulates, leading to the severe neurological manifestations of the disease. The disorder is inherited in an X-linked manner, and the syndrome occurs in approximately 1 in 10,000 males. Heterozygous females are usually asymptomatic.

Most children with the syndrome are normal at birth, but delayed motor development is evident in 3 to 4 months. Hyperreflexia, extensor plantar reflexes, sustained ankle clonus, and scissoring of the legs are characteristic. Extrapyramidal signs develop between 8 and 12 months and include dystonia, chorea, and athetoid movements of the head and feet. Approximately half the children have seizures. The most severe neurological defect is compulsive self-mutilation. Biting of the lips, buccal mucosa, and fingers is common. The children also may demonstrate aggressive behavior toward others. Elevation of uric acid leads to development of subcutaneous tophi and renal calculi. Death usually occurs by the second decade, often due to renal failure.

These children may require anesthesia for a variety of operative procedures. Complete dental extractions may be performed to decrease the patients ability to injure themselves. Operation is frequently required for treatment of renal calculi. Whenever a child with this disorder is scheduled for operation, the anesthesiologist must explain to the operating room personnel what to expect of a child with Lesch-Nyhan syndrome. Premedication with diazepam or midazolam may be helpful. These patients are prone to regurgitation and vomiting and may benefit from metoclopramide to speed gastric emptying. Ranitidine may be given to increase gastric pH. It may be necessary to administer an induction agent, such as intramuscular ketamine, or a rectal barbiturate before attempting to transport the child to the operating room. Rapid sequence induction should be considered. However, if self-mutilation has led to scarring of the mouth and difficulty with endotracheal intubation is anticipated, a rapid sequence induction is contraindicated. Administration of succinylcholine also may be inadvisable because of the potential for hyperkalemia. Atracurium may be the relaxant of choice in this condition.

Complex, poorly understood abnormalities of adrenergic responses have been described in association with the syndrome. The adrenergic pressor response may be diminished or absent. It is said that exogenous catecholamines should be administered with great caution. Some of the central nervous system effects of morphine may be secondary to morphine-induced release of the purine adenosine; therefore, the response to exogenously administered morphine may be modified.[50]

XANTHINURIA

Xanthinuria results from a deficiency of the enzyme xanthine oxidase, which catalyzes the oxidation of hypoxanthine to xanthine and xanthine to uric acid. At least half the patients are asymptomatic. However, urinary tract calculi do develop in a significant percentage of patients with the disorder. Muscle cramping following exercise and recurring polyarthritis are less common symptoms.

The anesthesiologist usually thinks of malignant hyperthermia in any patient with a history of muscle cramps. However, there is no reported case of malignant hyperthermia in a patient with this disorder. In the absence of other evidence of susceptibility to malignant hyperthermia, no modifications of anesthetic technique are indicated.

DISORDERS OF BILIRUBIN METABOLISM

Bilirubin is an orange pigment derived from the degradation of heme proteins. Following formation in the reticuloendothelial system, bilirubin is released into the circulation, where it binds to serum albumin and is rapidly cleared by the liver. The hepatic transport of bilirubin involves four distinct but interrelated steps: (1) uptake from the circulation; (2) intracellular binding or storage; (3) conjugation, primarily with glucuronic acid; and (4) biliary excretion. Several genetic disorders affecting bilirubin metabolism have been identified. Each disorder is characterized by varying degrees of hyperbilirubinemia of the unconjugated or conjugated type.

GLUCURONYL TRANSFERASE DEFICIENCY (CRIGLER-NAJJAR SYNDROME TYPES I AND II)

In Crigler-Najjar syndrome type I, there is virtually no hepatic glucuronyl transferase activity. The disease is usually associated with bilirubin encephalopathy or kernicterus. Serum bilirubin levels often reach 20 to 50 mg/dL, and survival past the neonatal period is uncommon. Phototherapy is employed but is not effective in older children. Plasmapheresis is the most efficient means of reducing the serum bilirubin level. There is a case report of liver transplantation in a 3-year-old child in whom the bilirububin rapidly declined to normal following the operation.[51]

Crigler-Najjar syndrome type II is almost always clinically benign, and the bilirubin level is usually below 20 mg/dL. The response to treatment with phenobarbital, which induces hepatic microsomal enzymes and reduces the bilirubin level, also distinguishes type II disease from type I disease.

GILBERT'S SYNDROME

Patients with Gilbert's syndrome have chronic, mild hyperbilirubinemia. Although the bilirubin levels rise during intercurrent illness, the serum bilirubin is usually less than 3 mg/dL and the course of the disease benign. Unconjugated hyperbilirubinemia without overt hemolysis should lead the clinician to suspect the diagnosis. Fatigue and abdominal discomfort are frequent complaints. The latter often lead to multiple diagnostic studies and to exploratory laparotomy. The disorder appears to be relatively common, with a suggested incidence of 5 percent.[52]

Anesthesiologists should be familiar with the characteristics of these disorders. Gilbert's disease should be considered in the differential diagnosis of postoperative jaundice. Elevated bilirubin levels in these patients are attributed to the stress of operation as well as preoperative fasting.[53] Some patients have erroneously been told that hyperbilirubinemia was due to "allergy" to the anesthetic agents employed.[54] The metabolism of morphine may not proceed normally. There is a case report of prolonged morphine effect in a patient with Gilbert's syndrome.[55] Although far fewer patients with Crigler-Najjar syndrome than Gilbert's syndrome will undergo anesthesia, the anesthesiologist should be aware of the implications of enzyme induction in patients with type II disease who are receiving phenobarbital therapy.

DUBIN-JOHNSON SYNDROME

The Dubin-Johnson syndrome is rarely detected prior to puberty. Conjugated hyperbilirubinemia and jaundice are characteristic. Bilirubin levels may be as high as 20 mg/dL and increase in the presence of intercurrent illness. Patients are usually asymptomatic but may complain of weakness and vague abdominal pain. Although the liver appears black on gross examination, it is normal histologically except for accumulation of a dense pigment within the lysosomes.[52] The exact nature of the pigment is unknown. The disorder is uncommon, although the incidence approaches 1:1300 in Persian Jews, in whom it is associated with deficiency of clotting factor VII.[52]

ROTOR'S SYNDROME

Also a benign disorder, Rotor's syndrome is characterized by chronic conjugated hyperbilirubinemia. In contrast to Dubin-Johnson syndrome, the liver is grossly as well as histologically normal.

PORPHYRIA

In porphyria, enzyme activity necessary for the heme biosynthetic pathway is deficient. Eight enzymes are involved in the synthesis of heme and several types of porphyria. In general, the porphyrias are classified as hepatic or erythroid, depending on the primary site of expression of the enzymatic defect. Only acute intermittent porphyria, the most common autosomal dominant form of acute hepatic porphyria, will be discussed.

Acute intermittent porphyria is due to deficiency of porphobilinogen deaminase (PBG deaminase) activity. Both symptomatic and asymptomatic heterozygotes have 50 percent or greater of normal PBG deaminase levels. It is of interest that approximately 90 percent of individuals who inherit the deficiency exhibit no clinical signs. The disorder is latent before puberty and more common in girls than boys. Hormonal and nutritional factors, as well as a variety of pharmacological agents, may exacerbate the disorder.

Abdominal pain is a hallmark of the disorder and is often the presenting symptom of an acute attack. Chest, back, and limb pain may also occur—with or without abdominal pain. Hypo- and hyperactivity of the urinary and gastrointestinal tracts are also features of the disorder. Tachycardia and hypertension are common, and in many patients hypertension is sustained between acute episodes.

Intermittent neurological dysfunction of undetermined etiology is the most significant feature of the disorder. Although motor neuropathies predominate, virtually any type of neuropathy may occur. The cranial nerves, particularly VII and X, may be involved. Patchy sensory neuropathy often accompanies motor neuropathy. Patients complain of paresthesias as well as numbness. Acute attacks can be accompanied by seizures. Hyponatremia, secondary to vomiting or inappropriate antidiuretic hormone release, may play a role in genesis of the seizures. Anxiety, restlessness, insomnia, depression, and paranoia often accompany acute episodes. Acute attacks, which often last days to months, can be precipitated by endogenous or exogenous environmental factors. Of primary interest to the anesthesiologist are the pharmacological agents reputed to induce acute attacks.

The primary drugs implicated in precipitating an episode of porphyria are the barbiturates. The barbiturates were introduced into clinical practice in 1903, and the first case of acute porphyria following barbiturate administration was described in 1906. Since that time, there have been numerous reports of neurological abnormalities and abdominal pain following anesthesia during which thiobarbiturates were administered.[56] The authors of one retrospective study, examining the outcome of patients who received thiopental, found that administration of the drug to patients not experiencing an acute attack at the time of operation did not precipitate symptoms in the postoperative period. However, porphyric symptoms were worse postoperatively in seven of ten patients who received thiopental and in two of four who did not receive the drug when an operation was performed during an acute episode.[57] Obviously, other factors may play a role in exacerbating porphyric symptoms. Nevertheless, it seems prudent to avoid administration of barbiturates to patients with acute intermittent porphyria.

Induction agents that have been used successfully include ketamine,[58, 59] etomidate,[60] and propofol.[61–64] Narcotics, inhalation anesthetic agents, muscle relaxants, and drugs used to reverse neuromuscular blocking agents appear to be safe. Regional anesthesia is usually avoided because of the propensity of these patients to develop neurological deficits postoperatively and the inability to differentiate whether the deficits are related to the underlying disease or are complications of the anesthetic.

It is essential that any preexisting neurological deficits be carefully documented. Electrolytes should be determined, particularly in patients who require an operation during an acute episode of porphyria, to rule out hyponatremia. Procedures should be deferred if possible in hyponatremic patients until the electrolyte disturbance is corrected. The period of perioperative fasting should be minimized and intravenous solutions containing glucose administered. Conventional therapy is indicated if hypertension or tachycardia occurs.

ALPHA$_1$-ANTITRYPSIN DEFICIENCY

Deficiency of alpha$_1$-antitrypsin results in a protease/protease inhibitor imbalance in the lung that results in destruction of the alveolar walls. Symptoms of lung disease do not usually appear until the third or fourth decade. Liver disease is, however, evident in 15 to 20 percent of infants with the deficiency. The disorder should be considered in the differential diagnosis of jaundice in infants and emphysema and liver disease in adults. Serum electrophoresis and immunological assays are required for diagnosis.

The most common inherited metabolic liver disease in children,[65] alpha$_1$-antitrypsin deficiency usually presents as "neonatal hepatitis syndrome," characterized by conjugated hyperbilirubinemia and elevated serum aminotransferases. Failure to thrive and hepatosplenomegaly may also occur. Approximately two thirds of the children with early symptoms recover.[66] At the present time, liver transplantation is the only therapy for patients with severe liver disease. The anesthetic considerations for these children are the same as for children with other types of liver disease. No agents or techniques are known to be contraindicated.

SUMMARY

Until recent years, many of the inborn errors of metabolism were considered untreatable. At present, it is possible only to speculate about the eventual role of gene replacement therapy.

However, the place of bone marrow and liver transplantation in treating children with several of these disorders is well established. It may be anticipated that many of the children who undergo successful transplantation will later come to operation for procedures commonly performed in "healthy" children. Thus, the anesthesiologist must be familiar with the sources of information regarding specific anesthetic implications of the genetic metabolic diseases.

REFERENCES

1. Garrod AE: Inborn Errors of Metabolism. 2nd ed. London, Oxford University Press, 1923.
2. Beaudet AL, Scriver CR, Sly WS, et al: Genetics and biochemistry of variant human phenotypes. *In* Scriver CR, Beaudet AL, Sly WS, Valle D (Eds.): The Metabolic Basis of Inherited Disease. 6th ed. New York, McGraw-Hill, 1989.
3. Pauling L, Itano HA, Singer SJ, Wells IC: Sickle cell anemia: A molecular disease. Science *110*:543, 1949.
4. Diseases of the genome—an interview with Victor A. McKusick, MD. JAMA *252*:1041, 1984.
5. Sandhoff K, Conzelmann E, Neufeld EF, et al: The G_{M2} gangliosidoses. *In* Scriver CR, Beaudet AL, Sly WS, Valle D (Eds.): The Metabolic Basis of Inherited Disease. 6th ed. New York, McGraw-Hill, 1989.
6. Scriver CR, Kaufman S, Woo SLC: The hyperphenylalaninemias. *In* Scriver CR, Beaudet AL, Sly WS, Valle D (Eds.): The Metabolic Basis of Inherited Disease. 6th ed. New York, McGraw-Hill, 1989.
7. Doherty LB, Rohr FJ, Levy HL: Detection of phenylketonuria in the very early newborn blood specimen. Pediatrics *87*:240, 1991.
8. Thompson GN, Butt WW, Shann FA, et al: Continuous venovenous hemofiltration in the management of acute decompensation in inborn errors of metabolism. J Pediatr *118*:879, 1991.
9. Whitington PF, Balistreri WF: Liver transplantation in pediatrics: Indications, contraindications, and pretransplant management. J Pediatr *118*:169, 1991.
10. Cohen A, O'Grady J, Mowat A, Williams R. Liver transplantation for metabolic disorders. Baillieres Clin Gastroenterol *3*:767, 1989.
11. Hers H-G, van Hoof F, de Barsy T: Glycogen storage diseases. *In* Scriver CR, Beaudet AL, Sly WS, Valle D (Eds.): The Metabolic Basis of Inherited Disease. 6th ed. New York, McGraw-Hill, 1989.
12. Malatack JJ, Finegold DN, Iwaatsuki S, et al: Liver transplantation in type I glycogen storage disease. Lancet *1*:1073, 1983.
13. Cox JM: Anesthesia and glycogen-storage disease. Anesthesiology *29*:1221, 1968.
14. Ellis FR: Inherited muscular disease. Br J Anaesth *52*:153, 1980.
15. McFarlane HJ, Soni N: Pompe's disease and anesthesia. Anaesthesia *41*:1219, 1986.
16. Selby R, Starzl TE, Yunis E, et al: Liver transplantation for type IV glycogen storage disease. N Engl J Med *324*:39, 1991.
17. Grunfeld JP, Ganeval D, Chanard J, et al: Acute renal failure in McArdle's disease. N Engl J Med *286*:1237, 1972.
18. Coleman P: McArdle's disease: Problems of anaesthetic management for Caesarean section. Anaesthesia *39*:784, 1984.
19. Edelstein G, Hirschman CA: Hyperthermia and ketoacidosis during anesthesia in a child with glycogen-storage disease. Anesthesiology *52*:90, 1980.
20. Hashimoto Y, Watanabe H, Satou M: Anesthetic management of a patient with hereditary fructose-1,6-diphosphatase deficiency. Anesth Analg *47*:503, 1978.
21. Steward DJ: Manual of Pediatric Anesthesia. 3rd ed. New York, Churchill Livingstone, 1990, Appendix I: Anesthetic implications of syndromes and unusual disorders.
22. Danner DJ, Elsas LJ: Disorders of branched chain amino acid and keto acid metabolism. *In* Scriver CR, Beaudet AL, Sly WS, Valle D (Eds.): The Metabolic Basis of Inherited Disease. 6th ed. New York, McGraw-Hill, 1989.
23. Berry GT, Heindenreich R, Kaplan P, et al: Branched-chain amino acid–free parenteral nutrition in the treatment of acute metabolic decompensation in patients with maple syrup urine disease. N Engl J Med *324*:175, 1991.
24. Delaney A, Gal TJ: Hazards of anesthesia and operation in maple-syrup urine disease. Anesthesiology *44*:83, 1976.
25. Mudd SH, Levy HL, Skovby F: Disorders of transsulfuration. *In* Scriver CR, Beaudet AL, Sly WS, Valle D (Eds.): The Metabolic Basis of Inherited Disease. 6th ed. New York, McGraw-Hill, 1989.
26. Parris WCV, Quimby CW: Anesthetic considerations for the patient with homocystinuria. Anesth Analg *61*:708, 1982.
27. Robinson BH: Lactic acidemia. *In* Scriver CR, Beaudet AL, Sly WS, Valle D (Eds.): The Metabolic Basis of Inherited Disease. 6th ed. New York, McGrawHill, 1989.
28. Roe CR, Coates PM: Acyl-CoA dehydrogenase deficiencies. *In* Scriver CR, Beaudet AL, Sly WS, Valle D (Eds.): The Metabolic Basis of Inherited Disease. 6th ed. New York, McGraw-Hill, 1989.
29. Katsuya H, Misumi M, Ohtani Y, Milke T: Postanesthetic acute renal failure due to carnitine palymityl transferase deficiency. Anesthesiology *68*:945, 1988.
30. Beilin B, Shulman D, Schiffman Y: Anaesthesia in myopathy of carnitine deficiency. Anaesthesia *41*:92, 1986.
31. Gibbs JM: A case of rhabdomyolysis associated with suxamethonium. Anaesth Intens Care *6*:141, 1978.
32. Mahley RW, Weisgraber KH, Innerarity TL, Rall SC: Genetic defects in lipoprotein metabolism: Elevation of atherogenic lipoproteins caused by impaired catabolism. JAMA *265*:78, 1991.
33. Brunzell JD: Familial lipoprotein lipase deficiency and other causes of the chylomicronemia syndrome. *In* Scriver CR, Beaudet AL, Sly WS, Valle D (Eds.): The Metabolic Basis of Inherited Disease. 6th ed. New York, McGraw-Hill, 1989.
34. Baines D, Keneally J: Anaesthetic implications of the mucopolysaccharidoses: A fifteen-year experience in a children's hospital. Anaesth Intens Care *11*:198, 1983.
35. Brosius FC, Roberts WC: Coronary artery disease in the Hurler syndrome. Am J Cardiol *47*:649, 1981.
36. Renteria VG, Ferrans VJ, Roberts WC: The heart in the Hurler syndrome. Am J Cardiol *38*:487, 1976.
37. Perks WH, Cooper RA, Bradbury S, et al: Sleep apnea in Scheie's syndrome. Thorax *35*:85, 1980.
38. Hopkins R, Watson JA, Jones JH, et al: Two cases of Hunter's syndrome—the anesthetic and operative difficulties in oral surgery. Br J Oral Surg *10*:286, 1973.
39. Kirkinshaw KJ: Anesthesia in a patient with an unstable neck—Morquio's syndrome. Anaesthesia *30*:46, 1975.

40. Lipson SJ: Dysplasia of the odontoid process in Morquio's syndrome causing quadriparesis. J Bone Joint Surg *59A*:340, 1977.
41. Pritzker MR, King RA, Kronenberg RS. Upper airway obstruction during head flexion in Morquio's disease. Am J Med *69*:467, 1980.
42. Jones AEP, Croley TF: Morquio syndrome and anesthesia. Anesthesiology *51*:261, 1979.
43. Kempthorne PM, Brown TCK: Anesthesia and the mucopolysaccharidoses: A survey of techniques and problems. Anaesth Intens Care *11*:203, 1983.
44. King DH, Jones RM, Barnett MB: Anaesthetic considerations and the mucopolysaccharidoses. Anaesthesia *39*:126, 1984.
45. Herrick IA, Rhone EJ: The mucopolysaccharidoses and anaesthesia: A report of clinical experience. Can J Anaesth *35*:67, 1988.
46. Theise ND, Ursell PC: Pulmonary hypertension and Gaucher's disease: Logical association or mere coincidence? Am J Pediatr Hematol Oncol *12*:74, 1990.
47. Carlson DU, Busuttil RW, Giudidi TA, Barranger JA. Orthotopic liver transplantation in the treatment of complications of Type I Gaucher disease. Transplantation *49*:1192, 1990.
48. Barranger JA, Ginns EI: Glucosylceramide lipidoses: Gaucher disease. *In* Scriver CR, Beaudet AL, Sly WS, Valle D (Eds.): The Metabolic Basis of Inherited Disease. 6th ed. New York, McGraw-Hill, 1989.
49. Mosnier JF, Degott C, Bedrossian J, et al: Occurrence of Fabry's disease in a renal allograft eleven years after successful renal transplantation. Transplantation *51*:759, 1991.
50. Larson LO, Wilkins RG: Anesthesia and the Lesch-Nyhan syndrome. Anesthesiology *63*:197, 1988.
51. Kaufman SS, Wood RP, Shaw BW, et al: Orthotopic liver transplantation for type I Crigler-Najjar syndrome. Hepatology *6*:1259, 1986.
52. Chiwdhury JR, Wolkoff AW, Arias IM: Hereditary jaundice and disorders of bilirubin metabolism. *In* Scriver CR, Beaudet AL, Sly WS, Valle D (Eds.): The Metabolic Basis of Inherited Disease. 6th ed. New York, McGraw-Hill, 1989.
53. Taylor S: Gilbert's syndrome as a cause of postoperative jaundice. Anaesthesia *39*:1222, 1984.
54. Hargreaves J: Anaesthesia and Gilbert's syndrome. Anaesthesia *40*:595, 1985.
55. Nishimura TG, Jackson SH, Cohen SN: Prolongation of morphine anaesthesia in a patient with Gilbert's disease: Report of a case. Can Anaesth Soc J *20*:709, 1973.
56. Dundee JW, McCleery WNC, McLouglin G: The hazard of thiopental anesthesia in porphyria. Anesth Analg *41*:567, 1962.
57. Mustajoki P, Heinonen J: General anesthesia in "inducible" porphyria. Anesthesiology *53*:15, 1980.
58. Rizk SF, Jacobson JH, Silvay G: Ketamine as an induction agent for acute intermittent porphyria. Anesthesiology *46*:305, 1977.
59. Bancroft GH, Lauria JI: Ketamine induction for cesarean section in a patient with acute intermittent porphyria and achrondroplastic dwarfism. Anesthesiology *59*:143, 1983.
60. Famewo CE: Induction of anaesthesia with etomidate in a patient with acute intermittent porphyria. Can Anaesth Soc J *32*:171, 1985.
61. Mitterschiffthaler G, Theiner A, Hetzel H, Fuith LC: Safe use of propofol in a patient with acute intermittent porphyria. Br J Anaesth *60*:109, 1988.
62. Cooper R: Anaesthesia for porphyria using propofol. Anaesthesia *43*:611, 1988.
63. McNeill MJ, Parikh RK, Moore MR: Propofol in acute porphyria. Anaesthesia *44*:532, 1989.
64. Haber JP, Malthe R: Propofol in acute porphyria. Anaesthesia *44*:932, 1989.
65. Ibarguen E, Gross CR, Savik K, Sharp HL: Liver disease in alpha-1-antitrypsin deficiency: Prognostic indicators. J Pediatr *117*:864, 1990.
66. Cox DW: Alpha$_1$-antitrypsin deficiency. *In* Scriver CR, Beaudet AL, Sly WS, Valle D (Eds.): The Metabolic Basis of Inherited Disease. 6th ed. New York, McGraw-Hill, 1989.

C H A P T E R

14 Orthopedic Diseases

HELEN M. HOLTBY, M.B., and JOHN E. S. RELTON, M.B.

Uncommon orthopedic problems in patients undergoing surgery include the congenital generalized diseases of bone and a variety of syndromes in which the bony manifestations are secondary to other major disorders.[1,2] The child with an uncommon orthopedic disease may present for surgical therapy to correct the primary disorder or a concomitant disease. Thus, a patient with radial aplasia may require closure of an atrial septal defect or repair of a cleft palate; or an achondroplastic child may present for tonsillectomy.

Table 14–1. INTERNATIONAL NOMENCLATURE FOR CONSTITUTIONAL DISEASES OF BONE

I. Osteochondrodysplasias
   a. Defects of growth of tubular bones and/or spine
      i. Identifiable at birth, e.g., achondroplasia, asphyxiating thoracic dystrophy, chondrodysplasia punctata
      ii. Identifiable in later life, e.g., spondylometaphyseal dysplasia (McKusick)
   b. Disorganized development of cartilage and fibrous components, e.g., cherubism, neurofibromatosis
   c. Abnormalities of density of cortical diaphyseal structure and/or metaphyseal modeling; e.g., osteogenesis imperfecta, osteopetrosis
II. Dysostoses: malformation of individual bones singly or in combination
   a. Dysostoses with cranial and facial involvement
   b. Dysostoses with predominantly axial involvement
   c. Dysostoses with predominant involvement of extremities
III. Idiopathic osteolyses
IV. Chromosomal aberrations
V. Primary metabolic abnormalities
   a. Calcium and/or phosphorus
   b. Complex carbohydrates
   c. Lipids
   d. Nucleic acids
   e. Amino acids
   f. Metals

There are also many acquired bone diseases of significance to anesthesiologists, such as juvenile rheumatoid arthritis, systemic lupus erythematosus, and the rarer forms of collagen vascular disease.[3] These are dealt with elsewhere in this volume.

The purposes of this chapter are to outline some of these rarer problems in orthopedic disease, to simplify the classification, and to make recommendations regarding management. There are few references in the literature concerning anesthetic management of specific syndromes,[4,5] but those that are available are listed, together with the surgical reports of management.

It must also be remembered that many children with orthopedic disease, particularly those with congenital disease, have had repeated hospitalization with its attendant psychological problems. They often undergo repeated surgical procedures and have to cope with significant disability in their daily lives.

GENERALIZED CONSTITUTIONAL DISEASES OF BONE AND CARTILAGE

The classification of generalized diseases of bone and cartilage is undergoing constant review and the nomenclature is confusing.[1,2] It includes a heterogeneous group of disorders whose pathogenesis in many cases remains unknown.

Table 14–1 shows an abbreviated form of the International Nomenclature for Constitutional Diseases of Bone first proposed in 1970,[3,6] revised in 1977,[7] and revised again in 1986.[8] The classification is based as far as possible on the pathophysiology of the various disorders as demonstrated radiologically; however, there remain many synonyms and eponyms, which add to the difficulties in reviewing the literature. Even within the classification there is great heterogeneity in the various syndromes, especially among the osteochondrodysplasias.

This section will review some of the more common syndromes and outline the problems that may face the pediatric anesthesiologist in dealing with children with orthopedic disease. General guidelines in dealing with the rarer forms also will be discussed.

OSTEOCHONDRODYSPLASIAS

The osteochondrodysplasias constitute three major groups (see Table 14–1) and include most of the numerous forms of dwarfism, of which over 100 have thus far been described. It should be noted that the term *dwarf* refers to those with disproportionate short stature and not those with growth retardation. Many of these conditions are exceptionally rare, with only one or two cases described. Even the most common form, achondroplasia, has an incidence of only 150 per million live births.[9] The other significant group of patients with dwarfism is children with metabolic abnormalities. The most important of these are the disorders of complex carbohydrate metabolism, and these are discussed in Chapter 13.

The first group, the chondrodystrophies, has been further divided into forms identifiable at birth and those identified in later life. Some of the syndromes identifiable at birth are lethal, either in utero or in the early neonatal period, and are mainly of interest to geneticists. The commonest cause of death is respiratory insufficiency arising from chest wall or tracheobronchial anomalies. However, there are occasional reports of survivors into childhood in some of these syndromes.[10, 11] Those forms of dwarfism in which survival into childhood is the exception include achondrogenesis, thanatophoric dwarfism, and the three forms of short rib syndrome.

ACHONDROPLASIA

This is the most common chondrodystrophy, with an incidence of 150 per million live births.[8, 11, 12] It is readily recognizable at birth by the classic clinical features of rhizomelic (proximal) shortening of the limbs, a relatively long trunk, a large head with frontal bossing, depression of the nasal bridge, and a relatively prominent mandible. Characteristically, the hands are tridentate, short, and broad. Achondroplasia is inherited as an autosomal dominant with little clinical variability. Over 80 percent of achondroplastic patients have no family history of the deformity and are considered new mutations.[12] The disorder may be associated with increased paternal age.

The clinical course of achondroplasia is characterized by respiratory, neurological, back, and lower limb problems. The evaluation of the separate and combined effects of neurological and respiratory impairment can be very difficult.[13, 14] Respiratory difficulties (obstructive sleep apnea, central apnea, hypoxia, cyanosis, or tachypnea) may arise as a manifestation of spinal cord compression or as a result of hypotonia, which is common in achondroplastic children.[15] Craniofacial anomalies, which predispose to upper airway obstruction, and thoracic dysplasia, which results in restrictive lung disease, also can occur. The problem of thoracic dysplasia is confined to children with achondroplasia. Obstructive sleep apnea is more common than central apnea.[15] A potential for tracheobronchial compression as a result of bony abnormality of the thorax also exists.[16, 17]

The neurological problems in achondroplasia take two basic forms. The first, hydrocephalus, has an uncertain incidence and an equally uncertain etiology. Megalencephaly is a usual finding: mildly dilated ventricles are very common and may be universal.[18] However, only a small proportion of patients develop hydrocephalus.[19] True hydrocephalus must be suspected if the head growth ceases to parallel the normal growth curve, albeit at above the 97th percentile. There are two postulated mechanisms for the development of hydrocephalus. Firstly, it may arise from stenosis of the foramen magnum secondary to occipital hypertrophy. Secondly, it has recently been reaffirmed that cerebral venous hypertension may also play a role.[20] This venous hypertension is reportedly caused by obstruction of the sigmoid sinus at the level of the jugular foramen. In two patients a further pressure gradient was found at the thoracic inlet. Support for this hypothesis is provided by one report of definitive operation (a venovenous bypass) that resulted in relief of the hydrocephalus.[21] It has also been suggested that the standard curves for head size in achondroplastic patients may be misleading as these were developed without reference to ventricular size and thus could include a population with undiagnosed hydrocephalus.[20] Whereas the role of foramen magnum stenosis in the development of hydrocephalus remains a topic for debate, its impact on the cervical cord is tangible.

The signs of cord compression may be subtle or overt. They consist of respiratory difficulties, cyanosis after crying, poor head control, and quadriparesis. The deep tendon reflexes may remain normal.[22, 23] Decompression by means of a suboccipital craniectomy is the treatment of choice. Failure to recognize spinal cord compression may be the cause of the high mortality in infant achondroplastic patients.[24]

The spine is also affected by abnormalities in the cervical region (odontoid hypoplasia and occipitalization of C1), which can compound the problem of cord compression. Farther down there is an abnormal configuration of the spinal canal, which tapers from top to bottom (in contrast to the normal taper from bottom to top). Thus the lumbar spinal cord occupies the entire canal in the lumbar spine. The characteristic lumbar lordosis, which may be accompanied by compensatory kyphoscoliosis, does not usually require surgical correction.[25]

The combination of a narrow spinal canal and bony abnormality may result in a neurological deficit in the lower limbs,[26] but this is extremely rare in the pediatric population.[27]

Anesthetic Implications. Reports of the anesthetic management of achondroplastic patients describe a number of actual and potential problems.[28–35] Two factors make achondroplasia the most likely syndrome to be encountered by the anesthesiologist. The first is obviously its prevalence and the second is that there are increasing numbers of reports of limb-lengthening techniques, such as those described by Ilizarov,[36] which often require several anesthetics.

The first considerations are of airway assessment and respiratory function. In view of the subtle changes in respiratory control that may herald cervicomedullary compression, a careful history must be taken and any positive findings followed up by additional investigation of both the neurological and respiratory systems. This may involve more sophisticated tests, such as pulmonary function studies (when the age and cooperation of the child permits), or CT and MRI studies as indicated. It is also important to assess the airway with reference to the ease of intubation. Most studies suggest that a majority of achondroplastic patients are easy to intubate. However, there is one case report of impossible direct laryngoscopy resulting from limitation of neck movement.[30] The cervical spine should be assessed in active flexion and extension for signs of instability. Extremes of motion of the neck must be avoided in the anesthetized patient. It has been suggested that weight may be the best guide for selecting the appropriate size of endotracheal tube, but the prudent approach is to have a variety of tube sizes available. In the child with significant thoracic deformity from either a small rib cage or severe kyphoscoliosis, the cardiovascular system should be evaluated for signs of pulmonary hypertension and cor pulmonale, although this is not common in early childhood. In view of the potential for both airway obstruction and inadequate ventilation when breathing spontaneously under anesthesia, the use of controlled ventilation is recommended. There are no reports regarding the use of laryngeal mask airways in achondroplasia, but this may well prove especially useful if there are difficulties with direct laryngoscopy.

Another consideration is the use of conduction anesthesia. This is most frequently used as an adjunct to general anesthesia in children.

Opinion is divided in case reports regarding the advisability of performing major regional blocks.[18, 19, 28, 35] However, lower limb neurological problems are rare in children (in contrast to cervical problems), and there have been no reports of serious complications. Technical difficulties with lumbar puncture or lumbar epidural catheter placement are common,[31, 32] as might be expected from the severe lumbar lordosis, although it is by no means impossible even using a midline approach. The greatest difficulty arises from the unpredictable level of blockade from a given dose of local anesthetic and a tendency for asymmetric levels of nerve block.[31] The use of a catheter and divided doses is recommended. There are no reports of the use of caudal anaesthesia, but the same difficulties regarding dose and level of nerve block may be expected. The use of caudal or epidural anesthesia for postoperative pain control in children has gained wide acceptance and may be particularly beneficial in limb-lengthening procedures that involve multiple osteotomies resulting in considerable postoperative pain.

Asphyxiating Thoracic Dystrophy (Jeune's Syndrome)

This disease was first described by Jeune in 1954. It is classified as a nonlethal form of dwarfism, although it has a 75 percent mortality in early life. The genetic pattern of this disorder is unclear, but it is probably autosomal recessive.[6, 11] Some of the difficulty arises because of the variety of clinical manifestations. There are 106 reported cases in the literature, of which 45 percent occur in siblings and 7 percent in the children of consanguineous unions.[37] A link may exist between it and the Ellis–van Creveld syndrome (chondroectodermal dysplasia),[38, 39] but there are many differences and it seems likely that they are separate entities.

The more severely affected infants have a stiff thorax that is small in all dimensions. The major features of the syndrome are thoracic abnormalities and renal dysfunction. Thoracic problems tend to dominate the case reports in part because renal failure tends to develop later in life, and only those children with less severe thoracic deformity survive long enough to acquire it. The typical chest wall deformity consists of a short, stiff thorax, with very short, stubby ribs and a prominent rib rosary in the midaxillary line. The ribs are horizontal and the clavicles high.

The hands and feet are short and broad, and there may be postaxial polydactyly. Limb shortening is variable.

This disease is of interest because it has been noted that respiratory function tends to improve with age,[40] and so attempts have been made to support these infants until they grow sufficiently.[37, 41, 42] Enlargement of the thorax by surgical intervention may increase lung compliance, which, in combination with long-term ventilatory support, may provide substantial improvement. In some cases it has been observed that the underlying lung appeared normal. However, pulmonary hypoplasia, cysts, and other abnormalities have been reported.[43]

Associated problems include pulmonary hypertension and occasional cardiac defects. Renal disease with proteinuria, hypertension, and uremia[44] is a significant cause of death in children surviving infancy. Hepatic fibrosis without portal hypertension, bile stasis, or involvement of liver parenchyma has been reported in late survivors.[37] Myocardial dysfunction may also occur, but it is not known whether this is a primary problem or arises as a result of chronic, severe respiratory impairment.

Anesthetic Implications. Serious difficulty may be encountered in ventilating these infants preoperatively and intraoperatively. There is a significant incidence of barotrauma.

Hypoxia and hypercapnia occur frequently even in children whose resting blood gases are relatively normal. The mechanical disadvantage of a horizontal, narrow rib cage causes asynchronous movements of the rib cage and abdominal muscles during crying, resulting in hypoxic spells. Pulmonary hypertension may contribute to an early demise.

The larynx has been noted to be small in both the children with the syndrome and their mothers.[42] One case is reported of management by long-term nasotracheal intubation (years) with surprisingly few complications.[41] In this case, no mention was made of endotracheal tube size. In a further series, seven children with Jeune's syndrome were anesthetized for a variety of procedures, notably bronchoscopy, thoracoplasty, and renal transplantation. The only intraoperative complication reported was one episode of laryngospasm that was followed by pneumothorax. Three of the four patients who underwent thoracoplasty required prolonged (months to years) postoperative ventilation. At least two of the children had tracheostomies, but endotracheal tube sizes were not mentioned in any of the cases.

Thus there are a number of special preoperative considerations for these patients. Respiratory function should be carefully assessed and the possibility of pulmonary hypertension considered. Despite the possibility of a small larynx and the risk of barotrauma, the likelihood of significant deterioration in ventilatory mechanics under general anesthesia makes a mask anesthetic with spontaneous ventilation inappropriate except for the briefest of cases.

Renal function should be checked, and all the implications of end-stage renal disease may apply. The difficulties of renal transplantation in small children are compounded by the fact that these children are small even before they develop growth retardation due to renal failure.

Chondroectodermal Dysplasia (Ellis–van Creveld Syndrome)

This disorder has features in common with asphyxiating thoracic dystrophy but is thought to be a separate entity. It was first described in 1940[45] and is inherited as an autosomal recessive. The largest incidence of the syndrome occurs in the Amish people of Lancaster County, Pennsylvania,[46] although over 40 other cases have been reported worldwide.

The skeletal abnormalities consist of polydactyly, mesomelic dwarfism, and a long narrow thorax; there are also abnormalities of the nails and teeth. Respiratory distress is common in the newborn period and is related to absence of cartilage in the tracheobronchial tree, which tends therefore to collapse and cause tension lobar emphysema.[47] Cardiac anomalies have been reported to affect as many as 60 percent of patients, but this may represent an overestimate[46] insofar as individuals with cardiac symptoms are more likely to seek medical attention. The most common abnormalities are atrial and ventricular septal defects, often with complete absence of the septum. Cleft mitral valve may also occur. Dental anomalies are common, and erupted teeth may be present at birth. Cleft lip and palate also can occur.

Anesthetic Implications. There are no reports of anesthetic experience with these children, and indeed the Amish people treated polydactyly by amputation, using string binding without benefit of surgeon or anesthesiologist!

A major consideration is the cardiorespiratory status. Physical examination may reveal significant heart disease preoperatively, which should be fully assessed so that antibiotic prophylaxis can be given and management plans formulated. There is a particular problem of airway collapse and emphysema in neonates and infants, and they should not be allowed to breathe spontaneously. Conversely, high airway pressures and short expiratory times during positive-pressure ventilation should be avoided because of barotrauma and gas trapping. Nitrous oxide should be avoided if emphysema is present.

CHONDRODYSPLASIA PUNCTATA

Chondrodysplasia punctata describes a heterogeneous group of disorders associated with radiographic stippling of the epiphyses and extraepiphyseal cartilage. There are several synonyms, eponyms (chondrodystrophia calcificans congenita, Conradi's disease, stippled epiphyses), and distinct genetic entities. There are probably at least three distinct forms.[8]

Over 100 cases have been described in the literature, revealing a variety of manifestations of multisystem involvement. The most constant characteristics include short stature, typical facies with hypertelorism, saddle nose, frontal bossing, high arched palate, micrognathia, short neck, and tracheal stenosis.[48] Additional findings that are less constant include renal anomalies, congenital heart disease,[49] and neurological abnormalities. In one study, all patients examined had major abnormalities of the central nervous system including Dandy-Walker malformation of the fourth ventricle.[50] Atlantoaxial instability may also occur as a result of odontoid hypoplasia.[51]

Anesthetic Implications. The facial abnormalities and tracheal stenosis make difficulty with the airway a distinct possibility. The presence of atlantoaxial instability demands extreme care at intubation.

Renal function should be checked preoperatively and any evidence of renal impairment noted and investigated. Examination may reveal significant cardiac anomalies, and antibiotic prophylaxis must be used when indicated. Hydrocephalus may be present with the concomitant danger of coning of the medulla during anesthesia.

OSTEOGENESIS IMPERFECTA

This is a connective tissue disorder primarily affecting bone. The earliest known case was probably that of Ivar the Boneless in the 9th century, and there are descriptions dating from the 16th century.[2, 52]

The etiology of the disorder is complex. Two basic types of inheritance exist (autosomal dominant or autosomal recessive), but there is considerable variation in clinical manifestation. The dominant forms of the disease tend to present later with fewer fractures. These would correspond to osteogenesis imperfecta tarda levis in the older literature but are now classified as Type I and Type IV osteogenesis imperfecta. Type II and Type III osteogenesis imperfecta are the more severe forms of the disease and show recessive inheritance. Type II corresponds to osteogenesis imperfecta congenita and is the most lethal form of the disease.

There is no consensus regarding its precise pathophysiology.[49] The basic defect appears to involve the synthesis of collagen. There is also evidence that there is some disturbance of high-energy phosphate metabolism, because there are abnormalities in platelet aggregation, increased oxygen consumption, evidence of generally elevated metabolic rates, and raised serum thyroxine levels.[54]

The classic triad of blue sclera, multiple fractures, and deafness is not constant,[53] with the latter being present in only about 10 percent of cases.

Type II osteogenesis imperfecta has an incidence of 1 in 20,000 to 1 in 60,000 live births. It may be diagnosed prenatally by means of ultrasound examination. At birth it may present as a stillbirth either from fractures in utero or from intracerebral hemorrhage due to the trauma of delivery on an unossified and fragile skull. If the infant survives, respiratory failure from severe thoracic involvement is a common cause of death in the neonatal period. This is also the commonest cause of death in Type III osteogenesis imperfecta, with few patients achieving adulthood.

Trivial trauma such as changing a diaper or the application of a blood pressure cuff may result in transverse subperiosteal fractures. Over time, gross deformity occurs, particularly in the long bones, due to repeated fractures that are painful and debilitating.

Other clinical findings are dentinogenesis imperfecta (discolored and brittle teeth), ligamentous laxity, scoliosis, cardiovascular anomalies, and an ill-defined bleeding diathesis that is probably secondary to platelet dysfunction.

Scoliosis is a very common finding and may arise in the cervical or thoracic spine. It is particularly difficult to treat.[55] However, there are case reports of successful surgical management.[53, 55]

The cardiovascular abnormalities include aortic and mitral regurgitation as a result of dilatation of the valvular annulus, abnormalities of the chordae tendineae, and cystic medial necrosis of the aorta.[56]

Management. The medical management of osteogenesis imperfecta has been disappointing. Calcitonin, anabolic steroids, and sodium fluoride do not provide any real benefit.

The surgical management has usually been directed toward correcting any deformity, particularly in the lower limbs, which tend to bear the brunt of the disorder. Ambulation is the key aim. The most commonly performed procedures are intramedullary nailing of the femur and Sofield's osteotomies with pin fixation[57] to correct tibial deformity. Harrington's instrumentations[41] and modified Dwyer's procedures have been performed to correct scoliosis.

Anesthetic Implications. The preoperative assessment of these children includes a review of the respiratory and cardiovascular systems, with particular emphasisis on the degree of chest wall deformity, which determines the severity of restrictive lung disease and subsequent cardiovascular problems. There is no correlation between the severity of the bone disease and the presence of valvular disease.[58] There are no reports of children with valvular disease of sufficient severity to require operation. A careful assessment of the airway and neck mobility also should be made. It is important to document old and new fractures preoperatively and check for fractures postoperatively. Finally, it should be ascertained whether or not the child has normal hearing. If not, the child should come to the operating room with a hearing aid in place. Deafness makes communication difficult. Repeated hospitalizations and chronic pain add psychological problems to the practical difficulties. These children have usually had several visits to the operating room. Recent fractures, even if undisplaced, are painful and so moving from bed to stretcher and then to the operating room table adds to the distress.

Once in the operating room, children with severe osteogenesis imperfecta constitute a major problem, since monitoring, positioning, establishment of intravenous access, and control of the airway all place them at risk of further fractures. The history of the individual child may be of benefit when considering the risk-benefit ratios of invasive monitoring rather than a blood pressure cuff, or the use of a tourniquet to provide good operating conditions for the surgeon. There are patients in whom the propensity for fractures is such that the use of a sphygmomanometer or a tourniquet is contraindicated; every aspect of their anesthetic has to be carefully reappraised.

Anesthesia may be induced by mask, taking particular care with fragile teeth and facial bones. This allows optimal conditions for establishing intravenous access without the use of a tourniquet. An arterial line may be placed (without extension of the wrist) for blood pressure measurement. Succinylcholine is contraindicated in these severely affected patients owing to the risk of fasciculation-induced fractures. Great care must be taken during laryngoscopy and intubation. The use of a mouth guard to protect the teeth is recommended. Maintenance of anesthesia may involve the use of intravenous or inhalational agents. There is one case report of likely malignant hyperthermia in a patient with osteogenesis imperfecta (no muscle biopsy was performed),[59] but generally the rises in temperature seen in these patients are thought to be part of the metabolic process of the disease.[60] The absence of respiratory acidosis is a significant factor in distinguishing between hyperthermia due to osteogenesis imperfecta and a true malignant hyperthermic reaction. However, it should be noted that the fever in patients with osteogenesis imperfecta may be severe and accompanied by extreme tachycardia and metabolic acidosis.[61] Muscle rigidity and masseter spasm are absent. It is possible that there is some association between the two disorders, but they are both so rare that, as yet, there is insufficient experience to suggest that patients with osteogenesis imperfecta are susceptible to malignant hyperthermia.

If there is severe chest wall deformity, then ventilation should be controlled. The anesthetic technique should also be modified in the presence of significant heart disease. Bleeding may be a particular problem in scoliosis operation, and excessive bleeding has also been reported following cardiopulmonary bypass. This is thought to be due to platelet abnormalities.

One report of anesthetic experience describes

the satisfactory use of intramuscular ketamine for repeated procedures on a 4-year-old child with severe osteogenesis imperfecta.[64] Other reports of open heart surgery on patients with osteogenesis imperfecta make no comment on the anesthesia but do describe problems with bleeding following cardiopulmonary bypass.[56, 63, 64]

OSTEOPETROSIS (ALBERS-SCHÖNBERG DISEASE)

Albers-Schönberg disease may present either in an autosomal recessive form, which usually results in death in infancy, or in an autosomal dominant form, which does not appear until early adulthood.

The usual presentation of the infantile type is a failure to thrive in the first few months of life. Frequently, petechiae or ecchymoses are seen, and the infant is pale and unwell. Megalencephaly or true hydrocephalus may be present. Abnormal eye movements are often seen, and examination may reveal optic atrophy. Variable degrees of hepatosplenomegaly occur.[3, 11, 49]

Radiological examination reveals a generalized skeletal density with disturbed mineralization at the growth plates similar to rickets. There is profound anemia, thrombocytopenia, and neutropenia. Serum calcium is frequently low despite an increase in calcium uptake from the gut.

Anesthetic Implications. It is important to assess the airway preoperatively, as osteomyelitis of the jaw is reported to occur frequently in osteopetrosis.[65] It may limit mouth opening, either as a result of trismus or joint destruction. A careful examination for sepsis should also be made since neutropenia renders the child more vulnerable to infection but less likely to have obvious signs or symptoms. A full blood count should be performed and the platelet count checked. If the proposed operation presents any risk of significant bleeding, then the platelet count should be at least 50,000/μL. Chronic compensated anemia may not need preoperative correction but will obviously reduce the allowable blood loss before transfusion.

The ionized calcium level should also be checked preoperatively since hypocalcemia predisposes the patient to arrhythmias, seizures, and inadequate reversal of neuromuscular blockade. Care must be taken when intubating and positioning patients with osteopetrosis because the bones are brittle and, despite their density, fracture easily.

GENERAL GUIDELINES FOR THE MANAGEMENT OF OSTEOCHONDRODYSPLASIAS

Since there are so many different syndromes classified under the general title of osteochondrodystrophies and many of them are rare, it seems useful to have a general plan for the preoperative assessment and intraoperative management of any patient with dwarfism.[66, 67] The Herculean task of remembering all the different syndromes, their synonyms, and eponyms is made even more difficult by the fact that many of the names have changed over time. It must also be realized that there are often single case reports (or no case reports) of anesthetic experience and that a good outcome in one particular instance is no guarantee of future success.

A number of problems are common to many of the dwarfing syndromes:

Odontoid Hypoplasia and/or Atlantoaxial Instability.[27, 66–70] Preoperatively, patients with these problems should have clinical and radiological examination of the cervical spine whenever possible, and great care should be taken when intubating them.

It should be remembered that the classic pyramidal tract signs and symptoms of cord compression are often not seen in infants and children. Suspicions should be raised by a history of cyanosis after crying or feeding, respiratory difficulties, poor head control, fatigue, and decreased exercise tolerance, all of which may appear before any pyramidal tract signs are detected.[19, 22, 68] Somatosensory evoked potentials may also be useful in evaluating spinal cord function.[13]

Surgical fusion of the cervical vertebrae is recommended for these patients. It may also be necessary in some patients (notably achondroplastics) to enlarge the foramen magnum.[71] The anesthetic considerations for these procedures include the problems of airway management with unstable cervical spines and the difficulties in positioning patients to provide adequate operating conditions. The use of the fiberoptic bronchoscope has alleviated some of the problems with intubation, especially with the improvement in resolution of the visual field.[72] In a review of the anesthetic experience of craniectomy for foramen magnum stenosis, all the major complications, with a single exception, occurred in patients operated on in the sitting position.[33] They include high spinal cord infarction, brachial plexus palsy, and macroglossia. A 60 percent incidence of venous air embolism was not included in the complications. In patients in the prone position there was one episode of air embolus, one accidental extubation, and one case in which the procedure was abandoned because of excessive bleeding (65 ml/kg). Thus, it would seem that there is little to recommend the sitting position in children requiring craniocervical surgical therapy.

The syndromes in which craniocervical problems are most commonly seen are (1) achondroplasia, (2) metatropic dysplasia, (3) diastrophic dysplasia (C2–C3 abnormalities), (4) chondrodysplasia punctata, (5) Kniest's syndrome, (6) spondyloepiphyseal dysplasia congenita, and (7) spondylometaphyseal dysplasia.

A majority of patients with abnormalities of the atlantoaxial joint are stable, though they may have limited neck mobility. Patients with quadriparesis may have overt or occult autonomic instability, rendering them susceptible to cardiac arrhythmias and acute changes in blood pressure. It may be difficult to wean such a patient from artificial ventilation.

Airway Problems. Many airway problems will be evident on examination of the child. Any individual with the problems described in the preceding paragraph must be approached with caution. A history of respiratory difficulties, especially sleep apnea or even severe snoring, should alert the anesthesiologist to the possibility of obstruction of the airway upon induction of anesthesia. This can often, though not invariably, be overcome with the use of an oropharyngeal airway and the use of gentle, positive end-expiratory pressure. The use of the laryngeal mask airway may be helpful under certain circumstances, and it has been used for awake intubation in one adult.[73] The techniques for management of the airway vary depending on both the patient and the proposed operation. A variety of methods have been described in adults and children.[72] The use of intravenous agents and the avoidance of the issue may be attractive, but vigilance is needed to ensure that the patient is maintaining a clear airway and adequate ventilation. This is often impossible in children with dwarfing syndromes because of the presence of tracheomalacia, bronchomalacia, chest wall anomalies, and restrictive lung disease.

The craniofacial abnormalities are dealt with separately (see Chapter 9), so the following list is far from exhaustive: mesomelic dysplasia, diastrophic dwarfism, Kniest's syndrome, spondyloepiphyseal dysplasia, metatropic dysplasia, chondrodysplasia punctata, camptomelic dysplasia, and osteogenesis imperfecta.

Thoracic Dystrophy. The asphyxiating thoracic dystrophy of Jeune is an obvious example of thoracic abnormality with short stature, but there are also a number of other syndromes in which the chest cavity is small and may also be noncompliant. Such patients may have problems with repeated chest infections, hypoxemia, increased work of breathing, and ultimately pulmonary vascular changes. Many die in the neonatal period. Conditions involving thoracic dystrophy include (1) asphyxiating thoracic dystrophy (Jeune), (2) metaphyseal chondrodysplasia (Jansen), (3) metaphyseal dwarfism, (4) achondroplasia, (5) Ellis–van Creveld syndrome, (6) lymphopenic agammaglobulinemia, (7) camptomelic dwarfism, and (8) Type II osteogenesis imperfecta.

Kyphoscoliosis. This occurs in a majority of dwarfing syndromes. In some cases, such as in achondroplasia, marked kyphosis and lordosis compound the structural problems of a small spinal canal, leading to neurological impairment. However, this is not common in the pediatric age group.

Cardiac Disease. Septal defects, patent ductus arteriosus, and other cardiac anomalies are associated with a number of dwarfing conditions: (1) Ellis–van Creveld syndrome, (2) Holt-Oram syndrome (described later), (3) metaphyseal chondrodysplasia, and (4) osteogenesis imperfecta. Pulmonary hypertension and cor pulmonale also may occur. The anesthetic management depends on the degree of physiological derangement. Antibiotic prophylaxis is indicated in patients undergoing operation when there is a risk of bacteremia.

Neurological Abnormalities. Macrocephaly and hydrocephalus are the commonest problems seen in children. Seizures also may occur. The combination of airway problems and hydrocephalus with intracranial hypertension presents a dilemma for the anesthesiologist.

Most dwarf children have normal intelligence. Motor delay is seen as a result of hypotonia in infancy. Psychosocial skills are often immature, in part due to the widely held perception that maturity is directly related to height.

Miscellaneous. Other problems to consider include renal dysfunction (Ellis–van Creveld) and bleeding diatheses (osteogenesis imperfecta). The risk of fractures and the possible difficulty in positioning the patient because of contractures also may arise (osteogenesis imperfecta and osteopetrosis). A careful preoperative assessment should reveal most of the significant problems and enable a plan of management to be formulated. One further consideration is that neither age nor weight[35] gives a reliable prediction of endotracheal tube size or length. No anesthetic drugs are contraindicated because of short stature per se, although airway problems or other complications may dictate a particular technique of management. A special effort should be made to treat children with short stature in an appropriate fashion for their age. This is particularly important in teenagers in whom the loss of autonomy associated with hospitalization is keenly felt. It then adds insult to injury to be treated like a member of the Munchkins.

DYSOSTOSES

The dysostoses are malformations of individual bones arising singly or in combination. The craniofacial dysostoses constitute a single group and are reviewed elsewhere (see Chapter 9). Several of these patients also exhibit axial involvement (for example, in Goldenhar's syndrome). Of the dysostoses with predominantly axial involvement, the Klippel-Feil syndrome is probably the most common. These disorders may present local problems (for example, intubation difficulties due to severely limited neck mobility) and systemic manifestations such as congenital heart disease and urinary tract abnormalities. Patients frequently require an operation for scoliosis arising from their structural vertebral abnormalities, particularly isolated hemivertebrae.

The dysostoses often present with predominant involvement of the extremities. The most commonly seen examples are syndactyly and polydactyly, which may be seen in combination with craniofacial or other abnormalities, as in Apert's syndrome or Carpenter's syndrome. Laryngeal abnormalities, particularly atresia, stenosis, or web, may occur.

The syndromes described next illustrate some of the potential problems that should be kept in mind in treating the child with a peripheral abnormality.

Radial Dysgenesis[74]

There are two types of radial dysgenesis. Either total absence or partial absence (usually of the distal portion) of the radius may occur, and the incidence of each type is about equal. Unilateral cases occur most frequently on the right side. The male:female ratio is about 3:2. This deformity is frequently associated with other defects, such as vascular and musculoskeletal abnormalities of the limb. It is rarely seen as an isolated defect (1 in 55,000 live births).

Radial and thumb aplasia may be associated with several chromosomal aberrations, notably trisomy 18 (1 in 6600 live births), chromosome 13q−, and trisomy 13. The combination of chromosomal abnormalities and radial dysgenesis usually implies multiple abnormalities, including congenital heart disease[75] and severe mental retardation. The life expectancy is usually less than 3 years. Two other syndromes with mental retardation and radial aplasia that may cause problems for the anesthesiologist, because of potential airway and intubation difficulties, are bird-headed dwarfism and Cornelia de Lange's syndrome. Varying degrees of mental retardation, microcephaly, and a characteristic facies occur in both these rare syndromes.

The association between craniofacial abnormalities and radial dysplasia is quite frequent. Some 7 percent of patients with radial aplasia have a cleft lip and palate. It is also seen in association with Treacher Collins syndrome, Goldenhar's syndrome, craniosynostosis, and abnormalities of the tracheobronchial tree, notably laryngeal atresia and laryngeal web.

Cardiac anomalies may also occur in two forms of heart-hand syndromes[76] (Holt-Oram syndrome and Lewis' upper limb cardiovascular syndrome). Holt-Oram syndrome is an autosomal dominant disorder with variable expressivity (usually worse in females) and consists of mild congenital heart disease (atrial septal defect in 70 percent of patients), combined with radial aplasia and abnormalities of the hand. Cardiac rhythm disturbances, both atrial and ventricular, are occasionally present, together with conduction defects. In Lewis' syndrome, which is also autosomal dominant, the cardiovascular anomalies are more variable but are usually nonfatal. There are multiple skeletal abnormalities of the upper limb.

Radial aplasia is seen with Fanconi's syndrome, which consists of pancytopenia with bone marrow hypoplasia, multiple congenital defects, and renal tubular acidosis usually secondary to cystinosis (see Chapter 7). Seventy percent of patients show abnormalities of the radius, 20 percent are mentally retarded, and a variable number have congenital heart disease and congenital hip dislocation. The pancytopenia does not usually become pronounced in childhood, although this is variable. Preoperative assessment of renal function, avoidance of renally excreted drugs, and correction of metabolic disturbances may be required. The pancytopenia may be severe enough to require reverse isolation and transfusion of blood components either preoperatively or intraoperatively.

A second hematological disorder associated with bilateral radial aplasia is the TAR syndrome (**t**hrombocytopenia, **a**bsent **r**adius), in which profound thrombocytopenia is seen in infancy. If at all possible, surgical therapy should be avoided in patients with the TAR syndrome until 1 year of age, by which time platelet counts usually have risen significantly. Episodic thrombocytopenia may be precipitated by minor illness or stress, and counts as low as 15,000 per ml are not unusual. This syndrome is autosomal recessive and has a high mortality (30 to 40 percent) in the first year of life as a result of intracranial hemorrhage.

Finally, radial aplasia is seen as part of the VATER association,[77] which is an unexplained grouping of abnormalities including *v*ertebral segmentation, congenital scoliosis, imperforate *a*nus, *t*racheo*e*sophageal fistula, *r*enal abnormalities, absent *r*adius, and congenital heart disease—most commonly *v*entricular septal defect. As the radial agenesis is the most obvious defect seen at birth, it should trigger a search for other anomalies. It has been noted that as the number of defects increases, so does the mortality.[78]

METABOLIC DISEASES OF BONE

A large number of metabolic disturbances, including the mucopolysaccharidoses, mucolipidoses, and disorders of glycogen synthesis and storage, show bony abnormalities as part of the disease process.[36] However, the orthopedic problems are rarely, if ever, of prime importance. Renal and endocrine disorders are also associated with derangements of calcium metabolism and abnormalities in bone growth, but, again, these rarely require the attention of the orthopedic surgeon and in any case are secondary to the ongoing primary disease process.

METABOLISM AND CONTROL OF CALCIUM[49, 79]

Bone is formed from calcium phosphate impregnated onto an organic matrix of collagen fibers and ground substance of glycosaminoglycans and glycoproteins. Calcium is the most prevalent electrolyte in the body, forming about 1.6 percent of the body weight in the adult.

The absolute and relative calcium content of the body increases rapidly from the seventh month in utero to adulthood. At 7 months, the calcium content of the fetus is 8 g, and this rises fourfold to some 30 g at term. It reaches 1100 g in the adult. About 99 percent of this calcium is fixed in the skeleton, with 1 percent remaining free as ionized calcium (0.4 percent) or bound to plasma proteins and chelating agents such as citrate (0.6 percent).

Calcium has many important functions; its primary importance (in bulk at least) is in the formation of ossified bone, providing a rigid framework for the body. However, it is also a critical factor in cellular membrane permeability and enzyme function throughout the body.

Calcium levels in the body are governed by intake, excretion, and mobilization of body stores, which can be modified by the hormonal influences of PTH (parathormone), calcitonin, and the active form of vitamin D. Calcium absorption is entirely from the gut and is modified by the activity of a transport protein whose synthesis is inhibited by renal insufficiency and decreased levels of vitamin D. Calcium is eliminated via the kidneys and the gut and to a limited extent through the skin.

Vitamin D is absorbed in the gut and transformed in the body to a number of active metabolites, of which the most significant is 1,25-dihydroxycholecalciferol. This is synthesized by the kidney from 25-hydroxycholecalciferol in response to decreased serum calcium levels. The effects of 1,25-dihydroxycholecalciferol are to increase calcium absorption from the gut, increase phosphate reabsorption in the kidney, and liberate calcium from bone. In turn, the conversion of vitamin D to its active form is regulated by PTH. The normal infant needs about 400 to 800 international units/day of vitamin D to prevent dietary rickets. Hypervitaminosis D (greater than 5000 units daily for several years) results in hypercalcemia with ectopic calcification and hypercalciuria with stone formation and renal damage. In children, the hypercalcemia may result in arrested growth with a permanent defect. Hypervitaminosis D during pregnancy may result in supravalvular aortic stenosis in the infant.

Parathormone is secreted by the parathyroid gland in response to a decrease in serum calcium. Its exact mechanism of action is unknown, but it increases the cell membrane permeability to calcium, increases levels of cyclic AMP, liberates calcium from bone by stimulation of the formation of osteoclasts, and increases tubular reabsorption of calcium while decreasing phosphate reabsorption. The net effect, therefore, is to increase serum calcium levels.

The third hormone involved in calcium homeostasis is calcitonin, discovered by Copp in 1962, which is secreted from the parafollicular cells of the thyroid gland. Hypercalcemia stimulates the secretion of calcitonin, which in turn affects direct inhibition of bone resorption. This occurs by a mechanism separate from the action of PTH that affects osteoclast and osteoblast activity.

Thus, many factors influence the maintenance of serum calcium levels within the normal range of 2.2 to 2.7 mmol/L. Derangements in this process lead to abnormalities of bone growth, disturbances of membrane and enzyme function, and renal impairment.

HYPOCALCEMIA

Hypocalcemia is very common in the newborn period, especially if the infant suffers fetal distress during delivery. The stores of calcium in the neonate are very small. A combination of respiratory alkalosis and elevated serum bicarbonate from overzealous resuscitation will tend to decrease further the serum ionized calcium level. Hypocalcemia also occurs with vitamin D deficiency states (whether absolute or relative) and in the various forms of hypoparathyroidism. DiGeorge's syndrome (thymic hypoplasia and hypoparathyroidism) is a rare cause of hypocalcemia. It is associated with major cardiovascular anomalies (transposition of the great vessels, tetralogy of Fallot, truncus arteriosus, and anomalous pulmonary veins) that are usually repaired in the neonatal period. A further complication associated with DiGeorge's syndrome is micrognathia. Tracheomalacia may arise as a result of a vascular ring.

Acute hypocalcemia decreases the threshold for neuronal excitability, leading to tetany and seizures. Prolongation of atrioventricular conduction in the heart gives rise to heart block. Delayed repolarization leads to a prolonged Q-T interval and ventricular dysrhythmias. Cardiac contractility and vasomotor tone are decreased, resulting in hypotension. Chronic hypocalcemia may be asymptomatic.

Anesthetic Implications. The use of potent inhalational anesthetics will increase the degree of hypotension and myocardial depression. Halothane may worsen the atrioventricular block and increase the risk of arrhythmia. The combination of hypocalcemia and cardiac dysfunction in DiGeorge's syndrome increases the risks of general anesthesia and precludes the use of inhalational agents. The tendency for tetanic contracture affects muscle of the vocal cords, so laryngospasm is a likely occurrence. This may be exacerbated by exogenous or endogenous catecholamines. Muscular weakness and difficulty in reversing neuromuscular blockade should be anticipated.

The commonest cause of hypocalcemia in the operating room is rapid or massive blood transfusion. This is a much more frequent problem in pediatrics than in adult practice and is in large part a function of size. Ten seconds may be the total time required to transfuse 25 ml of blood, and this may represent 10 percent of the circulating volume of a neonate.

Acute hypocalcemia is treated by the administration of intravenous calcium chloride or calcium gluconate. A continuous infusion may be needed, especially in neonates. The maintenance dose is 2 mmol/kg/24 hours. Hypokalemia and hypomagnesemia both exacerbate the effects of hypocalcemia and hinder efforts to restore normal calcium levels.

HYPERCALCEMIA

Hypercalcemia may arise as a result of hypervitaminosis D or hyperparathyroidism. Occasionally, patients (especially those with sarcoidosis) show hypersensitivity to vitamin D. Hypercalcemia may also be seen with lymphoproliferative disorders such as myeloma and is not uncommon during chemotherapy for malignant disease. Hyperparathyroidism commonly presents with a vague clinical picture and a history of renal calculi (see Chapter 7). Serum calcium levels of 3.5 mmol/L or higher are associated with abdominal pains, anorexia, nausea and vomiting, polyuria, dehydration, tachycardia, and hypertension (stones, bones, and abdominal groans!).

Treatment should be commenced immediately with rehydration of the patient, using a sodium-containing solution and administration of furosemide, 0.5 to 1.0 mg/kg every 4 to 6 hours to encourage the saline-induced calciuria. Potassium supplements will be required to avoid furosemide-induced hypokalemia. Steroids have been found to be useful in lymphoproliferative disorders and in the management of vitamin D intoxication. The cytotoxic antibiotic mithramycin has also been used and is extremely effective in the longer term but requires 48 to 72 hours to take effect. Calcium disodium edetate (EDTA) may also be used, but it is not recommended owing to the danger of an acute excessive fall in serum calcium.

Anesthetic Implications. Circulating volume must be restored, and an assessment of the degree of dehydration may be difficult owing to hypertension. Care must be taken with drug doses in the child with volume concentration. Potent inhalational agents may unmask a low circulating volume by causing vasodilatation.

Paralytic ileus may cause regurgitation and the possibility of aspiration at induction. A rapid sequence induction is therefore recommended.

METABOLISM AND CONTROL OF PHOSPHATE

Phosphate is an important constituent of high-energy bonds and modifies calcium concentrations in tissues. It is also a significant buffer of intracellular fluid and plays a primary role in renal excretion of hydrogen ions.

Phosphate is absorbed by an active process from the gut. This is modified by high concentrations of calcium or aluminum, which form insoluble salts and decrease absorption, and by vitamin D, which increases phosphate absorption. It is excreted via the kidneys. In children there is a net positive balance of phosphate, and the serum phosphate level is higher than in adults. This relative increase in phosphate increases the affinity of hemoglobin for oxygen, and a hypothesis has been proposed that this explains the physiological anemia of childhood.[80] Calcium and phosphate levels in blood are inversely related. A reduction in plasma phosphate levels permits increases in calcium levels and inhibits deposition of more bone salt. Conversely, elevated plasma phosphate levels facilitate the effects of calcitonin.

RICKETS

Rickets is a disorder of growing bone characterized by a decrease in bone anabolism and minimal mineralization of the new bone. The four principal causes of rickets are vitamin D deficiency, renal tubular insufficiency, chronic renal failure, and hypophosphatasia.

Simple deficiency of vitamin D is well recognized but still remains relatively frequent (compared, for example, with scurvy). Premature infants are particularly at risk because of diminished stores. The major concerns in anesthetizing such infants relate to their poor dentition and their general debility. They may present with muscular hypotonia, a hypochromic anemia, and other deficiency states. If vitamin D deficiency remains untreated, kyphoscoliosis may eventually develop. The serum calcium level is usually normal, but the phosphate level is low because of a compensatory elevation of parathormone levels. There is a high incidence of hyperchloremic acidosis secondary to renal phosphate loss. Supplementation with vitamin D, calcium, and phosphate is required for treatment. It is important not to supplement phosphate alone (despite the often normal serum calcium), since total body calcium is depleted and life-threatening hypocalcemia may occur with acute elevation of the serum phosphate level.

Rickets due to renal tubular insufficiency occurs in a number of disorders that result in either excess phosphate loss (most commonly) or excess calcium loss from the renal tubule. Simple hypophosphatemic vitamin D refractory rickets, hypophosphatemic vitamin D refractory rickets with aminoaciduria, and hypophosphatemic vitamin D refractory rickets with aminoaciduria and acidosis are all treated with large doses of vitamin D and phosphates.[81] The last two syndromes have been referred to as Fanconi's syndrome and are included together in some texts. Close supervision of children with this disorder is necessary to prevent vitamin D toxicity with its attendant risk of renal damage and hypercalcemia (see Chapter 7).

The surgical treatment of these patients includes correction of lower limb and pelvic deformities and treatment of kyphoscoliosis. It is important that vitamin D supplementation be discontinued 4 to 6 weeks preoperatively, since immobilization results in increased demineralization of bone, which may lead to dangerous levels of hypercalcemia and hypercalciuria. Obviously if children with this disorder present for emergency surgical therapy, urinary and serum calcium levels must be followed in the postoperative period and treatment instigated.

DISORDERS OF THE SPINE

Spinal disorders in children may be congenital or acquired. With the widespread use of vaccination against poliomyelitis and the increasing rarity of disseminated tuberculosis in the western world, the acquired forms are becoming relatively rare.

Congenital spinal disorders may be classified in several ways: by the resultant deformity (for example, kyphosis, scoliosis), by the location of the apex of the curve produced, or by the anatomical defect causing the deformity.

Associated anomalies are common in congenital disorders of the spine; the VATER association has already been described in the section on Radial Dysgenesis. In a series of 170 patients with congenital spinal deformities, 110 anomalies outside the vertebral column were seen.[82] There is an association between congenital cyanotic heart disease and scoliosis.[83, 84]

Some 20 to 30 percent of children with congenital spinal abnormalities have urogenital anomalies. Careful evaluation of the urogenital tract is essential to detect occult renal disease secondary to chronic obstruction.

Other problems that occur include facial anomalies (notably Goldenhar's syndrome), lung abnormalities, and gastrointestinal malformations. Scoliosis is the most frequent feature of spinal disease and often requires surgical treatment.

SCOLIOSIS

Scoliosis is derived from the Greek word meaning crooked. It can be defined as lateral deviation and rotation of a series of vertebrae from the midline anatomical position of the normal spinal axis. There are two fundamental types of scoliosis: functional (or postural) scoliosis, in which the curve is flexible and can be corrected by changes in posture, and structural scoliosis, in which the curvature is fixed. The classification of scoliosis on an etiological basis as outlined by Cobb is seen in Table 14–2. This may be further expanded by adding, for example, the different anatomical subsets of congenital vertebral anomalies leading to congenital scoliosis. The basic pathophysiology remains unknown, with the exception of those types of scoliosis secondary to neuromuscular disease in which the pathophysiological process may be due to muscular imbalance pulling the spinal column into abnormal configuration.

Congenital scoliosis is a lateral curve of the spine arising as a result of vertebral anomalies. Some anomalies cause so little deformity that they remain undetected, so the true incidence is unknown. Multiple anomalies are usually hereditary, whereas single ones are often sporadic. The scoliosis is often rigid and may be very difficult to treat. It is more common in girls than in boys. The prognosis is variable depending on the nature of the abnormality. The most severe form of scoliosis occurs when there is an unsegmented bar with an isolated contralateral hemivertebra. In such a case the spine deteriorates rapidly and may attain a curvature before 3 years of age.[85]

Table 14–2. CLASSIFICATION OF SCOLIOSIS

- Functional (postural)
- Structural
  - Congenital
  - Acquired
    - Idiopathic
      - Infantile
      - Juvenile
      - Adolescent
    - Neuromuscular
      - Poliomyelitis
      - Von Recklinghausen's disease
      - Friedreich's ataxia
      - Cerebral palsy
      - Syringomyelia
      - Myelodysplasias
      - Intraspinal tumor
      - Muscular dystrophies
      - Arthrogryposis multiplex congenita
    - Osteogenic
      - Postempyema, post-thoracoplasty, postirradiation, inflammatory conditions, rheumatoid, tuberculotic
      - Tumors, e.g., osteoid osteoma
      - Osteochondrodystrophies
      - Osteogenesis imperfecta
      - Scoliosis in congenital heart disease
      - Traumatic
      - Riley-Day syndrome (familial dysautonomia)
      - Congenital indifference to pain

Some 80 percent of cases requiring surgical correction are idiopathic in etiology, and 80 to 85 percent of these cases are in females. The incidence in North America is 4 per 1000 live births.[86] Infantile idiopathic scoliosis is infrequent in North America but almost as common as adolescent scoliosis in England.[87] The infant is usually male (90 percent of cases) with a left-sided curve that often disappears spontaneously, although in some cases there is rapid progression with severe deformity.[88] The adolescent, on the other hand, is usually female (85 percent) with a right-sided curve, but again only about 10 percent require active treatment. However, with an overall incidence of 4 per 1000, this constitutes a significant number of patients.

The neuromuscular forms of scoliosis can demonstrate rapid deterioration and often require both anterior and posterior fixation.[1] The commonest neuromuscular cause of scoliosis is cerebral palsy, and this can present some particular challenges in management. Cerebral palsy arises as a result of a neurological insult in utero or during the perinatal period. It results in a variety of clinical manifestations, most notably motor dysfunction leading to spastic diplegia, hemiplegia, or quadriplegia. The role

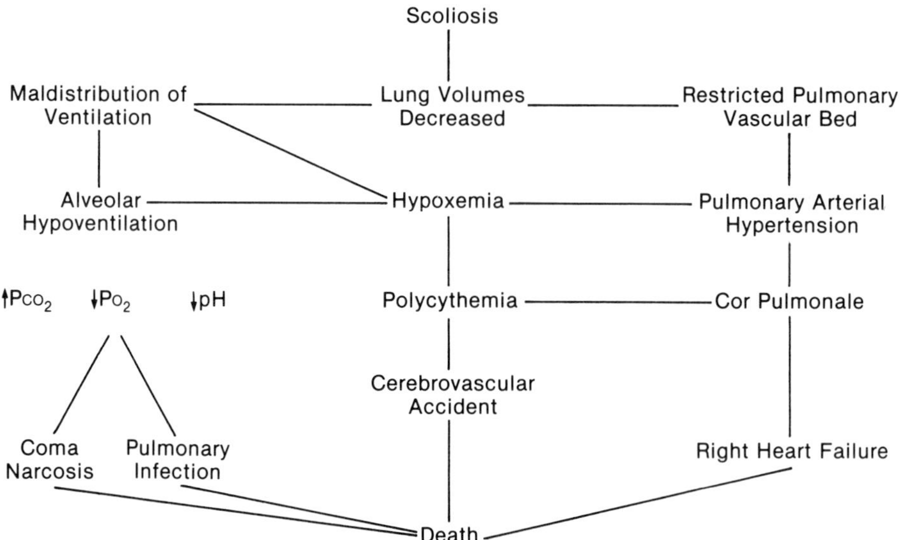

FIGURE 14–1. Pathophysiology of scoliosis. (Courtesy of Dr. Henry Levison.)

of scoliosis in producing lung pathology in these children is often difficult to assess because cooperation during pulmonary function tests may not be forthcoming. Many children with cerebral palsy also have difficulty swallowing, so frequent aspiration may exacerbate pulmonary problems.

Poliomyelitis is now a rare cause of scoliosis, although before the introduction of vaccination the incidence of paralytic scoliosis approached that of the idiopathic type. The curvature usually presents some 2 years after the acute illness and can increase rapidly if this period coincides with a growth spurt.[89]

In 10 percent of children with neurofibromatosis (von Recklinghausen's disease), a spinal curvature develops. This bears no relation anatomically to the location of neurofibromas and is most commonly a sharply angled thoracic kyphoscoliosis. These children require careful preoperative assessment to rule out pheochromocytoma, which although still rare is more common in patients with this disease than in the general population. (Pheochromocytoma has an incidence of 1:1000 hypertensive patients.) Probably less than 5 percent of pheochromocytomas are associated with neurofibromatosis. In children, sustained hypertension is the rule, rather than the episodic hypertension that is the classic presenting feature of pheochromocytoma.

Death from scoliosis has been recognized since the time of Hippocrates[4] and is due to cardiorespiratory failure. Associated neuromuscular weakness or congenital cardiac disease may add to this mortality.

Cardiorespiratory Pathophysiology

Severe scoliosis causes restrictive pulmonary disease (Fig. 14–1). This causes significant reduction in vital capacity and smaller reductions in total lung capacity and functional residual capacity. In children with idiopathic and congenital scoliosis, in contrast to adult patients, thoracic elastance remains normal.[90, 91]

The reduction in lung volumes leads to alveolar hypoventilation with increased intra-pulmonary shunt and hypoxemia. Although Vd/Vt ratios are elevated, the Pa_{CO_2} remains normal until late in the disease. Thus hypercapnia is an ominous sign. However, the response to carbon dioxide is impaired relatively early in the disease. Severe infantile scoliosis results in decreased alveolar development.[92]

Pulmonary hypertension is the result of prolonged hypoxia and low lung volumes and ultimately progresses to cor pulmonale and death. The signs of pulmonary hypertension (right ventricular enlargement, loud pulmonic second sound, and murmur of pulmonary insufficiency) should be sought in any patient with more than a 65-degree curvature and a long history of scoliosis.

The electrocardiographic changes of right ventricular hypertrophy and right atrial enlargement are late developments. These cardiorespiratory changes may be complicated by neuromuscular disease or cerebral palsy, resulting in inadequate cough and inability to clear secretions despite a relatively normal vital capacity. Cyanotic congenital heart disease accentuates the arterial hypoxemia and may hasten the onset of pulmonary hypertension. Cardiac failure per se will also complicate management. In severe cases of scoliosis, tracheal shortening or distortion may occur, and kinking of the pulmonary artery has been reported.[16]

Surgical correction of the deformity ideally should be performed before cardiorespiratory compromise has occurred. However, operation is often well tolerated despite striking reductions in vital capacity (below 35 percent of predicted values), particularly in the absence of neuromuscular disease.[93] Patients with a vital capacity of less than 30 percent of predicted values usually require postoperative mechanical ventilation. The indications and expected benefits should be weighed before proceeding with operation in the patient with this degree of respiratory impairment as it may lead to ventilator dependence, tracheostomy, and chronic hospitalization.

Surgical treatment of scoliosis generally does not result in any significant change in pulmonary function as determined by lung volume studies, although some improvement may occur in younger patients. Improvement in gas exchange has been demonstrated.[94, 95] Operation, however, does make a significant contribution to maintaining mobility in these children[1] and may help them retain a certain amount of independence by enabling them to continue to sit in a wheelchair.

ANESTHETIC CONSIDERATIONS

Preoperative Assessment. Preoperatively, the etiology of the scoliosis should be assessed and any associated abnormalities investigated. A majority of patients presenting for corrective operation have curves of less than 65 degrees (Cobb) and can be regarded as having normal lung function. Formal testing of pulmonary function should be performed in all cases with a greater curvature and particularly if there is associated neuromuscular disease. Patients with severe respiratory compromise should have their case reviewed by all medical personnel involved, especially the intensive care staff, and the patient should be warned about the possibility of postoperative ventilation. Premedication with narcotics or sedatives should be avoided in these patients.

The use of exoskeletal traction or body casts is fortunately now very rare but carries with it the potential for difficulty with intubation if the apparatus is not removed before induction. The use of an inhalation induction and fiberoptic intubation probably represents the simplest solution to this problem. Other potential problems to be reviewed preoperatively include the presence of flexion contractures, which are common in cerebral palsy and make vascular access and positioning difficult. The need for a wake-up test may also cause a modification in premedication and anesthetic technique.

A further consideration in the preoperative preparation of the patient with scoliosis is predonation of blood. This is becoming increasingly common. Protocols vary, but the basic requirements are (1) informed consent by the donor or legal guardian, (2) cooperation on the part of the child (some centers have a minimum age), (3) a minimum weight of 30 kg, (4) a minimum Hgb/Hct greater than 110 g/L/0.34, and (5) no medical contraindications—e.g., hemoglobinopathy or cardiovascular disease.

The usual routine is to collect blood on two or three occasions in the 3 weeks prior to operation (10 ml/kg to a maximum of 450 ml). Iron supplementation is given during this time and erythropoietin has been administered in some centers.

SURGICAL PROCEDURES IN SCOLIOSIS

The surgical approach to scoliosis may be anterior, posterior, or a combination of both. The anterior approach involves either thoracotomy or laparotomy and is usually reserved for those cases with rigid curves in the frontal and axial planes. The intervertebral disc is removed and instrumentation is placed that compresses the convex aspect of the curve. Dwyer's or Zielke's instrumentation is most commonly used.[96, 97]

The posterior approach involves a large incision, considerable bleeding, and all the concerns of the prone patient. The basic technique involves corrective stabilization followed by spinal fusion. A number of different forms of instrumentation have been developed; each carries its own risks and benefits. Harrington originated the technique in 1959.

Segmental instrumentation involves fixing the corrective rods at each level with wires passed anterior to each lamina. The risk of neurological damage is increased due to the wires, and the bleeding can be excessive. Stability is greatly improved, and better alignment of the spine can be achieved. This procedure is usually reserved for patients with neuromuscular disease. The Wisconsin system is used in some centers and is a combination of Luque's and Harrington's procedures. A more recent instrumentation is that developed by Cottrel and Dubousset.

Intraoperative Management

The intraoperative management of the patient for anterior stabilization involves all the considerations for thoracotomy or exploration of the retroperitoneum. It is not usually necessary to provide one-lung anesthesia for thoracotomy as adequate conditions are usually provided with simple retraction of the lung. The placement of the endotracheal tube must be checked after positioning the patient in the lateral position and frequently during the operation. This is necessary because the thoracic deformity can result in relative shortening of the trachea, and the surgical exposure will tend to encourage the endotracheal tube to descend down the right mainstem bronchus. Bleeding during anterior stabilization is not usually significant unless spinal osteotomy and wedge excision of vertebrae is performed. This can result in hemorrhage from the epidural and vertebral venous plexuses that can be difficult to control. The management of postoperative pain and avoidance of hypoventilation and atelectasis are important. The use of epidural narcotics may be very helpful, provided the patient is adequately monitored. Pain management is particularly difficult in the patient with cerebral palsy due to problems with communication.

The intraoperative management for the posterior approach includes all the considerations of the prone position, with particular emphasis on positioning, not only to avoid injury to the patient but also to minimize bleeding. The use of a suitable frame allows support of the shoulders and pelvis without compression of the chest or abdomen.[98] This avoids obstruction of the inferior vena cava and prevents engorgement of the vertebral venous plexus. It also enables adequate ventilation without high intrathoracic pressures and maintenance of functional residual capacity.

The control of blood loss and avoidance of homologous blood transfusion have been the subject of much research.[99] There are a number of ways of influencing blood loss by good anesthetic management, but it is also very important for the surgeon to infiltrate with epinephrine (1:500,000), operate as quickly as possible, pack those areas of the wound that are not in the field at any given moment, and dissect along tissue planes. Decortication of bone should be performed as late in the procedure as possible.

There are two main methods of reducing blood loss during the procedure. The first, acute hemodilution, involves phlebotomizing the patient and replacing the circulating volume with crystalloid or albumin.[100] The procedure is then performed at normotension, using hyperventilation to cause peripheral vasoconstriction. At the end of the procedure the blood is reinfused and the crystalloid is removed by diuresis. This technique has the advantage of simplicity and safety but may result in less than perfect conditions for the surgeon.

The second technique, induced hypotension, remains controversial despite several papers supporting its use.[101, 102] The concern arises because spinal cord damage is a major complication of scoliosis surgical therapy and in the prone position the spine is the highest point of the patient. Thus if the perfusion pressure is inadequate this area is the most vulnerable. However it does give very good conditions for the surgeon. If this technique is being considered there is evidence to suggest that nitroglycerin may be the agent of choice.[99, 103, 104] In some centers induced hypotension is used during dissection, and then the blood pressure is allowed to rise during spinal manipulation. Intraoperative blood losses can also be processed and returned to the patient to avoid homologous transfusion, but this involves a minimum recovery of 500 ml (which means a loss of about 1000 ml) and the use of expensive equipment. However, in the adolescent who can tolerate this loss before replacement, it offers the opportunity to avoid homologous transfusion, and the cost is comparable to that of banked blood.

Other anesthetic concerns during scoliosis operation include maintenance of body temperature, third space fluid losses, and the risk of air[105] or fat embolism.

The choice of anesthetic agents for maintenance depends in part on the choice of monitoring techniques. If somatosensory evoked potentials are used, then high concentrations of volatile anesthetic agents are contraindicated. If a wake-up test is used, it may be accomplished more easily by using a balanced technique with a low concentration of a volatile agent, a narcotic, and a muscle relaxant.[105–107]

Monitoring During Scoliosis Surgery

The risks of major blood loss, coagulopathy, respiratory complications, and neurological deficit make invasive monitoring necessary for scoliosis. The placement of an arterial line allows continuous monitoring of blood pressure (essential for cases using induced hypotension) and frequent blood sampling. A central venous pressure line is also useful as an indicator of intravascular volume. Measurement of urine output also gives an indication of intravascular volume and cardiac output.

The monitoring of spinal cord function is much more difficult and remains controversial. There are two methods of monitoring spinal cord function, and they may be used alone or in combination. The wake-up test is a one-time test of motor tract function, whereas somatosensory evoked potentials allow continuous monitoring of sensory pathways. The advantages of waking the patient after spinal distraction has occurred are threefold; it is simple to do, is reproducible, and provides a definitive test of motor function. The disadvantages are that it is often not appropriate for those patients most at risk (i.e., patients with neuromuscular scoliosis undergoing segmental instrumentation), it is not a continuous monitor, and the performance of the test itself carries a risk of complications, such as accidental extubation or venous air embolus.

Somatosensory evoked potentials involve the recording and interpretation of electrical impulses "evoked" by a distal stimulus. In scoliosis operation, the stimulus is commonly applied to one or both posterior tibial nerves. The impulses are recorded using either cortical or brain stem electrodes. Changes in both the duration and configuration of the evoked potentials can be used to assess spinal cord function. This form of monitoring has been used in scoliosis surgical therapy since 1977. It has the advantage of being a continuous monitor that is thought by its exponents to be predictable and reliable, although this view is not universally held.[108, 109] The disadvantages of the technique are that it is technically demanding and requires additional personnel in the operating room. It is expensive, and both false-negative and false-positive results occur. In addition, if brain stem recordings are made, it may be invasive, as it is necessary to introduce an electrode into the cervical epidural space.[110]

The incidence of neurological deficit is low (0.5 to 1 percent), but this is a devastating complication and all efforts to avoid it are worthwhile. At present, the use of evoked potentials can be viewed as an adjunct to the wake-up test. Improvements in technology are likely to lead to more widespread use of neurological monitoring, including motor evoked potentials, and this should further reduce the incidence of neurological complication.

FAT EMBOLISM

Fat embolism is a recognized complication of trauma, whether operative or accidental. It was first described in humans by Zenker in 1862, but despite over 100 years of experience with the entity a precise definition is not possible. This is due to controversy regarding both the origin of the fat and the precise pathophysiology of its effects. The presence of fat globules in the lungs and other tissues in patients dying of trauma varies from 46 to 100 percent in different series. However, the clinical incidence of the fat embolism syndrome is very much lower than this, varying from 1 to 6 percent in two reviews quoted by Wilkins.[111]

The fat embolism syndrome follows an initial episode of trauma, most commonly long bone fractures, and progresses within 48 hours to signs of cerebral impairment, fever, tachypnea, hypotension, and tachycardia. The onset of these symptoms in the early postoperative period (especially if a high fever is present) mimics the malignant hyperthermia syndrome. The pulmonary pathophysiological changes result in progressive hypoxia owing to shunting and hemorrhagic edema. The clinical picture becomes indistinguishable from that of adult respiratory distress syndrome. Fat globules usually can be demonstrated in either urine or sputum. At autopsy, fat can be seen in the pulmonary capillaries and in the systemic circulation involving the brain, liver, and kidneys. Coagulation abnormalities are common as a secondary event, and petechiae may be seen, typically on the upper part of the body.

Treatment of the syndrome includes supportive measures, such as intermittent positive-pressure ventilation with positive end-expiratory pressure. Hypoxic respiratory failure is the usual cause of death. Ethanol, either intravenously or by inhalation, has been advocated in the treatment of this syndrome,[112] but its use remains controversial. Heparin has also been administered,[113] although there are no clinical trials supporting its use and the side effects are particularly hazardous in the patient with multiple trauma. Steroids have also been recommended, based on reports of their use in three patients[114] and a prospective study in high-risk patients.[115]

The incidence of fat embolism in the pediatric population is unknown. A report from The Hospital for Sick Children, Toronto, suggested an incidence of less than 0.5 percent.[116] The presence of connective tissue disease in three of the nine cases was regarded as significant.

Two cases of fat embolism following spinal fusion have been reported,[117, 118] as has another case in an achondroplastic patient.[119]

Pediatric patients at risk for fat embolism include those with major long bone fractures, extensive crush injury, collagen vascular disease, or rickets, and any child undergoing procedures that involve compression of the intramedullary canal or extensive bony dissection. A high index of suspicion is necessary to make the diagnosis.

REFERENCES

1. Tachdjian MO: Pediatric Orthopedics. 2nd ed. Philadelphia, WB Saunders, 1990.
2. Behrman RE, Vaughan VC III (Eds.): Nelson Textbook of Pediatrics. 18th ed.: Philadelphia, WB Saunders, 1987.
3. McKusick VA: Heritable Disorders of Connective Tissue. St. Louis, CV Mosby, 1972.
4. Zauder HL (Ed.): Anaesthesia for Orthopaedic Surgery. Philadelphia, FA Davis, 1980.
5. Stehling L, Zauder HL: Anesthetic Implications of Congenital Anomalies in Children. New York, Appleton-Century-Crofts, 1980.
6. Bailey JA: Disproportionate Short Stature. Philadelphia, WB Saunders, 1973.
7. Second International Nomenclature of Constitutional Diseases of Bone. J Pediatr *93*:614, 1978.
8. Maroteaux P: International Nomenclature of Constitutional Diseases of Bones. Birth Defects *22*:1–54, 1986.
9. Orioli IM, Castilla EE, Barbosa Neto JG: The birth prevalence rates for the skeletal dysplasias. J Med Genet *23*:328, 1986.
10. Spranger J, Langer LO, Maroteaux P: Increasing frequency of a syndrome of multiple osseous defects. Lancet *2*:716, 1970.
11. Rimoin DL: The chondrodystrophies. Adv Hum Genet *5*:1, 1975.
12. Zellweger H, Taylor B: Genetic aspects of achondroplasia. Lancet *85*:8, 1965.
13. Reid CS, Pyeritz RE, Kopits SE, et al: Cervicomedullary compression in young patients with achondroplasia: Value of comprehensive neurologic and respiratory evaluation. J Pediatr *110*:522, 1987.
14. Todorov AB, Scott CI Jr, Warren AE, et al: Developmental screening tests in achondroplastic children. Am J Med Genet *9*:19, 1981.
15. Stokes DC, Phillips JA, Leonard CO, et al: Respiratory complications of achondroplasia. J Pediatr *102*:534, 1983.
16. Andrews TM, Myer CM III, Gray SP: Abnormalities of the body thorax causing tracheobronchial compression. Int J Pediatr Otorhinolaryngol *19*:139, 1990.
17. Stokes DC, Wohl ME, Wise RA, et al: The lungs and airways in achondroplasia. Do little people have little lungs? Chest *98*:145, 1990.
18. Dennis JP, Rosenberg HS, Alvord EC: Megalencephaly, internal hydrocephalus and other neurological aspects of achondroplasia. Brain *84*:427, 1961.
19. Cohen ME, Rosenthal AD, Matson D: Neurological abnormalities in achondroplastic children. J Pediatr *71*:367, 1967.
20. Steinbok P, Hall J, Flødmark O: Hydrocephalus in achondroplasia: The possible role of intracranial venous hypertension. J Neurosurg *71*:42, 1989.
21. Lundar T, Bakke SJ, Nornes H: Hydrocephalus in an achondroplastic child treated by venous decompression. J Neurosurg *73*:138, 1990.
22. Yamada H, Nakamura S, Masutaka T, et al: Neurological manifestations of paediatric achondroplasia. J Neurosurg *54*:49, 1981.
23. Hecht J, Butler IJ: Neurologic morbidity associated with achondroplasia. J Child Neurol *5*:84, 1990.
24. Hecht JT, Francomano CA, Horton WA, et al: Mortality in achondroplasia. Am J Hum Genet *41*:454, 1987.
25. Lutter LD, Lonstein GE, Winter RB, et al: Anatomy of the achondroplastic lumbar canal. Clin Orthop *126*:139, 1977.
26. Vogl H, Osbourne RL: Lesions of the spinal cord in achondroplasia. Arch Neurol Psychol *61*:644, 1949.
27. Bethem D, Winter RB, Lutter L, et al: Spinal disorders of dwarfism. J Bone Joint Surg *63A*:1412, 1981.
28. Cohen SE: Anesthesia for cesarean section in an achondroplastic dwarf. Anesthesiology *52*:264, 1980.
29. Bancroft GH, Lauria JI: Ketamine induction for cesarean section in a patient with acute intermittent porphyria and achondroplastic dwarfism. Anesthesiology *59*:143, 1983.
30. Mather JS: Impossible direct laryngoscopy in achondroplasia. Anaesthesia *21*:244, 1966.
31. Wardall GT, Frame WT: Extradural anaesthesia for caesarian section in achondroplasia. Br J Anaesth *64*:367, 1990.
32. Brimacombe JR, Caunt JA: Anaesthesia in a gravid achondroplastic dwarf. Anaesthesia *45*:132, 1990.
33. Mayhew JF, Katz J, Miner M, et al: Anaesthesia for the achondroplastic dwarf. Can Anaesth Soc J *33*:216, 1986.
34. Kalla GN, Fening E, Obiayo MO: Anaesthetic management of achondroplasia. Br J Anaesth *58*:117, 1986.
35. Watts LF, Finerman G, Wyatt GM: Anesthesia for dwarfs and other patients of pathological small stature. Can Anaesth Soc J *22*:703, 1975.
36. Bianchi Maiocchi A, Aronson J (Eds.): Operative Principles of Ilizarov. Baltimore, Williams and Wilkins, 1991.
37. Borland LM: Anesthesia for children with Jeune's syndrome. Anesthesiology *66*:86, 1987.
38. Hanissian AS, Riggs WW Jr, Thomas DA: Infantile thoracic dystrophy—a variant of Ellis–van Creveld syndrome. J Pediatr *71*:855, 1967.
39. Kozlowski K, Szmigiel C, Baylak A, et al: Difficulties in differentiation between chondroectodermal dysplasia and asphyxiating thoracic dystrophy. Aust Radiol *16*:401, 1972.
40. Langer LO Jr: Thoracic-pelvic-phalangeal dystrophy. Radiology *91*:447, 1968.
41. Zelt BA, LoSasso AM: Prolonged nasotracheal intubation and mechanical ventilation in the management of asphyxiating thoracic dystrophy: A case report. Anesth Analg *51*:342, 1972.
42. Barnes ND, Hull D, Miller AD, et al: Chest reconstruction in thoracic dystrophy. Arch Dis Child *46*:833, 1971.
43. Finegold MJ, Katzew H, Genieser NB, et al: Lung structure in thoracic dystrophy. Am J Dis Child *22*:153, 1971.
44. Herdman RC, Langer LO Jr: The thoracic asphyxiant dystrophy and renal disease. Am J Dis Child *116*:192, 1968.
45. Ellis RW, van Creveld S: A syndrome characterized by ectodermal dysplasia, polydactyly, chondrodysplasia and congenital morbus cordis. Arch Dis Child *15*:65, 1940.
46. McKusick VA, Egeland JA, Eldridge R, et al: Dwarfism in the Amish. 1. The Ellis–van Creveld syndrome. Bull Johns Hopkins Hosp *115*:306, 1964.
47. Moore TC: Chondroectodermal dysplasia (Ellis–van

Creveld syndrome) with bronchial malformation and neonatal tension lobar emphysema. J Thorac Cardiovasc Surg *46*:1, 1963.
48. Spranger JW, Opitz JM, Bidder V: Heterogeneity of chondrodysplasia punctata. Hum Genet *11*:190, 1971.
49. Maroteaux P: Bone Diseases of Children. Philadelphia, JB Lippincott, 1979.
50. Nyham WC, Sakati NO: Genetic and Malformation Syndromes in Clinical Medicine. Chicago, Year Book Medical Publishers, 1976.
51. Afshani E, Girdany BR: Atlanto-axial dislocation in chondrodysplasia punctata. Report of the findings in two brothers. Radiology *102*:399, 1972.
52. Hathaway WE, Johnson CC, Oh JE: Abnormalities of platelet function in osteogenesis imperfecta. Clin Res *18*:209, 1970.
53. King JD, Bobechko WP: Osteogenesis imperfecta. An orthopaedic description and surgical review. J Bone Joint Surg *53B*:72, 1971.
54. Cropp GV, Myers DN: Physiological evidence of hypermetabolism in osteogenesis imperfecta. Pediatrics *49*:375, 1972.
55. Gitelis S, Whiffen J, DeWald RL: The treatment of severe scoliosis in osteogenesis imperfecta. Clin Orthop *175*:56, 1983.
56. White NJ, Winearls CG, Smith R: Cardiovascular abnormalities in osteogenesis imperfecta. Am Heart J *106*:1416, 1983.
57. Sofield HA, Millar EA: Fragmentation realignment and intramedullary rod fixation of deformities of long bones in children. J Bone Joint Surg *34A*:500, 1952.
58. Gerlach PA, Rosensweig J, Ramanathan KB: Successful aortic valve replacement in osteogenesis imperfecta: With special emphasis on perioperative management. Can J Cardiol *3*:132, 1987.
59. Rampton AJ, Kelly DA, Shanahan EC, et al: Occurrence of malignant hyperpyrexia in a patient with osteogenesis imperfecta. Br J Anaesth *56*:1443, 1984.
60. Solomons CC, Yers DN: Hyperthermia of osteogenesis imperfecta and its relationship to malignant hyperthermia. *In* Gordon RA, Britt BA, Kalow W (Eds.): International Symposium on Malignant Hyperthermia. Springfield, Ill., Charles C Thomas, 1973.
61. Ryan CA, Al Ghamdi AS, Gayle M, et al: Osteogenesis imperfecta and hyperthermia. Anesth Analg *68*:811, 1989.
62. Oliverio RM: Anaesthetic management of intramedullary nailing in osteogenesis imperfecta. Report of a case. Anesth Analg *52*:232, 1973.
63. Wood SJ, Thomas J, Braimbridge MV: Mitral valve disease and open heart surgery in osteogenesis imperfecta tarda. Br Heart J *35*:103, 1973.
64. Weisinger B, Glassman E, Spencer FC, et al: Successful aortic valve replacement for aortic regurgitation associated with osteogenesis imperfecta. Br Heart J *37*:475, 1975.
65. Gupta DS, Gupta MK, Borle RM: Osteomyelitis of the mandible in marble bone disease. Int J Oral Maxillofac Surg *15*:201, 1986.
66. Berkowitz ID, Raja SN, Bender KS, et al: Dwarfs; Pathophysiology and anesthetic implications. Anesthesiology *73*:739, 1990.
67. Watts LF, Finerman G, Wyatt GM: Anesthesia for dwarfs and other patients of pathological small stature. Can Anaesth Soc J *22*:703, 1975.
68. Perovic MN, Kopits SE, Thompson RC: Radiological evaluation of the spinal cord in congenital atlantoaxial dislocation. Radiology *109*:713, 1973.
69. Shohat M, Lachuan R, Rimoin DI: Odontoid hypoplasia with vertebral cervical subluxation and ventriculomegaly in metatropic dysplasia. J Pediatr *114*:239, 1989.
70. Rodney GE, Callender CC, Harmer M: Spondyloepiphyseal dysplasia congenita. Anaesthesia *46*:648, 1991.
71. Aryanpur J, Hurko O, Francomano C, et al: Cranocervical decompression in pediatric patients with achondroplasia. J Neurosurg *73*:375, 1990.
72. McIntyre JW: The difficult tracheal intubation. Can J Anaesth *34*:204, 1987.
73. McCirrick A, Pracilio JA: Awake intubation: A new technique. Anaesthesia *46*:661, 1991.
74. Goldberg MJ, Meyer M: The radial clubhand. Orthop Clin North Am *7*:341, 1970.
75. Goldberg MJ, Ampola MG: Birth defect syndromes in which orthopedic problems may be overlooked. Orthop Clin North Am *7*:285, 1976.
76. Noonan JA: Association of congenital heart disease with syndromes or other defects. Pediatr Clin North Am *25*:797, 1976.
77. Quan L, Smith DW: The VATER association. Vertebral defects, anal atresia, T-E fistula with esophageal atresia, radial and renal dysplasia. A spectrum of associated defects. J Pediatr *82*:104, 1973.
78. Bany JE, Auldist AW: The Vater association: One end of a spectrum of anomalies. Am J Dis Child *128*:769, 1974.
79. Goodman AG, Gilman LS, Gilman A (Eds.): The Pharmacological Basis of Therapeutics. 6th ed. New York, Macmillan, 1980.
80. Card RT, Brain MC: The "anemia" of childhood: Evidence for a physiological response to hyperphosphatemia. N Engl J Med *288*:388, 1972.
81. Ferris B, Walker C, Jackson A: The orthopaedic management of hypophosphataemic rickets. J Pediatr Orthop *11*:367, 1991.
82. Kulns J, Homel R: Management of congenital scoliosis. Review of 170 cases. Arch Surg *65*:250, 1952.
83. Jordan GE, White RJ, Fischer KC, et al: The scoliosis of congenital heart disease. Am Heart J *84*:463, 1974.
84. Primiano F, Nussbaum E, Hirschfield S: Early echocardiographic and pulmonary function findings in idiopathic scoliosis. J Pediatr Orthop *3*:475, 1983.
85. McMaster MJ, Ohtsuka K: The natural history of congenital scoliosis. A study of 251 patients. J Bone Joint Surg *64A*:1128, 1982.
86. Shands AR, Eisberg HB: The incidence of scoliosis in the state of Delaware. J Bone Joint Surg *37A*:1249, 1955.
87. James JIP: The etiology of scoliosis. J Bone Joint Surg *52*:410, 1970.
88. Scott JC, Morgan TH: The natural history and prognosis for infantile idiopathic scoliosis. J Bone Joint Surg *37B*:400, 1955.
89. Keim HA: Scoliosis. CIBA Foundation Symposium, 1978.
90. Kafer ER: Respiratory and cardiovascular functions in scoliosis and the principles of anesthetic management. Anesthesiology *52*:339, 1980.
91. Nisbet HIA, Lamarre A, Levison H, et al: Thoracic elastance and its components in anaesthetized scoliotic children. J Bone Joint Surg *55A*:1721, 1973.
92. Davies G, Reid L: Effect of scoliosis on growth of alveoli and pulmonary arteries and on the right ventricle. Arch Dis Child *46*:623, 1971.
93. Jenkins JG, Bohn DJ, Edmonds JF, et al: Evaluation of pulmonary function in muscular dystrophy patients requiring spinal surgery. Crit Care Med *10*:645, 1982.
94. Sehir M, Brown JT, Kafer E, et al: Postoperative pulmonary function in children: Comparison of scoliosis with peripheral surgery. Am Rev Respir Dis *130*:46, 1984.

95. Shannon DC, Riseborough EJ, Kazemi H: Ventilation perfusion relationships following correction of kyphoscoliosis. JAMA *217*:579, 1971.
96. Dwyer AF, Schafer MF: Anterior approach to scoliosis; Results of treatment in fifty one cases. J Bone Joint Surg *56B*:218, 1974.
97. Zielke B: Ventral derotation spondylodesis. Preliminary report of fifty-eight cases. Beitr Orthop Traumatol *85*:103, 1978.
98. Relton JES, Hall JE: An operation frame for spinal fusion; A new apparatus designed to reduce haemorrhage during operation. J Bone Joint Surg *49B*:327, 1967.
99. Phillips WA, Hensinger RN: Control of blood loss during scoliosis surgery. Clin Orthop *229*:88, 1988.
100. du Toit G, Relton JES, Gillespie R: Acute haemodilutional autotransfusion in the surgical management of scoliosis. J Bone Joint Surg *60B*:178, 1978.
101. McNeill TN, DeWald RL, Kino KN, et al: Controlled hypotensive anaesthesia in scoliosis surgery. J Bone Joint Surg *56A*:1167, 1974.
102. Patel NJ, Patel BS, Parkin S, et al: Induced moderate hypotensive anesthesia for spinal fusion and Harrington rod instrumentation. J Bone Joint Surg *67A*:1384, 1985.
103. Jacobs HK, Lieponais VV, Bunch WH, et al: The influence of halothane and nitroprusside on canine spinal cord haemodynamics. Spine *7*:35, 1982.
104. Grundy BL, Nash CL Jr, Brown RH: Deliberate hypotension for spinal fusion. Prospective randomized study with evoked potential monitoring. Can Anaesth Soc J *29*:452, 1982.
105. Lang JA, Duncan PG, Dupuis PR: Fatal air embolism in an adolescent with Duchenne muscular dystrophy during Harrington instrumentation. Anesth Analg *69*:132, 1989.
106. Hall JE, Levine CR, Sudhir KG: Intraoperative awakening to monitor spinal cord function during Harrington instrumentation and spinal fusion. J Bone Joint Surg *60A*:533, 1978.
107. Pathak KS, Brown RH, Nash CL, et al: Continuous opioid infusions for scoliosis fusion surgery. Anesth Analg *62*:841, 1983.
108. Friedman WA, Grundy BL: Monitoring of sensory evoked potentials is highly reliable and helpful in the operating room. J Clin Monit *3*:38, 1987.
109. Michenfielder JD: Intraoperative monitoring of sensory evoked potentials may be neither a proven nor an indicated technique. J Clin Monit *3*:45, 1987.
110. Anderson SK, Hetreed MA, Longman BA: A technique for monitoring evoked potentials during scoliosis and brachial plexus surgery. Ann R Coll Surg Engl *72*:321, 1990.
111. Wilkins KE: Fat embolism. *In* Zauder HL (Ed.): Anaesthesia for Orthopaedic Surgery. Philadelphia, FA Davis, 1980.
112. Nice GW: Alcohol in fat embolism. J Kans Med Soc *75*:306, 1974.
113. Guenter CA, Braun TE: Fat embolism syndrome: Changing prognosis. Chest *79*:143, 1981.
114. Ashbaugh DG, Petty TL: Use of corticosteroids in treatment of respiratory failure. Surg Gynecol Obstet *123*:493, 1966.
115. Schonfeld S, Ploysonyang G, Dilisio R, et al: Fat embolism prophylaxis with corticosteroids. A prospective study in high-risk patients. Ann Intern Med *99*:438, 1983.
116. Drummond DS, Salter RB, Boone J: Fat embolism in children. Can Med Assoc J *101*:200, 1969.
117. Gittman JE, Buchanan TA, Fisher BJ, et al: Fatal fat embolism after spinal fusion for scoliosis. JAMA *249*:779, 1983.
118. Brown LP, Stehling LH: Fat embolism as a complication of scoliosis fusion. J Bone Joint Surg *56A*:1764, 1974.
119. Ganel A, Israeli A, Horoszowski H: Fatal complication of femoral elongation in an achondroplastic dwarf. Clin Orthop *185*:69, 1984.

CHAPTER

15 Skin and Connective Tissue Diseases

MICHAEL F. SMITH, M.D.

This chapter considers diseases of the skin and connective tissue in children. The more severe of these disorders are chronic, multisystemic in nature, and often debilitating. Treatment may involve prolonged medical support and repeated surgical interventions. Successful anesthetic management requires recognition of the relevant pathophysiological implications of each disorder and consideration of the psychological needs of anxious and often intolerant young patients enduring chronic illness.

It is appropriate that skin and connective tissue diseases be discussed in the same chapter. Connective tissue elements appear in the skin and in the stroma of most organ systems of the body and are vulnerable to similar underlying pathological mechanisms; thus, many of these diseases are closely related. The skin manifests changes that become a diagnostic clue for the recognition of systemic disease, just as observation of the skin is a valuable monitor for the anesthesiologist in assessing a patient's response during anesthesia and surgery.

For purposes of organization, skin diseases and connective tissue disorders are considered in separate sections within the chapter.

SKIN DISEASES

STRUCTURE AND FUNCTIONS OF NORMAL SKIN

The skin is a complex dynamic organ of many cell types and specialized structures. The outer layer of the skin, the epidermis, is an organized, stratified epithelium with appendages, notably hair follicles, apocrine sweat glands, and sebaceous glands, that project into the dermis. Two major zones can be identified: (1) the outer layer, called the stratum corneum, composed of nonviable desiccated squamous cells or keratinocytes that are continuously renewed in an orderly fashion from (2) basal germ cells known as the malpighian layer. The transit time of these cells is about 28 to 42 days.[1] Other cells within the basal epidermis include melanocytes, which synthesize the pigment melanin, and Langerhans cells, which are dendritic mesenchymal cells that function as the initial receptor for the cutaneous immune response to external antigens.

The dermal-epidermal junction serves to weld the epidermis to the underlying dermis and acts as a barrier to the movement of inflammatory and neoplastic cells into the epidermis.

The dermis, interposed between the epidermis and subcutaneous fat, forms a tough, viscoelastic supporting structure. This three-dimensional matrix of loose connective tissue is composed of the fibrous proteins collagen and elastin embedded in an amorphous gel of ground substance. It contains the epidermal appendages, blood vessels, lymphocytes, nerves, arrector pili muscles, and considerable amounts of bound water. The predominant cell is a spindle-shaped fibroblast that synthesizes the fibrillar proteins and the mucopolysaccharides of the ground substance. Other cells include phagocytic histiocytes or macrophages, mast cells, and motile leukocytes.

The subcutaneous tissue, or panniculus, is composed of lobules of fat cells divided by fibrous septa. These help anchor the dermis to the underlying fascia.

Intact, the skin provides an airtight, waterproof, elastic surface cover for the body and serves many crucial functions necessary to preserve life. It offers protection from chemical and mechanical injury and from ultraviolet light. Sensory organs aid further in the protection against injury. The surface film of lipid secretions from sebaceous glands creates an antiseptic layer, retarding the growth of microorganisms and reducing moisture loss from the epidermis.

The skin plays a major role in the regulation of body temperature, particularly in infants, who have a large surface area relative to their body mass. The gradient for heat loss by radiation is determined by skin blood flow, which may increase from basal levels of 50 ml/100 g/min to 200 ml/100 g/min under the sympathetic control of arteriovenous shunts in the dermis.[20] Further heat loss results from the evaporation of insensible water loss and of the hypotonic secretion of eccrine sweat glands.

Anesthesia affects the functions of the skin in several ways. The protective role of sensation is eliminated, and this may lead to injury, such as diathermy burns or nerve damage. Most anesthetic techniques and agents increase skin blood flow and significantly reduce the ability of children to maintain a normal body temperature. Under conditions in which cardiac output falls, skin perfusion is compromised, and its temperature will decrease. The use of anticholinergic drugs may reduce sweating sufficiently to cause hyperthermia.[20]

NEONATAL SKIN DISORDERS

Compared with that of the older child or adult, the skin of the neonate is thinner and less hairy, has weaker intercellular attachments, and is more sensitive to external irritants. It produces less sweat and sebaceous gland secretions.[6] Sweating on the face and trunk in a term infant is usually noted on the third to fifth day of life but in premature infants may be delayed until the 24th day. Depressed contact allergen reactivity may be explained by low levels of complement C_3 and C_4 in the neonate. The percutaneous adsorption of toxic substances is increased in premature infants and particularly in inflamed or ulcerated areas of skin.[6] These differences help explain the vulnerability of newborn infants to skin disease.

Toxic Erythema Neonatorum

Despite its dramatic descriptive name, toxic erythema neonatorum is a benign, asymptomatic, and self-limited cutaneous eruption of erythematous macules, papules, and pustules. It occurs in 50 to 70 percent of term infants.[6] Preterm infants are less affected. The skin lesions usually appear during the first 3 to 4 days of life. They may occur in numbers of a few to several hundred, anywhere on the body except the palms and soles. In more severe cases, urticarial wheals may develop. Smears of the pustular fluid show a predominance of eosinophils. Spontaneous recovery occurs within 2 days, and recurrences are rare. No treatment is required.

Apart from careful aseptic technique, there are no specific anesthetic considerations.

Herpes Simplex Neonatorum

A fetus may acquire herpes simplex virus infection on passage through the birth canal if the mother has an active herpetic cervicitis or vulvitis at the time of delivery. The previously healthy child becomes ill on day 4 to 8 of life and may develop erythematous or vesiculobullous lesions, which may recur, on the face, scalp, or upper trunk.[6, 21] The disseminated visceral involvement may initiate devastating pneumonitis, hepatitis, and meningoencephalitis and may be fatal.

Treatment must be aggressive and may include exchange transfusion from a donor with a history of a herpetic infection of the appropriate type, transfusion of type-specific immune globulin, and donor herpes virus–sensitive lymphocytes and monocytes. The use of intravenous adenosine arabinoside, vidarabine, and acyclovir has improved the outlook of neonatal herpes infections.

Anesthetic considerations include a careful assessment of hepatic function and the neurological status, especially with respect to intracranial pressure, which may be raised, and anticonvulsant therapy.

Erythema Desquamativum (Leiner Disease)

Leiner disease is a rare, possibly hereditary disorder thought to be a severe form of seborrheic dermatitis. It may occur in the first week of life but is usually seen in infants aged 2 to 4 months who are breast-fed; girls are affected more often than boys. It is characterized by the sudden onset of a generalized exfoliative erythemic dermatitis associated with intractable diarrhea, anemia, wasting, and recurrent local and systemic gram-negative infections (Fig. 15–1). The etiology is unknown, but in the familial form a defect in the opsonic activity of complement, leading to a functional deficiency of C_5, has been recognized.[3, 4]

Children with Leiner disease require intensive care, with correction of associated hypovolemia, anemia, sepsis, and secondary infections, usually pneumonia and meningitis. Temperature control is impaired. Intravenous access is difficult in infants who have generalized dermatitis and who may have severe cushingoid features. Adhesive tape should be used with caution. Despite aggressive supportive care with parenteral nutrition and fresh-frozen plasma, corticosteroids, and antibiotics, the mortality rate of this disease remains high.[22]

NEONATAL ICHTHYOSES

The ichthyoses represent a heterogeneous group of inherited keratinizing disorders in which there is increased epidermal germinal cell activity and a failure of separation of stratum corneum cells. The hyperkeratosis produces large amounts of scale of varying thickness on the skin surface. Except for ichthyosis vulgaris, which presents in early childhood and is less severe, all forms are usually obvious at birth. The most common immediate neonatal presentation of ichthyosis (1 in 300,000 births)[1] occurs in the *collodion baby,* often as a manifestation of lamellar ichthyosis. The child is encased in a dry, taut membrane resembling oiled parchment that fissures and then desquamates over the next several weeks.[8] Constriction of the chest and distortion of the face may compromise spontaneous respiration and the ability to feed.

Maintaining a warm, humidified environment is the most efficient means of hydrating the membrane and keeping it pliable.[1, 23] Respiratory function must be monitored, and adequate hydration and nutrition must be provided. Intravenous access is difficult. Skin infections at fissure sites and pneumonias must be aggressively treated with antibiotics. Temperature control is impaired.

The most severe presentation of this disorder is the rare *harlequin fetus,* in which the child is covered by thick plates of stratum corneum separated by fissures. Few babies survive beyond 1 week.[4, 6]

Other variants of ichthyosis in children may not present until the age of 3 months or more and may appear to be no more significant than dry skin. In the forms such as mild lamellar ichthyosis, ichthyosis vulgaris, or epidermolytic hyperkeratosis, the disorder is limited to the skin and is manifested as a buildup of considerable epidermal scale from massive hyperkeratosis (Fig. 15–2). Treatment is directed at reducing or softening the scale by the applica-

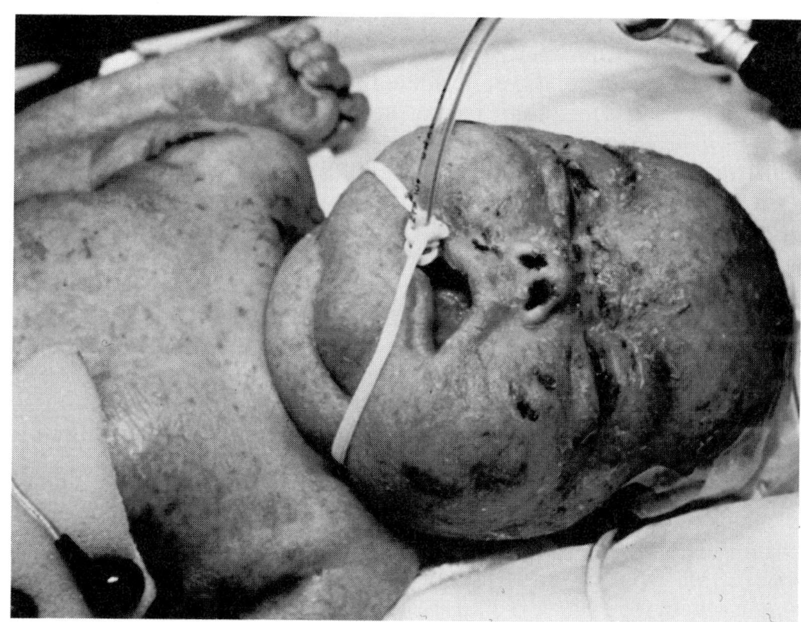

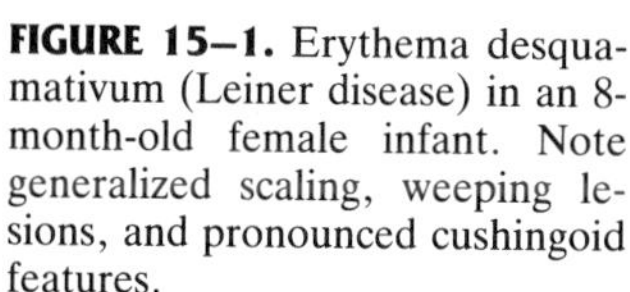

FIGURE 15–1. Erythema desquamativum (Leiner disease) in an 8-month-old female infant. Note generalized scaling, weeping lesions, and pronounced cushingoid features.

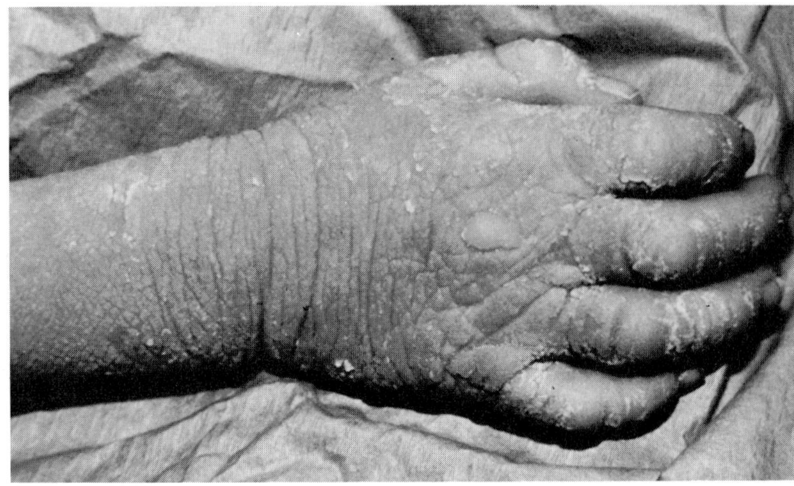

FIGURE 15–2. Epidermolytic hyperkeratosis in a 4-year-old boy. The accumulation of thickened epidermal scale has been softened by keratolytic and lubricant agents.

tion of lubricants or keratinolytic agents such as retinoic acid or salicylic acid. The oily base in some of these agents prevents adhesives from sticking to the skin. Intravenous cannulas, electrocardiograph electrodes, and endotracheal tubes must be tied or sutured in place. There are no other specific anesthetic considerations.

Sclerema Neonatorum and Subcutaneous Fat Necrosis of the Neonate

Sclerema neonatorum is an uncommon disorder that occurs in the first few weeks of life in premature, cold-stressed, or debilitated infants who have serious underlying sepsis, respiratory distress, gastroenteritis and dehydration, or congenital heart disease.[1, 3] It is a grave prognostic sign, characterized by an abrupt onset of diffuse, generalized hardening of the subcutaneous tissue of the trunk that spreads rapidly. The skin becomes waxy and stony in consistency, nonpitting, and cold.[8] Joint mobility and respiration are compromised. The child becomes sluggish and feeds poorly. The mortality of affected infants is 50 to 75 percent; death usually results from respiratory failure or secondary infections. In those who survive, the skin findings resolve without sequelae.[1, 24, 25] The etiology is unknown. Treatment is supportive and directed at the underlying disease.

Subcutaneous fat necrosis of the newborn infant is uncommon and usually occurs in healthy neonates in the first weeks of life.[26] The etiology is unknown, but excessive chilling and obstetrical trauma have been implicated. The lesions are sharply circumscribed, indurated plaques with overlying red to violaceous skin found on the thighs, buttocks, back, arms, and cheeks. This disorder is self limited, treatment is expectant, and resolution is spontaneous within a few weeks.

Management includes treatment of the underlying condition, supportive care in a warm environment with oxygen as required, and aggressive antibiotic control of infections. Systemic corticosteroids have been advocated.[6]

No specific anesthetic experience has been reported.

DEVELOPMENTAL ABNORMALITIES OF THE SKIN

Cutaneous Defects

Congenital Localized Absence of the Skin (Aplasia Cutis Congenita). This uncommon inherited defect in skin development is manifested at birth by single or multiple 1- to 2-cm ulcers, usually on the scalp. The depth of the ulcers is variable, but they may infrequently involve tissue deep to the dermis and even extend to the periosteum, skull, and dura. In its extreme, the defect may be staggering (Fig. 15–3). Associated defects are rare but include cleft lip and palate, vascular malformations, congenital heart disease, defects of the central nervous system, and trisomy 13 syndrome.[8] Bart has described the association of this disorder with epidermolysis bullosa.[27] Congenital localized absence of the skin in areas other than the scalp may in fact be a clinical expression of epidermolysis bullosa.

Small defects re-epithelialize spontaneously. Large or multiple lesions may be complicated

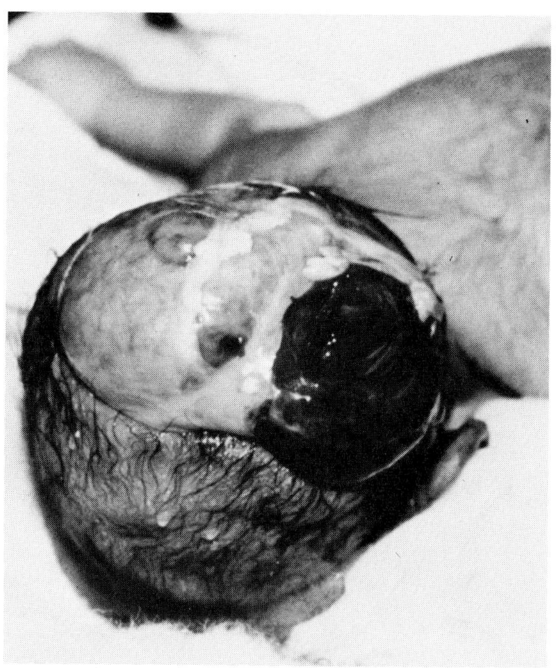

FIGURE 15–3. Aplasia cutis congenita in its extreme form in a prone newborn male infant. Note the total absence of cranial vault and dura and the partial infarction of the left cerebral cortex.

by secondary infection, massive hemorrhage, and meningitis. The repair may require excision, dural grafting, and rotation flaps to cover the defect.

The anesthesiologist must be aware of the possible association of this condition with epidermolysis bullosa and with other congenital anomalies described. Adequate blood products must be available for use during the closure of large defects.

Focal Dermal Hypoplasia (Goltz's Syndrome). Focal dermal hypoplasia is a rare, probably X-linked dominant disorder that occurs principally in girls and is usually lethal in males. It is characterized by the herniation of fat through thinned, partly deficient dermis, producing multiple papillomas. The papillomas usually involve the periorificial skin and the oral mucous membranes, but lesions in the oropharynx and peritonsillar regions have been described.[28–31] The skin may also show atrophy and linear hyperpigmentation. Associated anomalies include skeletal asymmetry and scoliosis, ocular abnormalities, dental defects, cardiac abnormality, small stature, and mental deficiency. The face may be oddly shaped. Surgical correction of the more disfiguring anomalies is often of value.

The airway must be evaluated preoperatively, but no difficulty in laryngoscopy has been reported. Apart from recognizing the associated abnormalities, no specific anesthetic recommendations are made.

Congenital Anhidrotic Ectodermal Dysplasia (Christ-Siemens-Touraine Syndrome). This rare, X-linked recessive disorder is seen with full expression only in males, although carrier females may be mildly affected. The ectodermal defect is manifested by the triad of absent sebaceous and sweat glands, few or no teeth, and hypotrichosis (absent hair).[28] The skin is dry, and heat loss by evaporation is impaired.[32] There may be virtual absence of mucous glands from the respiratory tract and esophagus. Respiratory infections are frequent. Body odor may be lacking. Affected children demonstrate the characteristic facies, which features a depressed bridge and root of the nose, prominent supraorbital ridges, large deformed ears, thick lips, and an underdeveloped maxilla and mandible.[32–34]

Affected infants may appear normal early in life, and the diagnosis may not be suspected until age 6 to 12 months, when the defective hair and teeth are recognized. The disorder ought to be suspected in a child presenting with pyrexia of unknown origin.[33] The prognosis is good, provided the child can be protected from the risks of hyperpyrexia secondary to infection, hot weather, or vigorous exercise. Drugs such as chlorpromazine, diazepam, and anticholinergics that may interfere with temperature control should be avoided. Survival to adulthood is common.

Several anesthetic considerations are important in the management of affected children. The abnormal facies and maxillary and mandibular underdevelopment may make airway management by mask awkward and laryngoscopy and intubation difficult. In some cases, regional anesthesia may be a reasonable alternative. When general anesthesia is required, fresh gases should be warmed and humidified. Lacrimation may be deficient, and the eyes should be protected by an ophthalmic ointment and taped closed. Careful monitoring of body temperature is necessary because of impaired thermoregulation.[33] Measures for cooling the patient, such as padded ice bags, cool intravenous solutions, or fans, should be available. Anticholinergic medication, although important in children, will reduce any available sweat production further and may contribute to hyperthermia.

In anticipation of postoperative chest infections, preoperative teaching and vigorous postoperative chest physiotherapy should be planned.[34]

VASCULAR MALFORMATIONS

Hemangiomas. Hemangiomas are quite common and occur in 10 percent of children under 1 year of age.[7] They usually appear shortly after birth and may vary considerably in number and size. Despite the marked overlap in their histology, they are usually classified as *capillary,* those composed of superficial, dilated capillaries with variable endothelial proliferation; as *cavernous,* consisting of large, blood-filled cavities that have compressed, single-layered endothelium and involve deeper tissues; or as *mixed.* They are characterized by an initial proliferative stage, in which there is rapid growth over the first 5 to 7 months of age, and then by an involuting phase, in which there is variable regression of the lesion size, with fibrosis and fat deposition. Cavernous hemangiomas are often composed of more mature vascular elements that are less likely to involute.[7]

The *strawberry nevus* is a capillary hemangioma that usually appears at 1 to 2 months of age on the face, scalp, or trunk and is more frequent in girls. These nevi are raised, bright red lesions rarely exceeding 5 cm in size. Spontaneous involution occurs in 95 percent by age 9 years, and fewer than 10 percent of patients have cosmetic defects that require plastic surgery. The association between subglottic hemangioma and cutaneous lesions must be considered in any infant who presents with any symptoms of stridor (see page 408).

Giant hemangiomas are often mixed capillary and cavernous lesions and are usually seen on the face and scalp. They may become very large and disfiguring. They may ulcerate, become secondarily infected, or bleed, or by compression they may interfere with vital functions. When such complications become severe, systemic corticosteroid therapy with prednisone, 2 to 4 mg/kg/24 hours, may produce significant regression in 2 to 3 weeks.[8, 35] For more benign lesions, compressive bandaging will often reduce the hemangioma size satisfactorily. Surgical therapy may be advised when involution has not begun by age 4 years and when arteriovenous fistulas have been demonstrated.[1, 36]

There may be significant problems in maintaining an airway by mask in children with distorting facial hemangiomas (Fig. 15–4). Laryngoscopy and intubation may be difficult and may traumatize upper airway components of the lesion. Even a minor procedure may precipitate considerable hemorrhage, and a reliable large-bore intravenous cannula is essential. For major procedures, the child must be in optimal hemodynamic and hemostatic condition prior to induction, and adequate blood products must be available.

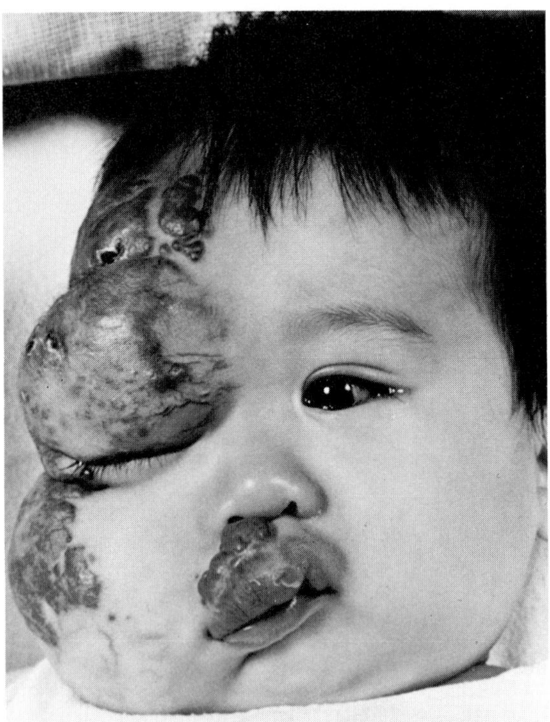

FIGURE 15–4. Mixed cavernous and capillary hemangioma of the face in a 14-month-old child. Remarkably, airway management by mask and laryngoscopy was not difficult.

Patients on systemic corticosteroids require additional coverage during the perioperative period.

Kasabach-Merritt Syndrome. In this syndrome, infants with giant hemangiomas, usually of the cavernous type, develop thrombocytopenia, hypofibrinogenemia, and a chronic consumption coagulopathy, which can precipitate acute hemorrhage and a sudden increase in the size of the lesion.[1] Platelets entrapped within the cavities are thought continuously to stimulate activation of the clotting mechanism.[37, 38] High-output cardiac failure may be aggravated by a secondary anemia. Volume resuscitation with blood products may be required, and repeated platelet administrations may be necessary to correct ongoing thrombocytopenia.

Systemic corticosteroid therapy is recommended as the treatment of choice, but radiotherapy and intralesional steroids have been reported to be successful.[35] Conservative management is preferred to surgical excision, which could precipitate disseminated intravascular coagulation.[12]

Diffuse Neonatal Hemangiomatosis. In this severe multisystemic disorder, multiple hemangiomas develop in the skin and most viscera, producing arteriovenous shunts and high-output congestive cardiac failure, complicated by thrombocytopenia and hemorrhage. The organ systems usually involved are the gastrointestinal tract and liver, central nervous system, and lungs. Few infants survive past 2 to 3 months of age, usually dying of cardiac failure, sepsis, respiratory obstruction, or central nervous system catastrophes.[9] Some response has been reported with systemic corticosteroids and radiotherapy. If cardiac failure cannot otherwise be controlled, some benefit from hepatic artery ligation is reported.[7]

These children are critically ill and deserve aggressive attempts to optimize their circulating blood volume, cardiac and respiratory status, and hemostatic mechanisms preoperatively. Central venous and arterial lines may be necessary for the evaluation of volume resuscitation and cardiovascular function. A reliable intravenous cannula is essential for perioperative blood product and fluid administration, and for postoperative intravenous alimentation when required.

Klippel-Trenaunay-Weber Syndrome. This noninherited condition is characterized by a variety of vascular malformations, including port wine nevus, venous varicosities, and arteriovenous aneurysms that develop in one or more extremities, usually the legs. Hypertrophy of regional soft tissues and bones occurs secondary to the increased limb blood flow (Fig. 15–5). There may be associated polydactyly and syndactyly. If the functional arteriovenous shunt is significant, high-output cardiac failure may develop.[7] The treatment for this otherwise benign disorder is usually conservative, but occasionally plastic reconstructive surgery and varicectomy are recommended.[40, 41]

It is important to recognize that children with Klippel-Trenaunay-Weber syndrome who have an increased cardiac output will not tolerate anesthetic agents that decrease myocardial contractility.

Sturge-Weber Syndrome (Encephalotrigeminal Angiomatosis). The diagnostic features of this syndrome are the presence of a port wine stain on the face in the distribution of the ophthalmic division of the trigeminal nerve and ipsilateral intracranial linear calcifications. Focal seizures and hemiparesis occur contralateral to the facial lesion. The vascular nevus is present at birth, but the neurological signs may not develop until later in childhood.[1, 8] Congenital glaucoma on the affected side is seen in 40 to 50 percent of patients.[7] Mental retardation is occasionally seen. In some cases, excision of the leptomeningeal angiomatosis is practical and of help in the treatment of seizures. Hemispherectomy may be indicated in some children under the age of 2 years.

TELANGIECTASIAS

Ataxia-Telangiectasia (Louis-Bar Syndrome). This autosomal recessive disorder presents as progressive cerebellar ataxia in children 12 to 18 months old. Oculocutaneous telangiectasia appears at about age 3 to 5 years on the conjunctiva and on the skin of the eyelids, face, ears, upper chest, and popliteal and antecubital

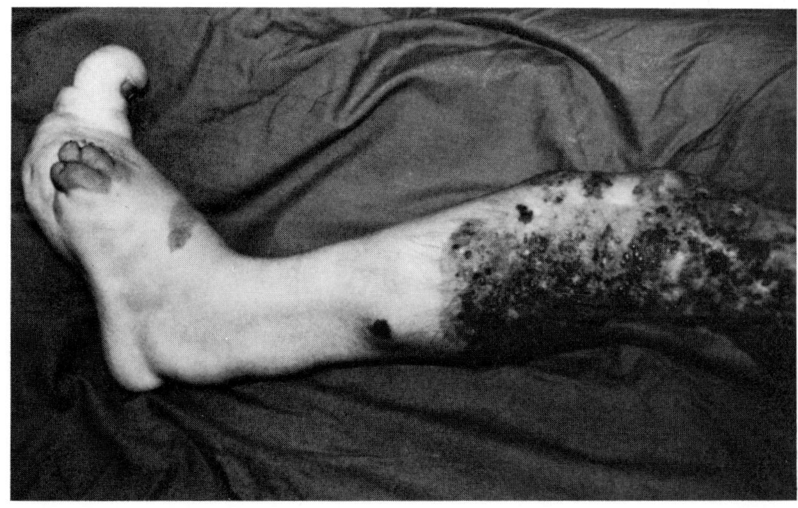

FIGURE 15–5. Klippel-Trenaunay-Weber syndrome in a 7-year-old boy demonstrating cutaneous phlebectasias and regional soft tissue and bone hypertrophy of the lower extremity.

fossae. Occasionally, café au lait spots are seen.[1] Deficiencies in the immune response are manifested by recurrent sinus and pulmonary infections and bronchiectasis, which may be fatal. Immunological deficiencies may include absent IgA and IgE and a flawed response to bacterial antigens.[4] Many children who survive to adolescence develop malignant lymphomas.[8] No specific treatment can be offered.

The principles of anesthetic management are directed at the complications of the disease, namely, the chronic pulmonary infections, bronchiectasis, and the development of lymphoreticular malignant tumors.

Hereditary Hemorrhagic Telangiectasia (Osler-Weber-Rendu Syndrome). Hereditary hemorrhagic telangiectasia is an autosomal dominant condition manifested by delicate ectatic vascular lesions in the skin, mucous membranes, and viscera. The telangiectasias are found most commonly in the nasal mucosa, lips, tongue, and gastrointestinal tract and less commonly in the bladder, bronchi, liver, and brain. Pulmonary lesions tend to resemble arteriovenous fistulae. The syndrome may present in childhood as repeated episodes of epistaxis. The diagnosis may be missed in the absence of a positive family history, because only at puberty do the skin lesions develop and subsequently increase in number. Infrequently the disease may present with gastrointestinal hemorrhage in infancy.[42]

Although clotting factors are normal, bleeding may be difficult to control. Hemorrhage is the most serious complication and may result in severe anemia. In an attempt to control mucosal bleeding, skin grafting to the nasal mucosa has been helpful although the telangiectasias continue to develop around the graft site.[43] Estrogen therapy to induce squamous metaplasia has had limited success. Embolization therapy and laser excision of the abnormal blood vessels has been helpful.

Prior to the induction of anesthesia, significant anemia or hypovolemia must be corrected. Care must be taken not to traumatize oral mucosal lesions during laryngoscopy. Nasal intubation is relatively contraindicated.

LYMPHANGIOMAS

Lymphangiomas are hamartomatous malformations composed of dilated lymph channels lined by normal lymph endothelium. There are four clinical types: simple lymphangiomas, lymphangioma circumscriptum, cavernous lymphangiomas, and cystic hygromas. They may vary greatly in size. The lesions are present at birth or develop in early infancy; they are usually slow growing, do not spontaneously involute, and are not radiosensitive. Lymphangiomas occur most commonly on the proximal limbs, shoulders, neck, tongue, and buccal mucosa. Symptoms are caused by compression of local structures. Surgical excision is often unsatisfactory, as recurrence of these lesions is frequent.

Cystic hygromas are uncommon, large, multiloculated cystic lymphangiomas, usually occurring on the neck, although the axilla, groin, and popliteal fossa are other reported sites (Fig. 15–6). They are frequently present at birth and may grow rapidly, infiltrating adjacent vessels, muscles, and nerves.[1] When cystic hygromas occur on the neck, intubation may be difficult, and tracheostomy is often required to protect the child from subsequent airway obstruction.[44, 45]

VESICULOBULLOUS DISORDERS

Common to all the vesiculobullous disorders is a disturbance of intraepidermal or dermal-

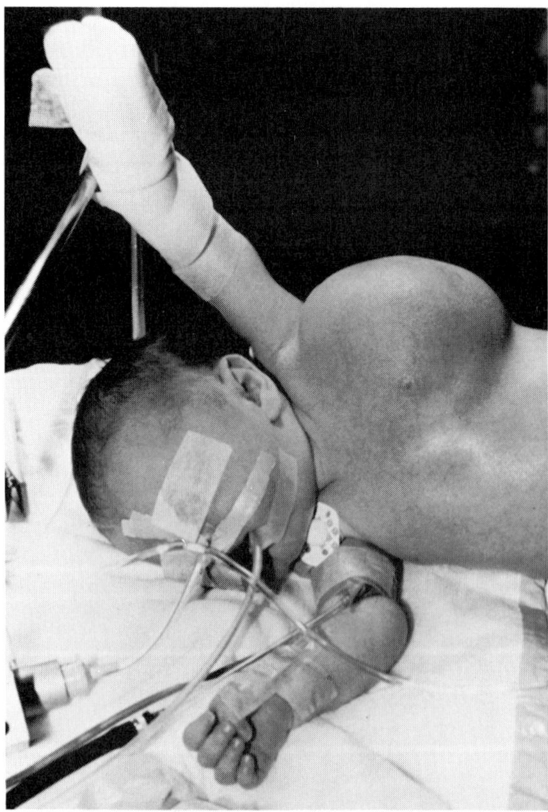

FIGURE 15–6. Recurrent cystic hygroma in the left axilla of a 10-month-old girl positioned for surgical excision.

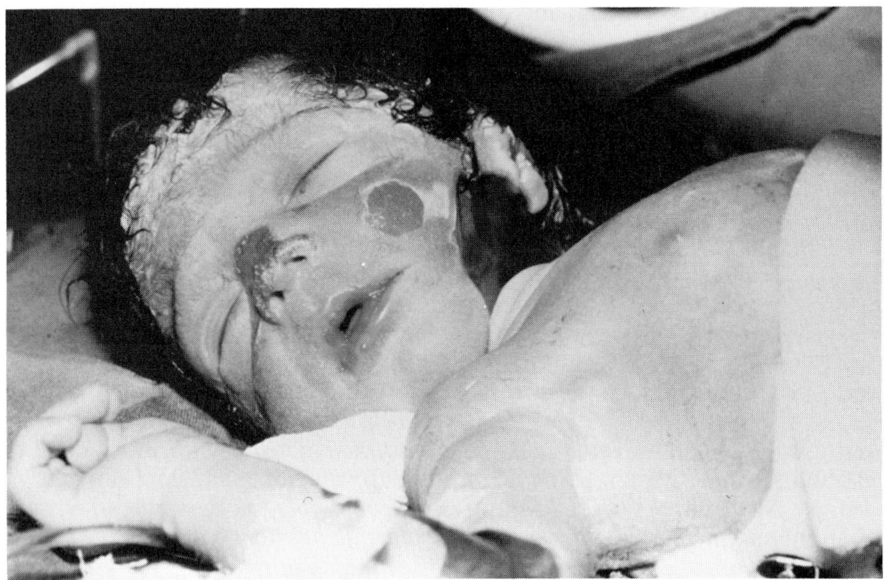

FIGURE 15–7. Junctional epidermolysis bullosa in a 3-month-old infant.

epidermal adherence with the subsequent accumulation of serous fluid within the cavities formed by tissue separation. Many pathological mechanisms lead to blister formation. A clinical sign, called Nikolsky's sign, is seen in many of these diseases. Layers of the epidermis or the dermal-epidermal junction itself separate with minor lateral or oblique friction forces, leading to the formation of blisters. These may occasionally be hemorrhagic.

Immunological techniques for diagnosis and for treatment evaluation have suggested that the immune system may feature in the pathogenesis of these disorders and explain their frequent association with connective tissue disorders such as systemic lupus erythematosus.

Epidermolysis Bullosa

Epidermolysis bullosa ia a rare subgroup of the mechanobullous diseases, characterized by blister formation initiated by minor trauma and heat to the skin. The various forms of epidermolysis bullosa are divided into scarring or nonscarring categories. The severity of the disease, however, is determined more by the extent of the bullous lesions and subsequent complications than by the presence of scarring alone, which merely reflects the depth of the cleavage plane.[3] Of the nearly 20 variants of this disease, only the more important will be reviewed.

The *nonscarring category* includes epidermolysis bullosa simplex, junctional epidermolysis bullosa (letalis), and Bart's syndrome.

Epidermolysis bullosa simplex is inherited as an autosomal dominant trait. The generalized form (Koebner's) presents in the neonate as intraepidermal blisters on the hands, feet, elbows, knees, legs, and scalp, but any skin surface may be involved. Intraoral lesions are minimal. Affected infants are usually vigorous; the lesions heal quickly without scarring, and exacerbations tend to decrease with age. Life span is normal. In the localized form (Weber-Cockayne), which presents in early childhood to adulthood, the bullae are limited to the hands and feet. There are no oral lesions. The incidence of both forms increases in warmer climates and in summer.[1, 46]

Junctional epidermolysis bullosa (letalis), an autosomal recessive disorder, presents at birth as severe subepidermal blisters on the scalp and extremities, which may eventually involve the entire cutaneous surface, sparing only the palms and soles[1, 8] (Fig. 15–7). Oral lesions are severe and may extend to the esophagus. The lesions heal slowly, often becoming secondarily infected and forming chronic granulomas, which may lead to scarring. A refractory anemia is common. The disease is progressive, and death from septicemia usually occurs in the early months or before age 2 years.

Bart described a syndrome of congenital localized absence of the skin and blistering, usually on the legs, with dystrophic nail changes. This variant may be a form of epidermolysis bullosa and has a good prognosis.[27]

The *scarring category* includes dystrophic epidermolysis bullosa, which has dominant and recessive forms.

Dystrophic epidermolysis bullosa, autosomal dominant form (Cockayne-Touraine), presents in early infancy with subepidermal bullae, usually limited to the hands, feet, and sacral area, which heal rapidly to leave soft, superficial wrinkled scars. Deformities are uncommon, and oral lesions are minor. The general health of children with this form and the prognosis are often good.

Dystrophic epidermolysis bullosa, autosomal recessive form (also polydysplastic, mutilans), although rare (1 in 300,000),[1] is the most incapacitating variant of the disorder. It presents at birth or in early infancy with severe, erosive, subepidermal bullae that heal slowly with atrophic scarring. All areas of the skin are vulnerable. Continuous mucous membrane involvement may be unrelenting, involving the mouth, pharynx, esophagus, and anus, and may cause severe feeding problems and nutritional deprivation, even in older children. Anemia and growth retardation are common. Repeat cycles of bulla formation and healing by scarring lead to strictures of the mouth, tongue, larynx, and esophagus and produce the mitten-hand deformity from digital fusion[46, 51] (Fig. 15–8). Joint contractures also occur. The overall prognosis is poor, and death usually occurs in the first three decades.

The underlying etiology of this disease is unknown. No specific effective treatment is available. Therapy is supportive and directed at skin care and at the management of complications such as anemia, malnutrition, and infections as they arise. Systemic corticosteroids are used in critical periods and may be palliative for such complications as esophageal strictures.[48, 50] Surgical intervention in these children is usually indicated for dental restorations, reconstructive procedures on the extremities, and the excision or grafting of corneal ulcers. Anesthesia may also be required for diagnostic esophagoscopy or cystoscopy.

Anesthetic Management. Children with epidermolysis bullosa demand careful preanesthetic assessment. They are often debilitated and in poor nutritional states. They may have chronic anemias, respiratory infections, sepsis, or fluid and electrolyte disturbances. Renal disease from secondary amyloidosis has been reported.[52] Hypercoagulable states have been described.[53] The extent of active disease, vulnerable skin areas, and contractures must be carefully identified. Good rapport with a young patient will encourage cooperation at induction and may avoid a traumatizing struggle. Premedication may be necessary and should be given orally. However, awake patients are able to transfer themselves, and this will avoid the potential trauma of even gentle handling. Perioperatively, steroid supplementation may be necessary, and the use of broad-spectrum antibiotics has been suggested.

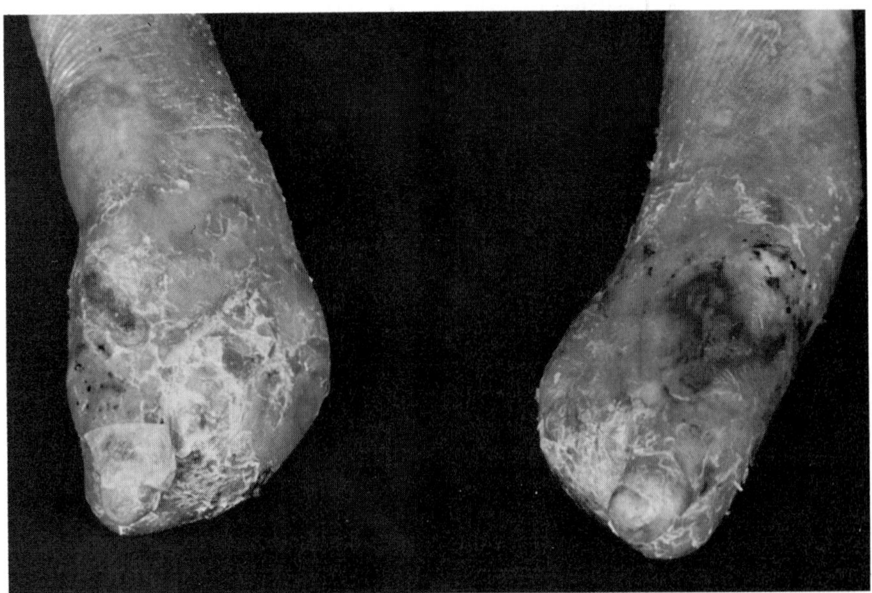

FIGURE 15–8. Dystrophic epidermolysis bullosa (recessive) in a 12-year-old boy demonstrating the classic mitten-hand deformity.

All personnel caring for these children must recognize the vulnerability of their skin to trauma. Friction is more harmful than perpendicular pressure. The bedding beneath the patient must be smooth, and adequate padding must be provided for pressure points when the patient is positioned. The removal of adhesive materials will cause skin loss, and where possible these materials should be avoided.

Monitoring is a considerable challenge and should be adequate but kept to a safe minimum. The skin on the arm can be protected from a blood pressure cuff by soft cotton padding. Nonadhesive ECG contacts or plates, axillary temperature probes, and weighted precordial stethoscopes should be used. The use of indwelling temperature probes and esophageal stethoscopes should be avoided. An atraumatic spray antiseptic and careful asepsis should be used for invasive procedures; intravenous and arterial lines should be secured in place by sutures and gauze bandaging. The eyes must be protected by an ophthalmic ointment but not taped shut. The operating room must be warm for small children, in whom thermoregulation may be significantly impaired.

General anesthesia is required for most procedures in children. A great variety of induction and maintenance techniques have been successfully used.[54–65, 69–80]

Intravenous induction should be used only in patients in whom clinical assessment predicts normal airway anatomy and an uncomplicated direct laryngoscopy for intubation. However, ketamine has been used intravenously and intramuscularly with good results for induction or as the sole agent.[54, 61–63] Induction is smooth, and the airway and ventilation are usually maintained adequately.[254]

The original reports of close association between epidermolysis bullosa and porphyria[51] have been overemphasized,[66] and more recently the association has been narrowed down to dystrophic epidermolysis bullosa involving skin only and porphyria cutanea tarda.[20, 68] Barbiturates have been used often and without incident for induction,[46, 69–72] but they should be avoided in the latter group of patients. Despite the theoretical risk of hyperkalemia in patients with extensive tissue injury, no complications have been reported using succinylcholine.[46–49, 69–73] There may be increased sensitivity to the nondepolarizing neuromuscular blocking agents.[61] Halothane probably remains the inhalational agent of choice.

When general inhalational anesthesia is required for induction because of potential airway or laryngoscopy difficulties, halothane is the agent of choice. Perioral scarring may restrict the opening of the mouth, the tongue may be distorted by adhesions,[72] and the larynx may be stenosed.[47, 51] The application of a face mask and finger support of the mandible may induce blister formation (Fig. 15–9). Inhalational induction may be achieved by delivering warmed and humidified anesthetic agents at high flows from a mask held just above the face. Several noncontact induction hoods or boxes have been proposed.[74, 75] Prior to mask or finger contact, the skin of the face and chin should be protected by 0.5 percent hydrocortisone cream or by cotton sponges soaked in saline, petroleum jelly (Vaseline), or other lubricant.[65, 73] The use of oropharyngeal airways is discouraged in most reports.[12]

When required, intubation should be performed very gently and with the patient sufficiently deeply anesthetized or paralyzed to facilitate the procedure. MacIntosh's blade is preferred, to minimize contact with the epiglottis.[76] The blade and endotracheal tube must be generously lubricated to reduce friction and a smaller tube than usual selected. The tube should be secured by soft flannel ties or by an external fixation device to avoid skin contact.[65] To avoid coughing, the patient may be extu-

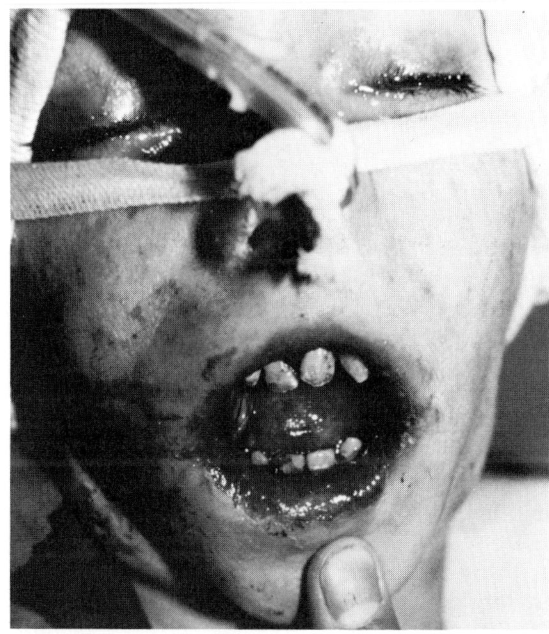

FIGURE 15–9. Dystrophic epidermolysis bullosa (recessive) in a 12-year-old boy. Note the ulceration of tongue and lips discovered after the removal of the dental dam following a 90-minute anesthesia for dental restorations.

bated deep (unless contraindicated) or following intravenous lidocaine, 1 to 1.5 mg/kg.

Fiberoptic laryngoscopy and intubation have not yet been described in patients with epidermolysis bullosa, but where airway anatomy is distorted this technique, carefully performed, may be very useful. A small-diameter, well-lubricated laryngoscope should be used to direct a warmed, softened endotracheal tube.

Preoperative airway obstruction from pharyngeal bullae has been described.[78] However, the literature is not very helpful in identifying the risk of intra- or postoperative airway obstruction following airway instrumentation and extubation.[46, 71, 73] James and Wark, in a retrospective study of 113 oral and 18 nasal intubations, reported only 3 cases of intraoral bullae formation directly attributable to intubation, and none caused postoperative airway problems.[70]

Despite the rarity of reports of postextubation airway problems from bullae or hemorrhage, such obstruction is a grave complication and all patients must be carefully observed in the postanesthetic period.

In recent years, there has been a great increase in the reports of regional blocks in children with epidermolysis bullosa for extremity and perineal surgery. Experiences with spinal, epidural, caudal, and brachial plexus techniques are described.[79–84] In appropriate patients, regional anesthesia offers significant advantages.

The patient must be carefully observed for airway problems throughout the postanesthetic recovery period.

Erythema Multiforme

The term *erythema multiforme* represents a spectrum of acute reactive, inflammatory diseases involving the skin and mucous membranes, ranging from a mild illness, erythema multiforme minor, to a severe, life-threatening condition, erythema multiforme major or the Stevens-Johnson syndrome.[85] The disorder is relatively common, accounting for up to 1 percent of dermatology outpatient visits. Although the disorder is rare in children under 3 years, more than 50 percent of patients are under age 20 years; 60 percent are males. Young adults and children, especially boys, present with the more severe form.

Many etiological factors have been implicated in the precipitation of erythema multiforme. Infections are the best documented and include viral infections with herpes simplex and adenovirus and *Mycoplasma* infections, particularly with *M. pneumoniae.* Drugs are associated with 60 percent of cases but are often falsely implicated because many are administered for the prodromal symptoms of the infections or of the disease itself.[1] These include the sulfonamides, penicillin, the hydantoin anticonvulsants, barbiturates, salicylates, hydralazine, and many others.[86] Erythema multiforme is seen in association with malignancies, usually lymphomas, and some connective tissue diseases, notably systemic lupus erythematosus.[87] The discovery of deposits of IgM, complement, and fibrin in dermal vessels suggests a hypersensitivity or immune complex etiology.[88]

Erythema multiforme minor presents with a nonspecific prodrome of malaise, low-grade fever, arthralgias, and symptoms of an upper respiratory tract infection, often in the spring and fall. The rash is usually symmetrical and distributed over the extensor surfaces of the extremities, including the palms and soles, the conjunctiva, and rarely the oral mucosa. The patient is usually asymptomatic, although the oral lesions may burn. The exanthem begins as dull, red macules that expand and then clear centrally, to form characteristic target or iris lesions. Urticarial plaques may be seen.[1] Occasionally the macules progress to vesicle formation in more severe cases. Successive crops of lesions may appear, but the rash rarely persists for more than 2 weeks. Apart from symptomatic measures, no specific treatment is required. Short-term corticosteroid therapy may be helpful in the more severe cases.

Erythema multiforme major (Stevens-Johnson syndrome)[67] is an uncommon but severe disease with a mortality rate, if untreated, of 5 to 15 percent.[1] Prodromal symptoms of malaise, fever, headache, sore throat, cough, chest pain, vomiting and diarrhea, myalgia, and arthralgia occur 1 to 14 days prior to the sudden onset of erosive bullous lesions on the skin and mucous membranes. The oral mucosa, lips, and bulbar conjunctiva are the most frequently and most severely involved areas (Fig. 15–10). The painful, erosive bullae may extend from the mouth and lips to the external nares, pharynx, esophagus, larynx, and tracheobronchial tree and involve the genital areas. Eating and breathing are uncomfortable and difficult. The ocular lesions include purulent conjunctivitis, corneal ulcerations, anterior uveitis, and staphylococcal panophthalmitis.[91] Blindness may ensue. Bullae in the visceral pleura may lead to pneumothorax,[92] and large pleural effusions may develop.[94, 95] Gastrointestinal tract ulceration and hemorrhage have occurred.[93] Poor nutrition, anemia, and fluid and electrolyte distur-

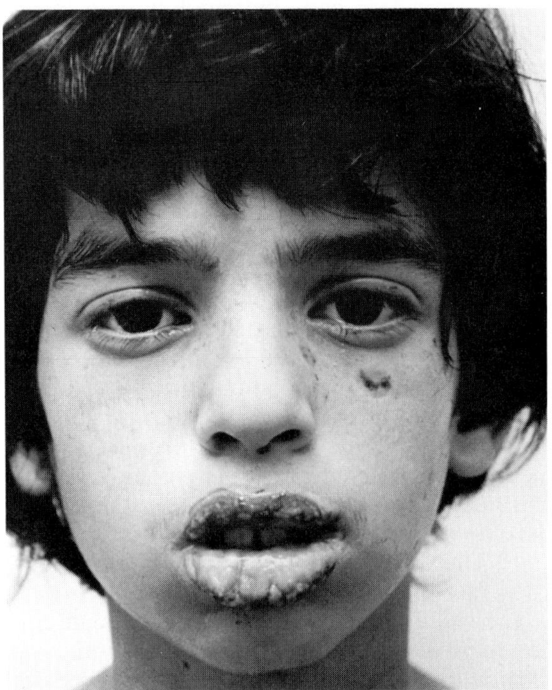

FIGURE 15–10. A mild example of Stevens-Johnson syndrome, demonstrating the oral lesions and conjunctivitis.

bances are frequent. Acute tubular necrosis, nephritis, and renal failure have been described. Cardiac involvement may be manifested by atrial fibrillation, pericarditis, and myocarditis.[96] Fatal complications usually arise from widespread epidermal necrolysis, respiratory obstruction, pulmonary infection, and septicemia.

The treatment of Stevens-Johnson syndrome is essentially supportive but requires hospital supervision. Precipitating infections and associated diseases should be treated, and implicated medications should be discontinued. Skin lesions are best managed with wet dressings and baths. Fluid and electrolyte disturbances must be corrected quickly. Intravenous alimentation may be required in younger children.[93] Secondary infections must be promptly treated with antibiotics. Systemic corticosteroids are usually administered in high doses during the stage of mucocutaneous extension and slowly tapered during the 1- to 3-week healing phase.[97] Resolution of the disease may take 2 to 7 weeks. Recurrences are seen in all forms of erythema multiforme in 25 percent of cases.

Anesthetic Management. Children with erythema multiforme present a major challenge to the anesthetist.[93–95] They are usually febrile and toxic and distressed by the painful lesions. Hypovolemia, anemia, and electrolyte disturbances must be corrected preoperatively. Percutaneous intravenous cannulation is preferred because cutdown incisions heal poorly and are vulnerable to infection. In very ill patients, no premedication is recommended.

Monitoring is important, but extreme care is required to avoid skin trauma. The arm may be protected from the blood pressure cuff by a soft roll, and a weighted precordial stethoscope may be used. ECG monitoring to identify dysrhythmias is necessary, but adhesive electrodes should not be used and the removal of electrodes must be gentle. Temperature should be monitored by an axillary probe; esophageal stethoscopes and nasal temperature probes should not be used. The presence of urethritis may discourage the use of urinary catheters. Appropriate physical means to control pyrexia (for example, cooling blankets) should be available.

If general anesthesia is required, airway maintenance poses many potential problems.[93–95] If obstructing bullae or edema compromises the upper airway, a tracheostomy (not without its own risks) may be required preoperatively.[12] The application of a face mask may denude affected skin, and the face must be protected by lubricated cotton or gauze sponges. The insertion of oral airways and laryngoscopy and intubation, however gentle, may traumatize existing bullae or laryngeal and tracheal mucosa sufficiently to initiate bleeding or bulla formation.

Induction techniques depend on the operation planned. Ketamine has been used as the sole agent.[93] Barbiturates are often implicated as a causal agent in erythema multiforme and should be avoided. Otherwise, a cautious inhalational induction is preferred. There are no reports of adverse reactions to neuromuscular blocking agents. Pancuronium or vecuronium is probably the nondepolarizing agent of choice. Because chest radiographs may not identify pleural bullae, positive-pressure ventilation should be avoided or used with the lowest possible peak airway pressure. Be alert to the possibility of pneumothorax. Corticosteroid coverage for the operative period likely will be required. The potential for postextubation airway obstruction is high in these patients, and close supervision must be provided.

Regional anesthesia may be a useful alternative if the overlying skin is clear and the child is cooperative.

Toxic Epidermal Necrolysis (Lyell's Disease)

Toxic epidermal necrolysis is a rare but extremely severe acute bullous eruption of the skin and mucous membranes that is seen in all age groups. The highest mortality rates (20 to 40 percent) are in young children and the elderly.[1, 3, 12] It may represent the most devastating variant of erythema multiforme.

A short prodrome of fever, malaise, and conjunctivitis usually precedes the acute development of mildly tender, diffuse erythema, which may be widespread. Nikolsky's sign (separation of the epidermis with lateral finger pressure) is present early. Confluent, flaccid bullae develop quickly and rupture, shedding large sheets of epidermis and leaving huge, denuded, erosive areas on the back, shoulders, and face. Severe mucous membrane lesions are common and involve the oropharynx, tongue, larynx, tracheobronchial tree, and esophagus, often resulting in tracheitis, pneumonia, and gastrointestinal hemorrhage.[1, 3] The course may be relentlessly progressive for 1 or more weeks and may be complicated by high fever, hypovolemia, electrolyte imbalance, secondary infections and septicemia, shock, renal impairment, and disseminated intravascular coagulation.[99, 100] Recovery is slow; healing may lead to scarring contractures of both skin and mucous membranes.

The etiological factors implicated in toxic epidermal necrolysis are similar to those responsible for erythema multiforme: drugs, including barbiturates, analgesics, and hydantoin anticonvulsants[86, 101, 102]; viral, bacterial, and fungal infections; vaccinations; radiation; and malignancies, notably lymphomas.[1, 8] Histological studies show necrosis of basal epidermal cell layers and subepidermal bulla formation.

The prognosis depends on the adequacy of treatment but is always guarded. High-dose systemic corticosteroid therapy, aggressive antibiotic control of secondary infections, and correction of fluid and electrolyte imbalance are mandatory. Local skin care, particularly of the mouth and eyes, is important.

The principles of anesthetic management in patients with toxic epidermal necrolysis are similar to those for erythema multiforme and epidermolysis bullosa. Careful attention must be paid to thermoregulation in small children.

Staphylococcal Scalded Skin Syndrome (Ritter Disease)

Staphylococcal scalded skin syndrome is an uncommon superficial cutaneous eruption manifested as widespread epidermolysis and intraepidermal desquamation.[1] It occurs in infants and young children either as a localized form, called bullous impetigo, or as a generalized form (Ritter disease).

Following a variable prodrome of malaise, conjunctivitis, or occult upper respiratory tract infection, a periorificial or generalized scarlatiniform rash appears that is exquisitely tender. Nikolsky's sign is present early. Within 48 hours, large, flaccid intraepidermal bullae develop, and sheets of epidermis separate. The moist erythematous base thus exposed usually dries quickly, with superficial desquamation (Fig. 15–11). Although the skin around the mouth and genitals is most commonly affected, mucosal involvement is rare. Healing is usually complete in 5 to 12 days, but a small number of patients may develop cellulitis, pneumonia, and septicemia.[1, 104, 105] The disease still carries a significant mortality rate of 2 to 3 percent.[1]

The syndrome is caused by the exotoxin epidermolysin, which is produced by infections with *Staphylococcus aureus* group II, phage type 71. It is distinct from toxic epidermal necrolysis,

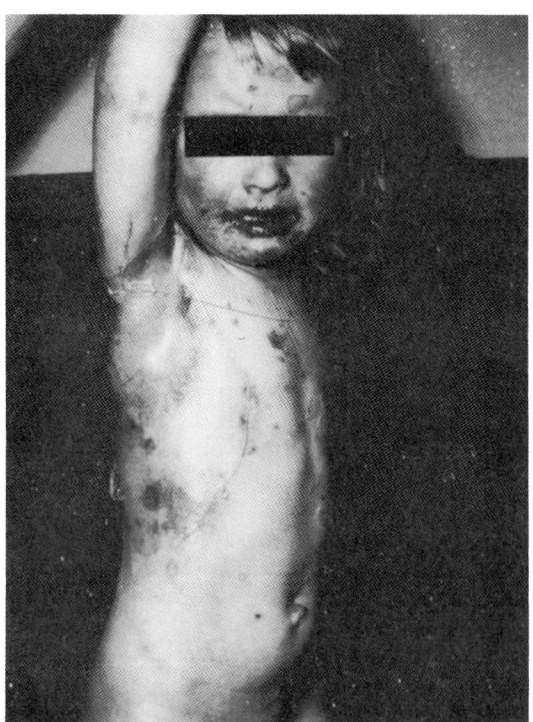

FIGURE 15–11. Staphylococcal scalded skin syndrome. Because the lesions so closely resemble scalds, mistaken allegations of child abuse have occasionally been made. (From Orkin, M., Maibach, H. I., Dahl, M. V. [eds.]. Dermatology. Norwalk, CT, Appleton & Lange, 1991.)

which is often drug-induced, because basal epidermal cell necrosis does not occur. Treatment requires strict isolation, the administration of penicillinase-resistant antibiotics, attention to hydration and electrolyte balance, and local skin care.[104, 105] The use of corticosteroids is considered only in those patients who become critically ill.

The anesthetic management of children with this disorder requires the preoperative correction of fluid and electrolyte disturbances and the recognition of complicating secondary infections such as pneumonia. Contact with involved skin is painful, and the patient must be handled gently. Anticholinergic agents should be used with caution because thermoregulation may be impaired. Temperature monitoring is mandatory.

No specific anesthetic technique is recommended, but local cutaneous infiltration should be avoided. When inhalational anesthesia is used, the face must be protected to prevent frictional trauma and bulla formation.[106] Adhesives should be avoided. Instrumentation of the airway must be cautious in the presence of mucosal involvement.

All equipment used should be regarded as septic and cleaned appropriately after use.[12]

Pemphigus, Pemphigoid, Dermatitis Herpetiformis, and Chronic Bullous Dermatosis of Childhood

The term pemphigus refers to a group of autoimmune bullous diseases involving the skin and mucous membranes, which all demonstrate the presence of serum antibodies directed against squamous epithelial intercellular substance.[107–109] The subsequent loss of cohesive epidermal cell bridges is called acantholysis and leads to intraepidermal bulla formation at varying depths.[1] Nikolsky's sign is frequently seen. Although pemphigus is most common in adults, three forms are recognized as occurring during childhood.

Pemphigus vulgaris most typically presents in the fourth and fifth decades of life and in people of Jewish and Mediterranean origin but has been reported in all races and in children as young as 3.5 years old.[111] A genetic link is suggested but has not been proved. In children, the disease is first manifested as painful oral ulcers and subsequently as large, flaccid, suprabasal bullae, most commonly on the scalp, face, and trunk. These lesions tend to enlarge and rupture, producing painful denuded areas that heal slowly. Oropharyngeal lesions may compromise adequate nutrition, and laryngeal lesions may cause hoarseness.[12] No other organ systems are primarily affected in children, but progressive disease may produce fluid and electrolyte disturbances or hypoalbuminemia and may be complicated by secondary infection and sepsis. Untreated, the mortality may reach 90 percent.[1] Pemphigus vulgaris has been found in association with thymomas and myasthenia gravis, lymphoid malignancies, and systemic lupus erythematosus.[112] An important differential diagnosis in children is erythema multiforme.

Pemphigus foliaceus is less common and less severe than pemphigus vulgaris. The cleavage plain is higher in the epidermis, and the bullae are superficial. They rupture easily to produce shallow erosions with scaling and crusting, which may be intensely pruritic. Common areas of involvement are the scalp, face, and upper chest, although generalized extension of the disease has been seen. Oral lesions are infrequent. A localized variant of this form, pemphigus erythematosus, presents as a lupus-like butterfly rash on the face. The prognosis is generally good.

Familial benign pemphigus (Hailey-Hailey disease) is inherited as an autosomal dominant trait and usually presents in the second decade as small pruritic vesicles on an erythematous base in the axilla, groin, and antecubital fossae. General health is not affected. Remissions occur, but there is little tendency to improvement with age.[1]

The successful treatment of pemphigus vulgaris requires prompt, high-dose systemic corticosteroid therapy, particularly during acute exacerbations. Local skin care with wet compresses is important. During critical periods with patients on steroids, secondary infections and fluid and electrolyte disturbances must be managed aggressively. Supplemental immunosuppressive agents, methotrexate, cyclophosphamide, and azathioprine have reduced maintenance steroid requirements.[114–116] Parenteral gold therapy has been a useful alternative in some patients.[1] Less severe forms of pemphigus respond well to lower doses of steroids; even topical preparations may be adequate.

Bullous pemphigoid is similar to but distinct from pemphigus, from which it is differentiated histologically by the presence of subepidermal bullae. It occurs rarely in children, in whom it presents as large, tense bullae over intertriginous areas, the flexor surfaces of the forearm, the groin, and the lower abdomen.[8, 118] Mucous membrane lesions are reported in 10 to 20 percent of cases and include the mouth, pharynx, esophagus, vagina, and anus. The bullae may rupture, leaving denuded areas, but these tend to heal well. Pruritus is less a feature, and the patient's general condition is good. The disease tends to be chronic but shows remissions and improvement over time.

Treatment includes systemic corticosteroids and immunosuppresive agents, but in lower doses than for pemphigus. Sulfapyridine and dapsone have been helpful.[117, 118]

Dermatitis herpetiformis is a chronic eruptive disease characterized by intensely pruritic, small, tense papules and vesicles grouped symmetrically over the extensor surfaces of the extremities, the buttocks, and the scalp. In the juvenile form, lesions may appear in the axillae and groin. The mucous membranes are usually spared. This disorder occurs in all age groups but most commonly in middle life. The etiology is unknown, but there is a strong association with celiac sprue (gluten-sensitive enteropathy), and an immunodeficiency mechanism is postulated.[1, 4] No cure is available, but effective suppression of the disease is possible by maintenance doses of sulfapyridine or dapsone.[4, 6]

Chronic bullous dermatosis of childhood (linear IgA dermatosis) is a noninherited disorder presenting in preschool children as deep, tense, 1- to 2-cm bullae on the lower trunk, perineum, and thighs, and occasionally on the scalp and face. This condition may resemble bullous pemphigoid and dermatitis herpetiformis but tends to be self-limiting and remits within 1 to 4 years of onset.[3, 4] Treatment includes a combination of corticosteroids, sulfapyridine, and dapsone.

Anesthetic Management. Evidence of the diseases associated with pemphigus must be sought and recognized in the preoperative assessment. These diseases include systemic lupus erythematosus, rheumatoid arthritis, lymphoid malignancies, thymoma, and myasthenia gravis. Each requires additional considerations for anesthetic management.[112] The effects of maintenance medications must be evaluated in relevant systems. Immunosuppressive agents may cause bone marrow suppression, hepatic dysfunction, and infiltrative pneumonitis. Sulfapyridine causes crystalluria and may impair renal function. Dapsone may induce a chronic hemolytic anemia[16] and a peripheral neuropathy.[12] Perioperative corticosteroid coverage usually will be required. In acute exacerbations, children with pemphigus may develop secondary infections, fluid and electrolyte disturbances, and hypovolemia.

No particular anesthetic techniques have been recommended in these patients, but local infiltration is contraindicated because of potential skin slough. In adults, the successful use has been reported of regional anesthesia by peridural catheter supplemented by ketamine,[120] and of a combination of ketamine and diazepam as sole agents.[121, 122]

When present, the facial, oropharyngeal, and laryngeal lesions produce difficulties for airway management similar to those in patients with epidermolysis bullosa, and the same principles apply. Skin surfaces must be carefully protected, and airway instrumentation, if required, must be cautious and gentle.

Acrodermatitis Enteropathica

Acrodermatitis enteropathica is a rare autosomal recessive disorder of zinc metabolism, presenting in the first year of life as an acral and periorificial vesiculobullous eruption, followed by alopecia, severe diarrhea, failure to thrive, and progressive cachexia.[1, 123] Associated manifestations include glossitis, stomatitis, and secondary bacterial and candidal infections. Untreated, the course is chronic and relapsing. Acute exacerbations may be fatal.

The metabolic defect appears to be related to the intestinal absorption of zinc, and oral zinc preparations rapidly abolish manifestations of the disease.[124]

Children with acrodermatitis enteropathica may be debilitated, nutritionally deprived, hypovolemic, anemic, and weak from muscle loss. The preoperative correction of treatable parameters should be undertaken. Under anesthesia, these children may show poor tolerance to inhalational agents and sensitivity to narcotics and neuromuscular blocking agents.

DISORDERS OF THE EPIDERMIS

Psoriasis

Psoriasis is a chronic papulosquamous dermatosis characterized by epidermal hyperplasia and increased epidermal turnover. The incidence varies from 0.1 to 3 percent, with equal frequency in males and females.[1] Presentation before age 16 years is reported in 30 to 45 percent of cases. The onset of psoriasis in childhood (mean age, 8.1 years) is associated with a strong family history and is twice as common in girls as in boys.[101, 126] The etiology includes both genetic and environmental factors.

The initial appearance and subsequent outbreaks of the eruption may follow epidermal injury (Koebner's reaction), infections, stress, cold weather, or withdrawal from corticosteroid therapy. The lesions are discrete erythematous papules and plaques covered with silvery scales, and they occur usually on the scalp, face, elbows, and knees. Pitting of the fingernails is characteristic. Mucosal lesions are rare. The increased blood flow to the subepidermal cutis in the generalized form, psoriatic erythroderma, has caused high-output cardiac failure in adults.[127, 128] Psoriatic lesions are culture-positive for *Staphylococcus aureus* in 30 percent of cases.[129] The arthropathy seen in 5 percent of adults with psoriasis is infrequently diagnosed in children and is rarely severe.[130, 131] Temporomandibular joint ankylosis has been reported in a 28-year-old man.[132] Hyperuricemia is seen in more extensive disease, but without gout.

The variant most commonly seen in children is guttate psoriasis, in which the lesions are small, teardrop plaques on the scalp, face, trunk, and proximal limbs (Fig. 15–12). There is frequently a history of prior streptococcal respiratory tract infection. Diaper psoriasis precedes chronic psoriasis in 17 percent of cases.[3] Neonatal psoriasis, although rare, is severe and recalcitrant and may be complicated by early joint involvement.[133] Children rarely develop the unusual manifestations of the disease, such as pustular psoriasis and psoriatic erythroderma.

The management of childhood psoriasis is conservative. Topical therapy with tar preparations, keratolytic agents, and low-dose ultraviolet light precedes the cautious addition of topical corticosteroids. Systemic steroids and methotrexate are avoided in children if possible. Prophylactic penicillin or tonsillectomy may reduce poststreptococcal guttatic flare-ups.[126]

Anesthetic considerations in children with psoriasis include the preoperative evaluation of the activity and extent of the disease, maintenance medications, and the identification of complications such as psoriatic arthropathy or high-output cardiac failure in psoriatic erythroderma.

No specific techniques are recommended, but several points deserve attention. It is important to prevent physical and chemical trauma to the skin, because further lesions may be precipitated. The handling and transfer of patients must be gentle. The use of adhesive tapes and ECG electrodes on areas of involved skin should be avoided if possible. The presence of *Staphylococcus aureus* in psoriatic skin demands careful aseptic techniques for intravenous cannulation and may contraindicate the use of regional blocks. Anesthetic and operating room equipment should be appropriately cleaned after use.

DISORDERS OF THE DERMIS

Ehlers-Danlos Syndrome

The Ehlers-Danlos syndrome is a heterogeneous group of inherited disorders of collagen

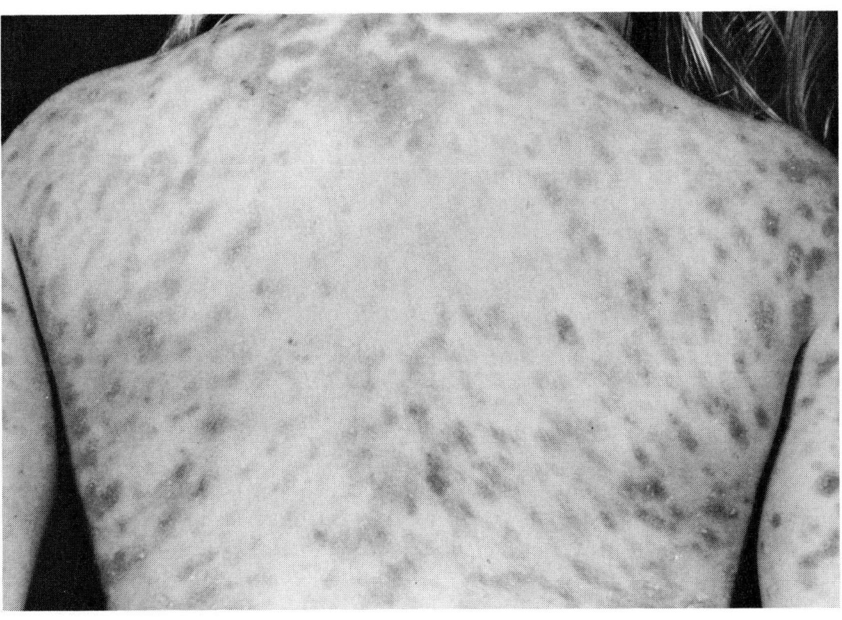

FIGURE 15–12. Guttate psoriasis in a 6-year-old girl.

synthesis. The clinical manifestations have been classified by Beighton and associates into eight distinct forms.[134] Characteristic clinical signs include hyperextensible skin, hypermobile joints, and excessive bleeding after minor trauma. The usual inheritance is autosomal dominant.

Premature birth is a frequent feature and is secondary to early rupture of the amniotic membranes, which share the connective tissue defect of the child. Transient postnatal hypotonia may predispose to pneumonia.[3] In all types, the skin is thin, hyperextensible, elastic, and very fragile. Minor trauma may result in lacerations that heal poorly, leaving thin, atrophic "cigarette paper" scars. Umbilical, femoral, and inguinal hernias are common and develop early. Joint hypermobility is manifested as congenital hip dislocation or later as spontaneous dislocations and kyphoscoliosis. Blood vessel walls are fragile, and minor trauma may induce ecchymoses or bleeding. Gastrointestinal hemorrhage and perforation are well-known complications. Varicose veins are common. The excessive bleeding, particularly in the ecchymotic form (type IV), may be explained by decreased collagen-platelet interaction, the failure of vessel constriction, and the absence of effective surrounding tissue tamponade.[135] Coagulation is usually normal, but the bleeding time is prolonged.

Cardiovascular manifestations of the disease may be minor but are unpredictable and potentially catastrophic in some patients. They include mitral valve prolapse, aortic insufficiency, conduction defects, and sudden death from spontaneous aortic aneurysm rupture.[136] Spontaneous pneumothorax has been reported.[137]

The management of Ehlers-Danlos syndrome is conservative. The potential complications of uncontrollable hemorrhage and wound dehiscence discourage invasive or surgical procedures unless absolutely necessary. The prognosis of this disorder, in the absence of arterial complications, is good, and life span may be normal.

The anesthetist must anticipate complications in managing patients with this disorder.[138] A coagulation screen, including bleeding time, should be obtained to identify the risk of excessive bleeding. Adequate blood products must be available even for minor procedures. Patients with cardiac murmurs should receive prophylactic antibiotics. Intramuscular premedication should be avoided. In the operating room, the patient must be transferred and positioned carefully to prevent skin and skeletal injuries.

Good intravenous access is mandatory but may be difficult and require surgical cutdown. Severe extravasation of intravenous fluid or hematoma formation may go unnoticed in these patients. Internal jugular or subclavian central venous lines may be complicated by mediastinal or pleural hematomas. Arterial cannulation may lead to aneurysm formation. Such invasive monitoring should be used only when essential.

Regional techniques have been used successfully despite the risk of hematoma but not reported in children.[138–140] Inhalational anesthesia by mask is the recommended technique for short, minor procedures. When intubation is required, the patient must be adequately relaxed so that airway instrumentation is smoothly accomplished, minimizing the risk of airway hematoma formation and temporomandibular joint dislocation. Peak ventilatory pressures must be kept as low as possible. Hypertension should be avoided or corrected early to reduce hemorrhage and the risk of aneurysm rupture. To minimize coughing at extubation, the endotracheal tube may be removed with the patient under deep anesthesia or after intravenous lidocaine, 1.5 mg/kg, has been administered.

Close postoperative monitoring of the patient's airway, ventilation, and blood pressure is mandatory.

Cutis Laxa

Cutis laxa is a rare congenital disorder of elastin synthesis, affecting the skin and internal organs. Inheritance may be autosomal recessive, X-linked recessive, or dominant. An acquired form, presenting later in life, may follow a febrile illness, a drug eruption, or erythema multiforme.[141] Skin biopsy specimens show deficient and disorganized elastin fibers in the dermis and vascular walls.

In all forms of the disease, the skin hangs on the body in loose, pendulous folds like an ill-fitting suit. The child looks prematurely wrinkled and aged. Unlike Ehlers-Danlos syndrome, the skin fails to recoil when released, but it does not bruise easily and heals normally. Hypermobile joints are not a feature. Infants may have a hoarse cry from vocal cord laxity.

Dominant cutis laxa may present only cosmetic problems, but the recessive forms may have multiple system manifestations. These include umbilical, inguinal, and obturator hernias, diaphragmatic atony, gastrointestinal and genitourinary tract diverticula, rectal prolapse, and generalized osteoporosis.[142] Severe cardiorespiratory complications include emphysema, peripheral pulmonary artery stenosis, pulmonary hypertension, cor pulmonale, and aneurysmal aortic dilatation. In the acquired form, severe occlusive coronary artery disease has been described in young children.[141]

No specific treatment is available, although anti-inflammatory agents and steroids may be useful in the acquired form. Complications are treated as they arise.

The chief anesthetic considerations in these children concern the severity of cardiac and pulmonary complications, in particular, cor pulmonale, aortic dilatation with valvular insufficiency, and coronary artery disease.

Pseudoxanthoma Elasticum

Pseudoxanthoma elasticum is a rare degenerative disorder of elastin tissue, involving the skin, eye, cardiovascular system, and gastrointestinal tract. It is inherited by autosomal dominant or recessive patterns and occurs in 1 per 160,000 to 1 per 1,000,000 population.[143] The diagnosis is often made after age 30 years, but many severely affected patients are children, and the disease has been reported in a 6-month-old infant.[144, 145]

The skin lesions usually appear in childhood as small yellow papules in linear or reticular patterns on the neck, axillary and inguinal folds, umbilical area, and the popliteal and antecubital fossae. The involved skin becomes lax, with poor elastic recoil, and hangs in folds. Ocular signs present as loss of visual acuity from amyloid streaks and retinal detachment.

The entire cardiovascular system is affected by the degenerative changes and calcification that develop in the arterial media. Peripheral pulses may be absent. Intermittent claudication and ischemic ulcers are frequent findings. Angina pectoris is seen in 8 percent of patients under age 20 years.[143] A triple aortocoronary bypass has been reported in an 18-year-old girl who had angina from age 11 years.[144] Dysrhythmias, renal hypertension, cerebrovascular occlusion, gastrointestinal and uterine hemorrhage, hypothyroidism, and psychotic depression have all been reported.[3, 8, 143]

There is no effective treatment. The prognosis varies considerably; despite reports of sudden death in children,[145] many patients seem to have normal longevity. Vascular surgery has often proved helpful.[146]

The primary anesthetic consideration in patients with pseudoxanthoma elasticum concerns the severity of cardiovascular complications. Even in children, a history of angina must be sought. An oral premedication to tranquilize young patients is desirable. Note that older patients may be taking maintenance tricyclic antidepressants.[143]

Monitoring must include electrocardiography and a precordial stethoscope. Blood pressure is best taken by a cuff and an ultrasonic Doppler probe. Arterial cannulation is difficult and may accelerate distal vascular ischemia, but it may be necessary in critically ill patients.[116] Myocardial oxygen supply and demand must be optimized by avoiding tachycardia and hypertension.

No specific anesthetic techniques or drugs are recommended.

DISORDERS OF SUBCUTANEOUS TISSUE

Lipodystrophy

The rare syndromes of partial and generalized lipodystrophy are characterized by the absence of subcutaneous fat over part of the body surface.

Partial lipodystrophy occurs more commonly in girls and presents before the age of 10 years as the progressive loss of subcutaneous fat from the face downward to the arms and upper trunk. The skin is normal, but the facies becomes cadaverous, and the muscles and veins of the trunk become prominent. Insulin-resistant diabetes mellitus develops in 20 percent of cases.[1] Many patients develop membranoproliferative glomerulonephritis, but the incidence of significant renal disease is unknown.

Congenital generalized lipodystrophy (Seip-Lawrence syndrome) is a progressive, multisystemic disorder inherited by an autosomal recessive trait. It may be present at birth as a generalized loss of subcutaneous fat or occur in early infancy. Associated features are prominent veins, hirsutism, and skin pigmentation. Hepatomegaly may be prominent even in infancy, secondary to fatty infiltration and cirrhosis. Skeletal growth is accelerated. With time, insulin-resistant nonketotic diabetes mellitus develops.[1, 8]

No specific treatment is available, but in older patients liposuction has been advocated.[147]

Anesthetic management requires attention to the control of associated diabetes mellitus and the recognition of coincident renal and hepatic dysfunction. Infants may become hypothermic easily and are vulnerable to hypoglycemia if glycogen stores are reduced.

ECZEMA

Eczema (Greek *eczein,* boiling over) is a generic term describing a particular inflammatory reaction pattern in the skin. The important forms of eczema in children are atopic dermatitis, contact dermatitis, and seborrheic dermatitis.

Atopic Dermatitis

Atopic dermatitis is a relatively common skin disorder (affecting 1 to 5 percent of children under age 5 years),[148] characterized by erythema, edema, intense pruritus, exudation, crusting, and scaling. There appears to be a genetic predilection. The onset is usually at age 2 to 3 months, with pruritic erythematous patches on the cheeks and subsequent extension to the face, neck, wrists, hands, and extensor aspects of the extremities. Constant scratching induces weeping and crusting. Secondary infection with staphylococci, beta-hemolytic streptococci, and herpes simplex virus is common and may be severe (Fig. 15–13). Remission tends to occur at age 3 to 5 years, but the disease may become relapsing and chronic.[3, 8] With increasing age, the involved areas of skin tend to dry and thicken.

About 80 percent of patients with atopic dermatitis have increased serum IgE levels, but a specific role for allergens, whether food or inhalants, is disputed.[8] Cell-mediated immunity is disordered. In a significant number of children contact dermatitis is provoked by application of a chemical or allergen to the skin surface. A significant number of children with atopic dermatitis subsequently develop reactive airway disease.[7]

The treatment of atopic dermatitis requires the avoidance of environmental precipitants. During acute flare-ups, therapy includes local care with wet dressings, antihistamines, topical corticosteroid cream, and systemic antibiotics for secondary infections.

Several considerations are important in the anesthetic management of children with atopic dermatitis. A careful history of allergies should be taken. The development of reactive airway disease in older children may favor the use of inhalational agents, such as halothane, to reduce bronchomotor tone. Affected skin sites should be avoided for intravenous cannulation, and the face, if actively involved, should be protected from mask pressure by saline-soaked gauze. Supplemental steroid coverage is rarely required.

Contact Dermatitis

Allergic contact dermatitis is a T-cell–mediated hypersensitivity reaction that is provoked by application of a chemical or allergen to the skin surface. Sensitization requires several days and becomes manifest as local, erythematous, intensely pruritic eczematous dermatitis on re-

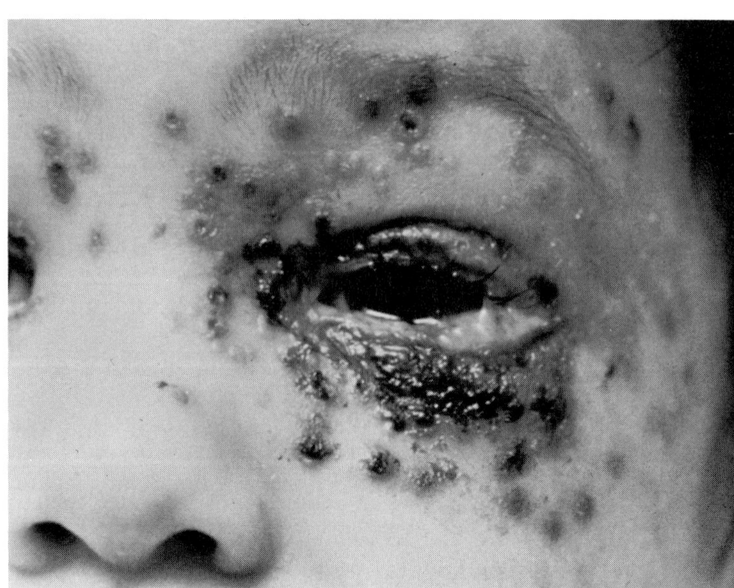

FIGURE 15–13. Atopic dermatitis in a 3-year-old girl complicated by secondary infection with herpes simplex virus.

exposure to antigen. If the reaction is severe, edema, vesicles, and bullae may develop.

Treatment requires removal of the allergen and the application of cool moist compresses. Antihistamines and topical corticosteroids are usually effective. In the acute massive bullous reactions, such as from poison ivy, a short course of systemic corticosteroids is very helpful.

Anesthetic considerations are similar to those for atopic dermatitis.

SEBORRHEIC DERMATITIS

Seborrheic dermatitis is a chronic inflammatory disorder that is manifested as dry, scaly, erythematous papular lesions. In children, it is most common in infancy and adolescence. Constitutional symptoms are infrequent and recovery is usual, even without treatment. Its severest clinical manifestation, erythema desquamativum (Leiner disease) was discussed on page 502.

Wiskott-Aldrich syndrome is an X-linked recessive disorder manifested by thrombocytopenia purpura, recurrent infections, and severe seborrheic dermatitis. The thrombocytopenia is present at birth. Bloody diarrhea is common, and a severe anemia develops early. Recurrent infections with pneumococcus, meningococcus, and *Haemophilus influenzae* begin at age 6 months. Recurrent pauciarticular arthritis may be seen.[9] A deficient immune response is postulated as the etiology of this syndrome.

Treatment is mainly supportive. Despite transfer factor therapy and bone marrow transplantations, survival past puberty is rare.[8]

Should these patients require surgical therapy, they present major challenges to the anesthetist, notably chronic debilitation, acute hypovolemia, anemia, coagulopathies, and secondary infections.

Letterer-Siwe disease is an acute, disseminated, and frequently fatal variant of histiocytosis X. It usually presents in infancy with seborrheic or eczematous eruptions on the scalp, postauricular folds, intertriginous areas, and diaper region. Major complications arise from involvement of bone, of the reticuloendothelial system, and of the central nervous system.[3, 8] Mandibular hypoplasia may occur and make laryngoscopy and intubation very difficult.

Menkes' syndrome is an inherited, neurodegenerative disorder associated with a copper enzyme deficiency state. Seborrheic dermatitis, generalized hypopigmentation, and sparse, kinky hair are frequent cutaneous features. Death from central nervous system complications usually occurs before age 2 years.[1, 3]

PHOTOSENSITIVITY

Photosensitivity denotes a qualitatively or quantitatively abnormal skin reaction to sunlight. Host factors are important, particularly normal melanin pigmentation, which reflects, absorbs, and scatters light. Photosensitivity may be a feature of some diseases, such as the porphyrias, or may be an exacerbating factor in others, such as erythema multiforme and connective tissue disorders, including systemic lupus erythematosus and dermatomyositis.[8]

Xeroderma pigmentosum is a rare autosomal recessive disorder characterized by severe photosensitivity, abnormalities of DNA repair, and the subsequent formation of cutaneous malignancies.[1, 3, 8] The more severe forms may have associated microcephaly, cerebellar ataxia, and mental retardation. By the age 3 years, exposed skin has become atrophic and scarred and develops telangiectasia and actinic keratoses. Basal and squamous cell carcinomas and malignant melanomas finally appear. Death from metastatic disease usually occurs between ages 7 and 20 years.

The rigorous avoidance of sunlight and the surgical excision of malignancies as they arise are the only treatments available.[150] There is a case report in the literature of a patient with xeroderma pigmentosum who had an obstructing carcinoma of the tongue and required a blind awake nasal intubation for airway management.[149]

Apart from care in handling involved skin and the recognition of metastatic disease, there are no specific anesthetic recommendations.

DISORDERS WITH PIGMENTARY CHANGE

NEUROFIBROMATOSIS (VON RECKLINGHAUSEN DISEASE)

Neurofibromatosis is a relatively common (1 per 3200 population)[151] autosomal dominant disorder characterized by café au lait spots and the appearance of neurofibromas in the skin, subcutaneous tissue, nervous system, bones, and internal organs. These tumors are overgrowths of the Schwann cells and endoneurium, which cover nervous tissue; their manifestations are greatly varied.

The presence of six or more café au lait spots (local areas of cutaneous hyperpigmentation) with a diameter of greater than 1.5 cm is usually diagnostic, but the disease is confirmed by the appearance of cutaneous and subcutaneous neurofibromas later in childhood. These tumors are usually soft, may be pedunculated, and may affect any area of the skin. Plexiform neuromas are less common but may be large and infiltrative and cause considerable disfigurement.[8]

Involvement of the central nervous system may approach 66 percent of cases and is associated with an increased incidence of gliomas and meningiomas.[12] Cranial nerves are frequent sites for neurofibromas. Acoustic neuromas cause deafness and vertigo, and optic neuromas may cause visual impairment. Pituitary and hypothalamic dysfunction may be manifested by growth disturbances and by precocious sexual development.[152] Spinal cord neuromas may cause paresis. A thoracic meningocele with vertebral anomalies has been reported.[153] Mild mental impairment is common, and seizure disorders are seen in 5 percent of patients.[8]

Hypertension may occur in children with neurofibromatosis. Pheochromocytoma is a possible association and must be excluded, but hypertension is also often secondary to extrinsic renal artery compression or to renal artery stenosis.[152, 159]

Skeletal complications occur in 30 to 50 percent of cases. Thoracic scoliosis, being the most common, is seen in 10 to 40 percent of cases.[154] Subperiosteal lesions may lead to pathological long bone fractures.

Neurofibromas arising from the larynx and pharynx are rare but have been reported in young children. Respiratory distress from airway obstruction, dysphonia, and dysphagia were the usual presentations. Tracheostomy may be required.[154, 156, 158]

Other manifestations of neurofibromatosis include genitourinary tract obstruction with uremia and the development of pulmonary interstitial fibrosis and honeycomb lung cysts. The lung changes usually occur only in adults older than 35 years.[157] Sarcomatous degeneration of neurofibromas occurs in 1 percent of patients but is rare in children.[8, 129]

In the absence of malignant change, life span may be normal. Surgical intervention in children with neurofibromatosis is required to correct scoliosis, resect painful subcutaneous nodules, repair renal artery stenosis, correct obstructive uropathy, and reduce pathological fractures.

Several considerations deserve attention in planning anesthetics for these children. The preoperative identification of upper airway lesions is mandatory. If obstructive symptoms have developed, tracheostomy may be required.[156]

Ventilatory function in the presence of scoliosis should be evaluated fully with pulmonary function tests. In patients who are hypertensive, laboratory investigations should include tests of urinary catecholamines, pituitary function, electrolytes, blood urea nitrogen, and creatinine.

The child should be positioned carefully, and all pressure points should be adequately protected. All basic monitoring is required. In patients who have pulmonary dysfunction or hypertension, an arterial line may be necessary.

Regional anesthesia has been used in older children, but technical difficulties from occult neurofibroma and back deformities may be encountered.[158]

When general anesthesia is required, no specific drugs are recommended. Of the inhalational agents, halothane may be more likely to cause dysrhythmias in patients with renal hypertension.[161] Patients with neurofibromatosis are reported to have increased sensitivity to both succinylcholine and nondepolarizing agents.[159, 160] High thoracic spinal lesions may predispose some patients to autonomic hyperreflexia.[12] Hypertensive crises should be quickly controlled.

Incontinentia Pigmenti (Bloch-Sulzberger Syndrome)

Incontinentia pigmenti is a rare multisystemic disorder inherited by an X-linked dominant gene, usually lethal in males. Skin lesions may be the only manifestation, but 80 percent of patients have additional neurological, ocular, and skeletal defects.[8, 162]

The skin lesions present in the first 2 weeks of life as erythematous streaks and streaks of vesicles on the trunk and limbs, followed by intermediate verrucous lesions that may persist for 6 months. Subsequently, irregular macules develop that contain patches of brown to slate gray pigment. The skin lesions usually resolve by adulthood.

The central nervous system manifestations include developmental retardation, cortical atrophy, degrees of spastic paresis, seizures, and hydrocephalus. Ocular complications include strabismus, cataracts, retinal detachment, and optic nerve atrophy. Blindness occurs in over 15 percent of cases. Skeletal anomalies are less common but include spina bifida, cleft lip and palate, dwarfism, and chondrodystrophy.

Pegged (conical) teeth are characteristic. Despite the partial anodontia and abnormal dentition, mandibular development is normal.[8, 12]

No anesthetic problems have been reported. Many of the patients are mentally impaired and blind. The operating room must be quiet for induction. No specific anesthetic drugs or techniques are recommended. Laryngoscopy and intubation are usually straightforward, but care must be taken because of the anomalous teeth.

Giant Congenital Melanocytic Nevus

These congenital lesions are relatively uncommon and occur in fewer than 1 in 20,000 neonates. They vary considerably in size but may cover a major anatomical area of the body, often the back, torso, or "bathing suit" region, and occasionally part of an extremity. They contain varying degrees of pigment, are often covered by dark, coarse hair, and have raised, verrucous borders (Fig. 15–14). Distribution on the head and neck is often associated with leptomeningeal melanocytosis, leading to seizure disorders and hydrocephalus.[7]

The major concern in these lesions is their potential for malignant degeneration. Malignant melanomas develop in 6 to 10 percent of these lesions, often in the first decade.[163–165] Optimal treatment requires staged, total surgical excision and the application of split-thickness skin grafts to cover the defects. Anesthetic considerations, therefore, relate to positioning and the preparation for potential blood loss.[166]

Peutz-Jeghers Syndrome

This autosomal dominant syndrome is characterized by intestinal polyps in association with a distinctive, freckle-like pigmentation of the skin around the mouth and in the oral cavity. The brown-to-black macules are present from birth or early infancy. The polyps develop singly or in groups from early infancy and throughout adult life.

The intestinal polyposis is not subject to malignant change, although other neoplasias are more common in these patients. The more frequent complications seen are intussusception, rectal prolapse, and gastrointestinal hemorrhage.

Multiple Lentigines Syndrome

The multiple lentigines syndrome was originally called the progressive cardiomyopathy lentiginosis syndrome, but the acronym LEOPARD syndrome is now used to describe its many features.

This disorder is an autosomal dominant trait characterized by multiple lentigines, which are flat, dark brown spots distributed over the whole body. The numbers increase with age. Associated features include hypertelorism, genital ab-

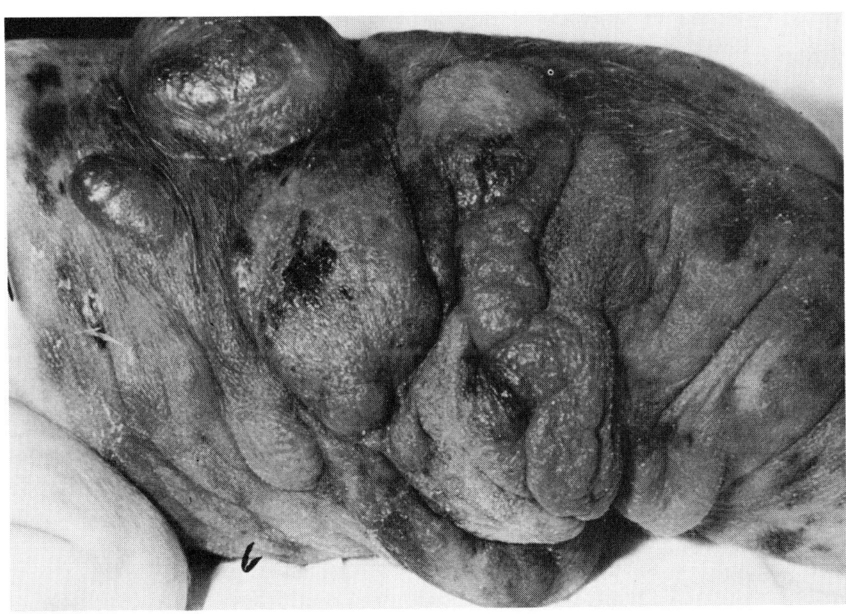

FIGURE 15–14. Giant congenital melanocytic nevus involving the torso and back of a prone 10-day-old infant.

normalities, growth retardation, deafness, and mental retardation.

The major concern for anesthesia is the frequent association of the lentigines syndrome with anatomical and/or conduction defects of the heart. Careful preoperative assessment and a cardiology consultation even in the absence of obvious disease is advised.[167]

URTICARIAL AND HYPERSENSITIVITY DISORDERS

Urticarial lesions are well-circumscribed, raised, pruritic, and erythematous areas of edema in the skin, limited to superficial layers of the dermis. When the edematous process is deeper, extending into the lower dermis and subcutaneous tissue, the lesion is referred to as angioedema.

Cold Urticaria

Cold urticaria is an uncommon disorder characterized by abrupt swelling of and edema in the skin on exposure to cold stimuli. It may be life-threatening when there is a local reaction to the ingestion of cold foods or when there is associated hypotension and cardiovascular collapse.[168] Cold challenge in these patients induces an IgE-dependent degranulation of mast cells and the release of histamine and other vasoactive mediators. Both acquired and familial forms are described.

A careful history of symptoms will identify the usual severity of the patient's reaction. Premedication with H_1 and H_2 histamine antagonists and steroids will not prevent the release of histamine but may attenuate many of its vascular effects.[168, 169, 200] The operating room, as well as the laryngoscope, intravenous solutions, and anesthetic gases, must be warmed. Warming blankets should be in place.

Inhalational anesthesia is probably the best choice in children. Those drugs known to cause histamine release should be avoided.[170–172, 195, 196] A fentanyl-metocurine combination, with the aforementioned premedication, was used without incident in a 47-year-old man with cold urticaria for cardiopulmonary bypass and hypothermia to 31°C.[168]

Hereditary Angioedema

Hereditary angioedema is an uncommon autosomal dominant disorder manifested by attacks of nonpruritic edema of the face, upper airway, extremities, and abdominal viscera and gastrointestinal tract. These attacks may occur spontaneously or following trauma. The underlying cause is a deficiency of C_1-esterase inhibitor or of normal amounts of a nonfunctional inhibitor, allowing uncontrolled complement activation and the formation of vasoactive mediators to proceed. Two thirds of patients are symptomatic before age 13 years. The mortality rate of untreated episodes from laryngeal edema has been reported to be as high as 30 percent.[173]

The disease may occur spontaneously or in response to blunt trauma or procedures, including tonsillectomy, dental manipulation, and endoscopy, that have initiated the syndrome in over half the cases. Emotional upset and anxiety may also provoke attacks.[176] Oropharyngeal and laryngeal edema occur in 64 percent of cases.[142] Abdominal pain is a frequent symptom, and accompanying diarrhea may cause hypovolemia. The onset is acute, and the edema lasts 24 to 72 hours.

The management of acute attacks requires large doses of epinephrine subcutaneously or by intravenous infusion[177–179] and fresh-frozen plasma.[174, 178] Antifibrinolytic agents also may be helpful. Corticosteroids and antihistamines are still used but are rarely effective alone.[171] Narcotics may be required for abdominal pain. If the airway is compromised, early intubation is advised before emergency tracheostomy becomes necessary.[180] Intraoperative angioedema has been managed with epsilon-aminocaproic acid.[181] Some controversy exists as to the effectiveness of epinephrine once the edema is established.[185]

Long-term prophylactic therapy with androgenic steroids like stanozolol, and the antifibrinolytic agents epsilon-aminocaproic acid and tranexamic acid, have had modest success.[1, 173]

The major priority in the anesthetic management of these patients is preoperative restoration of esterase inhibitor activity. For elective surgery, a 2- to 3-day course of an antifibrinolytic agent and an infusion of fresh-frozen plasma the day before operation is recommended. This treatment will restore the levels of C_1-esterase inhibitor to normal for 1 to 4 days. For emergency operation, an immediately preoperative infusion of fresh-frozen plasma may be sufficient.[174, 175]

Following preoperative preparation, many different anesthetic techniques have been reported, and there are few specific recommendations in the literature.[175–185] Effective premedication to reduce anxiety is important; antihistamines have been used.[177] Local infiltration for dental extractions,[176] a regional spinal block for genitourinary surgery,[177] and a hyoscine, thiopentone, succinylcholine induction for cesarean section[175] have been reported without problem.

In children, general anesthesia using a simple technique with inhalational agents may be preferred. Intubation is best avoided but, when required, must be performed gently to avoid upper airway trauma. Throat packs are discouraged.[20] Postoperative observation in an intensive care area is advised for 24 hours.[176]

Mastocytosis

Mastocytosis is a relatively rare disorder characterized by abnormal aggregates of mast cells in the dermis and in various organs of the body. Most cases are sporadic and occur in whites, with equal frequency in both sexes.[1] Local and systemic manifestations are due to the release of vasoactive mediators from the mast cell granules.

Urticaria pigmentosa is the most common form of the disease. It presents in children before the age of 2 years. The lesions are limited to the dermis and appear as yellow-to-brown macules, papules, or nodules distributed symmetrically over the skin, usually sparing the mucous membranes.[8] Occasionally, recurrent bullae are seen in infants. Pruritus may be intense. Isolated infiltrates (mastocytomas) occur in 10 percent of cases. The prognosis is good; spontaneous involution occurs by puberty in 50 percent of cases.

Systemic mastocytosis with disseminated, multisystemic involvement occurs in 5 to 10 percent of cases.[1, 8] Bone lesions are painful and may cause pathological fractures. Intestinal malabsorption, peptic ulceration, hepatic dysfunction, hepatosplenomegaly, and infiltrations in the kidneys, lymph nodes, and marrow may occur. Secondary anemia, thrombocytopenia, and coagulopathy are not infrequent. Pulmonary eosinophilic granulomas have been reported. The prognosis of systemic mastocytosis is guarded. Rarely, mast cell leukemia develops; this condition is rapidly fatal.[186, 187]

Episodic systemic symptoms are caused by mast cell degranulation and the release of histamine, prostaglandin D_2, and heparin into the circulation.[188] Forty to fifty percent of patients have attacks of flushing, pruritus, headaches, palpitations, abdominal colic, and occasionally vomiting and diarrhea[1] (Figs. 15–15 and 15–16). More severe attacks are accompanied by syncope and profound hypotension, which can progress to refractory shock and death. Bronchospasm is unusual but has been reported with salicylates.[188] Rarely, grand mal seizures are seen. Heparin release may induce a bleeding diathesis rarely found in patients without systemic disease. Factors precipitating mediator release include mechanical stimulation of skin lesions, psychological stress, extreme temperature changes, alcohol ingestion, and a variety of histamine-releasing medications such as the opiates, salicylates, atropine, muscle relaxants, dextran, and polymycin B, to name a few.

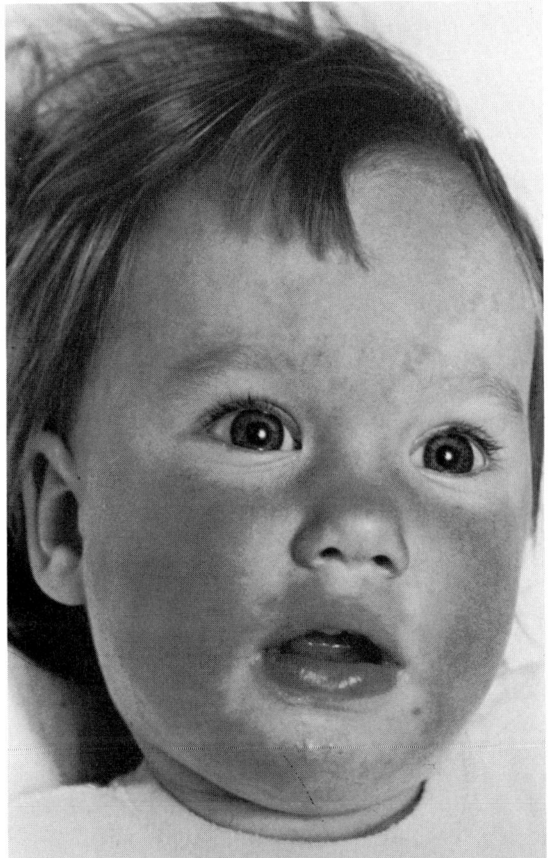

FIGURE 15–15. Histamine flush in a 14-month-old girl with mastocytosis.

No treatment is available to control the progress of the disease, although single mastocytomas may be excised. Symptomatic therapy provides variable results and includes H_1 and H_2 receptor antagonists, oral disodium cromoglycate, and the avoidance of triggering factors. Systemic corticosteroids have been used to treat the severe bullous eruptions that may occur in infants. Antimetabolites may have limited use in systemic disease.

Surgical intervention may be required for the

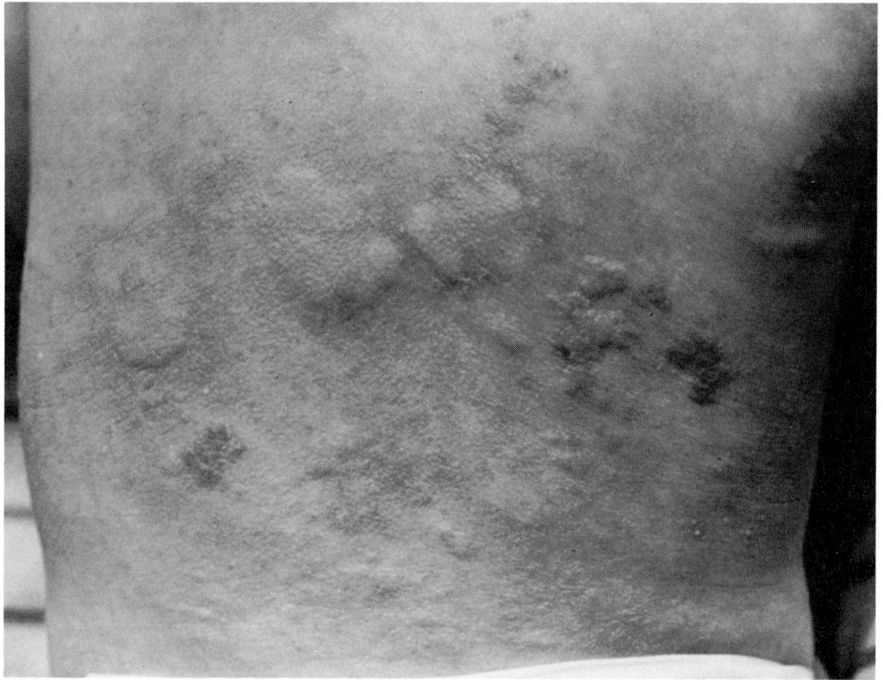

FIGURE 15–16. Urticarial lesions and flush in a 14-month-old girl with mastocytosis.

excision of isolated skin lesions, the reduction of pathological fractures, intestinal surgery for ulcers, or thoracotomy for pulmonary resection.[12] Even in unrelated and minor procedures, profound cardiovascular collapse has been reported.[189, 192, 194]

Anesthetic Management. The primary anesthetic consideration is the prevention of vasoactive mediator release and the prompt treatment of hypotension, should it occur. A preoperative history of syncope and precipitating factors may be very helpful. In patients who have serious disease, investigations must include hemoglobin, platelet count, coagulation screen, and serum electrolytes. Adequate blood products must be available when appropriate. Perioperative steroid coverage may be required.

A good rapport with the patient and adequate premedication will reduce anxiety levels in the operating room. Sedation should be given orally. H_1 and H_2 receptor antagonists and prostaglandin antagonists should be included for patients with systemic disease.[189, 190] Preoperative atropine should be avoided; glycopyrrolate may be safe, but no experience is reported.

The operating room must be warm and the temperature constant. The patient must be transferred and positioned carefully to avoid stimulation of skin lesions, bone pain, and pathological fractures.

No specific techniques are recommended. Both regional and general anesthesia have been reported.[190–194, 202] Thiopentone and pancuronium have both been shown to release histamine but have both been used.[197, 198] Succinylcholine is considered safe.[156] Rectal methohexital has been used without incident.[190] Demerol is the recommended analgesic, but fentanyl may also be free of histamine-releasing properties. The inhalational agents are probably most reliable in not releasing histamine.

In elective procedures in children, a cautious inhalational induction with halothane is the best choice. Reliable intravenous access should be obtained early. Oral lesions, if present, are minor so that intubation, if required, should not be difficult with the patient under halothane anesthesia and thus muscle relaxants can be avoided. However, glycopyrrolate and succinylcholine may be an appropriate combination. Vecuronium has been used. Monitoring must include pulse oximetry, an ECG, precordial stethoscope, and temperature probe. Blood pressure should be monitored by an arterial line for thoracotomy or major laparotomy.

In a retrospective study of 29 general anesthetics in children with isolated cutaneous mastocytosis, James and associates have suggested that major adverse reactions are not common and that a conservative approach with close monitoring is most appropriate.[192]

Should a hypotensive crisis occur, immediate resuscitative treatment with intravenous fluids, antihistamines, and sympathomimetics must be initiated. Epinephrine by infusion is reportedly the most effective vasopressor.[199] Transfusion reactions in these patients may be lethal.[12] Minor hemorrhage has been controlled by protamine.[190]

Vigilant care must be continued throughout the postoperative period.

ERYTHEMA NODOSUM

Erythema nodosum is a syndrome characterized by the development of inflammatory cutaneous nodules on the extremities. These nodules represent a hypersensitivity reaction to various antigens and involve the septal vessels of fat lobules. The disease affects females more than males (3:1), usually between the ages of 15 and 30 years.[1]

Following a variable prodrome of fever, malaise, and arthralgias, symmetrical crops of painful, indurated, red, hot, raised nodules appear on the extensor surfaces of the limbs, usually over the shins. After 2 to 3 weeks, the induration decreases and the violaceous colors subside, finally leaving a brown residuum. Joint involvement is usually minor, affecting the ankles most frequently with tender swelling and effusions. After 6 to 8 weeks, the disease becomes quiescent and rarely recurs.[1, 8]

Etiological factors include infections with tuberculosis, streptococci, *Brucella, Toxoplasma,* and some viruses. Drugs also have been implicated, in particular the sulfonamides, oral contraceptives, phenytoin anticonvulsants, and salicylates. Erythema nodosum is seen in association with other diseases, notably sarcoidosis (Löfgren's syndrome),[203] systemic lupus erythematosus, ulcerative colitis, regional ileitis,[204] and Behçet's syndrome.

Preoperatively, the underlying cause and associated diseases must be identified. If arthritis is a feature, the temporomandibular joints must be examined to determine whether laryngoscopy will be difficult. Care must be taken in transferring and positioning the patient. No specific anesthetic techniques are recommended. All contaminated anesthetic equipment should be appropriately cleaned.

MISCELLANEOUS SKIN DISORDERS

BEHÇET'S SYNDROME

Behçet's syndrome is traditionally described as a relatively rare mucocutaneous ocular disorder characterized by recurrent uveitis, aphthous stomatitis, and genital ulcerations. It is now well recognized to have serious manifestations in additional organ systems. Males are affected more than females (2.3:1). The average age of onset is 20 to 30 years, but the disease has been described in children.[1, 205, 206]

The oral lesions are recurrent, painful ulcers involving the lips, gums, tongue, pharynx, and larynx. Healing by scarring is not a usual complication but has been described.[207] Ocular lesions include recurrent uveitis, conjunctivitis, choroiditis, and optic atrophy; blindness may follow. The skin manifestations include papules, subcutaneous nodules, vesicles, pyoderma, and abscesses.

Central nervous system involvement may relapse and remit, and clinical signs include spastic paresis, ataxia, seizures, coma, and spinal cord lesions.[12] Cardiovascular manifestations include pericarditis, recurrent thrombophlebitis, superior and inferior vena caval obstruction, and arterial aneurysms.[208] A transient inhibition of fibrinolysis is recognized to coincide with the episodes of thrombophlebitis. Hemoptysis and obstructive pulmonary disease have been reported.[209] Renal dysfunction with anemia may progress to nephrotic syndrome secondary to glomerulonephritis or amyloidosis[206] (see Chapter 7).

The course of the disease is variable but is usually chronic and progressive. Treatment has included corticosteroids, immunosuppressants, and fibrinolytic agents, but it does not appear to alter the gradual deterioration of the patient's condition.[211]

The anesthetic management of patients with Behçet's syndrome requires attention to several points. Multiple systems are involved, and each deserves full assessment. Clinical appraisal of the upper airway should include pharyngoscopy, with the patient awake to identify oropharyngeal scarring that may make laryngoscopy and intubation difficult.[207] When this complication is suspected, intubation should be performed with the patient awake, using topical anesthesia and modest sedation, or under deep halothane anesthesia and breathing spontaneously. Once the airway is secured, no specific recommendations are reported. Aseptic techniques must be followed in the presence of active pyoderma.

MALIGNANT ATROPHIC PAPULOSIS (KOHLMEIER-DEGOS DISEASE)

Malignant atrophic papulosis is a rare, often fatal, multisystemic disease characterized by multiple infarcts in the skin, gastrointestinal tract, central nervous system, and other organs. It usually occurs in young adults but has been described in children.[212] The underlying pathology is an occlusive vasculitis of unknown etiology.

The skin lesions develop as porcelain white papules, which heal to form atrophic scars. Catastrophic complications arise from gastrointestinal lesions, which may result in bowel perforation and peritonitis, and from central nervous system infarcts, which may cause cerebral edema, increased intracranial pressure, and uncal herniation. Pleural effusions, restrictive pulmonary disease, constrictive pericarditis with effusions, and myocardial infarctions are also reported.[213] No effective treatment is available.[214]

Surgical intervention may be required for acute gastrointestinal perforation and peritonitis and occasionally for pulmonary decortication and pericardiectomy. Patients with this disease are critically ill, and most require aggressive preoperative fluid resuscitation. Invasive cardiovascular monitoring is advised, to provide optimal evaluation of compromised cardiac and pulmonary function. The maintenance of adequate venous return in the presence of constrictive pericarditis and pericardial effusion is mandatory. Those patients with increased intracranial pressure would benefit from a light narcotic with relaxant technique and hyperventilation.[12] Postoperative management should be provided in an intensive care unit.

Fabry's Disease (Angiokeratoma Corporis Diffusum Universale)

Fabry's disease is a sex-linked recessive inborn error of metabolism (alpha-galactosidase A deficiency), fully penetrant in males and characterized by the deposition of the glycolipid ceramide trihexoside in the blood vessels of skin, mucous membranes, eyes, heart, kidneys, liver, peripheral nerves, and brain (see Chapter 13).[215] The vascular reaction causes ischemia and degenerative change in the affected organs. The skin lesions are angiokeratomas: small ectasias of dermal vessels protruding into the epidermis. They appear at puberty on scrotal, sacral, and umbilical areas, elbows, thighs, fingers, lips, and mucous membranes of the mouth. They may, however, be absent. Hypohidrosis and hypotrichosis may occur.[12] Eye findings occur in late childhood as corneal opacities, conjunctival and retinal vessel tortuosity, and posterior capsular cataracts.

The disease presents in childhood as recurrent febrile episodes associated at first with weakness and then, in adolescence, with agonizing limb pain and paresthesias. Limitation of joint movement, including the temporomandibular joint, is seen but has not been explained. In early adulthood, symptoms of advancing organ system involvement appear. Neurological complications include presenile dementia, seizures, paralyses, and cerebrovascular accidents. Cardiac disease is manifest by angina pectoris, myocardial infarction, hypertension, dysrhythmias, and valvular disease (mitral insufficiency).[12, 216] Progressive renal failure with hypertension is a major cause of death by the fifth decade but has been reported in a 16-year-old.[217]

There is no specific treatment for this disease. Complications are treated as they arise. The paresthesias and acral pain have been controlled by oral diphenylhydantoin. Renal transplantation has had variable success.[218]

Anesthetic Management. The serious renal and cardiac complications of this disorder may not arise until early adulthood, but these systems must receive thorough evaluation even in children. A history of exercise intolerance or angina may be unlikely, but a chest radiograph and ECG should be obtained, and the hemoglobin, electrolytes, blood urea nitrogen, creatinine, and urinalysis should be reviewed. Restricted mouth opening is uncommon but must be identified preoperatively.

General anesthesia is usually required. Regional techniques in the presence of acral pain, paresthesias, and peripheral neuropathy are discouraged. All routine monitoring, including temperature probes, must be used. Anticholinergic agents may aggravate hypohidrosis and further impair thermoregulation. No specific anesthetic agents are recommended, but tachycardia and large blood pressure changes should be avoided.

Pyoderma Gangrenosum

Pyoderma gangrenosum is an unusual syndrome affecting any age group, characterized by unique skin ulcerations that appear most often on the lower extremities. Oral lesions have been described. The ulcers, which may be large, have purple, raised, tender, undermined borders with purulent granulating bases. There is frequent association with a variety of systemic diseases, notably ulcerative colitis, Crohn's disease, rheumatoid arthritis, some hematological malignancies, and Wegener's granulomatosis.[12, 363]

Treatment is directed at control of the underlying disease and local measures. Occasionally systemic corticosteroids and immunosuppressive agents are required.

CONNECTIVE TISSUE DISEASES

The connective tissues of the body arise from the differentiation of embryonic mesoderm and are adapted to a great number of diverse functions. They form the extracellular structures of support and movement—periosteum, bone, cartilage, fascia, and ligaments. They provide body coverings—the dermis, serosa, and internal organ capsules—and are major components in the structures of nourishment—blood vessels, the lymphatics, and the tracheobronchial tree. Connective tissue is composed of the fibrillar proteins collagen, elastin, and reticulin and a ground substance matrix.[1]

Collagen is the most abundant protein in human beings, constituting one third of total body protein, and is the principal fibrillar component of most connective tissue. The basic peptide is synthesized in fibroblasts and then undergoes postsynthetic, extracellular aggregation and cross-linking to form stable fibers of high tensile strength.[219] Elastin is synthesized in smooth muscle cells.[1] It is a highly branching fiber and lacks the tensile strength of collagen but displays much greater elasticity. With reticulin, elastin provides the major fibrillar component of connective tissue in blood vessels, muscles, and the parenchyma of internal organs.

The fibrous proteins are set in a ground substance matrix composed of glycosaminoglycans (mucopolysaccharides), which are long-chain carbohydrate polymers, maintained in stiffly extended configuration from the protein core by highly negatively charged molecular groups. A large amount of water and about half the plasma proteins are held within the spaces created by these molecules.[9]

The constant remodeling of connective tissue by degradation and regeneration is one of the primary reparative functions of the inflammatory process. In connective tissue disease, these tissues become the important focus of destruction or of degenerative change when the directed functions of acute inflammation are disturbed.

The etiology and pathogenesis of the connective tissue diseases are not fully understood. They all exhibit a variety of autoimmune phenomena in both the humoral and cellular immune systems, but the causal relationship of these phenomena to the inflammatory process is not always clear.[9, 220] However, in acute fulminant autoimmune disease, the most important therapeutic maneuver remains the use of anti-inflammatory agents.[221]

The connective tissue diseases usually present as clinically distinct entities, but their chronic and multisystemic features may produce considerable overlap in signs and symptoms. Precise diagnostic and laboratory criteria are lacking.

However uncommon some of these disorders may be, many of the patients require surgical intervention. Pediatric anesthesiologists, therefore, must have a good understanding of the systemic manifestations of each disease and of the secondary effects that medical management might induce.

JUVENILE RHEUMATOID ARTHRITIS (STILL DISEASE)

Juvenile rheumatoid arthritis is a chronic and extremely variable systemic disease characterized by synovitis and associated extra-articular manifestations.[8, 9] It is the most common of the pediatric connective tissue disorders. Its annual incidence is 9 to 15 cases per 100,000 population. Childhood-onset disease (prior to age 16 years) accounts for 5 percent of all patients with rheumatoid arthritis. Girls are twice as frequently affected as boys. All races and geographical regions are vulnerable. The etiology and pathogenesis are unknown, but infections, autoimmunity, and immunogenetic predisposition are considered possible causes.[9]

The pathology of adult and juvenile rheumatoid arthritis is similar. The synovitis is characterized by chronic, nonsuppurative, proliferative inflammation with hyperemia, edema, and an infiltration with lymphocytes and plasma cells. Joint effusions are common. Continuing synovitis may induce synovial hypertrophy and the progressive erosion and destruction of articular cartilage and contiguous bone. Although joint damage occurs much later and less commonly in juvenile-onset disease than in adults, joint subluxation, ankylosis, and deformity still represent end-stage disease in some patients. Rheumatoid nodules are seen less frequently in juvenile disease, and systemic complications over the long-term tend to be less severe.

Clinical Manifestations. The presentation of juvenile rheumatoid arthritis rarely occurs before the age of 6 months; the peak onset occurs between the ages of 1 and 3 years. The clinical picture of the disease falls into one of three broad clinical groups defined by the features that develop in the first 6 months of illness, namely polyarticular, pauciarticular, and systemic-onset disease.[222, 223]

Polyarticular-onset disease accounts for 40 percent of cases and may present at any time throughout childhood. Rheumatoid factor seronegativity is usual. The initial synovitis affects five or more joints and may be mild or fulminant, in which case the joints are warm, tender, swollen with effusions, painful, and stiff. The large joints are involved first: the knees, ankles, wrists, and elbows, and then the fingers. Hip involvement is frequent and may be severe, with destruction of the femoral head.

Cervical spine arthritis occurs in 60 to 70 percent of cases and is complicated by early apophyseal ankylosis. This leads to fusion en bloc of vertebrae, usually of C2 and C3, but several more levels commonly may be involved. Flexion deformities, loss of neck extension, and torticollis are common features. Atlantoaxial subluxation is a frequent radiological finding, but the incidence of significant instability is unknown. Nonetheless, neurological symptoms and complications are extremely rare in children.[9, 10, 224, 237]

Temporomandibular joint involvement often manifests as earache and occurs in 65 percent of cases.[225, 226] Grosfeld and associates report that 16 percent of patients develop reduced mouth opening, and 5 percent have severe secondary mandibular hypoplasia and retrognathia[226, 231] (Fig. 15–17). Cricoarytenoid arthritis, seen in 26 percent of adults, is uncommon in children,[227, 228] but it may occur. Presentation is usually with pain, dysphagia, hoarseness, stridor, or dyspnea and has led to airway obstruction.[229]

The systemic manifestations in polyarticular-onset disease are variable but not as acute or persistent as in systemic-onset juvenile disease. A low-grade fever, mild anemia, rheumatoid rash, minor hepatosplenomegaly, and lymphadenopathy are typical features. Clinically evident pericarditis or pleuritis is infrequent.

An important subgroup of children, usually girls who are rheumatoid factor–seropositive, present with polyarticular disease in late childhood. Their arthritis is characterized by rheumatoid nodules, erosive synovitis, and a chronic course very similar to that of adult-onset disease.

Pauciarticular-onset disease accounts for 50 percent of cases. It usually affects girls, is associated with rheumatoid factor seronegativity, and usually is found before the age of 4 years. The arthritis involves four or fewer joints and manifests as a low-grade inflammatory reaction affecting the knees, ankles, and elbows. The hips are spared. Only rarely are the temporomandibular joints or cervical vertebrae involved. Extra-articular manifestations are distinctly unusual, and the children are not systemically ill. This type of disease is prone to early remission.

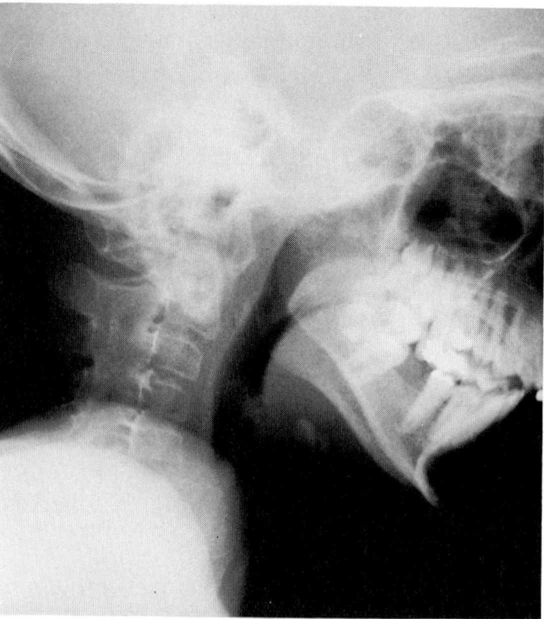

FIGURE 15–17. Juvenile rheumatoid arthritis in a 14-year-old boy. Note the fusion of cervical vertebrae from C2 inferiorly and the severe mandibular hypoplasia. Temporomandibular joint involvement was also present.

The concern in this group is the development of chronic uveitis, which occurs in 20 to 25 percent of cases and may persist for years. The major ocular sequelae are posterior synechiae, cataracts, glaucoma, visual impairment, and blindness in 10 to 20 percent of children affected.

Systemic-onset disease occurs in 10 to 15 percent of cases of juvenile rheumatoid arthritis, with equal frequency between girls and boys. It may present at any time throughout childhood. The severe systemic manifestations may precede the development of arthritis by months or years. Joint involvement is variable but usually follows the pattern of polyarticular disease. In some cases, the arthritis may become chronic and persist after the remission of systemic symptoms well into adulthood.

The diagnostic hallmark of systemic-onset disease is a high, spiking fever with the temperature rising to 39°C on a daily or twice daily pattern. The fever is almost always associated with the classic rash of juvenile rheumatoid arthritis, which is described as an evanescent, migratory, erythematous macular eruption on the trunk and proximal limbs.

Other visceral disease includes generalized lymphadenopathy and hepatosplenomegaly that may be quite impressive (Fig. 15–18). Abdominal pain is often a feature. Cardiac involvement occurs in 5 to 10 percent of cases, commonly as pericarditis associated with minor effusions and mild substernal discomfort.[230] It is not usually regarded as a bad prognostic sign in children.[9] Aortic valvular insufficiency has been described but is exceptional. Rarely, severe chest pain, dyspnea, and cardiac failure from pericardial tamponade have been reported.[232–234]

Pulmonary involvement is usually limited to transient pneumonitis and pleural effusions. Although diffuse interstitial fibrosis is described in children, the classic rheumatoid lung of adult disease is rare.[235, 236]

Anemia and transient proteinuria are common during periods of acute disease. Renal impairment is an unusual and late complication of juvenile disease, often occurring in association with amyloidosis. Both the vasculitis involving small and medium-sized vessels and the central and peripheral nervous system manifestations seen in adults are common in children.

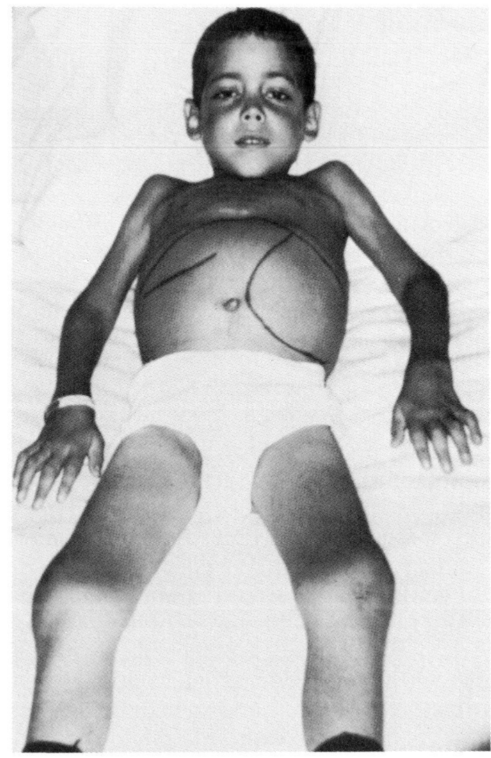

FIGURE 15–18. Systemic disease. Onset of severe systemic JRA at age 4 years in this 8-year-old boy. All major joints were involved. Note the cervical and axillary adenopathy and hepatosplenomegaly. (From Cassidy, J. T., Petty, R. E. Textbook of Pediatric Rheumatology. 2nd ed. New York, Churchill Livingstone, 1990.)

The systemic manifestations may be severe in some patients but usually run a self-limited course of several months. Recurrences are rare once adulthood is reached, although chronic arthritis may persist.

Course and Prognosis. Juvenile rheumatoid arthritis is rarely a life-threatening disease. It follows a course of remissions and exacerbations for several years, often causing little disability. The major morbidity of the polyarticular and systemic-onset types is chronic joint disease, which occurs in 10 to 25 percent of patients and may be complicated by severe joint destruction and permanent disability.[8] In pauciarticular-onset disease, the major concerns are the complications of chronic uveitis, as described earlier.

Treatment. There is no cure for juvenile rheumatoid arthritis. The principles of management are to preserve joint function and to control symptoms with as conservative a program as possible.

Aspirin is the most important drug used in the treatment of this disorder. It reduces the inflammatory arthritis and controls the fever and other systemic manifestations in 30 to 50 percent of patients. The chronic administration of salicylates to children is extremely safe.[9] However, the toxic signs of salicylism vary from drowsiness, metabolic acidosis, and ketosis in very young children to hyperventilation and respiratory alkalosis in older children. Salicylates induce irreversible platelet dysfunction, as demonstrated by an increased bleeding time, and may be responsible for unexpected surgical blood loss.[238, 239] Other hemorrhagic and hypersensitivity reactions are rare in children.

Of the nonsteroidal anti-inflammatory agents, only tolmetin and naproxen are available for use in children; they have proved to be very effective.[240] Acetaminophen is discouraged for long-term use because of possible interstitial nephritis.[9] The antimalarial drug hydroxychloroquine is used less frequently now in view of its retinal toxicity.

Parenteral gold salts provide remissions in some patients unresponsive to other conservative therapy, but the toxic effects of stomatitis, dermatitis, marrow suppression, and renal dysfunction seen in 25 percent of patients limit its widespread use. Penicillamine is similarly effective but may induce a lupus syndrome, dermatitis, thrombocytopenia, and proteinuria. The immunosuppressive and cytotoxic drugs are used in children only for life-threatening complications.

Although systemic corticosteroids dramatically suppress symptoms, they do not induce remissions, prevent joint damage, or alter the outcome of the disease in children. They are infrequently used for arthritic manifestations alone. Steroids may accelerate avascular necrosis of the femoral head and aggravate growth disturbances. The indications for their use are usually limited to the management of severe, unresponsive systemic complications such as pericarditis and deteriorating chronic uveitis. The lowest effective doses are sought, and gradual withdrawal is begun as soon as possible. The limited use of intra-articular steroid injections may be of help in selected active joints of some patients.

The management of chronic uveitis initially involves the use of a mydriatic agent to prevent posterior synechiae, and dexamethasone eye drops. Local injection of systemic corticosteroids may be required.

Physical therapy and occupational therapy provide essential training and rehabilitation programs to maintain muscle tone and joint function. Orthopedic splints help reduce joint subluxation and deformity that may complicate chronic, active disease. Surgical intervention is discouraged until the children are older and bone growth has ceased. Prophylactic synoviectomies are not beneficial in juvenile rheumatoid arthritis. Once the disease is quiescent, reconstructive procedures such as a total joint prosthesis for hips and knees are often very successful.[241]

Anesthetic Management. Juvenile rheumatoid arthritis is a multisystemic disease. Patients with this disease require thorough preoperative assessment.[242–244] The major challenge to the anesthesiologist in these children is usually airway management. Temporomandibular joint ankylosis, mandibular hypoplasia, and reduced neck extension can make effective application of a face mask difficult and direct laryngoscopy impossible[246] (see Fig. 15–17). Chronic or active cricoarytenoid arthritis can cause glottic narrowing and, if suspected, should be confirmed preoperatively by indirect laryngoscopy.[247–249] Atlantoaxial subluxation is common in children with polyarticular or systemic-onset disease, despite the infrequency of symptoms, and must be identified by flexion and extension radiographs of the cervical spine (Fig. 15–19).

Although systemic involvement is not usually as compromising in children as in adults, cardiovascular and respiratory dysfunction can be serious. All patients should have a chest radiograph, ECG, and, if indicated, pulmonary function tests. In systemic-onset disease, anemia is pronounced and may require correction prior to a major surgical procedure. Significant hepatosplenomegaly may compromise ventilation in small children. Hemostasis may be altered in patients on salicylates; a platelet count and bleeding time and coagulation studies will be helpful.[238, 239] Adequate blood products must be available. Renal impairment is seen rarely in children, but levels of serum electrolytes, blood urea nitrogen, and creatinine should be checked and a urinalysis performed. Perioperative corticosteroid supplementation must be arranged for those children on systemic therapy.

Modest sedative premedication may facilitate the induction of anesthesia in anxious and uncomfortable children. But, in those patients who have potentially difficult airways, conservative doses are advised. Patients with active disease may splint their painful joints fearfully. They must be transferred in the operating room gently and supported in a comfortable position, with adequate protection for pressure points created by contractures and deformities.

The safe position for atlantoaxial instability is extension of this joint, but exaggerated extension will increase the lordosis of lower segments of the cervical spine. Flexion of the neck must be avoided. Patients with unstable cervical spine should have a rigid neck collar applied to maintain neutral posture. Patients with difficult airways should have an intravenous infusion started prior to induction.

The choice of anesthetic technique in children with difficult airways is determined by the skill and experience of the anesthesiologist, assessment of the patient, and the nature of the surgical procedure. It may not be unreasonable for a skilled practitioner to provide inhalational anesthesia by mask for short, minor procedures. This is a judgmental decision, which carries the risk of airway obstruction, regurgitation, and pulmonary aspiration.

For major procedures, regional blocks have obvious advantages but are not always suited for young children. These procedures are relatively contraindicated in patients with peripheral neuropathies. D'Arcy and colleagues have reported good success with ketamine, nitrous oxide, and oxygen as the sole anesthetic agents for major joint operation in patients in whom direct laryngoscopy was not possible.[253] However, ketamine provides no guarantee against airway obstruction.[254]

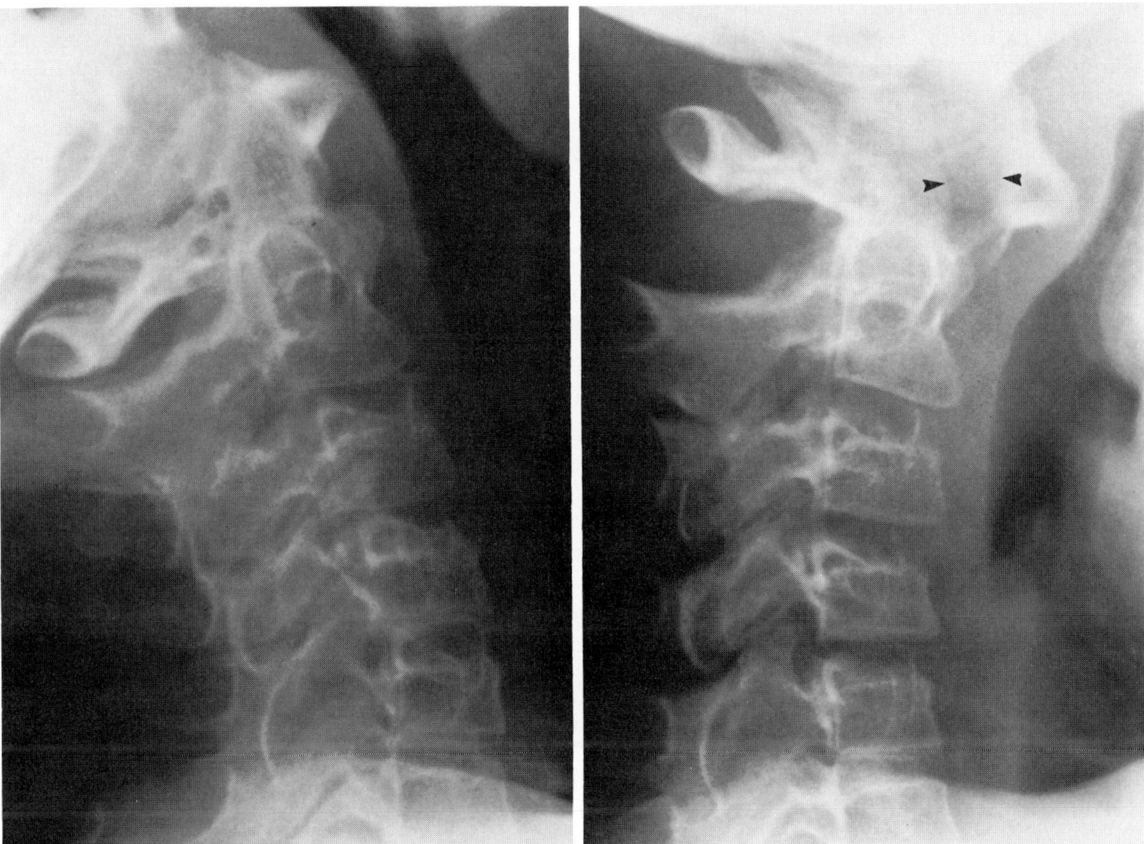

FIGURE 15–19. Extension and flexion radiographs of the cervical vertebrae in an 8-year-old girl with juvenile rheumatoid arthritis, demonstrating atlantoaxial instability in flexion. There is a 6-mm separation of the odontoid process from the body of C_1. She presented with acute aortic insufficiency and required aortic valve replacement.

The laryngeal mask airway (LMA) developed by Brain has been used successfully in the management of patients with juvenile rheumatoid arthritis who were difficult to intubate. However, some experience and skill are required for its use even in normal children. Therefore only those with expertise should attempt the use of the LMA in a patient with a difficult airway.[277–280]

In those children who have a difficult airway, endotracheal intubation is the preferred solution to airway management. However, intravenous induction with thiopentone and the use of muscle relaxants prior to intubation is a very dangerous practice. The complication of airway obstruction and the loss of spontaneous ventilation in a paralyzed patient whose larynx cannot be visualized may lead to disaster.

Historically, intubation in such patients has been accomplished blind, with sedation, or under inhalational or ketamine anesthesia, maintaining spontaneous ventilation. Hyperventilation, induced by adding 2 to 3 percent inspired carbon dioxide or 1 to 2 mg/kg doxapram intravenously, may facilitate laryngeal intubation in some cases.[259, 260] Cautious manipulation of the head and neck may be required. The use of various hooks, introducers, and retrograde catheters has been well described.[256–276] With skill and due care, these approaches remain appropriate for many practitioners.

In current practice, consideration should be given to the technique of fiberoptic nasal intubation as the safest management of patients who have abnormal airways.[261–270, 281–283] This can be performed even in young patients under cautious sedation, although general inhalational or ketamine anesthesia has been used frequently.

Details of technique and recipes for sedation are well described in the literature, but several points are worth emphasis. Preoperative metoclopramide and cimetidine or ranitidine may be advised to reduce the acidity and the volume of gastric contents.[251, 252] Preoperative intravenous fluid administration is recommended to assure adequate hydration. Atropine or glycopyrrolate should be given to dry secretions and protect against vagal reflexes. Sedation with incremental doses of intravenous midazolam, 0.05 mg/kg, and fentanyl, 0.5 μg/kg, or morphine, 0.05 mg/kg, is commonly used.

Effective topical anesthesia is critical to the procedure. The nasal mucosa can be anesthetized with 4 percent cocaine, 2 mg/kg, and lidocaine, administered to the pharynx and glottis first as a gargle, using up to 2 mg/kg of a 4 percent solution. The scope should be introduced by itself first and advanced slowly until the glottis is seen. Further topical anesthesia to the larynx and trachea is given via the working channel with lidocaine 2 percent to 5 mg/kg. Once the carina is seen, the tube with the bevel turned posteriorly is gently advanced over the scope into position. A smaller tube than usual should be used, particularly in patients with cricoarytenoid involvement. If all reasonable efforts at intubation fail, a tracheostomy may be necessary.

Once the airway is secured, several considerations remain. Patients with pulmonary disease or hepatosplenomegaly should have assisted or controlled ventilation.[242, 243] Cardiac reserve is reduced by myocarditis and valvular disease, and agents decreasing myocardial contractility will be tolerated poorly. Patients with secondary muscle atrophy may be sensitive to neuromuscular blocking agents. Gardiner and Holmes report low tolerance in adults to narcotics; all central nervous system depressants should be used with care.[244]

Extubation must be delayed until full recovery of neuromuscular function is verified and the child is awake. Postoperatively, close observation of the airway is mandatory and may warrant admission to an intensive care area.

SPONDYLOARTHROPATHIES

Juvenile Ankylosing Spondylitis

Juvenile ankylosing spondylitis is a chronic inflammatory disease characterized by progressive arthritis of the axial and peripheral skeleton with associated extra-articular manifestations. In 8 to 10 percent of adults with ankylosing spondylitis, onset occurred in childhood between the ages of 10 and 15 years.[9] The disorder in children may be almost as common as juvenile rheumatoid arthritis, but the age of onset is older at 10 years. Males predominate by a ratio of 6:1. Its strong familial incidence and close association with the antigen HLA-B27 suggest a genetically determined immune mechanism as an etiological factor.

In most children, juvenile ankylosing spondylitis presents in early adolescence, usually with peripheral arthritis first, affecting the hips, knees, and ankles. Occasionally, the shoulder and temporomandibular joints are involved. Enthesitis (inflammation and pain at the insertion of ligaments and tendons on bone) is a frequent symptom, particularly involving the heel and the tibial tuberosity. Subsequent deformity of the peripheral joints is uncommon, but destructive hip disease may develop and is the most severe peripheral joint complication.[9, 284] The pathological changes are very similar to those of rheumatoid arthritis.

The classic involvement of the sacroiliac joints and lumbodorsal spine produces low back pain and leads to early loss of lumbar spinal mobility. Chest exansion may be reduced by costovertebral and costosternal joint inflammation.[285] The ascending progression of axial skeletal changes to form the "bamboo spine" rigidity does not occur until much later in adulthood. Cervical involvement is rare in children, but atlantoaxial subluxation has been reported.[286]

Systemic manifestations at the disease onset are rare and develop to significant degrees only in adulthood. However, 20 percent of children develop acute, recurrent uveitis, which fortunately has no ocular sequelae. The cardiac complications seen in 4 to 10 percent of adults, notably pericarditis, conduction defects, and aortitis, are rare in children, but aortic insufficiency has been described.[287, 288] Clinical pulmonary fibrosis is rare in children. Amyloidosis, seen in 8 percent of adults, has not been described in juvenile ankylosing spondylitis.[9, 287]

The course of this disease is usually remitting and is frequently mild. In most cases, the prognosis is favorable if good posture is maintained and treatment begun early. Salicylates are usually effective for relief of pain; tolmetin has proved to be a useful alternative. Systemic corticosteroids are rarely indicated, but local steroid injection of sites of enthesitis may be helpful.

The anesthetic considerations for juvenile ankylosing spondylitis are similar to those for juvenile rheumatoid arthritis. Laryngoscopy is less a problem in children than in adults, but particular attention still should be directed to the evaluation of neck mobility, atlantoaxial instability, temporomandibular joint function, and systemic manifestations.[271, 286]

ACUTE RHEUMATIC FEVER

Acute rheumatic fever is an inflammatory disease that usually presents with joint and cardiac manifestations but may also affect the central nervous system, skin, and subcutaneous tissue. It occurs as a direct consequence of a prior upper respiratory tract infection with group A beta-hemolytic streptococci. Where antibiotic prophylaxis is available, the disease is now much less common, and the annual incidence has dropped to 10 per 100,000 population.[291] The peak incidence of first attacks occurs in the 5- to 15-year age group.

The precise pathological mechanism of acute rheumatic fever is not known. Host factors and hypersensitivity reactions may be important. Antistreptococcal antibodies have been shown to cross-react with antigens found in cardiac muscle and valves, suggesting an autoimmune etiology.[292] A subsequent exudative inflammatory reaction involves the connective tissue of each target organ.

Clinical Manifestations. The major clinical manifestations of acute rheumatic fever include arthritis, carditis, chorea, subcutaneous nodules, and erythema marginatum.

Joint symptoms are the most frequent presenting complaint and occur in 75 percent of cases as a migratory polyarthritis usually affecting the knees, ankles, elbows, and wrists. Pain may be severe but no permanent deformities develop, and the arthritis resolves in 3 to 4 weeks.

Carditis occurs in 40 to 50 percent of initial attacks, with the highest frequency in young children. Rheumatic valvular disease represents the only long-term complication of rheumatic fever. Carditis may be asymptomatic but may still lead to permanent valvular damage. Less frequently it is severe, and it has been fatal in the acute disease. Suggestive findings are tachycardia, cardiomegaly, a gallop rhythm, and the appearance of organic murmurs, usually a pansystolic murmur of mitral valvulitis and less commonly a murmur of aortic insufficiency. Pericarditis may produce chest pain, friction rubs, and effusions. Congestive failure may present as dyspnea, abdominal pain, and hepatomegaly.[8, 9] The manifestations of carditis may persist for 6 weeks to 6 months.

Chorea occurs in 10 to 15 percent of patients and is characterized by involuntary, purposeless movements associated with emotional lability (St. Vitus' dance). Treatment with barbiturates may be helpful. It usually subsides in 3 months. Painless, mobile, subcutaneous nodules appear over body prominences in 5 to 10 percent of cases and last 1 to 2 weeks. The classic rash, erythema marginatum, occurs in less than 5 percent of patients.

Minor clinical manifestations include fever, arthralgia, prolongation of the P-R interval, positive antistreptolysin O titer, and a previous history of rheumatic fever or heart disease. The Jones' criteria for diagnosis require the presence of two major or one major and two minor clinical manifestations.[293] Skin biopsies may help in the diagnosis.[294]

Treatment. Bed rest is important until the rheumatic process is quiescent, particularly in patients with carditis. Salicylates alone control the fever and arthritis dramatically. But in patients with carditis and cardiomegaly, prednisone, 2 mg/kg/24 hours, is preferred for 2 weeks and then gradually withdrawn and replaced by salicylates. Congestive failure is usually controlled by fluid restriction, but diuretics and digoxin may be needed. Penicillin is often begun in the acute attack and continued as long-term prophylaxis against streptococcal infections.

Surgical intervention is rarely indicated in first attacks but may be required subsequently for the correction of rheumatic mitral valvular disease, even in children. Both closed mitral valvotomy and mitral valve replacement, the latter usually for valvular insufficiency, have been reported in children.[295]

Anesthetic Management. Of major importance in the anesthetic management of children with acute rheumatic fever is the preoperative evaluation of cardiac function. Although uncommon, severe congestive cardiac failure may be precipitated by pericardial effusions, myocarditis, and valvular dysfunction. Recurrent disease may produce a variety of valvular lesions: mitral stenosis, mitral insufficiency, and aortic insufficiency. Atrial fibrillation may complicate mitral valve disease.[295] A cardiologist's consultation should be obtained, and a chest radiograph and ECG should be reviewed. The management of specific cardiac lesions is discussed in Chapter 6.

The presence of active arthritis and chorea and the medical therapy of each must be noted. Supplemental corticosteroid therapy may be required. Prophylactic antibiotic coverage for cardiac disease is mandatory. Laryngoscopy is not a reported problem in acute rheumatic fever. No specific recommendations of anesthetic drugs or technique have been made.

REITER SYNDROME

Reiter syndrome refers to the classic triad of urethritis, arthritis, and conjunctivitis. Other manifestations may include gastroenteritis and a mucocutaneous eruption. It is uncommon in children. Boys are affected more than girls by a 4:1 ratio. The disease often follows an enteritis caused by *Shigella, Yersinia,* or *Salmonella* infections in young children or following sexual contact in older children and adults.[296] There is a strong association with HLA-B27. Reiter syndrome has been described as a postinfectious or reactive arthritis.[7]

Joint involvement is generally pauciarticular; the large joints are affected, usually the knees and ankles. The severity of the arthritis may be remarkable. Enthesitis is common. Occasionally, the cervical spine and the temporomandibular, sacroiliac, and cricoarytenoid joints are affected.[297] The arthritis, urethritis, and conjunctivitis usually resolve within a few months. Joint complications are infrequent, but occasionally recurrent chronic arthritis may persist. Uncommonly, children may develop painless erythematous patches or ulcerations in the oropharynx. Scarring is not a feature.

The treatment for Reiter syndrome is relief of symptoms by salicylates and preservation of joint function with physiotherapy.

Apart from the evaluation of neck mobility and temporomandibular joint movement, there are no specific anesthetic considerations.

Arthritis of Inflammatory Bowel Disease

Between 10 and 20 percent of children with chronic ulcerative colitis or regional ileitis develop a spondylitis or a peripheral joint arthropathy, often coinciding with periods of active bowel disease.[9, 298] The affected children are usually over the age of 10 years.

The peripheral arthropathy is pauciarticular and involves the knees and ankles most commonly, although the temporomandibular joints and hands may be affected. The arthritis rarely lasts more than 2 months and responds well to salicylates or to prednisone, if required for control of the bowel disease. Functional loss in peripheral joints is most unusual. In contrast, the sacroiliac and lumbar spine disease tends to progress, despite good control of the bowel disorder. The spondylitis behaves very much like ankylosing spondylitis and may be accompanied by destructive hip disease.

The anesthetic considerations are similar to those for juvenile rheumatoid arthritis.

Psoriatic Arthropathy

Although psoriasis is relatively common in children, psoriatic arthropathy is rarely seen. The arthritis may precede the skin manifestations by several years, and early cases are frequently misdiagnosed. Girls affected outnumber boys by a ratio of 2.5:1. The usual age at onset of the joint symptoms is 9 to 10 years.[9, 131]

The arthritis is often pauciarticular, usually involving the distal interphalangeal joints of the hands, and is associated with flexor tendinitis of the wrists. The knees and small joints of the feet may be affected. Of children with the arthropathy, 25 percent develop sacroileitis. Cervical spine involvement, when it occurs, is not functionally restricting in children. The prognosis is generally good.

Symptomatic control is usually achieved with salicylates or tolmetin. Parenteral gold salts or systemic corticosteroids occasionally may be required.

The anesthetic considerations are similar to those for juvenile ankylosing spondylitis.

Arthritis of Immune Deficiency

The immunodeficiency diseases, in particular X-linked agammaglobulinemia, selective IgA deficiency, and complement component deficiencies, are associated with various forms of arthritis and connective tissue disorders. The incidence may be as high as 30 percent. The usual pattern of arthropathy is similar to that of juvenile rheumatoid arthritis, and the most common connective tissue disorder seen is systemic lupus erythematosus. The etiological implications of the close association of immune deficiency with autoimmune diseases is currently of intense interest.

The treatment of connective tissue disorders in patients with immune deficiency is the same as for uncomplicated disease, but corticosteroids and immunosuppressive agents must be used with extreme caution.

SYSTEMIC LUPUS ERYTHEMATOSUS

Systemic lupus erythematosus is an episodic, multisystemic disease characterized by widespread inflammatory changes of the blood vessels and connective tissues. The annual incidence of the disease is 0.6 to 1 per 100,000 population. Eighteen to twenty percent of cases present in childhood after the age of 8 years. Females are affected more often than males by an 8:1 ratio. The disease seems to be more prevalent in dark-skinned races. In children, the disease is usually more acute and more severe than in adults.[300] Although unpredictable, it is usually progressive and may be fatal if untreated.

The etiology of the disease is probably multifactorial. Although an altered immune response of genetic predisposition is a central feature, intercurrent viral infections, the hormonal changes of pregnancy, and environmental factors such as sunlight are associated with exacerbations of the disease.[299] A transient, lupus-like syndrome may develop following exposure to some drugs, notably hydralazine, isoniazid, the sulfonamides, procainamide, penicillamine, and the hydantoin anticonvulsants.[309]

The pathological lesions in systemic lupus include an immune complex–initiated necrotizing vasculitis, inflammatory cellular infiltrates of serosal tissues, and degenerative connective tissue changes. The antinuclear antibody is almost always present.

Clinical Manifestations. The onset of the disease in children before the age of 5 years is rare. The presentation may be insidious and episodic, or acute and rapidly fatal from cardiac, pulmonary, renal, and neurological complications or from secondary infection.[302, 314] Presenting features vary greatly, depending on which organ systems are involved. The usual constitutional symptoms of acute disease include fever, malaise, weakness, arthralgias, anorexia, and weight loss.

The mucocutaneous manifestations occur in most children at some stage. An erythematous butterfly rash over the nose and cheeks is highly suggestive of the disease. It may extend over the face, neck, shoulders, and trunk and may become bullous and secondarily infected.[304] Erythematous macules, secondary to dermal vasculitis, may appear anywhere on the skin.[8] Oral and nasal ulcerations occur in 50 percent of patients.[9] Raynaud's phenomenon, purpura, erythema nodosum, and erythema multiforme are associated skin features.

Arthralgias and migratory arthritis, affecting the small joints of the hands, wrists, elbows, shoulders, knees, and ankles, are common. The arthritis may be severely painful but is transient and almost never destructive. However, ischemic necrosis of the femoral heads does occur. Cricoarytenoid joint ankylosis has been described in an adult.[305]

Cardiac involvement may be severe. Pericarditis with friction rubs is most common. Myocarditis occurs in 25 percent of patients and is manifested as cardiomegaly, congestive failure, and dysrhythmias.[306] Verrucous endocarditis (Libman-Sacks), usually affecting the mitral valve, may develop in acute crises. Myocardial infarction is rare but has been described in children.[307] Pleuritic chest pain, pleural effusions, pulmonary infiltrates, pneumonitis, and secondary pneumonias may lead to later fibrosis.[236, 308] The necrotizing vasculitis may cause spontaneous pneumothorax or severe pulmonary hemorrhage[8, 9] (Fig. 15–20).

Central nervous system involvement is manifested as personality changes, seizure disorders, cerebrovascular accidents, and peripheral neuropathies.[309] Acute abdominal pain from inflammatory serositis may occur with vomiting and diarrhea. Mesenteric vasculitis, complicated by the infarction of bowel, may require emergency laparotomy.[310] Moderate hepatosplenomegaly and generalized lymphadenopathy occur in active disease. Anemia, with a hematocrit of less than 30, is seen in 50 percent of affected children. Leukopenia, thrombocytopenia, and coagulopathies occur frequently in active disease. Idiopathic thrombocytopenic purpura may be the initial presentation of systemic lupus.

Significant clinical renal involvement occurs in 75 percent of children. It is more severe than that seen in adults and develops within 2 years of the disease onset. The more severe forms of lupus nephritis, identified by renal biopsy, are diffuse proliferative glomerulonephritis and membranous glomerulonephritis. Nephrotic syndrome and hypertension are not uncommon. Renal failure may occur eventually in almost half the affected patients.[9]

Systemic lupus erythematosus may mimic many other rheumatic diseases. The diagnosis is based on clinical findings and confirmed by laboratory tests. Antinuclear antibodies are usually present but are not specific. Antibodies to DNA are specific but are present only in active disease. Serum hemolytic complement components are decreased in active disease and provide a good guide to the adequacy of treatment and remission.

Neonatal Lupus Erythematosus. Some infants of mothers with active disease will have transient lupus manifestations caused by the transplacental transfer of IgG autoantibodies. The most frequent clinical finding is a malar erythema, similar to adult discoid lupus. Transient thrombocytopenia, hemolytic anemia, and leukopenia have been described.[8, 9] No treatment is required; the abnormalities resolve spontaneously in a few months.

Congenital complete heart block is described in infants born to mothers with systemic lupus and some other rheumatic diseases.[315] Neonatal endocardial fibroelastosis has also been reported.[6]

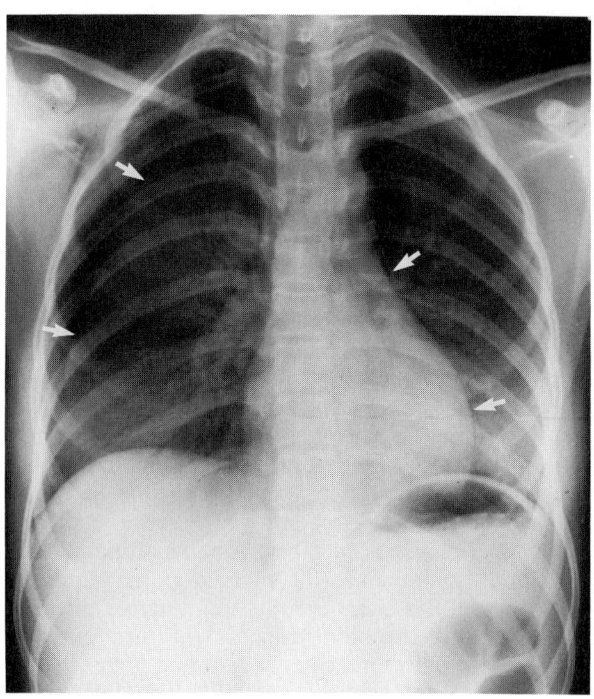

FIGURE 15–20. Chest radiograph of an 11-year-old girl with systemic lupus erythematosus in crisis, whose pulmonary vasculitis has produced a deteriorating pneumonitis complicated by spontaneous pneumothorax and pneumomediastinum *(arrows)*.

Sjögren's Syndrome. Sjögren's syndrome is a multisystemic disorder, characterized by the triad of the sicca syndrome (dry eyes and mouth), a connective tissue disease, usually systemic lupus erythematosus, and high titers of autoantibodies, which are often rheumatoid factors and antinuclear antibodies. Although it is rare in children, it usually presents as recurrent parotid swelling and as complaints of the sicca syndrome.[312] Lymphocytic infiltration is seen in the lacrimal and salivary glands; this may extend to involve the upper respiratory tract, larynx, stomach, and genitourinary tract. Systemic manifestations include achlorhydria, pancreatitis, chronic active hepatitis, nephropathy, lymphoma, and anemia.

The treatment of Sjögren's syndrome is symptomatic and includes artificial tears and increased air humidity.

Treatment. No specific treatment for lupus erythematosus is available. Patients should avoid excessive exposure to sunlight and the drugs associated with exacerbations. The objectives of medical treatment are to maintain clinical well-being and to slow the disease progression by suppressing the inflammatory process and the formation of immune complexes.

In mild disease without nephritis, salicylates and occasionally antimalarial drugs may be quite effective. Topical steroids often control the skin rash. In acute lupus crises, systemic corticosteroids are required in high doses (prednisone, 1 to 2 mg/kg/24 hours) for the control of carditis, neurological manifestations, and nephritis. Withdrawal to maintenance doses is not attempted for 4 weeks. The immunosuppressive agents azathioprine, cyclophosphamide, and chlorambucil are used with extreme caution when the nephritis is unresponsive to steroids.

Secondary infections during periods of active disease may be lethal and, when identified, must be treated aggressively.

Although remissions may occur in children, the usual course is one of chronic disease, extending over many years. The 5-year survival has now improved to 90 percent.[314] The major causes of death are secondary sepsis, nephritis, gastrointestinal hemorrhage and perforation, pulmonary hemorrhage, malignant hypertension, and carditis.[9]

Anesthetic Management. Systemic lupus erythematosus represents a chronic but episodic disease with potentially severe multiple organ dysfunction. Children with this disease may be acutely ill, febrile, weak, and debilitated and have secondary infections. Careful evaluation must be made of renal, cardiac, and pulmonary function and central nervous system manifestations. Joint mobility, particularly of the neck and temporomandibular joints, must be assessed. Erosive lesions of the nasal or oropharyngeal mucosa may make passage of an endotracheal tube difficult or traumatic but rarely compromise the airway. Patients with active disease are usually anemic and thrombocytopenic and may have a coagulopathy. Crossmatching for blood products may be difficult because of erythrocyte antibodies, but adequate blood products must be available.[8] Perioperative steroid coverage will likely be required. Antibiotic prophylaxis will be necessary in patients with endocarditis.

For general anesthesia, all usual monitors should be used. The anesthetic gases must be warmed and humidified. For patients with Sjögren's syndrome, the eyes should be protected by an ophthalmic ointment. Airway maintenance and laryngoscopy are not a reported problem in children, but care must be exercised in patients with facial bullae and erosive oropharyngeal mucous membrane lesions.

No specific anesthetic agents or techniques are recommended, but those drugs excreted via the kidney should be used with caution in the presence of renal impairment. Agents that depress myocardial contractility may be poorly tolerated in patients with carditis. Ventilation should be controlled in children with pulmonary involvement. The use of anticholinergic (drying) agents is discouraged in Sjögren's syndrome. Regional blocks are relatively contraindicated in patients with peripheral neuropathies.

DERMATOMYOSITIS

Juvenile dermatomyositis is a multisystemic disease characterized by acute and chronic nonsuppurative inflammation of striated muscle and skin. The incidence of the disease is 1 per 200,000 population. Childhood onset usually occurs between ages 5 and 9 years and accounts for 15 to 20 percent of cases.[9] Girls are affected twice as frequently as boys. Polymyositis, the same disease without cutaneous manifestations, is rare in children.

The etiology is unknown, but a cell-mediated immunological disturbance is responsible for some of the disease features. Photosensitivity, drug hypersensitivity, and infections also have been implicated. A necrotizing vasculitis of vessels in the skin, muscle, and subcutaneous tissue and occasionally in the gastrointestinal tract is the usual pathological finding in childhood dermatomyositis.

Clinical Manifestations. In children, the usual presenting feature is the insidious development of muscle weakness involving the proximal muscles of the hip and shoulder girdle. Muscle pain, tenderness, and stiffness are commonly associated with gait disturbances, fever, malaise, and weight loss.[315, 316] In 10 percent of cases, weakness of the palatal and pharyngeal muscles may cause dysphonia and dysphagia and lead to incompetent swallowing mechanisms and pulmonary aspiration.[317] Intercostal involvement may impair adequate ventilation. The healing of affected muscles by fibrosis may lead to incapacitating contracture deformities.

The hallmark of dermatomyositis is the skin rash, seen in 75 percent of affected children. The violaceous discoloration of the eyelids and occasionally the cheeks associated with periorbital and facial edema is pathognomonic. Generalized erythema may develop. Symmetrical, erythematous, atrophic changes are found over the extensor surfaces of joints of the hands, elbows, and knees. Nonpitting edema of the skin and subcutaneous tissue may be present. Mucosal ulcerations may develop secondary to local vasculitis. With resolution of the rash, varying pigmentation changes are subsequently observed in the skin. Raynaud's phenomenon is not seen in children.

Subcutaneous deposition of calcium (calcinosis) in response to tissue injury and fibrosis is a feature in 40 percent of children. The accumulations may be large and ultimately may protrude through the skin, producing sizable ulcerated and denuded areas. A transient, nondeforming arthritis develops occasionally. Modest hepatosplenomegaly and lymphadenopathy may be found. Infrequently, gastrointestinal ulceration and hemorrhage may cause anemia. Apart from aspiration pneumonitis, pulmonary involvement with interstitial fibrosis is rare in children.[318] Myocarditis and pericarditis are described but are also rare.[9]

The diagnosis is confirmed by the combination of muscle weakness, characteristic skin rash, elevated serum enzymes, notably the transaminases and creatine phosphokinase, and an abnormal electromyogram.

The course may be acute, with a mortality rate of 40 percent in untreated patients from complications of pharyngeal incompetence, respiratory weakness, and gastrointestinal hemorrhage, or may become slowly inactive over several years. Subsequent exacerbations are unusual. The associated malignancies (carcinomas) seen in 20 percent of adults do not occur in children.

Treatment. Functional recovery depends on the preservation of muscle strength and the prevention of deforming contractures. Ongoing physical therapy is important. In the acute phase, close scrutiny of the competence of swallowing and the adequacy of respiratory function is mandatory. Intubation and ventilatory support may be required.

Corticosteroids effectively suppress the inflammatory process and have reversed the earlier grim prognosis. Prednisone, 1 to 2 mg/kg/24 hours, is usually continued for 2 to 4 weeks before reduction to a maintenance dose is attempted. Steroids are often necessary for 1 to 2 years. Salicylates may be helpful in the relief of joint symptoms and myalgias. Rarely, immunosuppressive agents are required.

Anesthetic Management. The preoperative assessment of muscle weakness is mandatory. Palatal and pharyngeal weakness with incompetent swallowing may leave considerable mucus in the upper airway. The loss of respiratory reserve through muscle weakness may be complicated by aspiration pneumonitis. A forced vital capacity determination should be obtained and the chest radiograph reviewed. A facial rash, edema, and oral ulcerations must be identified. Patients with dermatomyositis may be anemic and generally debilitated. Perioperative corticosteroid coverage will usually be required.

Because of potential pharyngeal incompetence, general anesthesia with intubation is usually recommended.[10] Facial and oropharyngeal contractures do not occur and laryngoscopy should not be difficult. In the presence of active myositis, succinylcholine probably should be avoided, although in a recent case report its use in a child was not associated with problems.[319] Heightened sensitivity to nondepolarizing muscle relaxants has been observed; the shorter-acting agents should be used and only if necessary.[320, 321] Intolerance to narcotics may be pronounced; all sedatives must be used in modest doses. Ventilation should be assisted or controlled throughout the anesthetic.

Prior to extubation, the full return of neuromuscular function must be verified if relaxants were used, and the patient should be awake. If preoperative pulmonary function was significantly reduced, ventilatory support should be planned in an intensive care area following a major surgical procedure.

SCLERODERMA

Scleroderma is a chronic, multisystemic disorder of connective tissue affecting the skin, which becomes hardened and inelastic. Visceral involvement may be severe and affects heart, lungs, kidneys, gastrointestinal tract, and synovium. The disease is very uncommon in children, who account for only 1 to 3 percent of the total cases. The usual age of onset is 3 to 15 years; girls are predominantly affected, by a 5:1 ratio. In childhood, scleroderma usually presents as localized skin involvement alone, either in focal patches, *morphea,* or in linear patterns of distribution, *linear scleroderma.* Uncommonly seen in children is *progressive systemic sclerosis,* manifested by symmetrical skin involvement and severe visceral complications.

The affected tissues show perivascular infiltration with mononuclear cells and edema. Collagen fibers are thickened and have increased density. The disease progresses through stages of inflammation, fibrosis, and atrophy.[322] The etiology is unknown but may include an immune mechanism and an abnormality in collagen tissue.[323]

Clinical Manifestations. The skin and subcutaneous tissue involvement in morphea is patchy, and lesions are often found on an extremity. Initially these skin lesions are erythematous, with nonpitting edema, and have a shiny, atrophic appearance. Subsequent induration and scarring binds the skin to underlying structures. If extensive, this "hide-binding" may limit growth of the extremity or cause crippling contractures.

In systemic disease, the cutaneous features are similar, but distribution is symmetrical and involves the fingers, toes, distal extremities, trunk, and face. The indurative phase produces the characteristic masklike facies, with the loss of skin folds, a pinched nose, small, contracted mouth, and prominent teeth. Mouth opening is significantly reduced in 28 percent of adult patients.[324] Telangiectases of the face, lips, tongue, chest, and hands may develop. Accumulations of subcutaneous calcification may enlarge ultimately to ulcerate through the skin. Raynaud's phenomenon is a complaint in most patients.

Diffuse pulmonary fibrosis occurs in 60 percent of adults and children and presents as a dry cough or as exertional dyspnea.[9] Accompanying small airway disease is identified by a decreased maximal midexpiratory flow rate and increased closing capacities.[325] Thirty percent of patients have restrictive pulmonary disease, which may be complicated by pulmonary hypertension, cor pulmonale, and cardiac failure.[326–329]

Cardiac disease in adults with scleroderma is manifested by myocardial fibrosis with secondary conduction defects, dysrhythmias, right and left ventricular hypertrophy, and congestive failure. Angina pectoris with normal coronary arteries from presumed vasospastic phenomena is described.[330, 331] These features are not seen in children often, but pericardial effusions and cardiac failure do occur.

Renal dysfunction, presenting as proteinuria, hypertension, and azotemia, develops in 45 percent of patients within 3 years of the onset of disease. The underlying pathology is a microangiopathy.[9] Malignant hypertension develops in 7 percent of patients secondary to increased renin production.[9] The prognosis of renal complications is usually dismal.

Abnormalities in esophageal motility are found in the majority of patients and present as retrosternal dysphagia and pharyngeal reflux. Associated gastroesophageal reflux may be complicated by esophageal strictures in 25 percent of patients. Duodenal and small bowel pathology may cause diarrhea, constipation, and a malabsorption syndrome.

An inflammatory polyarthritis with juxta-articular osteoporosis, fibrosis, and contractures may develop involving the fingers (sclerodactyly), wrists, ankles, knees, and elbows. The mandible may be involved.[332] About 25 percent of children are anemic either from chronic disease or from repeated hemorrhage from telangiectasia. The malabsorption of vitamin K may lead to a coagulopathy.

Two similar disorders should be mentioned at this time:

Scleredema. This rare disorder is characterized by edematous induration of the face, neck, shoulders, thorax, and upper arms. In children, the disease is often preceded by a streptococcal infection. Systemic manifestations are uncommon, but minor cardiac abnormalities may occur. These include a diastolic gallop without failure and nonspecific ECG changes.[1, 9] Spontaneous resolution of the disease usually occurs within 6 months to 2 years.

Mixed Connective Tissue Disease. This uncommon overlap syndrome includes features of scleroderma, systemic lupus erythematosus, and dermatomyositis.[9] Common clinical manifestations include the edematous phase of scleroderma skin changes, the rash of dermatomyositis, Raynaud's phenomenon, myositis, anemia and thrombocytopenia, myocarditis, pericarditis, pleurisy, and Sjögren's syndrome. Severe renal disease is rare.[9, 333] High titers of antibodies to ribonucleoprotein are invariably found. Most manifestations of the disease respond rapidly to corticosteroids, and the prognosis of most patients is good.

Treatment. There is no specific treatment for scleroderma. Patients are advised to avoid cold and trauma. Joint mobility must be maintained by exercise and positions of function maintained by the use of splints. Lubricant creams may improve skin pliability.

Raynaud's phenomenon may be improved by sympathetic blocking agents such as reserpine, phenoxybenzamine, or methyldopa. Gastroesophageal reflux often requires antacids and cimetidine. Esophageal strictures may need surgical intervention. Cardiac failure usually can be controlled by digoxin and pericardial effusions by diuretics, although pericardiocentesis may be necessary. Some encouraging results from early treatment of renal failure with dialysis and transplantation have been reported.[334] Hypertension is usually managed with renin-suppressing agents such as captopril.[335]

Systemic corticosteroids are used for the suppression of the inflammatory contribution to pulmonary fibrosis and for acute myositis when it occurs. Very little response to steroids is seen in other features of the disease.

The prognosis of progressive systemic sclerosis depends on the severity of visceral organ involvement; the long-term outlook in children is guarded. Cardiac, renal, and pulmonary complications may cause death in 6 months to 10 years after the diagnosis is made.[9]

Anesthetic Management. Children with scleroderma may have severe multisystemic disease and require thorough preoperative assessment.

Of particular importance is the evaluation of the upper airway. Contracted perioral skin and a reduced mouth opening will make laryngoscopy difficult. Oropharyngeal telangiectasia should be identified. Pulmonary function tests should be obtained prior to major procedures. The cardiac complications of cor pulmonale, congestive failure, or pericardial effusion may have developed, and a history of angina pectoris in older children should be sought. A chest radiograph and ECG should be reviewed and renal and hepatic function assessed. Patients may be anemic and have a vitamin K–dependent coagulopathy secondary to malabsorption. Joints affected by active arthritis should be noted.

These patients may be on a variety of medications, notably antihypertensive drugs, sympathetic blocking agents, and systemic corticosteroids. Perioperative steroid supplementation may be required. Hypertensive patients may be volume contracted and will benefit from preoperative hydration. Premedication should include cimetidine and an antacid in the presence of gastroesophageal reflux.

The operating room should be kept warm and

the patient transferred carefully. In the presence of esophageal reflux, a relatively head-up position is advised.

Regional blocks have proved very successful in adults.[336–339] The prolonged analgesic effects reported may be useful in children for postoperative pain relief even if general anesthesia was required.[336]

When general anesthesia is required, all usual monitors should be applied. Blood pressure is best taken by cuff and Doppler probe. An arterial line may aggravate vasospastic phenomena and should be used only if necessary. Intravenous access may be difficult but should be obtained prior to induction. Intravenous injections may be painful and may provoke Raynaud's phenomenon.[339]

Patients who have limited mouth opening may require intubation awake with modest sedation, as for patients with juvenile rheumatoid arthritis (see page 532). In these patients, no relaxants should be used prior to successful intubation. In some children, an inhalational induction may be preferred. When laryngoscopy is performed in patients with a small mouth opening, avoid excessive retraction force as the corner of the mouth may tear.[340, 341] Cricoid pressure and a head-up position are recommended, even in elective operations.[255] Ketamine may be useful in some patients.[342]

With the airway under control, several recommendations remain. The anesthetic gases should be warmed and humidified. Ventilation should be assisted or controlled when pulmonary reserve is reduced. Hypovolemia and hypotension must be corrected quickly, particularly in hypertensive children, because any fall in renal blood flow may seriously compromise renal function.[9] Patients who were difficult to intubate should not be extubated until they are awake and have fully competent laryngeal reflexes.

SYSTEMIC VASCULITIS SYNDROMES

The inflammatory degeneration of vascular tissues produces a great variety of disease patterns that are determined by the location and the size of affected vessels. There may be considerable overlap among these syndromes and with the connective tissue diseases in which vasculitis is a feature, notably systemic lupus erythematosus, dermatomyositis, scleroderma, and less commonly rheumatoid arthritis.

The most common vasculitis syndrome in childhood is Henoch-Schönlein purpura, which affects small, nonmuscular blood vessels. The involvement of small and medium muscular vessels, referred to as polyarteritis nodosa, includes the variants infantile polyarteritis nodosa, Kawasaki's disease, and probably Wegener's granulomatosis; these are uncommon in children. Takayasu's arteritis affects the aorta and great vessels and is extremely rare in children.

Henoch-Schönlein Purpura (Anaphylactoid Purpura)

Henoch-Schönlein purpura is an acute, necrotizing vasculitis of small, nonmuscular blood vessels, clinically manifested as nonthrombocytopenic purpura, arthritis or arthralgias, abdominal pain, gastrointestinal hemorrhage, and nephritis. This syndrome is not rare and occurs most commonly in previously healthy children between the ages of 2 and 10 years. Boys are affected twice as frequently as girls.[9] The etiology is unknown, but important associations with allergies, drug sensitivities, and prior upper respiratory streptococcal infections are recognized. The vasculitis involves capillaries, small arterioles, and venules, which are surrounded by an acute inflammatory exudate of polymorphonuclear cells. Local edema and hemorrhage may occur at any site affected.

Clinical Manifestations. The onset is usually acute and presents with a purpuric rash over the buttocks and lower legs, which may extend to the arms and, less commonly, the face. The lesions appear in crops, and they are seen at different stages of resolution (Fig. 15–21). Nonpitting edema may involve the hands, feet, and upper face. Erythema multiforme and erythema nodosum may be associated conditions.[8]

Most children develop concurrent gastrointestinal symptoms, usually colicky abdominal pain and vomiting. Stools may show evidence of gross bleeding, and hematemesis may occur. Intestinal intussusception, infarction, and perforation are complications in less than 5 percent of cases but develop rapidly.[9] Most patients are anemic, but coagulation is normal.

Renal involvement occurs in about half the patients and is manifested by hematuria and proteinuria. In 5 percent of patients, the nephritis is complicated by progressive renal failure and hypertension. The central nervous system is affected infrequently, but this involvement is serious. Seizure disorders, paresis from intracranial hemorrhage, and coma may occur. Pulmonary involvement is most unusual but has been described in an adult.[343]

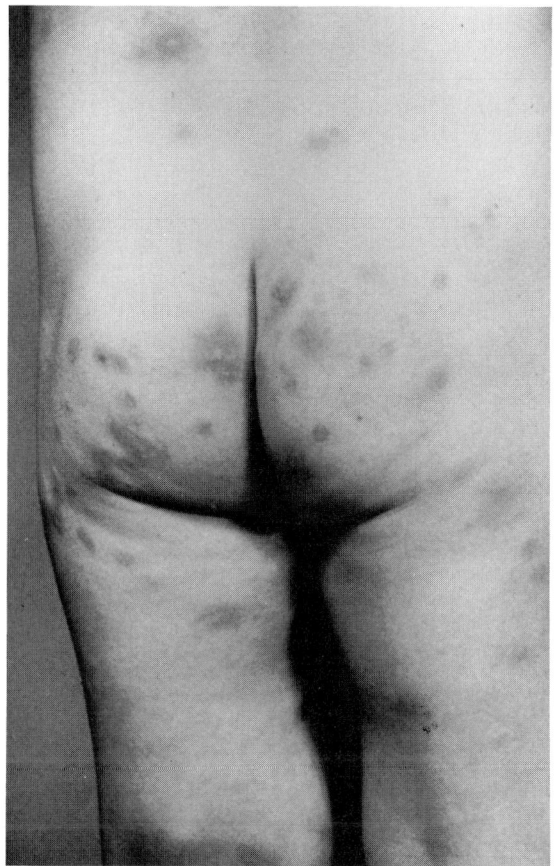

FIGURE 15–21. Henoch-Schönlein purpura in a 4-year-old boy. Note the purpuric lesions at different stages of resolution.

Arthritis or arthralgia occurs in 75 percent of patients, usually affecting knees and ankles, but elbows and hands may be involved. Joint swelling and tenderness are marked but are transient and nondeforming. Nonspecific constitutional symptoms of fever and malaise are usually present.

Treatment. No specific therapy is available; treatment is supportive and symptomatic. Identified allergens should be removed and streptococcal infections treated with antibiotics. Symptomatic relief of the arthralgias and fever by salicylates is usually adequate. Systemic corticosteroids are indicated only for life-threatening gastrointestinal hemorrhage or obstruction and for severe central nervous system manifestations.

In most children, resolution of the disease occurs within 4 weeks and the prognosis is excellent. Exacerbations may recur within 2 years. A major cause of morbidity is severe nephritis, which may progress to renal failure. In acute disease, death may occur from gastrointestinal hemorrhage or perforation, renal failure, or central nervous system complications.

Anesthetic Management. The children may be acutely ill, and they require careful preoperative assessment. The gastrointestinal complications of obstruction, intussusception, hemorrhage, perforation, and peritonitis demand aggressive resuscitation to correct anemia and hypovolemia. Adequate blood products must be available. Peripheral intravenous access may be difficult. Renal dysfunction, central nervous system signs, and acute arthropathies must be identified.

No specific anesthetic agents or techniques are recommended. However, when general anesthesia is required for such procedures as laparotomy, a rapid sequence induction and intubation should be planned. Patients who are hypovolemic will not tolerate potent myocardial depressants or peripheral vasodilatation. Intraoperative hypovolemia and hypotension must be corrected quickly; any decrease in renal blood flow may seriously jeopardize renal function in children with nephritis. In patients with cerebral vasculitis and increased intracranial pressure, a technique incorporating hyperventilation should be used. Postoperative care in an intensive care area is recommended.

POLYARTERITIS NODOSA

In polyarteritis nodosa, a necrotizing vasculitis involves the entire vessel wall thickness of medium and small muscular arteries of many organs. This manifests as tissue necrosis, vessel thrombosis, or aneurysm formation.[8, 9, 344] The clinical presentation and course of the disease may be extremely variable and are determined by the sites of the vascular disease. The most severe complications arise from involvement of the gastrointestinal tract, heart, kidneys, and central nervous system. The etiology is unknown, but associations with drug exposures, hepatitis B antigen, and streptococcal infections are described.[8, 9] It is a rare disease in children; boys and girls are affected equally with a peak age of onset between 9 and 11 years.

The onset of polyarteritis nodosa in children is often insidious, with vague constitutional symptoms of fever, malaise, weakness, and weight loss, but its ultimate progression is usually severe. Various purpuric or petechial skin lesions and joint symptoms may develop early. Gastrointestinal tract manifestations may present as an acute abdomen with colicky pain, hemorrhage, infarction, and perforation.[310]

Anemia is frequent. The nephritis is usually severe and is complicated by hypertension and early renal failure. Coronary vasculitis and myocarditis precipitate myocardial infarctions and congestive failure. Central nervous system involvement and peripheral neuropathies occur in 50 to 70 percent of patients.[9] Organic psychoses, seizures, hemiparesis, and coma are not uncommon. Pulmonary infiltrates produce a pneumonitis, and occasionally wheezing develops. Pharyngeal edema has been described in adults.[284]

Corticosteroids may suppress acute manifestations of the disease and prolong survival, but the overall prognosis is poor. Death usually results from renal failure, myocardial infarctions, or complications of hypertension.

Infantile Polyarteritis Nodosa. This variant of polyarteritis is a rare condition but is seen in infants less than 1 year of age with a characteristic clinical pattern. The illness begins with symptoms similar to those of a persistent viral upper respiratory tract infection with fever, rhinitis, conjunctivitis, and a macular erythematous skin rash, but subsequent internal organ involvement develops quickly. Cardiac manifestations include aneurysmal coronary artery vasculitis with cardiomegaly, congestive failure, pericarditis, and myocardial infarction. Severe nephritis with hypertension and renal failure, peripheral and central nervous system complications, and gastrointestinal crises reflect the severe widespread vasculitis.[8, 9, 346]

No effective treatment is available. Corticosteroids have not been beneficial; antiplatelet and antithrombotic agents may be more appropriate. Death often occurs within 1 month of the onset of the disease from myocardial infarction and renal complications.[9]

Anesthetic Management. These children are usually critically ill with multiple organ system dysfunction and demand careful preoperative assessment. Medical therapy may include corticosteroids, antihypertensive agents, and supportive treatment for myocardial failure with digoxin and diuretics. The correction of anemia and hypovolemia will be necessary.

Basic anesthetic considerations in children with polyarteritis nodosa are similar to those for Henoch-Schönlein purpura. However, several additional points should be stressed. Aggressive, invasive monitoring may be indicated. Small infants with acute abdomens are most safely intubated awake. Pulmonary involvement can be severe, and ventilation should be controlled. In view of the risk of coronary artery disease, myocardial oxygenation should be optimized by avoiding tachycardia and large swings in blood pressure. Lead II and/or lead V_5 should be monitored on the ECG.

Postoperative support in an intensive care area should be considered.

Mucocutaneous Lymph Node Syndrome (Kawasaki Disease)

The mucocutaneous lymph node syndrome is an acute febrile illness affecting primarily infants and children, characterized by a systemic vasculitis of small and medium muscular arteries. Although this syndrome is much less severe,

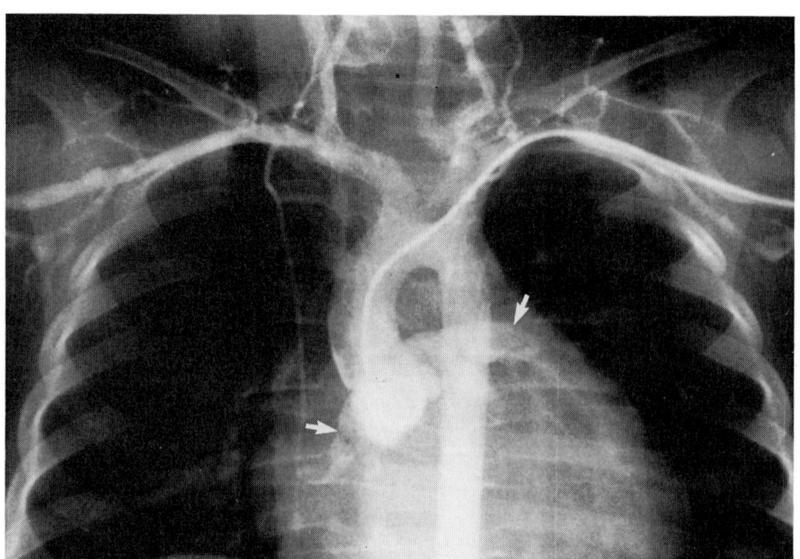

FIGURE 15–22. Kawasaki disease in a 4-year-old boy. Note the aneurysmal dilatation of the right and left coronary arteries *(arrows)*.

many features are similar to those of infantile polyarteritis nodosa, which may represent an extreme expression of this disease. Kawasaki disease is uncommon and is seen most frequently in Japanese children. However, an increasing incidence is now being recognized in North America.[9] Boys are affected more than girls by a ratio of 1.5:1; the peak age of onset is 1 to 4 years. The etiology is unknown; various viral and bacterial infections have been associated with the disease, but none have been proved to cause it.

Clinical Manifestations. The classic features of its presentation include an acute, high, and remittent fever that may cause febrile convulsions, accompanied by a skin rash that is usually erythematous and macular. Characteristic mucocutaneous changes include dry, red, fissuring lips; erythema of the oropharynx; and a strawberry tongue. Bilateral conjunctivitis is common. Painful, edematous induration of the hands and feet with subsequent desquamation of local skin during recovery is seen in 65 percent of patients.[9] Transient lymphadenopathy, usually involving the anterior cervical nodes, is common.[347–350]

Other clinical features may include a prodromal upper respiratory tract infection and variable pulmonary infiltrates. Abdominal pain from mesenteric vasculitis may be accompanied by watery diarrhea and dehydration. Central nervous system involvement may range from minor personality changes to the severe manifestations of aseptic meningitis. Large joint arthralgias are frequent. Hepatic dysfunction occurs in 10 percent of patients, but renal involvement is mild.

Cardiac complications represent the most serious manifestations of the disease and may be identified to some degree in 70 percent of patients.[348] Overt clinical myocarditis with conduction defects, dysrhythmias, pericarditis, mitral insufficiency, and congestive failure may be seen in 10 percent of patients. During the recovery period, coronary artery aneurysms are diagnosed in 15 percent of patients by two-dimensional echocardiography[349, 350] (Figs. 15–22 and 15–23). Myocardial infarction, coronary thrombosis, or rupture of the coronary aneurysms probably accounts for the early death described in 1.5 to 2.0 percent of affected children. The long-term prognosis of cardiac involvement is unknown.

The acute febrile stage lasts for 7 to 10 days and is followed by a subacute stage over the next 2 to 4 weeks. The subsequent recovery period may continue for months and possibly years.

Treatment. In the acute stage, careful monitoring of cardiac function is required in the hospital. High-dose salicylate therapy is used for its antiplatelet effects and to control the arthritis. In the acute phase, gamma globulin may decrease aneurysm formation.[349] Dipyridamole, a vasodilator, may be used in combination with salicylates. Corticosteroids may accelerate the development of coronary aneurysms and are generally contraindicated except for cautious use in patients with severe myocarditis. Successful aortocoronary bypass grafting has been performed for severe coronary disease in a 4-year-old boy.[351, 352]

Anesthetic Management. Of critical importance is the preoperative assessment of cardiac function and the identification of congestive failure, dysrhythmias, conduction defects, myocardial ischemia, coronary artery disease, and valvular dysfunction. The other major organ systems involved require careful review as well. Dehydration and electrolyte disturbances secondary to diarrhea must be corrected. The impli-

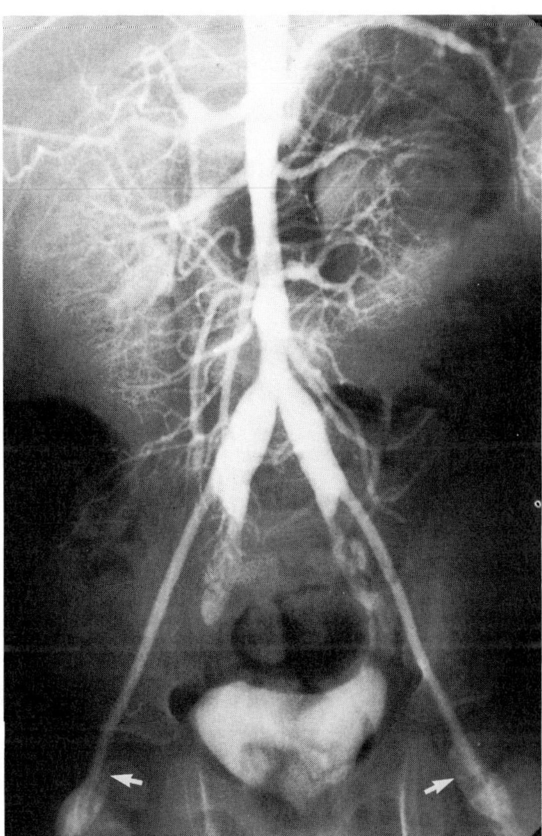

FIGURE 15–23. Severe, occlusive aortic and peripheral vascular disease in a 4-year-old boy with Kawasaki disease. Note the femoral artery aneurysms *(arrows)*.

cations of maintenance medications, which may include salicylates, digoxin, diuretics, narcotics for pain, and steroids, must be recognized. Cautious premedication may be required to facilitate a quiet induction.

No specific anesthetic drugs or techniques are recommended, but the approach should be similar to that for patients with coronary artery disease.[355] Induction should be smooth. Myocardial oxygen supply and demand should be optimized by avoiding tachycardia and acute swings in blood pressure. All usual monitors should be used at induction. ECG leads II and V_5 should be monitored to identify ischemic change in the myocardium. In some patients and for major procedures, full invasive monitoring may be required. Laryngoscopy must be gentle to avoid trauma to inflamed lips, tongue, and oropharynx. Ventilation should be controlled, and if significant central nervous system manifestations exist, hyperventilation may be indicated.

Repeat axillary and caudal nerve blocks in a 7-month-old infant with necrotizing angiitis from Kawasaki disease have been described. The resulting sympathetic blockade markedly improved peripheral blood flow.

Postoperative care for these patients may be best provided in an intensive care area.

Takayasu Arteritis (Pulseless Disease)

This uncommon disorder is characterized by a segmental arteritis involving the aorta, its major branches, and the pulmonary arteries. It predominantly affects young women more than men by an 8:1 ratio. Twenty percent of patients are less than 20 years of age, and the disease has been described in young children.[292] The etiology is unknown.

The characteristic pathology is a focal or diffuse loss of muscular and elastic tissue in the arterial wall, with subsequent extensive fibrosis of the media. Giant cells are frequently seen in the areas of destruction. Aneurysmal dilatation, rupture, stenosis, and occlusion may occur in affected vessels. Pulses to the upper extremity may be absent, and the blood pressure in the legs may exceed that in the arms (hence, the terms pulseless disease and reverse coarctation). Seventy-five percent of patients develop myocardial failure, ventricular strain, or coronary artery involvement.[357] The impairment of renal blood flow leads to secondary hypertension; the interruption of cerebral blood flow may cause neurological disturbances.

Over half of affected children present with an acute onset of fever and hypermetabolic symptoms, including night sweats, anorexia, and weight loss. Arthritis and anemia are frequent features. However, the disease may be asymptomatic; in these cases, disorders of peripheral pulses or hypertension may be the first indications of its presence.[355]

Treatment. Anti-inflammatory agents usually alleviate symptoms of the disease; corticosteroids may have a beneficial effect in acute periods. Hypertension may require aggressive medical management with renin-inhibiting agents and vasodilators. Anticoagulants may be useful in the chronic, occlusive phase. Good results with surgical endarterectomy, bypass grafting, and radiological dilatation angioplasty have been reported, but these procedures are not advised in patients with acute disease.[356] The prognosis of the disease is variable, but slow progression is the usual rule.

Anesthetic Management. The cardiovascular system must be evaluated preoperatively to identify the cardiac complications of failure and myocardial ischemia and to assess the extent of reduced peripheral pulses. Secondary renal hypertension and its medical management should be noted. Coincident anemia may require correction prior to operation.

All usual monitors are required.[357–359] ECG leads II and V_5 best identify ischemic changes. The true blood pressure may be difficult to measure in extremities with reduced peripheral pulses even when an indwelling cannula is used. Warner and associates recommend the use of a balloon-tipped flow-directed pulmonary artery catheter for a major operation in patients with absent pulses. Cardiac output, wedge pressures, and mixed venous gases can then be measured.[357]

Anesthetic techniques and drugs should be chosen that will preserve the balance of myocardial oxygen supply and demand and are appropriate for patients with hypertension and coronary artery disease. Premedication will be helpful. Diazepam, fentanyl, and pancuronium have been used in adults.[357] A careful inhalation induction may be more suitable for some children. Care should be taken to prevent, or quickly correct, hypovolemia and secondary hypotension, which will jeopardize vital organ perfusion.

Wegener Granulomatosis

Wegener granulomatosis is a rare syndrome in children. Destructive granulomatous lesions in the upper airway and lungs are associated with a necrotizing angiitis most prominent in the lungs and kidneys. In a more widespread form, the skin, heart, central nervous system, gastrointestinal tract, and joints may be involved. When the lesions are limited to the upper respiratory tract and the vasculitis is minimal, the disorder is called *lethal midline granuloma.* The onset usually occurs between ages 25 and 50 years, but it has been described in a 1-year-old child. It occurs predominantly in males by a ratio of 2:1.[360] The etiology is unknown, but an association with drug sensitivity and allergy is reported.[8]

Clinical Manifestations. The clinical presentation usually begins with nasal congestion and discharge and respiratory symptoms of cough, hemoptysis, and pleuritic chest pain. Fever, malaise, and weight loss are frequent. The progressively destructive lesions may cause obliteration of the nasal sinuses, perforation of the orbit and palate, and ulcerations or narrowing of the pharynx, larynx, and trachea. A complicating tracheoesophageal fistula is described in an adult.[361] Pulmonary infiltrates, obstructive airway disease due to granuloma formation, and reduced lung volumes are common.[362] Pleural effusions, pneumothorax, and massive pulmonary hemorrhage are described.[9]

In the presence of necrotizing glomerulonephritis, uremia and renal failure may develop rapidly but usually without hypertension. Cardiac involvement with coronary vasculitis, conduction defects, valvular distortion, and congestive failure has been described but is uncommon. Arthritis involving the larger joints, splenomegaly, anemia, and peripheral neuropathy may be seen.

The prognosis of untreated disease is grim. Death from pulmonary complications or renal failure may occur in months. However, the immunosuppressive agents cyclophosphamide, azathioprine, and chlorambucil may arrest the disease and permit long-term survival. Corticosteroids may also suppress the vasculitis if used in early stages.

Anesthetic Management. Preoperative evaluation of midfacial anatomy and the upper airway to identify ulcerations and obstructing lesions is imperative. Preoperative tracheostomy may rarely be required. Pulmonary complications must be recognized, and pulmonary function tests should be obtained when indicated. Renal impairment and cardiac dysfunction must be noted. The complications of immunosuppressive agents, namely anemia, leukopenia, thrombocytopenia, and hepatic dysfunction with coagulopathy, should be corrected if possible. Perioperative steroid coverage may be required.

In the operating room, intravenous access should be obtained early, and all usual monitors should be used. In patients with upper airway lesions, Lake recommends the use of regional techniques when appropriate.[365] When general anesthesia is required in children with lesions obstructing the airway, intubation must be performed gently, avoiding trauma to the lesions. A smaller tube than usual may be required. Laryngoscopy should be done with the patient awake, cautiously sedated, or under inhalational anesthesia with spontaneous ventilation maintained. Fiberoptic laryngoscopy and intubation may be indicated.

An anesthetic technique appropriate for patients with ischemic myocardial disease should be used, avoiding tachycardia and large swings in blood pressure. Intraoperative blood loss and hypovolemia must be corrected quickly. Ventilation should be controlled, but pressures must be kept as low as possible.

Careful postoperative observation for airway obstruction is mandatory.

Goodpasture Syndrome

Patients with Goodpasture syndrome develop episodic intra-alveolar pulmonary hemorrhage in association with glomerulonephritis. The disorder is probably a distinct clinical entity but may have some overlap with polyarteritis nodosa, although generalized vasculitis is not a feature. The pulmonary lesion is thought to be the primary defect. Electron microscopy has demonstrated endothelial cell gaps and thickened alveolar septa. The renal disease arises secondary to the development of the cross-reactive anti–basement membrane antibodies. The etiology is unknown, but the syndrome has occurred in association with drug sensitivities, hepatitis, rheumatoid arthritis, and scleroderma.[9] Young adult men are predominantly affected; 90 percent of cases occur in males. Goodpasture syndrome is unusual in patients less than 16 years of age but has been described in children.[366, 367]

The early clinical presentation may be insidious but is eventually characterized by hemoptysis, nephritis, and anemia. Dyspnea, wheezing, fever, malaise, and weakness are usual associated symptoms. The chest radiograph demonstrates perihilar flocculent infiltrates, which may extend out to the peripheral lung fields. In time, pulmonary fibrosis may develop.[367] The nephritis is usually complicated by azotemia and renal failure, but hypertension is rare.[9] The recurrent pulmonary hemorrhages lead to a chronic anemia in most patients.

The progression of the disease is variable but often rapid; death usually occurs from pulmonary hemorrhage, asphyxia, or uremia. Corticosteroids and immunosuppressive agents may prolong survival in some patients; plasmapheresis has been shown to be of some benefit in others.[366]

Anesthetic Management. Particular attention should be directed to the evaluation of pulmonary and renal function. A chest radiograph should be reviewed; arterial blood gases, hemoglobin, electrolytes, blood urea nitrogen, and creatinine should be measured; and a urinalysis should be obtained. Preoperative transfusion may be required if the anemia is severe, and adequate blood products must be available for the operating room. Elective surgery should be postponed during periods of pulmonary hemorrhage. Perioperative corticosteroid supplementation may be necessary.

No specific anesthetic techniques or drugs are recommended. If pulmonary fibrosis has produced significant restrictive disease, ventilation should be controlled with an increased FIO_2, small tidal volumes, and an increased ventilatory rate.

MISCELLANEOUS CONNECTIVE TISSUE DISORDERS

MARFAN SYNDROME

Marfan syndrome is a familial disorder of connective tissue inherited as an autosomal dominant trait, with prominent manifestations in the skeletal, ocular, cardiovascular, and pulmonary systems.[9, 368] The prevalence of the syndrome is about 4 to 6 cases per 100,000 population. The underlying pathology involves a defect in collagen synthesis or maturation and results in connective tissue elements of decreased tensile strength and elasticity. An inborn error of metabolism is presumed, but not yet identified; the etiology remains unknown.

Clinical Manifestations. There is considerable variance in the clinical expression of Marfan syndrome; the diagnosis may be made in infancy or not recognized until later in life.

Skeletal abnormalities may be pathognomonic. Patients are usually tall and thin from excessive longitudinal bone growth and have long, "spidery" fingers (arachnodactyly). Body segments are disproportionate, and arm span usually exceeds body height. The face is long, narrow, and asymmetrical, often with a prognathic jaw; a high-arched palate is common. Atlantoaxial instability, thoracolumbar scoliosis, pectus excavatum and carinatum, slipped epiphysis of the femoral head, and talipes equinovarus may occur with varying degrees of severity.

Joint hypermobility is a relatively consistent feature. Pain, effusions, and even dislocation may occur after minor trauma. Peripheral muscular hypotonia may account in part for the high frequency of inguinal, umbilical, femoral, and even diaphragmatic hernias.

The most important ocular complication (seen in 50 to 80 percent of patients) is dislocation of the lens from weakened suspensory ligaments. This may be complicated by secondary glaucoma. Most patients are myopic and may develop retinal detachments. Visual impairment is frequent.

The cardiovascular manifestations represent the greatest threat to patients with Marfan syndrome. These complications result from the degeneration of elastic fibers in the vascular media, referred to as cystic medial necrosis. Subsequent dilatation of the mitral annulus, aortic root, and aortic arch leads to valvular dysfunction and to aneurysm formation, which may be complicated by dissection and rupture. Aortic root dilatation can be identified early in childhood and variably progresses to aortic regurgitation in later years. Mitral valve prolapse is equally common in children. Mitral regurgitation may be severe and require prosthetic valvular replacement; it is the leading cause of cardiovascular morbidity in these children.[369] Sixty percent of patients have auscultatory evidence of aortic or mitral regurgitation or systolic clicks. Ventricular strain, cardiomegaly, congestive failure, or angina pectoris may develop before the fourth decade.[4]

Restrictive pulmonary disease may result from severe kyphoscoliosis or pectus excavatum. The forced vital capacity is consistently low in these patients.[368] Diffuse and bullous emphysema with a "honeycomb" appearance on the chest radiograph may be complicated by spontaneous pneumothorax.[370] Compression of the left mainstem bronchus by an enlarged left atrium has been described in children.[371]

Skin manifestations, striae, are minor. Wound healing and scar formation are normal.

Treatment. No specific treatment is available. Beta-adrenergic blockade with propranolol has been used to reduce cardiac and great vessel wall tension and thereby limit the complications of vascular dilatation, but the results have not been encouraging. The indications for surgical intervention vary greatly but include hernia repairs, scoliosis correction, retinal detachment procedures, thoracotomy for pneumothorax, aneurysm repairs, and prosthetic valvular replacements.[370]

Anesthetic Management. These children require careful preoperative assessment to identify the cardiac complications of valvular dysfunction, cardiac failure, and aortic aneurysm and the pulmonary complications of emphysema, bronchogenic bullae, and decreased respiratory reserve. Medications for cardiac failure and propranolol therapy should be continued if good control has been established.[12] Prophylactic antibiotic coverage should be arranged for those patients with cardiac lesions.

The patient must be transferred gently in the operating room and positioned carefully to avoid stress on joints and to prevent intraoperative dislocations. All usual monitors are required for induction. Intravenous access should be obtained early. Additional invasive monitors should be reserved for major cases and high-risk patients because of the potential for vascular complications.

No specific anesthetic recommendations are reported, but the induction and maintenance technique used should avoid hypertension and tachycardia to prevent aneurysm rupture and to preserve myocardial oxygenation.[373] When intubation is required, laryngoscopy must be gentle to avoid soft tissue trauma, cervical spine injury, and temporomandibular joint damage. Ventilation may be assisted or controlled, but peak airway pressures should be kept as low as possible to minimize the risk of pneumothorax. The appropriate equipment to treat this possible complication should be readily available.

SARCOIDOSIS

Sarcoidosis is a multisystemic disorder of variable clinical severity, characterized by the development of noncaseating granulomas in the lungs, liver, spleen, lymph nodes, bones, eyes, and skin. It occurs in all races and regions of the world, but in North America it is more common in rural communities and among blacks; women are more frequently affected than men. The diagnosis is usually made between the ages of 20 and 50 years. It does occur in children but is uncommon under the age of 10 years.

The etiology of sarcoidosis is unknown, but evidence suggests a host reaction pattern determined by an abnormal immune response to some initiating factor. The reactive granulomas do not undergo central necrosis but heal by fibrosis. The original granuloma contracts and becomes hyalinized to leave a small, dense scar.[374]

Clinical Manifestations. The disease onset is usually insidious; many patients are asymptomatic despite extensive organ involvement. Constitutional symptoms in more acute presentations include fever, malaise, anorexia, weight loss, and abdominal pain.

Pulmonary involvement is most common and eventually develops in 85 to 90 percent of patients.[375, 376] Even in asymptomatic patients, pulmonary function tests show early changes of restrictive disease, with decreased vital capacity and functional residual capacity. Ventilation and perfusion abnormalities develop, compliance falls as fibrosis increases, and finally a progressive obstructive component complicates the clinical picture. A dry cough and exertional dyspnea are common complaints in late disease. Typical chest x-ray findings are bilateral hilar and paratracheal lymphadenopathy with scattered parenchymal infiltrates. The pulmonary adenopathy may compress and partially obstruct large bronchi.[310] In severe cases, pulmonary fibrosis may be complicated by cor pulmonale and right ventricular failure.

Upper airway involvement has been reported in 1 to 5 percent of adults as mucosal infiltration of the nose, pharynx, tonsils, and larynx.[374] Laryngeal lesions are usually supraglottic and have symptoms of obstruction rather than hoarseness.

Disseminated disease may affect almost every organ system. Significant cardiac involvement occurs in 5 percent of cases; conduction defects, paroxysmal tachyarrhythmias, and congestive failure may develop. Hepatic dysfunction, splenomegaly, and generalized lymphadenopathy can occur. Painless parotid gland enlargement is fairly common. Other manifestations described include skin lesions very similar to those of erythema nodosum, interstitial nephritis, renovascular hypertension, central nervous system symptoms, and peripheral neuropathies. A destructive chronic uveitis and a peripheral arthritis may develop that usually involves the ankles, knees, wrists, and hands.[9]

The characteristic features of rare patients under the age of 1 year include arthritis, skin lesions, and uveitis.

Laboratory findings may include anemia and thrombocytopenia, a polyclonal hypergammaglobulinemia, positive rheumatoid factor (which correlates with the degree of pulmonary involvement),[12] hypercalciuria, and hypercalcemia. The diagnosis is confirmed by tissue biopsy and often by a positive Kveim's test.

The treatment of sarcoidosis is symptomatic and supportive. Anti-inflammtory agents, particularly corticosteroids, may be required to suppress acute manifestations. The prognosis in children is unpredictable; remissions do occur, but the course is often chronic with slowly progressive obstructive pulmonary disease.[8, 377]

Anesthetic Management. Although some patients are symptom-free, significant systemic disease may be established and careful preoperative assessment is important. The upper airway must be evaluated for obstructing nasal or laryngeal lesions and ankylosis of the temporomandibular joints. A history of exertional dyspnea, auscultation of the chest, and a review of the chest radiograph are important. Pulmonary function tests may be required to quantify lung volumes and the relative degree of restrictive and obstructive respiratory disease. Preoperative arterial blood gases on room air may be very helpful. Cardiac involvement in children is uncommon, but an ECG should be obtained. Hepatic and renal dysfunction should be identified. Perioperative corticosteroid supplementation may be required.

No specific anesthetic drugs or techniques are recommended. All usual monitors, including the ECG, must be used for induction. If a difficult laryngoscopy is anticipated, relaxants should be avoided until the airway is secured. If laryngeal or epiglottic lesions are found, a smaller endotracheal tube than predicted may be required. Anesthetic gases must be warmed and humidified.

In the presence of significant pulmonary disease, ventilation should be assisted or controlled and an increased FIO_2 used. Patients with restrictive disease may require small tidal volumes and an increased respiratory rate.

RELAPSING NODULAR NONSUPPURATIVE PANNICULITIS (WEBER-CHRISTIAN DISEASE)

This rare, recurrent, febrile illness is characterized by subcutaneous and visceral fat necrosis. The areas of fatty tissue inflammation and degeneration heal with fibrosis and occasionally with calcification. The etiology is unknown, but infections, drug reactions (bromides and iodides), and hypersensitivity are suggested. The disorder may represent a vasculitis or be the presenting sign of a connective tissue disease. It has been associated with pancreatic disease and with corticosteroid withdrawal. A similar but localized and transient disorder, subcutaneous fat necrosis, is seen in some neonates on exposure to cold (see page 504). Adults are predominantly affected, but Weber-Christian disease has been reported in all age groups, including infants.[378]

Clinical Manifestations. Weber-Christian disease may exhibit crops of subcutaneous nodules that are tender, erythematous, and warm and appear on the thighs, abdomen, and arms. Fever, associated with arthralgias and myalgias, is a common feature. Individual lesions regress without scarring over days or weeks, leaving brown atrophic areas, but recur. The disorder may continue in this fashion for months.

Systemic features depend on the severity of the visceral sites affected. Pericardial fat involvement with subsequent fibrosis can lead to constrictive pericarditis with a fixed, low cardiac output. Mesenteric disease may cause abdominal pain and tenderness. Hepatosplenomegaly has been reported.[8] An association with coagulopathy and hemolytic anemia has been reported.[379] Central nervous system or meningeal fat necrosis may provoke a seizure disorder. Acute adrenal insufficiency from adrenal infarction has been reported secondary to retroperitoneal panniculitis.[12]

The treatment is symptomatic and supportive. Anti-inflammatory agents and corticosteroids are usually effective for most manifestations of the disease.

Anesthetic Management. The preoperative identification of systemic complications is mandatory. Constrictive pericarditis, seizure disorders, and adrenal insufficiency must be recognized. Perioperative corticosteroid supplementation may be required for some patients.

Care must be taken to protect the patient's subcutaneous tissue and skin from heat, cold, trauma, and pressure, which may precipitate new lesions. The operating room, intravenous solutions, and anesthetic equipment should be warm. Anesthetic gases should be warmed and humidified.

Patients who have constrictive pericarditis require high venous filling pressures. Adequate preoperative hydration and volume resuscitation are critically important. Reliable intravenous access must be available for operative and postoperative fluid administration. Bradycardia and agents that depress myocardial contractility will be tolerated poorly. Invasive cardiovascular monitoring may be required in patients with severe disease.

No specific anesthetic drugs or techniques are recommended. No contraindication has been reported to the use of inhalational agents, whose biodegradation releases bromide and fluoride ions.[12]

Eosinophilic Fasciitis

This unusual and rare syndrome is characterized by painful inflammation and induration of the skin, subcutaneous tissue, and fascia of the upper or lower extremities. The inflammation occasionally may extend to the trunk and face. The characteristic feature on biopsy is a thickened fascia with perivascular infiltration by eosinophils, histiocytes, and lymphocytes.[9] The disorder frequently has followed heavy physical exertion. It is most often seen in adults but has been reported in children.[380] Some clinicians feel that this syndrome is a variant of scleroderma.

There are no systemic manifestations, although musculoskeletal contractures may develop.[8] Raynaud's phenomenon is absent. Small doses of corticosteroids markedly improve symptoms. The disorder is usually self-limited; spontaneous resolution often occurs in less than 3 to 4 years, but the long-term prognosis is unknown.

Children with eosinophilic fasciitis may require perioperative corticosteroid supplementation. Significant facial involvement may reduce the mobility of the temporomandibular joint and create a small mouth opening. As a result, laryngoscopy and intubation may be difficult. In these patients, the recommended approach to airway management is similar to that described for juvenile rheumatoid arthritis (see page 532).

IMPLICATIONS OF CORTICOSTEROID THERAPY

The corticosteroid drugs are the most potent anti-inflammatory agents used in the treatment of skin and connective tissue diseases. The beneficial effects of topical and systemic steroid therapy must be weighed against the potentially serious complications that may arise from their use. Perioperative steroid management is a shared responsibility of the pediatrician and the anesthetist and deserves special attention at this time.

The anti-inflammatory and immunosuppressive actions of the corticosteroids are multiple and complex.[16, 381–386] Steroids maintain the integrity of capillary endothelium, reducing edema and cellular infiltration, and stabilize cellular and lysosomal membranes. They inhibit the migration of immunocompetent cells to areas of inflammation. Steroids interfere with phagocytosis and antigen processing by lymphocytes and macrophages. The inflammatory response of the antigen-antibody complex is also reduced. Cell-mediated immunity is modified substantially.

Prolonged suppressive therapy with corticosteroids in the supraphysiological dose range is associated with many complications and side effects that have significant anesthetic implications (Table 15–1). The more important of these in children include growth retardation, osteoporosis, protein-wasting, iatrogenic Cushing's syndrome, sodium and water retention, hypertension, metabolic alkalosis, gastrointestinal irritation, susceptibility to infections, and carbohydrate intolerance. Accelerated coronary artery disease may be seen after 10 years of therapy.[9] Cataracts, myopathies, and psychoses are frequent. Surgical patients on steroids have increased morbidity and prolonged recovery times. Typical problems include poor tissue healing complicated by wound dehiscence, he-

Table 15–1. COMPLICATIONS OF CORTICOSTEROID THERAPY

Endocrine
Suppression of hypothalamic-pituitary-adrenal axis
Growth disturbances
Metabolic
Glucose intolerance; diabetes mellitus
Hyperosmolar nonketotic coma
Hyperlipidemia
Centripetal obesity
Gastrointestinal
Gastric hemorrhage
Gastric and duodenal ulceration
Intestinal perforation
Pancreatitis
Suppression of Immune Response
Secondary bacterial, viral, and fungal infections and parasitic infestation
Renal
Sodium and water retention and edema
Hypokalemic alkalosis
Cardiovascular
Hypertension
Accelerated coronary artery disease
Musculoskeletal
Myopathy
Osteoporosis, vertebral compression fractures
Aseptic necrosis, especially of femoral head
Ophthalmological
Posterior subcapsular cataracts
Glaucoma
Inhibition of Fibroplasia
Impaired wound healing
Subcutaneous tissue atrophy
Central Nervous System
Steroid-induced neuroses, psychoses

matomas, and infections. The latter may present as localized abscesses or as septicemia and shock.

One of the most common and potentially hazardous complications of corticosteroid therapy is the suppression of the hypothalamic-pituitary-adrenal (HPA) axis. Biochemical evidence of HPA axis suppression has been demonstrated with 5 days to 2 weeks of therapy and has been shown to persist for up to 12 months.[381–383]

The degree of HPA axis suppression is determined by the duration of treatment, dose of steroid required, potency of the drug used, and schedule of administration. The reduction of the dose and discontinuance of therapy, as permitted by the disease response, is attempted as early as possible. Alternate-day therapy has been shown to allow recovery of the HPA axis and an improvement of some other complications.[381, 382] Suppression of the HPA axis in children has been described following the systemic absorption of topical steroids when the area of application is large and when potent agents are used, especially under occlusive dressings.[387, 388]

Graber and colleagues defined the recovery of the HPA axis after withdrawal of therapy in patients who had been on steroids for at least 1 year.[392] For the first month after withdrawal, depressed function of both the pituitary and adrenal glands persists. During the second to fifth months, corticotropin levels rise to above normal, but the adrenal output of cortisol remains low. From the fifth to ninth months, cortisol output is normal but only with continuing high corticotropin levels. After 9 months, full recovery of adrenal function can be demonstrated.

During periods of stress, such as infection, trauma, and major surgical procedures, the endogenous production of cortisol normally rises from two- to sevenfold above base levels for at least 72 hours.[343, 390, 407, 417] In theory, if this demand is not met, acute adrenal insufficiency may be precipitated and the patient's depressed stress response may progress to cardiovascular collapse and death. Such perioperative catastrophes have been reported, although some disagreement exists on the documentation of these cases.[394, 395]

The role that corticosteroid hormones play in cardiovascular homeostasis is not clearly defined. Steroids appear to be involved in synthesis and release of endogenous catecholamines and in the cardiovascular response to these catecholamines.[397] They also influence the homeostatic fluid shift response to acute hemorrhagic challenge.[398]

However, cortisol is not the prime factor in the maintenance of arterial pressure in the perioperative period in glucocorticoid-treated patients.[399, 400] Postoperative cardiovascular collapse has rarely been associated with low plasma cortisol, and a low plasma cortisol level alone is not a sufficient condition to produce hypotension.[401–403] Provided adequate fluid and electrolyte homeostasis is maintained perioperatively, circulatory collapse is rarely encountered even when steroid coverage is omitted.[404] Meyers has reported depressed neuromuscular transmission in patients with adrenocortical insufficiency.[406]

Despite this controversy, supplemental corticosteroids are provided to prevent the risk of unrecognized acute adrenal insufficiency. Most investigators recommend steroid coverage for patients who have been treated with supraphysiological steroid doses for more than 5 days in the previous 9 months, or who currently require maintenance therapy.

If there is time preoperatively, the functional reserve of the HPA axis should be evaluated by the patient's response to the rapid ACTH stimulation test or metyrapone test. If the reserve is normal, no steroid coverage is necessary. If it is borderline, coverage is preferred. Acute supplemental steroids, even if unnecessary, can be withdrawn without difficulty as the acute stress resolves.

Many protocols for steroid coverage have been proposed.[407–419] Work with adults by Plumpton and associates (1969) advocated the use of high-dose steroid supplementation in the range of 400 mg per 24 hours.[407]

Current recommendations for adults call for more moderate doses, as described by Baxter and Tyrell.[413] For major procedures, hydrocortisone hemisuccinate, 100 mg, is given intramuscularly on call to the operating room and continued intravenously at 50 mg every 6 hours for 24 hours. The dose is then reduced to 25 mg every 6 hours for 24 hours and finally withdrawn slowly over the following 3 to 5 days. For minor procedures, the same initial protocol is followed but discontinued after 24 hours. For short diagnostic procedures, a single preoperative dose of hydrocortisone hemisuccinate, 100 mg, should be adequate. If at any postoperative time hypotension, fever, or other complications arise, then the full supplemental coverage of 200 to 400 mg per 24 hours should be reinstituted immediately.

Several recent studies have recommended lower dose schedules for steroid supplementa-

Table 15–2. PERIOPERATIVE STEROID REPLACEMENT FOR MAJOR SURGICAL PROCEDURES

1. Hydrocortisone hemisuccinate, 50 mg/m^2 intravenously, 1 hour preoperatively
2. Hydrocortisone hemisuccinate, 25 mg/m^2 intravenously, q6h for 24 to 72 hours, depending on the length and extent of the operation
3. If the postoperative course is satisfactory, the supplemental steroid dose may be tapered to maintenance levels over the next 5 days
4. If hypotension, fever, or other complications arise, increase the hydrocortisone dosage to 50 mg/m^2 for 24 hours
5. Doses for all children may be calculated proportionate to body surface area

tion that provide much more physiological levels of serum cortisol. These protocols call for a total dose over 24 hours of about 125 mg of hydrocortisone in adults. The supplemental steroids are then decreased after 72 hours. No problems were encountered.[417–420]

Intramuscular cortisone acetate has been used frequently and without problems to provide steroid coverage. However, the administration of this preparation should be commenced at least 48 hours preoperatively because plasma cortisol levels are very slow to rise when steroids are administered by the intramuscular route.[407–414]

Kenny and colleagues demonstrated that daily cortisol production rates are equivalent in children and adults when corrected for body surface area, and they found the 24-hour output to be 11.8 ± 2.5 mg/m^2/24 hours.[415] An approximate dose for steroid coverage in children can be extrapolated from the adult protocols by comparing body surface areas (Table 15–2).[420] The use of body weight to calculate steroid doses may provide inadequate coverage in younger children and infants.

Acknowledgments

I thank my wife, Connie, for her tolerance and support during the preparation of this chapter and my father, Dr. Foster Smith, for his continuing interest in anesthesia and for his example. I am also indebted to Mrs. Margaret Cutler for her help in producing the manuscript.

REFERENCES

SKIN AND CONNECTIVE TISSUE DISORDERS—GENERAL

1. Orkin M, Maibach HI, Dahl MV (eds): Dermatology. Norwalk, Conn., Appleton and Lange, 1991.
2. Arnold HL, Odom RB, James WD (eds): Andrew's Diseases of the Skin. Clinical Dermatology. 8th ed. Philadelphia, WB Saunders, 1990.
3. Schachner LA, Hansen RC (eds): Pediatric Dermatology. New York, Churchill Livingstone, 1988.
4. Jordan RE (ed): Immunologic Diseases of the Skin. Norwalk, Conn., Appleton and Lange, 1991.
5. Callen JP, Jorizzo J, Greer K, et al (eds): Dermatological Signs of Internal Disease. Philadelphia, WB Saunders, 1988.
6. Maibach HI, Boisits EK (eds): Neonatal Skin. Vol 1: Structure and Function. New York, Marcel Dekker, 1982.
7. Rasmussen JE (ed): Symposium on pediatric dermatology. Pediatr Clin North Am *30* (3 and 4), 1983.
8. Rudolph AM (ed): Rudolph's Pediatrics. 19th ed. Norwalk, Conn., Appleton and Lange, 1991.
9. Cassidy JT, Petty RE: Textbook of Pediatric Rheumatology. 2nd ed. New York, Churchill Livingstone, 1990.
10. Kelly WN, Harris ED, Ruddy S, Sledge CB (eds): Textbook of Rheumatology. 3rd ed. Philadelphia, WB Saunders, 1989.
11. McCarty DJ (ed): Arthritis and Allied Conditions. A Textbook of Rheumatology. 11th ed. Philadelphia, Lea and Febiger, 1989.
12. Katz J, Benumof JL, Kadis LB (eds): Anesthesia and Uncommon Diseases. 3rd ed. Philadelphia, WB Saunders, 1990.
13. Gregory GA (ed): Pediatric Anesthesia. 2nd ed. New York, Churchill Livingstone, 1989.
14. Stoelting RK, Dierdorf SF (eds): Anesthesia and Co-Existing Disease. New York, Churchill Livingstone, 1983.
15. Motoyama EK, Davis PJ (eds): Smith's Anesthesia for Infants and Children. 5th ed. St. Louis, CV Mosby, 1990.
16. Felig P, Baxter JD, Broadus AE, et al (eds): Endocrinology and Metabolism. New York, McGraw-Hill, 1981.
17. Kaplan SA (ed): Symposium on pediatric endocrinology. Pediatr Clin North Am *26*(1), 1979.
18. Dickerman JD, Lucey JF (eds): Smith's The Critically Ill Child: Diagnosis and Medical Management. 3rd ed. Philadelphia, WB Saunders, 1985.
19. Gorlin RJ, Pinborg JJ, Cohen MM (eds): Syndromes of the Head and Neck. 2nd ed. New York, McGraw-Hill, 1976.
20. Smith GB, Shribman AJ: Anaesthesia and severe skin disease. Anaesthesia *39*:443, 1984.

NEONATAL AND DEVELOPMENTAL ABNORMALITIES

21. Amstey MS, Lewin EB, Meyer MR: Herpesvirus infection in the newborn. Its treatment by exchange transfusion and adenosine arabinoside. Obstet Gynecol *47*(Suppl):33, 1976.
22. Weston WL, Humbert JR: Failure of fresh plasma in Leiner disease. Arch Dermatol *113*:233, 1977.
23. Rane RE, Baden HP: The ichthyoses—a review. J Am Acad Dermatol *8*:285, 1983.
24. Benedek TG, Rodnan GP: The early history and nomenclature of scleroderma and its differentiation from sclerema neonatorum and scleroedema. Semin Arthritis Rheum *12*:52, 1982.
25. Jardine D, Atherton DJ, Trompeter RS: Sclerema neonatorum and subcutaneous fat necrosis of the newborn in the same infant. Eur J Pediatr *150*:125, 1990.

26. Fretzin DF, Arias AM: Sclerema neonatorum and subcutaneous fat necrosis of the newborn. Pediatr Dermatol *4*:112, 1987.
27. Bart BJ: Epidermolysis bullosa and congenital localized absence of skin. Arch Dermatol *101*:78, 1970.
28. Freire-Maia N, Pinheiro M: Ectodermal Dysplasias: A Clinical and Genetic Study. New York, Alan R. Liss, 1984.
29. Temple IK, MacDowal P, Baraitser M, Atherton DJ: Focal dermal hypoplasia (Goltz syndrome). J Med Genet *27*:180, 1990.
30. Lawlor F, Holmes SC: Focal dermal hypoplasia in the neonate. J R Soc Med *82*:165, 1989.
31. Goltz RW, Henderson RR, Hitch JM, et al: Focal dermal hypoplasia syndrome. A review of the literature and report of two cases. Arch Dermatol *101*:1, 1970.
32. Rietschel RL: Anhidrotic ectodermal dysplasia and heat loss: Management. Dermatology *18*:370, 1979.
33. Ramchander V, Jankey N, Ramkissoon R, et al: Anhidrotic ectodermal dysplasia in an infant presenting with pyrexia of unknown origin. Clin Pediatr *17*:51, 1978.
34. Beahrs JO, Lillington GA, Rosan RC, et al: Anhidrotic ectodermal dysplasia: Predisposition to bronchial disease. Ann Intern Med *74*:92, 1971.
35. Edgerton MT: The treatment of hemangiomas: Special reference to the role of steroid therapy. Ann Surg *183*:517, 1976.
36. Ryan TJ, Cherry GW (eds): Vascular Birth Marks. Pathogenesis and Management. Oxford, Oxford University Press, 1987.
37. Meeks EA, Jay JB, Heaton LD: Thrombocytopenic purpura occurring with large hemangioma. Am J Dis Child *90*:349, 1955.
38. Kasabach HH, Merritt KK: Capillary hemangioma with extensive purpura. Am J Dis Child *59*:1063, 1940.
39. Keller L, Bluhm JF: Diffuse neonatal hemangiomatosis. Cutis *23*:295, 1979.
40. Gloviczki P, Hollier LH, et al: Surgical implications of Klippel-Trenaunay syndrome. Ann Surg *197*:353, 1983.
41. Telander RL, Kaufman BH, Gloviczki P, et al: Prognosis and management of lesions of the trunk in children with Klippel-Trenaunay syndrome. J Pediatr Surg *19*:417, 1984.
42. Mestre JR, Andres JM: Hereditary hemorrhagic telangiectasia causing hematemesis in an infant. J Pediatr *101*:577, 1982.
43. Ulso C, Vase P, Stoksted P: Long-term results of dermatoplasty in the treatment of hereditary haemorrhagic telangiectasia. J Laryngol Otol *97*:223, 1983.
44. Weller RM: Anaesthesia for cystic hygroma in a neonate. Anaesthesia *29*:588, 1974.
45. MacDonald DJF: Cystic hygroma. Anaesthesia *21*:66, 1966.

EPIDERMOLYSIS BULLOSA

46. Reddy ARR, Wong DHW: Epidermolysis bullosa. A review of anaesthetic problems in case reports. Can Anaesth Soc J *19*:536, 1972.
47. Cohen SR, Landing BH, Isaacs H: Epidermolysis bullosa associated with laryngeal stenosis. Ann Otol Rhinol Laryngol *87*:25, 1978.
48. Milne B, Rosales JK: Anaesthesia for correction of esophageal stricture in a patient with recessive epidermolysis bullosa dystrophia: Case report. Can Anaesth Soc J *27*:169, 1980.
49. Becker MH, Swingard CA: Epidermolysis bullosa dystrophica in children. Radiological manifestations. Radiology *90*:124, 1968.
50. Katz J, Grybowski JD, Rosenbaum HM, et al: Dysphagia in children with epidermolysis bullosa. Gastroenterology *52*:259, 1967.
51. Ramadass T, Thangavelu TA: Epidermolysis bullosa and its E.N.T. manifestations. Two case reports. J Laryngol Otol *92*:441, 1978.
52. Malaga S, Fernandez Toral J, Santos F, et al: Renal amyloidosis complicating a recessive epidermolysis bullosa in childhood. Helv Paediatr Acta *38*:167, 1983.
53. Tio TH, Waardenburg PJ, Vermeulen HJ: Blood coagulation in epidermolysis bullosa hereditaria. Arch Dermatol *88*:76, 1963.
54. Hamann RA, Cohen PJ: Anesthetic management of a patient with epidermolysis bullosa dystrophica. Anesthesiology *34*:389, 1971.
55. Wright JT: Epidermolysis bullosa: Dental and anesthetic management of two cases. Oral Surg Oral Med Oral Pathol *57*:155, 1984.
56. Bloch MS, Gross BD: Epidermolysis bullosa dystrophica recessive: Oral surgery and anesthetic implications. J Oral Maxillofac Surg *40*:753, 1982.
57. Lanier PA, Posnick WR, Donly KJ: Epidermolysis bullosa—dental management and anesthetic considerations: Case report. Pediatr Dent *12*:246, 1990.
58. Wright JT: Comprehensive dental care and general anesthetic management of hereditary epidermolysis bullosa. A review of fourteen cases. Oral Surg Oral Med Oral Pathol *70*:573, 1990.
59. Holzman RS, Worthen HM, Johnson KL: Anaesthesia for children with junctional epidermolysis bullosa (letalis). Can J Anaesth *34*:395, 1987.
60. Kubota Y, Norton ML, Goldenberg S, et al: Anesthetic management of patients with epidermolysis bullosa undergoing surgery. Anesth Analg *40*:244, 1961.
61. Lee C, Nagel EL: Anesthetic management of a patient with epidermolysis bullosa dystrophica. Anesthesiology *43*:122, 1975.
62. LoVerme SR, Oropollo AT: Ketamine anesthesia in dermatolytic bullous dermatosis (epidermolysis bullosa). Anesth Analg *56*:398, 1977.
63. Idvall J: Ketamine monoanesthesia for major surgery in epidermolysis bullosa: Case report. Acta Anaesth Scand *31*:658, 1987.
64. Hager R, Landenberg C: Anesthetic management in patients with epidermolysis bullosa dystrophica. Anaesthesia *43*:482, 1988.
65. Marshall BE: A comment on epidermolysis bullosa and its anaesthetic management for dental operations. A case report. Br J Anaesth *35*:724, 1963.
66. Spargo PM, Smith GB: Epidermolysis bullosa and porphyria (letter). Anaesthesia *44*:79, 1989.
67. Dundee JW, Riding JE: Barbiturate narcosis in porphyria. Anaesthesia *10*:55, 1955.
68. Prince DG, Swart E: Epidermolysis bullosa. Anaesthesia *23*:707, 1968.
69. Tomlinson AA: Recessive dystrophic epidermolysis bullosa. The anaesthetic management of a case for major surgery. Anaesthesia *38*:485, 1983.
70. James I, Wark H: Airway management during anesthesia in patients with epidermolysis bullosa dystrophica. Anesthesiology *56*:323, 1982.
71. Pratilas V, Biezunski A: Epidermolysis bullosa manifested and treated during anesthesia. Anesthesiology *43*:581, 1975.
72. Young DA, Hardwick PB: Anaesthesia for epidermolysis bullosa dystrophica. A report of multiple anaesthetics in one patient. Anaesthesia *23*:264, 1968.

73. Berryhill RE, Benumof JL, Saidman LJ, et al: Anesthetic management of emergency cesarean section in a patient with epidermolysis bullosa dystrophica polydysplastica. Anesth Analg *57*:281, 1978.
74. Fisk GC, Kern IB: Anaesthesia for oesophagoscopy in a child with epidermolysis bullosa—a case report. Anaesth Intens Care *1*:297, 1973.
75. Petty WC, Gunther RC: Anesthesia for nonfacial surgery in polydysplastic epidermolysis bullosa (dystrophic). Anesth Analg *49*:246, 1970.
76. Wilson F: Epidermolysis bullosa: A rare disease of anaesthetic interest. Br J Anaesth *31*:26, 1959.
77. Haber RM, Ramsay CA, Boxall LBH: Assessment of a treatment for epidermolysis bullosa. Can Med Assoc J *131*:10, 1984.
78. Fisher GC, Ray DA: Airway obstruction in epidermolysis bullosa (letter). Anaesthesia *44*:449, 1989.
79. Yee LL, Gunter JB, Manley CB: Caudal epidural anesthesia in an infant with epidermolysis bullosa. Anesthesiology *70*:149, 1989.
80. Boughton R, Crawford MR, Vonwiller JB: Epidermolysis bullosa—a review of 15 years' experience, including experience with combined general and regional anesthetic techniques. Anesth Intensive Care *16*:260, 1988.
81. Kelly RE: Regional anesthesia in children with epidermolysis bullosa dystrophica (letter). Anesthesiology *68*:469, 1988.
82. Kelly RE, Koff HD, Rothans KO, et al: Brachial plexus anesthesia in eight patients with recessive dystrophic epidermolysis bullosa. Anesth Analg *66*:1318, 1987.
83. Kaplan R, Strauch B: Regional anesthesia in a child with epidermolysis bullosa. Anesthesiology *67*:262, 1987.
84. Broster T, Placek R, Eggers JW Jr: Epidermolysis bullosa: Anesthetic management for cesarian section. Anesth Analg *66*:341, 1987.

ERYTHEMA MULTIFORME

85. Chandra JJ, Callen JP: Erythema multiforme and the Stevens-Johnson syndrome. South Med J *71*:566, 1978.
86. Pollack MA, Burk PG, Nathanson G: Mucocutaneous eruptions due to antiepileptic drug therapy in children. Ann Neurol *5*:262, 1979.
87. Rallison ML, Carlisle JW, Lee RE Jr, et al: Lupus erythematosus and Stevens-Johnson syndrome. Am J Dis Child *101*:725, 1961.
88. Kazmierowski JA, Wuepper KD: Erythema multiforme: Immune complex vasculitis of superficial cutaneous microvasculature (abstract). Clin Res *25*:282, 1977.
89. Stevens AM, Johnson FC: A new eruptive fever associated with stomatitis and ophthalmia. Am J Dis Child *24*:526, 1922.
90. Costello MJ: Erythema multiforme exudativum. J Invest Dermatol *8*:127, 1947.
91. Taffee AG: The Stevens-Johnson syndrome. Br J Clin Pract *29*:169, 1975.
92. Broadbent RV: Stevens-Johnson disease presenting with pneumothorax. Rocky Mount Med J *64*:69, 1967.
93. Cucciara RF, Dawson B: Anesthesia in Stevens-Johnson syndrome: Report of a case. Anesthesiology *35*:537, 1971.
94. Madan R, Chawla R, Dhar P, et al: Anesthesia in Stevens-Johnson syndrome. Indian Pediatr *26*:1038, 1989.
95. Kalhan SB, Ditto SR: Anesthetic management of a child with Stevens-Johnson syndrome. Cleve Clin J Med *55*:467–469, 1988.
96. Schartum S: Stevens-Johnson syndrome with cardiac involvement: Report of two cases. Acta Med Scand *179*:729, 1966.
97. Rasmussen JE: Erythema multiforme in children: Response to treatment with systemic corticosteroids. Br J Dermatol *95*:181, 1976.
98. Alexander MK, Cope S: Erythema multiforme exudativum major (Stevens-Johnson syndrome). J Pathol Bacteriol *68*:373, 1954.

TOXIC EPIDERMAL NECROLYSIS

99. Krumlowsky FA, Del Greco F, Herdson PB, et al: Renal disease associated with toxic epidermal necrolysis. Am J Med *57*:817, 1974.
100. Lyell A: Toxic epidermal necrolysis (the scalded skin syndrome): A reappraisal. Br J Dermatol *100*:69, 1979.
101. Stuttgen G: Toxic epidermal necrolysis provoked by barbiturates. Br J Dermatol *88*:291, 1973.
102. Hunter JAA, Davison AM: Toxic epidermal necrolysis associated with pentazocine therapy and severe reversible renal failure. Br J Dermatol *88*:287, 1973.
103. Orfanos CE, Schaumberg-Lever G, Lever SF: Dermal and epidermal types of erythema multiforme. Arch Dermatol *109*:682, 1974.
104. Rasmussen JE: Toxic epidermal necrolysis: A review of 75 cases in children. Arch Dermatol *111*:1135, 1975.
105. Melish ME, Glasgow LA: Staphylococcal scalded skin syndrome: The expanded clinical syndrome. J Pediatr *78*:958, 1971.
106. Dominguez Perez F, Candela Toha AM, et al: Anesthesia in a patient with toxic epidermal necrolysis (Spanish). Rev Esp Anestesiol Reanim *36*:350, 1989.

PEMPHIGUS

107. Oranje AP, van Joost T: Pemphigoid in children. Pediatr Dermatol *6*:277, 1989.
108. Burge S, Wojnarowska F, Marsden A: Chronic bullous dermatosis of childhood persisting into adulthood. Pediatr Dermatol *5*:246, 1988.
109. Roberts LJ, Sonthiemer RD: Chronic bullous dermatosis of childhood: Immunopathologic studies. Pediatr Dermatol *4*:6, 1987.
110. Schiltz JR, Michel B, Papay R: Pemphigus antibody interaction with human epidermal cells in culture. J Clin Invest *62*:778, 1978.
111. Berger BW, Maier HS, Kantor I, et al: Pemphigus vulgaris in a 3½ year old boy. Arch Dermatol *110*:941, 1974.
112. Krain LS: The association of pemphigus with thymoma or malignancy: A critical review. Br J Dermatol *90*:397, 1974.
113. Izumi AK, Shmunes E, Wood MG: Familial benign chronic pemphigus. Arch Dermatol *104*:177, 1971.
114. Lever WF: Immunosuppressants and prednisone in pemphigus vulgaris. Arch Dermatol *113*:1236, 1977.
115. Lever SF: Methotrexate and prednisone in pemphigus vulgaris. Arch Dermatol *106*:491, 1972.
116. Roenigk HH, Deodhar S: Pemphigus treatment with azathioprine. Arch Dermatol *107*:353, 1973.
117. Cotterill JA, Barker DJ, Millard JG: Plasma exchange in the treatment of pemphigus vulgaris. Br J Dermatol *98*:243, 1978.
118. Piamphongsant T, Chaikittisilpa S, Kullavanijaya P: Bullous pemphigoid in childhood: Report of three cases and a review of literature. Int J Dermatol *16*:126, 1977.

119. Hamilton DV, McKenzie AW: Bullous pemphigoid and primary biliary cirrhosis. Br J Dermatol *99*:447, 1978.
120. Jeyaram C, Torda TA: Anesthetic management of cholecystectomy in a patient with buccal pemphigus. Anesthesiology *40*:600, 1974.
121. Prasad KK, Chen L: Anesthetic management of a patient with bullous pemphigoid. Anesth Analg *69*:537, 1989.
122. Vatashsky E, Aronson HB: Pemphigus vulgaris: Anaesthesia in the traumatized patient. Anaesthesia *37*:1195, 1982.
123. Nelder KH, Hagler L, Wise WL, et al: Acrodermatitis enteropathica. A clinical and biochemical survey. Arch Dermatol *110*:711, 1974.
124. Portnoy B, Molokhia M: Acrodermatitis enteropathica treated by zinc. Br J Dermatol *91*:701, 1974.

EPIDERMAL AND DERMAL DISORDERS

125. Farber EM, Nall ML: The natural history of psoriasis in 5600 patients. Dermatologica *148*:1, 1974.
126. Nyfors A, Lemholt K: Psoriasis in children. A short review and a survey of 245 cases. Br J Dermatol *92*:437, 1975.
127. Fox RH, Shuster S, et al: Cardiovascular, metabolic and thermoregulatory disturbances in patients with erythrodermic skin diseases. Br Med J *1*:619, 1965.
128. Shuster S: High-output cardiac failure from skin disease. Lancet *1*:1338, 1963.
129. Aly R, Maibach HI, Mandel A: Bacterial flora in psoriasis. Br J Dermatol *95*:603, 1976.
130. Bachmann E, Clemmensen OJ, Dyrbye M, et al: Joint involvement in psoriasis: scintigraphic, radiologic and clinical findings. Dermatologica *166*:250, 1983.
131. Lambert JR, et al: Psoriatic arthritis in children. Clin Rheum Dis *2*:339, 1976.
132. Stimson CW, Leban SG: Recurrent ankylosis of the temporomandibular joint in a patient with chronic psoriasis. J Oral Maxillofac Surg *40*:678, 1982.
133. Lerner MR, Lerner AB: Congenital psoriasis—report of 3 cases. Arch Dermatol *105*:598, 1972.
134. Beighton P, Price A, Lord J, et al: Variants of the Ehlers-Danlos syndrome. Ann Rheum Dis *28*:228, 1969.
135. Karaca M, Cronberg L, Nilsson IM: Abnormal platelet collagen reaction in Ehlers-Danlos syndrome. Scand J Haematol *9*:465, 1972.
136. Cabeen WR Jr, Reza MJ, Kovick RB, et al: Mitral valve prolapse and conduction defects in Ehlers-Danlos syndrome. Arch Intern Med *137*:1227, 1977.
137. Smit J, Alberts C, Balk AG: Pneumothorax in Ehlers-Danlos syndrome. Consequence or coincidence? Scand J Resp Dis *59*:239, 1978.
138. Dolan P, Sisko R, Riley E: Anesthetic considerations for Ehlers-Danlos syndrome. Anesthesiology *52*:266, 1980.
139. Abouleish E: Obstetric anaesthesia and Ehlers-Danlos syndrome. Br J Anaesth *52*:1283, 1980.
140. Yamashita M, Narita M, Ishihara H, et al: Uterine rupture in a case of Ehlers-Danlos syndrome type N—anesthetic considerations. Middle East J Anesthesiol *9*:277, 1987.
141. Muster AJ, Bharati S, Herman JJ, et al: Fatal cardiovascular disease and cutis laxa following acute febrile neutrophilic dermatosis. J Pediatr *102*:243, 1983.
142. Sakati NO, Nyhan WL: Congenital cutis laxa and osteoporosis. Am J Dis Child *137*:452, 1983.
143. Krechel SL, Remirez-Inawat RC, Fabian LW: Anesthetic considerations in pseudoxanthoma elasticum. Anesth Analg *60*:344, 1981.
144. Bete JM, Banas JS Jr, Moran J, et al: Coronary artery disease in an 18 year old girl with pseudoxanthoma elasticum: Successful surgical therapy. Am J Cardiol *36*:515, 1975.
145. Wilhelm K, Pauer K: Sudden death in pseudoxanthoma elasticum. Med J Aust *2*:1363, 1972.
146. Carter DJ, Woodward DA, Vince FP: Arterial surgery in pseudoxanthoma elasticum. Postgrad Med J *52*:291, 1976.
147. Mole B: Possibilities of treatment of lipodystrophies with ambulatory liposuction (French). Ann Dermatol Venereol *15*:867, 1988.
148. Walker RB, Warin RP: The incidence of eczema in childhood. Br J Dermatol *68*:182, 1956.
149. Meger RJ: Awake blind nasal intubation in a patient with xeroderma pigmentosum. Anaesth Intensive Care *10*:64, 1982.
150. Lynch HT, Frichot BC, Lynch JF: Cancer control in xeroderma pigmentosum. Arch Dermatol *113*:193, 1977.

DISORDERS WITH PIGMENTARY CHANGES

151. Riccardi VM: Pathophysiology of neurofibromatosis. IV. Dermatologic insights into heterogeneity and pathogenesis. J Am Acad Dermatol *3*:157, 1980.
152. Wander JV, Das Gupta TK: Neurofibromatosis. Curr Probl Surg *14*:11, 1977.
153. Leech RW: Intrathoracic meningocele and vertebral anomalies in a case of neurofibromatosis. Surg Neurol *9*:55, 1978.
154. Chaglassian JH, Riseborough EJ, Hall JE: Neurofibromatous scoliosis. Natural history and results of treatment in thirty-seven cases. J Bone Joint Surg *58*:695, 1976.
155. Cohen SR, Landing BH, Isaacs H: Neurofibroma of the larynx in a child. Ann Otol Rhinol Laryngol *87*:29, 1978.
156. Chang-Lo M: Laryngeal involvement in von Recklinghausen's disease; A case report and review of the literature. Laryngoscope *87*:435, 1977.
157. Sagel SS, Forrest JV, Askin FB: Interstitial lung disease in neurofibromatosis. South Med J *68*:647, 1975.
158. Fisher MM: Anaesthetic difficulties in neurofibromatosis. Anaesthesia *30*:648, 1975.
159. Yamashita M, Matsuki A, Oyama T: Anaesthetic considerations on von Recklinghausen's disease. Abnormal response to muscle relaxants. Anaesthetist *26*:317, 1977.
160. Magbagbeola JAO: Abnormal responses to muscle relaxants in a patient with von Recklinghausen's disease. Br J Anaesth *42*:710, 1970.
161. Krishna G: Neurofibromatosis, renal hypertension and cardiac dysrhythmias. Anesth Analg *54*:542, 1975.
162. Carney RG: Incontinentia pigmenti. A world statistical analysis. Arch Dermatol *112*:535, 1976.
163. Hendrickson MR, Ross JC: Neoplasms arising in congenital giant nevi. Am J Surg Pathol *5*:109, 1981.
164. Greeley PW, Middleton AG, Curtin JW: Incidence of malignancy in giant pigmented nevi. Plast Reconstr Surg *36*:26, 1965.
165. Rhodes AR, Sober AJ, Day CL, et al: The malignant potential of small congenital nevocellular nevi. J Am Acad Dermatol *6*:230, 1982.
166. Backman ME, Kopf AW: Iatrogenic effects of general anesthesia in children: Considerations in treating large congenital nevocytic nevi. J Dermatol Surg Oncol *12*:363, 1986.

167. Rodrigo MR, Cheng CH, Tai YT, O'Donnell D: LEOPARD syndrome. Anaesthesia *45*:30, 1990.

URTICARIAL AND HYPERSENSITIVITY DISORDERS

168. Johnston WE, Moss J, Philbin DM, et al: Management of cold urticaria during hypothermic cardiopulmonary bypass. N Engl J Med *306*:219, 1982.
169. Philbin DM, Moss J, Akins CW, et al: The use of H_1 and H_2 histamine antagonists with morphine anaesthesia: A double-blind study. Anesthesiology *55*:292, 1981.
170. Moss J, Rosow CE, Savarses JJ, et al: Role of histamine in the hypotensive action of D-tubocurarine in humans. Anesthesiology *55*:19, 1981.
171. Lorenz W, Doenicke A, Meyer R, et al: Histamine release in man by propanidid and thiopentone: Pharmacological effects and clinical consequences. Br J Anaesth *44*:355, 1972.
172. Gerecke WB, Imasato Y, Keats AS: Histamine release by drugs used in association with anesthesia in man. Abstracts of Scientific Papers. Annual Meeting of the American Society of Anesthesiologists, 1969, p 127.
173. Frank MM, Gelfand JA, Atkinson JP: Hereditary angioedema: The clinical syndrome and its management. Ann Intern Med *84*:580, 1976.
174. Jaffe CJ, Atkinson JP, Gelfand JA, et al: Hereditary angioedema: The use of fresh frozen plasma for prophylaxis in patients undergoing oral surgery. J Allergy *55*:386, 1975.
175. Hopkinson RB, Sutcliffe AJ: Hereditary angioneurotic oedema. Anaesthesia *34*:183, 1979.
176. Gibbs PS, LoSasso AM, Moorthy SS, et al: The anesthetic and perioperative management of a patient with documented hereditary angioneurotic edema. Anesth Analg *56*:571, 1977.
177. Abada ROP, Owens WD: Hereditary angioneurotic edema, an anesthetic dilemma. Anesthesiology *46*:428, 1977.
178. Cohen G, Peterson A: Treatment of hereditary angioedema with fresh frozen plasma. Ann Allergy *30*:690, 1972.
179. Roth M, Schreier L, Cutter R: Adrenalin treatment for hereditary angioneurotic edema. Ann Allergy *35*:175, 1975.
180. Hamilton AG, Bosley ARJ, Bowen DJ: Laryngeal oedema due to hereditary angioedema. Anaesthesia *32*:265, 1977.
181. Johns ME, Vanselow MA, Boles R: Hereditary angioneurotic edema. Treatment with epsilon-aminocaproic acid during surgery. Arch Otolaryngol *99*:388, 1974.
182. Rothbach C, Green RL, Levine MI, et al: Prophylaxis of attacks of hereditary angioedema. Am J Med *66*:681, 1979.
183. Wall RT, Frank M, Hahn M: A review of 25 patients with hereditary angioedema requiring surgery. Anesthesiology *71*:309, 1989.
184. Wingtin LN, Hardy F: Epidural block during labour in hereditary angioneurotic edema (letter). Can J Anaesth *36*:366, 1989.
185. Spargo PM, Smith GB: Hereditary angioneurotic edema, tracheal intubation and airway obstruction (letter). Can J Anaesth *34*:540, 1989.
186. Poppers PJ: Anesthetic implications of hereditary angioneurotic oedema. Can J Anaesth *34*:76, 1987.
187. Wyre HW, Henrichs WD: Systemic mastocytosis and pulmonary eosinophilic granuloma. JAMA *239*:856, 1978.
188. Cooper AJ, Winkelmann RK, Wiltsie JC: Hematologic malignancies occurring in patients with urticaria pigmentosa. J Am Acad Dermatol *7*:215, 1982.
189. Roberts LJ, Sweetman BJ, Lewis RA, et al: Increased production of prostaglandin D_2 in patients with systemic mastocytosis. N Engl J Med *303*:1400, 1980.
190. Scott HW, Parris WCV, Sandidge PC, et al: Hazards in operative management of patients with systemic mastocytosis. Ann Surg *197*:507, 1983.
191. Coleman MA, Liberthson RR, Crone RK, et al: General anesthesia in a child with urticaria pigmentosa. Anesth Analg *59*:704, 1980.
192. James PD, Krafchik BR, Johnston AE: Cutaneous mastocytosis in children: Anesthetic considerations. Can J Anaesth *34*:522, 1987.
193. Greenblatt EP, Chen L.: Urticaria pigmentosa: An anesthetic challenge. J Clin Anesth *2*:108, 1990.
194. Hosking MP, Warner MA: Sudden intraoperative hypotension in a patient with asymptomatic urticaria pigmentosa. Anesth Analg *66*:344, 1987.
195. Rosow CE, Moss J, Philbin DJ, et al: Histamine release during morphine and fentanyl anesthesia. Anesthesiology *56*:93, 1982.
196. Moss J, Rosow CE: Histamine release by narcotics and muscle relaxants in humans. Anesthesiology *59*:330, 1983.
197. Brown TP: Thiopentone anaphylaxis—case report. Anaesth Intensive Care *3*:257, 1975.
198. Buckland RW, Avery RF: Histamine release following pancuronium. A case report. Br J Anaesth *45*:518, 1973.
199. Roberts LJ, Turk JW, Oates JA: Shock syndrome associated with mastocytosis: Pharmacological reversal of the acute episode and therapeutic prevention of recurrent attacks. Adv Shock Res *8*:145, 1982.
200. Roberts LJ II, Marney SR Jr, Oates JA: Blockade of the flush associated with metastatic gastric carcinoid by combined H_1 and H_2 receptor antagonists: Evidence for an important role of H_2 in human vasculature. N Engl J Med *300*:236, 1979.
201. Manchikanti L, Kraus JW, Edds SP: Cimetidine and related drugs in anesthesia. Anesth Analg *61*:595, 1982.
202. Parris WCV, Sandidge PC, Petrinely G: Anaesthetic management of mastocytosis. Anesthesiol Rev *8*:32, 1981.
203. Hannuksela M; Erythema nodosum with special reference to sarcoidosis. Ann Clin Res *3*(Suppl 7):1, 1971.
204. Jacobs WH: Erythema nodosum in inflammatory disease of the bowel. Gastroenterology *37*:286, 1959.

MISCELLANEOUS DISORDERS

205. Lehner T: Progress report: Oral ulcerations and Behçet's syndrome. Gut *18*:491, 1977.
206. Penza R, Brunetti L, Franciosa G, et al: Renal amyloidosis in a child with Behçet's syndrome. Int J Pediatr Nephrol *4*:35, 1983.
207. Turner ME: Anaesthetic difficulties associated with Behçet's syndrome. Br J Anaesth *44*:100, 1972.
208. Roguin N, Haim S, Reshef R, et al: Cardiac involvement and superior vena caval obstruction in Behçet's disease. Thorax *33*:375, 1978.
209. Ahonen AV, Stenius-Aarniala BSM: Obstructive lung disease in Behçet's syndrome. Scand J Respir Dis *59*:44, 1978.
210. Mason RM, Barnes CG: Behçet's syndrome with arthritis. Ann Rheum Dis *28*:95, 1969.

211. Chajeh T, Fainarn M: Behçet's disease: Report of 41 cases and review of literature. Medicine *54*:179, 1975.
212. Horner FA, Myers GJ, Stumpf DA, et al: Malignant atrophic papulosis (Kohlmeier-Degos disease) in childhood. Neurology *26*:317, 1976.
213. Pierce RN, Smith GJW: Intrathoracic manifestations of Degos' disease. Chest *73*:79, 1978.
214. Black MM: Malignant atrophic papulosis (Degos' disease). Int J Dermatol *15*:405, 1976.
215. Taaffe A: Angiokeratoma corporis diffusum. The evolution of a disease entity. Postgrad Med J *53*:78, 1977.
216. Rowe JW, Carralis DG: Accelerated atrioventricular conduction in Fabry's disease. Angiology *29*:562, 1978.
217. Sheth KJ, Roth DA, Adams MB: Early renal failure in Fabry's disease. Am J Kidney Dis *2*:651, 1983.
218. Buhler RF, Theil G, Dubach UC, et al: Kidney transplantation in Fabry's disease. Br Med J *3*:28, 1973.

CONNECTIVE TISSUE DISEASE

219. Prockop J, Kiviriko KI, Tuderman L, et al: The biosynthesis of collagen and its disorders. N Engl J Med *301*:13, 77, 1979.
220. MacKay IR, Burnet FM: Autoimmune Diseases: Pathogenesis, Chemistry and Therapy. Springfield, Ill., Charles C Thomas, 1964, p 16.
221. Rees AJ: Autoimmunity and autoimmune disease. Br J Anaesth *51*:13, 1979.

JUVENILE RHEUMATOID ARTHRITIS

222. Schaller JG: The diversity of juvenile rheumatoid arthritis: A 1976 look at the subgroup of chronic arthritis. Arthritis Rheum *20*(Suppl):52, 1977.
223. Calabro JJ, Katz RM, Malty BA: A critical appraisal of juvenile rheumatoid arthritis. Clin Orthop *74*:101, 1971.
224. Smith PH, Sharp J, Kellgren JH: Natural history of rheumatoid cervical subluxations. Ann Rheum Dis *31*:222, 1972.
225. Martis CS, Kara Kasis DT: Ankylosis of the temporomandibular joint caused by Still's disease. Oral Surg *35*:462, 1973.
226. Grosfeld O, Czarnecka B, Drecka-Kuzan K, et al: Clinical investigations of the temporomandibular joint in children and adolescents with rheumatoid arthritis. Scand J Rheum *2*:145, 1973.
227. Lofgren RH, Montgomery WW: Incidence of laryngeal involvement in rheumatoid arthritis. N Engl J Med *267*:193, 1962.
228. Montgomery WW: Cricoarytenoid arthritis. Laryngoscope *73*:801, 1963.
229. Jacobs JC, Hui RM: Cricoarytenoid arthritis and airway obstruction in juvenile rheumatoid arthritis. Pediatrics *59*:292, 1977.
230. Svantesson H, Bjorkhem G, Elborgh R: Cardiac involvement in juvenile rheumatoid arthritis. A follow-up study. Acta Paediatr Scand *72*:345, 1983.
231. Brewer E: Juvenile rheumatoid arthritis—cardiac involvement. Arth Rheum *20*(Suppl):231, 1977.
232. Majeed HA, Kvasnicka J: Juvenile rheumatoid arthritis with cardiac tamponade. Ann Rheum Dis *37*:273, 1978.
233. Scharf J, Levy J, Benderly A, et al: Pericardial tamponade in juvenile rheumatoid arthritis. Arthritis Rheum *19*:760, 1976.
234. Zvaifler NJ, Weintraub AM: Aortitis and aortic insufficiency in the chronic rheumatic disorders—a reappraisal. Arthritis Rheum *6*:241, 1963.
235. Walker WC, Wright V: Rheumatoid pleuritis. Ann Rheum Dis *26*:467, 1967.
236. Divertie MB: Lung involvement in the connective-tissue disorders. Med Clin North Am *48*:1015, 1964.
237. Espada G, Babini JC, Maldonado-Cocco JA, Garcia-Morteo O: Radiologic review: The cervical spine in juvenile rheumatoid arthritis. Semin Arthritis Rheum *17*:185, 1988.
238. Davies DW, Steward DJ: Unexpected excessive bleeding during operation: Role of acetyl salicylic acid. Can Anaesth Soc J *24*:452, 1977.
239. Amrein PC, Ellman L, Harris WH: Aspirin-induced prolongation of bleeding time and perioperative blood loss. JAMA *245*:1825, 1981.
240. Gewanter HL, Baum J: The use of tolmetin sodium in systemic onset juvenile rheumatoid arthritis. Arthritis Rheum *24*:1316, 1981.
241. Ansell BM, Arden GP, McLennan I: Valgus knee deformities in children with juvenile polyarthritis treated by epiphyseal strapping. Arch Dis Child *45*:388, 1970.
242. Jenkins LC, McGraw RW: Anaesthetic management of the patient with rheumatoid arthritis. Can Anaesth Soc J *16*:407, 1969.
243. Edelist G: Principles of anaesthetic management in rheumatoid arthritic patients. Anesth Analg *43*:227, 1965.
244. Gardiner DL, Holmes F: Anaesthetic and postoperative hazards in rheumatic arthritis. Br J Anaesth *33*:258, 1961.
245. Reginster JY, Damas P, Franchimont P: Specific risks of anesthesia in patients with osteoarticular disease. Acta Anaesth Belgica *2*:105, 1984.
246. Taylor RC, Way WL, Hendrixson R: Temporomandibular joint problems in relation to the administration of general anesthesia. J Oral Surg *26*:327, 1968.
247. Funk D, Raymon F: Rheumatoid arthritis of the cricoarytenoid joints: An airway hazard. Anesth Analg *54*:742, 1975.
248. Goldhagen JL: Cricoarytenoiditis as a cause of acute airway obstruction in children. Ann Emerg Med *17*:532, 1988.
249. Phelps JA: Laryngeal obstruction due to cricoarytenoid arthritis. Anesthesiology *27*:518, 1966.
250. Roelofse JA, Shipton EA: Difficult intubation in a patient with rheumatoid arthritis. SA Med J *64*:679, 1983.
251. Goudsouzian N, Cote CJ, Liu LM, et al: The dose-response effects of oral cimetidine on gastric pH and volume in children. Anesthesiology *27*:518, 1966.
252. Salem MR, Wong AY, Mani M, et al: Premedicant drugs and gastric juice pH and volume in pediatric patients. Anesthesiology *44*:216, 1976.
253. D'Arcy EJ, Fell RH, Ansell BM, et al: Ketamine and juvenile chronic polyarthritis (Still's disease). Anaesthesia *31*:624, 1976.
254. Careson IW, Moore J, Balmer JP, et al: Laryngeal competence with ketamine and other drugs. Anesthesiology *38*:128, 1973.
255. Salem MR, Wong AY, Fizzotti GF: Efficacy of cricoid pressure in preventing aspiration of gastric contents in paediatric patients. Br J Anaesth *44*:401, 1972.
256. Salem MR, Mathrubhutham M, Bennett EJ: Difficult intubation. N Engl J Med *295*:879, 1976.
257. France NK: Management of the difficult intubation. *In* Gregory GA (ed): Pediatric Anesthesia. New York, Churchill Livingstone, 1983, p 825.

258. Pelton DA, Daly M, Cooper PD, et al: Plasma lidocaine concentrations following topical aerosol application to the trachea and bronchi. Can Anaesth Soc J *17*:250, 1970.
259. Davies JAH: Blind nasal intubation using doxapram hydrochloride. Br J Anaesth *40*:361, 1968.
260. Salem MR, Wong AY, Kiam D, et al: Difficult intubation in children: Evaluation of two techniques. Abstracts of scientific papers. American Society of Anesthesiologists Meeting, 1977.
261. Rucker RW, Silva WJ, Worcester CC: Fiberoptic bronchoscopic nasotracheal intubation in children. Chest *76*:56, 1979.
262. Stiles CM: A flexible fiberoptic bronchoscope for endotracheal intubation of infants. Anesth Analg *53*:1017, 1974.
263. Alfery DD, Ward CF, Harwood IR, et al: Airway management for a neonate with congenital fusion of the jaws. Anesthesiology *51*:340, 1979.
264. Stool SE: Intubation techniques of the difficult airway. Pediatr Infect Dis J *7*:S154, 1988.
265. Teale C, Muers MF, Pearson SB: Local anesthesia for fiberoptic bronchoscopy (letter). Thorax *45*:646, 1990.
266. Shelley MP, Wilson P, Norman J: Sedation for fiberoptic bronchoscopy. Thorax *44*:679, 1989.
267. Tassonyi E, Lehman C, Gunning K, et al: Fiberoptically guided intubation in children with gangrenous stomatitis. Anesthesiology *73*:348, 1990.
268. Khoo ST: Anaesthesia for fiberoptic bronchoscopy in children (letter). Anaesthesia *45*:248, 1990.
269. Kleeman PP, Jantzen JP, Bonfils P: The ultra-thin bronchoscope in the management of the difficult paediatric airway. Can J Anaesth *34*:606, 1987.
270. Fan LL: Transnasal fiberoptic endoscopy in children with obstructive apnea. Crit Care Med *12*:590, 1984.
271. Munson ES, Cullen SC: Endotracheal intubation in a patient with ankylosing spondylitis of the cervical spine. Anesthesiology *26*:365, 1965.
272. Rosenberg MB, Levesque PR, Bourke DL: Use of the LTA kit as a guide for endotracheal intubation. Anesth Analg *56*:287, 1977.
273. Waters DJ: Guided blind endotracheal intubation. Anaesthesia *38*:128, 1963.
274. Berry FA: The use of a stylet in blind nasotracheal intubation. Anesthesiology *61*:469, 1984.
275. Fox DJ, Matson MD: Management of the difficult pediatric airway in an austere environment using the light wand. J Clin Anesth *2*:123, 1990.
276. Stone DJ, Stirt JA, Kaplan MJ, et al: A complication of lightwand-guided nasotracheal intubation. Anesthesiology *61*:780, 1984.
277. Brain AIJ: Three cases of difficult intubations overcome by the laryngeal mask airway. Anaesthesia *40*:353, 1985.
278. Smith BL: Brain airway in anaesthesia for patients with juvenile chronic arthritis (letter). Anaesthesia *43*:421, 1988.
279. Johnston DF, Wrigley SR, Ross PJ, Jones HE: The laryngeal mask airway in pediatric anaesthesia. Anaesthesia *45*:924, 1990.
280. Mason DG, Bingham RM: The laryngeal mask airway in children. Anaesthesia *45*:760, 1990.
281. Hemmer D, Lee TS, Wright BD: Intubation of a child with a cervical spine injury with aid of a fiberoptic bronchoscope. Anaesth Intensive Care *10*:163, 1982.
282. Berthelsen P, Prytz S, Jacobsen E: Two-stage fiberoptic nasotracheal intubation in infants; A new approach to difficult pediatric intubation. Anesthesiology *63*:457, 1985.
283. Sutherland AD, Sale JP: Fiberoptic awake intubation—a method of topical anaesthesia and orotracheal intubation. Can Anaesth Soc J *33*:502, 1986.

SPONDYLOARTHROPATHIES

284. Ladd JR, Cassidy JT, Martel W: Juvenile ankylosing spondylitis. Arch Rheum *14*:579, 1971.
285. Schaller J, Bitnum S, Wedgwood RJ: Ankylosing spondylitis with childhood onset. J Pediatr *74*:505, 1969.
286. Reid GD, Hill RH: Atlantoaxial subluxation in juvenile ankylosing spondylitis. J Pediatr *93*:531, 1978.
287. Applerough D, Gottlieb NL: Pulmonary manifestations of ankylosing spondylitis. J Rheumatol *2*:446, 1975.
288. Reid GD, Patterson MWH, Patterson AC, et al: Aortic insufficiency in association with juvenile ankylosing spondylitis. J Pediatr *95*:78, 1979.
289. Calin A, Porta J, Fries JF, et al: Clinical history as a screening test for ankylosing spondylitis. JAMA *237*:2613, 1977.
290. Brewerton DA, Hart FD, Nicholls A, et al: Ankylosing spondylitis and HL-A27. Lancet *1*:904, 1973.
291. DiSciascio G, Taranta A: Rheumatic fever in children: A review. Am Heart J *99*:635, 1980.
292. Van de Rijn I, Zabriske JB, McCarty M: Group A streptococcal antigens cross-reactive with myocardium. J Exp Med *146*:579, 1977.
293. Stollerman GH, Markowitz M, et al: Jones criteria (revised) for guidelines in the diagnosis of rheumatic fever (Committee report). Circulation *32*:664, 1965.
294. Troyer C, Grossman ME, Silvers DN: Erythema marginatum in rheumatic fever: Early diagnosis by skin biopsy. J Am Acad Dermatol *8*:724, 1983.
295. John S, Bashi VV, Mairaj PS, et al: Mitral valve replacement in the young patient with rheumatic heart disease. J Thorac Cardiovasc Surg *86*:209, 1983.
296. Felman YM, Nikitas JA: Reiter's syndrome. Cutis *31*:152, 1983.
297. Singsen BH, Bernstein BH, et al: Reiter's syndrome in childhood. Arthritis Rheum *20*(Suppl):402, 1977.
298. Lindsley CB, Schaller JB: Arthritis associated with inflammatory bowel disease in children. J Pediatr *84*:16, 1974.

SYSTEMIC LUPUS ERYTHEMATOSUS

299. Brunner CM, Davis JS: Immune mechanisms in the pathogenesis of systemic lupus erythematosus. Bull Rheum Dis *26*:854, 1976.
300. Wallace DJ, Dubois EL (eds): Dubois' Lupus Erythematosus. 3rd ed. Philadelphia, Lea and Febinger, 1987.
301. Lee SL, Chase PH: Drug-induced systemic lupus erythematosus: A critical review. Semin Arthritis Rheum *5*:83, 1975.
302. Fish AJ, Blau EB, Westberg NG, et al: Systemic lupus erythematosus within the first two decades of life. Am J Med *62*:99, 1977.
303. Koster-King K, Kornreich HK, et al: The clinical spectrum of systemic lupus erythematosus in childhood. Arthritis Rheum *20*(Suppl):287, 1977.
304. Kettler AH, Bean SF, Duffy JO, Gammon WR: Systemic lupus erythematosus presenting as a bullous eruption in a child. Arch Dermatol *124*:1083, 1988.
305. Sourander LB, Pulkinen K: Simultaneous occurrence of ankylosis of cricoarytenoid joints with dyspnea and lupus erythematosus syndrome in rheumatoid arthritis. Acta Rheum Scand *8*:255, 1962.
306. del Rio A, Vazquez JJ, Sobrino JA, et al: Myocardial

involvement in systemic lupus erythematosus. Chest *74*:414, 1978.
307. Ishikawa S, Segar WE, Gilbert EF, et al: Myocardial infarct in a child with systemic lupus erythematosus. Am J Dis Child *132*:696, 1978.
308. Matthay RA, Schwarz MI, Petty TL, et al: Pulmonary manifestations of systemic lupus erythematosus: Review of twelve cases of acute lupus pneumonitis. Medicine *54*:397, 1975.
309. Bennahum DA, Messner RP: Recent observations on central nervous system lupus erythematosus. Semin Arthritis Rheum *4*:253, 1975.
310. Zizic TM, Classen JN, Stevens MB: Acute abdominal complications of systemic lupus erythematosus and polyarteritis nodosa. Am J Med *73*:525, 1982.
311. Davis S, Furie BC, Griffin JH, et al: Circulating inhibitors of blood coagulation associated with procainamide-induced lupus erythematosus. Am J Hematol *4*:401, 1978.
312. Bernstein B, Koster-King K, et al: Sjögren's syndrome in childhood. Arthritis Rheum *20*:361, 1977.
313. Esscher E, Scott JS: Congenital heart block and maternal systemic lupus erythematosus. Br Med J *1*:1235, 1979.
314. Walravens PA, Chase HP: The prognosis of childhood systemic lupus erythematosus. Am J Dis Child *130*:929, 1976.

DERMATOMYOSITIS

315. Winkelmann RK: Dermatomyositis in childhood. Clin Rheum Dis *8*:353, 1982.
316. Rose AL: Childhood polymyositis. A follow up study with special reference to treatment with corticosteroids. Am J Dis Child *127*:518, 1974.
317. Metheny JA: Dermatomyositis. A vocal and swallowing disease entity. Laryngoscope *88*:147, 1978.
318. Olsen GN, Swenson EW: Polymyositis and interstitial lung disease. Am Rev Respir Dis *105*:611, 1972.
319. Johns RA, Finholt DA, Stirt JA: Anaesthetic management of a child with dermatomyositis. Can Anaesth Soc J *33*:71, 1986.
320. Ganta R, Campbell IT, Mostafa SM: Anaesthesia and acute dermatomyositis/polymyositis. Br J Anaesth *60*:854, 1988.
321. Ueki M, Tosaki Y, Ogli K, Uefuji T: Anesthetic management of a patient with dermatomyositis—clinical observation of the effect of muscle relaxants (Japanese). Masui *38*:1505, 1989.

SCLERODERMA

322. Siegel RC: Scleroderma. Med Clin North Am *61*:283, 1977.
323. Fleischmajer R: The pathophysiology of scleroderma. Int J Dermatol *16*:310, 1977.
324. Weisman RA, Calcaterra TC: Head and neck manifestations of scleroderma. Ann Otol *87*:332, 1978.
325. Guttadauria M, Ellman H, Emmanuel G, et al: Pulmonary function in scleroderma. Arthritis Rheum *20*:1071, 1977.
326. Ritchie B: Pulmonary function in scleroderma. Thorax *19*:28, 1964.
327. Iliffe GD, Pettigrew NM: Hypoventilatory respiratory failure in generalized scleroderma. Br Med J *286*:337, 1983.
328. Russell DC, Maloney A, Muir AL: Progressive generalized scleroderma: Respiratory failure from primary chest wall involvement. Thorax *36*:219, 1981.
329. Young RH, Mark GJ: Pulmonary vascular changes in scleroderma. Am J Med *64*:998, 1978.
330. Bulkley BH, Ridolfi RL, Salyer WR, et al: Myocardial lesions of progressive systemic sclerosis. Circulation *53*:483, 1976.
331. Clements PJ, Furst DE, Cabeen W, et al: The relationship of arrhythmias and conduction disturbances to other manifestations of cardiopulmonary disease in progressive systemic sclerosis. Am J Med *71*:38, 1981.
332. Caplan HI, Benny RA: Total osteolysis of the mandibular condyle in progressive systemic sclerosis. Oral Surg *46*:362, 1978.
333. Singsen BH, Bernstein BH, Kornreich HK, et al: Mixed connective tissue disease in childhood. J Pediatr *90*:893, 1977.
334. LeRoy EC, Fleischmann RM: The management of renal scleroderma—experience with dialysis, nephrectomy, transplantation. Am J Med *64*:974, 1978.
335. Lopez-Ovejero JA, Saal SD, D'Angelo WA, et al: Reversal of vascular and renal crises of scleroderma by oral angiotensin-converting enzyme blockade. N Engl J Med *300*:1417, 1979.
336. Thompson J, Conklin KA: Anesthetic management of a pregnant patient with scleroderma. Anesthesiology *59*:69, 1983.
337. Neill RS: Progressive systemic sclerosis. Prolonged sensory blockade following regional anaesthesia in association with reduced response to systemic analgesics. Br J Anaesth *52*:623, 1980.
338. Lewis GBH: Prolonged regional analgesia in scleroderma. Can Anaesth Soc J *21*:495, 1974.
339. Eisele JH, Reitan JA: Scleroderma, Raynaud's phenomenon and local anesthetics. Anesthesiology *34*:386, 1971.
340. Davidson-Lamb RW, Finlayson MCK: Scleroderma. Complications encountered during dental anaesthesia. Anaesthesia *32*:893, 1977.
341. Lim J, Wong KL, Wang CT, et al: Anesthesia for scleroderma—a case report (English). Ma Tsui Hsueh Tsa Chi *27*:197, 1989.
342. Birkhan J, Heifetz M, Haim S: Diffuse cutaneous scleroderma: An anaesthetic problem. Anaesthesia *27*:89, 1972.

SYSTEMIC VASCULITIS SYNDROMES

343. Kathuria S, Chejfec G: Fatal pulmonary Henoch-Schönlein syndrome. Chest *82*:654, 1982.
344. Reimold EW, Weinberg AG, Fink CW, et al: Polyarteritis in children. Am J Dis Child *130*:534, 1976.
345. Martin TH: Pharyngeal edema associated with arteritis. Can Med Assoc J *101*:229, 1969.
346. Roberts FB, Feterman GH: Polyarteritis nodosa in infancy. J Pediatr *63*:519, 1963.
347. Kawasaki T, Kosaki F, Okawa S, et al: A new infantile acute febrile mucocutaneous lymph node syndrome (MLNS) prevailing in Japan. Pediatrics *54*:271, 1974.
348. Melishe ME: Kawasaki syndrome (the mucocutaneous lymph node syndrome). Annu Rev Med *33*:569, 1982.
349. Rowe RD, Rose V: Kawasaki disease: Canadian update. Can Med Assoc J *132*:25, 1985.
350. Bell DM, Brink EW, Nitzin JL, et al: Kawasaki syndrome: Description of two outbreaks in the United States. N Engl J Med *304*:1568, 1981.
351. Wada J, Endo M, Takao M, et al: Mucocutaneous lymph node syndrome. Successful aortocoronary bypass homograft in a 4 year old boy. Chest *77*:443, 1980.
352. Ohe Y, Iwabuchi K, Takeuchi Y: Anesthesia for aorto-

coronary bypass graft in children with Kawasaki disease (Japan). Masui *38*:777, 1989.
353. Edwards WT, Burney RG: Use of repeated nerve blocks in management of an infant with Kawasaki's disease. Anesth Analg *67*:1008, 1988.
354. McNiece WL, Krishna G: Kawasaki disease—a disease with anesthetic implications. Anesthesiology *58*:269, 1983.
355. Feld LG, Weiss RA, Weiner S, et al: Takayasu's arteritis. Asymptomatic presentation in a two-year-old boy. NY State J Med *83*:229, 1983.
356. Pokrovsky AV, Sultanaliev TA, Spiridonov AA: Surgical treatment of vasorenal hypertension in nonspecific aortoarteritis (Takayasu's disease). J Cardiovasc Surg *24*:111, 1983.
357. Warner MA, Hughes DR, Messick JM: Anesthetic management of a patient with pulseless disease. Anesth Analg *62*:532, 1983.
358. Ramanthan S, Gupta V, Chalon J, et al: Anesthetic considerations in Takayasu arteritis. Anesth Analg *58*:247, 1979.
359. Gaida BJ, Gervais HW, Mauer D, et al: Anesthesiology problems in Takayasu's syndrome (German). Anaesthesist *40*:1, 1991.
360. Beckman A, Grahne B, Holopainen B, et al: Wegener's granulomatosis in childhood. A clinical report based on 3 cases. Int J Pediatr Otorhinolaryngol *1*:145, 1979.
361. Kulis JC, Nequin ND: Tracheo-esophageal fistula due to Wegener's granulomatosis. JAMA *191*:148, 1965.
362. Fauci AS, Haynes BF, Katz P, et al: Wegener's granulomatosis: Prospective clinical and therapeutic experience with 85 patients for 21 years. Ann Intern Med *98*:76, 1983.
363. Thomas RHM, Payne CMER, Black MM: Wegener's granulomatosis presenting as pyoderma gangrenosum. Clin Exp Dermatol *7*:523, 1982.
364. Landman S, Burgener F: Pulmonary manifestations in Wegener's granulomatosis. Am J Roentgenol Radium Ther Nucl Med *122*:750, 1974.
365. Lake CL: Anesthesia and Wegener's granulomatosis: Case report and review of the literature. Anesth Analg *57*:353, 1978.
366. Simonsen H, Brun C, Thomsen OF, et al: Goodpasture's syndrome in twins. Acta Med Scand *212*:425, 1982.
367. Proskey AJ, Weatherbee L, Easterling RE, et al: Goodpasture's syndrome. A report of five cases and review of the literature. Am J Med *48*:162, 1970.

MISCELLANEOUS CONNECTIVE TISSUE DISORDERS

368. Pyeritz RE, McKusick VA: The Marfan syndrome: Diagnosis and management. N Engl J Med *300*:772, 1979.
369. Sisk HE, Zahka KG, Pyeritz RE: The Marfan syndrome in early childhood: Analysis of 125 patients diagnosed at less than 4 years of age. Am J Cardiol *52*:355, 1983.
370. Hall JR, Pyeritz RE, Dudgeon DL, et al: Pneumothorax in the Marfan syndrome: Prevalence and therapy. Ann Thorac Surg *37*:500, 1984.
371. Bolande RP, Tucker AS: Pulmonary emphysema and other cardiorespiratory lesions as part of the Marfan syndrome. Pediatrics *33*:356, 1964.
372. Newbold SG, Shafer AD, Goodwin CD, et al: Stage III Wilm's tumour of a solitary kidney in a patient with Marfan's syndrome: A 5-year survival. J Pediatr Surg *17*:841, 1982.
373. Wells DG, Podolakin W: Anaesthesia and Marfan's syndrome: Case report. Can J Anaesth *34*:311, 1987.
374. Miglets AW, Viall JH, Kataria YP: Sarcoidosis of the head and neck. Laryngoscope *87*:2038, 1977.
375. Snider GI, Doctor LR: The mechanics of ventilation in sarcoidosis. Am Rev Respir Dis *89*:897, 1964.
376. Johnson RL, Lawson WH, Wilcox WCN: Alveolar capillary block in sarcoidosis. Clin Res *9*:196, 1961.
377. Kendig EL, Brummer DL: The prognosis of sarcoidosis in children. Chest *70*:351, 1976.
378. Hendricks WM, Ahmad M, Gratz E: Weber-Christian syndrome in infancy. Br J Dermatol *98*:175, 1978.
379. Spivak JL, Lindo S, Coleman M: Weber-Christian disease complicated by consumption coagulopathy and microangiopathic hemolytic anemia. Johns Hopkins Med J *126*:344, 1970.
380. Britt WJ, Duray PH, Dahl MV, et al: Diffuse fasciitis with eosinophilia: A steroid-responsive variant of scleroderma. J Pediatr *97*:432, 1980.

CORTICOSTEROID THERAPY

381. Axelrod L: Glucocorticoid therapy. Medicine *55*:39, 1976.
382. Melby JC: Systemic corticosteroid therapy: Pharmacology and endocrinologic considerations. Ann Intern Med *81*:505, 1974.
383. Thorn GW: Clinical considerations in the use of corticosteroids. N Engl J Med *274*:775, 1966.
384. Kaplan SR, Calabresi P: Immunosuppressive agents. N Engl J Med *289*:952, 1973.
385. Chabner BA, Myers CE, Coleman CN, et al: The clinical pharmacology of antineoplastic agents. N Engl J Med *292*:1107, 1159, 1975.
386. Schein PS, Winokur SH: Immunosuppressive and cytotoxic chemotherapy: Long-term implications. Ann Intern Med *82*:84, 1975.
387. Munro DD: The effect of percutaneously absorbed steroids on hypothalamic-pituitary-adrenal function after intensive use in in-patients. Br J Dermatol *94*(Suppl 12):67, 1976.
388. Wilson L, Williams DI, Marsh SD: Plasma corticosteroid levels in out-patients treated with topical steroids. Br J Dermatol *88*:373, 1973.
389. Laaksonen AL, Sunell JE, Westeren H, et al: Adrenocortical function in children with juvenile rheumatoid arthritis and other connective tissue disorders. Scand J Rheumatol *3*:137, 1974.
390. Mohler JL, Michael KA, Freedman AM, et al: The serum and urinary cortisol response to operative trauma. Surg Gynecol Obstet *161*:445, 1985.
391. Hedner P, Kullberg G, Bostedt I: Recovery of the hypothalamus-pituitary-adrenal axis after short-term high dose corticosteroid treatment in neurosurgical practice. Acta Neurochir *73*:157, 1984.
392. Graber AL, Ney RL, Nicholson WE, et al: Natural history of pituitary-adrenal recovery following long-term suppression with corticosteroids. J Clin Endocrinol Metab *25*:11, 1965.
393. Cope CL: The adrenal cortex in internal medicine (I). Br Med J *2*:47, 1966.
394. Fraser CG, Preuss FS, Bigford WD: Adrenal atrophy and irreversible shock associated with cortisone therapy. JAMA *149*:1542, 1952.
395. Roberts JC: Operative collapse after corticosteroid therapy—a survey. Surg Clin North Am *50*:363, 1970.
396. Sury MR, Russell GN, Heaf DP: Hydrocortisone myopathy (letter). Lancet *2*:515, 1988.
397. Kehlet H, Nikki P, et al: Plasma catecholamines during

surgery in unsupplemented glucocorticoid treated patients. Br J Anaesth *46*:73, 1974.
398. Barton RN, Passinghem BJ: Early responses to hemorrhage in the conscious rat: Effects of corticosterone. Am J Physiol *243*:R416, 1982.
399. Weatherill D, Spence AA: Anaesthesia and disorders of the adrenal cortex. Br J Anaesth *56*:741, 1984.
400. Kehlet H, Binder C: Adrenocortical function and clinical course during and after surgery in unsupplemented glucocorticoid-treated patients. Br J Anaesth *45*:1043, 1973.
401. Oyama T: Hazards of steroids in association with anaesthesia. Can Anaesth Soc J *16*:361, 1969.
402. Mulvihill SJ, Fonkalsrud EW: Complications of excessive operative fluid administration in children receiving steroids for inflammatory bowel disease. J Pediatr Surg *19*:247, 1984.
403. Bovill JG, Sebel PS, Fiolet JW, et al: The influence of sufentanil on endocrine and metabolic response to cardiac surgery. Anesth Analg *62*:391, 1983.
404. Ishihara H, Ishida K, Matsuki A, et al: Adrenocortical response to general anaesthesia and surgery. Can Anaesth Soc J *26*:186, 1979.
405. Traynor C, Hall GM: Endocrine and metabolic changes during surgery: Anaesthetic implications. Br J Anaesth *53*:153, 1981.
406. Meyers EF: Partial recovery from pancuronium neuromuscular blockade following hydrocortisone administration. Anesthesiology *46*:148, 1977.
407. Plumpton FS, Besser GM, Cole PV: Corticosteroid treatment and surgery. Anaesthesia *24*:3, 1969.
408. Black GW, Montgomery DAD: Adrenal disease. *In* Vickers MD (ed): Medicine for Anaesthetists. Oxford, Blackwell Scientific Publications, 1982, p 451.
409. Fass B: Glucocorticoid therapy for non-endocrine disorders: Withdrawal and "coverage." Pediatr Clin North Am *26*:251, 1979.
410. Olin R: When should you consider a cortisone prep? Medical Times *100*:64, 1972.
411. Morse WI: Carrying the patient on steroids through surgery. NS Med Bull *45*:185, 1966.
412. Solem JH, Lund I: Surgery in patients treated with cortisone or cortisone-like steroids. Oslo City Hosp J *19*:3, 1969.
413. Baxter JD, Tyrell JB: The adrenal cortex. *In* Felig P, Baxter JD, Broadus AE, et al (eds): Endocrinology and Metabolism. New York, McGraw-Hill, 1981, p 462.
414. Fariss BL, Hane S, Shinsako J, et al: Comparison of absorption of cortisone acetate and hydrocortisone hemisuccinate. J Clin Endocrinol Metab *47*:1137, 1978.
415. Kenny FM, Preeyasombat C, Midgeon CJ: Cortisol production rate. II. Normal infants, children and adults. Pediatrics *37*:34, 1966.
416. Gran L, Pahle JA: Rational substitution therapy for steroid-treated patients. Anaesthesia *33*:59, 1978.
417. Kehlet H: A rational approach to dosage and preparation of parenteral glucocorticoid substitution therapy during surgical procedures. Acta Anaesth Scand *19*:260, 1975.
418. Symreng T, Karlberg BE, Kagendal B, et al: Physiological cortisol substitution of long-term steroid-treated patients undergoing major surgery. Br J Anaesth *53*:949, 1981.
419. Korolenko OA, Aliakin LN: Anesthesiologic tactics in the case of children with rheumatoid arthritis receiving hormonal therapy (Russian). Anesteziol Reanimatol *6*:58, 1989.
420. Cassidy JT, Petty RE: Preventing acute adrenal insufficiency. *In* Cassidy JT, Petty RE: Textbook of Pediatric Rheumatology. 2nd ed. New York, Churchill Livingstone, 1990, p 76.

CHAPTER

16 Immune Disorders

FREDERICK A. BURROWS, M.D.,
BERNARD M. BRAUDE, M.B., and MILTON GOLD, M.D.

The host-defense mechanism, or immune response, is a multicomponent system divided into two major groups, the innate and the adaptive. The innate system is nonspecific and acts similarly on all different foreign antigens. It consists of mechanical barriers such as the external skin and the internal mucous membranes lining the gastrointestinal and respiratory tracts; secreted products such as the stomach acids, lysozyme in tears, and sebaceous gland secretions; and inflammatory cells such as the macrophage and polymorphonuclear leukocytes.

The adaptive system (Fig. 16–1) is a more powerful back-up defense mechanism. Its response to individual foreign antigens is very specific. Since it is capable of recognizing previously encountered antigens, its response to them is accelerated. The primary cells involved in this process are the B cells, which are involved in antibody response (humoral immunity), and the T cells, which are mediators of cellular immunity. The humoral response protects against extracellular bacteria; the cellular response is directed against intracellular bacteria, viruses, fungi, and mycobacteria. The immune response is supported by other cells such as macrophages, neutrophils, eosinophils, basophils, and mast cells, as well as by a collection of soluble proteins, collectively called the *complement system.*

As a consequence of the immunological process, allergic responses, autoimmune phenomena, and transplant rejection may occur. Dysfunction of the immune response (or immunodeficiencies) also can occur, and it can have consequences not only for the patient but also for the anesthetist. Understanding these anesthetic implications requires a basic understanding of the normal development and function of the immune system.

These immunodeficiencies can be classified as either primary or secondary (Table 16–1). This chapter deals with the primary immunodeficiencies; with the acquired immunodeficiency syndrome (AIDS) in children (a secondary immunodeficiency); with graft-versus-host disease; and with complement-mediated disorders.

THE IMMUNE SYSTEM

COMPONENTS

LYMPHOCYTES

Lymphocytes are the main effector cells of the immune system. Two populations exist: agranular small lymphocytes and large granular lymphocytes, also called *natural killer* (NK)

References are arranged under subject headings in the bibliography at the end of the chapter.

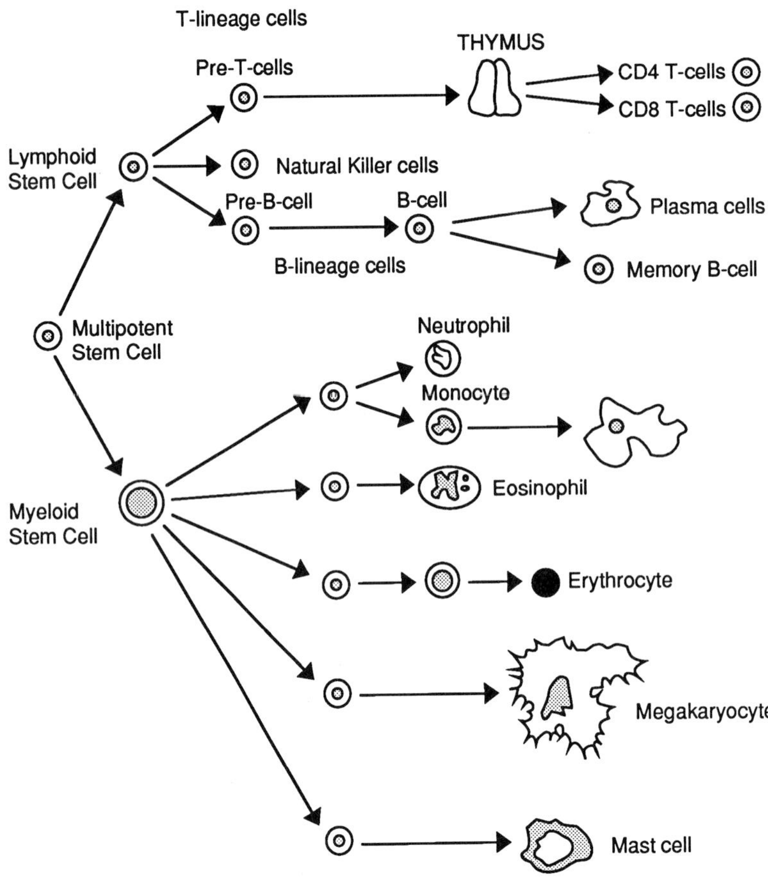

FIGURE 16–1. Derivation of cells of the immune system. Pleuripotent stem cells are derived from the yolk sac and ultimately reside in the bone marrow. Lymphocytes are derived from a lymphoid stem cell, whereas monocytes and macrophages are derived from myeloid stem cells. Lymphocytes can be divided into B-lineage and T-lineage cells. (Modified from Nelson DL: Cellular interactions in the human immune response. *In* Stiehm ER (ed): Immunological Disorders in Infants and Children. 3rd edition. Philadelphia, WB Saunders, 1989, pp 15–28.)

cells. The small lymphocyte population consists of T cells and B cells: T cells constitute 65 percent of the peripheral blood lymphocytes; B cells, 5 to 15 percent; non-T, non-B large granular lymphocytes (formerly called null cells), the remainder.

T Cells

T cells arise from pluripotent stem cells of mesenchymal origin (Fig. 16–2). Precursor cells differentiate and mature after entering the thymus. On leaving the thymus, T cells travel throughout the body in the bloodstream and seed the spleen, lymph nodes, intestinal Peyer's patches, and appendix. T cells remain only transiently in these locations and then leave through the efferent lymphatic vessels, reentering the blood stream. Mature T cells express surface antigens acquired in the thymus, which permits the identification of subpopulations of T cells. Since surface antigens can be identified by monoclonal antibodies, they have assisted in defining subpopulations of T cells. A unified nomenclature for these surface antigens has been developed: they are now referred to as *clusters of differentiation* (CD). CD4 and CD8 antigens are important: they enable the distinction of T cells with so-called helper or inducer functions (CD4) from those with suppressor or cytotoxic functions (CD8).

T-helper cells undergo blast transformation and cell division when they interact with processed antigens presented on the surfaces of macrophages, dendritic cells, and Langerhans' cells in the skin. The activated T-helper cells produce cytokines. Those cytokines that come from lymphocytes are called *lymphokines;* since some act on other white blood cells they are also known as *interleukins*. Interleukin–2 (IL–2) promotes proliferation and stimulation of other T cells (such as CD8 cells) and B cells; IL–3 stimulates neutrophils, eosinophils, basophils, mast cells, and monocytes; IL–4 stimulates B cells to produce immunoglobulins, including IgE. IL–5 and IL–6 also affect T and B cells. Newer interleukins, IL–7 to IL–10, have also been described, but their function has not been fully characterized. Other cytokines with broader power than the interleukins have been described, for example, interferon gamma (IFN-γ), which acts on macrophages; tumor necrosis factor, and granulocyte-monocyte colony-stimulating factor (GM-CSF)

T cells thus produce soluble factors that engage other T and B cells in the immune response (Fig. 16–3). This response, established by the T-helper cell, is countered by activation of the T-suppressor cell, which dampens the immune response. T cells alone can control gram-negative bacterial, viral, fungal, protozoal, and mycoplasmal infections, reject grafts of foreign tissues, and cause delayed hypersensitivity reactions. These immune responses are referred to as *cellular immunity*.

Natural Killer Cells

Natural killer cells are a class of cytotoxic lymphocytes that do not require immunological specific activation to function; rather, their activity is induced by interferon. These cells play a role in resistance to tumor growth and host defense against viruses.

B Cells

The multipotent stem cells that give rise to the T cells also give rise to the B-cell lineage (see Fig. 16–2). Development begins in the fetal liver and continues in the bone marrow when hematopoiesis shifts to that site with later development. During this development immunoglobulin-gene rearrangement occurs, determining the specific immunoglobulin the cell will produce.

After formation, B cells enter the bloodstream and migrate to lymphoid follicles in the spleen, lymph nodes, Peyer's patches, and other lymphoid tissues. Like T cells, B cells recirculate through the lymphatic and circulatory systems; unlike T cells, they are short-lived. Their short life is offset by their high level of production.

The surface antigens of B cells enable them to recognize and thus interact with T cells. Such interaction is a requirement for antigen activation of the resting B cell. Activation of a B cell occurs both after antigen interaction with B-cell surface antibody molecules and on interaction

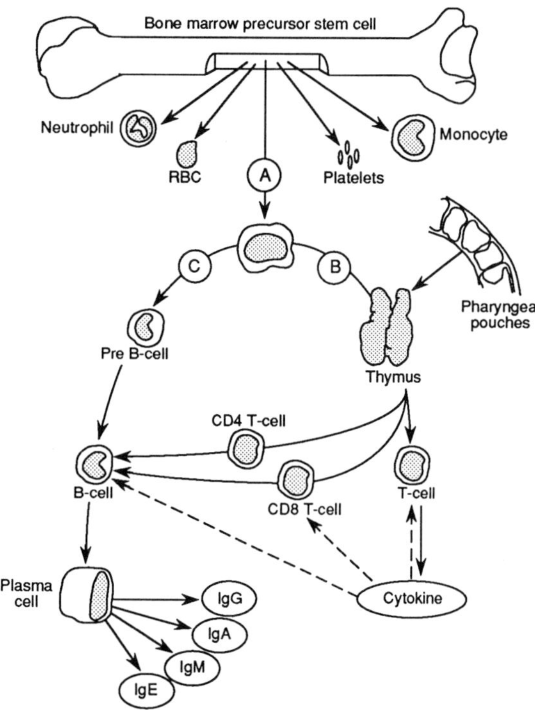

FIGURE 16–2. Derivation of cells in the T- and B-cell lineage. Lymphocytes are derived from a lymphoid stem cell. Defects along pathway A result in combined T- and B-cell immunodeficiencies. Defects along pathway B or C result in T- and B-cell deficiencies, respectively. The hatched lines represent suspected interactions. (Modified from Fireman P: Immunology of allergic disorders. *In* Fireman P, Slavin RG (eds.): Atlas of Allergies. New York, Gower Medical Publishing, 1991, pp 1.1–1.24.)

Table 16–1. CLASSIFICATION OF IMMUNODEFICIENCIES

Primary Immunodeficiencies	Neoplastic and hematological diseases
B-lymphocyte (antibody) syndrome	Lymphoma, leukemia, myeloma, neutropenia, aplastic anemia, sickle cell disease
T-lymphocyte (cell-mediated) deficiency	Metabolic diseases
Combined T- and B-lymphocyte deficiency	Protein losing enteropathy, nephrotic syndrome, diabetes, malnutrition
Phagocytic deficiency	Trauma and surgery
Complement deficiency	Burns, splenectomy, anesthesia
Secondary Immunodeficiencies (Incomplete Listing)	Miscellaneous
Infectious diseases	Lupus erythematosus, chronic hepatitis, Down's syndrome
Acquired immunodeficiency	
Therapeutic agents	
Steroids, radiation, immunosuppressive agents, antilymphocyte (T-cell) serum	

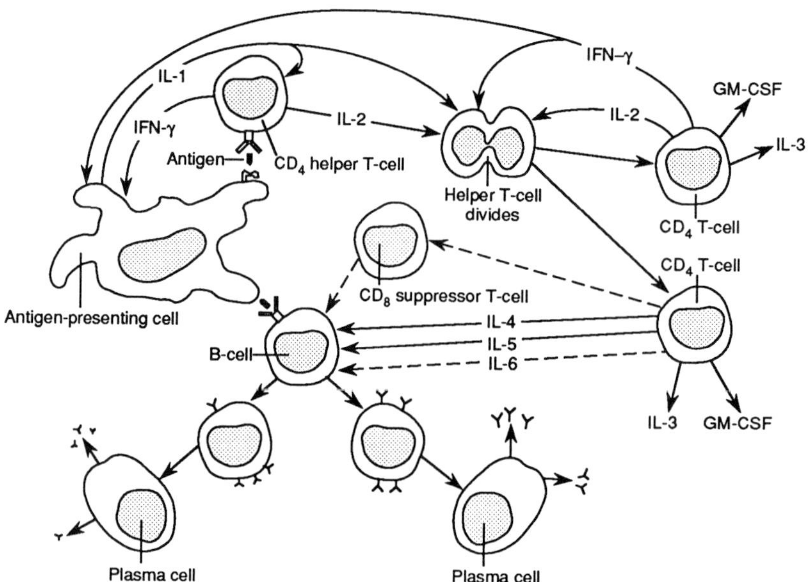

FIGURE 16–3. T-cell, B-cell, and macrophage interactions in tissue producing the immune reaction to foreign allergens. The *antigen-presenting cell* is a macrophage that processes foreign antigen and then interacts with T cells. The binding of the processed antigen to the T cell stimulates the cell to produce cytokines such as interferon gamma (IFN-γ), which stimulate the macrophage to synthesize and release several other cytokines, including interleukin (IL)-1. This acts on the antigen-activated T cells, stimulating synthesis and release of IL-2.

IL-2 induces the T cells to proliferate, differentiating into various populations. The CD4 T-helper cells consist of two subpopulations, H_1 and H_2. IL-2 promotes proliferation and stimulation of the T cells, B cells, and natural cytotoxic killer cells. IL-3 stimulates neutrophils, eosinophils, basophils, mast cells, and monocytes. IL-4, IL-5, and IL-6 act on B cells to promote immunoglobulin synthesis. The granulocyte-monocyte colony–stimulating factor (GM-CSF) promotes the activities and functions of the neutrophils and monocytes. The hatched lines represent suspected interactions. (Modified from Fireman P: Immunodeficiency and allergic disorders. *In* Fireman P, Slavin RG (eds): Atlas of Allergies. New York, Gower Medical Publishing, 1991, pp 17.1–17.19.)

with a T-helper cell (Fig. 16–3). The B cell then enlarges and undergoes differentiation into a plasma cell capable of secreting thousands of identical antibodies per second. These plasma cells, which rarely divide and are short-lived, engage in humoral immunity: elimination of gram-positive bacteria, neutralization of toxins, and immediate allergic reactions.

IMMUNOGLOBULINS

Normal antibody activities of the various groups of immunoglobulins are presented in Table 16–2. Antibodies function to bind antigen. This binding has several different possible results, depending upon the particular antibody and antigen. Antibodies neutralize toxic substances. For example, tetanus toxin is neutralized by antibodies because it is an antigenic determinant. Antibodies that facilitate the phagocytosis of particulate antigens are important in opsonization. In opsonization, antibodies combine with the foreign antigenic determinant. The free portion of the antibody combines with receptors on the surface of the phagocytes, thus

Table 16–2. ANTIBODY ACTIVITIES OF IMMUNOGLOBULINS

	IgG_1	IgG_2	IgG_3	IgG_4	IgM	IgA	sIgA	IgE
Antibody activity	+	+	+	+	+	+	+	+
Viral neutralization	+	+	+	±	+	−	+	−
Toxin neutralization	+	?	?	?	−	?	?	−
Bactericidal activity (gram-negative)	−	−	−	−	+	−	−	−
Antibodies to polysaccharide antigen	±	+ +	−	−	−	−	−	−

Modified from Fireman P: Immunology of allergic disorders. *In* Fireman P, Slavin RG (eds): Atlas of Allergies. New York, Gower Medical Publishing, 1991, pp 1.1–1.24.

greatly enhancing their ability to ingest the antigens. Antibodies also can facilitate complement activation by either the classic or the alternative pathway (see page 595). Such complement activation can result in the release of factors that facilitate chemotaxis, function as anaphylatoxins, or assist in cell lysis.

Immunoglobulin M (IgM) is the first immunoglobulin formed in response to an antigenic challenge and is distributed primarily in the vascular space. It is a polymer, a pentamer consisting of five individual immunoglobulins linked by disulfide bonds and a joining (J) chain. IgM does not cross the placenta. It is extremely efficient in activating complement in agglutination and in opsonic activity.

Immunoglobulin G (IgG) is the major immunoglobulin found in blood. It has a long life and is the only immunoglobulin that can cross the placenta, thus making it suitable for use in passive immunization. There are four subgroups of IgG (IgG_1, IgG_2, IgG_3, IgG_4), each of which has a unique biological behavior.

Immunoglobulin A (IgA) exists in two forms. In blood, it exists as a monomer (IgA). In secretions, in which IgA serves its primary function, secretory IgA (sIgA) exists as a dimer joined by a J chain and is protected from proteolysis by a secretory component, a peptide acquired from the epithelial cells through which sIgA must pass to reach the duct or lumen into which it is secreted. IgA protects mainly the secretory surfaces of the gastrointestinal tract, respiratory tract, and eyes: it immobilizes microorganisms or prevents their attachment to mucosal surfaces, or both.

The bond between immunoglobulin E (IgE) and its surface receptors on mast cells and basophils exposes its antigen-binding sites. Interaction of antigen with these receptors results in the release of pharmacologically active mediators from the cell, which can cause asthma, hay fever, and anaphylaxis.

Immunoglobulin D (IgD) functions as a receptor on B-cell surfaces. It is believed to be important in directing antigen to the B-cell surfaces, thus facilitating initial immunization.

When an individual receives an antigen, IgM appears first, followed in a few days by IgG. If the individual is reexposed to the same antigen, an amnestic response occurs: the IgM response is similar to that of the initial response, but the IgG antibody appears sooner and rises to a higher level. The speed of this secondary response explains why infections often are minimal or do not occur at all.

GENERAL ANESTHETIC CONSIDERATIONS IN IMMUNODEFICIENCY SYNDROMES

Our current understanding of the mechanisms by which the human body resists microbial agents has accrued over the last 30 years. Although the effects of anesthetic agents and surgical procedures on the immune system of the normal patient have been described in the literature, there has been very little investigation of the effects of anesthesia and operations on the immune system of the patient with an underlying defect. Because of this, it is largely impossible to recommend specific anesthetic techniques that will have a less depressant effect on an already compromised immune system. Many of the immunological syndromes do have associated abnormalities that may be affected by the choice of anesthesia. These implications will be discussed in relation to the particular syndromes. There are, however, essentials of anesthetic management for immunosuppressed patients that can be discussed together. These relate to their increased susceptibility to infection.

The major manifestation of immunodeficiency is increased susceptibility to infection: increased frequency of infections, increased severity of infections, prolonged duration of infection, repeated infections without a symptom-free interval, increased dependency on antibiotics, unexpected or severe complications of infections, or infection with an unusual organism, usually an opportunistic one. Table 16–3 summarizes some of the common clinical findings for patients with immunodeficiencies that the anesthetist should consider during the preanesthetic history and physical evaluation of these patients. These include features that are common to several disorders, grouped according to their relative frequency. Certain clinical patterns seen in patients with primary immunodeficiencies are characteristic for age of onset, type of infection, gender, and other clinical findings (Table 16–4).

B-cell immunodeficiencies manifest clinically with one or more of the following: recurrent pneumonia and otitis media, pharyngitis-tonsillitis, sinusitis, bronchiectasis, conjunctivitis, rhinitis, meningitis, septicemia, persistent infectious diarrhea and viral encephalitis, viral hepatitis, cholangitis, paralytic poliomyelitis, mycoplasmal arthritis, and chronic cystitis and urethritis. Classically, recurrent infections are due to encapsulated bacteria such as *Streptococcus pneumoniae, Staphylococcus aureus, Hae-*

Table 16–3. CLINICAL FEATURES OF IMMUNODEFICIENCY

Usually Present
Recurrent upper respiratory infections
Severe bacterial infections
Persistent infections with incomplete or no response to therapy
Often Present
Failure to thrive or growth retardation
Infection with an unusual organism
Skin lesions (rash, seborrhea, pyoderma, necrotic abscesses, alopecia, eczema, telangiectasia)
Recalcitrant thrush
Diarrhea and malabsorption
Persistent sinusitis
Recurrent bronchitis, pneumonia
Evidence of autoimmunity
Paucity of lymph nodes and tonsils
Hematological abnormalities: aplastic anemia, hemolytic anemia, neutropenia, thrombocytopenia
Occasionally Present
Weight loss, fevers
Chronic conjunctivitis
Lymphadenopathy
Hepatosplenomegaly
Severe viral disease
Arthralgia or arthritis
Chronic encephalitis
Recurrent meningitis
Pyoderma gangrenosa
Adverse reaction to vaccines
Bronchiectasis
Delayed umbilical cord detachment
Chronic stomatitis or peridontitis

Modified from Stiehm ER: Immunodeficiency disorders: General considerations. *In* Stiehm ER (ed.): Immunologic Disorders in Infants and Children. 3rd edition. Philadelphia, WB Saunders, 1989.

mophilus influenzae, Neisseria meningitidis, and *Pseudomonas aeruginosa.* Other less common bacteria, viruses, protozoa, and mycoplasmas have also been responsible for recurrent infections. Serious enteroviral syndromes such as chronic encephalitis, dermatomyositis, and vaccine-induced paralytic poliomyelitis have also been associated with B-cell immunodeficiencies. A list of opportunistic infections is presented in Table 16–5.

T-cell immunodeficiencies are associated both with severe infections produced by organisms that cause common illnesses in normal children and with a variety of opportunistic infections from organisms that rarely cause disease in normal children (Table 16–5). There are also several infections unique to immunodeficient children. Chronic diarrhea is caused by *Cryptosporidium* sp., *Giardia lamblia,* and rotaviruses. Chronic pulmonary infections are caused by respiratory syncytial viruses, parainfluenza viruses, cytomegalovirus, and adenoviruses.

Immunodeficient patients may require anesthesia and operation for both disease-related and non disease-related conditions. When an immunodeficient patient requires operation, the anesthesiologist and surgeon should consult with the physician managing the immunodeficient state to optimize the patient's condition before the procedure.

The respiratory system is frequently involved in these patients' infections. This involvement can range from mild, recurrent upper respiratory infections to recurrent pneumonias and bronchiectasis. Assessment of the status of the respiratory system, therefore, is very important. Acute infections should be aggressively treated and eradicated if time and antibiotic sensitivities permit. Before operation, patients should be taught the techniques of physiotherapy, incentive spirometry, coughing, deep breathing, and bronchodilator therapy that they will need after the operation. Pulmonary function tests should be performed to establish baseline values and assess the adequacy of therapy.

Viral infections may increase airway resistance for up to 5 weeks after infection. If possible, surgical therapy should be delayed for this period, especially in view of the adverse effect of viral infection on respiratory defense mechanisms against bacteria.

Since chronic respiratory disease may produce right-sided heart failure, the patient's cardiac status should be assessed before anesthesia and operation. Appropriate drug therapy should be instituted if necessary.

Since treatment with certain antibiotics can result in renal insufficiency, the possibility of impaired renal function must be considered. The involvement of other organ systems, for example, hepatic or cerebral abscesses, must also be evaluated. It is emphasized that involvement of one organ can produce effects in other organs, especially when cardiac or hepatic disease is present.

The preanesthetic use of prophylactic antibiotics has been advocated, particularly when bacteremia is possible (as in airway manipulation or abscess drainage). Meticulous antiseptic technique is required for all procedures requiring skin puncture, such as intravenous access, invasive monitors, and bladder catheterization. Such monitors and lines should be discontinued as soon as possible to minimize the risk of infection at these sites. Anesthetic equipment coming into direct contact with the patient should be sterile. The anesthesiologist should use aseptic technique in handling these patients.

Guidelines have been established for the use of regional anesthetic techniques in immunosup-

Table 16–4. CHARACTERISTIC CLINICAL PATTERNS OF SOME PRIMARY IMMUNODEFICIENCIES

Features	Diagnosis
In Newborns and Young Infants (0–6 months)	
Hypocalcemia, heart disease, unusual facies	Thymic hypoplasia (DiGeorge syndrome)
Delayed umbilical cord detachment, leukocytosis, recurrent infections	Granulocyte glycoprotein deficiency
Diarrhea, pneumonia, thrush, failure to thrive	Severe combined immunodeficiency
Maculopapular rash, alopecia, lymphadenopathy, hepatosplenomegaly	Severe combined immunodeficiency with graft-versus-host disease
Melena, draining ears, eczema	Wiskott-Aldrich syndrome
Mouth ulcers, neutropenia, recurrent infections	Immunodeficiency with hyper-IgM
In Infancy and Young Children (6 months–5 years)	
Paralytic disease following oral poliovirus immunization	X-linked agammaglobulinemia
Recurrent cutaneous and systemic staphylococcal infections, coarse features	Hyper-IgE syndrome
Recurrent cutaneous staphylococcal infections in fair, red-headed girls	Job's variant of the hyper-IgE syndrome
Persistent thrush, nail dystrophy, endocrinopathies	Chronic mucocutaneous candidiasis
In Older Children and Adults (over 5 years)	
Progressive dermatomyositis with chronic echovirus encephalitis	X-linked agammaglobulinemia
Sinopulmonary infections, neurological deterioration, telangiectasia	Ataxia telangiectasia
Oculocutaneous albinism, recurrent infection	Chédiak-Higashi syndrome
Lymphadenopathy, dermatitis, pneumonia, osteomyelitis	Chronic granulomatous disease

Modified from Stiehm ER: Immunodeficiency disorders: General considerations. *In* Stiehm ER (ed): Immunologic Disorders in Infants and Children. 3rd edition. Philadelphia, WB Saunders, 1989.

pressed patients in the presence of infection, but no recommendations concerning their use in an immunosuppressed patient have been made. Nevertheless, though controversial, these techniques in immunosuppressed patients may be indicated and desirable. Meticulous antiseptic technique will minimize the risk of introducing infection. Indwelling catheters should be removed as soon as possible, since they may increase that risk.

To minimize the risk of infection after surgery, further precautions should be taken. Immunodeficient patients may require reverse (i.e., protective) isolation (discussed later) after operation, not to protect them against infection from endogenous organisms but to decrease their risk of acquiring infections from others in the postanesthetic recovery room or the ward. Because many immunodeficient patients requiring anesthesia and operation harbor organisms that are resistant to antibiotic therapy, they may pose a hazard to operating room personnel and

Table 16–5. INFECTIONS IN THE B-CELL AND T-CELL IMMUNODEFICIENT PATIENT

B-Cell Immunodeficiencies	Encapsulated bacteria (*Streptococcus pneumoniae, Staphylococcus aureus, Haemophilus influenzae, Neisseria meningitidis, Pseudomonas aeruginosa); Campylobacter* sp., *Ureaplasma urealyticum, Mycoplasma pneumoniae* Viruses (enterovirus, rotavirus) Protozoa (*Giardia lamblia; Cryptosporidium* sp.; *Pneumocystis carinii)*
T-Cell Immunodeficiencies	Encapsulated bacteria (*Streptococcus pneumoniae, Staphylococcus aureus, Haemophilus influenzae)* Facultative intracellular bacteria (*Mycoplasma tuberculosis,* other *Mycobacterium* sp., *Listeria monocytogenes); Escherichia coli, Pseudomonas aeruginosa, Enterobacter* sp., *Klebsiella* sp., *Serratia marcescens, Salmonella* sp., *Nocardia* sp. Viruses (cytomegalovirus, herpes simplex virus, varicella-zoster virus, Epstein-Barr virus, rotaviruses, adenoviruses, enteroviruses, respiratory syncytial virus, measles virus, vaccinia virus, parainfluenza viruses) Protozoa (*Pneumocystis carinii, Toxoplasma gondii, Cryptosporidium* sp.) Fungi (*Candida* sp., *Cryptococcus neoformans, Histoplasma capsulatum)*

Modified from Cherry JD, Feigin RD: Infection in the compromised host. *In* Stiehm ER (ed.): Immunologic Disorders in Infants and Children. 3rd edition. Philadelphia, WB Saunders, 1989.

patients operated on later in the same operating room (see below). After operation, these immunodeficient patients may require isolation.

Universal Precautions

Since it is recognized that we cannot rely on patient history and physical examination to identify those patients (immunodeficient or otherwise) who are infected with blood-borne pathogens, the anesthesiologist must regard all patients as being potentially infected. Such pathogens common to immunodeficient patients include human immunodeficiency virus, hepatitis B virus, non-A,non-B hepatitis virus, herpes simplex, cytomegalovirus, and many bacteria.

In 1983, the Centers for Disease Control (CDC) published their initial *Guideline for Isolation Precautions in Hospitals*, containing a section entitled "Blood and Body Fluid Precautions." The recommendations in this section outline blood and body fluid precautions that should be taken when a patient is known or suspected to be infected with blood-borne pathogens. They note that the human immunodeficiency virus (HIV) is much less readily transmitted than is the hepatitis B virus (HBV).

In August 1987, the CDC published their recommendations that blood and body fluid precautions be used consistently for all patients, regardless of their status for blood-borne infection. This extension of blood and body fluid precautions to all patients is referred to as the *Universal Blood and Body Fluid Precautions* or *Universal Precautions.*

Universal precautions are intended to prevent health care workers' and all patients' parenteral, mucous membrane, and nonintact skin exposures to blood-borne pathogens. Immunization with HBV vaccine is recommended as an important adjunct to universal precautions for hospital care workers who are exposed to blood.

In June 1988, an update to universal precautions addressed the following specific issues:

1. Identification of body fluids to which universal precautions apply
   - blood and other body fluids containing visible blood
   - semen, vaginal secretions
   - cerebrospinal fluid, synovial fluid, pleural and peritoneal fluid, pericardial fluid, amniotic fluid
   - human breast milk, only in the perinatal transmission of HIV to the nursing neonate
   - *not* feces, nasal secretions, sputum, sweat, tears, urine, and vomitus, unless they contain visible blood
   - *not* saliva, except in the dental setting, where saliva is likely to be contaminated with blood
2. Use of protective barriers (e.g., gloves, masks, protective eyewear [safety glasses], face shields, and protective clothing [gowns or aprons]) to reduce the risk of exposure to potentially infective materials
3. Use of gloves for phlebotomy
4. Selection of gloves (latex or vinyl)
5. Waste management programs

The principles of universal precautions include

1. Routine use of appropriate barrier precautions (e.g., gloves, masks, protective eyewear, face shields, gowns, aprons)
2. Handwashing immediately after gloves are removed
3. Precautions for use and disposal of needles and sharp instruments
4. Refraining from all direct patient care and from handling patient care equipment and devices used for invasive procedures while health care workers have exudative lesions or weeping dermatitis

Guidelines for the prevention of the transmission of HIV and HBV to health care workers (including paramedic and emergency medical technicians) and public safety workers (including fire service, law enforcement, and correctional facility personnel) are addressed in the context of their activities. Because of their length and complexity, these guidelines are not presented here but can be found in the sources in the Bibliography under "Universal Precautions."

Recommendations recently have been updated for exposure-prone invasive procedures, including dental, obstetrical, and gynecological procedures. Additional precautions are prudent to prevent HIV and HBV transmission during procedures that have been linked to health care worker-to-patient HBV transmission or that are considered exposure-prone. Special care is required in the disinfection and sterilization of instruments and reusable equipment used for invasive procedures.

Reverse Isolation

Over the past decade, innovative immunosuppressive and chemotherapeutic regimens have permitted successful outcomes in children with the underlying host-risk factors unique to many of the disorders outlined in this chapter. Improvement and refinement in surgical techniques have made anesthesiologists and operating room personnel more aware of the factors that determine the types and site of potential infection in this group of patients.

Current controversy centers on which elements of the protective environments are most useful in preventing infections in compromised hosts. Several viruses (e.g., influenza, parainfluenza) may be transferred from the health care worker with an upper respiratory infection to the patient.

Simple protective isolation (reverse precautions) is performed to avoid these risks. It is emphasized, however, that practicing the basic concepts of infection control is the most important principle. All patients require measures to prevent cross-contamination by observing good clothing, handwashing, and decontamination practices. Not all immunodeficient patients will require reverse isolation techniques, but for those who do, there are implications for normal anesthetic management.

Although there are variations from institution to institution, in general reverse isolation is used in patients with severely immunodeficient bone marrow transplant (aplastic anemia) or severe combined immune deficiency (SCID) syndromes to minimize the patients' risk of acquiring infections from other patients or staff. Other less stringent protective practices are used for other less compromised states (e.g., leukemias). Infection control experts should be consulted to ensure compliance with specific protocols of an institution.

Anesthetic equipment that will be used on these patients will require sterilization or special cleansing, depending upon the type of equipment. The attending anesthesiologist must follow approved sterile technique, which includes wearing a mask, sterile gown, and gloves, and practicing strict handwashing technique. The attending health care workers must understand each patient's underlying immune status and be aware of the specific institutional policies. The availability of an assistant greatly facilitates charting and handling any nonsterile materials. If any of the staff are suffering from a cold, cold sore, or any other infective process, they should not work in a room with a reverse isolation patient.

The operating room must be totally prepared before the patient is called. The patient should travel directly from the ward into the operating theater to decrease the risk of cross-contamination during the preoperative period. Since transport through construction areas has been associated with infection by *Aspergillus,* such areas should be avoided. Application and insertion of monitors requires the use of sterile monitors and technique. Venipuncture and fingersticks for blood samples should be done with care to avoid the formation of hematomas that can serve as a nidus of infection.

After the procedure, patients usually recover either in the operating theater or on the ward in their own rooms. Under certain circumstances, if facilities are appropriate, the patient may recover in the postanesthetic recovery area. If the patient requires admission to an intensive care unit after the operation, sufficient notice must be given to enable the intensive care staff to arrange appropriate accommodation.

PRIMARY IMMUNODEFICIENCY DISEASES

Syndromes of immunological dysfunction may involve solely B cells, solely T cells, or both types of cells. Generally, T-cell disorders present a more unfavorable prognosis than B-cell disorders; the prognosis of combined disorders is even worse.

In this section we review the primary and secondary disorders of immunological function, in the context of the relevant issues for anesthesiologists whenever possible. The classification and nomenclature of diseases used in this discussion conforms to that accepted by the World Health Organization.

B-LYMPHOCYTE (ANTIBODY) DEFICIENCIES

X-Linked Agammaglobulinemia

Panhypogammaglobulinemia is a term that describes a deficiency of the three major classes of immunoglobulins: IgG, IgM, and IgA. There are several forms of the disease: autosomal recessive, sporadic, and late onset. Congenital X-linked agammaglobulinemia (Bruton's disease), which is the best defined of these syndromes, is discussed here in detail.

Males affected with Bruton's disease demonstrate a lack of IgA and IgM in their serum and of IgA in their secretions. IgG levels are normal at birth because of placental transfer, but these levels decrease as maternal IgG is diluted and catabolized. Levels of IgG are low thereafter.

These patients lack B cells in their blood and plasma cells in their blood and tissues. Investigation of their bone marrow indicates the presence of B-lymphocyte precursors, implying that the defect involves their failure to differentiate into mature B cells. T-cell function, as assessed by in vitro techniques and by delayed hypersensitivity skin responses, is normal.

Patients appear normal until 4 months of age, during which time their underlying immune deficiency has been hidden by placentally transferred maternal IgG. After this period, recurrent infections are common. The respiratory tract is most often affected. Recurrent otitis media and sinusitis occur in the upper airway, which is also characterized by a decreased amount of pharyngeal lymphoid tissue, with small or absent tonsils and adenoids. Lower airway diseases include bouts of pneumonia and bronchitis that produce a chronic pulmonary disease with bronchiectasis, pulmonary fibrosis, and eventual cor pulmonale. Common infecting organisms include *Streptococcus pneumoniae, Haemophilus influenzae,* and staphylococci. With normal T-cell system function, most patients recover promptly from viral infections. There are exceptions to this, however, notably the ECHO virus, which affects 10 percent of patients. It can produce an acute fatal encephalitis or a prolonged deterioration with chronic viremia.

Other systems are less commonly involved. *Giardia lamblia* infection of the gastrointestinal tract may occur and produce severe diarrhea with lack of weight gain. Treatment with metronidazole is usually effective, but about 10 percent of all patients develop an enteropathy that resembles Crohn's disease. Significant amounts of protein may be lost into the gut from this enteropathy, the etiology of which is uncertain. It has been suggested that the enteropathy may occur as the result of a bacterial overgrowth, since antibiotic therapy seems helpful in some cases.

A dermatomyositis-like syndrome is also described in these patients. This is thought to be of viral etiology and is characterized by transient rashes that lack the normal distribution of dermatomyositis and by a firm, peripheral edema. Elevation of serum IgE occurs frequently with this condition and is associated with eczema, recurrent skin infections, and an increased incidence of allergic phenomena.

An autoimmune disease resembling rheumatoid arthritis is present in about 10 percent of these patients. This disease is distinguishable from true rheumatoid arthritis by a lack of rheumatoid factor. The presence of *Ureaplasma* species in effusions suggests an infectious etiology. Knees and ankles are most commonly affected. In some patients with gastrointestinal manifestations, the spine may be involved as well. The symptoms usually respond to IgG replacement.

Anesthetic Considerations. Patients with panhypogammaglobulinemia are at increased risk for bacterial infection, require strict sterile technique, and may require reverse isolation during their anesthetic management. Chronic pulmonary disease is common and may result in severe debilitation with cor pulmonale. The cardiopulmonary system requires careful evaluation and optimization of pulmonary and cardiac status before surgical therapy. The presence of otitis media and sinusitis may contraindicate use of nitrous oxide. Preoperative prophylactic antibiotic therapy is advised.

Autoimmune features of the disease may result in difficulty in positioning the patient for anesthesia and operation. Although temporomandibular joints and the cervical spine are rarely involved, their function should be evaluated. The serum protein and electrolyte levels of patients with spinal dysfunction should be assessed, since enteropathy frequently accompanies spinal involvement and results in significant loss of serum into the gut. Hypoproteinemia can affect drug disposition. Bowel infections should be treated appropriately.

If musculoskeletal and skin involvement occurs with a resultant dermatomyositis-type lesion, the use of succinylcholine may produce an acute increase in serum potassium.

Viral central nervous system (CNS) infections are not uncommon; any change in the level of consciousness should alert the physician to a possible CNS infection and elevation of intracranial pressure. Anesthetics in these circumstances should be chosen to avoid further increases in intracranial pressure.

Since these patients suffer from chronic infections, including those caused by *Staphylococcus, Streptococcus pneumoniae,* and *Haemophilus influenzae,* anesthetic equipment requires appropriate cleaning or disposal after use.

X-Linked Hypogammaglobulinemia with Growth Hormone Deficiency

A defect with B-cell dysfunction, X-linked hypogammaglobulinemia with growth hormone deficiency has currently been described in only one family: panhypogammaglobulinemia is present in three members, while the fourth demonstrates some B-cell function with normal IgM and IgA. Cellular immunity and T-cell function are normal. The growth hormone defect is manifested by short stature, retarded bone age, small phallus, and delayed onset of puberty. The origin of the basic defect is unknown, but it may result from a block in B-cell differentiation. The reason for the association of the growth hormone defect with the hypogammaglobulinemia is unclear.

AUTOSOMAL RECESSIVE AGAMMAGLOBULINEMIA

Autosomal recessive agammaglobulinemia has been applied to a form of agammaglobulinemia presenting in female patients that is indistinguishable from X-linked agammaglobulinemia. This disorder is believed to be the same as X-linked agammaglobulinemia, a defect of the precursor to B-cell differentiation.

IMMUNOGLOBULIN DEFICIENCY WITH INCREASED IGM (AND IGD)

The occurrence of immunoglobulin deficiency with increased IgM suggests an X-linked inheritance, but the etiology of this disorder is unclear. Affected boys have decreased levels of IgG, elevated levels of IgM, and in some instances elevated levels of IgD. The syndrome is characterized by severe pyogenic infections, autoimmune disorders, and lymphoproliferative disorders. T-cell function is normal. Acquired forms of the disease and its occurrence in females have been demonstrated. Treatment involves IgG replacement.

SELECTIVE IMMUNOGLOBULIN A DEFICIENCY

IgA is the main immunoglobulin that protects the respiratory system, gastrointestinal tract, and other secreting areas. A deficiency of IgA is the most common primary defect of specific immunity. Its incidence is reported to be 1 in 400 to 1 in 3000, depending upon the ethnic group. Its inheritance has been variously reported as autosomal dominant and autosomal recessive. It has also been reported as a rare complication of the congenital rubella syndrome. Its occurrence, however, is primarily sporadic.

IgA-deficient patients possess normal serum levels of IgG and IgM and have been demonstrated to possess IgA-bearing B cells in their blood. In vitro lymphocyte testing reveals that these cells are able to differentiate into plasma cells but fail to synthesize and release normal amounts of IgA. The etiology of this disorder is not entirely clear, but some patients have T cells that suppress the production of IgA but not IgG or IgM.

Most patients with IgA deficiency are healthy. Others usually have symptoms of infections, autoimmunity, allergy, or malignancy. Recurrent respiratory infections may occur in the form of sinusitis, bronchitis, or pneumonia. Diarrhea caused by *Giardia* or other infections may occur, and some patients become chronic salmonella carriers. Susceptibility to viral infections is less well-documented. Many patients have no excess infections, most likely because of the potential of IgG and IgM antibodies to protect mucosal surfaces or, possibly, because of associated changes in other immunoglobulins. Patients with associated low IgG_2 levels and normal total serum IgG tend to have an increased susceptibility to infections as compared with those patients with IgA deficiency but normal IgG_2 levels.

There is a high incidence of autoimmune syndromes in patients with IgA deficiency (Table 16–6). This association is apparently due to the absorption of dietary proteins through IgA-unprotected intestinal mucosa and results in a stimulus to antibody production against normally nonabsorbed antigen. Some of the antibodies can be involved in major transfusion reactions.

Low IgA levels are positively correlated with atopic disorders. This correlation is possibly due to the decreased presence of IgA, which normally would incorporate foreign antigens into antigen-antibody complexes. When this fails to occur, these foreign antigens are incorporated into IgE and IgG complexes.

IgA-deficient patients have an increased risk of malignancy. Primarily of gastrointestinal and lymphoreticular origin, malignancies occur at a rate of two to four times normal.

Anesthetic Considerations. As with panhy-

Table 16–6. AUTOIMMUNE SYNDROMES ASSOCIATED WITH SELECTIVE IGA DEFICIENCY

Autoimmune Syndromes	Percentage Affected
Rheumatoid arthritis	30
Systemic lupus erythematosus	15
Thyroiditis	10
Pernicious anemia	10
Dermatomyositis	<1
Sjögren's syndrome	<1
Addison's disease	<1
Pulmonary hemosiderosis	<1
Hemolytic anemia	<1
Thrombocytopenia	<1

pogammaglobulinemia, patients with selective IgA deficiency exhibit increased susceptibility to infections. Since the respiratory system and gastrointestinal tract are commonly involved, management should follow that described previously. Similarly, because of their high incidence of autoimmune syndromes (Table 16–6), all such patients should be carefully assessed. The presence of Addison's disease requires steroid supplementation. Dermatomyositis, which is more common in children than in adults, is a contraindication to the use of succinylcholine. Hemolytic anemia and thrombocytopenia occur and require assessment.

Since patients demonstrate a higher incidence of atopic disorders than the normal population, a complete history must be obtained and appropriate management undertaken. In many cases, owing to the underlying nature of the disease, the agents producing allergic reactions will be unknown to the patient or parents, so careful vigilance is necessary.

The presence of antibodies to IgG, IgM, and especially IgA, which may occur in as many as 40 percent of patients, can induce severe transfusion reactions. Matching blood can be extremely difficult and may require a longer period than usual to establish a safe cross-match. The emergency administration of type O, Rh-negative blood is dangerous for this reason.

Selective Deficiency of Secretory Component

Secretory component is a protein produced by epithelial cells in secretory surfaces. It is believed that the secretory component assists in the transport of IgA from its site of synthesis in plasma cells at the lamina propria and possibly prevents the IgA from proteolysis during its transport to the secretory surface. In at least two clinical situations the deficiency of the secretory component (as distinct from IgA deficiency states caused by the lack of IgA on secretory surfaces) may be important. The first of these is a state of chronic diarrhea, which may produce dehydration and electrolyte imbalance in poorly managed patients. The second is suggested by a study that demonstrated a deficiency of the secretory component in 62.5 percent of children with sudden infant death syndrome (SIDS).

Patients with a selective deficiency of secretory component lack IgA in their secretions, but their serum IgA levels are normal. Because of this lack of IgA on secretory surfaces, these patients also exhibit signs and symptoms of infection and atopic disorders similar to those seen in patients with selective IgA deficiency.

Anesthetic Considerations. The presence of chronic diarrhea necessitates evaluation of the state of hydration and serum electrolyte balance. Intravenous hydration is advisable during any period of fasting before operation. The higher incidence of SIDS in patients with this disorder requires careful postoperative monitoring for apnea in an intensive care unit or other area with personnel trained in managing apnea.

Since these patients are also subject to infections and atopic disorders, their management is similar to that discussed for those with IgA deficiency.

Selective Immunoglobulin M Deficiency

Any individual deficient in IgM has serum IgM levels lower than two standard deviations below the normal for age, not a complete absence of IgM. This deficiency is called selective when it is associated with otherwise normal serum immunoglobulin levels and with normal cell-mediated immunity. It occurs with a frequency of 1 in 1000, usually in males. Although in adults it is most commonly secondary to lymphoma, primary cases are well described. Current evidence suggests a genetic etiology, since studies have demonstrated that relatives, especially fathers, have decreased levels of serum IgM. Several hypotheses have attempted to explain the decreased serum IgM. It may represent T-cell suppression of the differentiation of B cells into mature plasma cells: B cells bearing IgM have been found in the blood of some patients. It may represent selective failure of IgM monomers to polymerize or a premature switch of IgM to IgG and IgA production.

Affected infants are extremely prone to septicemia, particularly with encapsulated organisms, such as pneumococci and meningococci. Each patient differs in susceptibility; this difference is due to a varying ability to produce IgM. These patients must undergo aggressive antibiotic therapy at the first sign of infection and possibly should receive continuous prophylactic antibiotics. Associated with this disorder is an increased frequency of Whipple's disease, regional enteritis, and lymphoid nodular hyperplasia.

Anesthetic Considerations. Because patients with this disorder are extremely susceptible to infection and septicemia is not uncommon, their anesthetic management requires very careful sterile technique, and they may require reverse isolation. Prophylactic antibiotic therapy is advisable and should be commenced preoperatively. Associated regional enteritis may result in hemoglobin and protein loss and serum electrolyte imbalance. These conditions need to be assessed and managed.

Immunoglobulin G Deficiencies

Although a complete lack of all IgG components (IgG_1, IgG_2, IgG_3, and IgG_4) is not seen, selective subgroup deficiencies do occur in patients with IgG deficiencies. In normal individuals, IgG_1 predominates, and IgG_4 levels may be low enough to be undetected. In IgG-subgroup deficiency, total serum IgG is normal, but subgroup deficiencies can be detected as abnormalities of electrophoretic mobility.

Although selective deficiencies of a particular subclass are not associated with particular clinical syndromes, some antibodies are preferentially made in a particular subclass (see Table 16–2). Clinically, the patients manifest an increased susceptibility to infections similar to that characteristic of patients with panhypogammaglobulinemia.

Anesthetic Considerations. Sterile techniques and reverse isolation are advised during perioperative management, together with the administration of prophylactic antibiotics.

Transient Hypogammaglobulinemia of Infancy

By definition, transient hypogammaglobulinemia of infancy is a transient condition that resolves in the first to second year of life. Although common, occurring in 18 percent of patients with a primary immunodeficiency, it is rare as a clinical problem and is found in less than 0.01 percent of the patients with immune disorders studied.

The disorder is characterized by a lower than normal serum IgG level. IgM and IgA levels are frequently normal. On antigenic stimulation, good antibody responses are usually demonstrated but T-cell function is depressed, as shown by a deficient response of the B cell to T-cell–dependent stimulation. It is believed that the syndrome may represent delayed maturation of the normal humoral response. Clinically, the patients suffer recurrent infections that vary in frequency or severity with the individual patient.

There are two groups of patients with transient hypogammaglobulinemia, those with and those without immunodeficient relatives.

Since patients recover spontaneously in the first to second year of life, treatment with immunoglobulins is usually reserved for those demonstrating severe recurrent infections.

MEDICAL MANAGEMENT OF ANTIBODY DEFICIENCY SYNDROMES

Acute bacterial infections require antibiotic therapy; this treatment must be aggressive in IgM-deficient patients because of their tendency to develop septicemia. Prophylaxis may consist of continuous treatment with an antibiotic such as cotrimoxazole, which has been advocated for patients with IgM-deficient states.

Prophylaxis, however, depends primarily upon IgG replacement by intramuscular injection of immune serum globulin (ISG), which contains 150 mg of IgG per ml. ISG is administered with an initial loading dose of 1.4 ml/kg, followed every 4 weeks by 0.7 ml/kg. The aim of this treatment is to achieve a serum level of 300 mg/dl.

Although ISG can be administered intravenously, it then requires additional processing to become aggregate-free. The presence of such aggregates may activate complement, causing anaphylaxis by the production of vasoactive kinins. A variety of products that process ISG by physical and chemical means are now available. These products permit the administration of large amounts of immunoglobulin that bring IgG levels in the blood to nearly normal levels not obtainable with intramuscular injections. The recommended dose is 100 mg/kg per month, which provides an increase of about 200 mg/dl in the serum IgG level after equilibration. The IgG level decreases progressively until the next injection, but it is possible to maintain a normal level even at the nadir by increasing the dose.

An alternative to the use of ISG is the use of plasma. Plasma contains 10 mg/ml of IgG and provides protection at a dose of 1.5 ml/kg every 21 days. In addition, plasma provides IgA and IgM, which are not provided by ISG. For patients with associated malabsorption syndromes, plasma has the advantage of providing a range of proteins. The main disadvantage of plasma is the risk of serum hepatitis. This risk can be minimized by restricting the number of donors and by careful screening of the plasma.

Approximately 20 percent of patients receiving intramuscular ISG develop reactions at some stage. Complement activation from aggregates in the injectate, which produce vasoactive kinins, is considered the most likely cause. These reactions vary in severity from mild limb and back pain to anaphylaxis. They usually occur within 30 minutes of administration. Mild reactions resolve spontaneously within 3 to 4 hours and require no treatment.

It is important to realize that the optimal dose and optimal serum levels of ISG have yet to be determined. Likewise, there is no information available about the efficacy of ISG in the prevention of long-term complications of immunoglobulin deficiency, such as chronic sinopulmonary disease.

T-LYMPHOCYTE (CELL-MEDIATED) DEFICIENCIES

B-cell production of antibodies is normal in few diseases involving deficiency of cell-mediated immunity because of the required interaction of T-helper cells with B cells for most antibody responses in humans. Because of this association, T-cell compromise results in deficient antibody production by B cells and, consequently, clinical features of combined T-cell and B-cell disease.

Thymic Hypoplasia (DiGeorge Syndrome)

Embryologically, the thymus and the parathyroids are derived from the third and fourth pharyngeal pouches. DiGeorge syndrome is characterized by the failure of the third and fourth pouches to develop normally, with subsequent failure of the development of the thymus and parathyroids. To confirm the diagnosis, T-cell dysfunction and parathyroid-hormone deficiency must be demonstrated. Other features that are variably present include abnormalities of the heart and great vessels and micrognathia, low-set ears, and short philtrum.

Hypoplastic parathyroid glands result in low parathormone levels and hypocalcemia. The spectrum of clinical expression of the immunological problem ranges from minimal thymic involvement to B-cell deficiency. Patients are at increased risk for infections by *Candida, Pneumocystis,* and numerous other organisms that may produce chronic diarrhea.

DiGeorge syndrome may be diagnosed as early as the first week of life, when tetany or evidence of cardiac failure may become apparent. If the symptoms are mild, diagnosis may not be made until cardiac evaluation is carried out or until a surgical procedure, when the absence of a thymus is apparent.

Treatment of the disorder depends upon its severity. In those with minimal thymic hypoplasia, spontaneous acquisition of normal T-cell function is possible. Thymic transplantation and transplantation of thymus cells in a millipore chamber also have been effective and suggest the involvement of the soluble factors in normal T-cell function. Hypocalcemia may respond to enteral calcium supplementation with vitamin D. Parathyroid hormone injections may be necessary.

Anesthetic Considerations. Patients with thymic hypoplasia present anesthetic challenges. The presence of decreased serum ionized calcium has several implications. Management of such patients requires ready access to determinations of serum calcium and arterial blood gas levels. The low initial serum ionized calcium and the patients' reduced ability to respond to further decreases in serum ionized calcium (because of parathyroid deficiency) make these patients susceptible to symptomatic hypocalcemia. This may be secondary to the presence of citrate in blood transfusions or alkalosis induced by hyperventilation. Hypocalcemia can produce tetanic seizures, cardiac depression, and prolongation of nondepolarizing neuromuscular block. Treatment of low calcium levels requires the administration of intravenous calcium. Flashburg and colleagues reported low normal serum ionized calcium levels throughout the anesthetic course of management of such a patient, but they were able to manage the problem by monitoring the acid-base balance and level of serum ionized calcium.

Since cardiovascular anomalies may involve both the heart and the great vessels, a patient's cardiac status needs to be assessed carefully. Common abnormalities include transposition of the great vessels, interrupted aortic arch, truncus arteriosus, tetralogy of Fallot, and anomalous pulmonary venous drainage. Cardiac anomalies may be manifested as cardiac failure, which may be accentuated in the presence of low serum ionized calcium levels.

Upper airway problems may occur because of the small jaw, and in the presence of a vascular ring anomaly, which is not uncommon in this syndrome, tracheomalacia may become apparent after the repair of the vascular ring.

Although infections in patients with intact immunoglobulins are usually viral or fungal, severe forms of the syndrome may present with associated B-cell dysfunction. In these cases, susceptibility to bacterial infections may be a problem. Such patients are subject to chronic interstitial pneumonitis; consequently, their pulmonary status requires careful assessment. It may not be possible to eradicate pulmonary infections fully before surgery.

To prevent infection in these patients, anesthesiologists must use sterile technique, particularly when establishing intravenous access and invasive monitoring, to minimize the risk of introducing a source of infection. The need for invasive monitoring should be carefully considered; all lines should be removed as soon as they are no longer necessary. Perioperative prophylactic antibiotic therapy is advisable. Blood for transfusion should be irradiated to prevent graft-versus-host disease. The use of reverse isolation procedures may be indicated for patients with severe forms of the syndrome.

Chronic Mucocutaneous Candidiasis

Chronic mucocutaneous candidiasis comprises a group of diseases, all of which involve chronic infection of the skin and mucosa with *Candida albicans.* Various subdivisions of this group of diseases are based upon the presence or absence of endocrinopathy and laboratory abnormalities.

Endocrine abnormalities, which may manifest at any time, include hypothyroidism, hypoadrenalism, hypoparathyroidism, hypopituitarism, and pernicious anemia. The presence of autoantibodies in some patients implies a possible autoimmune mechanism to the endocrine disorders.

Patients may demonstrate normal serum immunoglobulins or selective IgA deficiency. Anticandidal antibodies are usually high. T-cell numbers and function are usually normal except for a decreased reactivity to *Candida.*

Clinical Features. Onset occurs in infancy, with either endocrine abnormalities or the appearance of candidal lesions as the first symptom. The mouth, lips, scalp, eyelashes, vagina, and nails are the most common sites of involvement; systemic spread of *Candida* is very rare.

Treatment. The iron metabolism of patients with chronic mucocutaneous candidiasis is abnormal. The resultant anemia improves after treatment with oral or intravenous iron. Most patients require intravenous antifungal agents: amphotericin and ketoconazole are extremely effective. Ketoconazole, which is less toxic than amphotericin, is currently replacing it as the most commonly used therapeutic agent. Recurrences of the condition are frequent when the treatment is discontinued. Such relapses frequently can be treated with topical ketoconazole or clotrimazole. Transfer factor, leukocyte infusions, and thymosin all have been used in treatment with variable success.

All patients must be investigated for endocrinopathies and appropriate therapy initiated. Cases of sudden death during minor infections have been reported. These are likely due to an adrenal crisis.

Anesthetic Considerations. Although these patients suffer from a very mild immunodeficiency affecting B cells and T cells, and infections with organisms other than *Candida* are rare, anesthesiologists should use sterile technique when handling these patients. Since a selective IgA deficiency may be present, these patients are at risk for transfusion reactions if blood products containing IgA are given. Because of this, full cross-matching of blood is required and may be difficult.

Patients must be carefully assessed for the presence of endocrinopathies and treated appropriately. Since endocrinopathies can become manifest at any time, previously normal assessments must be discounted and further studies performed.

Several effects of the amphotericin many of these patients may have received for treatment of the candidiasis may complicate their perioperative management. Acute administration may produce anaphylaxis. Long-term treatment can produce thrombocytopenia and leukopenia, which are not usually present in patients with chronic mucocutaneous candidiasis. A normochromic normocytic anemia may occur because of a decrease in erythropoietin activity. Amphotericin may produce hepatic toxicity; however, more recent work has raised questions about whether this is directly related to therapy with this drug. Amphotericin produces a decrease in renal function in 80 percent of patients. Function usually returns to normal upon completion of therapy, but some individuals who have received a complete course have residual glomerular dysfunction. In those currently undergoing treatment, mild renal tubular acidosis and hypokalemia are frequently present, and supplemental potassium may be required to correct serum potassium levels before anesthesia. Hypomagnesemia is also observed and may require correction.

Purine Nucleoside Phosphorylase Deficiency

Purine nucleoside phosphorylase (PNP) deficiency is a rare enzyme defect. This deficiency results in the intracellular accumulation of deoxyguanosine triphosphate, which inhibits ribonucleotide reductase, which in turn limits cell division. The urine and blood of patients with PNP contain increased amounts of inosine, guanosine, deoxyguanosine, and guanosine triphosphate.

A deficiency in PNP causes a much more severe defect in T-cell function than in B-cell function because T cells divide more rapidly. Levels of immunoglobulins and the percentage of B cells are usually normal. As the disease increases in severity, B cells become affected because of a decrease in normal B-cell to T-cell interactions, and immunoglobulin function may become impaired.

This immunodeficiency may not be demonstrated at birth. Neonates and infants may have normal lymphocyte counts and in vitro function yet become symptomatic with decreasing T-cell function before 18 months of age. Symptoms occur between 7 months and 7 years of age. Early problems include recurrent upper respiratory infections and a Coombs'-positive hemolytic anemia, suggesting the beginning of impaired regulation of antibody responses. Later, if vaccinia or varicella infections occur, they may be fatal. Graft-versus-host disease may occur if nonirradiated blood is administered.

Laboratory confirmatory findings should demonstrate a deficiency of PNP in red cell lysates; mutant forms of the enzyme may be present. Spot or 24-hour urine studies that demonstrate purine excretion also help confirm the diagnosis.

The response to therapy is uncertain. Irradiated red cell infusions, injections of thymus extracts, and uridine or deoxycytidine treatments have been tried with variable success.

Anesthetic Considerations. The problems and precautions necessary in the anesthetic management of patients with immunodeficiency have been discussed previously. If low hemoglobin levels because of an autoimmune hemolytic process necessitate transfusions, the blood should be irradiated to kill donor lymphocytes; otherwise graft-versus-host disease may result. Death caused by transfusion with nonirradiated blood has been reported in a patient with PNP deficiency.

COMBINED B- AND T-LYMPHOCYTE DEFICIENCIES

Severe Combined Immunodeficiency Syndrome (SCIDS)

Severe combined immunodeficiency syndrome, commonly referred to as SCIDS, is inherited as an autosomal recessive or X-linked recessive trait; consequently most of the patients (75 percent) are male. The cause appears to be a primary T-cell abnormality that secondarily produces a failure of normal embryogenesis of the thymic epithelium. Infants become ill during the first few months of life, exhibiting a marked failure to thrive. Moniliasis of the oropharynx, larynx, and skin can be extensive, but systemic candidiasis is rare. Pneumonitis is frequent, usually interstitial, and caused by *Pneumocystis carinii.* These two features, plus intractable diarrhea, form the characteristic triad of findings in this disease.

Patients are extremely vulnerable to overwhelming viral infections such as varicella, herpes, and cytomegalovirus, which are fatal if contracted by an untreated patient. Smallpox vaccination is contraindicated. Many infants in the first few days of life have a morbilliform rash caused by an abortive graft-versus-host reaction (see page 586) to maternally transferred lymphocytes. A profound lymphopenia is common (less than 1000 lymphocytes per cubic millimeter). Other hematological abnormalities include thrombocytosis and anemia. Monocytosis and eosinophilia may occur in response to overwhelming infection, such as occurs with *Pneumocystis* pneumonia. The disorder is usually fatal in the first few years of life.

Current treatment consists of transplants of fetal liver cells, or of implants of fetal thymus or thymic epithelium. Most successful has been bone marrow transplantation. This originally required donations of bone marrow from HLA-identical siblings, but the procedure is now possible with parental haploidentical marrow. Successful transplantation depends upon the removal of the T cells from the donated marrow to prevent the recipient from developing graft-versus-host disease caused by the T cells. Thus, the therapeutic possibilities for bone marrow transplantation have been extended.

Anesthetic Considerations. Because patients are extremely vulnerable to infection and are frequently chronically infected, their pulmonary and nutritional status must be assessed. These patients require strict sterile technique and may require reverse isolation procedures. Sites for intravenous access and access sites for other invasive monitors should be very carefully prepared with antiseptic solutions. Postoperatively, monitoring lines and intravenous lines should be discontinued as early as possible to decrease the risk of infection.

The use of blood products adds the risk of graft-versus-host disease. Since lymphocytes in blood from blood banks are viable for 3 weeks, blood transfused into such patients should be irradiated before transfusion to kill the lymphocytes. If the patient has anemia, irradiated blood may be required preoperatively.

Serum proteins and electrolytes must be checked if the patient has diarrhea. Intravenous therapy may be necessary to prevent dehydration during fasting before operation.

Severe Combined Immunodeficiency with Adenosine Deaminase Deficiency

Severe combined immunodeficiency with adenosine deaminase deficiency, a variant of severe combined immunodeficiency, results from a deficiency of the enzyme adenosine deaminase. This disorder is inherited in an autosomal recessive pattern. Adenosine deaminase converts adenosine and deoxyadenosine to inosine and deoxyinosine, thus functioning as a purine-salvage pathway enzyme. It is present in most cells, including erythrocytes and lymphocytes. In its absence, ATP, cyclic AMP, and their deoxy analogues increase to toxic levels. This results in inhibition of ribonucleotide reductase, which impairs reduction of other nucleoside diphosphates and causes inhibition of DNA synthesis. No other organ system is affected by this deficiency. The reason for this specificity is unclear.

The features of this disorder are similar to those of severe combined immunodeficiency, except that at birth lymphocyte function is usually normal. After birth, a gradual deterioration of lymphocyte function occurs. Definitive diagnosis is by means of enzyme-level determination in erythrocytes. Without treatment most patients die by 2 years of age.

The disease is most satisfactorily treated with bone marrow transplantation. In the absence of a suitable bone marrow donor, transfusions of frozen irradiated red blood cells have been used as a source of adenosine deaminase. These transfusions are thought to supply a level of enzymes sufficient to protect the lymphocytes from the accumulation of the toxic products that inhibit DNA. A recent development is the application of gene therapy to correct this disease.

Combined Immunodeficiency with Predominant T-Cell Defect

First described in 1964, combined immunodeficiency with predominant T-cell defect, also known as Nezelof's syndrome, consists of a predominant T-cell defect. B-cell function is also abnormal: B cells produce normal serum concentrations of immunoglobulins, but they function abnormally. This disorder has been observed in children with congenital viral infections (for example, cytomegalovirus). It is not as rapidly fatal as severe combined immunodeficiency, but affected persons have a poor long-term prognosis.

Wiskott-Aldrich Syndrome

Wiskott-Aldrich syndrome is an X-linked recessive disorder with an incidence of 4 per 1 million live births. It is characterized by thrombocytopenia, eczema, and recurrent infections. Immunodeficiency is progressive: abnormal immunological findings become increasingly common with increasing age. Serum IgG is usually normal, IgM reduced, and IgA and IgE elevated. Normal antibody responses with IgG and IgA are usually present, whereas those with IgM have an impaired ability to form antibodies active against bacterial polysaccharides. With time, increases in IgA and decreases in IgM occur, and abnormalities of the lymphoid tissues develop.

Deficiencies of cell-mediated immunity are variable, depending upon the age of the patient. Mild T-cell dysfunction is apparent but is less than that ascribed to other T-cell–deficient states. With increasing age, patients become anergic and are slow to reject foreign skin grafts.

Thrombocytopenia is present (less than 50,000/μl); the platelets are small and deficient in adenosine diphosphate (ADP), so they fail to aggregate normally. The abnormalities of platelet size are secondary features; they disappear after splenectomy.

Clinically, patients with Wiskott-Aldrich syndrome demonstrate early onset eczema with an unusual atopic distribution. Thrombocytopenia may lead to bloody diarrhea and intracranial hemorrhage. The patients are susceptible to a wide range of infections, including otitis media and externa, pneumonitis, and septicemia. They are particularly susceptible to infections by herpes simplex, as well as other opportunistic organisms. Twenty percent experience renal problems, including hematuria, proteinuria, increased levels of blood urea nitrogen, and decreased creatinine clearance.

Few patients survive into their teens. Infection is responsible for 60 percent of deaths, bleeding for 27 percent, and malignancy for 5 percent.

Medical Management. Bone marrow transplantation has been successful in the treatment of patients with Wiskott-Aldrich syndrome, but, unlike treatment for patients with combined immunodeficiency diseases, it is necessary to destroy the recipient's own stem-cell population. This requires the use of large doses of cyclophosphamide or high-level irradiation before transplantation, which increases the mortality and morbidity of the procedures.

Those patients without tissue-type-matched siblings undergo therapy with intravenous transfer factor or thymosin. Although increased anergic response, increased platelet counts, and decreased bleeding tendencies have provided symptomatic improvement, survival does not appear to be prolonged.

Splenectomy has been successful in decreasing the risk of bleeding, particularly intracranial hemorrhage. This improvement is due in part to an increase in platelet numbers and in part to improved function. However, splenectomy also increases susceptibility to infection (particularly pneumoccocal). This increased susceptibility in patients with an underlying immunodeficiency is an indication for long-term prophylactic antibiotic therapy.

Antiviral agents may be of value in the treatment of associated herpes simplex or varicella infections. Intravenous gammaglobulin therapy may successfully inhibit both viral and bacterial infections.

Antibiotics should be given promptly with each infection to prevent complications and to prevent overwhelming sepsis with *Streptococcus pneumoniae, Haemophilus influenzae,* and certain gram-negative organisms. Some patients may require continuous antibiotics.

Systemic steroids should be avoided unless needed to control autoimmune hemolytic anemia. Local steroids are often necessary to control severe eczema.

Anesthetic Considerations. To minimize the risk of infection because patients present with a combined immunodeficiency picture, antibiotic prophylaxis is necessary preoperatively, as is the use of sterile technique.

Thrombocytopenia with platelet counts of less than 50,000/μl, is frequently present, and this level is insufficient for even minor surgical procedures, particularly when combined with failure of proper platelet aggregation. These patients may be anemic as well as thrombocytopenic and therefore may require transfusions of red blood cells and platelets before operation. Since these patients demonstrate dysfunction of cell-mediated immunity, blood products should be irradiated before transfusion to prevent graft-versus-host disease.

The presence of bloody diarrhea, as well as serving as a focus for blood loss, may result in electrolyte imbalance, which should be assessed and corrected before operation. Twenty percent of patients demonstrate decreased renal function, with an elevated level of blood urea nitrogen and decreased creatinine clearance. Consequently, renal function, should be adequately evaluated preoperatively.

The patients suffer from chronic and recurrent pulmonary infections because of their immunodeficient status; therefore their pulmonary status should be optimized. The presence of chest infections may be an indication that an operation should be delayed, especially when improvement with therapy is expected and the operation is not urgent.

ATAXIA-TELANGIECTASIA SYNDROME

Ataxia-telangiectasia syndrome is an autosomal recessive disorder with an incidence of 2 to 3 per 100,000 live births. This disorder is characterized by a progressive ataxia, chronic sinopulmonary disease, ocular and cutaneous telangiectasia, endocrine abnormalities, and variable B-cell and T-cell deficiencies. An embryological fault producing abnormalities in mesodermal-endodermal interactions causing telangiectasia, lymphoid abnormalities, and neurological disease underlies the disorder.

The ataxia is a result of progressive neuronal degeneration in the cerebellar cortex. Purkinje's cells, granular cells, and the neurons of the dentate and olivary nuclei are particularly affected. Anterior horn cell degeneration and posterior column demyelination characterize spinal cord involvement. Schwann's cells of the peripheral nerves degenerate, and this, in conjunction with spinal cord involvement, produces a progressive muscle weakness.

The telangiectases are venous rather than arterial, and bleeding is rarely a significant problem. The bulbar conjunctivae, the bridge of the nose, the ears, and the shoulders are the areas primarily affected. Other dermatological changes include progeric changes with premature graying of hair, skin atrophy, pigmentary changes with vitiligo or café au lait spots, multiple senile keratoses, and basal cell carcinoma.

Endocrine abnormalities, such as ovarian hypoplasia, elevated gonadotropins, and cytoplasmic vacuoles in the anterior pituitary, also occur. Biochemically, ataxia-telangiectasia cells have increased susceptibility to breakage upon exposure to X-radiation or ultraviolet light. There appears to be a defect of DNA excision repair as well, but the cause of this failure of repair has not yet been established.

The immunological defect is a variable and progressive B-cell and T-cell defect. The B-cell defect consists of low or absent serum IgE and IgA. IgG is usually normal, and IgM levels are elevated. T-cell defects result in lymphopenia. Cell-mediated immunity is often normal in younger children, but by 12 years of age there is a decrease in delayed hypersensitivity, which continues to worsen with time.

Clinical Features. Cerebellar ataxia is usually the presenting symptom of ataxia-telangiectasia syndrome, which becomes apparent as the child begins to walk. Later there is progressive muscle weakness, dysarthria, nystagmus, intention tremor, increased drooling, and choreoathetosis. Intellectual development is normal until the age of 9 years, after which development ceases. Patients with this syndrome generally have placid and agreeable temperaments.

Recurrent infections are common, affecting particularly the respiratory tract. Recurrent sinopulmonary infection leading to bronchiectasis and pneumonia is the most common cause of death.

Malignancies are the second leading cause of death in these patients and most commonly affect the lymphoreticular system.

Medical Treatment. Treatment of this disorder is at present unsatisfactory. Some improvement in lymphocyte function has been demonstrated after thymus grafting or thymosin treatment, but the neurological course of the disease has remained unaffected.

Anesthetic Considerations. Patients present a variable B-cell and T-cell defect. Since they are immunodepressed as a result, preoperative prophylactic antibiotic therapy and sterile technique to prevent infection are necessary. Chronic and recurrent pulmonary infections are common, so the pulmonary status should be optimized before surgery. Similarly, hemoglobin and hematocrit levels should be assessed.

The problem of excessive drooling in these patients may be controlled with an anticholinergic premedicant.

Although usually emotionally agreeable and cooperative, these patients will be apprehensive about needles: despite their older chronological age, their mental age tends to plateau at 9 years of age.

Succinylcholine should be avoided, since these patients suffer from progressive muscle weakness caused by peripheral nerve and anterior horn cell degeneration, and they are subject to marked elevations in serum potassium when given depolarizing muscle relaxants.

SECONDARY IMMUNODEFICIENCY SYNDROMES

ACQUIRED IMMUNODEFICIENCY SYNDROME

Acquired immunodeficiency syndrome (AIDS) was first described in children in 1982. Since that time its incidence has been increasing steadily. It is estimated that there were over 4000 pediatric cases in the United States in 1993. Several thousand more children will be infected with the human immunodeficiency virus (HIV) but will not be classified as having AIDS because they do not fully meet the Centers for Disease Control (CDC) criteria (Tables 16–7 and 16–8) for classification. As the numbers of children with AIDS increase, increasing numbers of children with this disease can be expected for surgical therapy for disease-related and -unrelated conditions. Since the modes of transmission, as well as the clinical spectrum of the disease, differ between the adult and pediatric population (Table 16–9), pediatric AIDS is defined as occurring in children under 13 years of age. The form of AIDS that children over age 13 years have is so strikingly similar to that of adults that

Table 16–7. PEDIATRIC AIDS CLASSIFICATION: CENTERS FOR DISEASE CONTROL CRITERIA

Class	Description
P-O	Indeterminate infection (not tested or noninterpretable test results: includes infants born to HIV-positive mothers)
P-1	Asymptomatic infection A Normal immune function B Abnormal immune function C Immune function not tested
P-2	Symptomatic infection A Nonspecific findings (ARC) B Progressive encephalopathy C Lymphoid interstitial pneumonitis D Secondary infectious diseases D–1 Opportunistic infections (AIDS) D–2 Recurrent bacterial infections D–3 Recalcitrant infections, specifically *Candida* and herpes E Secondary malignancy E–1 Those listed in CDC definition of AIDS E–2 Others F Other diseases possibly due to HIV infection (hepatitis, cardiopathy, nephropathy, anemia, thrombocytopenia, dermatologic disease)

Modified from CDC: Classification system for human immunodeficiency virus (HIV) infection in children under 13 years of age. MMWR *36*:225, 1987.

Table 16–8. CDC DEFINITION OF HIV INFECTION IN CHILDREN LESS THAN 13 YEARS OF AGE

1. Children <15 months of age with perinatal infection have *one* of the following:
   a. HIV in blood or tissue confirmed by culture or other laboratory detection method
   b. Symptoms meeting CDC case definition for AIDS
   c. Antibody to HIV (repeatedly reactive screening test plus positive confirmatory test result) and evidence of both cellular and humoral immunodeficiency (↑ immunoglobulin levels, ↓ absolute CD4 T-cell count, absolute lymphopenia, ↓ CD4-to-CD8 T-cell ratio) *and* symptoms (class P2, Table 16–9)
2. Older perinatally infected children or children who acquired infection through another mode of transmission have *one* of the following:
   a. HIV in blood or tissues confirmed by culture or other laboratory detection method
   b. Antibody to HIV (repeatedly reactive screening test plus positive confirmatory test result)
   c. Symptoms meeting CDC case definition for AIDS

Modified from CDC: Classification system for human immunodeficiency virus (HIV) infection in children under 13 years of age. MMWR *36*:225, 1987.

these children are included in the adult statistics. This section deals primarily with pediatric AIDS.

The etiological agent of AIDS is a T-lymphotropic retrovirus. Infection occurs in specific CD4 receptor-positive T cells (helper cells). The CD8 (suppressor) T cells are not affected. It appears that the monocyte or macrophage is the host cell that is initially infected with HIV and subsequently serves as the vehicle of viral replication and persistent infection. As the virus replicates, T lymphocytes are damaged or destroyed, resulting in a cell-mediated immunity. HIV infection of previously immunocompetent cells may result in immunodeficiency by several mechanisms. Direct cell damage and subsequent death lead to T-cell depletion. Cytotoxic but uninfected T cells may destroy infected cells and result in a reduced number of CD4 T cells and therefore a decrease in the CD4-to-CD8 T-cell ratio. Defects in macrophages, monocytes, neutrophils, and complement pathways all have been described. Abnormal immunological findings in the HIV-infected child are presented in Table 16–10. At least two distinct variants of HIV have been identified: HIV-1 and HIV-2. Each variant is capable of producing AIDS. HIV-1 is the most common variant in Africa, Europe, and North and South America, but both variants have been identified in the blood supply in North America.

Eighty percent of HIV-infected children become infected by perinatal exposure to maternal HIV, most likely transplacental in origin: they are born of mothers either who have frank AIDS or who belong to a high-risk group (prostitutes, drug abusers, and sexual consorts of drug abusers). Other sources of infection include blood transfusions (13 percent) and blood products for coagulation disturbances (5 percent).

Serological Testing and Limitations in Diagnosis. There are two methods of detection of HIV infection. The first method consists of the direct determination of the presence of virus particles or antigen in blood or tissues by various labor-intensive laboratory procedures. These techniques are impractical in the clinical setting, and negative results are hard to interpret. The enzyme-linked immunosorbent assay (ELISA),

Table 16–9. CLINICAL MANIFESTATIONS OF CHILDREN WITH AIDS

Features More Common in Children Than in Adults
Failure to thrive
Chronic interstitial pneumonitis
Recurrent bacterial infections
Parotitis
Dysmorphic syndrome
Features Common to Both Children and Adults
Neurological abnormalities
Opportunistic infections
Hepatosplenomegaly
Diffuse adenopathy
Chronic or recurrent diarrhea
Chronic or recurrent fevers
Chronic eczematoid rash
Chronic mucocutaneous candidiasis
Clubbing of digits
Progressive renal disease
Cardiomyopathy
Hepatitis
Features More Commonly Described in Adults
Neoplasms (including Kaposi's sarcoma and lymphomas)

From Prober CG, Gershon AA: Medical management of newborns and infants born to seropositive mothers. *In* Pizzo PA, Wilfert CM (eds): Pediatric AIDS: The Challenge of HIV Infection in Infants, Children, and Adolescents. Baltimore, Williams & Wilkins, 1991. © 1991, the Williams & Wilkins Co., Baltimore.

Table 16–10. LABORATORY ABNORMALITIES IN SYMPTOMATIC PEDIATRIC HIV-INFECTED PATIENTS

Hypergammaglobulinemia
Hypogammaglobulinemia*
Total lymphopenia
CD4 lymphopenia
Reversed CD4:CD8 T-cell ratio (<1.0)†
Neutropenia
Anemia

*Rare in comparison with hypergammaglobulinemia.
†Late manifestation.

an indirect method of serological testing for the antibody to HIV, is the most commonly used method because of its low cost, simplicity, and suitability for large scale use. The ELISA measures antibodies to all viral proteins. When its results are repeatedly positive, they must be confirmed by the more specific Western blot technique or radioimmunoprecipitation assay, which detects antibodies against specific HIV-associated antigens. A new assay to detect HIV proviral DNA sequences in infected lymphocytes (polymerase chain reaction) shows promise as a means of diagnosing HIV infection early in infancy. The ELISA screening for HIV-1, however, does not always reveal the presence of antibodies to HIV-2.

There are problems associated with the diagnosis of HIV in children less than 15 months of age. During pregnancy there is passive transplacental transmission of the HIV maternal antibody; therefore all children born to an HIV-positive mother will test positive for the first 6 to 15 months of life. But only 30 to 40 percent of children of HIV-positive mothers are truly infected with HIV and will begin to make their own antibodies and develop AIDS. Therefore, the presence of antibody to HIV is not a reliable indicator of infection in children less than 15 months of age (see Table 16–8), but if the antibody persists beyond 15 months, the child must be presumed to be infected. The CDC's initial criteria for the diagnosis of AIDS in children less than 15 months of age was restrictive because of concern about excluding children with congenital immunodeficiency. More recently, the CDC criteria have been revised. The current CDC criteria (see Table 16–7) for a child with AIDS ranges from children with asymptomatic infections to those with severe life-threatening symptoms. In all cases there must be some evidence of altered immune function; being infected with HIV alone is insufficient for a diagnosis of AIDS.

Clinical Spectrum of the Disease. Of the children born of HIV-positive mothers who eventually develop AIDS, 20 percent develop symptoms during the first year of life. The remainder develop AIDS at a constant rate of 8 percent per year; children born with exposure to HIV infection develop AIDS at a median age of 4.8 years. There appear to be two distinct groups of children with AIDS: those who develop the disease early at a median of 4.1 months and those with a longer incubation who develop the disease at a mean of 6.1 years. The reasons for these differences are not clear.

Several clinical profiles seen in children with AIDS are summarized below.

Pulmonary Syndromes. Pulmonary disease is the leading cause of morbidity and mortality in children with HIV infection and is often the first manifestation of HIV infection. *Pneumocystis carinii,* cytomegalovirus, and *Mycobacterium avium-intracellulare* are the common opportunistic infections. *Streptococcus pneumoniae, Haemophilus influenzae,* and respiratory syncytial virus represent the more typical pediatric bacterial and viral infections common to, and more severe in, this group of patients.

Pneumocystis carinii infection in HIV-infected children follows a much more virulent course with a poorer prognosis than in HIV-infected adults. In HIV-infected children, the presence of a normal lymphocyte count does not protect them from this organism, as it does in HIV-infected adults.

Another cause of chronic interstitial disease with progressive alveolar-capillary block has been termed *lymphoid interstitial pneumonitis* or *pulmonary lymphoid hyperplasia.* This entity is uncommon in adults. It consists of interstitial and peribronchiolar infiltration with lymphocytes and plasma cells. It is slowly progressive: the patient develops dyspnea, bronchospasm, and chronic hypoxia.

Infectious pneumonias can be treated with specific antibiotics. Lymphoid interstitial pneumonitis may respond to treatment with steroids and bronchodilators.

Cardiac Syndromes. Cardiac findings can be present in children with asymptomatic HIV infection and those with advanced AIDS symptoms. Therefore, all HIV-infected children should have a preanesthetic cardiological evaluation. The HIV directly affects cardiac myocytes. Cardiac abnormalities can include left and right ventricular dysfunction, pericardial effusions, and dysrhythmias. Cardiac function variably demonstrates increased or depressed contractility. An autonomic neuropathy producing exaggerated heart rate and blood pressure responses to certain medications has also been described.

Renal Syndromes. Like the HIV-infected adult patient, 5 to 10 percent of HIV-infected children develop nephrotic signs of proteinuria, hypoalbuminemia, and edema. Microscopic analysis demonstrates focal glomerulosclerosis or mesangial hyperplasia. In some children these changes may progress to produce severe renal failure.

Neurological Syndromes. Neurological involvement is common and appears to be due to a direct infection of the brain by HIV across the blood-brain barrier. Electron microscopy has

Table 16–11. INDICATIONS FOR AND EFFECTS OF MEDICATIONS GIVEN TO HIV-INFECTED CHILDREN

Drug	Indication	Toxicity
AZT (retrovir, zidovudine)	Antiretroviral	Anemias, neutropenia, thrombocytopenia, myopathy, nausea, vomiting
ddC (2′,3′ dideoxycytidine)	Antiretroviral	Neutropenia, thrombocytopenia, peripheral neuropathy
Acyclovir (Zovirax)	Antiviral (herpes simplex)	Renal failure, marrow suppression, encephalopathy, abnormal liver function tests
Ganciclovir (DHPG)	Antiviral (CMV)	Neutropenia, thrombocytopenia, hypotension, nausea, vomiting, renal failure, abnormal liver function tests
Bactrim (trimethoprim-sulfamethoxazole)	*Pneumocystis carinii* pneumonia (treatment, prophylaxis)	Fever, rash, marrow suppression
Pentamidine	*Pneumocystis carinii* pneumonia (treatment, prophylaxis)	Renal failure, hypotension, hypoglycemia, marrow suppression, abnormal liver function tests, rash, bronchospasm (nebulized)
Dapsone	*Pneumocystis carinii* pneumonia (prophylaxis)	Rash, hemolytic anemia, nephrotic syndrome
Amphotericin B	Antifungal	Renal failure, hypokalemia, anemia, nausea, vomiting, fever, chills
Ketoconazole	Antifungal	Nausea, vomiting, hepatitis, thrombocytopenia

From Schwartz D, Schwartz T, Cooper E, et al: Anaesthesia and the child with HIV infection. Can J Anaesth *38*:626, 1991 (with permission).

demonstrated the presence of viral particles in multinucleated giant cells and macrophages in the brain, and the virus has been isolated from cerebrospinal fluid. These children demonstrate a progressive encephalopathy with developmental delay, progressive motor dysfunction, and behavioral changes. Decreased brain growth produces microcephaly. Pathologically, cerebral atrophy, ventriculomegaly, and calcification of the basal ganglia and periventricular white matter occur. These children have a very poor prognosis. A less severe static encephalopathy has also been demonstrated in HIV-infected children. These children display nonprogressive cognitive and motor impairment.

Gastrointestinal Syndromes. HIV-infected children frequently demonstrate what has been classically described as a wasting syndrome. This failure to thrive is associated with chronic or recurrent diarrhea, either as a direct effect of HIV on the gastrointestinal tract or as the result of a secondary opportunistic infection such as mucocutaneous candidiasis, which occurs in over 75 percent of these patients. Hepatosplenomegaly and hepatitis are other gastrointestinal manifestations of HIV infection.

Infectious Syndromes. Bacterial infections are common and recurrent. They include otitis media, cellulitis, urinary tract infection, osteomyelitis, pneumonia, meningitis, and sepsis. The causative agents include the usual pathogens in the pediatric population such as *Streptococcus pneumoniae, Haemophilus influenzae,* and *Salmonella.* Opportunistic infections with *Pneumocystis,* cytomegalovirus, *Mycobacterium,* herpes, and *Candida* also occur and can result in pneumonitis, hepatitis, enteritis, and esophagitis.

Hematological Syndromes. In the HIV-infected child, all cell lines can be depressed either as a result of the HIV infection or secondary to therapy (Table 16–11). An autoimmune process similar to idiopathic thrombocytopenic purpura has been associated with the HIV infection in these patients.

Lymphadenopathy/Parotitis. Lymphadenopathy and parotitis are common presenting features in the HIV-positive child. They may present together or as separate entities. Although they may remain the only manifestation of disease in an infected child, they may be associated with the later onset of pulmonary disease.

Embryopathy. A characteristic dysmorphic syndrome in children with congenital HIV infection has been reported. This syndrome consists of ocular hypertelorism, prominent forehead, flat nasal bridge, mild obliquity of the eyes, long palpebral fissures, short nose, triangular philtrum, and patulous lips.

Other Manifestations. Secondary malignancies occur in children, although more common in the adult HIV-infected patient. Kaposi's sarcoma is rare in the pediatric population, but lymphomas have been reported with increased frequency.

Indications for Surgical Therapy. The current indications for operation in the HIV-infected child are primarily diagnostically and therapeutically related to the infection (Table 16–12). As the numbers of HIV-infected children increase and treatment and survival improve, more of these children can be expected to be seen for surgical procedures for AIDS-related and -unrelated conditions.

ANESTHETIC CONSIDERATIONS

Preanesthetic Assessment. Because HIV infection can produce damage in most organ systems, HIV-infected children require careful and thorough preanesthetic assessment. The preanesthetic history from the chart and the patient (parents or guardian) can provide information about prior HIV-related problems, such as cardiac, pulmonary, and neurological involvement, and any specific treatment they might have required. Previously unrecognized symptoms may also become apparent. It is important to elicit information about concurrent drug therapy. Patients with lymphoid interstitial pneumonitis perhaps are being or may have been treated with steroids and require perioperative steroid coverage. Such patients also may be receiving acute or chronic bronchodilator therapy or may benefit from such treatment perioperatively. Many of the other medications used in the treatment of AIDS have side effects that have implications on anesthetic management (see Table 16–11).

Physical examination should be directed to careful evaluation and documentation of the preanesthetic status. Careful examination of the heart and lungs is necessary to detect any underlying dysfunction that may not have been previously identified. Oral candidiasis is common and difficult to eradicate. It often extends into the esophagus and is associated with gastroesophageal reflux. Since this increases the potential for gastric aspiration, appropriate precautions must be taken. Cytomegalovirus and herpes may also cause esophagitis and sometimes coexist with *Candida.*

Additional preanesthetic laboratory evaluations of hematological, hepatic, and renal function may be required. A chest radiograph can provide information about pulmonary and cardiac involvement and may indicate the need for further pulmonary and cardiac evaluation.

Anesthetic Management. Universal precautions to protect both patient and anesthesiologist are necessary. The incidence of seroconversion after needle puncture from an HIV-infected patient is 0.5 percent; it is very important to appreciate that HIV is not transmitted by casual contact. The CDC's guidelines for the protection of the health care worker and patient are presented earlier in the chapter.

The presence of and potential for end-organ damage requires careful titration of anesthetic agents in these patients, since their ability to eliminate agents by hepatic and renal mechanisms may be impaired and their response to various anesthetic agents may be enhanced. The administration of an anesthetic to these patients requires that oxygen saturations, end-tidal carbon dioxide concentrations, cardiovascular status, and urinary output be carefully monitored in accordance with the anesthetic agents, concentrations, and fluids being administered. Because of the immunosuppressed state of these patients, the use of sterile technique is necessary when intravenous access and invasive monitoring are established.

Table 16–12. SURGICAL PROCEDURES FOR HIV-INFECTED CHILDREN

Surgical Procedure	Boston City Hospital (*n = 20 patients)*	Johns Hopkins Hospital (*n = 21 patients)*
Central venous catheter placement	11	23
Gastrostomy tube	8	—
Bronchoscopy	3	—
Lung biopsy	5	11
Lymph node, rectal or liver biopsy	5	
Myringotomy tube insertion	2	3
Incision and drainage of soft tissue abscess	—	6
Incision and drainage of perirectal abscess	—	4
Inguinal and umbilical hernia repair	—	3
Diverting colostomy	—	2
Nissen fundoplication	—	1
Colostomy closure		1
Other	4	
Total	38	54

Modified from Schwartz D, Schwartz T, Cooper E, et al: Anaesthesia and the child with HIV infection. Can J Anaesth *38*:626, 1991; and Beaver BL, Hill JL, Vachon DA, et al: Surgical intervention in children with human immunodeficiency virus infection. J Pediatr Surg *25*:79, 1990.

Table 16–13. PROCEDURES ASSOCIATED WITH A HIGH RISK OF GVHD

Procedure	Groups at High Risk
Bone marrow transplantation	Patients receiving no GVHD prophylaxis; older patients; recipients of HLA-nonidentical bone marrow; recipients of bone marrow from allosensitized donors
Solid-organ transplantation (organs containing lymphoid tissue)	Recipients of small bowel transplants
Transfusion of unirradiated blood products	Neonates and fetuses; patients with congenital immunodeficiency syndromes; patients receiving immunosuppressive chemoradiotherapy; patients receiving directed blood donations from partially HLA-identical, HLA-homozygous donors

From Ferrara JLM, Deeg HJ: Graft-versus-host disease. Reprinted with permission of the New England Journal of Medicine, *324*:667, 1991.

Local or regional anesthesia, as opposed to general anesthesia, is usually the preferred technique. Although in some instances the type of operation or preference of the patient may preclude the use of a certain technique, there may be certain advantages to the use of local or regional techniques in such immunodepressed patients. It has been suggested that after local or regional techniques, the depression of cell-mediated immunity, evident after the administration of a general anesthetic, is not present, although the advantages of local or regional anesthesia based on these considerations are currently theoretical.

Patient Management. The CDC's universal precautions (see earlier) should be followed in the anesthetic management of patients and equipment since HIV has been recovered from both wet and dry environments for 3 to 7 days after inoculation.

GRAFT-VERSUS-HOST DISEASE

Graft-versus-host disease (GVHD) occurs in patients with severely impaired cell-mediated immunity who have received allogeneic immunocompetent lymphocytes (mature T cells). For the development of GVHD, three requirements must be met: the graft must contain immunologically competent T cells, the recipient must express tissue antigens that are not present in the transplant donor, and the recipient must be incapable of mounting an effective T-cell response to destroy the transplanted cells.

In the recipient, the donor T cells attack the recipient's major histocompatibility antigens. The requirement for recipient T-cell depression is most commonly seen in allogeneic bone marrow transplantation: recipients have usually received immunosuppressive doses of chemotherapy and radiation before marrow infusion that in turn depress their own immune systems. Graft-versus-host disease may also occur in patients with cancer who are receiving cytotoxic (and immunosuppressive) chemotherapy and require blood transfusions. Recipients of solid-organ grafts are treated with immunosuppressive drugs to prevent rejection of the transplanted organ and thereby become susceptible to attack by T cells present in the donor graft. Graft-versus-host disease can occur in fetuses who have received maternofetal transfusions and in neonates who have been given exchange transfusions. Immunocompetent recipients who are heterozygous for HLA proteins will not reject lymphocytes that are transfused from a donor who is homozygous for one of the recipients' haplotypes; these lymphocytes then may recognize the recipients' second haplotype. On this basis, GVHD may develop in patients undergoing operation who receive blood transfusions, even though they are not immunocompromised (Table 16–13).

Graft-versus-host disease can be subdivided into acute, chronic, and syngeneic forms, the features of which are similar.

ACUTE GVHD

Symptoms of GVHD generally begin within 5 to 30 days after an immunodeficient patient has received immunocompetent lymphocytes. The incidence of the disease ranges from less than 10 percent to more than 80 percent, depending on the degree of histoincompatibility, number of T cells in the graft, patient's age, and prophylactic regimen. The principal target organs include the immune system, skin, liver, and intestine. Initially there is skin involvement: lymphocytes infiltrate the dermis and epidermis with symptoms that resemble the scalded skin syndrome. Later there is liver involvement accompanied by periportal necrosis of hepatocytes, fever, and gastrointestinal mucosal degeneration with diarrhea. Coagulation studies and bleeding time may become abnormal, and hepatic failure with ascites and encephalopathy may develop in severe cases. Other problems include hemolytic anemia, granulocytopenia with aplastic anemia, cough, and pulmonary infiltrates as a result of lymphocyte infiltration and necrosis of the bronchial mucosa. In infants, the administration of 50 ml of blood containing completely mismatched lymphocytes may be fatal. Those receiving incompletely but partially matched lymphocytes do better.

Chronic GVHD

Chronic GVHD was initially defined as a GVHD syndrome presenting more than 100 days after bone marrow transplantation, whether it presents as an extension of acute GVHD after a disease-free interval or with no preceding disease. Chronic GVHD is characterized by scaling erythroderma, alopecia, and failure to thrive as well. Chronic cholestatic liver disease occurs in 80 percent of patients and often resembles acute GVHD; it rarely progresses to cirrhosis. Severe mucositis of the mouth and esophagus can result in weight loss and malnutrition. Gastrointestinal involvement is infrequent. Chronic GVHD also produces a sicca syndrome, with atrophy and dryness of mucosal surfaces caused by lymphocytic destruction of exocrine glands that usually affects the eyes, mouth, airways, skin, and esophagus. The hematopoietic system may also be affected. Thrombocytopenia is an unfavorable prognostic factor.

Syngeneic GVHD

A GVHD-like syndrome that is usually self-limited and predominantly affects the skin can occur in recipients of syngeneic or autologous transplants. The disease usually resolves promptly with the administration of glucocorticoids and is not life-threatening. Virtually all patients in whom this syndrome develops after syngeneic transplantation have been prepared with intensive conditioning regimens, usually involving irradiation.

IMPLICATIONS

In the chronic and acute forms of GVHD, there is increased susceptibility to both bacterial and viral infections. Latent infections such as cytomegalovirus may become active and fulminant. *Pneumocystis carinii* pneumonia also is common.

PROPHYLAXIS AND TREATMENT

Prophylaxis and treatment of GVHD is aimed at eliminating or preventing the activation of donor T cells. Glucocorticoids and methotrexate have been used alone or in combination to prevent donor T-cell proliferation and activation.

Removing all T cells from the donor bone marrow is the most effective method of preventing GVHD. This can be accomplished by physical separation (lectin agglutination) or by treatment with monoclonal antibodies directed at T cells.

When a patient with T-cell dysfunction is transfused with blood, it is important to remember that lymphocytes in blood from blood banks are viable for up to 3 weeks. Blood transfused into patients with T-cell dysfunction, therefore, should be irradiated before transfusion to kill the lymphocytes.

Antithymocyte or antilymphocyte globulin has been used to treat established GVHD, but success with this approach has been limited. The use of monoclonal antibodies to treat GVHD is increasing and most certainly will be a mainstay of therapy in the future. Recently, commercial gamma globulin preparations given intravenously have also benefited patients with GVHD.

THE PHAGOCYTIC SYSTEM AND ASSOCIATED DISEASES

Phagocytes are either mononuclear or polymorphonuclear. They arise from a pluripotent stem cell in the bone marrow and other hematopoietic tissue (Fig. 16–4, and see also Fig. 16–1). Phagocytes are produced in numbers equal to those of erythrocytes, but they have a much shorter half-life, which accounts for their lower absolute numbers.

Mononuclear phagocytes (monocytes) have a circulating half-life of 70 hours. A large reserve of monocytes exists in the bone marrow and is marginated in the circulation. When monocytes are released, they are immature. After a period in the circulation they leave the blood compartment to become the fixed macrophages of the spleen, liver, lungs, lymph nodes, intestine, and central nervous system. With maturation their

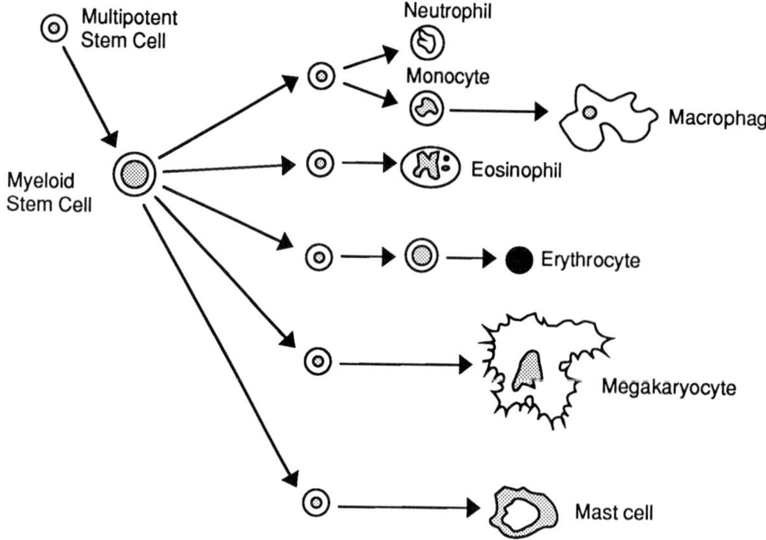

FIGURE 16–4. Derivation of cells in the myeloid-cell lineage. Cells are derived from a myeloid stem cell producing monocytes, free and fixed macrophages, and neutrophils. (Modified from Nelson DL: Cellular interactions in the human immune response. *In* Stiehm ER (ed): Immunological Disorders in Infants and Children. 3rd edition. Philadelphia, WB Saunders, 1989, pp 15–28.)

phagocytic activity increases. Fixed macrophages demonstrate morphological and metabolic characteristics that are unique to and dependent upon the resident organ system. Circulating mononuclear cells migrate into areas of inflammation and are responsible for walling off an infectious process and for granuloma formation.

Polymorphonuclear leukocytes (PMNs) (neutrophils, basophils, eosinophils) have a circulating half-life of 6 to 10 hours. As in the case of monocytes, a large reservoir of PMNs is stored in the bone marrow and marginated in the circulation. Polymorphonuclear leukocytes are released into the circulation as highly differentiated mature cells, where they circulate for 4 to 10 hours and then, like monocytes, migrate into tissues.

The functions of phagocytes are complex. Phagocytes enter the circulation from the bone marrow or marginated pool in response to inflammatory stimuli, producing a sharp increase in absolute numbers. Inflammation also stimulates rapid multiplication of precursor cells and rapid differentiation. In the area of inflammation, phagocytes adhere to the vascular endothelium and enter the tissues by diapedesis. Once in the tissues, they migrate toward the affected area by moving up a concentration gradient of chemotactic substances (chemotaxis). Once the phagocytes reach the affected area and make contact with the infecting organism, adherence, endocytosis, and killing of the infecting organism occur.

The properties of the foreign particles may contribute to the activity of phagocytes, including spontaneous activation of complement by the alternate pathway, as occurs with some yeasts, and production of a hydrophobic surface, a surface charge, and surface sugars. Opsonins are specific antibacterial antibodies and components of complement that neutralize antiphagocytic factors on bacterial surfaces and serve as ligands binding bacteria to phagocytes. The interaction of bacteria with such opsonins enhances phagocytosis. Phagocytic cells have membrane receptors for portions of the antibodies and for the activated fragments of complement.

Once such recognition and adherence occur, endocytosis follows: certain contractile proteins are activated to form a pseudopod that surrounds the organism. When the cell membrane completely surrounds the particle, a phagocytic vacuole is formed. Cytoplasmic granules contribute their contents to this phagosome and thus stimulate oxidative metabolism.

Phagocytosis is associated with a burst of oxygen consumption. This is associated with a tenfold increase in glucose consumption by the hexose monophosphate pathway. Oxygen is univalently reduced to form a superoxide radical, then hydrogen peroxide and hydroxyl radicals, and finally water (Fig. 16–5). Halides are oxidized. The interaction of reactive oxygen molecules, myeloperoxidase, which originates from the cytoplasmic granules, and halides rapidly kills most bacterial and fungal organisms. Oxygen-reduced pyridine nucleotides and oxidases are essential for this response.

Defects in phagocytic function, either singly or in combination, may occur at one or more of

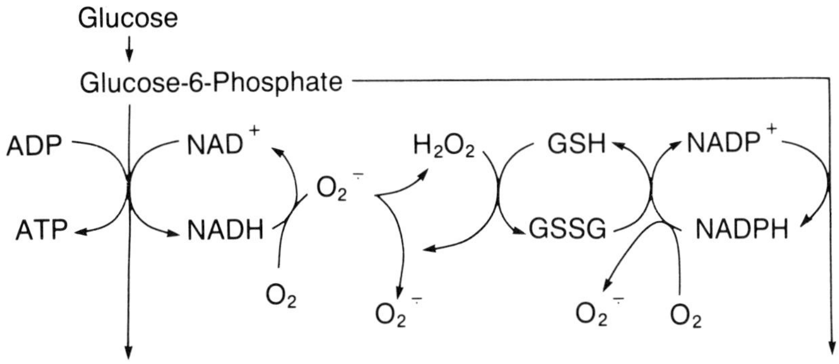

Glucose
Glucose-6-Phosphate
ADP
ATP
NAD^+
NADH
$O_2^{\overline{\cdot}}$
O_2
H_2O_2
$O_2^{\overline{\cdot}}$
GSH
GSSG
$NADP^+$
NADPH
$O_2^{\overline{\cdot}}$
O_2

FIGURE 16–5. Oxidative response of the hexose monophosphate pathway with phagocytosis, demonstrating the production of hydrogen peroxide (H_2O_2) and superoxide radical ($O_2^{\overline{\cdot}}$), which are responsible for the bactericidal activity of the cells. ADP, Adenosine diphosphate; GSH, reduced glutathione; ATP, adenosine triphosphate; GSSG, oxidized glutathione; NAD^+, oxidized nicotinamide adenine dinucleotide; $NADP^+$ oxidized nicotinamide adenine dinucleotide phosphate; NADPH, reduced nicotinamide adenine dinucleotide phosphate.

these steps. Table 16–14 describes the susceptibilities to infection that occur with different defects.

DISORDERS OF POLYMORPHONUCLEAR LEUKOCYTES

Disorders of Bactericidal Function (Table 16–15)

Chronic Granulomatous Disease of Childhood. Chronic granulomatous disease (CGD) is a genetic disorder characterized by recurrent and chronic bacterial or fungal infections. It is a disorder of phagocytic cells in which bactericidal capacity is defective owing to an abnormal oxidative metabolic response during phagocytosis. Humoral and cell-mediated responses are unaffected, and cells are morphologically normal.

Table 16–14. INCREASED SUSCEPTIBILITY WITH SPECIFIC DEFECTS

Defects	Increased Susceptibility to
Bactericidal	
Chronic granulomatous disease	Catalase-producing bacterial and fungal infections
Myeloperoxidase deficiency	Candidiasis, bacterial infections, or none
Chemotaxis	
Hyperimmunoglobulin E (Job's syndrome)	*Staphylococcus aureus* infection of skin and nodes
Lazy leukocyte syndrome	Upper respiratory tract infections and stomatitis
Mixed Disorders	
Chédiak-Higashi syndrome	Gram-positive coccal infections
Other	
Neutropenia, congenital or acquired	Bacterial infections

The inheritance pattern of CGD appears to be X-linked. In males, patients are either normal or affected. In females, heterozygous and homozygous states occur. As a group, female heterozygotes have low levels of bactericidal activity, but there is considerable variability, and normal levels of bactericidal activity do not exclude heterozygosity.

The onset of CGD may occur at any age from infancy to adulthood. Diagnosis can now be made in utero from fetal cells obtained at amniocentesis. The presentation of the syndrome is variable; Table 16–16 lists some of the clinical manifestations that may occur.

Patients demonstrate increased susceptibility to both bacterial and fungal infections. *Staphylococcus aureus, Serratia marcescens,* and *Klebsiella* are common infecting organisms. The syndrome is characterized by recurrent and chronic

Table 16–15. DISORDERS OF BACTERICIDAL FUNCTION

Chronic granulomatous disease
Myeloperoxidase deficiency
Glucose-6-phosphatase deficiency
Glutathione peroxidase deficiency
Down's syndrome
Bilobed PMN nucleus
Chédiak-Higashi syndrome

Table 16–16. CLINICAL MANIFESTATIONS OF CHRONIC GRANULOMATOUS DISEASE

System	Disease
Skin	Eczematous dermatitis
	Granulomas
	Pyoderma
Ear-nose-throat	Otitis
	Rhinitis
	Sinusitis
Cardiopulmonary	Pericarditis
	Mediastinitis
	Pneumonia
	Focal lung abscess
	Diffuse persistent pulmonary infiltrates
Gastrointestinal	Ulcerative stomatitis
	Esophagitis
	Antral granuloma or thickening with obstruction
	Subphrenic abscess
	Focal liver abscess
	Miliary liver abscesses
	Granulomatous ileitis/colitis
	Vitamin B_{12} malabsorption
	Steatorrhea
	Perianal fistulas
Genitourinary	Renal abscess
	Pyelonephritis
	Cystitis
	Dysuria of unknown cause
Endocrine	Septic thyroiditis with thyrotoxicosis
Neurological	Meningitis
	Epidural abscess
Hematological	Granulocytosis
	Hypochromic/microcytic anemia
Immunological	Diffuse hypergammaglobulinemia
	Lymphadenopathy
	Suppurative lymphadenitis
	Splenomegaly
	Urticaria, arthralgias, costochondritis
Musculoskeletal	Osteomyelitis
	Septic arthritis
	Pyomyositis

microabscesses of lymph nodes and liver, osteomyelitis, and chronic pneumonitis.

Pneumonitis is frequent, with *Staphylococcus aureus,* gram-negative bacilli, and *Aspergillus fumigatus* as causative agents. In spite of appropriate therapy, chronic infiltrates and residual pulmonary changes are frequent. The presence of circulating immune complexes is common and can produce arthralgias, urticaria, and costochondritis. Female heterozygotes demonstrate an increased incidence of systemic lupus erythematosus.

Pathogenesis. As previously described (see page 588), neutrophils normally metabolize oxygen to produce superoxide anion and hydrogen peroxide. After ingestion of a foreign organism, production of oxygen metabolites by the hexose monophosphate pathway and their accumulation occur in the phagosome. Myeloperoxidase, delivered into the phagosome by degranulation, and hydrogen peroxide kill the phagocytized microbe. Many microorganisms produce catalase, which is capable of catabolizing hydrogen peroxide, but neutrophils normally produce hydrogen peroxide in amounts sufficient to overwhelm this catalase and enable normal bactericidal capacity. In patients with chronic granulomatous disease, the oxygen metabolites, including hydrogen peroxide, are not produced by the neutrophils. Although some microorganisms produce hydrogen peroxide themselves, those that produce catalase (catalase-positive) are able to catabolize the produced hydrogen peroxide and therefore are not killed. Catalase-negative cells such as *Streptococcus* are unable to break down the hydrogen peroxide produced by the microbe itself, which, in association with the myeloperoxidase delivered, is sufficient to enable its own destruction.

This disorder is termed *granulomatous* because the phagocytozed bacteria elicit a granulomatous response common to intracellular pathogens in tissues such as lymph nodes, liver, bone marrow, and lung that contain many macrophages. Histologically, the lesions consist of polymorphonuclear, lymphocytic, macrophage, and plasma cell infiltration.

Medical Management. Currently no satisfactory treatment is available to correct the defect in bactericidal activity; management is aimed at the prophylaxis of infections. Many infections, if detected and treated early, respond to conservative therapy such as oral antibiotics. More severe infections require hospitalization and intravenous antibiotics; frequently, broad-spectrum antibiotic coverage is used when the offending organism cannot be identified. Once phagocytozed into neutrophils, the bacteria are segregated from most antibiotics. Agents such as chloramphenicol and rifampin have been advocated in many of these cases because of their ability to diffuse into neutrophils and kill phagocytozed bacteria.

Granulocyte transfusion therapy has been used with success in these patients, but such therapy is difficult. This is due to a lack of the normally present Kell's antigens on the erythrocytes and leukocytes of these patients, which increases their susceptibility to transfusion reactions.

Glucocorticoid therapy has been tried but appears to offer no advantages.

Medical and surgical management have considerably improved the course and prognosis of this disorder over the past few years.

Anesthetic Considerations. Careful attention must be paid to sterile techniques. Patients with CGD frequently harbor chronic infections or abscesses and may have draining sinuses from previous surgical therapy. The high incidence of resistant organisms in these individuals who have been treated with numerous antibiotics makes isolation necessary.

The cardiopulmonary status needs assessment. Pericarditis has been reported, and pneumonitis and chronic pulmonary changes are common. Pulmonary function tests, arterial blood gases, and a current chest radiograph must be obtained preoperatively.

Obstruction of the gastric antrum by granuloma formation is frequent. Such obstruction may produce nausea and vomiting and may delay gastric emptying; thus, patients with CGD must be managed to avoid potential aspiration during induction of anesthesia.

The lack of the normally present Kell's antigens on the erythrocytes and leukocytes complicates blood transfusion. There is a high risk of transfusion reactions. The use of blood products containing red blood cells or leukocytes or both requires careful cross-matching. Such matching may require a longer than normal period. Similarly, emergency blood (type O, Rh negative) should be used only when absolutely necessary and then with extreme caution. Concurrent drug therapy must be assessed for potential interactions with anesthetic agents. Many antibiotics are known to interact with muscle relaxants.

These considerations are some of the more common problems associated with chronic granulomatous disease. Table 16–16 delineates some of the other clinical manifestations of chronic granulomatous disease that have been reported.

Myeloperoxidase Deficiency. Myeloperoxidase deficiency is an autosomal recessive disorder characterized by the absence of myeloperoxidase in the granules of neutrophils and monocytes. This enzyme potentiates the bactericidal effectiveness of hydrogen peroxide, and its absence produces a bactericidal defect in neutrophils. The impairment is less severe than that which occurs in chronic granulomatous disease. This syndrome is relatively common in the population (1 in 4000), but because patients may not appear as unusually susceptible to infections, it may not be as readily recognized as is chronic granulomatous disease.

Glucose-6-Phosphate Dehydrogenase Deficiency. Glucose-6-phosphate dehydrogenase (G6PD) deficiency is a relatively common inborn error of metabolism that primarily affects erythrocytes. Profound deficiencies of the enzyme (values less than 5 percent of normal) are rare, however, and it is only these profound deficiencies that affect neutrophil function. Such a deficiency produces a defect similar to chronic granulomatous disease, with recurrent infections and granulomatous lesions.

Glucose-6-phosphate dehydrogenase generates reduced pyridine nucleotide NADPH by the hexose monophosphate pathway, which is necessary for converting oxygen to superoxide and for maintaining intracellular levels of reduced glutathione. Patients with G6PD that is 25 percent of normal usually have normal leukocyte bactericidal activity.

Glutathione Peroxidase Deficiency. Glutathione peroxidase is involved in the glutathione-dependent reduction of hydrogen peroxide to water. Its deficiency results in intracellular accumulation of hydrogen peroxide after the initial increase in hexose monophosphate pathway activity after phagocytosis. This accumulation results in injury or death of cells and produces neutropenia.

DISORDERS OF CHEMOTAXIS

Movement of PMNs to the site of infection within the first few hours of inoculation is critical for the elimination of invading bacteria. Abnormal locomotion has been identified in many patients with recurrent serious infections. Such abnormal movement may result from cellular abnormalities or conditions with abnormal PMN chemotaxis; these are listed in Table 16–17.

Hyperimmunoglobulin E Syndrome (Job's Syndrome). Abnormal PMN chemotaxis, called hyperimmunoglobulin E syndrome (Job's syn-

Table 16–17. CELLULAR DEFECTS OF CHEMOTAXIS

Chédiak-Higashi syndrome
Shwachman's syndrome
Panhypogammaglobulinemia
Lazy leukocyte syndrome
Hyperimmunoglobulin E and A
Down's syndrome
Wiskott-Aldrich syndrome
Chronic renal failure
Acrodermatitis enteropathica
Mannosidosis
Leukemia
Kartagener's syndrome
Anchor disease
Ichthyosis

drome), has been identified in patients with extremely elevated levels of IgE. These patients present with recurrent severe staphylococcal infection, cellulitis, or subcutaneous or deep muscle abscesses, frequently without pain or local signs of inflammation. Eczema and atopic dermatitis are common. The association of staphylococcal infections, defective phagocytic cell chemotaxis, eczema, and hyperimmunoglobulin E is common in this disease, although the degree of each individual abnormality is variable. Patients with Job's syndrome frequently, but not always, have red hair. They generally develop severe bacterial infections within the first months of life. Pulmonary involvement is common, and pneumatoceles may develop and require surgical removal.

Although *Staphylococcus aureus* is the most commonly seen organism, others such as *Cryptococcus* and *Pneumocystis carinii* may be present and produce serious infection, suggesting an associated dysfunction of cell-mediated immunity.

Immotile Cilia Syndrome (Kartagener's Syndrome). Patients with immotile cilia syndrome (Kartagener's syndrome) demonstrate abnormal ciliary function and abnormal polymorphonuclear leukocyte motility. Immotile cilia syndrome is an autosomal recessive trait with an incidence of 1 in 4000. There are several consequences of this disorder, most of which are related to abnormal ciliary function. Chronic otitis media and sinusitis are common in children because of impaired clearance of bacteria from the sinuses, middle ear, and eustachian tubes. Males are sterile because of inadequate spermatozoal movement. Chronic bronchitis caused by abnormal mucociliary clearance is common in children. Bronchiectasis is usually a late complication. Wheezing is common and is due to inadequate clearance of antigens from the lungs. Situs inversus is a usual finding in these patients and may be due to failure of ciliary-like activity during embryonal development. The presence of abnormal neutrophil chemotaxis further increases the susceptibility to infection. Associated abnormal ciliary function and neutrophil locomotion suggest a common physiological basis for these cellular activities.

Medical Management. Currently treatment is symptomatic and includes aggressive treatment of otitis media, sinusitis, and pulmonary infections with antibiotics, physiotherapy, and bronchodilators. *Haemophilus* and *Pneumococcus* are common infecting organisms. The prognosis is unknown, but morbidity caused by bronchiectasis is considerable.

Anesthetic Considerations. Patients with Kartagener's syndrome are at increased risk of infection and are likely to harbor pathogens. Their pulmonary status is of primary concern and must be optimized before surgery. Physiotherapy, bronchodilator therapy, and antibiotic coverage must be provided.

The presence of chronic otitis media and sinusitis may represent a contraindication to the use of nitrous oxide.

The presence of chronic infective processes demands that these patients be isolated to prevent cross-contamination. Careful cleaning of the room and equipment after the procedure and use of disposable equipment when possible are indicated.

The neutrophil dysfunction increases susceptibility to infection even at sites that are not influenced by the ciliary dysfunction. Strict aseptic techniques are therefore necessary.

Shwachman's Syndrome. Patients with Shwachman's syndrome suffer pancreatic insufficiency and metaphyseal dyschondroplasia and are susceptible to recurrent infections because of depressed neutrophil chemotaxis. This syndrome is rare and is inherited in an autosomal recessive pattern. It is, however, the second most common cause of pancreatic insufficiency in children, after cystic fibrosis. Unlike the case in cystic fibrosis, the secretions in Shwachman's syndrome are normal. In addition to impaired chemotaxis, neutropenia, thrombocytopenia, and hypoplastic anemia are present. The latter two are rarely a problem. The decreased number of cells seems to represent an arrest of maturation in the bone marrow. Musculoskeletal abnormalities are common: metaphyseal dyschondroplasia produces short stature. Ribs also may be affected, and in some patients the thoracic cage may be narrow enough to impair respiration.

Medical Management. No specific treatment for Shwachman's syndrome is available. Early in life, patients require pancreatic supplements, but this treatment may not be necessary for life, since the malabsorption syndrome may improve. Most patients survive infancy, and their subsequent prognosis is usually good.

Anesthetic Considerations. Infants suffer from malabsorption, and serum proteins may be depressed. These factors may affect drug distribution. Thrombocytopenia and anemia may be present and require correction before a surgical procedure. Musculoskeletal abnormalities may produce problems with positioning, and the involvement of the rib cage may decrease chest wall compliance and compromise

Table 16–18. CIRCULATING INHIBITORS OF CHEMOTAXIS

Wiskott-Aldrich syndrome
Chronic mucocutaneous candidiasis
Rheumatoid arthritis
IgA myeloma
Hodgkin's disease

ventilatory parameters intraoperatively. The presence of neutrophil dysfunction requires consideration.

Lazy Leukocyte Syndrome. Patients with lazy leukocyte syndrome have normal neutrophils in the bone marrow. These cells display normal phagocytosis and bacterial killing, but their locomotion is defective. This defect affects their migration from the bone marrow to the circulation, producing neutropenia, and from the circulation to sites of inflammation. Patients with this syndrome are susceptible to upper respiratory infections and stomatitis.

Inhibitors of Chemotaxis. Patients with circulating inhibitors of chemotaxis present a clinical picture similar to that of patients with cellular defects of chemotaxis. Table 16–18 lists conditions in which circulatory inhibitors have been demonstrated. Circulating inhibitors include a lymphocyte-derived chemotactic factor that is found in the serum of patients with Wiskott-Aldrich syndrome. Inhibitors of chemotaxis are present in normal plasma, but their levels are elevated in certain conditions such as Hodgkin's disease. Polymeric IgA may inhibit normal chemotaxis in individuals with elevated levels of this immunoglobulin.

Deficiency of Chemotactic Factors. The absence of normal chemotactic factors can affect the efficiency of chemotaxis. The majority of these factors are derivatives of the complement system of proteins and will be discussed below. Other causes are presented in Table 16–19; all are rare.

MIXED FUNCTIONAL DEFECTS

Chédiak-Higashi Syndrome. Chédiak-Higashi syndrome (CHS) is an autosomal recessive immunological disorder of neutrophil function. This immunological disorder consists of defects in chemotaxis, lysosomal degranulation, and intracellular killing. Giant cytoplasmic lysosomes are identified in leukocytes, lymphocytes, erythrocytes, and fibroblasts, as well as in neurons and renal tubular epithelium. In neutrophils, these granules appear to contain normal lysosomal enzymes, peroxidase, and acid phosphatase. Phagocytosis is normal, but degranulation of the lysosomes into the phagosome is inhibited. It has been suggested that the abnormalities seen in these patients may be produced by altered microtubular function, which is necessary for normal chemotaxis and degranulation.

Table 16–19. DEFICIENT PRODUCTION OF CHEMOTACTIC FACTOR

Absent C_5
Hageman's factor abnormality
Abnormal activation of C_3
Systemic lupus erythematosus
Immunoglobulin deficiency

Patients with CHS are characterized by abnormal pigment of skin, hair, and eyes (partial oculocutaneous albinism), photophobia, and nystagmus. Neurological abnormalities may be present and include long tract signs, cerebellar involvement, peripheral neuropathies, and mental retardation.

The defect in neutrophil function results in frequent bacterial or fungal infections of the upper and lower respiratory tract and skin. Viral infections are handled normally.

Initially in infancy, infections are minor and respond to appropriate antibiotic therapy. Later, an accelerated phase occurs: it is associated with lymphoid infiltration of all tissues, anemia, neutropenia, refractory infections, and hemorrhage, which is associated with thrombocytopenia and defective platelet function, all of which require supportive therapy. Infections require aggressive antibiotic management, and many become refractory to therapy. Steroids, cytotoxic drugs, and splenectomy are used to induce remission but are rarely successful. The disease is commonly fatal in early childhood, and death is most often secondary to infection.

Recent studies have demonstrated that normal microtubular function is regulated by 3′,5′-guanosine monophosphate (cyclic GMP). Agents that increase neutrophil cyclic AMP have improved neutrophil function and have been used successfully in patients with CHS, but the long-term implications are unclear.

Anesthetic Considerations. Patients with CHS present several potential problems for the anesthesiologist. Their susceptibility to recurrent respiratory infections may have compromised their pulmonary status. Chronic respiratory infections may occur and be resistant to therapy. Vigorous therapy is required postoperatively to prevent serious complications. During the progression of the disease, and particularly during the accelerated phase, anemia and thrombocytopenia with defective platelet function may be present and require therapy. This may contraindicate certain techniques (for example, epidural anesthesia, intramuscular injections). The presence of peripheral neuropathies caused by the disease (discussed earlier) or its treatment (see later) is a contraindication to the use of depolarizing muscle relaxants. Renal function may be impaired because of the involvement of the renal tubular epithelium. Concurrent antibiotic medication must be assessed, optimized, and evaluated for possible interaction with anesthetic agents. Supplemental steroid therapy may be required. The implications of cytotoxic agents, if in use, should be considered. Vincristine is commonly used. It may produce a peripheral neuropathy, different in etiology from that described earlier, and an autonomic dysfunction. Because of the patients' susceptibility to infections, aseptic techniques are mandatory. It is best to avoid techniques (such as epidural anesthesia) in which any complicating infection is likely to be devastating. The presence of chronic infections, many of which are resistant to antibiotic therapy, requires that anesthetic equipment be carefully cleaned before use with other patients and that, when possible, disposable equipment be used.

Postoperatively these patients may require reverse or barrier isolation or both.

Actin Dysfunction. A defect in the actin filaments has been associated with recurrent bacterial infections with the formation of pus. The PMNs exhibit profoundly depressed chemotactic and phagocytic abilities. Bactericidal abilities are normal.

Bilobed PMN Nucleus Syndrome. A bilobed PMN nucleus, intermittent neutropenia, deficient specific granules, defective bactericidal activity against *Staphylcoccus aureus*, and impaired chemotaxis form the constellation of features of bilobed PMN nucleus syndrome, a rare disorder. Phagocytosis and other bactericidal activity are normal.

DISORDERS OF MONONUCLEAR LEUKOCYTES

Few functional defects of mononuclear leukocyte cells have been identified or well characterized. Those that have been described are similar to those seen in PMN leukocytes. Mononuclear leukocytes demonstrate depressed chemotaxis under conditions in which PMN chemotaxis is depressed. This includes allergic conditions with elevated immunoglobulin E, and the Wiskott-Aldrich syndrome (see Table 16–17). The anesthetic considerations are the same as described for defects of PMN.

THE COMPLEMENT SYSTEM AND ASSOCIATED DISEASES

The complement system is a system of soluble proteins that interact with each other in a sequential fashion. It serves as the primary humoral effector system of inflammation against infection (Table 16–20). The complement system works via either the classical or the alternate pathway (Fig. 16–6). Twenty components and regulators compose the complement system; all are proteins; and together they make up 10 percent of the globulin fraction of serum.

The components of the classical pathway are assigned numbers corresponding to the order of their discovery, not necessarily the same as their order of activation. Fragments of the component proteins resulting from their cleavage are assigned small letters (a, b, c, d, or e). With the exception of C2, released fragments are designated by "a," and the part of the component retained in the protein complex is assigned "b." An activated component is designated by a bar,

Table 16–20. ACTIVITIES OF COMPLEMENT IN HOST DEFENSE AGAINST INFECTION

Components or Fragments	Functional Activity
C14, C1423	Neutralization of viruses
C4a, C3a, C5a	"Anaphylatoxin" (capillary dilation)
C5a	Chemotaxis of neutrophils, monocytes, eosinophils
C3b	Opsonization
C3b	Enhancement of cell-mediated cytotoxicity
C3b	Stimulation of production of B cell lymphokines
C3b, C3d	Enhanced induction of antibody formation
C3e	Induction of granulocytosis
Bb	Macrophage adherence and spreading
C5	Opsonization of fungi
C1–6 (? additional components)	Inactivation of endotoxin
C1–9	Lysis of viruses, virus-infected cells, tumor cells, mycoplasma, protozoa, spirochetes, and bacteria

From Johnston RB Jr: Complement and associated diseases. *In* Behrman RE, Vaughan VC III (eds): Nelson Textbook of Pediatrics. 13th edition. Philadelphia, WB Saunders, 1987.

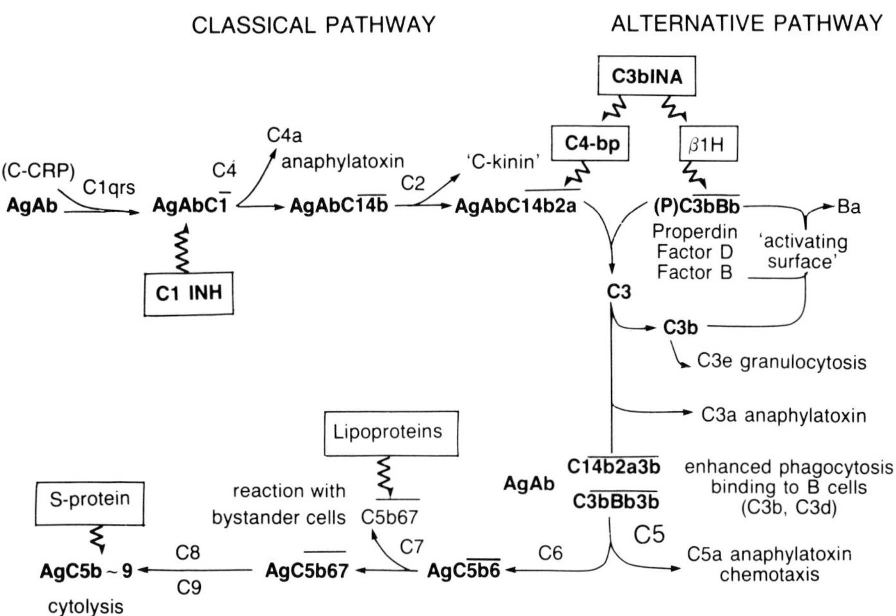

FIGURE 16–6. Sequence of activation of the components of the classical pathway of complement and interaction with the alternate pathway. Regulator proteins are each enclosed in a box. Ag, Antigen (bacterium, virus, tumor cell, or erythrocyte); Ab, antibody (IgG or IgM classes only); C-CRP, C carbohydrate–C-reactive protein; C1 INH, C1 inhibitor; C3b INA, C3b inactivator; C4–bp, C4–binding protein. (From Johnston RB Jr: Complement and associated diseases. *In* Behrman RE, Vaughan VC III [eds]: Nelson Textbook of Pediatrics. 12th edition. Philadelphia, WB Saunders, 1983.)

for example, $C\bar{1}$. Components of the alternate pathway have been assigned letters B, D, and P (properdin). Factor 8 has an active form $B\bar{b}$. The common feature of these pathways is that they both serve to activate C3.

Complement in association with antibody is necessary for the bactericidal capacity of serum. This is demonstrated by the fact that when complement is destroyed by heating serum, bactericidal capacity is lost even when antibody remains active.

CLASSICAL PATHWAY ACTIVATION

The combination of antigen with antibody, produces a conformational change in the antibody, exposing a binding site for the C1 component of the cascade. C1 is a trimolecular complex. It is bound by the C1q subunit to the Fc portion of the antibody. This produces a conformational change in the C1 component that results in the activation of the C1s component, an esterase. The third subunit (C1r) acts to bind the two reactive subunits. A second substance, C-reactive protein, also can initiate the binding of C1. Elevated in certain inflammatory states, C-reactive protein is not an antibody but a protein that can react with C-carbohydrates on microorganisms. It can combine with only a few organisms, but it does have the potential of initiating inflammation in the absence of antibody.

C4 and C2 are next bound, producing $\overline{C14b2a}$. C4a is released. This is an anaphylatoxin that induces mast cells to release mediators of immediate hypersensitivity. With the binding of C2, a kinin-like peptide is released that can increase vascular permeability and edema via action on postcapillary venules. C4b enables immune adherence of the complex to neutrophils, monocytes, and erythrocytes (known as immune adherence). C3 is activated next. The fixation of C3b enables adherence of the antibody-antigens to cells with C3b receptors, including neutrophils, monocytes, macrophages, B lymphocytes, and erythrocytes. This fixation is extremely important in phagocytosis by the phagocytic cells. The released C3a fragment has anaphylatoxin activity. C3b is broken down by C3b inactivator to produce C3d, which remains bound, and C3c, which is released. C3c is cleaved to C3e, which induces the release of granulocytes from the bone marrow.

C3 may also be activated by $\overline{C3bBb}$ of the alternate pathway (see below). The action of $\overline{C14b2a3b}$ or $\overline{C3bBb3b}$ on C5 releases C5a, an anaphylatoxin and chemoattractant for neutrophils, monocytes, and macrophages. C6 is bound to C5b but serves to stabilize the com-

Table 16–21. CONGENITAL DEFICIENCIES OF THE COMPLEMENT SYSTEM

Deficient Component*	Probable Inheritance†	Associated Clinical Findings‡
C1q	Not known	Recurrent infections, dermatitis, CGN
C1q dysfunction	AR (CD)	SLE syndrome
C1r	AR (CD)	CGN, SLE syndrome
C1s	Not known	SLE
C4	AR (CD)	SLE or SLE syndrome, discoid lupus erythematosus
C2	AR (CD)	SLE or SLE syndrome; MPGN; H-S purpura; dermatomyositis; septicemia, especially pneumococcal
C3	AR (CD)	Pyogenic infections, absence of expected neurophilia; CGN
C5	AR (CD)	SLE; pyogenic infections; gonococcal, meningococcal infections
C5 dysfunction	AD	Pyoderma, septicemia, Leiner's disease
C6	AR (CD)	Gonococcal, meningococcal infections; SLE syndrome
C7	AR (CD)	Sclerodactyly; chronic nephritis; gonococcal, meningococcal infections
C8	AR (CD)	Gonococcal, meningococcal infections; SLE syndrome
C8 dysfunction	Not known	Meningococcal infections
C9	AR (CD)	Meningococcal infections
C1 INH×	AD	Angioedema, SLE
C3b INA×	AR (CD)	Pyogenic infections

*INA = inactivator; INH = inhibitor.
†AD = autosomal dominant; AR (CD) = autosomal recessive, co-dominant (heterozygotes have approximately half-normal serum levels).
‡CGN = chronic glomerulonephritis; H-S = Henoch-Schönlein; MPGN = membranoproliferative glomerulonephritis; SLE = systemic lupus erythematosus.
From Johnston RB Jr: Complement and associated diseases. *In* Behrman RE, Vaughan VC III (eds): Nelson Textbook of Pediatrics. 13th edition. Philadelphia, WB Saunders, 1987.

plex, not undergoing cleavage. The $\overline{\text{C5b6}}$ complex next dissociates from the parent complex (C5 convertase) and combines with C7. The $\overline{\text{C5b67}}$ complex attaches to the cell membrane and binds C8 and C9. The complex breaks the integrity of the cell membrane by forming a hole, producing cell lysis.

ALTERNATE PATHWAY ACTIVATION

The alternate pathway can be activated by several mechanisms. C3b can bind to B to form C3bB, which is then cleaved by D to form $\overline{\text{C3bBb}}$. This becomes an efficient C3 convertase producing more C3b. C3 alone may bind to B to be cleaved to $\overline{\text{C3Bb}}$, which is analogous to but less active than $\overline{\text{C3bBb}}$. Cleavage of B releases Ba, which has chemotactic activity. P (properdin) can bind to $\overline{\text{C3bBb}}$, preventing decay-disassociation of B.

Other mechanisms for alternate pathway activation include activation of thrombin, plasmin, trypsin, or leukocyte proteases.

REGULATORY MECHANISMS

Regulatory mechanisms exist to protect the host. C1 inhibitor (C1 INH) inhibits C1s activity and therefore the cleavage of C2 and C4. The short half-life of C2 effectively limits the activity of the complexes in which it takes a part. The $\overline{\text{C3bBb}}$ of the alternate pathway has a short half-life, but this is increased by binding to properdin. C3a and C5a activity is controlled by a deactivating enzyme. C3b inactivator (C3b INA) is important in that it serves as a means of controlling both pathways. β1H increases the inactivation of C3b by C3b INA, and C4 binding protein accelerates cleavage of C4b by C3b INA.

INHERITED DISORDERS OF THE COMPLEMENT SYSTEM

Deficiencies or dysfunction of all components of the complement system have been described (Table 16–21). Not all the deficiencies are associated with increased susceptibility to infection. Depending upon the particular component, patients may present with histories of (1) autoimmune disease, (2) recurrent bacterial infection, or (3) angioedema. Overlap of symptoms does occur.

AUTOIMMUNE PHENOMENON

Deficiencies of certain components of the classical activities pathway are associated with an increased incidence of rheumatic diseases. Patients with C1q, C1r, C1s, C2, C4, and C1 INH deficiencies present with rheumatic diseases but with a lower susceptibility to bacterial infection as occurs in other component deficiencies. This implies that alternate pathway activation may be sufficient for host protection. This results in C3 activation, which is required for opsonization of foreign organisms, which in turn promotes phagocytosis by neutrophils and macrophages. Deficiencies of C5, C6, C7, and C8 cause an increased susceptibility to infection that is likely to be due to impairment of complement mediated cytolysis by the C5–C9 complex, decreasing resistance to infections (especially with *Neisseria*).

The etiology of the increased incidence of rheumatic diseases is unclear. It has been postulated that the classical activating pathway is in some way responsible for the clearance of immune complexes and that impairment of this function may predispose to rheumatic disease. A genetic basis linking complement genes with histocompatibility genes has also been suggested as a possible mechanism for the association.

BACTERIAL INFECTIONS

Complement factor 3 can be activated by either the classical or alternative pathways, and because of this, a defect in either pathway can be compensated for to some extent. Defects or deficiencies in C3 or beyond, however, result in a significant increase in the susceptibility to bacterial infection. Congenital absence of C3 is associated with recurrent pyogenic infections such as pneumococcal pneumonia and meningococcal meningitis. C3 is required for the opsonization of foreign organisms through production of C3b. Likewise, production of C3e causes an increase in neutrophil count, and C3 activation of C5 produces C5a, which is a chemotactic factor. Therefore, the lack of C3 reduces the efficiency of phagocytosis. Patients with deficiencies of C5, C6, C7, or C8 appear to be unusually susceptible to systemic *Neisseria* infections. This implies that complement-mediated serum bacteriolysis is an important factor in resistance to these organisms. Patients with a deficiency of C3b inactivator have a congenital deficiency of the regulatory protein of the C3 convertase of the alternate pathway. Such a deficiency allows continuous activation of C3 convertase, causing a decrease of C3 owing to its high rate of catabolism. These patients suffer the same symptoms as those that occur in C3 deficiency.

Medical Management. Certain complement defects may be treated by plasma infusions to replace components. C5 abnormalities are due to a dysfunction rather than a deficiency, and repeated plasma infusions may be used to deter infections. In those with deficiencies rather than dysfunction of components, infusions of foreign complement components introduce a risk of antibody formation to these complement factors if long-term replacement therapy is attempted. Although replacement therapy may be used for a short period, most of the primary diseases of the complement system can receive only supportive management. The exact diagnosis of the defect is important. Patients with some defects are extremely susceptible to infections and require earlier and more aggressive intervention than others. Such patients should be immunized against bacterial antigens when possible.

Anesthetic Considerations. Because most of the disorders of complement result in some increase in susceptibility to infection, these patients should be treated with careful aseptic technique as previously described. Although many of the disorders can be treated only in supportive fashion, it is important to determine the specific defect. Associated disorders may have significant anesthetic implications that may demand varying techniques.

HEREDITARY ANGIONEUROTIC EDEMA

Hereditary angioneurotic edema (HAE) is a rare, genetically determined (autosomal dominant) disorder of complement regulation. This disorder involves deficiency of the alpha globulin (C1 inhibitor) that inhibits the activated first component of complement. Consequently, there is excessive consumption of C4 with low levels of this component during and between attacks. Clinical presentations are episodic and are characterized by swelling of the extremities, face, and bowel wall, leading to severe morbidity in many patients. Involvement of the upper airway with resultant asphyxia is a major cause of mortality. The differential diagnosis at the time of first presentation is discussed under Urticaria and Angioedema in Chapter 17.

The onset of the disorder is usually in the second or third decade, although symptoms may present at an advanced age. The diagnosis is established by demonstrating low levels of C1 inhibitor (5 to 30 percent of normal) and of C4.

During attacks, levels of C2 are also depressed. In about 15 percent of cases, C1 inhibitor levels are reported to be normal by immunological measurements but low by functional assays. Inhibitor is present but functionally inactive.

Attacks can occur spontaneously (without an apparent cause) but more commonly can be attributed to physical or emotional trauma. During an attack, levels of C1 inhibitor and C4 and C2, the substrates of C1s, are depressed. The levels of other complement components are normal. A vasoactive peptide that increases local vascular permeability is generated during the attack and accounts for the development of the subepithelial edema. The nature of the peptide produced is not clear. It may be derived by the breakdown of C2, which produces the "C-kinin." It has also been postulated that trauma may activate Hageman's factor, which interacts with other cofactors initiating fibrinolysis, converting plasminogen to plasmin (Fig. 16–7). Plasmin activates C1 with subsequent breakdown of C2 and release of "C-kinin." Recently, however, it has been suggested that activation of the plasma kallikrein system may induce attacks of HAE. C1 inhibitor also normally inhibits activated Hageman's factor and kallikrein, enzymes that participate in the generation of bradykinins. Minor damage to the vascular interna may first facilitate the formation of activated Hageman's factor locally and promote the activation of plasma kallikrein and the release of kinins, such as bradykinin, that can enhance vascular permeability and produce edema.

The cutaneous edema is not painful or itchy, nor is it accompanied by redness of the skin. Edema of the small bowel causes severe abdominal cramps and bilious vomiting. Colonic involvement produces a profuse watery diarrhea. Laryngeal edema is the most severe manifestation, and in the past up to 25 percent of patients with laryngeal involvement have died from respiratory obstruction.

Medical Management. For patients who suffer infrequent and mild attacks, no ongoing therapy may be indicated. In more severe cases, for many years prophylaxis was effected by the use of plasmin inhibitors such as epsilon-aminocaproic acid (EACA) or anabolic steroids such as methyltestosterone. However, side effects made therapy with these agents unsatisfactory. EACA therapy is associated with muscle discomfort caused by a reversible increase of serum enzymes, such as creatinine phosphokinase and aldolase. The drug is also an antifibrinolytic agent, and as such may cause thrombotic episodes that may lead to serious consequences. Side effects of methyltestosterone include cholestatic jaundice, suppression of endogenous androgen production, and masculinization in women.

Danazol and stanozolol have been found to be extremely effective in preventing attacks of

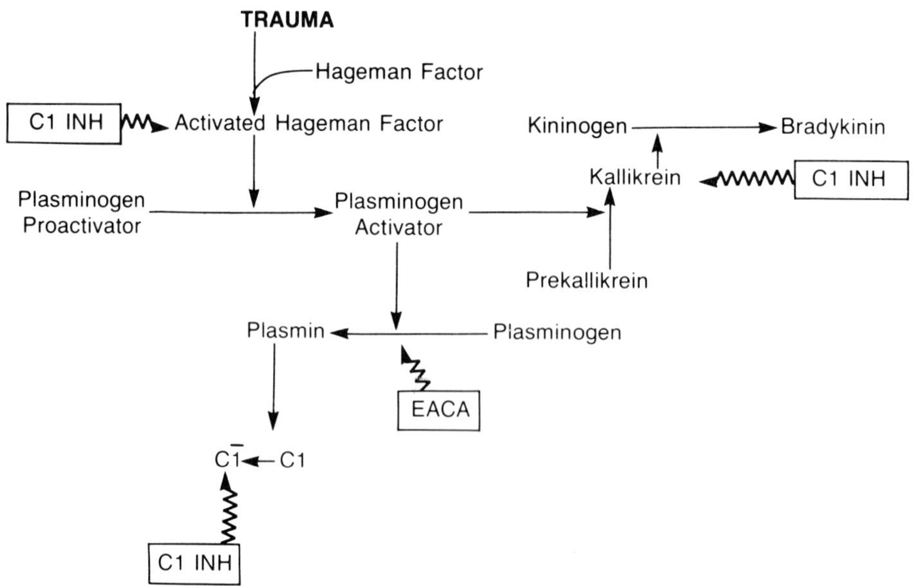

FIGURE 16–7. The pathogenesis of hereditary angioneurotic edema by the production of bradykinin and activated complement factor 1. The sites of action of C1 INH and EACA are demonstrated. C1 INH, Complement factor 1 inhibitor; EACA, epsilon aminocaproic acid; C1̄, complement factor 1; C1̄, activated complement factor 1.

HAE. They suppress the pituitary ovarian axis by inhibiting the output of gonadotropins from the pituitary gland and interfere with hormonal target tissue interactions. The only hormonal activity other than pituitary inhibition is mild androgenic activity, which is dose-related. It is the androgenic activity that stimulates the synthesis of normal C1 inhibitor in patients with C1 inhibitor deficiency, without the side effects of methyltestosterone. Danazol also increases C4 synthesis by an anabolic effect.

By raising levels of C1 inhibitor, these agents provide more effective regulation of C1 activation, Hageman's factor, and kallikrein. Adverse effects of treatment with such attenuated steroids include impairment of the growth rate in children (this has resulted in the preferential use of EACA in children in some centers), masculinization in women, and a reversible disturbance of liver function.

Management of ongoing episodes can be difficult. Often patients with involvement of the head and neck do not require hospitalization. Many episodes will resolve without treatment, and most others will respond to measures such as antihistamines or adrenergic agents or both. Failure of response or progression of symptoms will require hospitalization. The suggestion of airway involvement necessitates close observation, as these patients are in a high-risk category for death, and airway support by tracheostomy or intubation may be necessary.

The use of fresh frozen plasma (FFP) to supply active C1 inhibitor has been debated for many years as a treatment for ongoing episodes of HAE. The use of FFP reportedly has been sufficient to arrest an attack of HAE in progress, but well controlled studies have not been performed. The controversy arises in the treatment of ongoing attacks, because, in addition to C1 inhibitor, C2 and C4 are also supplied, and these may serve as additional substrates during an attack. The use of FFP also carries the risks associated with transfusion, such as hepatitis.

Recently, trials evaluated the replacement of C1 inhibitor protein partly purified from pooled plasma. In asymptomatic patients the administration of C1 inhibitor protein produced increases in C4 activity, indicating biological activity of the infused C1 inhibitor. Of greatest interest is that the administration of the C1 inhibitor during acute abdominal or laryngeal attack of HAE resulted in abatement of symptoms in addition to increased C4 activity. The initial treatment of the pooled plasma in preparing the concentrate is with 20 percent polyethylene glycol, which serves to precipitate C1 esterase, C2 and C4, and hepatitis B virus if present. Therefore the risk of transfusion-associated hepatitis B is minimized. This preparation, then, may offer safe, effective replacement therapy and may provide a means of controlling an attack of HAE that is in progress.

Anesthetic Considerations. The problem faced in the management of patients is that attacks of HAE may be induced by physical or emotional trauma, both of which are present in the perioperative period.

Preoperatively, several aspects of these patients require special attention. The upper respiratory tract requires careful evaluation so that any evidence of edema in the early postoperative period may be quickly identified. Many patients require intubation, which can produce local trauma. Even if minimal, this trauma may be sufficient to induce an attack of HAE. The importance of this is demonstrated by the mortality rate of 25 to 30 percent for those with upper airway involvement. Attacks involving the gastrointestinal tract may produce a watery diarrhea, which necessitates careful evaluation of fluid and electrolyte status. Concurrent medications may involve drugs with attenuated androgen function. These drugs may affect hepatic function, and liver function tests, therefore, should be included preoperatively.

Levels of C1 inhibitor and C4 should be assessed preoperatively. Fifteen percent of patients have normal C1 inhibitor levels, but this C1 inhibitor is nonfunctional, and this can be demonstrated by depressed C4 levels in the presence of normal C1 inhibitor levels. In long-term management, doses are generally reduced to the lowest level required to prevent attacks, regardless of the measured C1 inhibitor, because many of the side effects of androgen therapy can be annoying to patients, such as virilization in females.

For surgical therapy, the ideal is to have the C1 inhibitor and C4 as near as possible to normal levels. For elective operation, the full therapeutic dose of androgen (danazol, 200 mg orally TID) should be resumed for 7 to 10 days preoperatively, with monitoring of C1 inhibitor and C4 levels. Such androgen treatment also results in the formation of a functional C1 inhibitor in patients who have the variant form of the disease with an antigenically intact but functionally inactive C1 inhibitor. Plasmin inhibitors such as epsilon-aminocaproic acid and tranexamic acid also provide effective prophylactic treatment but are rarely used today because of their significant toxicities.

If an untreated patient requires emergency

operation, 5 to 10 ml/kg of FFP is recommended to increase the concentration of C1 inhibitor. As discussed, if an attack of HAE has already started, FFP administration is controversial because it provides not only C1 inhibitor but also complement compounds that could worsen the attack. Partly purified C1 inhibitor is effective in acutely increasing C1 inhibitor levels without the addition of further complement compounds. It is also very effective in terminating ongoing episodes of HAE. Various doses have been suggested; interruption of attacks of HAE has been successful with infusions of 1000 plasma equivalents of C1 inhibitor, although up to 3000 plasma equivalents have been used.

The ability to elevate C1 inhibitor and C4 to normal levels has greatly assisted our management of the airway of these patients. Danazol pretreatment and FFP have been demonstrated to prevent attacks of HAE in patients undergoing oral surgical therapy. Thus general anesthesia with an endotracheal tube may be safe when C1 inhibitor and C4 levels have been demonstrated to be normal. If concern exists, the avoidance of oropharyngeal airways and endotracheal tubes is suggested. Conduction anesthesia has been successfully carried out in these patients.

Postoperatively, patients require monitoring in the intensive care unit for a period of time, depending upon the type and extent of surgery. C1 inhibitor levels and C4 levels decrease toward pretreatment levels by 36 hours, and patients require early recommencement of androgen therapy or intravenous supplementation. Vital signs need to be closely monitored. With acute attacks, use of the partly purified C1 inhibitor may be successful in their treatment. The development of imminent pharyngeal edema requires endotracheal intubation or tracheotomy.

Associated Conditions. Systemic lupus erythematosus and lymphoid cancers have been described in association with HAE.

SECONDARY DISORDERS OF THE COMPLEMENT SYSTEM

Defects in complement also are seen secondary to or in association with a primary disorder.

The association of rheumatic disorders with certain complement deficiencies has been discussed. Primary systemic rheumatic disorders are frequently associated with depressed concentrations of serum C1q, C4, and C3. In those conditions, the response to therapy may be demonstrated by the return of complement levels to normal. In more localized rheumatic disorders, the serum levels of complement are frequently normal but synovial fluid will demonstrate decreased complement levels.

Certain renal diseases demonstrate alterations of serum complement levels. Poststreptococcal glomerulonephritis demonstrates depression of C3. An immunoglobulin G autoantibody termed nephritic factor is present in these cases. It serves to stabilize the $\overline{\text{C14b2a}}$ complex (the classical pathway C3 convertase) resulting in C3 deficiency due to catabolism. A similar situation is demonstrated in patients with chronic membranoproliferative glomerulonephritis and partial lipodystrophy. In these cases, the nephritic factor is once again an IgG autoantibody but is directed against $\overline{\text{C3bBb}}$ (the alternate pathway 3 convertase), again producing a C3 deficiency. Increased susceptibility to infection occurs when C3 levels decrease to below 10 percent of normal.

The frequency of pneumococcal infections in association with sickle cell disease and in patients who have undergone splenectomy can be explained in part by an as yet not fully defined defect of the alternate pathway.

Anesthetic Considerations. The anesthetic considerations in these patients are related to their primary disease, but additionally they demonstrate increased susceptibility to infection.

REFERENCES

INTRODUCTION—THE IMMUNE SYSTEM

Cantor H, Gershon RK: Immunological circuits: Cellular composition. Fed Proc *38*:2058, 1979.

Cantrell DA, Smith KA: The interleukin–2 T-cell system: A new cell growth model. Science *224*:1312, 1984.

de Freitas AA, Coutinho A: Very rapid decay of mature B lymphocytes in the spleen. J Exp Med *154*:994, 1981.

Dinarello CA: An update on human interleukin–1: From molecular biology to clinical relevance. J Clin Immunol *51*:287, 1985.

Engleman EG, Benike CJ, Grumet FC, et al: Activation of human T lymphocyte subsets: Helper and suppressor/cytotoxic T cells recognize and respond to distinct histocompatibility antigens. J Immunol *127*:2124, 1981.

Fireman P: Immunology of allergic disorders. *In* Fireman P, Slavin RG (eds): Atlas of Allergies. New York, JB Lippincott, 1991, pp 1.1–1.24.

Gathings WE, Lawton AR, Cooper MD: Immunofluorescent studies of the development of pre-B cells, B lymphocytes and immunoglobulin isotype diversity in humans. Eur J Immunol 7:804, 1977.

Gillis S: Interleukin 2: Biology and chemistry. J Clin Immunol *3*:1, 1983.

Härfast B, Huddlestone JR, Casali P, et al: Interferon acts directly on human B lymphocytes to modulate immunoglobulin synthesis. J Immunol *127*:2146, 1981.

Howard JC, Hunt SV, Gowans JL: Identification of marrow-derived and thymus-derived small lymphocytes in the lymphoid tissue and thoracic duct lymph of normal rats. J Exp Med *135*:200, 1972.

Jett JR, Mantovani A, Herberman RB: Augmentation of human monocyte-mediated cytolysis by interferon. Cell Immunol *54*:425, 1980.

Julius MH. Cellular interactions involved in T-dependent B-cell activation. Immunol Today *3*:295, 1982.

Krensky AM, Burakoff SJ: Basic science seminar: Cytotoxic T-lymphocyte response to HLA antigens. J Pediatr *102*:814, 1983.

Lachman LB: Human interleukin 1: Purification and properties. Fed Proc *42*:2639, 1983.

Lawrence HS: Transfer factor. Adv Immunol *11*:195, 1969.

Leonard WJ, Depper JM, Robb RJ, et al: Characterization of the human receptor for T-cell growth factor. Proc Natl Acad Sci USA *80*:6957, 1983.

Nelson DL, Rubin LA, Kurman CC, et al: An analysis of the cellular requirements for the production of soluble interleukin–2 receptors in vitro. J Clin Immunol *6*:114, 1986.

Ortaldo JR, Pestka S, Slease RB, et al: Augmentation of human K-cell activity with interferon. Scand J Immunol *12*:365, 1980.

Reinherz EL, Kung PC, Goldstein G, et al: Discrete stages of human intrathymic differentiation: Analysis of normal thymocytes and leukemic lymphoblasts of T-cell lineage. Proc Natl Acad Sci USA *77*:1588, 1980.

Rosen FS, Cooper MD, Wedgwood RJP: The primary immunodeficiencies. (First of two parts.) N Engl J Med *311*:235, 1984.

Rosen FS, Wedgwood RJ, Aiuti F, et al: Primary immunodeficiency diseases. Report prepared for the WHO by a scientific group on immunodeficiency. Clin Immunol Immunopathol *28*:450, 1983.

Stiehm ER: Immunodeficiency disorders: General considerations. *In* Stiehm ER (ed): Immunologic Disorders in Infants and Children. 3rd ed. Philadelphia, WB Saunders, 1989, p 829.

Thomas Y, Rogozinski L, Irigoyen OH, et al: Functional analysis of human T cell subsets defined by monoclonal antibodies. IV. Induction of suppressor cells within the $OKT4^+$ population. J Exp Med *154*:459, 1981.

Tonegawa S: Somatic generation of antibody diversity. Nature *302*:575, 1983.

Toy JL: The interferons. Clin Exp Immunol *54*:1, 1983.

Weissman IL: Thymus cell migration. Studies on the origin of cortisone-resistant thymic lymphocytes. J Exp Med *137*:504, 1973.

Welsh RM: Natural killer cells and interferon. CRC Crit Rev Immunol *5*:55, 1984.

Welsh RM, Biron CA, Bukowski JF, et al: Role of natural killer cells in virus infections of mice. Surv Synth Pathol Res *3*:409, 1984.

GENERAL ANESTHETIC CONSIDERATIONS IN IMMUNODEFICIENCY SYNDROMES

Altemeier WA (ed), Committee on Control of Surgical Infections: Manual of Control of Infection in Surgical Patients. Philadelphia, JB Lippincott, 1984.

Appel GB, Neu HC: The nephrotoxicity of antimicrobial agents. N Engl J Med *296*:663, 1977.

Committee on Infections within Hospitals, American Hospital Association: Infection Control in the Hospital. Chicago, American Hospital Association, 1979.

Green GM, Jakab GJ, Low RB, et al: Defense mechanisms of the respiratory membrane. Am Rev Respir Dis *115*:479, 1977.

Hall WJ, Douglas RG Jr, Hyde RW, et al: Pulmonary mechanics after uncomplicated influenza A infection. Am Rev Respir Dis *113*:141, 1976.

Levine AS, Siegel SE, Schreiber AD, et al: Protected environments and prophylactic antibiotics. A prospective controlled study of their utility in the therapy of acute leukemia. N Engl J Med *288*:477, 1973.

Schimpff SC, Greene WH, Young VM, et al: Infection prevention in acute nonlymphocytic leukemia. Laminar air flow room reverse isolation with oral, nonabsorbable antibiotic prophylaxis. Ann Intern Med *82*:351, 1975.

UNIVERSAL PRECAUTIONS

Campbell, B: Universal precautions: A Health and Welfare Canada perspective. Dimens Health Serv *65*(7):10, 1988.

Centers for Disease Control: Recommendations for prevention of HIV transmission in health-care settings. MMWR *36*:(Suppl 2):1, 1987.

CDC: Update. Universal precautions for prevention of transmission of human immunodeficiency virus, hepatitis B virus, and other bloodborne pathogens in health-care settings. MMWR *37*:377, 1988.

CDC: Guidelines for prevention of transmission of human immunodeficiency virus and hepatitis B virus to health-care and public-safety workers. MMWR *38*(Suppl 6S):1, 1989. (An erratum appears in MMWR *38*:746, 1989.)

CDC: Recommendations for preventing transmission of human immunodeficiency virus and hepatitis B virus to patients during exposure-prone invasive procedures. MMWR *40*:1, 1991.

Garner JS, Simmons BP: Guideline for isolation precautions in hospitals. Infect Control *4*:245, 1983.

REVERSE ISOLATION

Abrahm J: Management of the immunocompromised host. Med Clin North Am *68*:617, 1984.

Arnow PM, Andersen RL, Mainous PD, et al: Pulmonary aspergillosis during hospital renovation. Am Rev Respir Dis *118*:49, 1978.

Blaha M, Merka V: Prevention of infectious complications in immunologically compromised patients. Part I: Reverse isolation. Sb Ved Pr Lek Fak Karlovy Univerzity Hradci Kralove *31*:299, 1988.

Buckner CD, Clift RA, Sanders JE, et al: Protective environment for marrow transplant recipients. Ann Intern Med *89*:893, 1978.

Carlson JAK, Middleton PJ, Szymanski MT, et al: Fatal rotavirus gastroenteritis. An analysis of 21 cases. Am J Dis Child *132*:477, 1978.

Garibaldi RA: Reduction of nosocomial infection during pediatric intensive care by protective isolation (letter). N Engl J Med *322*:553, 1990.

Heidt PJ: Management of bacterial and fungal infections in bone marrow transplant recipients and other granulocytopenic patients. Cancer Detect Prev *12*:609, 1988.

Jarvis WR, Middleton PJ, Gelfand EW: Significance of viral infections in severe combined immunodeficiency disease. Pediatr Infect Dis J *2*:187, 1983.

Lee JJ, Marvin JA, Heimbach DM, et al: Infection control in a burn center. J Burn Care Rehabil *11*:575, 1990.

Nauseef WM, Maki DG: A study of the value of simple protective isolation in patients with granulocytopenia. N Engl J Med *304*:448, 1981.

Ogden AF, Steuber CP, Mahoney DH Jr, et al: Bone marrow transplantation in childhood leukemia using reverse isolation techniques. Med Pediatr Oncol *18*:1, 1990.

Pizzo PA, Levine AS: The utility of protected-environment

regimens for the compromised host: A critical assessment. *In* Brown EB (ed): Progress in Hematology, Vol X. New York, Grune & Stratton, 1977, p 311.

van den Broek PJ: Infection control during neutropenia. J Hosp Infect *11* (Suppl A):7, 1988.

Yonekura S, Nagao T, Komatsuda M, et al: [Studies of intestinal microbial flora in post-BMT (bone marrow transplantation) patients under a protected environment] (in Japanese). Kansenshogaku-Zasshi *64*:963, 1990.

X-LINKED AGAMMAGLOBULINEMIA

Fu SM, Hurley JN, McCune JM, et al: Pre-B cells and other possible precursor lymphoid cell lines derived from patients with X-linked agammaglobulinemia. J Exp Med *152*:1519, 1980.

Hoffman T, Winchester R, Schulkind M, et al: Hypoimmunoglobulinemia with normal T cell function in female siblings. Clin Immunol Immunopathol 7:364, 1977.

Mease PJ, Ochs HD, Wedgwood RJ: Successful treatment of echovirus meningoencephalitis and myositis-fasciitis with intravenous immune globulin therapy in a patient with X-linked agammaglobulinemia. N Engl J Med *304*:1278, 1981.

Ochs HD, Ament ME, Davis SD: Giardiasis with malabsorption in X-linked agammaglobulinemia. N Engl J Med *287*:341, 1972.

Ochs HD, Davis SD, Wedgwood RJ: Immunologic responses to bacteriophage $\phi\chi$ 174 in immunodeficiency diseases. J Clin Invest *50*:2559, 1971.

Pearl ER, Vogler LB, Okos AJ, et al: B lymphocyte precursors in human bone marrow: an analysis of normal individuals and patients with antibody-deficiency states. J Immunol *120*:1169, 1978.

Saulsbury FT, Bernstein MT, Winkelstein JA: *Pneumocystis carinii* pneumonia as the presenting infection in congenital hypogammaglobulinemia. J Pediatr *95*:559, 1979.

Saulsbury FT, Winkelstein JA, Yolken RH: Chronic rotavirus infection in immunodeficiency. J Pediatr *97*:61, 1977.

Schwaber J, Lazarus H, Rosen FS: Bone marrow-derived lymphoid cell lines from patients with agammaglobulinemia. J Clin Invest *62*:302, 1978.

Stuckey M, Quinn PA, Gelfand EW: Identification of *Ureaplasma urealyticum* (T-strain mycoplasma) in a patient with polyarthritis. Lancet *2*:917, 1978.

Wedgwood RJ: X-linked agammaglobulinemia. *In* Seligson D (ed): CRC Handbook Series in Clinical Laboratory Science. Section F, Vol I, Part 1. Cleveland, CRC Press, 1977, p 41.

Wright PF, Hatch MH, Kasselberg AG, et al: Vaccine-associated poliomyelitis in a child with sex-linked agammaglobulinemia. J Pediatr *91*:408, 1977.

X-LINKED HYPOGAMMAGLOBULINEMIA WITH GROWTH HORMONE DEFICIENCY

Fleisher TA, White RM, Broder S, et al: X-linked agammaglobulinemia with isolated growth hormone deficiency. N Engl J Med *302*:1429, 1980.

AUTOSOMAL RECESSIVE AGAMMAGLOBULINEMIA

Hoffman T, Winchester R, Schulkind M, et al: Hypoimmunoglobulinemia with normal T cell function in female siblings. Clin Immunol Immunopathol 7:364, 1977.

Rosen FS, Cooper MD, Wedgwood RJP: The primary immunodeficiencies. (First of two parts.) N Engl J Med *311*:235, 1984.

IMMUNOGLOBULIN DEFICIENCY WITH INCREASED IgM (AND IgD)

Schwaber JF, Lazarus H, Rosen FS: IgM-restricted production of immunoglobulin by lymphoid cell lines from patients with immunodeficiency with hyper IgM (dysgammaglobulinemia). Clin Immunol Immunopathol *19*:91, 1981.

SELECTIVE IMMUNOGLOBULIN A DEFICIENCY

Atwater JS, Tomasi TB: Suppressor cells and IgA deficiency. Clin Immunol Immunopathol *9*:379, 1978.

Cunningham-Rundles C, Brandeis WE, Good RA, et al: Milk precipitins, circulating immune complexes, and IgA deficiency. Proc Natl Acad Sci USA 75:3387, 1978.

Cunningham-Rundles C, Pudifin DJ, Armstrong D, et al: Selective IgA deficiency and neoplasia. Vox Sang *38*:61, 1980.

Koistinen J: Selective IgA deficiency in blood donors. Vox Sang *29*:192, 1975.

Lawton AR, Royal SA, Self KS, et al: IgA determinants on B-lymphocytes in patients with deficiency of circulating IgA. J Lab Clin Med *80*:26, 1972.

Ogra PL, Coppola PR, MacGillivray MH, et al: Mechanisms of mucosal immunity to viral infections in γA immunoglobulin-deficiency syndromes. Proc Soc Exp Biol Med *145*:811, 1974.

Oxelius V-A, Laurell A-B, Lindquist B, et al: IgG subclasses in selective IgA deficiency. N Engl J Med *304*: 1476, 1981.

Paganelli R, Levinsky RJ, Atherton DJ: Detection of specific antigen within circulating immune complexes: Validation of the assay and its application to food antigen-antibody complexes formed in healthy and food-allergic complexes. Clin Exp Immunol *46*:44, 1981.

Soothill JF, Hayes K, Dudgeon JA: The immunoglobulins in congenital rubella. Lancet *1*:1385, 1966.

Taylor B, Norman AP, Orgel HA, et al: Transient IgA deficiency and pathogenesis of infantile atopy. Lancet *2*:111, 1973.

van Loghem E: Familial occurrence of isolated IgA deficiency associated with antibodies to IgA. Evidence against a structural gene defect. Eur J Immunol *4*:57, 1974.

Vyas GN, Fudenberg HH: Immunobiology of human anti-IgA: a serologic and immunogenetic study of immunization to IgA in transfusion and pregnancy. Clin Genet *1*:45, 1970.

Waldmann TA, Broder S, Krakauer R, et al: Defect in IgA secretion and in IgA specific suppressor cells in patients with selective IgA deficiency. Trans Assoc Am Physicians *89*:215, 1976.

SELECTIVE DEFICIENCY OF SECRETORY COMPONENT

Strober W, Krakauer R, Klaeveman HL, et al: Secretory component deficiency. A disorder of the IgA immune system. N Engl J Med *294*:351, 1976.

SELECTIVE IMMUNOGLOBULIN M DEFICIENCY

Faulk WP, Kiyasu WS, Cooper MD, et al: Deficiency of IgM. Pediatrics *47*:399, 1971.

Hobbs JR: IgM deficiency. Birth Defects *11*(1):112, 1975.

Hobbs JR, Milner RDG, Watt PJ: Gamma-M deficiency predisposing to meningococcal septicaemia. Br Med J *4*:583, 1967.

IMMUNOGLOBULIN G DEFICIENCIES

Spiegelberg HL: Biological activities of immunoglobulins of different classes and subclasses. Adv Immunol *19*:259, 1974.

TRANSIENT HYPOGAMMAGLOBULINEMIA OF INFANCY

Hayakawa H, Iwata T, Yata J, et al: Primary immunodeficiency syndrome in Japan. I. Overview of a nationwide survey on primary immunodeficiency syndrome. J Clin Immunol *1*:31, 1981.
Rieger CHL, Nelson LA, Peri BA, et al: Transient hypogammaglobulinemia of infancy. J Pediatr *91*:601, 1977.
Tiller TL Jr, Buckley RH: Transient hypogammaglobulinemia of infancy: Review of the literature, clinical and immunologic features of 11 new cases, and long-term follow-up. J Pediatr *92*:347, 1978.

MEDICAL MANAGEMENT OF IMMUNODEFICIENCY DISEASES

Ammann AJ, Ashman RF, Buckley RH, et al: Use of intravenous gamma-globulin in antibody immunodeficiency: Results of a multicenter controlled trial. Clin Immunol Immunopathol *22*:60, 1982.
Buckley RH: Replacement therapy in immunodeficiency. *In* Thompson R (ed): Recent Advances in Clinical Immunology I. Edinburgh, Churchill Livingstone, 1977.
Norman ME, Hansell JR, Holtzapple PG, et al: Malabsorption and protein-losing enteropathy in a child with X-linked agammaglobulinemia. Clin Immunol Immunopathol *4*:157, 1975.
Nydegger UE (ed): Immunotherapy: A Guide to Immunoglobulin Prophylaxis and Therapy. London, Academic Press, 1981.
Soothill JF: Reactions to immunoglobulin. *In* Hypogammaglobulinaemia in the United Kingdom. MRC Special Report Series 310. London, H. M. Stationery Office, 1971.

THYMIC HYPOPLASIA (DiGEORGE'S SYNDROME)

Cleveland WW: Immunological reconstitution in the DiGeorge syndrome by fetal thymic transplant. Birth Defects *11*(1):352, 1975.
Conley ME, Beckwith JB, Mancer JFK, et al: The spectrum of the DiGeorge syndrome. J Pediatr *94*:883, 1979.
Denlinger JK, Nahrwold ML, Gibbs PS, et al: Hypocalcaemia during rapid blood transfusion in anaesthetized man. Br J Anaesth *48*:995, 1976.
DiGeorge AM: Congenital absence of the thymus and its immunologic consequences: Concurrence with congenital hypoparathyroidism. Birth Defects *4*(1):116, 1968.
Flashburg MH, Dunbar BS, August G, et al: Anesthesia for surgery in an infant with DiGeorge syndrome. Anesthesiology *58*:479, 1983.
Freedom RM, Rosen FS, Nadas AS: Congenital cardiovascular disease and anomalies of the third and fourth pharyngeal pouch. Circulation *46*:165, 1972.
Hong R, Ammann AJ, Huang SW, et al: Cartilage-hair hypoplasia: effect of thymus transplants. Clin Immunol Immunopathol 7:15, 1972.
Kahn RC, Jascott D, Carlon GC, et al: Massive blood replacement: correlation of ionized calcium, citrate, and hydrogen ion concentration. Anesth Analg *58*:274, 1979.
Kelley RI, Zackai EH, Emanuel BS, et al: The association of the DiGeorge anomalad with partial monosomy of chromosome 22. J Pediatr 101:197, 1982.
Lobdell DH: Congenital absence of the parathyroid glands. Arch Pathol *67*:412, 1959.
Lux SE, Johnston RB Jr, August CS, et al: Chronic neutropenia and abnormal cellular immunity in cartilage-hair hypoplasia. N Engl J Med *282*:231, 1970.
McKusick VA, Cross HE: Ataxia-telangiectasia and Swiss-type agammaglobulinemia. Two genetic disorders of the immune mechanism in related Amish sibships. JAMA *195*:739, 1966.
Steele RW, Limas C, Thurman CB, et al: Familial thymic hypoplasia. Attempted reconstitution with fetal thymus in a Millipore diffusion chamber. N Engl J Med *287*:787, 1972.
Waud BE, Waud DR: Interaction of calcium and potassium with neuromuscular blocking agents. Br J Anaesth *52*:863, 1980.

CHRONIC MUCOCUTANEOUS CANDIDIASIS

Arulanantham K, Dwyer JM, Genel M: Evidence for defective immunoregulation in the syndrome of familial candidiasis endocrinopathy. N Engl J Med *300*:164, 1979.
Fischer A, Ballet J-J, Griscelli C: Specific inhibition of in vitro Candida-induced lymphocyte proliferation by polysaccharide antigens present in the serum of patients with chronic mucocutaneous candidiasis. J Clin Invest *62*:1005, 1978.
Higgs JM, Wells RS: Chronic mucocutaneous candidiasis: Associated abnormalities of iron metabolism. Br J Dermatol *86* (Suppl 8):88, 1972.
Kirkpatrick CH: Transfer factor and defense against infectious disease. *In* Amos DB, Schwartz RS, Janicki BW (eds): Immune Mechanisms and Diseases. New York, Academic Press, 1979.
Sande MA, Mandell GA: Antimicrobial agents: Miscellaneous antibacterial agents; Antifungal and antiviral agents. *In* Gilman AG, Goodman LS, Gilman A (eds): Goodman and Gilman's The Pharmacological Basis of Therapeutics. 6th ed. New York, Macmillan, 1980.
Valdimarsson H, Higgs JM, Wells RS, et al: Immune abnormalities associated with chronic mucocutaneous candidiasis. Cell Immunol *6*:348, 1973.

PURINE NUCLEOSIDE PHOSPHORYLASE DEFICIENCY

Cohen A, Coyle D, Martin DW Jr, et al: Abnormal purine metabolism and purine overproduction in a patient deficient in purine nucleoside phosphorylase. N Engl J Med *295*:1449, 1976.
Cohen A, Gudas LJ, Ammann AJ, et al: Deoxyguanosine triphosphate as a possible toxic metabolite in the immunodeficiency associated with purine nucleoside phosphorylase deficiency. J Clin Invest *61*:1405, 1978.
Gelfand EW, Dosch HM, Biggar WD, et al: Partial purine nucleoside phosphorylase deficiency. Studies of lymphocyte function. J Clin Invest *61*:1071, 1978.
Gelfand EW, Lee JJ, Dosch HM: Selective toxicity of purine deoxynucleosides for human lymphocyte growth and function. Proc Natl Acad Sci USA *76*:1998, 1979.
Giblett ER, Ammann AJ, Wara DW, et al: Nucleoside-phosphorylase deficiency in a child with severely defective T-cell immunity and normal B-cell immunity. Lancet *1*:1010, 1975.
Rich KC, Arnold WJ, Palella T, et al: Cellular immune deficiency with autoimmune hemolytic anemia in purine

nucleoside phosphorylase deficiency. Am J Med *67*:172, 1979.

Sandman R, Ammann AJ, Grose C, et al: Cellular immunodeficiency associated with nucleoside phosphorylase deficiency. Immunologic and biochemical studies. Clin Immunol Immunopathol *8*:247, 1977.

Staal GEJ, Stoop JW, Zegers BJM, et al: Erythrocyte metabolism in purine nucleoside phosphorylase deficiency after enzyme replacement therapy by infusion of erythrocytes. J Clin Invest *65*:103, 1980.

Stoop JW, Zegers BJM, Hendrickx GFM, et al: Purine nucleoside phosphorylase deficiency associated with selective cellular immunodeficiency. N Engl J Med *296*:651, 1977.

SEVERE COMBINED IMMUNODEFICIENCY

Gatti RA, Meuwissen HJ, Allen HD, et al: Immunological reconstruction of sex-linked lymphopenic immunological deficiency. Lancet *2*:1366, 1968.

Githens JH, Fulginiti VA, Suvatte V, et al: Grafting of fetal thymus and hematopoietic tissue in infants with immune deficiency syndromes. Transplantation *15*:427, 1973.

Haynes BF, Warren RW, Buckley RH, et al: Demonstration of abnormalities in expression of thymic epithelial surface antigens in severe cellular immunodeficiency diseases. J Immunol *130*:1182, 1983.

Hong R, Santosham M, Schulte-Wissermann H, et al: Reconstruction of B and T lymphocyte function in severe combined immunodeficiency disease after transplantation with thymic epithelium. Lancet *2*:1270, 1976.

Keightley RG, Lawton AR, Cooper MD, et al: Successful fetal liver transplantation in a child with severe combined immunodeficiency. Lancet *2*:850, 1975.

Levey RH, Klemperer MR, Gelfand EW, et al: Bone-marrow transplantation in severe combined immunodeficiency syndrome. Lancet *2*:571, 1971.

O'Reilly RJ, Dupont B, Pahwa S, et al: Reconstitution in severe combined immunodeficiency by transplantation of marrow from an unrelated donor. N Engl J Med *297*:1311, 1977.

Rádl J, Dooren LJ, Eijsvoogel VP, et al: An immunological study during post-transplantation follow-up of a case of severe combined immunodeficiency. Clin Exp Immunol *10*:367, 1972.

Reinherz EL, Geha R, Rappeport JM, et al: Reconstitution after transplantation with T-lymphocyte–depleted *HLA* haplotype–mismatched bone marrow for severe combined immunodeficiency. Proc Natl Acad Sci USA *79*:6047, 1982.

Reisner Y, Kapoor N, Kirkpatrick D, et al: Transplantation for severe combined immunodeficiency with HLA-A,B,D,DR incompatible parental marrow cells fractionated by soybean agglutinin and sheep red blood cells. Blood *61*:341, 1983.

SEVERE COMBINED IMMUNODEFICIENCY WITH ADENOSINE DEAMINASE DEFICIENCY

Carson DA, Kaye J, Seegmiller JE: Lymphospecific toxicity in adenosine deaminase deficiency and purine nucleoside phosphorylase deficiency: Possible role of nucleoside kinase(s). Proc Natl Acad Sci USA *74*:5677, 1977.

Chen S-H, Ochs HD, Scott CR, et al: Adenosine deaminase deficiency. Disappearance of adenine deoxynucleotides from a patient's erythrocytes after successful marrow transplantation. J Clin Invest *62*:1386, 1978.

Hirschhorn R: Clinical delineation of adenosine deaminase deficiency. *In* Elliot K, Whelan J (Eds.): Enzyme Defects and Immune Dysfunction. Ciba Foundation Symposium, 68. Amsterdam, Excerpta Medica, 1979.

Hirschhorn R, Beratis N, Rosen FS, et al: Adenosine deaminase deficiency in a child diagnosed prenatally. Lancet *1*:73, 1978.

Hirschhorn R, Roegner-Maniscalco V, Kuritsky L, et al: Bone marrow transplantation only partially restores purine metabolites to normal in adenosine deaminase-deficient patients. J Clin Invest *68*:1387, 1981.

Ito K, Sakura N, Usui T, et al: Screening for primary immunodeficiencies associated with purine nucleoside phosphorylase deficiency or adenosine deaminase deficiency. J Lab Clin Med *90*:844, 1977.

Parkman R, Gelfand EW, Rosen FS, et al: Severe combined immunodeficiency and adenosine deaminase deficiency. N Engl J Med *292*:714, 1975.

Polmar SH: Enzyme replacement and other biochemical approaches to the therapy of adenosine deaminase deficiency. *In* Enzyme Defects and Immune Dysfunction. Ciba Foundation Symposium, 68. Amsterdam, Excerpta Medica, 1979.

Polmar SH, Wetzler EM, Stern RC, et al: Restoration of in-vitro lymphocyte responses with exogenous adenosine deaminase in a patient with severe combined immunodeficiency. Lancet *2*:743, 1975.

COMBINED IMMUNODEFICIENCY WITH PREDOMINANT T-CELL DEFECT

Ammann AJ: Is there an acquired immune deficiency syndrome in infants and children? Pediatrics *72*:430, 1983.

Lawlor GI Jr, Ammann AJ, Wright WC Jr, et al: The syndrome of cellular immunodeficiency with immunoglobulins. J Pediatr *84*:183, 1974.

Nezelof C, Jammet ML, Lortholary P, et al: L'hypoplasie hereditaire du thymus: Sa place et sa responsabilité dans une observation d'aplasie lymphocytaire, normoplasmocytaire et normoglobulinemique du nourrisson. Arch Franc Pediatr *21*:897, 1964.

Schimke RN, Bolano C, Kirkpatrick CH: Immunologic deficiency in the congenital rubella syndrome. Am J Dis Child *118*:626, 1969.

WISKOTT-ALDRICH SYNDROME

Cooper MD, Chase HP, Lowman JT, et al: Immunologic defects in patients with Wiskott-Aldrich syndrome. Birth Defects *4*(1):378, 1968.

Kuramoto A, Steiner M, Baldini MG: Lack of platelet response to stimulation in the Wiskott-Aldrich syndrome. N Engl J Med *282*:475, 1970.

Lum LG, Tubergen DG, Corash L, et al: Splenectomy in the management of the thrombocytopenia of the Wiskott-Aldrich syndrome. N Engl J Med *302*:892, 1980.

Parkman R, Rappeport J, Geha R, et al: Complete correction of the Wiskott-Aldrich syndrome by allogeneic bone-marrow transplantation. N Engl J Med *298*:921, 1978.

Perry GS III, Spector BD, Schuman LM, et al: The Wiskott-Aldrich syndrome in the United States and Canada (1892–1979). J Pediatr *97*:72, 1980.

Spitler LE: Transfer factor therapy in the Wiskott-Aldrich syndrome. Results of long-term follow-up in 32 patients. Am J Med *67*:59, 1979.

ATAXIA-TELANGIECTASIA SYNDROME

Biggar WD, Good RA: Immunodeficiency in ataxia-telangiectasia. Birth Defects *11*(1):271, 1975.

Boder E: Ataxia-telangiectasia: some historic, clinical and pathologic observations. Birth Defects *11*(1):255, 1975.
McFarlin DE, Strober W, Waldmann TA: Ataxia-telangiectasia. Medicine *51*:281, 1972.
Paterson MC, Smith PJ: Ataxia telangiectasia: An inherited human disorder involving hypersensitivity to ionizing radiation and related DNA-damaging chemicals. Annu Rev Genet *13*:291, 1979.
Trompeter RS, Layward L, Hayward AR: Primary and secondary abnormalities of T cell subpopulations. Clin Exp Immunol *34*:388, 1978.

ACQUIRED IMMUNODEFICIENCY SYNDROME

Arden J: Anesthetic management of patients with AIDS (letter). Anesthesiology *64*:660, 1986.
Beaver BL, Hill JL, Vachon DA, et al: Surgical intervention in children with human immunodeficiency virus infection. J Pediatr Surg *25*:79, 1990.
Belman AL: Neurologic manifestations of HIV infection in children. *In* ACTS, International Conference. Paris, France, 1989, p 177.
Brun-Vezinet F, Rey MA, Katlama C, et al: Lymphadenopathy-associated virus type 2 in AIDS and AIDS-related complex. Clinical and virological features in four patients. Lancet *1*:128, 1987.
Centers for Disease Control: CDC revision of the case definition of acquired immunodeficiency syndrome for national reporting—United States. MMWR *34*:373, 1985.
CDC. Classification system for human immunodeficiency virus (HIV) infection in children under 13 years of age. MMWR *36*:225, 1987.
Connor E, Gupta S, Joshi V, et al Acquired immunodeficiency syndrome—associated renal disease in children. J Pediatr *113*:39, 1988.
Cooper ER, Pelton SI, LeMay M. Acquired immunodeficiency syndrome: a new population of children at risk. Pediatr Clin North Am *35*(6):1365, 1988.
Epstein LG, Sharer LR, Goudsmit J. Neurologic and neuropathologic features of human immunodeficiency virus infection in children. Ann Neurol *23* (Suppl):S19, 1988.
Ginzburg HM, Hrainer J, Reis E: A review of epidemiologic trends in HIV infection of women and children. Pediatric AIDS and HIV Infection: Fetus to Adolescent *1*:11, 1990.
Greene ER: Spinal and epidural anesthesia in patients with acquired immunodeficiency syndrome (letter). Anesth Analg *65*:1090, 1986.
Grody WW, Cheng L, Lewis W: Infection of the heart by human immunodeficiency virus. Am J Cardiol *66*:203, 1990.
Husson RN, Comeau AM, Hoff R: Diagnosis of human immunodeficiency virus infection in infants and children. Pediatrics *86*:1, 1990.
Leibovitz E, Rigaud M, Pollack H, et al: *Pneumocystis carinii* pneumonia in infants with the human immunodeficiency virus with more than 450 CD4 T lymphocytes per cubic millimeter. N Engl J Med *323*:531, 1990.
Lipshultz SE, Chanock S, Sanders SP, et al: Cardiovascular manifestations of human immunodeficiency virus infection in infants and children. Am J Cardiol *63*:1489, 1989.
Marcus R. CDC Cooperative Needlestick Surveillance Group. Surveillance of health care workers exposed to blood from patients infected with the human immunodeficiency virus. N Engl J Med *319*:1118, 1988.
Marion RW, Wiznia AA, Hutcheon G, et al: Human T-cell lymphotropic virus Type III (HTLV-III) embryopathy. A new dysmorphic syndrome associated with intrauterine HTLV-III infection. Am J Dis Child *140*:638, 1986.
McDougal JS, Martin LS, Cort SP, et al: Thermal inactivation of the acquired immunodeficiency syndrome virus, human T lymphotropic virus-III/lymphadenopathy-associated virus, with special reference to antihemophilic factor. J Clin Invest *76*:875, 1985.
Medlock MD, Tilleli JT, Pearl GS: Congenital cardiac toxoplasmosis in a newborn with acquired immunodeficiency syndrome. Pediatr Infect Dis J *9*:129, 1990.
Phillips AJ, Spence AA: Zidovudine and the anaesthetist (editorial). Anaesthesia *42*:799, 1987.
Pizzo PA, Wilfert CM (eds): Pediatric AIDS: The Challenge of HIV Infection in Infants, Children, and Adolescents. Baltimore, Williams & Wilkins, 1991, p 813.
Resnick L, Veren K, Salahuddin SZ, et al: Stability and inactivation of HTLV-III/LAV under clinical and laboratory environments. JAMA *255*:1887, 1986.
Rubinstein A, Bernstein LJ, Charytan M, et al: Corticosteroid treatment for pulmonary lymphoid hyperplasia in children with the acquired immune deficiency syndrome. Pediatr Pulmonol *4*:13, 1988.
Scannel KA: Surgery and human immunodeficiency virus disease. J Acquir Immune Defic Syndr *2*:42, 1989.
Schwartz D, Schwartz T, Cooper E, et al: Anaesthesia and the child with HIV infection. Can J Anaesth *38*:626, 1991.
Steinherz LJ, Brochstein JA, Robins J: Cardiac involvement in congenital acquired immunodeficiency syndrome. Am J Dis Child *140*:1241, 1986.
Stevenson GW, Hall SC, Rudnick S, et al: The effect of anesthetic agents on the human immune response. Anesthesiology 72:542, 1990.
Strauss J, Abitbol C, Zilleruelo G, et al: Renal disease in children with the acquired immunodeficiency syndrome. N Engl J Med *321*:625, 1989.
Williams I, Mindel A, Weller I (eds): AIDS. Philadelphia, JB Lippincott, 1989, p 92.

GRAFT-VERSUS-HOST DISEASE

Anderson KC, Weinstein HJ: Transfusion-associated graft-versus-host disease. N Engl J Med *323*:315, 1990.
Beschorner WE, Saral R, Hutchins GM, et al: Lymphocytic bronchitis associated with graft-versus-host disease in recipients of bone-marrow transplants. N Engl J Med *299*:1030, 1978.
Ferrara JLM, Deeg HJ: Graft-versus-host disease. N Engl J Med *324*:667, 1991.
Grebe SC, Streilein JW: Graft-versus-host reactions: A review. Adv Immunol *22*:119, 1976.
Hess AD, Fischer FC: Immune mechanisms in cyclosporine-induced syngeneic graft-versus-host disease. Transplantation *48*:895, 1989.
Lerner KG, Kao GF, Storb R, et al: Histopathology of graft-vs.-host reaction (GvHR) in human recipients of marrow from HL-A-matched sibling donors. Transplant Proc *6*:367, 1974.
Spitzer TR. Transfusion-induced graft-vs.-host disease. *In* Burakoff SJ, Deeg HJ, Ferrara J, et al (eds): Graft-Vs.-Host Disease: Immunology, Pathophysiology, and Treatment. New York, Marcel Dekker, 1990, p 539.
Tsoi M-S, Storb R, Jones E, et al: Deposition of IgM and complement at the dermoepidermal junction in acute and chronic cutaneous graft-vs-host disease in man. J Immunol *120*:1485, 1978.

THE PHAGOCYTIC SYSTEM AND ASSOCIATED DISEASES

Babior BM: Oxygen-dependent microbial killing by phagocytes. (First of two parts.) N Engl J Med *298*:659, 1978.

Fliedner TM, Cronkite EP, Killmann SÅ, et al: Granulocytopoiesis. II. Emergence and pattern of labeling of neutrophilic granulocytes in humans. Blood *24*:683, 1964.

Mauer AM, Athens JW, Ashenbrucker H, et al: Leukokinetic studies. II. A method for labelling granulocytes in vitro with radioactive diisopropylfluorophosphate (DFP[32]). J Clin Invest *39*:1481, 1960.

Metcalfe D: Transformation of granulocytes to macrophages in bone marrow colonies in vitro. J Cell Physiol *77*:277, 1971.

Nathan CF, Murray HW, Cohn ZA: The macrophage as an effector cell. N Engl J Med *303*:622, 1980.

Quesenberry P, Levitt L: Hematopoietic stem cells. (First of three parts.) N Engl J Med *301*:755, 1979.

Stossel TP: Phagocytosis. (Second of three parts.) N Engl J Med *290*:774, 1974.

CHRONIC GRANULOMATOUS DISEASE OF CHILDHOOD

Ament ME, Ochs HD: Gastrointestinal manifestations of chronic granulomatous disease. N Engl J Med *288*:382, 1973.

Boxer LA, Baehner RL: Defects in neutrophil leukocyte function. *In* Franklin EC (ed): Clinical Immunology Update. New York, Elsevier/NorthHolland, 1981, p 357.

Clark RA, Klebanoff SJ: Chronic granulomatous disease. Studies of a family with impaired neutrophil chemotactic, metabolic and bactericidal function. Am J Med *65*:941, 1978.

Curnette JT, Whitten DM, Babior BM: Defective superoxide production by granulocytes from patients with chronic granulomatous disease. N Engl J Med *290*:593, 1974.

Dupree E, Smith CW, MacDougall NLT, et al: Undetected carrier state in chronic granulomatous disease. J Pediatr *81*:770, 1972.

Gold SB, Hanes DM, Stites DP, et al: Abnormal kinetics of degranulation in chronic granulomatous disease. N Engl J Med *291*:332, 1974.

Griscom NT, Kirkpatrick JA Jr, Girdany BR, et al: Gastric antral narrowing in chronic granulomatous disease of childhood. Pediatrics *54*:456, 1974.

Johnston RB Jr, Baehner RL: Chronic granulomatous disease: correlation between pathogenesis and clinical findings. Pediatrics *48*:730, 1971.

Lazarus GM, Neu HC: Agents responsible for infection in chronic granulomatous disease of childhood. J Pediatr *86*:415, 1975.

Lobo MC, Mandell GL: Treatment of experimental Staphylococcal infection with rifampicin. Antimicrob Agents Chemother *2*:195, 1972.

Marsh WL, Øyen R, Nichols ME, et al: Chronic granulomatous disease and the Kell blood group. Br J Haematol *29*:247, 1975.

Mills EL, Rholl KS, Quie PG: X-linked inheritance in females with chronic granulomatous disease. J Clin Invest *66*:332, 1980.

Newberger PE, Cohen HJ, Rothchild SB, et al: Prenatal diagnosis of chronic granulomatous disease. N Engl J Med *300*:178, 1979.

Philippart AI, Colodny AH, Baehner RL: Continuous antibiotic therapy in chronic granulomatous disease: Preliminary communication. Pediatrics *50*:923, 1972.

Quie PG, White JG, Holmes B, et al: *In vitro* bactericidal capacity of human polymorphonuclear leukocytes: Diminished activity in chronic granulomatous disease of childhood. J Clin Invest *46*:668, 1967.

Raubitschek AA, Levin AS, Stites DP, et al: Normal granulocyte infusion therapy for aspergillosis in chronic granulomatous disease. Pediatrics *51*:230, 1973.

Windhorst DB, Page AR, Holmes B, et al: The pattern of genetic transmission of the leukocyte defect in fatal granulomatous disease of childhood. J Clin Invest *47*:1026, 1968.

MYELOPEROXIDASE DEFICIENCY

Lehrer RI, Cline MJ: Leukocyte myeloperoxidase deficiency and disseminated candidiasis: The role of myeloperoxidase in resistance to *Candida* infection. J Clin Invest *48*:1478, 1969.

Salmon SE, Cline MJ, Schultz J, et al.: Myeloperoxidase deficiency. Immunologic study of a genetic leukocyte defect. N Engl J Med *282*:250, 1970.

GLUCOSE-6-PHOSPHATASE DEFICIENCY

Cooper MR, DeChatelet LR, McCall CE, et al: Complete deficiency of leukocyte glucose–6-phosphate dehydrogenase with defective bactericidal activity. J Clin Invest *51*:769, 1972.

GLUTATHIONE PEROXIDASE DEFICIENCY

Boxer LA, Oliver JM, Spielberg SP, et al: Protection of granulocytes by vitamin E in glutathione synthetase deficiency. N Engl J Med *301*:901, 1979.

Oliver JM, Spielberg SP, Pearson CB, et al: Microtubule assembly and function in normal and glutathione synthetase–deficient polymorphonuclear leukocytes. J Immunol *120*:1181, 1978.

Spielberg SP, Boxer LA, Oliver JM, et al: Oxidative damage to neutrophils in glutathione synthetase deficiency. Br J Haematol *42*:215, 1979.

HYPERIMMUNOGLOBULIN E SYNDROME

Gallin JI: Abnormal chemotaxis: cellular and humoral components. *In* Bellanti JA, Dayton DH (Eds.): The Phagocytic Cell in Host Resistance (Conference). New York, Raven Press, 1975, p 227.

Gallin JI, Wright DG, Malech HL, et al: Disorders of phagocyte chemotaxis. Ann Intern Med *92*:520, 1980.

Hill HR, Quie PG: Raised serum IgE levels and defective neutrophil chemotaxis in three children with eczema and recurrent bacterial infections. Lancet *1*:183, 1974.

Miles AA, Miles EM, Burke J: The value and duration of defence reactions of the skin to the primary lodgement of bacteria. Br J Exp Pathol *38*:79, 1957.

Schopfer K, Baerlocher K, Price P, et al: Staphylococcal IgE antibodies, hyperimmunoglobulinemia E and *Staphylococcus aureus* infection. N Engl J Med *300*:835, 1979.

Snyderman R, Pike MC: Disorders of leukocyte chemotaxis. Pediatr Clin North Am *24*(2):377, 1977.

Steerman RL, Snyderman R, Leiken SL, et al: Intrinsic defect of the polymorphonuclear leucocyte resulting in impaired chemotaxis and phagocytosis. Clin Exp Immunol *9*:939, 1971.

IMMOTILE CILIA SYNDROME

Afzelius B: A human syndrome caused by immotile cilia. Science *193*:317, 1976.

Eliasson R, Mossberg B, Camner P, et al: The immotile-cilia syndrome. A congenital ciliary abnormality as an etiologic factor in chronic airway infections and male sterility. N Engl J Med *297*:1, 1977.

Fischer TJ, McAdams JA, Entis GN, et al: Middle ear ciliary defect in Kartagener's syndrome. Pediatrics *62*:443, 1978.
Pedersen H, Mygind N: Absence of axonemal arms in nasal mucosa cilia in Kartagener's syndrome. Nature *262*:494, 1976.
Rooklin AR, McGeady SJ, Mikaelian DO, et al: The immotile cilia syndrome: A cause of recurrent pulmonary disease in children. Pediatrics *66*:526, 1980.
Sturgess JM, Chao J, Wong J, et al: Cilia with defective radial spokes. A cause of human respiratory disease. N Engl J Med *300*:53, 1979.

SCHWACHMAN'S SYNDROME

Aggett PJ, Cavanagh NPC, Matthew DJ, et al: Schwachman's syndrome. A review of 21 cases. Arch Dis Child *55*:331, 1980.
Burke V, Colebatch JH, Anderson CM, et al: Association of pancreatic insufficiency and chronic neutropenia in childhood. Arch Dis Child *42*:147, 1967.
Schussheim A, Choi SJ, Silverberg M: Exocrine pancreatic insufficiency with congenital anomalies. J Pediatr *89*:782, 1976.
Shmerling DH, Prader A, Hitzig WH, et al: The syndrome of exocrine pancreatic insufficiency, neutropenia, metaphyseal dysostosis and dwarfism. Helv Paediatr Acta *24*:547, 1969.

LAZY LEUKOCYTE SYNDROME

Miller ME, Oski FA, Harris MB: Lazy leukocyte syndrome. A new disorder of neutrophil function. Lancet *1*:665, 1971.

DEFICIENCY OF CHEMOTACTIC FACTORS

Gallin JI, Quie PG (eds): Leukocyte Chemotaxis: Methods, Physiology and Clinical Implications. New York, Raven Press, 1978.
Gallin JI, Wright DG, Malech HL, et al: Disorders of phagocyte chemotaxis. Ann Intern Med *92*:520, 1980.
Hill HR, Quie PG: Raised serum IgE levels and defective neutrophil chemotaxis in three children with eczema and recurrent bacterial infections. Lancet *1*:183, 1974.
Schopfer K, Baerlocher K, Price P, et al: Staphylococcal IgE antibodies, hyperimmunoglobulinemia E and *Staphylococcus aureus* infections. N Engl J Med *300*:835, 1979.
Snyderman R, Pike MC: Disorders of leukocyte chemotaxis. Pediatr Clin North Am *24*(2):377, 1977.

CHÉDIAK-HIGASHI SYNDROME

Blume RS, Wolff SN: The Chédiak-Higashi syndrome: Studies in four patients and a review of the literature. Medicine *51*:247, 1972.
Boxer LA, Watanabe AM, Rister M, et al: Correction of leukocyte function in Chédiak-Higashi syndrome by ascorbate. N Engl J Med *295*:1041, 1976.
Clark RA, Kimball HR: Defective granulocyte chemotaxis in the Chédiak-Higashi syndrome. J Clin Invest *50*:2645, 1971.
Dent PB, Fish LA, White JG, et al: Chédiak-Higashi syndrome. Observations on the nature of the associated malignancy. Lab Invest *15*:1634, 1966.
Gallin JI, Elin RJ, Hubert RT, et al: Efficacy of ascorbic acid in Chédiak-Higashi syndrome (CHS): Studies in humans and mice. Blood *53*:226, 1979.
Leader RW: The Chédiak-Higashi anomaly—an evolutionary concept of disease. Natl Cancer Inst Monogr *32*:337, 1969.
Malawista SE: Microtubules and the mobilization of lysosomes in phagocytizing human leukocytes. Ann NY Acad Sci *253*:738, 1975.
Oliver JM: Impaired microtubule function correctable by cyclic GMP and cholinergic agonists in the Chédiak-Higashi syndrome. Am J Pathol *85*:395, 1976.
Root RK, Rosenthal AS, Balestra DJ: Abnormal bactericidal, metabolic, and lysosomal functions of Chédiak-Higashi syndrome leukocytes. J Clin Invest *51*:649, 1972.
Stossel TP, Root RK, Vaughan M: Phagocytosis in chronic granulomatous disease and the Chédiak-Higashi syndrome. N Engl J Med *286*:120, 1972.

ACTIN DYSFUNCTION

Boxer LA, Hedley-Whyte ET, Stossel TP: Neutrophil actin dysfunction and abnormal neutrophil behavior. N Engl J Med *291*:1093, 1974.

BILOBED PMN NUCLEUS

Komiyama A, Morosawa H, Nakahata T, et al: Abnormal neutrophil maturation in a neutrophil defect with morphologic ahnormality and impaired function. J Pediatr *94*:19, 1979.
Strauss RG, Bove KE, Jones JF, et al: An anomaly of neutrophil morphology with impaired function. N Engl J Med *290*:478, 1974.

DISORDERS OF MONONUCLEAR LEUKOCYTES

Altman LC, Synderman R, Blaese RM: Abnormalities of chemotactic lymphokine synthesis and mononuclear leukocyte chemotaxis in Wiskott-Aldrich syndrome. J Clin Invest *54*:486 1974.
Rogge JL, Hanifin JM: Immunodeficiencies in severe atopic dermatitis. Depressed chemotaxis and lymphocyte transformation. Arch Dermatol *112*:1391, 1976.
Synderman R, Buckley RH: Defects of monocyte chemotaxis in patients with hyperimmunoglobulinemia E and undue susceptibility to infection (abstract). J Allergy Clin Immunol *55*:102, 1975.

HEREDITARY ANGIONEUROTIC EDEMA

Abda RP, Owens WD: Hereditary angioneurotic edema, an anesthetic dilemma. Anesthesiology *46*:438, 1977.
Donaldson VH, Rosen FS, Bing DH: Role of the second component (C2) and plasmin in kinin release in hereditary angioneurotic edema (H.A.N.E.) plasma. Trans Assoc Am Phys *90*:174, 1977.
Fabriani JE, Paulin P, Simkin G, et al: Hereditary angioedema: Therapeutic effect of danazol in C4 and C1 esterase inhibitors. Ann Allergy *64*:388, 1990.
Frank MM, Gelfand JA, Atkinson JP: Hereditary angioedema: The clinical syndrome and its management. Ann Intern Med *84*:580, 1976.
Gadek JE, Hosea SW, Gelfand JA, et al: Replacement therapy in hereditary angioedema: Successful treatment of acute episodes of angioedema with partly purified C_1 inhibitor. N Engl J Med *302*:542, 1980.
Gelfand JA, Sherins RJ, Alling DW, et al: Treatment of hereditary angioedema with danazol: Reversal of clinical and biochemical abnormalities. N Engl J Med *295*:1444, 1976.
Gibbs PS, LoSasso AM, Moorthy SS, et al: The anesthetic

and perioperative management of a patient with documented hereditary angioneurotic edema. Anesth Analg *56*:571, 1977.

Hosea SW, Santaella KL, Brown EJ, et al: Long-term therapy of hereditary angioedema with danazol. Ann Intern Med *93*:809, 1980.

Jaffe CJ, Atkinson JP, Gelfand JA, et al: Hereditary angioedema: the use of fresh frozen plasma for prophylaxis in patients undergoing oral surgery. J Allergy Clin Immunol *55*:386, 1975.

Landerman NS: Hereditary angioneurotic edema. I. Case report and review of the literature. J Allergy *33*:316, 1962.

Michel RG, Hudson WR, Pope TH: Angioneurotic edema: A review of modern concepts. Arch Otolaryngol *101*:544, 1975.

Ohela K, Rasanen JA, Wager O: Hereditary angioneurotic edema. Genealogical and immunological studies. Ann Clin Res *5*:174, 1973.

Pence HL, Evans R, Gurnsey LH, et al: Prophylactic use of epsilon aminocaproic acid for oral surgery in a patient with hereditary angioneurotic edema. J Allergy Clin Immunol *53*:298, 1974.

Poppers PJ: Anesthetic implications of hereditary angioneurotic edema. Can J Anaesth *34*:76, 1987.

Rothbach C, Green RL, Levine MI, et al: Prophylaxis of attacks of hereditary angioedema. Am J Med *66*:681, 1979.

Schapira M, Silver LD, Scott DF, et al: Prekallikrein activation and high-molecular-weight kininogen consumption in hereditary angioedema. N Engl J Med *308*:1050, 1983.

Wall RT, Frank M, Hahn M: A review of 25 patients with hereditary angioedema requiring surgery. Anesthesiology *71*:309, 1989.

SECONDARY DISORDERS OF THE COMPLEMENT SYSTEM

Berkel AI, Loos M, Sanal O, et al: Clinical and immunologic studies in a case of selective complete C1q deficiency. Clin Exp Immunol *38*:52, 1979.

Colten HR: Biosynthesis of complement. Adv Immunol *22*:67, 1976.

Corry JM, Polhill RB Jr, Edmonds SR, et al: Activity of the alternate complement pathway after splenectomy: Comparison to activity in sickle cell disease and hypogammaglobulinemia. J Pediatr *95*:964, 1979.

Fearon DT: Complement. J Allergy Clin Immunol *71*:520, 1983.

Fearon DT, Austin KF: The alternate pathway of complement: A system for host defense to microbial infection. N Engl J Med *303*:259, 1980.

Halbwachs L, Leveille M, Lesavre PH, et al: Nephritic factor of the classical pathway of complement: Immunoglobulin G autoantibody directed against the classical pathway C3 convertase enzyme. J Clin Invest *65*:1249, 1980.

Hyatt AC, Altenburger KM, Johnston RB Jr, et al: Increased susceptibility to severe pyogenic infections in patients with an inherited deficiency of the second component of complement. J Pediatr *98*:412, 1981.

Johnston RB Jr: Complement and associated diseases. *In* Behrman RE, Vaughan VC III (eds): Nelson Textbook of Pediatrics. 12th ed. Philadelphia, WB Saunders, 1983, pp 516–518.

Johnston RB Jr, Stroud RM: Complement and host defense against disease. J Pediatr *90*:169, 1977.

Lachman PJ, Rosen FS: Genetic defects of complement in man. Semin Immunopathol *1*:399, 1978.

Sissons JGP, West PJ, Fallows J, et al: The complement abnormalities of lypodystrophy. N Engl J Med *294*:461, 1976.

CHAPTER

17 Allergic Diseases

JERROLD LERMAN, M.D.

URTICARIA AND ANGIOEDEMA

Urticaria and angioedema are cutaneous disorders that may result in fulminant cardiorespiratory collapse during anesthesia. In addition, the anesthesiologist may be called on to assist in the management of acute medical emergencies in these patients.

Urticaria is a cutaneous eruption characterized by diffusely distributed, raised wheals of varying size, shape, and number, which are red or pale in color and blanch under pressure. Urticarial lesions (commonly known as hives) are intensely pruritic and appear within minutes after a trigger stimulus. They usually resolve in 24 hours or less.

Angioedema is a generalized cutaneous eruption characterized by a single giant wheal that is neither erythematous nor pruritic. This lesion may cause a stinging, burning, or tingling sensation. In angioedema, the lesion appears slowly, evolving over a few hours, and resolves slowly over hours or days. Angioedema may occur on any part of the body but is most common on the face, extremities, and genitalia. It may affect the mucous membranes of the upper airway, larynx, bronchi, gastrointestinal tract, and genitourinary tract. If laryngeal edema develops, the presenting signs may include hoarseness, stridor, dyspnea, and respiratory failure. Laryngeal edema, however, is a rare complication of urticaria and angioedema. Angioedema rarely affects the brain and meninges, conjunctiva, cornea, or uveal tract. Systemic angioedema may cause vomiting, diarrhea, and fluid sequestration. Severe fluid and electrolyte imbalance may result in cardiovascular instability and seizures.

The incidence of urticaria and angioedema in infants and children is about 3.4 percent. Up to 20 percent of young adults experience at least one episode of urticaria or angioedema by college age. Urticaria is noted more frequently in patients who have a history of eczema and hay fever; it is 2.5 times more frequent in patients who have a history of asthma.

Urticaria and angioedema may occur either individually or together. When they appear together, urticaria is the predominant skin disorder. The "acute" form of these disorders is defined arbitrarily as an isolated episode lasting less than 6 weeks. The "chronic" form is defined as involving lesions that last 6 weeks or longer. The acute form is commonly a single, nonrecurrent episode that occurs more frequently in atopic children. The chronic form occurs as infrequently as once or twice per year or as often as many times per day. Eighty percent of all cases of urticaria and angioedema are idiopathic, without any known etiology, and 70 percent resolve completely within 1 year (90 percent within 5 years).

The lesions of urticaria and angioedema result

References are arranged under subject headings in the bibliography at the end of the chapter.

from the triple response described by Lewis: first, a red reaction results from precapillary sphincter dilatation; second, an axon reflex results in an erythematous flare from arteriolar dilatation; and third, a wheal is formed by a serum transudate. The triple response is a result of the release of histamine and other mediators from the mast cells and basophils. Many mediators are capable of producing a triple response, including histamine liberators such as anaphylatoxin, trypsin, and acetylcholine and direct effectors such as serotonin, bradykinin, and kallikrein. Histamine is the most important mediator for the formation of urticarial lesions, although acetylcholine is predominant in cholinergic urticaria. In urticaria the lesions occur principally in the dermis, whereas in angioedema the lesions occur in the deep dermal and subcutaneous layers. In urticaria, irritation of the superficial cutaneous nerve endings results in pruritus, whereas in angioedema this does not occur.

PATHOPHYSIOLOGY

The wheals of urticaria and angioedema are transient, evanescent lesions mediated by substances that produce edema, erythema, and pruritus. The most common mediators include histamine, serotonin, bradykinin, eosinophil chemotactic factor of anaphylaxis (ECF-A), arachidonic acid metabolites, and C3 and C5 fragments.

Histamine is released from preformed granules within mast cells and basophils and causes erythema (vasodilation), edema (increased vascular permeability), and pruritus (irritation of the nerve endings). Histamine is also chemotactic for eosinophils. Other factors, such as the metabolites of arachidonic acid, are synthesized and released after the mast cells are stimulated. SRS-A (slow-reacting substance of anaphylaxis) causes bronchial smooth muscle constriction and increases vascular permeability; prostaglandin E_1 (PGE_1) or PGE_2 may cause both pain and the triple response.

Platelet-activating factor (PAF) is also released from mast cells. PAF increases vascular permeability and, more importantly, stimulates the release of serotonin from platelets present at the site of action.

Serotonin is present in platelets in high concentrations. It is released after activation of PAF, which itself is derived from mast cells. Serotonin probably amplifies the principal mast cell degranulation and directly causes erythema.

The importance of SRS-A and PAF in these reactions in humans is not completely understood.

Acetylcholine causes vasodilation and erythema when injected into the dermis. It may modulate mediator release from mast cells, although its role in humans has not been fully elucidated.

The activation of complement is responsible in part for the genesis of the lesions in urticaria and angioedema. Both C3 and C5 are products of complement activation and are potent anaphylatoxins. They adhere to the surface of mast cells (even in the absence of antibodies) and cause the mast cells to degranulate and release histamine. C5a is a more potent anaphylatoxin than C3a. C5a also increases vascular permeability and is a chemotactic factor for neutrophils, eosinophils, and mononuclear cells.

Bradykinin is another important mediator that is released during urticaria and angioedema. Bradykinin is the end-product of a chain of converting enzymes and their products. When a small quantity of Hageman's factor is activated, it in turn activates kallikrein. Kallikrein converts kininogen to the vasoactive peptide bradykinin. Bradykinin is a potent vasodilator and increases vascular permeability to the same extent as histamine. At high serum concentrations, bradykinin may cause profound hypotension. It also irritates nerve endings, causing a burning pain in the area of the lesions.

The vasoactive mediators may be released by one of two mechanisms: immunological or nonimmunological. The immunological mechanism includes the classic type I, II, or III allergic reactions. Type I reactions, the immediate hypersensitivity reactions, are those in which an inhaled, ingested, or parenterally administered trigger binds to IgE on the surface of mast cells and results in the release of histamine and other mediators.

Type II reactions, the cytotoxic mechanism, occur when IgG or IgM binds to an antigen on a cell surface and activates complement. ABO blood type incompatibility is an example of such a reaction. Type III reactions are those in which antigen-antibody complexes (IgG, IgM, or IgA) deposit in target tissues, activate complement, and release mast cell mediators through the action of C3a and C5a. Serum sickness is mediated by such a mechanism.

Nonimmunological stimuli are very important in the pathogenesis of urticaria and angioedema. Table 17–1 lists those important factors considered responsible for this mechanism of action.

The final common pathway for mediator re-

Table 17–1. NONIMMUNOLOGICAL CAUSES OF URTICARIA

Drugs
Food
Physical urticarias
Cold
Cholinergic
Pressure
Dermographia
Solar
Vibratory
Mastocytosis
Hereditary diseases
Hereditary angioedema
C3b inactivator deficiency
Familial cold urticaria
Urticaria, deafness, amyloidosis syndrome
Malignancy
Idiopathic

lease is degranulation of mast cells. The message from cell surface to degranulation follows a series of steps that likely involve changes in membrane potential, cyclic nucleotide concentrations, and sodium and calcium transmembrane fluxes. This is important in the drug management of this disorder.

ETIOLOGY

The etiology of urticaria and angioedema is diverse. A brief description of some of the more relevant causes is given here.

Drugs. The most common cause of urticaria and angioedema is the administration of drugs: oral, rectal, or parenteral. Drugs cause urticaria and angioedema by one of five possible mechanisms: (1) type I IgE hypersensitivity reaction, (2) type III antigen-antibody reaction, (3) direct histamine release from mast cells, (4) complement activation, and (5) alteration in arachidonic acid metabolism.

Those drugs commonly responsible for urticaria and angioedema include codeine, morphine, demerol, penicillin, aspirin and nonsteroidal anti-inflammatory drugs, diuretics, and hormones.

A careful history may give clues about the drug responsible for the urticaria or angioedema. Because more than one drug may be taken concurrently, this may be difficult. All drugs must be stopped if possible and then reintroduced one at a time to determine which is responsible. Skin testing is useful only for IgE-mediated urticaria and angioedema and has many false-positive reactions. The radioallergosorbent test (RAST) measures IgE concentration following administration of a drug. However, this test is available only on a limited basis and has many false-negative results.

Blood. Urticaria and angioedema may occur in response to a blood transfusion, because of (1) ABO incompatibility, (2) type II complement-mediated cytotoxic reaction, (3) type I and III reactions, particularly after administration of fresh-frozen plasma, factor VIII, and cryoprecipitate, and (4) trace concentrations of haptens in the blood.

Food. Food may cause urticaria and angioedema by type I (IgE-mediated) hypersensitivity reaction or through a direct effect on histamine release. Food dyes (tartrazine) and additives such as sodium benzoate are responsible for urticaria in up to 15 percent of patients.

Infections and Infestations. Urticaria and angioedema have been reported after most bronchial, viral, fungal, and parasitic diseases. Viral respiratory infections are a major cause of urticaria in children. Approximately 25 percent of patients with hepatitis and 6 percent with infectious mononucleosis have urticaria during their illnesses. Most infections cause acute urticaria and angioedema; only rarely do infections cause chronic manifestations. Infections may induce urticaria through type III and, less commonly, type I allergic reactions.

Physical Urticarias. Physical stimuli may cause urticaria by releasing histamine, and this effect is reproducible. Other mediators that may be responsible for this type of urticaria include serotonin and ECF-A.

Cold Urticaria and Angioedema. Cold-induced urticaria and angioedema are precipitated by changes in temperature, either warm or cold. The mediators responsible for the reaction include histamine and ECF-A. Cold-induced urticaria and angioedema may occur as isolated lesions or in association with other diseases such as cold agglutination, cryoglobulinemia, cryofibrinogenemia, and paroxysmal hemoglobinemia of the Donath-Landsteiner type. The lesions in cold-induced urticaria may be either focal or diffuse and can be associated with systemic symptoms such as nausea, vomiting, headache, tachycardia, and syncope. To test for cold urticaria, an ice cube is placed on the volar aspect of the forearm for 4 minutes, and the site is observed for 10 minutes. The therapy for cold-induced urticaria is cyproheptadine (Periactin), an antihistamine, in a dose of 0.2 mg/kg/day.

Cholinergic Urticaria. In this type of urticaria, stimuli such as exercise, sweating, heat, and anxiety cause acetylcholine release from parasympathetic (and sympathetic) nerve fibers.

Acetylcholine causes the release of vasoactive mediators such as histamine and ECF-A. Intradermal injection of 100 μl of methacholine will produce a wheal and flare response in patients with cholinergic urticaria. Effective therapy includes hydroxyzine (Atarax), 1 to 3 mg/kg/day in divided doses.

Pressure Urticaria and Angioedema. Pressure-induced urticaria and angioedema occur under the pressure points of the body. Lesions may begin within minutes or up to 24 hours after stimulation. Fever, chills, and nausea may occur in the delayed form. The diagnosis is verified by the appearance of lesions at the sites of pressure. The therapy is to avoid pressure on body points by such techniques as the use of padding. Antihistamines are relatively ineffective, although theophylline and corticosteroids do work in some patients.

Dermographia. This variety of urticaria results from stroking the skin. The wheal and flare response occurs immediately after stroking and resolves within 30 minutes. In approximately 50 percent of patients, dermographia is IgE-mediated. It is seen in 5 percent of normal patients, in some patients with chronic idiopathic urticaria, and in mastocytosis. Therapy for dermographia includes antihistamines.

Melkersson's Syndrome. This rare syndrome is associated with angioedema of the face, peripheral facial nerve palsy, and lingua plicata.

Urticaria-Deafness-Amyloidosis Syndrome. This very rare inherited syndrome begins in adolescence with frequent but brief attacks of an urticaria-like rash. This syndrome is associated with progressive nerve deafness, hyperglobulinemia, nephropathy, and amyloidosis.

Systemic Diseases. A small number of systemic diseases may be associated with urticaria and angioedema. Serum sickness, a type III allergic reaction, is one. Among the many causes of serum sickness are drugs, including penicillin, cephalosporins, and sulfonamides. Serum sickness is usually self-limiting and resolves once the drugs are discontinued.

The connective tissue disorders, juvenile rheumatoid arthritis, acute rheumatic fever, and lupus erythematosus may be associated with the skin lesions of urticaria and angioedema. The patients have multisystemic signs and symptoms associated with the connective tissue disorder, which simplifies the diagnosis of the urticarial lesions.

Urticaria and angioedema may be associated with lymphomas and carcinomas, but there are relatively few cases in the pediatric literature. Urticaria is rarely associated with thyrotoxicosis. Urticaria pigmentosa and systemic mastocytosis are discussed later in the chapter.

Idiopathic Urticaria and Angioedema. Thorough investigation will result in a diagnosis in only 5 to 20 percent of patients. The remainder have chronic urticaria or angioedema of unknown etiology. This disease occurs most frequently in women in their third or fourth decade and is benign, without associated systemic manifestations or complications. It is rare in childhood.

ANESTHETIC MANAGEMENT

Acute self-limited urticaria in patients under anesthesia does not usually require therapy. However, if the urticaria is generalized, immediate management may be required to prevent circulatory and respiratory collapse. This most commonly occurs in hereditary angioneurotic edema. Therapeutic management includes epinephrine, H_1 and H_2 antihistamines, theophylline, and other sympathomimetics. For the drug doses required, refer to the sections on Anaphylaxis, Mastocytosis, and Asthma later in this chapter. H_1 and H_2 blockers may act synergistically to reduce the size of the wheal and flare response to intradermal histamine. However, up to 50 percent of patients do not respond completely to combined H_1 and H_2 antihistamine therapy. Antihistamines bind to the histamine receptors on the effector cells. They reduce the severity of pruritus and the evolving lesions. However, antihistamines do not speed the resolution of lesions that are already present. Steroids have been used with varying success.

Urticaria may occur at the site of intravenous blood transfusion. This reaction may be treated with parenteral H_1 antihistamines. The blood transfusion may be continued. If signs of the systemic manifestations of a transfusion reaction develop, such as fever, cyanosis, hypotension, and oliguria, then the blood transfusion should be stopped and the blood returned to the blood bank for further cross-matching. Resuscitation should include oxygen, H_1 and (if necessary) H_2 antihistamines, sympathomimetics, and fluids.

Preoperative Assessment. The diagnosis of urticaria and angioedema is often made before the anesthesiologist contacts the patient. The precipitating causes and the local and systemic manifestations of the lesions must be carefully enumerated and recorded. Most of the nonsystemic forms manifest local reactions only and do not present life-threatening problems during anesthesia. However, if any of the systemic disorders are responsible for the skin lesions, then a careful history and physical examination for the stigmata of rheumatoid arthritis, lupus erythematosus, lymphoma, carcinoma, and systemic mastocytosis must be performed. In all cases, previous medical records must be obtained to examine the course of the previous anesthetics. Careful questioning to elicit a history of recent steroid administration must be documented on the preoperative record.

Intraoperative Course. The principal goal of the management of patients with urticaria and angioedema under anesthesia is to avoid all trigger stimuli. Those drugs that are known to trigger urticaria should be avoided. Furthermore, it is advisable to avoid those drugs that may release histamine (see the section on Anaphylaxis later in this chapter). If temperature is the trigger of urticaria, then the operating room should be warmed before the patient arrives, and all facilities for maintaining temperature control should be made available. All pressure points should be padded. Specific considerations for patients with systemic illness associated with urticaria depend on the individual disease.

ASTHMA

Asthma is a chronic disorder of the tracheobronchial tree, characterized by paroxysmal increases in airway resistance of varying degree and duration that are partially or totally reversible, either spontaneously or pharmacologically. The defect in asthma is a hyperresponsiveness of the airways to both endogenous and exogenous stimuli. The clinical spectrum of asthma ranges from occasional wheezing to chronic debilitating episodes of airway obstruction and shortness of breath, which may progress in some cases to respiratory failure (status asthmaticus).

Asthma is one of the most common chronic diseases afflicting children. The prevalence varies with age: it is most common in young children, less common in adolescents, and again more common in adults. Asthma affects 0.06 to 12 percent of children in different populations, with a predominance in boys. This large variation may be attributable to differences in geographic location (0.06 percent in Sweden) and in the criteria for diagnosis (12 percent includes those children who wheeze only during respiratory infections). Recent data (1973–1986) suggest that the prevalence of asthma in children 5 to 12 years of age has increased from 5.5 percent in 1973 to 12 percent in 1988 in Wales. Asthma accounts for 11 percent of all chronic diseases in children under 17 years of age and for approximately 23 percent of all school days missed because of chronic diseases in the United States.

About 70 percent of asthmatic children experience wheezing by 3 years of age. Of those children with mild asthma beginning before 10 years of age, most will be symptom-free by adulthood. In contrast, of those children with moderate-to-severe asthma beginning between 3 and 10 years of age, approximately one third will continue to wheeze during adulthood. Some of this latter group may then become incapacitated.

The number of hospital admissions for asthma has been increasing steadily for children less than 14 years of age during the 15-year period from 1970 to 1985. The admission rate for infants and children 0 to 4 years of age slightly exceeded that for children aged 5 to 14 years in 1975, but by 1985 the difference in admission rate was fourfold. This has been attributed to the increasing prevalence of severe asthma in childhood.

Over the past decade, the mortality from asthma around the world has been gradually increasing. Mortality is currently approximately 1.1 per 100,000 children, and is 1 to 2 percent in children with chronic severe asthma. Mortality is more frequent in those under 5 years and between 10 and 14 years of age. The increased mortality in children less than 5 years of age is consistent with the increased hospital admissions for severe asthma in this age group. Although the etiology of this most disturbing trend remains elusive, several possible explanations have been suggested: underestimation of the severity of the asthma, polypharmacy, overdoses with beta-agonists, underusage of corticosteroids, patient education, and other factors.

ETIOLOGY

Asthma may be classified into the following groups based on its causes: (1) extrinsic (allergic), (2) intrinsic (nonallergic, infectious, idiopathic), (3) exercise-induced, (4) aspirin-induced, (5) occupational, and (6) mixed.

Extrinsic Asthma. Extrinsic asthma is caused by either IgE- or cytotoxic IgG-activated mast cell and basophil mediator release (type I allergic reaction). In infants and children, extrinsic asthma may be heralded by atopic dermatitis (eczema), allergic rhinitis, and food intolerance. It is reported to occur in up to 50 percent of infants and children with a history of eczema.

Furthermore, of those children with two mildly atopic parents, 50 percent will have mild atopy, 25 percent will have severe atopy, and 25 percent will be spared. This suggests an autosomal codominant pattern of inheritance. Although skin testing is used to detect allergic tendencies, it may be unreliable, particularly in children under 4 years of age.

Intrinsic Asthma. Intrinsic asthma is a diagnosis of exclusion, in which no allergic etiology is detectable. Intrinsic asthma occurs more commonly in adolescents and adults than in children and is often associated with respiratory tract infections. Asthmatic bronchitis refers to wheezing associated with viral infections, usually in children under 3 years of age. The viruses responsible for these infections in younger children are the respiratory syncytial virus and the parainfluenza B virus; in older children and adults the most common causative viruses are the rhinovirus and influenza A virus.

The mechanism of wheezing during a viral respiratory infection is unclear. Asthmatic bronchitis presents with signs of an upper respiratory infection (rhinorrhea and nasal congestion) that progresses to coughing and wheezing. The characteristic upper respiratory infection usually lasts longer than expected and is more debilitating than expected. Bacterial infections have never been identified as the cause of asthmatic bronchitis in children. Inflammation of the nasal passages and systemic signs such as fever may be present. A significant percentage of children with asthmatic bronchitis progress to asthma.

Intrinsic asthma causes reflex bronchoconstriction, which may be attenuated by inhaled atropine. This suggests that intrinsic asthma may be mediated by a reflex cholinergic pathway. Airways are hyperresponsive to inhalational challenges with methacholine and histamine.

Exercise-Induced Asthma. Exercise-induced asthma (EIA) occurs in 90 percent of children with asthma and 40 percent of children with allergic rhinitis. EIA can occur after as little as 5 minutes of exercise and lasts between 20 minutes and several hours. The mechanism postulated for EIA is a decrease in the temperature of the airways and possibly hyperventilation. This results in the release of mediators and reflex bronchospasm. Patients respond favorably to cromolyn sodium, beta-adrenergic inhalers, and theophylline.

Aspirin-Induced Asthma. This syndrome is a triad of aspirin sensitivity, hyperplastic rhinitis (associated with polyps and sinus infections), and asthma. It is more frequent in adults than in children. Some patients manifest only part of the triad of symptoms. Aspirin tolerance extends to all nonsteroidal anti-inflammatory agents, including tartrazine. Tartrazine (yellow dye No. 5) is present in many foods (ice cream, gelatins, beverages) and drugs. It is prudent to check the contents of all drugs prior to administration in any patient with a known sensitivity to aspirin. The mechanism of aspirin-induced wheezing is unclear, but may be mediated through increased synthesis of prostaglandins (PGF_{2a}, PGD_2) and leukotrienes (including slow-reacting substance of anaphylaxis, SRS-A).

Occupational Asthma. This rare form of asthma is seen infrequently in pediatric practice. Once the patient is removed from the stimulus, the asthma resolves.

Mixed Asthma. Any combination of the preceding forms of asthma may be found in any one individual. Treatment follows the general therapeutic guidelines.

PATHOGENESIS

Airway hyperresponsiveness is the hallmark of asthma. It causes bronchoconstriction in response to a challenge of inhaled, physical, or pharmacological stimuli. There is evidence to suggest that airway hyperreactivity may originate from either an imbalance of the autonomic neural control or mast cell dysfunction. Neural control of the tracheobronchial tree influences the bronchomotor tone through four possible pathways: (1) $beta_2$-adrenergic hyperreactivity, (2) nonadrenergic inhibitory pathways decreasing bronchomotor tone, (3) alpha-adrenergic hyperreactivity, or (4) cholinergic hyperreactivity increasing bronchomotor tone.

Although sympathetic innervation of the tracheobronchial tree is scant, the sympathetic nervous system has a strong influence on bronchomotor tone through the first messenger pathway, hormones. Epinephrine is the most important circulating hormone in asthma. The $beta_2$-adrenergic receptor activates membrane-bound adenyl cyclase to produce 3′5′-cyclic AMP (cAMP) (second messenger). An increase in cAMP exerts two effects on bronchomotor tone: (1) it diminishes the release of mediators from mast cells and basophils, and (2) it decreases the tone of the smooth muscle of the airways. cAMP is metabolized by phosphodiesterase, a pathway that may be pharmacologically important in the mechanism of action of theophylline. It has been suggested that $beta_2$-hyporeactivity may be responsible for bronchial hyperreactivity in asthmatics. Although the cAMP response to beta$_2$-agonist stimulation in some atopic and asthmatic models is blunted, there is no evidence in humans that beta$_2$-hyporesponsiveness is the mechanism responsible for bronchial hyperreactivity.

The nonadrenergic nervous system is an incompletely defined alternate nervous pathway that was recognized first for its ability to relax the gastrointestinal smooth muscle. Activation of this nervous pathway relaxes the smooth muscle of the airway. Although inhibition of this pathway may cause an increase in bronchomotor tone, there is no experimental evidence linking the nonadrenergic pathway to the pathogenesis of asthma in humans.

Alpha-adrenergic stimulation causes a small increase in bronchomotor tone. Airway hyperreactivity in asthma may be in part dependent on an alpha-adrenergic hyperresponsiveness.

The cholinergic pathway, carried by vagal fibers in the lung, primarily controls the tone of the central airways (larynx and bronchi). Stimulation of the cholinergic receptors increases cytoplasmic cGMP (a second messenger). The effects of cGMP are opposite to those of cAMP: cGMP increases the release of mediators from mast cells and basophils, and it increases bronchomotor tone. Inhalation of methacholine (a cholinergic agonist) has been shown to increase bronchomotor tone in the asthmatic patient.

The afferent and efferent pathways for the cholinergic fibers have been well defined. The vagal afferent pathway begins at the irritant receptors in the lung, synapses in the central nervous system, and returns through vagal efferent pathways. This afferent irritant pathway may be important in understanding the mechanism by which drugs and foreign bodies (for example, endotracheal tubes) precipitate rapid reflex increases in bronchomotor tone.

Mast cell dysfunction may result in hyperresponsive airways in allergic patients or in patients with intrinsic asthma. When the membrane surface of the mast cell is activated, a number of intermediary events begin that culminate in the release of the mediators of anaphylaxis: (1) vasoactive mediators: histamine 1, 2, and 3, lipid mediators (platelet-activating factor [PAF] and arachidonic acid metabolites [leukotrienes]), and adenosine; (2) chemoattractant mediators: eosinophil chemotactic factor of anaphylaxis (ECF-A), neutrophil chemotactic factor (NCF-A), and PAF; and (3) enzymatic mediators. PAF is released not only from the mast cell but also from polymorphonuclear leukocytes.

In the asthmatic patient, arachidonic acid is liberated by either phospholipase A_2 or by the action of phospholipase C from membrane phospholipids. Adrenal corticosteroids may reduce bronchospasm by preventing the activation of phospholipase A_2 and thus the release of arachidonic acid. Prostaglandins may be synthesized after activating cyclo-oxygenase, lipoxygenase, H_1 receptors, bradykinin, leukotrienes, prostaglandin-generating factor, and smooth muscle bronchoconstriction. Cyclo-oxygenase metabolizes arachidonic acid into a number of prostaglandins. PGD_2 is the major prostaglandin synthesized in mast cells, and PGE_2 is the major prostaglandin from polymorphonuclear white cells. PGI_2 (prostacyclin) is synthesized in vascular endothelium, and thromboxane A_2 originates in platelets. PGD_2, PGF_2, and thromboxane A_2 cause bronchoconstriction, whereas PGE_2 and PGI_2 cause bronchodilatation. PGD_2 causes vasodilatation. In a parallel pathway, lipoxygenase metabolizes arachidonic acid into leukotrienes C, D, and E. Leukotrienes C_4, D_4, and E_4 combine to form SRS-A, an important mediator of bronchoconstriction. In addition, leukotriene D increases vascular permeability and is a vasodilator, and leukotriene B has chemotactic activity for granulocytes.

Increased cytoplasmic calcium may in part cause bronchial hyperreactivity, although supportive evidence is weak. Verapamil or nifedipine may prove to be of value in the treatment of pediatric asthma.

Mediator Action. Histamine interacts with three receptors: H_1, H_2, and H_3. The H_1 receptor mediates smooth muscle contractile responses and edema formation. The H_2 receptor contributes to mucus secretion and vasodilatation. The H_3 receptor regulates histamine release in the brain and possibly its synthesis in other tissues. Histamine (via H_1 receptors), adenosine, bradykinin, leukotrienes C_4, D_4, and E_4, PGD_2, PGF_2, and thromboxane A_2 all produce bronchoconstriction. Adenosine may augment allergen-induced histamine release. Histamine, bradykinin, leukotrienes C_4, D_4, and E_4, and PGE increase capillary permeability, which reduces intravascular volume and may produce edema, syncope, and, if severe, cardiac arrest. Histamine can stimulate the submucosal glands (via cholinergic receptors). In decreasing order of potency, leukotriene D, leukotriene C, PGF_2, PGD_2, PGI_2, and PGE_1 stimulate secretions of the mucous glands. With prolonged mucus production and bronchoconstriction, desquamated cells of the tracheobronchial tree and secretions may become inspissated (forming Charcot-Leyden crystals) and plug the airways. This may worsen ventilation/perfusion mismatch. Inspissated secretions in the mold of bronchioles (Curschmann's spirals) may be seen if the sputum is examined.

PATHOPHYSIOLOGY

The clinical signs and symptoms of asthma result from a triad of pathophysiological changes in the tracheobronchial tree: (1) a reduction in the diameter of the airways, (2) inflammatory thickening of the bronchial mucosa, and (3) accumulation of tenacious secretions. Bronchospasm results from smooth muscle constriction and causes narrowing of the central airways; it is responsible for most acute episodes of asthma. Chronic inflammation and the accumulation of tenacious secretions also narrow the diameter of the peripheral airways and are responsible for the chronic changes seen in asthma. Because both the pathophysiological changes in the tracheobronchial tree and the primary site of airway involvement vary from child to child, the therapeutic management must be carefully individualized.

The pathophysiological changes in asthma affect all indices of pulmonary function. Because of physiological differences in the respiratory system, children are more susceptible than adults to the effects of asthma on respiratory function. Bronchospasm and the inflammatory airway changes of asthma increase static lung volumes (residual volume, functional residual capacity, and total lung capacity).

Approximately 50 percent of the total airway resistance in infants resides in the peripheral airways, in contrast to only 20 percent in adults. Thus, small changes in the caliber of the peripheral airways will significantly affect the airway resistance in infants; furthermore, the smooth muscle present in the terminal bronchioles of infants may not be responsive to therapeutic drugs or other interventions. Air trapping transiently compensates for the constricted airways by keeping airways open (that is, increasing functional residual capacity above closing volume). Closing volume, however, is proportionally greater in infants than in adults because of the increased chest wall compliance (noncalcified horizontal ribs) and the decreased lung compliance (reduced elastin, a reduced number of alveoli, and compression of the lung by a protuberant abdomen). Because the functional residual capacity is similar in infants and adults, infants are at a disadvantage compared with adults when lung volume falls, because this leads to early airway closure, V/Q mismatch, and intrapulmonary shunting.

Air trapping results in a reduced chest compliance and an increased physiological dead space. It increases the lung volumes and shifts ventilation up the compliance curve where compliance is reduced. This increases the work of breathing, which is compensated to some extent by activation of the accessory muscles of respiration and augmented diaphragmatic activity. The accessory muscles of respiration, however, are poorly developed in the infant and may not respond adequately. In infants, the diaphragm works at a mechanical disadvantage because it is flat and has few fatigue-resistant fibers. As a consequence, the diaphragm of the infant may fatigue much more rapidly than that of the adult. These factors all reduce the pulmonary reserve for gas exchange, predisposing infants and children to pulmonary insufficiency during asthma. The increased work of breathing also increases oxygen consumption and carbon dioxide production. All these problems tend to increase the arterial carbon dioxide tension, worsen ventilation/perfusion mismatch, and decrease arterial oxygenation.

Ventilation/perfusion mismatch results from an altered distribution of ventilation (because of bronchospasm), air trapping, atelectasis from retained secretions, and an increased pulmonary artery pressure. Atelectasis may be prominent in children with asthma because children have smaller airways and a greater concentration of mucous glands than adults. Furthermore, interalveolar and interlobular gas exchange may be impaired because the pores of Kohn and canals of Lambert are poorly developed. The proportionately greater metabolic rate and decreased surface area for gas exchange in infants and children reduce their capacity to tolerate significant increases in ventilation/perfusion mismatch.

Pulmonary artery pressure becomes elevated secondary to the increased pulmonary arteriolar resistance (alveolar vessels) that results from marked air trapping. The increased pulmonary artery pressure may reverse hypoxic pulmonary vasoconstriction and worsen the ventilation/perfusion mismatch. Furthermore, pulmonary hypertension may cause right ventricular strain and cor pulmonale. The reduced cardiac output during hypoxemia and hypercapnia may prove fatal.

PREOPERATIVE MANAGEMENT

HISTORY

The purposes of the preoperative assessment are to develop a clear understanding of the severity of the asthma, to determine whether the child is currently experiencing bronchospasm, and to ascertain whether further therapeutic intervention is warranted before proceeding with anesthesia. All this information is necessary for planning an optimal anesthetic regimen. As in most pediatrics cases, it is imperative that a full history of the child's illness be obtained from the parents.

The anesthesiologist should determine the age of onset of wheezing, the periodicity of the wheezing, and factors associated with the wheezing (such as viral respiratory infections, exercise, cold weather, and eczema). A history of eczema, allergies to food, and allergies to drugs (particularly aspirin) should be obtained; this history should extend back to infancy. If respiratory infections are a recurrent problem, a history of these infections should be taken, indicating their periodicity, the date and duration of the last infection, whether hospital admission was required, and whether continued cough and sputum were present. If cough or sputum is persistent, it is important to know whether either of these symptoms has changed or worsened recently. The association of drug administration with the onset of wheezing should be clarified.

It is important to document the severity of bronchospasm during each attack and the therapy required to relieve the bronchospasm. This should include information on whether the child visited or was admitted to hospital, was placed in intensive care, received drug treatment (with or without parenteral drugs), or required artificial ventilation or intubation.

It is important to review previous anesthetic records, to determine the severity of the asthma prior to and the reactivity of the airways during anesthesia. It is also important to determine whether there were any intraoperative or postoperative anesthetic complications attributable to the asthma.

A detailed history of all recent drug therapy should be obtained. One should determine time course, dose, side effects, and efficacy of all drug therapy. For those children taking aminophylline, monitoring of the blood concentration of theophylline (normal range is 10 to 20 μg/ml) is preferred for judging the adequacy of the therapy. The use of steroids by inhalation or orally must be included in the drug history.

Physical Examination

The physical examination should focus on the respiratory and cardiovascular systems. The child with acute asthma may breathe with nasal flaring, be tachypneic, and be sitting upright, unable to lie down because of shortness of breath. Respiration may be labored and require the use of the sternomastoid accessory muscles. Lower rib flaring may be present. The chest appears hyperinflated, with an increased anteroposterior diameter, and is hyperrespondent to percussion. On auscultation, breath sounds are diminished. High-pitched expiratory wheezing is heard throughout the chest. Occasionally, compression of the chest between the stethoscope and a hand placed on the back produces wheezing in the patient with latent asthma. As the severity of the bronchospasm increases, inspiratory breath sounds disappear, and expiratory wheezing decreases until no air movement is audible. Bronchial breathing may indicate a pneumonic process. The complete absence of air entry on one side of the chest, with hyperresonance, suggests a pneumothorax. The signs of severe acute asthma with impending respiratory failure (hypoxia and hypercapneic narcosis) include central nervous system depression (manifest by glassy-eyed staring, a slow response to auditory or visual stimuli, and confusion) and shallow respirations without audible air entry. Peripheral cyanosis may be present.

The cardiovascular responses to asthma include tachycardia and a weak, thready pulse. Dehydration is not uncommon during an acute asthmatic attack. Pulsus paradoxus (a greater than 10 mm Hg decrease in systolic blood pressure during inspiration) is present with the more severe cases. Occasionally bradycardia occurs.

Chronic hypoxemia and pulmonary hypertension may result in right ventricular strain, cor pulmonale, and cardiovascular collapse. These are rare in children. The signs of right heart failure include an elevated jugular venous pressure, hepatomegaly, hepatojugular reflux, peripheral edema, and pleural effusion. Dehydration, manifested by depressed fontanelles, sunken eyes, dry mouth, loss of skin turgor, and oliguria, may complicate a protracted episode of asthma or chronic respiratory infection.

Laboratory Tests

Hemoglobin and hematocrit are increased in proportion to the degree of chronic hypoxemia and the extent of dehydration. An eosinophil concentration of between 5 and 40 percent may be present. A sample for urinalysis may be difficult to obtain because of oliguria. However, if one can be obtained, it usually has a high specific gravity and often contains protein as a result of infection and fever.

Chest radiographs will indicate hyperinflation (flat diaphragm) and increased lung markings (peribronchial cuffing) and may demonstrate prominent pulmonary arteries, which are indicative of pulmonary hypertension. X-ray films are not usually helpful in the diagnosis of acute exacerbations of asthma. They may, however, be useful in the diagnosis of complications of asthma: atelectasis, pneumonia, pneumothorax, pneumomediastinum, or pleural effusions.

In mild asthma, the arterial blood gas levels may indicate mild hypocapnia and hypoxemia at rest. In severe cases, hypercapnia, respiratory acidosis, and occasionally metabolic acidosis may occur.

The electrocardiogram may indicate right bundle branch block, atrial or ventricular premature beats, right ventricular hypertrophy pattern, or cor pulmonale.

Pulmonary function testing (PFT) is usually restricted to children over 6 years of age and often involves only spirometry. Such testing in asthma will indicate an obstructive pattern during episodes of acute asthma, with increases in lung volumes (RV, FRC, TLC) and decreases in flow rates (FEV_1, FVC) and lung compliance. A minimum increase of 10 to 15 percent in flow rates after bronchodilator therapy indicates reversibility of the disease. Flow volume loops may be used to indicate reductions in both static lung volumes and flow rates and to differentiate wheezing from other causes.

Drug Therapy

Bronchodilators and anti-inflammatory drugs may be administered by four routes: orally, rectally, parenterally, or inhalation. Oral administration is restricted to therapy for chronic asthma. This route of drug administration suffers from the problems of incomplete gastrointestinal absorption and the first-pass effect of the liver. The rectal route is rarely used for the treatment of asthma in North America. Parenteral administration is useful during anesthesia. Aminophylline, isoproterenol, and steroids are the only bronchodilators currently administered by this route. Bronchodilators also may be delivered to their site of action by inhalation. This path is direct, maximizes the concentration of drug at the site of action, and minimizes systemic side effects. Inhalants are available in either a prepared aerosol delivered via a fluorocarbon propellant generator or a liquid form delivered by jet nebulizer. The prepared aerosol is more difficult to administer to smaller children, but both preparations may be used during anesthesia.

The mass median aerodynamic diameter of aerosols should be approximately 3.5 to 5 μm for bronchial deposition. The dose of bronchodilators required for maximal bronchodilatation is unknown, although the total dose delivered to the lung determines the responses.

Sympathomimetic drugs comprise first-line drug therapy for the treatment of mild asthma. As symptoms increase in frequency, cromoglycate or nedocromil may be added. If cromoglycate and nedocromil are ineffective, inhaled steroids may be substituted. As the severity of the asthma increases, theophylline may be added to the treatment regimen.

Beta-Agonists. The beta-agonist sympathomimetics are among the most commonly used bronchodilators. Beta-agonist drugs combine with the membrane-bound receptors to activate magnesium-dependent cAMP and convert ATP to cAMP. This prevents the release of the stored mediators of bronchoconstriction. Beta-receptors are divided into two types: $beta_1$, responsible for chronotropy, inotropy, and lipolysis; and $beta_2$, responsible for smooth muscle relaxation (bronchodilatation, vasodilatation), attenuating histamine release, increasing mucociliary clearance, and skeletal muscle tremor.

The preferred bronchodilators should activate $beta_2$-receptors and exert minimal effects on the $beta_1$-receptors. Sympathomimetic bronchodilators are divided into several categories: catecholamines, noncatecholamines, resorcinols, saligenins, and others (Table 17–2).

Bronchodilators are delivered by oral, inhalational, and parenteral routes. The parenteral route is limited to administration of the catecholamines (epinephrine), albuterol (Canadian), and theophylline. The oral route is reserved primarily for theophylline. Most beta-agonist medication is administered by inhalation. Two delivery systems may be used: pressurized aerosol canister (metered-dose inhaler, MDI) or jet nebulizer. Although many held that the latter was more effective than the former in children, recent evidence disputes this notion. MDI aerosols contain a beta-agonist, a fluorocarbon, and a surfactant (oleic acid or lecithin) pressurized to 400 kPa. Actuation of a canister ejects a fixed dose of beta-agonist that is inhaled by the patient. Most aerosol is deposited in the oropharynx or is exhaled; less than 10 percent reaches the lower airways in adults and even less in children and infants. Two different methods of inhaler placement are used: open and

Table 17–2. STRUCTURE-FUNCTION RELATIONSHIPS OF ADRENERGIC BRONCHODILATORS

Classification Generic Name, Proprietary Name	Molecular Structure	Major Receptor Activity	Current Availability: *Oral*	*Inhale*	*Inject*	Approximate Duration of Effect (Hr)
Ephedrine	–CH–CH–NH–CH_3; OH, CH_3	α,β_1,β_2	TAB LIQ	No	No	2–3
Catecholamines						
Epinephrine Adrenalin Primatine Mist Bronkaid Mist	HO, HO–; –CH–CH_2–NH–CH_3; OH	α,β_1,β_2	No	MDI	Yes	<1
Isoproterenol Isuprel Medihaler-Iso Norisodrine	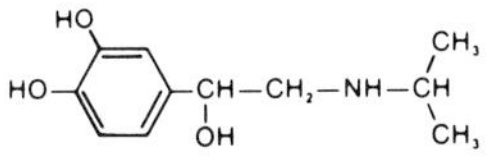 HO, HO–; –CH–CH_2–NH–CH(CH_3)(CH_3); OH	β_1,β_2	TAB LIQ	MDI NEB	Yes	1–2
Isoetharine Bronkosol Bronkometer	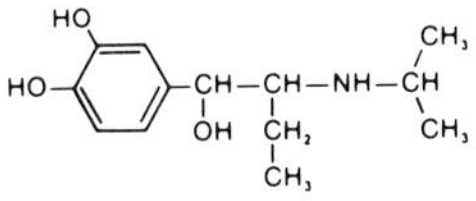 HO, HO–; –CH–CH–NH–CH(CH_3)(CH_3); OH, CH_2–CH_3	$(\beta_1),\beta_2$	No	MDI NEB	No	3
Resorcinols						
Metaproterenol Alupent Metaprel	HO, HO; –CH–CH_2–NH–CH(CH_3)(CH_3); OH	β_2	TAB LIQ	MDI NEB	No	3–5
Terbutaline Brethine Brethaire Bricanyl	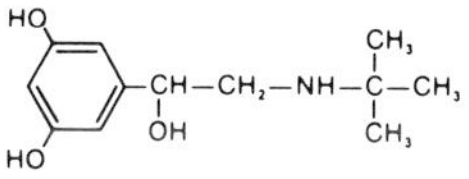 HO, HO; –CH–CH_2–NH–C(CH_3)(CH_3)–CH_3; OH	β_2	TAB LIQ*	MDI	Yes	4–6
Fenoterol Berotec	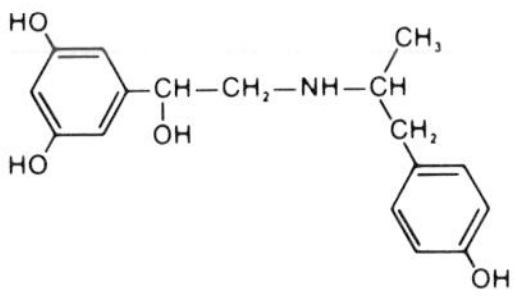 HO, HO; –CH–CH_2–NH–CH(CH_3)–CH_2–(ring)–OH; OH	β_2	No	MDI*	No	4–6
Saligenin						
Albuterol Proventil Ventolin	CH_2OH, HO–; –CH–CH_2–NH–C(CH_3)(CH_3)–CH_3; OH	β_2	TAB LIQ	MDI Powder NEB	Yes*	4–6
Miscellaneous						
Bitolterol Tornalate	CH_3–(ring)–O–C–O–; CH_3–(ring)–O–C–O–(ring)–CH–CH_2–NH–C(CH_3)(CH_3)–CH_3; OH	β_2	No	MDI NEB*	No	6–8
Pirbuterol Maxair	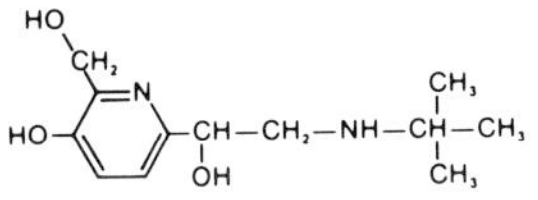 HO–CH_2, =N, HO–; –CH–CH_2–NH–CH(CH_3)(CH_3)–CH_3; OH	β_2	No	MDI	No	4–6
Procaterol Pro-Air	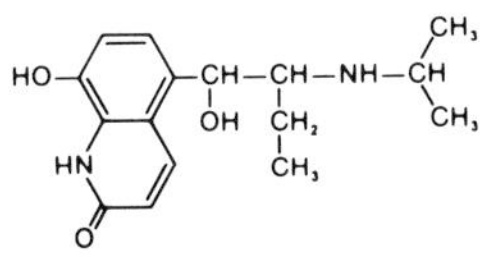 HO–; HN, O; –CH–CH–NH–CH(CH_3)(CH_3); OH, CH_2–CH_3	β_2	TAB* LIQ*	MDI*	No	6–8

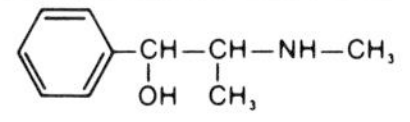

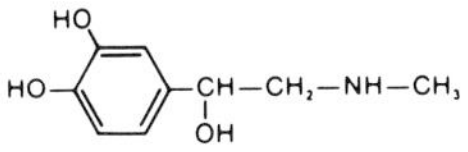

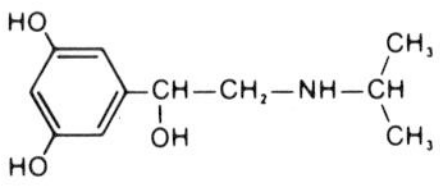

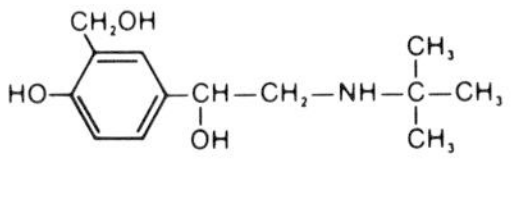

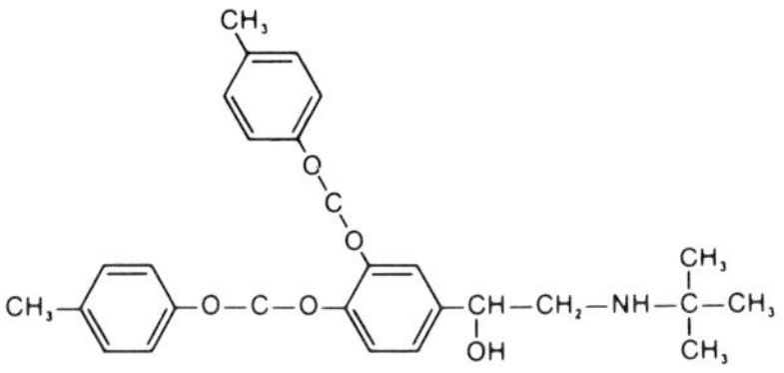

*Not currently available in the United States.

TAB = tablet; LIQ = liquid, syrup, or suspension; MDI = metered dose inhaler; NEB = nebulizer solution.

Reprinted from Meltzer DL, Kemp JP: $Beta_2$-agonists: Pharmacology and recent developments. J Asthma *28*:179, 1991, by courtesy of Marcel Dekker, Inc., N.Y.

closed mouth. Each has its own advantages and disadvantages. More recently, spacers have become available to increase the proportion of small-diameter aerosol delivered to the lung. As concerns for the impact of chlorofluorocarbons on the ozone layer increase, pressurized canisters are gradually being replaced by negative pressure–activated powder canisters. These may prove to be somewhat more difficult for infants and children less than 2 years of age.

Paradoxical bronchoconstriction has been reported after inhalation of beta-agonists. This has occurred after both MDI aerosols and nebulized solutions. This effect has been attributed to the nonactive ingredients in the inhalant: chlorofluorocarbons, surfactant, and, for nebulized solutions, osmolarity of and preservatives in bronchodilator solution.

Catechols. Epinephrine, isoproterenol, and isoetharine are 3,4-dihydroxybenzene rings with substituted amine side chains. Bulky substitutions on the *N*-terminus of the side chain increase their beta activity and decrease their alpha activity. Bulky substitutions on the carbons on the side chains decrease $beta_1$ activity to a greater extent than $beta_2$ activity. The catechols are inactivated by reuptake into the presynaptic membrane and metabolized to a lesser extent by the monoamine oxidase (MAO) enzymes and catechol-*O*-methyl transferase (COMT). Because of the presence of MAO in the gastrointestinal tract, catechols are inactivated by metabolic pathways when the drugs are ingested.

Epinephrine has alpha, $beta_1$, and $beta_2$ activity, although $beta_2$ activity is the primary beta effect in vivo. In addition to the beta activity, the alpha activity shrinks mucosal congestion. The *l*-isomer is considered to be the active form. The dose of epinephrine for adults is 0.1 to 0.3 ml of 1:1000 solution and for children, 0.02 to 0.10 ml/kg of 1:10,000 solution (2 to 10 μg/kg) administered subcutaneously. This dose can be repeated every 30 minutes. The onset of bronchodilatation occurs within 5 to 10 minutes and lasts up to 60 minutes. Subcutaneous and intravenous epinephrine are reserved for acute, severe asthmatic episodes and allergic reactions. Epinephrine should not be administered intravenously for the treatment of acute bronchospasm without intensive monitoring because of the high risk of ventricular fibrillation and cardiac arrest.

Isoproterenol is a catechol devoid of alpha activity because of the bulky *N*-terminus substitutions. It has both $beta_1$ and $beta_2$ properties but is dose-limited because of its $beta_1$ chronotropic stimulation. Its short duration of action is caused by reuptake and metabolism by COMT. Isoproterenol may be administered by inhalation (0.5 ml of 0.5 to 1 percent solution); in this form it has an onset of action within 1 to 2 minutes, peaks within 5 minutes, and lasts for 10 to 30 minutes. When it is administered by the intravenous route to children, an initial infusion dose of 0.1 μg/kg/min is recommended. The dose is increased until either the bronchospasm is relieved or the heart rate reaches 200 beats per minute. The intravenous regimen for isoproterenol has been found to be very effective in children with severe asthmatic episodes and borderline respiratory failure within the intensive care setting. Caution must be exercised when using isoproterenol by inhalation, since rebound bronchospasm, ventricular fibrillation, and death have been reported.

Isoetharine, which contains a substituted side chain, has one tenth the $beta_2$ activity and one three hundredth the $beta_1$ activity of isoproterenol. It is metabolized primarily by COMT and is resistant to MAO enzymes. It is available by aerosol only (340 μg/puff). One to four puffs every 4 hours should provide a therapeutic response. Peak activity is at 15 minutes, and duration is less than 2 hours.

Noncatecholamines. Ephedrine is a noncatecholamine sympathomimetic with alpha, $beta_1$, and $beta_2$ activity. Because its mechanism of action is predominantly indirect (through the release of norepinephrine), the effects of ephedrine decrease with frequently repeated doses. It is associated with a significant incidence of side effects, including central nervous system irritability (headaches, tremors, restlessness, and weakness), palpitations, tachycardia, and hypertension. Although ephedrine is currently used, newer $beta_2$ selective bronchodilators are slowly replacing it. The dosage of oral ephedrine ranges from 15 to 45 mg, depending on the age of the patient. The time of action is from 30 minutes to 3 hours. Seventy percent of ephedrine is excreted in the urine unchanged.

Resorcinols. The resorcinols include metaproterenol, terbutaline, and fenoterol. Metaproterenol (Alupent or orciprenalin) is a 3,5-dihydroxyphenyl group with a bulky amine substituted side chain. This combination confers $beta_2$ receptor selectivity, although the overall beta activity is 10 to 40 times less than that of isoproterenol. Metaproterenol may be taken orally (10 to 20 mg for an adult), with a duration of action of 2 to 5 hours; by inhalation from a pressurized canister (650 μg/puff), up to 8 puffs per day for an adult; or by nebulized aerosol (metaproterenol sulfate 5 percent) 0.01 and 0.02 ml/kg in preschool children. The puff delivery has a very rapid onset of action. This drug, like all resorcinols, is resistant to metabolism by COMT and MAO. Metaproterenol has equivalent bronchodilating activity to isoproterenol but produces more cardioacceleration than other $beta_2$ selective agents.

Terbutaline is a synthetic resorcinol that is similar in structure to metaproterenol. The tertiary butyl substitution on the *N*-terminal side chain further reduces the $beta_1$ activity. Compared with metaproterenol, terbutaline is twice as potent a bronchodilator, with double the duration of action and fewer side effects. Terbutaline has been effective in combination with theophylline, although seizures have been reported. Terbutaline causes skeletal muscle tremor and sinus tachycardia, and, if given parenterally, myocardial ischemia, ventricular tachycardia, and pulmonary edema. Terbutaline is available for oral use (2.5 to 5 mg per day for children over 12 years of age) or for subcutaneous use (0.25 mg every 30 minutes to a maximum of 0.5 mg within 4 hours).

Fenoterol hydrobromide (Berotec) is a synthetic sympathomimetic similar to metaproterenol, with a 4-hydroxyphenyl substitution on the *N*-terminal side chain. Compared with ephedrine, fenoterol has a faster onset of action and a longer duration of activity and is a more potent bronchodilator. When compared with salbutamol and terbutaline, fenoterol has more $beta_1$-agonist activity. It is available by inhalation at 200 μg/puff; one puff has approximately four times the bronchodilator effect of 1 puff of salbutamol. Optimal bronchodilation occurs after 5 mg by mouth, with a peak action at 2 hours and a duration of 6 hours. Side effects include tachycardia and tremor.

Several recent studies have focused on the possible relationship between $beta_2$-agonist inhalants and death. As with isoproterenol, some have proposed that the increasing death rate from asthma may be due to the beta-agonist fenoterol. Despite the attractiveness of this explanation, others continue to pursue other explanations.

Saligenins. Salbutamol (Ventolin, albuterol) has a molecular structure similar to that of isoproterenol, with a $CH_2(OH)$ substitution at position 3 of the benzene ring. This has the effect of reducing the beta activity, $beta_1$ more than $beta_2$. Salbutamol is devoid of alpha activity. It is almost as potent a bronchodilator as isoproterenol and has only 10 to 20 percent of the chronotropic effect. Salbutamol may be administered by inhalation, 100 μg per puff, 1 to 2 puffs every 4 hours (maximum 8 puffs per day). It has a maximal effect within 15 minutes and a duration of up to 5 hours. Orally, it can be taken at 1 to 4 mg every 6 to 8 hours in adults and has a maximal effect after 2 to 4 hours. Nebulized salbutamol appears to be effective in children, including those less than 2 years of age. In children 5 to 17 years of age with severe, acute asthma, 0.15 mg/kg of nebulized salbutamol every 20 minutes for successive doses was no more effective than a lower dose of 0.05 mg/kg.

Salbutamol has minimal chronotropic side effects. However, when it is administered orally, it may cause tremor, loss of appetite, headache, and nausea. Excessive use or overdose may cause electroencephalographic abnormalities and convulsions. When albuterol is administered by aerosol, tremor is common. However, the severity of the tremor in children 4 to 14 years usually requires no therapy.

In studies comparing salbutamol, terbutaline, and metaproterenol, all three were found to be effective when taken orally, although metaproterenol exhibited less $beta_2$ selectivity than the other two. Skeletal muscle tremors were reported after all three drugs when they were given orally but not after they were given by the inhalational route; this direct $beta_2$ effect varies among patients and the three drugs.

Theophylline. Theophylline, a dimethylated xanthine, has been a principal drug in the treatment of asthma. However reevaluation of its effects in acute asthma using meta-analysis failed to support its role as a primary therapeutic modality. In contrast, its role in chronic asthma appears justified.

It has been suggested that theophylline may relieve bronchospasm by relaxing bronchial smooth muscle. Four possible mechanisms of action have been proposed: (1) inhibition of phosphodiesterase (increasing cAMP), (2) decrease in cytosolic intracellular calcium concentration, (3) inhibition of adenosine bronchoconstriction, and (4) antagonism of prostaglandin synthesis. However, theophylline does not act by the first two pathways at serum levels of less than 50 μg/ml. Adenosine inhibition is currently believed to be the primary mechanism in bronchodilation.

Theophylline affects many organ systems. It increases diaphragmatic contractility and sensitizes the brain stem to carbon dioxide. This latter effect is used to prevent apnea in premature infants. Theophylline increases cerebrovascular resistance, decreases cerebral blood flow, and stimulates the central nervous system, causing irritability, tremors, and seizures. At serum concentrations greater than 15 μg/ml, theophylline triggers the vomiting center.

Theophylline affects the cardiovascular system by increasing chronotropy and by inducing arrhythmias at high serum concentrations. It dilates both the coronary vessels and peripheral arteriolar and venous vessels and also increases both right and left ventricular contractility. It dilates the renal arteries and causes a transient diuresis. At the neuromuscular junction, theophylline antagonizes the nondepolarizing blockade by pancuronium.

Serum concentrations above 20 μg/ml are toxic. The toxic side effects increase in proportion to the serum concentration. At concentrations below 20 μg/ml, theophylline induces minor gastrointestinal upset and central nervous system irritation. These minor disturbances usually subside within 7 to 10 days of therapy. At concentrations between 20 and 35 μg/ml, toxic side effects of headache, nausea, irritability, insomnia, vomiting, gastric bleeding, and diarrhea are seen. Above 35 μg/ml, seizures, cardiac arrhythmias, and death are not uncommon.

Severe toxicity and death may occur in sick children receiving excess intravenous or rectal theophylline. The symptoms of irritability may suddenly progress to seizures and brain damage. However, seizures may occur without prior signs of impending toxicity. The mechanism of brain damage may be severe cerebral vasoconstriction with the associated neuronal hypoxia. These toxic effects are enhanced in the presence of ephedrine.

Mild seizures may respond to diazepam, phenytoin (Dilantin), phenobarbital, or thiopentone. However, at higher serum concentrations, theophylline-induced seizures may be resistant to all forms of therapy. The definitive preventive management is to maintain serum levels below 20 μg/ml.

Markedly increased serum concentrations should be treated first by stopping the theophylline. Whether theophylline was administered orally or intravenously, the stomach may be lavaged with charcoal every 4 hours to remove it. A persistently increased serum concentration may be reduced by charcoal hemoperfusion or, less efficiently, by peritoneal dialysis. Protracted vomiting from toxic concentrations of theophylline may result in dehydration in children. Vomiting, dehydration, and a renal diuresis together suggest toxicity.

Cardiac arrhythmias occur less commonly in children than in adults. Tachycardia, ventricular ectopic beats, and severe hypotension (especially following infusion through a central venous line) may occur. Ventricular ectopic beats respond to cessation of the theophylline and intravenous lidocaine.

The pharmacokinetics of theophylline are well known. The optimal bronchodilator effect of theophylline occurs between serum concentrations of 10 and 20 μg/ml, although some patients have full therapeutic benefit from serum concentrations as low at 5 μg/ml, particularly following acute loading doses. The volume of distribution is fairly constant: 0.6 L/kg in neonates and premature infants, and 0.45 L/kg in children and adults. Theophylline freely crosses the placenta and reaches 90 percent of the serum concentration in the cerebrospinal fluid of premature infants. Approximately 40 percent is albumin-bound in neonates, compared with 60 percent in older age groups. Ninety percent is eliminated by the microsomal mixed-function oxidase enzyme system in the liver. Metabolism is reduced in premature infants and neonates to approximately 50 percent that in adults and is greatest in older children and adolescents. There is no first-pass effect by the liver. The remaining 10 to 15 percent of theophylline is excreted unchanged by the kidney.

Theophylline clearance is reduced in neonates, in patients with heart and liver failure or severe pneumonia, and in association with the administration of cimetidine, propranolol, erythromycin, and macrolide antibiotics. In animals, hypercapnia or hypoxia reduces metabolism. In patients in whom clearance is decreased, the dose should be reduced. In contrast, in patients receiving phenobarbital or intravenous infusions of isoproterenol, the clearance of theophylline may be increased. However, this latter effect may not be of major clinical importance.

Theophylline is available in a wide variety of preparations for oral, rectal, and intravenous administration. Slow-release oral preparations (elixirs, uncoated tablets, and bead-filled capsules [50 or 60 mg each]) and rectal solutions may be administered every 6 to 8 hours to infants or every 4 to 6 hours to children and adults with high metabolic rates. Children may use the elixirs or the bead-filled capsules sprinkled over their food. Uncoated tablets should be given only to older children. If the tablets are crushed, the absorption of theophylline may be increased. Rectal solutions are useful because they are packaged with a calibrated syringe for accurate dosing. They may be used preoperatively in patients who are fasting or vomiting and can be repeated but should be stopped after

36 hours of continuous therapy because of the mucosal irritation that may occur from the alkaline pH of the solutions. Suppositories of theophylline are erratically and incompletely absorbed and are not recommended.

If theophylline is required during anesthesia to relieve bronchospasm in a patient who had not received the drug recently, then 7.5 mg/kg should be given intravenously over 15 to 30 minutes. This will provide a serum concentration of approximately 15 μg/ml. If the loading dose is administered too rapidly, transient toxic serum concentrations may result. If the patient had received theophylline recently and still develops bronchospasm, then a blood sample should be taken for serum concentration, and 2.5 mg/kg should be administered over 30 minutes. After an appropriate loading dose is administered, therapeutic serum concentrations should be maintained by infusion at the rates listed in Table 17–3.

Serum theophylline concentrations should be monitored serially after 4 to 6 hours of therapy and every 12 hours until stable serum concentrations are achieved.

Enprofylline (propylxanthine) is a new, potent bronchodilator with fewer side effects than theophylline has. Seizures and cardiac arrhythmias are less common with enprofylline, although headaches have been common. This drug is currently under investigation and not available for clinical use.

New Beta-Agonists. Three new beta-agonists will be available in the near future. Procaterol (see Table 17–2) is the most potent bronchodilator, being ten times more potent than comparable agonists. It will be available for administration by oral and inhalational routes. There are no clinical data supporting its superiority over comparable agonists. Future development in beta-agonist bronchodilator therapy is not likely to focus on increased potency but rather on longer duration of action and fewer side effects. Two new beta-agonists, formoterol and salmeterol, have two to three times the duration of action of currently available agonists. Formoterol is 5 to 15 times more potent than salbutamol when administered by inhalation. It is available as 12 and 24 μg/puff. In studies in older children, it proved to be superior to salbutamol as a long-acting bronchodilator in childhood asthma. The role of these new drugs in the management of childhood asthma will await the results of clinical trials.

Table 17–3. INFUSION RATES TO MAINTAIN THERAPEUTIC SERUM THEOPHYLLINE LEVELS

	Theophylline (mg/kg/hr)
Neonates	0.13
Infants (2–6 mos)	0.4
Infants (6–11 mos)	0.7
Children (1–9 yrs)	0.8
Children (9–16 yrs) to adults (smokers)	0.6
Adults (nonsmoking, healthy)	0.4
Elderly and adults with cor pulmonale	0.25
Cardiac failure, liver dysfunction	0.1

Corticosteroids. Corticosteroids are second-line drug therapy for the treatment of asthma and are indicated for failure of conventional therapy (optimal inhaled aerosols and aminophylline); for acute exacerbations of asthma, including status asthmaticus; or for chronic asthma (1 to 10 percent of children with asthma), or to reduce the dose of the first-line bronchodilators. They modify bronchospasm by four possible mechanisms: (1) potentiating the beta-adrenergic system, (2) inhibiting the release of the mediators of bronchoconstriction and inflammation, (3) changing leukocyte kinetics and function, and (4) thinning mucus and reducing mucosal edema. The importance of steroids in asthma and anesthesia relates to (1) the treatment of severe asthma in the perioperative period, and (2) protection against relative hypoadrenalism during anesthesia.

Corticosteroids may be administered to children by three routes: oral, inhalation, and parenteral. Oral administration of steroids may be indicated for one of two reasons: daily steroids for a brief period after an acute exacerbation and alternate-day oral therapy for continued use. The oral steroid preparation is usually prednisone, which is available in a syrup (1 mg/ml) for children. It is administered in the morning as a single daily dose to minimize adrenal suppression. The usual dose for acute exacerbations is about 30 mg (1 to 2 mg/kg) for a 10-year-old for 1 week and then gradually tapered over a 10-day period. Although prednisone, 7.5 mg/m^2/day, usually causes minimal side effects, doses as small as 4 to 6 mg/m^2/day have been reported to suppress growth. Alternate-day prednisone in a single morning daily dose is less likely to suppress adrenal function or cause growth retardation, osteoporosis, or cushingoid symptoms.

Several formulations of corticosteroids for inhalation are available. These include beclomethasone dipropionate, budesonide, triamcinolone, and flunisolide. The choice of corticosteroid is determined in part by its relative risk-benefit ratio. This ratio depends on the topical-to-systemic potency (i.e., the more systemic effects, the greater risk). The relative topical-to-systemic potency is budesonide>beclomethasone>flunisolide ≈ triamcinolone. Because of systemic side effects, these drugs are not recommended for first-line antiasthmatic therapy in children. However, in moderate-to-severe asthma, inhaled corticosteroids are recognized as very beneficial and recommended for optimal therapy.

Beclomethasone dipropionate (BD) (Beclovent) is the most commonly used steroid aerosol. BD is administered by inhalation to the tracheobronchial tree and is rapidly absorbed. Approximately 59 μg of BD is available per puff, and of this, 50 percent reaches the airways. The other 50 percent is swallowed and may be absorbed through the gastrointestinal tract. There is a significant first-pass metabolism in the liver. It has been suggested that less than 1000 μg daily is required for the maximal steroid effect. Systemic absorption is reported to be minimal with BD, with few systemic effects when the dose is restricted to less than 1000 μg. However, adrenal-hypothalamic axis suppression has been reported with doses in excess of 400 μg daily in children but not at prescribed doses of ≤ 400 μg daily. It has been suggested that doses of less than 13 μg/kg/day of BD do not suppress the adrenal-hypothalamic axis. A similar degree of adrenal suppression is seen with 20 to 40 mg of prednisone every other day. Local side effects commonly reported include oral and esophageal moniliasis and hoarseness. My opinion is that additional preoperative parenteral steroids should be used in children receiving steroids by inhalation.

Budesonide has a greater topical-to-systemic potency ratio than has BD, although its clinical superiority over BD has not been clearly established. Few studies compared beclomethasone with flunisolide and none with triamcinolone in adults. There are no comparisons in children.

Parenteral steroids may be useful in the treatment of acute asthma and status asthmaticus. However, steroids may need at least 3 to 4 hours for the onset of action and up to 24 hours to improve pulmonary function (FEV_1). The delayed action is consistent with the time that may be required for protein synthesis. Steroid therapy for an acute attack should begin with a short-acting form such as hydrocortisone, 1 to 2 mg/kg bolus, followed by 0.5 mg/kg/h, or methylprednisolone, 2 to 3 mg/kg/day in four divided doses. Therapy should be continued for 24 hours, at which time an oral preparation should be introduced (1 to 2 mg/kg of prednisone) as one daily dose in the morning. This should be continued for 5 to 7 days and then tapered over 7 to 10 days.

Prophylactic steroids should be administered in the perioperative period if the child is currently receiving steroids or has taken steroids for at least 1 week in the previous 6 months. During the stress of operation, adrenal steroid production may increase two- to sevenfold. Patients who are receiving steroids or recently (less than 1 year ago) received steroids may be unable to mount an adrenal response to the stress of surgery and develop relative adrenal insufficiency. To prevent hypotension and shock, parenteral steroids should be administered. One successful regimen is 1.5 mg/kg of hydrocortisone as a slow intravenous infusion in the preoperative period, followed by the same dose every 8 hours. Recently, this dose of steroids has been reduced to hydrocortisone, 0.4 mg/kg in the preoperative period, followed by an intravenous infusion of 1.5 mg/kg over 24 hours. This infusion is then tapered over the subsequent 72 hours.

Steroids are required because the adrenergic receptors of vascular smooth muscle are hyporesponsive to catecholamines. Consequently, if the blood pressure falls, the vascular smooth muscle is unable to compensate by constricting. Parenteral steroids enhance the vascular smooth muscle response to catecholamines and prevent or reverse the hypotension.

Cromolyn. Cromolyn sodium, a sodium salt of the bis-cromones, is believed to prevent bronchospasm by inhibiting mediator release from mast cells, although the precise mechanism is unclear. It has no direct bronchodilating properties nor direct sympathomimetic activity and is effective only when given prophylactically, that is, before mediator release. Because cromolyn is not lipid-soluble, it is poorly absorbed (approximately 1 percent) by the gastrointestinal tract. It is administered by inhalation only in asthma. Two vehicles are available: the turbo-inhaler and the pressurized canister. The turbo-inhaler delivery system is difficult for young children with asthma to use; therefore it had limited application until a nebulized form of cromolyn solution (20 mg in a 1 percent solution) became available.

Approximately 10 percent of cromolyn is absorbed from the distal airways in the lung. It has an onset of action of 10 to 20 minutes, and a duration of action of approximately 6 hours. Its action is terminated by excretion of the unchanged drug in the urine (50 percent) and in the liver (50 percent). Cromolyn is optimally effective when administered 10 minutes prior to the stimulus.

Cromolyn is a very safe drug with a very low incidence of side effects, which include hyperventilation, hoarseness, dry mouth, nasal congestion, and rarely bronchospasm. Other rare side effects include nausea, vomiting, facial dermatitis, and joint swelling. Hypersensitivity to cromolyn powder may present as laryngeal edema, urticaria, angioedema, or anaphylaxis. There have been no reports of hematological, renal, or hepatic dysfunction from its use in children.

Cromolyn is indicated for prophylaxis against exercise-induced, IgE-mediated, and intrinsic asthmas, as well as type III delayed reactions. Although cromolyn reduces the theophylline requirement in children with asthma, it is not indicated for the treatment of acute asthma or status asthmaticus already in evolution.

Contraindications to cromolyn sodium include known hypersensitivity to the drug and eosinophilic pneumonitis.

Ketotifen. Ketotifen, a benzocycloheptathiophen derivative, is an antiasthmatic and antianaphylactic drug that is effective as a prophylactic agent only. Ketotifen may act by antagonizing histamine, inhibiting phosphodiesterase, blocking calcium channels, inhibiting mediator release, or antagonizing slow-reacting substance of anaphylaxis (SRS-A). It is effective in reducing bronchoconstriction in patients with allergic and aspirin-induced asthma. In children, 1 mg/kg of ketotifen may be effective when administered orally twice daily, although one recent study in children 1 to 3 years old failed to prove its effectiveness over placebo. In one study, there were no side effects or complications from this drug. Ketotifen appears to be effective in preventing asthma in children.

Anticholinergics. The use of anticholinergic agents in pediatric asthma is limited. They may reduce bronchomotor tone in the central airways (as described earlier), mucous gland secretions, and the size of the bronchial vascular bed. To effect these changes, anticholinergic drugs are administered by intravenous or intramuscular injection or by inhalation. Intravenous or intramuscular atropine (0.01 to 0.02 mg/kg) is commonly used by pediatric anesthesiologists for preventing bradycardia and drying secretions in the airways. However, the parenteral use of atropine in the treatment of chronic asthma is both impractical because of its short half-life and complicated with extensive side effects. Anticholinergic agents for bronchospasm are available by inhalation (Sch 1000 or ipratropium bromide), and these have fewer side effects than parenteral atropine. Ipratropium bromide has been shown to be effective for asthma triggered by irritant inhalation and in 50 percent of patients with exercise-induced asthma. Glycopyrrolate has also been used by inhalation in asthma with similar success.

Atropine causes a dose-related toxicity leading to tachycardia, restlessness, headache, constipation, urine retention, dry and hot skin, delirium, coma and arrhythmias, which may culminate in death. Ingestion of 10 mg of atropine has been fatal in children. I believe that an absolute maximal dose of oral or parenteral atropine in children is approximately 50 μg/kg in divided doses.

The dose of nebulized ipratropium bromide is about 50 μg/kg in children. Ipratropium bromide produces comparable bronchodilatation when compared with isoproterenol and metaproterenol by inhalation. The side effects of ipratropium are fewer compared with parenteral atropine. Xerostomia is a common complaint. Ipratropium bromide, in contrast to the beta-blockers, does not cause tremor or restlessness in recommended doses.

ANESTHETIC MANAGEMENT

During the preoperative visit, a decision about whether or not to proceed with surgical therapy is made. If the operation is elective and the child has not been optimally treated for asthma, then it must be delayed and therapy optimized. If the operation is a life-saving emergency procedure, the relative risks of operation and anesthesia must be discussed with both the parents and the surgeon, with therapy for control of the asthma instituted immediately. If the operation can be delayed a short while, immediate therapy for cases of severe asthma may be effective. If operation cannot be delayed, as safe an anesthetic as possible must be administered.

Premedication may be administered for bronchodilatation and/or sedation. Children should receive their routine oral bronchodilators on the morning of the operation with a sip of water. Inhaled bronchodilators should also be given on the morning of surgery and, if necessary, repeated prior to transfer to the operating room. If the child is currently receiving steroids or has received steroids for at least 1 week in the past 6 months, an intravenous infusion of hydrocortisone hemisuccinate (1.5 mg/kg) should be commenced about 1 hour before operation.

Atropine (0.02 mg/kg) or glycopyrrolate (0.01 mg/kg) may be administered intramuscularly 45 minutes before surgery for antisialorrhea, bronchodilatation, and suppression of the afferent irritant vagal pathways in the lung.

Sedation may be indicated for those children in whom asthma is precipitated by anxiety. Midazolam, 0.5 mg/kg, may be given orally in a syrup 10 to 15 minutes before operation to children 1 to 10 years of age. An alternative is diazepam (0.15–0.20 mg/kg) 1 to 2 hours before operation. If the child is extremely anxious, methohexital (15 mg/kg of a 1 percent solution with 0.02 mg/kg of atropine) may be given per rectum 10 minutes before operation to children 1 to 6 years of age. In adolescents and adults, the major tranquilizer promethazine (Phenergan) has been suggested as a premedication (25 mg/70 kg intramuscularly) for both its sedating and antisialogogue effects. Although controversial, the combination of a narcotic such as meperidine and promethazine has been recommended for premedication of older patients with lung disease. The preoperative use of H_2 antagonists is theoretically contraindicated in asthma, because stimulation of H_2 receptors is thought to inhibit the feedback control of mediator release and antagonize the effects of histamine on the H_1 receptors and possibly increase bronchoconstriction. The order of H_2 receptor antagonists from greatest to least likely to augment bronchoconstriction is cimetidine>ranitidine>famotidine.

The choice of anesthetic techniques includes local, regional, and general. In children, local infiltration for a surgical procedure is often extremely difficult. Regional anesthesia is becoming increasingly popular: caudal, spinal, and axillary blocks may be used. A spinal block may be effective for a lower abdominal or lower extremity procedure. However, if preservation of an adequate vital capacity for an effective cough is important, evidence suggests that regional techniques may not have advantages over general anesthesia.

If general anesthesia is undertaken, intubation of the trachea should be avoided if possible, since a foreign body in the airway is one of the most potent triggers for bronchospasm. Therefore, anesthesia should be given by mask or via total intravenous anesthesia (propofol) whenever possible.

Anesthesia may be induced by either an intravenous or inhalational route. Thiopentone theoretically releases more histamine than methohexitone or ketamine, although there are no controlled clinical studies in asthmatics to support this theory. In clinical doses, thiopentone does not block irritant-induced reflex bronchoconstriction, although there is evidence that thiopentone is relatively safe in asthmatic patients. Methohexitone does not release histamine in vitro and may be useful as an induction agent in asthmatics, although one anaphylactoid reaction to rectal methohexital has been reported. Ketamine relaxes the airways through activation of the sympathetic system (beta-adrenergic agonist action), blockade of endogenous catecholamine reuptake, and depression of afferent irritant vagal pathways. In the dog model, ketamine protects against antigen-induced bronchospasm better than thiopentone. Propofol is a new total intravenous anesthetic that does not trigger airway reflex response in vivo, but there have been few trials in known asthmatics. In studies in children, propofol has not triggered bronchospasm.

The inhalational agents halothane, enflurane, and isoflurane all prevent and reverse bronchospasm. The mechanism is thought to involve blockade of the irritant vagal pathways within the central nervous system. It is therefore important that a deep level of anesthesia is established before the trachea is intubated. Although it has been suggested that halothane produces bronchoconstriction by its beta$_2$-agonist action, there is no evidence to support this theory. However, halothane is associated with an increased incidence of arrhythmias in dogs pretreated with theophylline, compared with enflurane or isoflurane in the same model. Despite this caution, halothane remains the most commonly used inhalational agent in pediatric asthma. Isoflurane is associated with an increased incidence of breathholding, coughing, and laryngospasm compared with halothane and enflurane in children and may be less desirable for use in asthmatics for these reasons. Nonetheless, ventricular arrhythmias may occur in children with high therapeutic blood levels of theophylline during halothane anesthesia, and in this situation isoflurane may be the preferred agent. In a recent report, three adults in status asthmaticus who were refractory to medical therapy responded dramatically to isoflurane and enflurane. Studies in children are required before the preferred inhalational anesthetic is identified.

Narcotics release histamine, which may be responsible for narcotic-induced bronchospasm and should be avoided. Although H_1 antihistamines block the hypotensive effects of narcotics, they are ineffective in preventing narcotic-induced bronchospasm. For a complete discussion of narcotic and histamine release, see the following section on Mastocytosis.

Neuromuscular blocking drugs may release histamine, and some cause bronchoconstriction. Of the muscle relaxants currently available, vecuronium is least likely to induce bronchoconstriction. A detailed discussion is found in the section on Mastocytosis.

If possible, intubation should be performed while the patient is at a deep level of general anesthesia. This blocks the irritant reflex afferent vagal pathways from the lung. Deep anesthesia may be accomplished with high concentrations of an inhalational agent or during a lighter level of anesthesia supplemented with intravenous lidocaine. Lidocaine blocks the irritant reflex vagal pathways from the lungs and, as suggested by studies in animals, may directly relax bronchial smooth muscle. Intravenous lidocaine is preferred to aerosol lidocaine because it removes the need for prior laryngoscopy and avoids use of a high-pressure chlorofluorocarbon.

During anesthesia, ventilation may become difficult, resulting in rapid arterial oxygen desaturation and clinical signs of cyanosis. This may necessitate differentiating a tight chest as a result of light anesthesia from that due to bronchospasm. The former is relieved after administration of muscle relaxants or deep anesthesia, whereas the latter is unaffected by muscle relaxants but is relieved by a deeper level of anesthesia.

Anesthetic gases should be humidified, particularly in smaller children, in whom inspissated secretions may plug the smaller diameter endotracheal tube. Humidification is also recommended for prolonged anesthesia and in those children with chest infections in whom suctioning and chest physiotherapy are required to remove secretions.

If bronchospasm occurs during anesthesia, the differential diagnosis outlined in Table 17–4 should be considered.

If the child is not intubated, management includes assisted ventilation with 100 percent oxygen and increasing concentrations of halothane. If the diagnosis is asthmatic bronchospasm and the bronchospasm is severe, the child should be ventilated with 100 percent oxygen. In cases of severe asthmatic bronchospasm, inhalational therapy is often ineffective, and parenteral therapy is then required. Severe bronchospasm requires tracheal intubation to ensure adequate alveolar ventilation and supplementation with parenteral bronchodilators such as theophylline or isoproterenol.

Table 17–4. DIFFERENTIAL DIAGNOSIS OF WHEEZING

	Intraoperative	Nonoperative
Upper airway obstruction	Endobronchial intubation Obstructed endotracheal tube Carinal irritation Secretions in the airway Foreign body in the airway Aspiration	Foreign body in the airway Croup Epiglottitis Tracheal stenosis or malacia Extrinsic compression of trachea (tumor, cyst, nodes, vascular)
Lower airway disease	Pneumothorax Aspiration	Bronchiolitis Bronchiectasis Cystic fibrosis Pneumonia
Cardiac	Pulmonary edema	Pulmonary edema

If the child is intubated and the diagnosis is asthmatic bronchospasm, the child should be hyperventilated with 100 percent oxygen and increasing concentrations of halothane. If the bronchospasm is not relieved, aerosol ventolin should then be administered into the tracheal tube, with the realization that less than 10 percent of the actuated dose enters the lungs. Further therapy with intravenous theophylline or isoproterenol may be required. Isoproterenol in doses beginning with 0.1 μg/kg/min may be administered intravenously (see Table 17–8, p. 633). Subcutaneous, slow intravenous, or endotracheal epinephrine must be administered cautiously in the presence of halothane.

At the end of anesthesia, neuromuscular blockade must be completely reversed. Although neostigmine may increase bronchomotor tone, the addition of an anticholinergic agent such as atropine or glycopyrrolate will minimize this effect. The trachea should be extubated while the child is deeply anesthetized and breathing spontaneously or when the child is wide awake. There have been no controlled clinical studies comparing the effects of these two extubation techniques on the incidence of airway reflex responsiveness after anesthesia. The decision to extubate the child under deep anesthesia or awake depends on the expertise of the anesthesiologist, the severity of the asthma, and preexisting problems that may predispose the child to regurgitation.

In the postanesthetic room, children should receive humidified oxygen. Careful attention should be paid to auscultating the chest for evidence of bronchospasm. If bronchospasm develops, then ventolin should be administered by inhalation. If this treatment is insufficient, consideration should be given to parenteral theophylline. Postoperative sedation should be used with caution, particularly if ventilation or oxygenation is impaired. Regional anesthesia may be used to prevent postoperative pain.

MASTOCYTOSIS

Mastocytosis, a disorder of unknown etiology, is defined histologically as an abnormal proliferation of mast cells in the skin (urticaria pigmentosa) or, less frequently, in both the skin and systemic tissues (systemic mastocytosis). This rare disorder (0.01 to 0.1 percent of new dermatology clinic patients) presents with cutaneous signs at birth in 11 percent of cases and by 2 years of age in 50 to 80 percent of the cases. The inheritance pattern for mastocytosis is thought to be multifactorial, although autosomal dominant patterns with variable penetrance have been suggested. The prognosis of the disease in the pediatric age group is excellent, with resolution of the disease in 50 percent of the children by puberty. Mast cell leukemia is a rare complication of systemic mastocytosis, usually of the adult-onset type.

Urticaria pigmentosa is the most common form of mastocytosis in the pediatric age group. This disorder is characterized by a single or multifocal eruption of reddish-brown macules, papules, or nodules 1 to 3 cm in diameter on the trunk or, less commonly, on the extremities. These lesions appear and disappear over a period of time. They can coalesce and give the appearance of "leopard skin." In infancy, vesicular or bullous lesions are characteristic. Mastocytomas also may appear in early infancy in as many as 10 percent of all patients with urticaria pigmentosa as solitary reddish-brown or yellow nodules on the trunk or extremities. Rarely, yellow papules (xanthelasmoidea) resembling xanthomas are also present in infants with urticaria pigmentosa. The erythrodermic and diffuse cutaneous forms of mastocytosis are rare and suggest the possibility of systemic involvement, particularly in adults.

Systemic mastocytosis, which occurs in approximately 10 percent of all cases, complicates urticaria pigmentosa infrequently in infants and children. However, when present it can involve bone (15 percent of pediatric cases), the gastrointestinal tract, the liver (48 percent of cases), the spleen, and to a lesser extent lymph nodes, thymus, and pancreas. Systemic mastocytosis rarely involves cardiac, renal, pulmonary, and meningeal tissues. Systemic complications of mastocytosis result from the dense proliferation of large numbers of mast cells, which engorge the organ and compromise function. When bone is involved, local bone pain and tenderness are common. Invasion of the bone marrow (myelolisthesis) may replace bone marrow precursors and result in pancytopenia. Direct infiltration of the gastric, small bowel, and rectal mucosae may cause anorexia, nausea, vomiting, diarrhea, and hematemesis. A resultant malabsorption syndrome can cause vitamin B_{12} deficiency and hypocalcemia.

Peptic ulcers are present in 5 percent of patients with systemic mastocytosis. Extensive infiltration of the liver can produce hepatic dysfunction, resulting in a decrease in the serum concentrations of the liver-dependent coagulation factors, albumin, and cholesterol. If portal hypertension develops, splenomegaly, anemia, and bleeding may ensue. The hematological manifestations include anemia and decreased eosinophil chemotaxis. Bleeding may occur because of a reduced concentration of the liver-dependent coagulation factors, thrombocytopenia, or from systemic heparin released from mast cells during degranulation. Infrequently, polycythemia rubra vera is associated with urticaria pigmentosa.

DIAGNOSIS

Urticaria pigmentosa is usually diagnosed by the characteristic skin lesions, the presence of circumferential erythema when the lesions are firmly stroked (Darier's sign is positive in 92 percent of cases), dermographism (wheals in 50 percent of cases), or the presence of vesicles and bullae in infants and children when uninvolved skin is firmly stroked. The diagnosis is confirmed by a skin biopsy, which reveals densely packed mast cells (in addition to eosinophils, plasma cells, and lymphocytes) in the perivascular regions of the dermis. The peripheral blood smear usually shows a leukocytosis; mast cells are rarely present.

The local and systemic manifestations of mastocytosis result from the clinical effects of the products of degranulation: histamine, heparin, and possibly prostaglandin D_2 (Table 17–5). Two thirds of those patients with isolated urticaria pigmentosa are asymptomatic. However, approximately one third of these patients experience pruritus and intermittent episodes of flushing of the face and upper torso. Less commonly, bruising, blistering, and bleeding occur. These symptoms may be precipitated by exer-

Table 17–5. MAST CELL MEDIATORS

Mediator	Pharmacological Effect
Preformed mediators	
Histamine (H_1)	Bronchoconstriction, increased capillary permeability
Eosinophil chemotactic factor (ECF)	Eosinophil chemotaxis
Neutrophil chemotactic factor (NCF)	Neutrophil chemotaxis
Heparin	Anticoagulation, inhibition of complement activation
Immediately synthesized mediators	
Leukotrienes C, D, E (slow-reacting substance)	Bronchoconstriction, increased capillary permeability
PGD_2, PGF_2	Bronchoconstriction
Thromboxane A_2, PGE_1, PGE_2	Bronchodilation, increased capillary permeability
Platelet activating factor (PAF)	Platelet aggregation and degranulation

cise, stress, wide swings in temperature, or drugs such as aspirin and codeine.

Systemic mastocytosis should be thought of when the aforementioned symptoms complicate either isolated mastocytosis or extensive cutaneous infiltrations (with bullous, erythrodermic, or diffuse cutaneous forms). Furthermore, systemic mastocytosis should be suspected when the mastocytosis syndrome of headache, fever, flushing, dyspnea, palpitations, syncope, nausea, vomiting, diarrhea, hepatosplenomegaly, or bone pain occurs alone or in combination with cutaneous lesions such as isolated mastocytoma, extensive bullae, erythroderma, or diffuse cutaneous eruptions.

Histamine concentrations have been measured in both the urine and serum of patients with mastocytosis. Urine concentrations of histamine and 1-methyl-4-imidazolacetic acid (the major metabolite of histamine) may be significantly increased in these patients. However, urine concentrations may fluctuate and do not remain consistently increased. The severity of mastocytosis does not correlate with the urine concentration of histamine. The serum concentration of histamine is not usually increased in patients with mastocytosis, although recent data suggest the contrary. Serum histamine is consistently increased during sudden degranulation of mast cells. During this period, the serum concentration neither predicts the likelihood of the disease nor reliably correlates with the severity of the disease; nor does it reflect the tissue concentration of histamine.

Carcinoid syndrome is the major differential diagnosis from systemic mastocytosis. Patients with carcinoid syndrome have symptoms similar to those of systemic mastocytosis—palpitations, diarrhea, syncope, and flushing. However, carcinoid syndrome differs from systemic mastocytosis in that the major urinary metabolite in carcinoid syndrome, 5-hydroxy-indoleacetic acid, is rarely present in urticaria pigmentosa, and a skin biopsy in carcinoid syndrome reveals extensive argentaffin cell (rather than mast cell) infiltration in the dermis. Additionally, antiserotonin drugs are therapeutic in carcinoid syndrome and not mastocytosis. Right-sided heart disease may be present in carcinoid syndrome but not in mastocytosis.

PATHOPHYSIOLOGY

The local and systemic manifestations of mastocytosis result from the extensive degranulation of mast cells producing histamine, heparin, and prostaglandin D. In mastocytosis, the concentrations of mediators in mast cells and the extent of degranulation of the mast cells are similar to those of mast cells from unaffected individuals. The mediators released (Table 17–5) cause both local (cutaneous) and systemic effects. The local effects are described on page 525. Systemic effects include respiratory (bronchoconstriction and increased mucus secretions), cardiovascular (hypotension, arrhythmias, increased capillary permeability, and shock) and gastrointestinal (vomiting, diarrhea, and bleeding).

Mast cells release mediators in response to either immunological or nonimmunological triggers. The immunological triggers may be either a type I (IgE) hypersensitivity reaction or a complement-mediated reaction. Although immunological triggers may be present, there is no evidence that allergy, atopy, or asthma is associated with either urticaria pigmentosa or mastocytosis. Nonimmunological triggers of mast cell degranulation (Table 17–6) are probably responsible for the release of mast cell mediators in mastocytosis. The mechanism responsible for the release during a nonimmunological trigger is unclear, but drugs, wide fluctuations in temperature, vomiting, psychogenic stimulation, and skin irritation have been implicated. Drugs remain the most common nonimmunological trigger of mast cell degranulation in mastocytosis.

Anesthetic drugs must be carefully selected to minimize the risk of mast cell degranulation. In the experimental model, the extent of mast

Table 17–6. NONIMMUNOLOGICAL TRIGGERS OF MAST CELL DEGRANULATION

Physical stimuli
Temperature fluctuations
Cutaneous stimulation
Trauma
Psychogenic stimulus
Calcium ionophor A23187
Drugs
Codeine, morphine
D-Tubocurarine, gallamine, dexamethonium
Polymyxin B, dextran
Adenosine phosphate
Alcohol
Radiographic dyes

cell degranulation by drugs is proportional to the peak serum concentration of histamine. Incremental doses of drugs release histamine in a graded response. The release of histamine has been shown to be proportional to the logarithmic concentration of a number of drugs, including morphine and D-tubocurarine. This graded response suggests that all drugs should be administered in small incremental doses to minimize the release of histamine. Although this model may not accurately reflect the response to these drugs in vivo, the serum concentration of histamine remains the only method currently available for comparing the effects of drugs on mast cell degranulation.

The release of histamine in response to intravenous drugs varies with age. Three groups of children, ages 1 to 4, 5 to 9, and 10 to 15 years, were challenged with D-tubocurarine. There was a highly significant increase in local histamine release with increasing age. This suggests that older children (10 to 15 years) are more likely to release histamine in response to a trigger than are younger children.

General anesthetic drugs have a varied effect on histamine release. The inhalational agents halothane, enflurane, and isoflurane do not release histamine and actively relax the airways in a dose-dependent manner. Rare episodes of bronchospasm have been reported following exposure to enflurane. Of the intravenous drugs currently available for induction of anesthesia, both thiopentone and methohexitone are reported to release histamine in at least 75 percent of responders within 10 minutes of administration, although recent data suggest that methohexital releases significantly less histamine from mast cells in vitro. Ketamine and etomidate are the only intravenous agents that do not release histamine. The effect of propofol on mast cell degranulation and histamine release is unknown.

Anticholinergic drugs theoretically attenuate mast cell degranulation by decreasing cytoplasmic cGMP concentration. Atropine and glycopyrrolate do not increase the serum concentration of histamine. In contrast, scopolamine is reported to induce mast cell degranulation.

Muscle relaxants have a variable effect on histamine release. D-Tubocurarine causes a moderate release of histamine in a dose-dependent manner. Succinylcholine, metocurine, and atracurium mildly stimulate release of histamine, whereas gallamine, pancuronium, and vecuronium do not to any extent.

Neostigmine in doses of up to 0.4 mg/kg (10 times the clinical dose) does not release histamine from mast cells.

The effect of narcotics is unclear. Demerol has been the narcotic of choice for many years in allergic and asthmatic patients, because it does not release clinically significant quantities of histamine. Morphine, however, is avoided in allergic patients because it does release histamine and thus may precipitate bronchospasm. In contrast, fentanyl and sufentanil do not release significant quantities of histamine in doses of 100 μg/kg and 15 μg/kg, respectively, and recent research suggests that butorphanol also does not. There are no studies on the effect of alfentanil on histamine release. Demerol, fentanyl, and sufentanil are probably safe to use in these patients.

TREATMENT

There is no known cure for urticaria pigmentosa or mastocytosis. Therapy is often unnecessary in children with asymptomatic skin lesions. If, however, the lesions cause persistent pruritus or wheals or are bothersome in some other way, or if systemic manifestations of mastocytosis occur, then therapy is indicated. This may be divided into three categories: (1) symptomatic, (2) curative, and (3) therapy for malignancies.

SYMPTOMATIC THERAPY

The systemic manifestations of mastocytosis result from the release of large quantities of mediators, most commonly histamine. Histamine exerts its physiological effects through two functional receptors, H_1 and H_2. Stimulation of H_1-receptors results in contraction of smooth muscle (as in bronchoconstriction), an increased spacing between the tightly packed endothelial cells (as in increased vascular permeability and edema), and stimulation of nerve end-organs (as in pruritus). Stimulation of H_2-receptors results in changes in the cellular cyclic nucleotides, increased gastric acid secretion, and reduced leukocyte function. The overall effect of histamine on a particular organ depends on which histamine receptor is more dominant in that organ.

Antihistamines block the systemic manifestations of histamine by blocking its tissue uptake. They are most effective when given prophylactically. There is recent evidence that antihistamines may stabilize the mast cell membrane and thereby attenuate the release of histamine.

H_1 and H_2 antihistamines may be used in combination to attenuate the systemic manifestations of mastocytosis. H_1 antihistamines alone are unsatisfactory. The H_2 antihistamines cimetidine (2–4 mg/kg PO or IV) and ranitidine (1 mg/kg IV) have each been successful in controlling gastrointestinal problems. The combination of H_1 and H_2 antihistamines appears more effective than either drug used singularly to control the systemic manifestations. Anecdotal reports vary concerning this combination therapy for symptomatic control. There have been no controlled studies comparing combination antihistamine therapy to the individual therapies.

Both H_1 and H_2 antihistamines may cause side effects and toxicity even within the dose range recommended for children. H_1 antihistamines produce drowsiness, incoordination, dizziness, tinnitus, blurred vision, and tremor, although the new generation of H_1 antihistamines (ketotifin, terfenadine, astemizole, and others) sedate patients to a far less degree. Furthermore, this second generation of H_1 antihistamines is well absorbed by the oral route, with administration half-lives of between 4.5 hours and 9.5 days. Some children become hyperactive, irritable, and excitable but only rarely progress to convulsions. Toxic doses of antihistamines may disturb the autonomic nervous system, resulting in cardiorespiratory arrest. The treatment of an overdose of an H_1 antihistamine includes supportive therapy, gastric emptying and lavage, anticonvulsants, and, if necessary, hemodialysis.

Although H_2 antihistamines have not been used for an extended period of time in pediatrics, data are available from studies in adults. H_2 antihistamines cause gastrointestinal disturbances, headache, and rash in less than 2 percent of adults. Cimetidine may lower the threshold for histamine-induced bronchospasm. Hepatic and renal complications have been reported in addition to leukopenia and altered moods. The latter complications appear to be reversible upon cessation of the drug.

Disodium cromoglycate is a membrane-stabilizing drug that has been used with moderate success in patients with urticaria pigmentosa and systemic mastocytosis. The dose of oral disodium cromoglycate is up to 100 mg/kg/day. Large doses of cromoglycate are required since only 1 percent of the oral preparation reaches the systemic circulation. The oral preparation of cromoglycate appears most effective for the gastrointestinal symptoms of mastocytosis but is also reported to relieve both the cutaneous and central nervous system manifestations.

Ketotifen is a new antihistamine and antianaphylactic drug currently under investigation for use in patients with urticaria pigmentosa and mastocytosis. Preliminary data suggest that ketotifen acts by inhibiting mediator release, blocking calcium channels, and indirectly by activating beta-agonist receptors. Studies suggest that ketotifen may be as effective as disodium cromoglycate in preventing histamine release in mastocytosis.

The indications for aspirin and other nonsteroidal anti-inflammatory drugs in the treatment of mastocytosis are unclear. These drugs inhibit prostaglandin synthesis and may attenuate systemic manifestations but have been contraindicated because of reports of severe hypotension following their use. The current recommendations are that aspirin and other noninflammatory drugs may be used with mastocytosis provided they are administered only after the patients are adequately blocked with H_1 and H_2 antihistamines, and only in small incremental doses.

Curative Therapy

Isolated skin lesions in infants and children usually resolve spontaneously but may require surgical excision. PUVA (a combination of oral 8-methoxypsoralen and long-wave ultraviolet radiation) has been used with moderate success.

Therapy for Malignant Complications

Malignancy is extremely rare in mastocytosis, particularly in pediatric patients. If a malignancy occurs, it may be either leukemia or a benign neoplasm that became malignant. Because these lesions are rare and quite variable, no specific chemotherapeutic regimen has been recommended.

ANESTHETIC MANAGEMENT

PREOPERATIVE

A careful history of the signs and symptoms of the systemic manifestations of mastocytosis is important. Because massive amounts of histamine may be released in any patient with urticaria pigmentosa or urticaria, specific triggers such as drugs, anxiety, and others listed in Table 17–6 must be identified and carefully avoided.

Physical examination should begin with the dermatological system, noting the areas of skin involvement and in particular the presence of vesicular or bullous lesions on the face. The respiratory, cardiovascular, hepatic, and neurological systems should be examined for the systemic manifestations of mastocytosis. Laboratory investigations should include a routine hemoglobin assay, urinalysis, platelet count, and a coagulation screen (prothrombin time and partial thromboplastin time).

Premedication should include an H_1 and H_2 antihistamine (Table 17–7). H_1 and H_2 antihistamines have been effective in attenuating the clinical manifestations of mastocytosis in chronically treated children. These drugs should be administered orally about 1.5 hours prior to operation. For children who are anxious about the operation, diazepam, 0.2 mg/kg, should be administered orally 2 hours before the procedure.

INTRAOPERATIVE

The anesthetic technique must be tailored to the patient, the operation, and the anesthesiologist. The three anesthetic techniques are local, regional, and general. There are reports of mast cell degranulation with local and regional techniques. General anesthesia is the technique most commonly used.

To manage these patients successfully during operation, regardless of anesthetic technique, it is imperative to avoid all the triggers of mast cell degranulation. Because large changes in temperature may precipitate mast cell degranulation, the operating room should be warmed to a comfortable temperature before the patient arrives. Ancillary warming equipment, including a blood warmer, heater-humidifier, and warming blanket, should be available. The routine anesthetic monitors, including an electrocardiogram, blood pressure cuff, core temperature probe, and precordial stethoscope, must be present. Nonallergenic tape should be used where possible in these children to avoid dermographism, wheals, and bullae.

Resuscitation equipment and drugs must be available in the operating room before induction of anesthesia. The life-threatening complications of mastocytosis are profound hypotension (shock) and intense bronchospasm. Profound hypotension must be treated immediately with a balanced salt solution (Ringer's lactate or normal saline, 10 to 20 ml/kg initially), epinephrine infusion, and diphenhydramine (Table 17–8). If the response to this is poor, then repeated boluses of balanced salt solution or colloid may be infused, as well as further doses of epinephrine. Isolated mild bronchospasm may respond to halothane or a beta$_2$-agonist by inhalation. Intense bronchospasm may require further beta$_2$-agonist by inhalation in 100 percent oxygen, intravenous theophylline, and isoproterenol (see Table 17–8 and the section on Asthma earlier in this chapter).

The drugs used during general anesthesia in these patients should have either no effect or only a minimal effect on histamine release. Nevertheless, we recommend that general anesthesia be induced with either an inhalational induction (halothane, nitrous oxide, and oxygen) or an intravenous induction (methohexital or ketamine). If an intravenous cannula is not in place before induction of anesthesia, then intravenous access should be established immediately after induction, and intravenous atropine, 0.02 mg/kg, should be administered. Pancuronium, vecuronium, or succinylcholine may be used to provide muscle relaxation.

If there are no lesions on the face, anesthesia may be maintained with an inhalational agent administered by a soft mask. However, if there are bullous or vesicular lesions on the face, endotracheal intubation can be used to avoid exacerbations from physical irritation by the

Table 17–7. ANTIHISTAMINES IN PEDIATRICS

Drug	Dose*	$\tau_{1/2}$ (Hours)	τ_{max} (Hours)
Diphenhydramine (Benadryl)	5 mg/kg/day in divided doses	3.4†	2.5†
Chlorpheniramine (Chlor-Trimeton)	0.35 mg/kg/day in divided doses	9.6–13	2.5
Promethazine (Phenergan)	0.3 mg/kg/day in divided doses		
Hydroxyzine (Atarax)	2–4 mg/kg/day in 4 divided doses	7	2

*Oral drug dose
†Adult data.

Table 17–8. RESUSCITATION REGIMEN

Drug	Dilution	Dose	Maximum Dose	Frequency
Epinephrine (Adrenalin)	1:10,000	0.02–0.1 ml/kg SC or IV or in ETT (2–10 μg/kg)	0.5 mg	q 5–10 min
Diphenhydramine (Benadryl)	50 mg/ml	1–2 mg/kg IV	50 mg	Bolus
		5 mg/kg/day IV or PO		q 6 h
Isoproterenol (Isuprel)	1 mg in 250 ml Ringer's lactate	3 μg/kg IV	100 μg	Bolus
		0.05–0.5 μg/kg/min IV	2 μg/kg/min	Continuous
Aminophylline	500 mg in 500 ml of D5W/ 0.2%	5–7 mg/kg	Serum levels <20 μg/ml	Infusion over 20 min
		0.1–1 mg/kg/h*		Infusion
Atropine		20 μg/kg IV, IM, or SL	1.0 mg	q 20 min

ETT = endotracheal tube; SL = sublingual
*As in Table 17–3.
Adapted from Edmonds J, Surh L, Banks J: Resuscitation Card. Resuscitation Committee. Toronto, The Hospital for Sick Children, 1984.

mask. The tracheal tube should be secured with a 2-inch wide flannel tie around the tracheal tube and the patient's neck. For premature infants, neonates, and older infants, the caliber of the tracheal tubes is too small to secure with a flannel tie. In these cases, we recommend that nonallergenic tape be used and the tube supported with a bite block. Supplemental narcotics, including meperidine, fentanyl, or sufentanil, may be used safely during operation. All neuromuscular blockade should be reversed at the completion of anesthesia, with extubation when the patient is completely awake.

Postoperative

In the postoperative period, analgesia must be restricted to small doses of those drugs that do not release histamine: meperidine, acetaminophen, and fentanyl. Codeine, which is commonly used in the postoperative period for analgesia in children, should not be given. If fentanyl is used, it should be given as an infusion only in the postanesthetic recovery room or intensive care unit, where continuous monitoring of respiratory rate is possible.

Postoperative fever may be treated with either oral or rectal acetaminophen (10–20 mg/kg for infants and young children). Although aspirin had been considered contraindicated in these patients, its use has been recommended recently. However, aspirin should be used cautiously in the immediate postoperative period, since it may cause postoperative bleeding.

ERYTHEMA MULTIFORME

Erythema multiforme is an inflammatory cutaneous syndrome that occurs in all age groups. It is usually benign, although in the more severe form of the disease (Stevens-Johnson syndrome), death has been reported in as many as 18 percent of cases. Death results from extensive respiratory, skin, and infectious complications.

Erythema multiforme is classified into two types: (1) erythema multiforme minor, which is a self-limiting, mild cutaneous syndrome, and (2) erythema multiforme major (or Stevens-Johnson syndrome). The latter may present with the same cutaneous findings as the minor type but is distinguished by the sudden onset of a febrile illness associated with severe lesions of the mucocutaneous membranes (stomatitis and conjunctivitis) and possibly toxic epidermal necrolysis. Toxic epidermal necrolysis is associated with an approximate 50 percent mortality.

ERYTHEMA MULTIFORME MINOR

In one third of patients, the onset of the minor form of erythema multiforme is heralded by an upper respiratory tract infection. The characteristic skin lesion is a target lesion, which begins as a round, erythematous macule and evolves into a papule with circumferential pallor within a few days. The center of the papule undergoes epidermal necrosis, leaving a pale center and an erythematous ring. The papules may coalesce into plaques with a central vesicle, bulla, or dry skin. The skin lesions are symmetrically distributed over the dorsal surfaces of the hands, nailfolds, and extensor surfaces (elbows and knees), and are particularly prominent in areas of sun exposure and physical trauma (Koebner's phenomenon). These lesions may cause pruritus and burning and usually resolve within 2 to 4 weeks, leaving areas of hyperpigmentation.

ERYTHEMA MULTIFORME MAJOR (STEVENS-JOHNSON SYNDROME)

The major form is a much more severe disease; systemic manifestations include fever, malaise, headache, sore throat, cough, chest pain, vomiting, and diarrhea, which occur up to 2 weeks before the onset of mucocutaneous lesions. The characteristic bullous lesion appears quite suddenly on the oral mucosa, lips, and conjunctiva. Other ocular problems include bilateral purulent conjunctivitis, corneal ulcers, and panophthalmitis. Atrial fibrillation and myocarditis also may be present.

The skin lesions may evolve into large bullae or extensive areas of toxic epidermal necrolysis, which have a tendency to become infected and slough. They develop slowly and may take up to 6 weeks to heal completely.

Mucosal involvement may include the oropharynx, nasopharynx, tracheobronchial tree, esophagus, and genitourinary tract. Extensive ulceration of the respiratory tree has been reported. This has been complicated by pneumonia, pleural effusions, and bronchopleural fistulas.

Histological examination reveals an accumulation of mononuclear cells in the upper dermis. In the major form, there may be severe epidermal skin damage with necrosis and exfoliation of large areas of full-thickness epidermis.

Erythema multiforme is associated with four underlying causes: (1) drugs, (2) *Mycoplasma pneumoniae* infections, (3) recurrent herpes simplex viral infections, and (4) neoplasms.

The major form is one of the most severe cutaneous reactions associated with drugs. Sulfa drugs (such as thiazides), barbiturates, penicillins, and diphenylhydantoin have been implicated. The eruption may occur from hours to weeks after exposure.

Antecedent infections are the second most common cause of erythema multiforme major. *Mycoplasma pneumoniae* or recurrent herpes simplex may herald an eruption.

Two mechanisms have been proposed to explain the pathogenesis of this disorder: an immune complex response or a generalized hypersensitivity reaction.

TREATMENT

Treatment of the minor form of erythema multiforme includes topical soaks with hydrogen peroxide and antihistamines for pruritus, although antihistamines may trigger the major form. There is no indication for topical or systemic steroids in the treatment of the minor form of erythema multiforme.

The major form must be managed more aggressively, with special consideration to the presence of toxic epidermal necrosis, bullous lesions, and ocular complications. This includes control of fluids, temperature, and infections (avoiding penicillin). High-dose steroids have been used in cases of Stevens-Johnson syndrome with extensive exfoliative epidermal necrosis, although the indications for this therapy remain controversial. Prednisone, 1 to 2 mg/kg, may be administered orally (or a comparable dose parenterally) and then tapered quickly over a short period of time.

ANESTHETIC MANAGEMENT

Preoperative assessment should include a careful inquiry for a recent chest infection and for drug reactions or allergies. Reduced exercise tolerance, shortness of breath, or chest pain suggests respiratory or cardiovascular involvement. Recent administration of systemic steroids will require parenteral steroids preoperatively.

The physical examination should assess the severity of the cutaneous and mucosal lesions. If extensive epidermal necrolysis is present, intravenous access may be difficult to establish, the fluid balance and electrolyte concentrations may be abnormal, and the patient's temperature may be difficult to control. If the epidermis is diffusely necrotic, sterile precautions must be used. When extensive oral mucosal lesions are present, care must be exercised in manipulating the airway. In this case, intubation should be avoided if possible. Specific findings in the respiratory system include evidence of lower airway infection, bullous lung disease, or bronchopleural fistulas. Chest tubes may be present in patients with the latter two findings. The cardiac system should be examined for evidence of arrhythmias or cardiac decompensation (myocarditis or pericarditis). Evidence of systemic illness, including fever, dehydration, and electrolyte imbalance, may predispose to renal insufficiency.

Laboratory investigations should include hematocrit, urinalysis, and electrolytes. Depending on the severity of systemic involvement, a chest radiograph, blood gas measurement, and electrocardiogram may be indicated.

Premedication, if required, should be administered orally, rectally, or intravenously. Intramuscular or subcutaneous injections should be avoided because of the risk of bullous epidermal reactions. Preoperative steroids are indicated if the patient is currently receiving them or has received them in the previous 6 months.

All patients with Stevens-Johnson syndrome are susceptible to exfoliative skin reactions from minimal trauma. As a result, all monitors must be adapted to minimize this complication. The blood pressure cuff should be well padded and the electrocardiogram fitted with needles rather than sticky pads. A precordial stethoscope should be gently placed on the chest without strong adhesives during the induction period. An esophageal stethoscope may be used to monitor the heart sounds and air entry if the trachea is intubated. All pressure points (for example, elbows, heels) should be well padded after the patient is positioned.

The airway should be maintained with minimal intervention. Consideration should be given to local or regional anesthetic techniques, although direct infiltration of drugs may result in bullous formation. Anesthesia may be maintained with a neurolept or inhalational technique. If an inhalational technique is used, gentle application of a padded mask is suggested. Padding for the mask in such cases may include soft cotton or muslin soaked with hydrocortisone cream.

Tracheal intubation is sometimes necessary. In these cases, care should be taken to avoid trauma to pharyngeal and glottic structures. An uncuffed tracheal tube, a half size smaller than required, will help minimize the laryngeal trauma. The tube may be secured with a flannel strip around the neck. When the larynx cannot be visualized and airway obstruction develops, a tracheotomy may be required.

Anesthesia may be induced with an inhalational induction or ketamine. All barbiturates must be avoided. If the oral lesions are extensive, visualization of the laryngeal inlet may be difficult. In this case, an inhalational induction with halothane and oxygen is indicated. Anesthesia may be maintained with any combination of inhalational agents (halothane, isoflurane, enflurane, or nitrous oxide), intravenous agents (excluding barbiturates), and neuromuscular blocking drugs. The administration of penicillin, sulfonamides, streptomycin, and chloramphenicol must be carefully avoided at all times.

Mild postoperative pain may be controlled with rectal acetaminophen. If the pain is severe, an intravenous bolus or infusion of narcotics may be required. Salicylates should not be used because they may trigger reactions and cause platelet dysfunction and postoperative bleeding.

ANAPHYLAXIS

Anaphylaxis, which means "backward protection," is a clinical syndrome resulting from the sudden release of cytoplasmic mediators from mast cells and basophils. It may be immune-mediated or nonimmunologically mediated. Immune-mediated anaphylaxis is either IgE-mediated or complement-mediated (by C3 and C4 or the alternate pathway). Nonimmunological anaphylaxis (often referred to as anaphylactoid) depends on either arachidonic acid metabolites or direct release of cytoplasmic mediators. Regardless of etiology, anaphylaxis commonly involves four organ systems: skin, cardiovascular, respiratory, and gastrointestinal. The spectrum ranges from a minor reaction involving only the skin to fatal anaphylaxis with cardiovascular or respiratory collapse or both.

The reported incidence of anaphylaxis varies. The incidence of anaphylaxis to drugs at induction of anesthesia ranges from 1 in 1000 to as low as 1 in 30,000, with a 3 to 4 percent mortality. Reactions to penicillin, one of the most common triggers, may occur as frequently as 7 per 1000 patients with a fatality rate of approximately 0.1 per million cases. Anaphylaxis causing death occurs in approximately 0.4 per million patients. The risk of anaphylaxis increases with the duration and frequency of exposures to the triggering agent. Parenteral administration is more likely to induce problems than oral or rectal administration. Recent data suggest that a history of atopy does not predispose patients to anaphylaxis.

ETIOLOGY

IgE-Mediated Anaphylaxis. The immunoglobulin IgE is synthesized in B lymphocytes and comprises less than 0.001 percent of the circulating immunoglobulins in healthy individuals. Between 1000 and 5000 IgE molecules are fixed to the surfaces of mast cells and basophils. When an antigen bridges two IgE molecules, cell membrane receptors are approximated. This activates a membrane-bound methyltransferase enzyme that, with the aid of cAMP, facilitates the transmembrane influx of calcium ions. An increased cytoplasmic concentration of calcium induces degranulation of the mast cells and basophils, with the release of cytoplasmic mediators.

The serum concentration of IgE depends on age. IgE is present in only trace concentrations in the fetus. After birth, the serum concentration of IgE increases very slowly for the first 2 or 3 years of life (to 10 percent of the serum concentration in adults) and then increases to a maximum between 10 and 15 years of age. It decreases gradually between 20 and 80 years of age.

IgE-mediated anaphylaxis is responsible for most reactions to antibiotics (for example, penicillin, cephalosporin, and vancomycin), some anesthetic drugs (for example, thiopentone, local anesthetics, muscle relaxants, steroids), foreign proteins (for example, insulin, chymopapain, protamine, vasopressin, ACTH), and foods. This type of anaphylaxis occurs in both atopic and nonatopic individuals with similar frequencies.

Latex products have recently been associated with anaphylaxis during surgical procedures. These allergic reactions are IgE-mediated, occur more frequently in children, particularly those with a history of sensitivity to latex (rubber) gloves or rubber balloons or who have a history of spina bifida or congenital myologic defects, and may be life-threatening. In one large series, sensitization to latex occurred during repeated rectal or urethral manipulations with latex products that some have postulated led to submicroscopic mucosal tears and thus, a portal of entry for latex allergens. Subsequent exposure to latex results in allergic reactions. The large number of recent reports of latex sensitivity has been attributed in part to an abbreviated curing period of the latex. The severity of the reactions varies from none or mild (skin contact to latex) to severe life-threatening anaphylaxis (latex gloves used during intra-abdominal or thoracic surgery). Signs of an allergic response begin at least 40 minutes after induction of anesthesia with the classical signs of anaphylaxis: (1) respiratory (increased airway pressure and arterial oxygen desaturation), (2) cardiovascular (hypotension), and (3) cutaneous (urticaria). First-line therapy is to withdraw the source of the latex allergen. Surgical gloves should be changed to a nonlatex material such as one of the following: Neonlon (Deseret Medical Inc., Sandy, Utah), Dispos-a-Glove (Surgikos Co., Montreal, Quebec) or Elastyren (Hermal Pharmaceutical Laboratories Inc., Oak Hill, New York). Second-line therapy includes epinephrine as the treatment of choice for anaphylaxis. Since these reactions often persist, an infusion of epinephrine may be required (see Management section). Skin prick and RAST testing to latex usually confirm the diagnosis of latex allergy.

Repeat operation in children with known sensitivity to latex has been performed without latex products. Empirical prophylactic drug regimens have also been used (i.e., diphenhydramine, ranitidine, and hydrocortisone) successfully, although a prospective clinical trial is required.

Immune Complex–Mediated Anaphylaxis. This type of anaphylaxis occurs after the administration of blood or plasma or their byproducts or other volume expanders such as dextran and other collodion substitutes. Protein complexes in blood may activate complement, which degranulates mast cells and basophils.

Arachidonic Acid Metabolism. Aspirin and the nonsteroidal anti-inflammatory drugs (NSAIDs) may trigger anaphylaxis. Although the mechanism of this is unclear, it has been suggested that these drugs act either by inhibiting cyclo-oxygenase and therefore prostaglandin synthesis, or by disruption of the enzymes in the lipoxygenase pathway involved in arachidonic acid metabolism. The serum concentration of histamine is normal, and complement is usually decreased. Anaphylaxis, urticaria, and angioedema following ingestion of aspirin or NSAIDs may occur in up to 1 percent of the general population, with a possible familial predisposition. The incidence of these reactions in asthmatic patients is between 1 and 20 percent, also with a possible familial predisposition. Such patients are also cross-sensitive to NSAIDs, tartrazine, and benzoate-containing compounds. An anaphylactic reaction in the asthmatic person begins slowly, with rhinorrhea and flushing of the upper torso, and progresses to the development of bronchospasm, hypotension, and rarely cyanosis. Symptoms may continue for several hours before abating.

Direct Mast Cell–Degranulating Drugs. Anaphylaxis following administration of some drugs results in direct degranulation of mast cells and basophils, causing a massive release of histamine and activation of complement in otherwise normal patients. Drugs reported to cause anaphylaxis in this manner include muscle relaxants (D-tubocurarine, gallamine, succinylcholine, and pancuronium), narcotics (morphine, codeine, and meperidine), thiopentone, methohexitone, local anesthetics (para-aminobenzoic acid esters), steroids (hydrocortisone and methylprednisolone), and radiocontrast media.

Miscellaneous Causes. Idiopathic anaphylaxis is defined as recurrent anaphylaxis of unknown etiology. Exercise-induced anaphylaxis is a recently defined syndrome in which anaphylaxis occurs after exercise if affected patients ingest trigger foods before exercising. Neither of these two syndromes is well defined.

CLINICAL MANIFESTATIONS

The clinical signs and symptoms of anaphylaxis vary from individual to individual, and from attack to attack. Symptoms may occur almost immediately or up to 1 hour after exposure to the trigger. The more acute the onset, the more severe is the reaction. The signs and symptoms may begin with erythema, pruritus, cramps, and presyncope. Urticaria and angioedema may also occur and last up to 24 hours. Early upper respiratory symptoms, which include hoarseness, dyspnea, and in the older child and adult the sensation of a lump in the throat, may herald laryngeal edema and impending upper airway obstruction. Laryngeal edema is a major cause of fatal anaphylaxis, and respiratory complications are responsible for up to 70 percent of cases of fatalities. Early lower respiratory tract symptoms include dyspnea, wheezing, and bronchospasm.

In some cases, severe and intractable bronchospasm leads to hypoxia and cardiac arrest, which are frequently fatal. Death may occur within minutes of the attack or as long as days or weeks later. Cardiovascular complications alone are responsible for 24 percent of fatal anaphylaxis. Gastrointestinal symptoms include nausea, vomiting, acute cramps, and severe diarrhea. Minor associated problems include nasal, ocular, and palatal pruritus, fecal or urinary incontinence, sneezing, diaphoresis, and disorientation.

PATHOLOGICAL FINDINGS

The triad of pathological findings in severe anaphylaxis includes angioedema of the upper airway, bronchospasm of the lower airway, and vasodilatation and circulatory collapse. Approximately 66 percent of cases of fatal anaphylaxis develop angioneurotic or laryngeal edema and upper airway obstruction. Laryngeal edema results from interstitial swelling in the lamina propria of the hypopharynx, larynx, and epiglottis. In cases of delayed death, pathological findings in the lower airway are common, with 25 to 50 percent of patients showing changes of pulmonary hyperinflation. Less commonly, atelectasis, pulmonary hemorrhage, and edema are found.

Circulatory collapse is attributed to marked peripheral vasodilatation, which leads to reduced venous return and hypotension. Occasionally, cardiac arrhythmias and myocardial ischemia may occur.

Anaphylaxis may also affect other organs. Congestion of the liver, spleen, and stomach has been reported.

Laboratory and radiological tests for anaphylaxis are nonspecific. The plasma concentration of histamine is increased, clotting times may be prolonged, and the serum concentration of complement is abnormal in some patients. Plasma tryptase and chymase, two enzymes released from mast cells, recently have been used as mast cell markers in anaphylaxis. Although histamine peaks within 10 minutes, plasma levels return to normal by 30 to 60 minutes. In contrast, tryptase levels peak 1 to 2 hours after the reaction and decrease with a half-life of 2 hours. Despite advances in our understanding of these plasma markers, none of these tests is diagnostic of anaphylaxis.

Investigations may be performed to detect allergy to drugs. Intradermal skin testing is commonly used. Pediatric patients will not accept repeated skin punctures. Furthermore, the results of intradermal testing are quite variable in children. During an anaphylactic reaction, blood may be taken for measurement of the serum concentration of histamine, IgE antibody, and the C_3 and C_4 complement fractions.

The passive transfer test provided a very accurate means to detect allergies by transferring serum from an allergic patient to a second individual and then testing that individual for the Prausnitz-Küstner reaction. However, the risk of transferring viral infections has made this test obsolete.

An assay for detecting antibodies to the trigger may be used. The coprecipitation test and the radioallergosorbent test (RAST) are two such tests. Other studies that may be done include the leukocyte histamine release and IgE inhibition tests.

DIFFERENTIAL DIAGNOSIS

The syndrome of a precipitous eruption of urticaria or angioedema and paroxysmal airway obstruction and circulatory collapse is virtually diagnostic of anaphylaxis. A vasovagal episode, as may occur after injection of a drug in an awake patient, may mimic anaphylaxis without the signs of urticaria or angioedema. In such a case, the patient often feels faint, perspires, and becomes pale. Laryngeal edema is rare, and the blood pressure does not change. Patients with hereditary angioedema (HAE) do not commonly exhibit urticaria or hypotension, and there is usually a family history of the disease. The definitive diagnosis of HAE is based on the isolation of C1a inhibitor, the slow response to androgens, and resistance to treatment with epinephrine. Less common syndromes that must be differentiated from anaphylaxis include serum sickness, cold urticaria, insulin anaphylaxis, adrenal insufficiency, and massive hemorrhage. Serum sickness usually has a slow onset—1 to 3 weeks after antigenic exposure—and is associated with fever, edema, lymphadenopathy, nephritis, arthritis, and neuritis. Cold urticaria is associated with a history of cold exposure and the development of urticaria. Insulin anaphylaxis must be differentiated from hypoglycemic shock; during anesthesia, this can be done only on the basis of the serum glucose concentration or the presence of urticaria and angioedema. Occasionally an occult massive hemorrhage may be difficult to distinguish from anaphylaxis; urticaria and angioedema, if present, suggest anaphylaxis.

PATHOGENESIS

Histamine is the principal endogenous mediator responsible for the signs and symptoms of anaphylaxis in humans. It causes bronchoconstriction, vasodilatation, and increased leak of serum from venules.

Other mediators may be involved in the pathogenesis of anaphylaxis. SRS-A, slow-reacting substance of anaphylaxis, is important in animal models of anaphylaxis but as yet has an indefinite role in humans. SRS-A is composed of leukotrienes C, D, and E and potentiates histamine action, constricting the bronchial airways. Leukotriene C is a vasoconstrictor, and leukotriene D is a potent vasodilator.

Platelet-activating factor (PAF, acetyl glyceryl ether phosphorylcholine) is also important in animal models of anaphylaxis. Platelet factor 4 is released after antigen-induced bronchospasm in humans. Other mediators that may be involved include eosinophil and neutrophil chemotactic factors, heparin, and digestive lysozymal enzymes.

Non-IgE–mediated anaphylaxis depends upon complement activation and the release of C3a and C5a, but the precise mechanism remains to be elucidated. C3a and C5a cause bronchospasm, hypotension, and vasogenic edema.

MANAGEMENT DURING ANESTHESIA

When anaphylaxis occurs during anesthesia, it is usually unexpected. Severe reactions culminate in cardiorespiratory collapse and may rapidly prove fatal. Every effort must be made to preclude such an attack. If anaphylaxis develops, the diagnosis should be made quickly so that treatment may begin, because the longer the delay, the more likely it is that the outcome will be fatal.

Preoperative evaluation of every patient must include a careful history of allergies to either prescribed or over-the-counter drugs. A review of the previous anesthetic record and medical chart may reveal information about previous anaphylactic reactions. A Medic-Alert bracelet may be the only information available in the unconscious patient.

For those patients at high risk for anaphylaxis because of previous reactions to the same drug or trigger, prophylactic preoperative treatment is indicated. H_1 antihistamines (0.5 to 1.0 mg/kg of diphenhydramine orally or subcutaneously), together with H_2 antihistamines (4 to 6 mg/kg of cimetidine orally), have been used effectively to attenuate allergic reactions. These antihistamines block the peripheral manifestations of systemic histamine release, as may be demonstrated in the case of histamine release following morphine administration. Cromolyn also may be effective by limiting histamine release. High-dose steroids (30 mg/kg of methylprednisolone sodium succinate) will prevent histamine release from mast cells and mediators. Steroids have been used in combination with antihistamines for prophylaxis against anaphylactic reactions. Steroids may also act by reducing the arachidonic acid metabolites that are responsible for nonimmunological anaphylaxis. There is also evidence that the administration of NSAIDs (such as ibuprofen), together with steroids, further prevents the release of histamine from mast cells. Ketotifen has been effective in the prevention of anaphylaxis in corticosteroid-dependent adults with idiopathic anaphylaxis. Its future role remains to be established.

If a drug known to cause anaphylaxis must be administered, it should be administered slowly. This will minimize peak serum levels and thus minimize the release of histamine from mast cells and basophils and attenuate an anaphylactic response. Whenever possible another drug should be substituted for one known to cause anaphylaxis.

Life-threatening anaphylaxis presenting as paroxysmal angioneurotic edema (laryngeal edema), bronchospasm, or cardiorespiratory collapse following administration of a trigger must be immediately recognized. The dose of the trigger must be minimized. If the trigger has been administered via an extremity, placement of a tourniquet may help prevent further absorption until the reaction is under control. If the reaction is life-threatening, the anesthetic and the operation should be stopped. The goals of initial therapy include maintenance of adequate alveolar ventilation and oxygenation, attenuation of mediator release, and restoration of cardiac output. Angioneurotic edema and laryngeal edema are immediate life-threatening risks since patency of the airway may be lost. The trachea should be intubated, and the lungs should be ventilated with 100 percent oxygen.

Epinephrine is the principal drug for the treatment of anaphylaxis. It should be administered by slow intravenous infusion or, less optimally, intramuscularly or subcutaneously, 2 to 10 μg/kg. Since the duration of anaphylaxis often exceeds that of a single dose of epinephrine, a continuous infusion of epinephrine may be required: infusion rates range from 0.05 to 2 μg/kg/min. Epinephrine attenuates the release of mediators and restores the cardiac output and blood pressure. It probably acts by increasing cAMP and thereby decreasing the release of mediators. H_1 antihistamines such as diphenhydramine (0.5 to 1.0 mg/kg) may be effective for persistent or slowly developing angioneurotic edema. H_2 antihistamines may also work. Antihistamines appear to act by blocking the binding of histamine to histamine receptors. The role of steroids in the treatment of laryngeal edema and anaphylaxis remains controversial.

If bronchospasm develops, immediate therapy is required. One hundred percent oxygen should be administered with assisted positive-pressure ventilation. Epinephrine is the drug of choice in the previously indicated dose. When bronchospasm is not immediately reversed, 5 to 6 mg/kg of aminophylline should be infused over 15 to 30 minutes, followed by a continuous infusion of 0.9 mg/kg/h or less (see Table 17–3). The use of theophylline in these cases must be carefully monitored by measurement of the serum concentration, particularly in the presence of cimetidine, because cimetidine blocks hepatic metabolism of theophylline. To attenuate the persistent bronchospasm, hydrocortisone, 3 to 4 mg/kg intravenously, is also recommended.

Circulatory collapse may result in cardiac arrest from severe hypotension, myocardial ischemia, or arrhythmias. Anaphylaxis causes extreme vasodilatation and peripheral edema with an acute decrease in blood volume. Therapy includes the administration of 100 percent oxygen, placing the patient in the Trendelenburg position, and administration of large volumes of crystalloid or colloid solutions to restore the blood volume. The immediate therapy for hypotension includes parenteral epinephrine, as discussed. If bradycardia occurs, atropine, 0.02 mg/kg intravenously, should be administered. The same dose should be given intramuscularly if venous access is not available. A vasopressor such as metaraminol (0.5 mg intravenously for children less than 10 kg, and 1.0 mg for those over 10 kg) may be required to support the blood pressure, particularly if there is concern over administering repeated doses of epinephrine in the presence of halothane. Although alpha-agonists theoretically may cause mediator release by increasing intracellular cGMP, the need for these agents to maintain the circulation overrides this theoretical disadvantage. Secondary therapy includes steroids and H_1 antihistamines for persistent anaphylaxis, although their contribution to a successful outcome remains to be established.

Occasionally, drugs that are known allergens must be administered to very allergic patients. This may precipitate an acute anaphylactic reaction. The severity of allergic and anaphylactic reactions may be attenuated if the trigger agent is administered orally rather than parenterally. However, anaphylactic reactions to oral drugs have been reported. If the patient is very allergic, a small "test" dose may be administered and the patient observed before administering the full drug dose. Both H_1 antihistamines and prednisone may prevent anaphylactic reactions to radiocontrast dyes, protamine, and chymopapain.

REFERENCES

URTICARIA AND ANGIOEDEMA

Beall GN: Urticaria: A review of laboratory and clinical observations. Medicine *43*:131, 1964.

Benveniste J, Kamoun P, Polonsky J: Aggregation of human platelet activating factor from human and rabbit basophils (abstract). Fed Proc *34*:985, 1975.

Boggs PB, Ellis CN, Grossman J, et al: Double-blind, placebo-controlled study of terfenadine and hydroxyzine in patients with chronic idiopathic urticaria. Ann Allergy *63*:616, 1989.

Champion RH, Roberts SOB, Carpenter RG, et al: Urticaria and angiooedema. Br J Dermatol *81*:588, 1969.

Clark RAF, Gallin JI, Kaplan AP: The selective eosinophilic chemotactic activity of histamine J Exp Med *172*:1462, 1975.

Collins-Williams C: Urticaria and angioedema. *In* Kelley VC (ed): Practice of Pediatrics. Vol 2. Philadelphia, Harper & Row, 1984.

Harvey RP, Schocket AL: The effect of H_1 and H_2 blockade on cutaneous histamine release in man. J Allergy Clin Immunol *65*:136, 1980.

Holgate ST: The mast cell and its function in allergic disease. Clin Exp Allergy *21*:(Suppl 3)11, 1991.

Kaplan AP: Urticaria and angioedema. *In* Middleton E, Reed CE, Ellis EF (eds): Allergy: Principles and Practice. Vol 2. St. Louis, CV Mosby, 1983.

Kettle K: Melkersson's syndrome: Report of 5 cases, with special reference to pathologic observations. Arch Otolaryngol *46*:341, 1947.

Paul E, Reinel D, Ulrich R, Kohler ME: Comparison of efficacy and tolerability of terfenadine administered once daily versus twice daily in patients with chronic idiopathic urticaria. Ann Allergy *63*:34, 1989.

Plant M: Histamine, H_1 and H_2 antihistamines, and immediate hypersensitivity reactions. J Allergy Clin Immunol *63*:371, 1975.

Schneider SB, Atkinson JP: Urticaria and angioedema. *In* Fitzpatrick TB, Eisen AZ, Wolff K, et al (eds): Update: Dermatology in General Medicine. New York, McGraw-Hill, 1983, p 61.

Sheffer AL: Urticaria and angioedema. Pediatr Clin North Am *22*:193, 1975.

Sly RM: Urticaria and angioedema. *In* Berman BA, MacDonnell KF (eds): Differential Diagnosis and Treatment of Pediatric Allergy. Boston, Little, Brown, 1981.

Smith GB, Shribman AJ: Anesthesia and severe skin disease. Anaesthesia *39*:443, 1984.

ASTHMA

Anderson HR: Increase in hospital admissions for childhood asthma: Trends in referral, severity, and readmissions from 1970 to 1985 in a health region of the United Kingdom. Thorax *44*:614, 1989.

Andersson KE, Persson CG: Extrapulmonary effects of theophylline. Eur J Respir Dis *61*(Suppl 109):17, 1980.

Aranda JV, Turmen T: Methylxanthines in apnea of prematurity. Clin Perinatol *6*:87, 1979.

Aublier M, DeTroyer A, Sampson M, et al: Aminophylline improves diaphragmatic contractility. N Engl J Med *305*:249, 1981.

Avner SE: Beta-adrenergic bronchodilators. Pediatr Clin North Am *22*:121, 1975.

Baran D: A comparison of inhaled budesonide and beclomethasone dipropionate in childhood asthma. Br J Dis Chest *81*:170, 1987.

Becker AB, Simmons FER: Formoterol, a new long-acting selective β_2-agonist, decreases airway responsiveness in children with asthma. Lung (Suppl):99, 1990.

Bentur L, Kerem L, Canny G, et al: Response of acute asthma to a $beta_2$ agonist in children less than two years of age. Ann Allergy *65*:122, 1990.

Bernstein IL, Johnson CL, Tse CST: Therapy with cromolyn sodium. Ann Intern Med *89*:228, 1978.

Berstrand H: Phosphodiesterase inhibition and theophylline. Eur J Respir Dis *61*(Suppl 109):37, 1980.

Bierman CW, Pearlman DS: Asthma. *In* Kendig EL Jr, Chernick V (eds): Disorders of the Respiratory Tract in Children. 4th ed. Philadelphia, WB Saunders, 1983.

Bory C, Baltassat P, Rorthault M, et al: Metabolism of theophylline to caffeine in premature newborn infants. J Pediatr *94*:988, 1981.

Boutros AR, Weisel M: Comparison of effects of three anaesthetic techniques on patients with severe pulmonary obstructive disease. Can Anaesth Soc J *18*:296, 1971.

Bukowsky M, Nakatsu K, Munt PW: Theophylline reassessed. Ann Intern Med *101*:63, 1984.

Bundgaard A, Bach-Mortensen N, Schmidt A: The effect of sodium cromoglycate delivered by Spinhaler and by pressurized aerosol on exercise-induced asthma in children. Clin Allergy *12*:601, 1982.

Burney PGJ, Rona RJ: Has the prevalence of asthma increased in children? Evidence from the national study of health and growth 1973–1986. Br Med J *300*:1306, 1990.

Burr ML, Butland BK, King S, Vaughn-Williams E: Changes in asthma prevalence: Two surveys 15 years apart. Arch Dis Child *64*:1452, 1989.

Chang TMS, Espinosa-Melendez E, Francoeur TE, et al: Albumin-collodion activated charcoal hemoperfusion in the treatment of severe theophylline intoxication in a 3-year-old patient. Pediatrics *65*:811, 1980.

Church MK: The role of basophils in asthma. 1. Sodium cromoglycate on histamine release and content. Clin Allergy *12*:223, 1982.

Crago RR, Bryan AC, Laws AK, et al: Respiratory flow resistance after curare and pancuronium, measured by force oscillation. Can Anaesth Soc J *19*:697, 1972.

Craps LP, Ney UM: Ketotifen: Current views on its mechanism of action and their therapeutic implications. Respiration *45*:411, 1984.

Dawson A, Simon RA: Bronchospastic disorders: An overview. *In* Dawson A, Simon RA (eds): The Practical Management of Asthma. Orlando, Fla., Grune and Stratton, 1984.

Dees SC: Asthma. *In* Kendig EL Jr, Chernick V (eds): Disorders of the Respiratory Tract in Children. 3rd ed. Philadelphia, WB Saunders, 1977.

Delaney JC: The effect of ketotifen on aspirin-induced asthmatic reactions. Clin Allergy *13*:247, 1983.

Dorow P, Schiess W: Influence of ketotifen on the airway responsiveness in asthmatics. J Asthma *21*:81, 1984.

Downes H, Gerber N, Hirshman CA: I.V. lignocaine in reflex and allergic bronchoconstriction. Br J Anaesth *52*:873, 1980.

Downes H, Hirshman CA: Lidocaine aerosols do not prevent allergic bronchoconstriction. Anesth Analg *60*:28, 1981.

Downes JJ, Wood DW, Harwood I, et al: Intravenous isoproterenol infusion in children with severe hypercapnia due to status asthmaticus: Effects on ventilation, circulation and clinical score. Crit Care Med *1*:65, 1973.

Ellis EF: Asthma. *In* Middleton E, Reed CE, Ellis EF (eds): Allergy: Principles and Practice. St. Louis, CV Mosby, 1978.

Ellis EF, Koysooko R, Levy G: Pharmacokinetics of theophylline in children with asthma. Pediatrics *58*:542, 1976.

Ellul-Micallef R, Fenech FF: Effect of intravenous prednisolone in asthmatics with diminished adrenergic responsiveness. Lancet *2*:1269, 1975.

Falliers CJ: Cromolyn sodium (disodium cromoglycate) prophylaxis. Pediatr Clin North Am *22*:141, 1975.

Falliers CJ: Corticosteroids for childhood asthma: Systemic and topical treatment. J Asthma *20*:475, 1983.

Fanta CH, Rossing TH, McFadden ER: Glucocorticoids in acute asthma—a critical controlled trial. Am J Med *74*:845, 1983.

Fanta CH, Rossing TH, McFadden ER Jr: Treatment of acute asthma: Is combination therapy with sympathomimetics and methylxanthines indicated? Am J Med *80*:5, 1986.

Feld LH, Negus JB, White PF: Oral midazolam preanesthetic medication in pediatric outpatients. Anesthesiology *73*:831, 1990.

Feldman CH, Sher TN, Hutchison VE, et al: Fenoterol dose-response study in children with asthma. J Allergy Clin Immunol *73*:356, 1984.

Fisher DM, Robinson S, Brett CM, et al: A comparison of enflurane, halothane and isoflurane for diagnostic and therapeutic procedures in children with malignancies. Anesthesiology *63*:647, 1985.

Friedman MS: Psychological factors associated with pediatric asthma death: A review. J Asthma *21*:97, 1984.

Friegang B, Ashford DR: Adrenal cortical function after long-term beclomethasone aerosol therapy in early childhood. Ann Allergy *64*:342, 1990.

Gal P, Roop C, Robinson H, et al: Theophylline-induced seizures in accidentally overdosed neonates. Pediatrics *65*:547, 1980.

Gal TJ, Suratt PM, Lu J: Glycopyrrolate and atropine inhalation: Comparative effects on normal airway function. Am Rev Respir Dis *129*:871, 1984.

Geller-Bernstein C, Sneh N: The management of bronchial asthma in children under the age of 3½ years using Intal (sodium cromoglycate) administered by Spinhaler. Clin Allergy *10*:503, 1980.

Giacoia G, Jusko WJ, Menke J, et al: Theophylline pharmacokinetics in premature infants with apnea. J Pediatr *89*:829, 1976.

Godfrey S: The place of a new aerosol steroid, beclomethasone dipropionate, in the management of childhood asthma. Pediatr Clin North Am *22*:147, 1975.

Goudsouzian NG, Young ET, Moss J, Liu LMP: Histamine release during the administration of atracurium and vecuronium in children. Br J Anaesth *56*:1229, 1986.

Graff-Lonnevig V, Browaldh L: Twelve hours' bronchodilating effect of inhaled formoterol in children with asthma: A double-blind cross-over study versus salbutamol. Clin Exp Allergy *20*:429, 1990.

Grainger J, Woodman K, Pearce N, et al: Prescribed fenoterol and death from asthma in New Zealand, 1981–7: A further case-control study. Thorax *46*:105, 1991.

Gran L, Pahle JA: Rational substitution therapy for steroid-treated patients. Anaesthesia *33*:59, 1978.

Greenwood C: The pharmacology of ketotifen. Chest *82*:45S, 1982.

Gross NJ, Skomedin MS: Anticholinergic antimuscarinic bronchodilators. Am Rev Respir Dis *129*:856, 1984.

Hardy CC, Robinson C, Tattersfield AE, et al: The bronchoconstrictor effect of inhaled prostaglandin D_2 in normal and asthmatic men. N Engl J Med *311*:209, 1984.

Henderson WR, Shelhamer JH, Reingold DB, et al: Alpha-adrenergic hyperresponsiveness in asthma: Analysis of vascular and pupillary responses. N Engl J Med *300*:642, 1979.

Hendles L, Weinberger M: Theophylline. *In* Middleton E, Reed CE, Ellis EF (eds): Allergy: Principles and Practice. Vol I. St. Louis, CV Mosby, 1983, p. 535.

Hilman B: Aerosol deposition and delivery of therapeutic aerosols. J Asthma *28*:239, 1991.

Hirschman CA: Airway reactivity in humans. Anesthesiology *58*:170, 1983.

Horrobin DF, Manku MS, Franks DJ, et al: Methylxanthine phosphodiesterase inhibitors behave as prostaglandin antagonists in a perfused rat mesentery artery preparation. Prostaglandins *13*:33, 1977.

Jacobs MH, Senior RM, Kessler G: Clinical experience with theophylline: Relationship between dosage, serum concentration and toxicity. JAMA *235*:1983, 1976.

Katz RM, Rachelefsky GS, Siegel SC, et al: Theophylline administration in children with asthma: Optimal pulmonary function and possible tolerance to chronic administration. Ann Allergy *50*:23, 1983.

Kemp JP: Adrenergic bronchodilators, old and new. J Asthma *20*:45, 1983.

Kerrebijn ICF: Use of topical corticosteroids in the treatment of childhood asthma. Am Rev Respir Dis *141*:577, 1990.

Kingston HGG, Hirschman CA: Perioperative management of the patient with asthma. Anesth Analg *63*:844, 1984.

Kline LE: Sympathomimetic agents. *In* Dawson A, Simon RA (eds): The Practical Management of Asthma. Orlando, Fla., Grune and Stratton, 1984.

Koga Y, Iwatsuki N, Hashimoto Y: Direct effects of H_2-receptor antagonists on airway smooth muscle and on responses mediated by H_1- and H_2-receptors. Anesthesiology *66*:181, 1987.

Konig P: The use of cromolyn in the management of hyperreactive airways and exercise. J Allergy Clin Immunol *73*:686, 1984.

Konig P: Inhaled corticosteroids—their present and future roles in the management of asthma. J Allergy Clin Immunol *82*:297, 1988.

Landay RA, Gonzalez MA, Taylor JC: Effect of phenobarbital on theophylline disposition. J Allergy Clin Immunol *62*:27, 1978.

Law CM, Marchant JL, Honour JW, et al: Nocturnal adrenal suppression in asthmatic children taking inhaled beclomethasone dipropionate. Lancet *1*:942, 1986.

Letarte L, duSouich P: Influence of hypercapnia and/or hypoxemia and metabolic acidosis on theophylline kinetics in the conscious rabbit. Am Rev Respir Dis *129*:762, 1984.

Levy G, Koysooka R: Pharmacokinetic analysis of the effect of theophylline on pulmonary function in asthmatic children. J Pediatr *86*:789, 1975.

Lichtenstein LM, Gillespie E: Inhibition of histamine release controlled by the receptor. Nature *244*:287, 1973.

Lofdahl C-G, Svedmyr N: Formoterol fumarate, a new β_2-adrenoceptor agonist. Acute studies of selectivity and duration of effect after inhaled and oral administration. Allergy *44*:264, 1989.

Lonnerholm G, Foucard T, Lindstrom B: Dose, plasma concentration, and effect of oral terbutaline in long-term treatment of childhood asthma. J Allergy Clin Immunol *73*:508, 1984.

Matthys H: Inhalation delivery of asthma drugs. Lung (Suppl) 645, 1990.

Mazer B, Figueroa-Rosario W, Bender B: The effect of albuterol aerosol on fine-motor performance in children with chronic asthma. J Allergy Clin Immunol *86*:243, 1990.

McFadden ER Jr: Pathogenesis of asthma. J Allergy Clin Immunol *73*:413, 1984.

McLaughlin ET, Bethea LN, Wittig HJ: Comparison of the bronchodilator effect of oral fenoterol and ephedrine in asthmatic children. Ann Allergy *49*:191, 1982.

Meltzer DL, Kemp JP: Beta$_2$-agonists: Pharmacology and recent developments. J Asthma *28*(3):179, 1991.

Menendez R, Kelly HW: Theophylline therapy. J Asthma *20*:455, 1983.

Middleton E Jr: The biochemical basis for the modulation

of allergic reactions by drugs. Pediatr Clin North Am *22*:111, 1975.

Mislap RL, Krauss AN, Auld PAM: Oxygen consumption in apneic premature infants after low-dose theophylline. Clin Pharmacol Ther *28*:536, 1980.

Mitenko PA, Ogilvie RI: Rational intravenous doses of theophylline. N Engl J Med *289*:600, 1973.

Mueller RA: Recent developments in the physiology of bronchomotor tone and the pharmacology of bronchodilators. Int Anesthesiol Clin *15*:137, 1977.

Nathan RA, Segall N, Glover GC, et al: The effects of H_1 and H_2 antihistamines on histamine inhalation challenges in asthmatic patients. Am Rev Respir Dis *120*:1251, 1979.

Nelson DR, Sachs MI, O'Connell EJ: Approaches to acute asthma and status asthmaticus in children. Mayo Clin Proc *64*:1392, 1989.

Newhouse MT, Lam A: Management of asthma and chronic airflow limitations: Are methyl xanthines obsolete? Lung (Suppl) 634, 1990.

Nicklaus RA: Perspective on asthma mortality—1989. Ann Allergy *63*:578, 1989.

Nussbaum E, Eyzaguirre M, Galant SP: Dose-response relationship of inhaled metaproterenol sulfate in preschool children with mild asthma. Pediatrics *85*:1072, 1990.

Oyama T: Hazards of steroids in association with anaesthesia. Can Anaesth Soc J *16*:361, 1979.

Parnass SM, Feld JM, Chamberlin WH, Segil LJ: Status asthmaticus treated with isoflurane and enflurane. Anesthesiology *66*:193, 1987.

Patel KR: Sodium cromoglycate in histamine and methacholine reactivity in asthma. Clin Allergy *14*:143, 1984.

Pearce N, Crane J: Beta agonists and asthma mortality: Deja vu. Clin Exp Allergy *21*:401, 1991.

Pollock J, Kiechel F, Cooper D, et al: Relationship of serum theophylline concentration to inhibition of exercise-induced bronchospasm and comparison with cromolyn. Pediatrics *60*:840, 1977.

Popa VT: Clinical pharmacology of adrenergic drugs. J Asthma *21*:183, 1984.

Prenner BM: Safety, efficacy and bronchodilator sparing effects of nebulized cromolyn sodium solution in the treatment of asthma in children. Ann Allergy *49*:186, 1982.

Ramsdale EH, Otis J, Kline PA, et al: Prolonged protection against methacholine-induced bronchoconstriction by the inhaled β_2-agonist formoterol. Am Rev Respir Dis *143*:998, 1991.

Ravin MB: Comparison of spinal and general anesthesia for lower abdominal surgery in patients with chronic obstructive pulmonary disease. Anesthesiology *35*:319, 1971.

Salmon B, Wilson NM, Silverman M: How much aerosol reaches the lungs of wheezing infants and toddlers? Arch Dis Child *65*:401, 1990.

Schuh S, Parkin P, Rajan A, et al: High- versus low-dose, frequently administered, nebulized albuterol in children with severe, acute asthma. Pediatrics *83*:513, 1989.

Schuhl JF, De Cuesta DH: A double-blind trial comparing disodium cromoglycate (DSCG) and ketotifen in extrinsic asthma. Clin Allergy *11*:401, 1981.

Sears MR, Taylor DR, Print CG, et al: Regular inhaled beta-agonist treatment in bronchial asthma. Lancet *2*:1391, 1990.

Selcow JE: Cromolyn therapy in children. J Allergy *20*:361, 1983.

Shapiro GG: Corticosteroids in the treatment of allergic disease: Principles and practice. Pediatr Clin North Am *30*:955, 1983.

Sherman B, Weinberger M, Chen-Walden H, et al: Further studies of the effects of inhaled glucocorticoids on pituitary-adrenal function in healthy adults. J Allergy Clin Immunol *69*:208, 1982.

Shnider SM, Paper EM: Anesthesia for the asthmatic patient. Anesthesiology *22*:886, 1961.

Siegel SC: Bronchial asthma. *In* Kelley VC (ed): Practice of Pediatrics. Philadelphia, Harper and Row, 1984.

Simons FER, Friesen FR, Simons KJ: Theophylline toxicity in term infants. Am J Dis Child *134*:39, 1980.

Sly RM: Current theories of the pathophysiology of asthma. J Asthma *20*:419, 1983.

Snell NJC: Adverse reactions to inhaled drugs. Respir Med *84*:345, 1990.

Somani SM, Khanna NN, Bada HS: Caffeine and theophylline serum/CSF correlation in premature infants. J Pediatr *96*:1091, 1980.

Spector SL, Gomez MG: Dose-response effects of albuterol aerosol compared with isoproterenol and placebo aerosols: Response to albuterol, isoproterenol and placebo aerosols. J Allergy Clin Immunol *59*:280, 1977.

Stevenson DD: Anticholinergic agents. *In* Dawson A, Simon RA (eds): The Practical Management of Asthma. Orlando, Fla., Grune and Stratton, 1984.

Summers QA: Inhaled drugs and the lung. Clin Exp Allergy *21*:259, 1991.

Symreng T, Karlberg BE, Kagedal B, et al: Physiological cortisol substitution of long-term steroid-treated patients undergoing major surgery. Br J Anaesth *53*:949, 1981.

Szefler SJ: Practical considerations in the safe and effective use of theophylline. Pediatr Clin North Am *30*:943, 1983.

Taylor RH, Lerman J: High-efficiency delivery of salbutamol with a metered-dose inhaler in narrow tracheal tubes and catheters. Anesthesiology *74*:360, 1991.

Tinkelman DG: The scope and state of pediatric asthma. J Asthma *20*:331, 1983.

Tinkelman DG, Berkowitz RB, Cole WQ III: Aerosols in the treatment of asthma. J Asthma *28*(4):243, 1991.

Tserng K, King KC, Takieddine FN: Theophylline metabolism in premature infants. Clin Pharmacol Ther *29*:594, 1981.

Urthaler F, James TN: Both direct and neurally mediated components of the chronotropic actions of aminophylline. Chest *70*:24, 1976.

Varsano I, Volvovitz B, Malik H, Amir Y: Safety of 1 year of treatment with budesonide in young children with asthma. J Allergy Clin Immunol *85*:914, 1990.

Volvovitz B, Varsano I, Cumella JC, Jaber L: Efficacy and safety of ketotifen in young children with asthma. J Allergy Clin Immunol *81*:526, 1988.

von Berg A, Berdel D: Efficacy of formoterol metered aerosol in children. Lung (Suppl) 90, 1990.

Wasserman SI: Mast cell–mediated inflammation in asthma. Ann Allergy *63*:546, 1989.

Webb-Johnson DC, Andrews JL: Bronchodilator therapy. N Engl J Med *297*:476, 1977.

Weinberger M, Hendles L, Ahrens R: Clinical pharmacology of drugs used for asthma. Pediatr Clin North Am *28*:61, 1981.

Weinberger MM: Use of ephedrine in bronchodilator therapy. Pediatr Clin North Am *22*:121, 1975.

Weinberger MM, Bronsky EA: Evaluation of oral bronchodilator therapy in asthmatic children. J Pediatr *84*:421, 1974.

Weinberger MM, Bronsky EA: Interaction of ephedrine and theophylline. Clin Pharmacol Ther *17*:585, 1975.

White PF: Propofol: Pharmacokinetics and pharmacodynamics. Semin Anesth 7:4, 1988.

White VA, Kumagai LF: Preoperative endocrine and metabolic considerations. Med Clin North Am *63*:1321, 1979.

Wyatt R, Waschek J, Weinberger M, et al: Effects of inhaled beclomethasone dipropionate and alternate-day

prednisone on pituitary-adrenal function in children with chronic asthma. N Engl J Med *299*:1387, 1978.
Yarborough J, Mansfield LE, Ting S: Metered dose inhaler induced bronchospasm in asthmatic patients. Ann Allergy *55*:25, 1985.
Zeiger RS: Special considerations in the approach to asthma in infancy and early childhood. J Asthma *20*:353, 1983.
Zwillich CW, Sutton FD, Neff TA, et al: Theophylline-induced seizures in adults: Correlation with serum concentrations. Ann Intern Med *82*:784, 1975.

MASTOCYTOSIS

Ammann RW, Vetter P, Deyhle P, et al: Gastrointestinal involvement in systemic mastocytosis. Gut *17*:107, 1976.
Basta SJ, Savarese JJ, Ali HH, et al: Histamine releasing potencies of atracurium, dimethyl tubocurarine, and tubocurarine. Br J Anaesth *55*:105S, 1983.
Basta SJ, Savarese JJ, Ali HH, et al: Vecuronium does not alter serum histamine release within the clinical dose range. Anesthesiology *59*:A273, 1983.
Bristow MR, Ginsburg R, Harrison DC: Histamine and the human heart: The other receptor system. Am J Cardiol *49*:249, 1982.
Broitman SA: Mastocytosis and intestinal malabsorption. Am J Med *48*:382, 1970.
Businco L, Cantani A, Businco E, et al: Systemic mastocytosis in a 5-year-old child: Successful treatment with disodium cromoglycate. Clin Allergy *14*:147, 1984.
Campbell EW, Hector D, Gossain V: Heparin activity in systemic mastocytosis. Ann Intern Med *90*:940, 1979.
Caplan RM: The natural course of urticaria pigmentosa. Analysis and follow-up of 112 cases. Arch Dermatol *87*:146, 1963.
Christophers E, Honigsmann H, Wolff K, et al: PUVA—treatment of urticaria pigmentosa. Br J Dermatol *98*:701, 1978.
Coleman MA, Liberthson RR, Crone RK, et al: General anaesthesia in a child with urticaria pigmentosa. Anesth Analg *59*:704, 1980.
Colten HR: Mediators of allergic response. *In* Kelley VC (ed): Practice of Pediatrics. Vol 2. Philadelphia, Harper and Row, 1984.
Czarnetzki BM, Behrendt H: Urticaria pigmentosa: Clinical picture and response to oral disodium cromoglycate. Br J Dermatol *105*:563, 1981.
Demis DJ: The mastocytosis syndrome: Clinical and biological studies. Ann Intern Med *59*:194, 1963.
DiBacco RS, De Leo VA: Mastocytosis and the mast cell. J Am Acad Dermatol *7*:709, 1982.
Ellis JM: Urticaria pigmentosa: Report of a case with autopsy. Arch Pathol *48*:426, 1949.
Fine J: Mastocytosis. Int J Dermatol *19*:117, 1980.
Flacke JW, Van Etten A, Flacke WE: Greatest histamine release from meperidine among four narcotics: Double-blind study in man. Anesthesiology *59*:A51, 1983.
Friedman BS, Steinberg SC, Meggs WJ, et al: Analysis of plasma histamine levels in patients with mast cell disorders. Am J Med *87*:649, 1989.
Galletly DC, Treuren BC: Anaphylactoid reactions during anaesthesia: Seven years' experience of intradermal testing. Anaesthesia *40*:329, 1985.
Gay MW, Noojin RO, Finley WH: Urticaria pigmentosa discordant in identical twins. Arch Dermatol *102*:29, 1970.
Gerrard DM, Ko C: Urticaria pigmentosa: Treatment with cimetidine and chlorpheniramine. J Pediatr *94*:843, 1979.
Greenwood C: The pharmacology of ketotifen. Chest *82*:45S, 1982.
Hermens JM, Ebertz JM, Hanifin JM, et al: Comparison of histamine release in human skin mast cells induced by morphine, fentanyl, and oxymorphone. Anesthesiology *62*:124, 1985.
Hirschowitz BI, Groarke MB: Effect of cimetidine on gastric hypersecretion and diarrhea in systemic mastocytosis. Ann Intern Med *90*:769, 1979.
Hirshman CA, Edelstein RA, Eastman CL, et al: Histamine release by barbiturates in human mast cells. Anesthesiology *61*:A352, 1984.
Hosking MP, Warner MA: Sudden intraoperative hypotension in a patient with asymptomatic urticaria pigmentosa. Anesth Analg *66*:344, 1987.
Karlin JM: The use of antihistamines in allergic disease. Pediatr Clin North Am *22*:157, 1975.
Klaus SN, Winkelman RK: Course of urticaria pigmentosa in children. Arch Dermatol *86*:86, 1962.
Lerno G, Slaats G, Coenen E, et al: Anaesthetic management of systemic mastocytosis. Br J Anaesth *65*:254, 1990.
Lewis RA, Austen KF: Mastocytosis—clinical mediators and therapeutic intervention. *In* Fitzpatrick TB, Eisen AZ, Wolff K, et al (eds): Update: Dermatology in General Medicine. New York, McGraw-Hill, 1983, p 197.
Lorenz W, Doeniche A: Anaphylactoid reactions and histamine release by IV drugs used in surgery and anesthesia. *In* Watkins J, Ward AM (eds): Adverse Response to IV Drugs. New York, Grune and Stratton, 1978, p 83.
Lucaya J, Perez-Candela V, Aso C, et al: Mastocytosis with skeletal and gastrointestinal involvement in infancy. Radiology *131*:363, 1979.
Manchikanti L, Kraus JW, Edds SP: Cimetidine and related drugs in anesthesia. Anesth Analg *61*:595, 1982.
Miller RD, Rupp SM, Fisher DM, et al: Clinical pharmacology of vecuronium and atracurium. Anesthesiology *61*:444, 1984.
Mishima S, Yamamura T: Anaphylactoid reaction to pancuronium. Anesth Analg *63*:865, 1984.
Moss J, Rosow CE: Histamine release by narcotics and muscle relaxants in humans. Anesthesiology *59*:330, 1983.
Moss J, Rosow CE, Savarese JJ, et al: Role of histamine in the hypotensive action of D-tubocurarine in humans. Anesthesiology *55*:19, 1981.
Nightingale DA, Bush GH: A clinical comparison between D-tubocurarine and pancuronium in children. Br J Anaesth *45*:63, 1973.
Orkin M, Good RA, Clawson CC, et al: Bullous mastocytosis. Arch Dermatol *101*:547, 1970.
Parker F, Odland GF: The mastocytosis syndrome. *In* Fitzpatrick TB, Eisen AZ, Wolff K, et al (eds): Dermatology in General Medicine. New York, McGraw-Hill, 1979, p 772.
Philbin DM, Moss J, Akins CW, et al: The use of H_1 and H_2 histamine antagonists with morphine anesthesia: A double-blind study. Anesthesiology *55*:292, 1981.
Rimmer SJ, Church MK: The pharmacology and mechanisms of action of histamine H_1-antagonists. Clin Exp Allergy *20*(Suppl 2):3, 1990.
Roberts LJ II, Sweetman BJ, Lewis RA, et al: Increased production of prostaglandin D_2 in patients with systemic mastocytosis. N Engl J Med *303*:1400, 1980.
Rockoff AS: Urticaria pigmentosa in identical twins. Arch Dermatol *114*:1227, 1978.
Rosenbaum KJ, Strobel GE: Anesthetic considerations in mastocytosis. Anesthesiology *38*:398, 1973.
Rosow CE, Moss J, Philbin DM, et al: Histamine release during morphine and fentanyl anesthesia. Anesthesiology *56*:93, 1982.
Rosow CE, Philbin DM, Keegan CR, et al: Hemodynamics and histamine release during induction with sufentanil or fentanyl. Anesthesiology *60*:489, 1984.
Sagher F, Even-Paz Z: Mastocytosis and the Mast Cell.

Chicago, Year Book Medical Publishers, 1968, pp 14–120, 148–338.
Schachner L, Press S: Vesicular bullous and pustular disorders in infancy and childhood. Pediatr Clin North Am *30*:609, 1983.
Scott RPF, Savarese JJ, Basta SJ, et al: Atracurium: Clinical strategies for preventing histamine release and attenuating the hemodynamic response. Br J Anaesth *57*:550, 1985.
Siler JN, Mager JG, Wyche MQ: Atracurium: Hypotension, tachycardia and bronchospasm. Anesthesiology *62*:645, 1985.
Simone JV, Hayes WT: Bullous urticaria pigmentosa with bleeding. J Pediatr *78*:160, 1971.
Simons FER: New H_1-receptor antagonists: Clinical pharmacology. Clin Exp Allergy *20*(Suppl 2):19, 1990.
Simons FER, Simons KJ: Second-generation H_1-receptor antagonists. Ann Allergy *66*:5, 1991.
Soter NA, Austin KF, Wasserman SI: Oral disodium cromoglycate in the management of systemic mastocytosis. N Engl J Med *303*:465, 1979.
Sutter MC, Beaulieu G, Birt AR: Histamine liberation by codeine and polymyxin B in urticaria pigmentosa. Arch Dermatol *86*:217, 1962.
Watkins J: Adverse anaesthetic reactions. Anaesthesia *40*:797, 1985.
Williams JG: H_2 receptor antagonists and anaesthesia. Can Anaesth Soc J *30*:264, 1983.
Wyre HW, Hendrichs WD: Systemic mastocytosis and pulmonary eosinophilic granuloma. JAMA *239*:856, 1978.

ERYTHEMA MULTIFORME

Bean SF, Quezada RK: Recurrent oral erythema multiforme: Clinical experience with 11 patients. JAMA *249*:2810, 1983.
Bedi TR, Pinkus H: Histopathologic spectrum of erythema multiforme. Br J Dermatol *95*:243, 1976.
Collins-Williams C: Urticaria and angioedema. *In* Kelley VC (ed): Practice of Pediatrics. Vol 2. Philadelphia, Harper and Row, 1984.
Cucchiara RF, Dawson B: Anesthetic in Stevens-Johnson syndrome: Report of a case. Anesthesiology *35*:537, 1971.
Edmond BJ, Huff JL, Weston WL: Erythema multiforme. Pediatr Clin North Am *30*:631, 1983.
Ginsburg CM: Stevens-Johnson syndrome in children. Pediatr Infect Dis *1*:155, 1982.
Lever WF, Schaumburg-Lever G: Histopathology of the Skin. 6th ed. Philadelphia, JB Lippincott, 1983, p 122.
Lyell A: A review of toxic epidermal necrolysis in Britain. Br J Dermatol *79*:662, 1967.
Smith GB, Shribman AJ: Anaesthesia and severe skin disease. Anaesthesia *39*:443, 1984.
Szefler SJ, Ellis EF: Adverse reactions to drugs. *In* Kelley VC (ed): Practice of Pediatrics. Vol 2. Philadelphia, Harper and Row, 1984.

ANAPHYLAXIS

Anderson JR, Poblis A, Slavin R: Fatal case of aminophylline intoxication. Arch Intern Med *143*:559, 1983.
Barnard JH: Studies of 400 Hymenoptera sting deaths in the United States. J Allergy Clin Immunol *52*:259, 1973.
Beaupre PN, Roizen MF, Cahalan MK, et al: Hemodynamic and two-dimensional transesophageal echocardiographic analysis of an anaphylactic reaction in a human. Anesthesiology *60*:482, 1984.
Beavan MA: Anaphylactoid reactions to anesthetic drugs. Anesthesiology *55*:3, 1981.
Bleeker ER, Smith PL, Kagy-Sobotka A: Physiologic manifestations of human anaphylaxis. J Clin Invest *66*:1072, 1980.
Bochner BS, Lichtenstein LM: Anaphylaxis. N Engl J Med *324*:1785, 1991.
Burman D, Hodson AK, Wood CBS, et al: Acute anaphylaxis, pulmonary edema, and intravenous hemolysis due to cryoprecipitate. Arch Dis Child *48*:483, 1973.
Chaffee FH, Sertipane GA: Aspirin intolerance. I. Frequency in allergic population. J Allergy Clin Immunol *53*:193, 1974.
Church MK, El-lati S, Okayama Y: Biological properties of human skin mast cells. Clin Exp Allergy *21*(Suppl 3):1, 1991.
Clarke RSJ, Dundee JW, Garrett RT, et al: Adverse reactions to intravenous anaesthetics. Br J Anaesth *47*:575, 1975.
Criep LH, Woehler TR: The heart in human anaphylaxis. Ann Allergy *29*:399, 1971.
Delage C, Irey NS: Anaphylactic deaths: A clinicopathologic study of 43 cases. J Forensic Sci *17*:525, 1972.
Driggs RL, O'Day RA: Acute allergic reaction associated with methohexital anaesthesia: Report of six cases. J Oral Surg *30*:906, 1972.
Dykewicz MS, Wong S, Patterson R, Harris KE: Evaluation of ketotifen in corticosteroid-dependent idiopathic anaphylaxis. Ann Allergy *65*:406, 1990.
Edde RR, Burtis BB: Lung injury in anaphylactoid shock. Chest *63*:639, 1973.
Evans JM, Keogh JAM: Adverse reactions to intravenous anaesthetic induction agents. Br Med J *2*:735, 1977.
Fisher MM: Severe histamine mediated reaction to intravenous drugs used in anaesthesia. Anaesth Intensive Care *3*:180, 1975.
Fisher MM: Intradermal testing after severe histamine reactions to intravenous drugs used in anaesthesia. Anaesth Intensive Care *4*:97, 1976.
Fisher MM: The management of acute anaphylaxis. *In* Watkins J, Ward AM (eds): Adverse Response to Intravenous Drugs. New York, Grune and Stratton, 1978, p 145.
Fisher MM, Munro I: Life-threatening anaphylactoid reactions to muscle relaxants. Anesth Analg *62*:559, 1983.
Frank MM, Gelfand JA, Atkinson JP: Hereditary angioedema: The clinical syndrome and its management. Ann Intern Med *84*:580, 1976.
Gerber AC, Jong W, Zbinden S, et al: Severe intraoperative anaphylaxis to surgical gloves: Latex allergy, an unfamiliar condition. Anesthesiology *71*:800, 1989.
Gold M, Swartz JS, Braude BM, et al: Intraoperative anaphylaxis: An association with latex sensitivity. J Allergy Clin Immunol *87*:662, 1991.
Goldberg M: Systemic reactions to intravascular contrast media. Anesthesiology *60*:46, 1984.
Greenberger PA, Patterson R, Simon R, et al: Pre-treatment studies of high-risk patients requiring radiographic contrast media studies. J Allergy Clin Immunol *67*:185, 1981.
Hammerschmidt DE, Harris PD, Wayland H, et al: Complement-induced granulocyte aggregation in vivo. Am J Pathol *102*:146, 1981.
Hammerschmidt DE, White JG, Cradoch PR, et al: Corticosteroids inhibit complement-mediated granulocyte aggregation: A possible mechanism for their efficacy in shock states. Clin Invest *63*:798, 1979.
Haneshiro PK, Weil MH: Anaphylactic shock in man: Report of two cases with detailed hemodynamics and metabolic studies. Arch Intern Med *119*:129, 1967.
Heimlich EM, Siegel SC: Anaphylaxis. *In* Kelley VC (ed): Practice of Pediatrics. Philadelphia, Harper and Row, 1984.

Henry DA, MacDonald IA, Kitchingham G, et al: Cimetidine and ranitidine: Comparison of effects on hepatic drug metabolism. Br Med J *281*:775, 1980.

Horowitz L: Atopy as a factor in penicillin reactions. N Engl J Med *292*:1243, 1975.

James LP, Austen KF: Fatal systemic anaphylaxis in man. N Engl J Med *270*:597, 1964.

Kelly JF, Patterson R: Anaphylaxis—course, mechanisms and treatment. JAMA *227*:1431, 1974.

Kelly JF, Patterson R, Lieberman P, et al: Radiographic contrast media studies in high-risk patients. J Allergy Clin Immunol *62*:181, 1978.

Knauer KA, Adkinson NF Jr: Clinical significance of IgE. *In* Middleton E, Reed CE, Ellis EF (eds): Allergy: Principles and Practice. St. Louis, CV Mosby, 1983, p 673.

Knauer KA, Lichtenstein LM, Adkinson NF Jr, et al: Platelet activation during antigen-induced airway reactions in asthmatic subjects. N Engl J Med *304*:1404, 1981.

Larsen EC, Walters AJ, Lang JH: An experimental basis for histamine release in contrast material reactions. Radiology *110*:49, 1974.

Levy JH, Rockoff MA: Anaphylaxis to meperidine. Anesth Analg *61*:301, 1982.

Lorenz W, Doenicke A: Anaphylactoid reactions and histamine release by intravenous drugs used in surgery and anaesthesia. *In* Watkins J, Ward AM (eds): Adverse Response to Intravenous Drugs. New York, Grune and Stratton, 1978, p 83.

McManus LM, Hannahan DJ, Demopoules CA, et al: Pathobiology of the intravenous infusion of acetyl glyceryl ether phosphorylcholine (AGEPC), a synthetic platelet-activating factor (PAF), in the rabbit. J Immunol *124*:2919, 1980.

Miller WL, Doppman JL, Kaplan AP: Renal arteriography following systemic reaction to contrast material. J Allergy Clin Immunol *56*:291, 1975.

Moss J, McDermott DJ, Thisted RA, et al: Anaphylactic/anaphylactoid reactions in response to Chymodiactin (chymopapain). Anesth Analg *63*:253, 1984.

Orange RP, Donsky GJ: Anaphylaxis. *In* Middleton E, Reed CE, Ellis EF (eds): Allergy: Principles and Practice. St. Louis, CV Mosby, 1978.

Philbin DM, Moss J, Atkins CW, et al: The use of H_1 and H_2 histamine antagonists with morphine anesthesia: A double-blind study. Anesthesiology *55*:292, 1981.

Ring J, Messmer K: Incidence and severity of anaphylactoid reactions to colloid volume substitutes. Lancet *1*:466, 1977.

Schwartz LB, Yunginger JW, Miller J, et al: Time course of appearance and disappearance of human mast cell tryptase in the circulation after anaphylaxis. J Clin Invest *83*:1551, 1989.

Settipane GA, Klein DE, Boyd GK: Relationship of atopy and anaphylactic sensitization: A bee sting allergy model. Clin Allergy *8*:259, 1978.

Sheffer AL, Austen KF: Exercise-induced anaphylaxis. J Allergy Clin Immunol *66*:106, 1980.

Slater JE: Rubber anaphylaxis. N Engl J Med *320*:1126, 1989.

Small P, Satin R, Palayew MJ, et al: Prophylactic antihistamines in the management of radiographic contrast reactions. Clin Allergy *12*:289, 1982.

Steschulte DJ, Orange RP, Austen KF: Detection of slow reacting substance of anaphylaxis (SRS-A) in plasma in guinea pigs during anaphylaxis. J Immunol *111*:1585, 1973.

Stoelting RK: Allergic reactions during anesthesia. Anesth Analg *62*:341, 1983.

Swartz J, Brande BM, Gilmour RF, et al: Intraoperative anaphylaxis to latex. Can J Anaesth *37*:589, 1990.

Szefler SJ, Ellis EF: Adverse reactions to drugs. *In* Kelley VC (ed): Practice of Pediatrics. Philadelphia, Harper and Row, 1984.

Tannenbaum H, Ruddy S, Schur PH: Acute anaphylaxis associated with serum complement depletion. J Allergy Clin Immunol *56*:226, 1974.

Wasserman SI: Anaphylaxis. *In* Middleton E Jr, Reed CE, Ellis EF (eds): Allergy: Principles and Practice. Vol 2. St. Louis, CV Mosby, 1983, p 689.

Watkins J, Udnoon S, Taussig PE: Mechanisms of adverse response to intravenous agents in man. *In* Watkins J, Ward AM (eds): Adverse Response to Intravenous Drugs. New York, Grune and Stratton, 1978, p 71.

Westacott P, Ramachandran PR, Jancelewicz Z: Anaphylactic reaction to thiopentone. Can Anaesth Soc J *31*:434, 1984.

CHAPTER

18 Diseases of Blood

WILLIAM R. HAIN, M.B.† and SUSAN E. F. JONES, M.B.

Diseases of the blood are so diverse in etiology, pathophysiology, treatment, and prognosis that a text devoted to them must range widely in approach.

Four aspects of diseases of the blood have special implications for the anesthesiologist: reduced oxygen carriage, hemolysis of red cells, bleeding diathesis, and susceptibility to thrombosis.[1]

In any particular disorder one or more of these features may require attention in preoperative planning, in choice of agents and techniques for anesthesia, and in postoperative care. The anesthetic management appropriate to each is in some cases well documented (as in sickle cell disease). In others (for example, aplastic anemia), recommendations given are based upon the known features of the disease, considered in conjunction with accepted anesthetic practice and known drug activity.

The normal range of hemoglobin concentrations for a particular subject differs according to sex, age, race, and the laboratory concerned. A patient with a hemoglobin concentration below the range accepted as normal is suffering from anemia.

Classification of anemias may be based upon etiology,[2, 3] as summarized in Table 18–1.

†Deceased

Table 18–1. CLASSIFICATION OF ANEMIAS

1. Impaired production of red cells
   a. Stem cell, e.g., aplastic anemias, chronic renal failure
   b. Disturbance of proliferation and maturation of differential erythroblasts, e.g., iron deficiency anemia, vitamin B_{12}/folic acid deficiency, marrow infiltrations
2. Shortened red cell survival
   a. Red cell abnormalities, e.g., sickle cell disease, spherocytosis
   b. Extrinsic factors: splenomegaly, toxic agents, bacterial agents
3. Anemia of blood loss
   a. Acute
   b. Chronic

APLASTIC ANEMIAS

Aplastic anemias are rare and may be congenital or, more frequently, acquired. The incidence of fatal aplastic anemia has been estimated as 1.1 per million up to the age of 9 years.[4]

The low hemoglobin concentration is due to the absence or reduction in number of erythroblasts. Most often other formed elements of blood are also deficient, so that neutropenia and thrombocytopenia are usually present. Pure red cell aplasia occurs but is exceedingly rare.

Congenital causes of aplastic anemia include Fanconi's anemia,* dyskeratosis congenita, and occasionally Schwachman's syndrome.[5]

Acquired forms of aplastic anemia may result from drugs, toxic agents, or infections. Antimetabolites and cytotoxic agents cause marrow depression in all individuals, but other drugs will do so only in some patients. Among ac-

*Autosomal recessive trait, low birth weight, poor growth, and skeletal, cardiac, and urogenital anomalies.[5]

quired aplastic anemias, that due to chloramphenicol is the most common, accounting for half the cases in one survey.[4] Indeed, patients receiving chloramphenicol are at a risk 13 times greater than the population at large of developing aplastic anemia. The inhalation of aromatic hydrocarbons, as in "glue sniffing," also can be causative.[2] Frank aplastic anemia may occur during viral hepatitis.

Clinical Manifestations. The pancytopenia of constitutional aplastic anemia does not usually appear until 4 to 7 years of age in boys and 6 to 10 years in girls. Exceptions have been recorded, rarely. A relatively low birth weight is usual, but anemia is not present at birth or in the neonatal period.

Activity is usually normal during the insidious onset of the disease, and bruising, purpura, and hemorrhage are often the presenting symptoms.[4] There is no associated splenomegaly, hepatomegaly, or lymphadenopathy. Liability to infection is frequently found. Radiological investigation may show retarded bone age.

Treatment. In children with severe aplastic anaemia the prognosis is poor with supportive care alone. Infections should be treated promptly with broad-spectrum antibiotics and transfusions of leukocyte-depleted blood products given when clinically indicated.

Curative treatment is by allogeneic bone marrow transplantation or by immune suppression. Transplantation is the method of choice,[6] especially in severe cases, but suitable family donors may not be immediately available.[7] Immune suppression can be achieved in the less severe cases using antilymphocyte globulin in the original instance and cyclosporin for relapses.[5]

Children with Fanconi's anemia may respond to oral androgens, but bone marrow transplantation is also indicated in most of these patients.[5]

Anesthetic Management. Bone marrow puncture will be required to establish the diagnosis, and general anesthesia of brief duration is often needed. Affected patients receiving therapy may require incidental surgical procedures.

Preoperative assessment should establish the presence or absence of any other congenital defects and their nature and severity. Any intercurrent infections should be defined and appropriate therapy instituted. The duration of administration and dosage of steroid hormones must be noted. The degree of cardiovascular compensation for a low hemoglobin level requires assessment. Cardiac murmurs require elucidation, and the possibility of congenital heart disease should be investigated. Consultation with a hematologist, a full blood picture, and a coagulogram all should be obtained before any but the most urgent operation is undertaken. Severe neutropenia alone may warrant prophylactic antimicrobial therapy.

Preoperative blood transfusion should be undertaken only if absolutely required, because sudden rises in blood oxygen content may further depress the marrow and discourage erythropoiesis.[8, 9] Nevertheless, a generous allowance should be made when ordering cross-matched blood to replace perioperative blood losses. When repeated transfusions of blood or platelets have been given previously, the patient should be screened for antibodies. Should an adverse reaction (for example, urticaria or angioneurotic edema) appear, intravenous doses of antihistamines and corticosteroids may be beneficial.

Thrombocytopenia (discussed later) usually coexists, and platelet concentrates should be readily available.

Whenever coagulation defects are present, intramuscular injections should be avoided and premedication by alternative routes chosen. It also is important to avoid the risk of respiratory depression. Although there are isolated reports of blood dyscrasia related to diazepam,[10] and falls in the white cell counts of patients on regular phenothiazine therapy are common,[11] such drugs are probably not contraindicated if given for oral premedication. A distressed, struggling child utilizes oxygen rapidly, and hence suitable premedication is often indicated.

Steroid therapy may require supplementation perioperatively. Patients with congenital heart disease will require prophylactic antibiotic therapy.

A smooth induction of anesthesia is desirable. Instrumentation of the airway, with the attendant risk of trauma and hemorrhage, should be avoided whenever possible. However, a reliable airway is essential, and endotracheal intubation should be gently performed whenever it is advantageous. Many local analgesia techniques, especially spinal and epidural analgesia, are contraindicated if a bleeding diathesis is present. For bone marrow puncture and for other short procedures, patients may be allowed to breathe spontaneously, but high concentrations of inspired oxygen should be assured.

Recently, deep sedation with propofol has proved most useful when combined with local analgesia for bone marrow aspiration and biopsy.

Nitrous oxide depresses the bone marrow even after relatively short exposures,[12] and it might be desirable to avoid this agent in patients with known or suspected aplastic anemia (see later section on Megaloblastic Anemia and Nitrous Oxide). An oxygen-air mixture is probably the ideal vehicle for inhalation agents, and monitoring transcutaneous oxygen saturation may be helpful, particularly in smaller infants, in ensuring appropriate arterial oxygenation while avoiding any potential bone marrow depressant effects of hyperoxia.

For a major surgical procedue in which intermittent positive-pressure ventilation is required, careful endotracheal intubation is essential. Modest positive end-expiratory pressure should secure optimal hemoglobin saturation at minimum FIO_2. Normocapnia is desirable.

Optimal cardiovascular performance should be maintained, so that oxygen transport is maintained despite a low hemoglobin level. In general, fluid replacement therapy should be adequate to maintain blood volume and cardiac output. Circulatory overload must be avoided, however, especially in patients with coexisting cardiac defects.

Induced hypotension cannot be recommended in anemic patients, despite any potential for reduction in operative blood loss.[13]

Postoperative analgesia should be achieved by intravenous drugs initially and orally thereafter. Postoperative blood investigations must include hemoglobin estimation. Special care must be taken to promote postoperative cardiovascular stability and to avoid impaired pulmonary function. Postoperative hypoxemia should be anticipated and oxygen therapy administered using a mask, nasal prongs, or headbox (Fig. 18–1) as appropriate and tolerated. The anesthetic considerations for bone marrow transplantation are detailed on page 656.

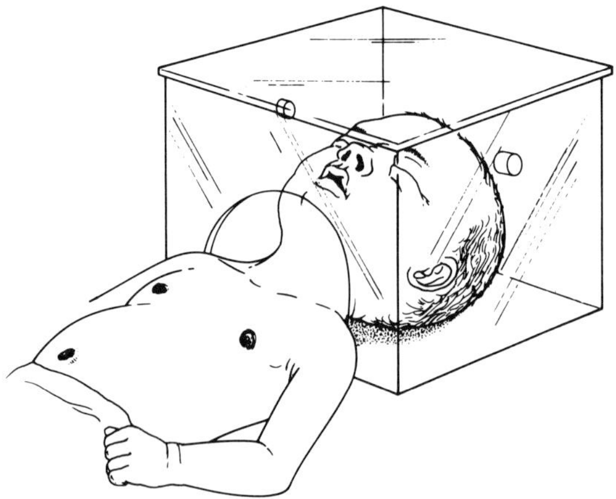

FIGURE 18–1. Infant headbox. Ports allow ingress of air/oxygen mixture and of leads for oxygen partial pressure monitoring. Transparent material is used to maintain visibility. The lid is readily removed if urgent access is required.

CHRONIC RENAL FAILURE

Chronic renal failure affects two to three children per million of total population per year in Britain. A normochromic, normocytic anemia is invariably present, due to a decreased rate of production and shortened life span of red cells. Iron deficiency and megaloblastic and hemolytic anemias also may be present, for which iron and folic acid may be prescribed.

Blood transfusion is avoided when possible, but it may be necessary when a patient's hemoglobin level falls below 6 g/dl consistently. At low hemoglobin levels there are compensatory increases in 2,3-diphosphoglycerate (2,3-DPG) levels and cardiac output, permitting adequate tissue oxygenation.[3, 14] Blood for transfusion should be screened for hepatitis B, cytomegalovirus, and HIV, and it may be advisable to immunize patients against hepatitis B.

Recently recombinant erythropoietin has been used to treat the anemia of chronic renal failure, mostly in transfusion-dependent patients. It may take some weeks to achieve hemoglobin levels of 10 g/dl, but the need for transfusion is decreased and in many instances no further transfusion is necessary.[15] In about one third of children receiving erythropoietin, hypertension is worsened and adjustment of drug therapy is necessary.

Although anemia in patients with chronic renal failure needs to be considered, the anesthetic management of these patients is principally dictated by other aspects of the condition. (See Chapter 7 on the renal system.)

IRON DEFICIENCY ANEMIA

The most common anemia of childhood is that due to iron deficiency. It is most prevalent in children under 3 years of age, especially in lower socioeconomic groups. Children from developing countries are frequently anemic, and any nutritional deficiency in these children may be compounded by hookworm infestation.[16]

Iron deficiency anemia may be due to deficient intake of iron (nutritional), deficient absorption (secondary), and excessive blood losses (from infestation or associated with a bleeding tendency).

Children over 3 years of age in Western countries usually have adequate iron intake with a good mixed diet. Gastrointestinal investigation may be warranted if the anemia is unresponsive to an improved diet and iron supplements.

Clinical Manifestations. Anemia may be discovered incidentally by the anesthesiologist in reviewing the results of preoperative screening tests. Direct questioning of parents may reveal that the patient dislikes iron-rich foods or is anorectic. Other symptoms may include irritability, listlessness, gastrointestinal upsets, pica, or susceptibility to infections. The nails, palms, conjunctivae, and mucous membranes may reveal extreme pallor, and slight splenomegaly may be found. Cardiac enlargement or a "hemic" murmur may be present.

Atrophic glossitis and angular cheilitis may be present early in iron deficiency, even without overt anemia.[17]

Treatment. Simple nutritional iron deficiency anemia is treated by attention to diet and by oral iron therapy. Other nutritional deficiencies (such as vitamin B_{12} and folate deficiencies) may coexist and require supplementary therapy. Noncompliance with, or gastrointestinal problems from, oral therapy may be indications for parenteral iron (iron dextran or iron sorbitol). These may be given intramuscularly or intravenously, but complications have been reported with these techniques.

The response to treatment depends upon the capacity of the marrow to produce hemoglobin, not upon the dosage of any iron medication. A reticulocytosis occurring within 1 week and becoming maximal at about 2 weeks indicates a satisfactory response to therapy. Hemoglobin levels may rise 1 to 1.5 g/dl per week.[18] When iron deficiency is secondary to another disease, treatment must be directed also at the primary cause; this may include diet therapy for celiac disease or chemotherapy for hookworm. In later childhood a peptic ulcer, polyp, or hemangioma may be responsible for the anemia and require anesthesia for surgical treatment.

The child whose anemia is severe, producing fatigue, dyspnea on exertion, palpitations, sustained tachycardia, or frank heart failure requires urgent but cautious infusion of packed red cells. Furosemide may be required concurrently to minimize the risk of cardiovascular overload.

Anesthetic Management. No precise hemoglobin level has been established below which it is unsafe to anesthetize the anemic patient.[3] An oxygen-carrying capacity of 50 percent of normal may be satisfactory, provided other factors affecting tissue oxygenation are optimal.[19]

Major elective surgical therapy should be postponed until the nature of the anemia is clarified and treatment successful. Mild anemia (a hemoglobin level of 9 to 10 g/dl) is not an absolute contraindication to a minor surgical procedure in an otherwise fit child. Iron therapy can be given postoperatively. For a major operation of an urgent nature, severe anemia can be corrected by transfusion of red cells 48 hours or more prior to operation. Alternatively, and in cases of a milder nature, blood can be more conveniently transfused at the time of operation. Losses due to operation also must be taken into account. Whole blood is suitable when operative loss is brisk and extensive and a concentrated red cell transfusion when blood loss is much less, as it reduces the risk of circulatory overload.

Cyanosis is usually discernible when more than 5 g/dl of circulating hemoglobin is in the reduced form. It follows that in patients with very low hemoglobin levels, absence of cyanosis cannot be regarded as a sign of adequate oxygenation of the blood. Furthermore, serious iron deficiency anemia is found more frequently among populations with heavy skin pigmentation in whom the recognition of cyanosis is often difficult.

Premedication should not cause respiratory depression. Preoxygenation is desirable, and induction may be by any appropriate means provided hypoxia is avoided. The hyperkinetic circulation, which compensates for serious anemia, is associated with delay in reaching the required alveolar concentrations of inhalation agents.[9] Halothane and some narcotics (for example, fentanyl) have a slowing effect on the heart and may depress this hyperkinetic circulation.

During maintenance, inspired oxygen concentrations of 50 percent are recommended; higher concentrations of oxygen will not increase the blood oxygen content significantly. Measurement of oxygen saturation by means of pulse oximetry is essential in the anemic patient. The pulse oximeter reading is acceptably accurate in patients with a hematocrit as low as 15, but below this level the monitor becomes increasingly unreliable.[20] Blood gas analysis during a major operation, especially if the circulating blood volume is less than adequate, may be necessary. Cardiovascular performance should be closely monitored and preserved at optimal levels.

The patient with simple iron deficiency anemia presents no particular contraindication to the use of local analgesic techniques, since no bleeding tendency or neurological sequelae need be anticipated. Hence the risk of respiratory depression following narcotic analgesic drugs can be avoided by the substitution, when practicable, of local analgesic techniques both to supplement light general anesthesia and to prevent postoperative pain.

Severe anemia can delay wound healing and increase susceptibility to infection. Serial hemoglobin investigations in the few days postoperatively may indicate the need to give further blood transfusions.

MEGALOBLASTIC ANEMIAS

VITAMIN B_{12} DEFICIENCY

Juvenile pernicious anemia is very rare. It may result from (1) genetic inability to secrete intrinsic factor (which may be present from 7 months of age onward); (2) the formation of antibodies to intrinsic factor, with gastric atrophy and possibly other exocrine gland abnormality; (3) a specific defect of vitamin B_{12} absorption associated with proteinuria; (4) extensive surgical resection of the terminal ileum; or (5) infestation by *Diphyllobothrium latum* (fish tapeworm)

Clinical Manifestations. Pallor, fatigue, and glossitis may be present, though their occurrence and severity will depend upon the age of the patient and the duration of the anemia. The splenomegaly and slight jaundice seen in adult pernicious anemia is usually absent in childhood. Subacute combined degeneration of the cord may supervene.[21] Treatment consists of parenteral hydroxycobalamin. The dose depends on the etiology.

FOLIC ACID DEFICIENCY

Infants who are premature or fed only on goat's milk or other folate-poor diets (such as the diet for patients with phenylketonuria) may develop megaloblastic anemia. Malabsorption syndromes and leukemic and hemolytic anemias also may be associated with folic acid deficiency. However, iron deficiency is the usual cause of the anemia of celiac disease.[4]

Folate deficiency can accompany the dialysis of patients with chronic renal disease, severe infection and diarrhea, and co-trimoxazole therapy.[22]

Drugs associated with folic acid deficiency also include the anticonvulsants sodium phenytoin and primidone, barbiturates, methotrexate, and pyrimethamine.

Clinical Manifestations. Symptoms of folic acid deficiency include anorexia, failure to thrive, weakness, liability to infection, and gastrointenstinal disturbances. The sore tongue and mouth of tropical sprue are seldom seen in temperate climates. Hemorrhagic manifestations can occur secondary to thrombocytopenia, and infection can occur from neutropenia.

Treatment with folic acid is usually given by mouth but can be given parenterally. No improvement in hemoglobin concentration is expected in the first week of therapy. Occasionally blood transfusion may be required.[23] Any other accompanying deficiencies require diagnosis and treatment.

Anesthetic Management. Patients known to be receiving a folate-poor diet, suffering from malabsorption, or receiving therapy with the aforementioned drugs should be assessed particularly carefully for their hematological status. Pallor and gingival hypertrophy may alert the anesthesiologist to megaloblastic anemia.

Diagnosis and successful treatment should precede nonurgent surgery.

For urgent surgery, a small blood transfusion may be needed to initiate treatment. Severely affected patients may have heart failure and pulmonary edema; particular care in transfusion is necessary.

Close attention should be paid to plasma potassium levels pre-, peri-, and postoperatively in the child who is in the early days of treatment for megaloblastic anemia. Falls of nearly 1.0 mEq/L on average have been noted in patients during vitamin B_{12} or folate treatment, with levels as low as 2.5 mEq/L in some cases.[24] The hypokalemia is not usually believed to be of clinical significance.[25] However, based on comparison of patients with megaloblastic anemia with a group of patients with iron deficiency anemia, it has been concluded that megaloblastic anemia is a much more dangerous condition, possibly since purine synthesis is deranged throughout the body.[24, 25]

The management of anesthesia for the child with megaloblastic anemia will be governed by the foregoing and by the general considerations that apply also to patients with anemia. In particular, any bleeding tendency contraindicates intramuscular injections and many local analgesic techniques.

MEGALOBLASTIC ANEMIA AND NITROUS OXIDE

The administration of nitrous oxide is associated with inhibition of methionine synthetase activity. There is consequent impairment of

DNA synthesis, with inactivation of vitamin B_{12} and a risk of megaloblastic anemia. Chemical changes indicative of this tendency have been demonstrated after as little as 1 to 2 hours of nitrous oxide administration.[12] The changes are related to the duration of exposure to nitrous oxide and were more common in sick patients than in others who had had uncomplicated surgery,[26] but they were not seen at all in patients who had not been given anesthesia.

Folinic acid is effective in preventing the development of bone marrow toxicity when given repeatedly in large amounts. The dose suggested for adults is 60 mg in divided doses at the beginning of anesthesia and 12 hours later.[27]

Such protection notwithstanding, it might be prudent to avoid nitrous oxide in patients whose bone marrow function is depressed, provided alternative agents are available to produce anesthesia that is at least equally safe and effective.

MARROW INFILTRATIONS: THE LEUKEMIAS

Acute leukemia is the commonest form of marrow infiltration in childhood. It accounts for more than half of all cancers diagnosed in children under 15 years of age[28] and is one of the commonest causes of death in the first 4 years of life, despite improved results of treatment. There are geographical, racial, and gender differences in the incidence, with white males being the most frequently affected.[29] The peak incidence worldwide is at 2 to 4 years of age.

The etiology is still largely unknown, but ionizing radiation and chemotherapy have been established in some instances, and exposure to infective agents and chemicals have been considered.[29, 30] Chromosomal disorders such as Down's syndrome, Klinefelter's syndrome, and Fanconi's anemia are associated with leukemia in about 3 percent of cases.[30]

Acute lymphocytic (or lymphoblastic) leukemia (ALL) is more common in childhood than acute myeloid leukemia (AML) and has a better prognosis. In both there is a malignant proliferation of hemic precursor cells, primarily affecting the bone marrow but also involving the peripheral blood and other tissues, especially the reticuloendothelial system.

Clinical Manifestations. Although marked differences in specific clinical features in response to therapy and in prognosis distinguish the different leukemias, the general features are similar, as all involve profound disruption of bone marrow function.

The presentation is nonspecific, usually within 6 weeks of onset of signs and symptoms. Failure to "throw off" a mild respiratory infection, pallor, irritability, lassitude, anorexia, fever, and a bleeding tendency with bruising or bone pain are common features. There may be generalized lymphadenopathy, hepatomegaly, or splenomegaly (unlike a typical aplastic anemia). Sepsis, even septicemia, may be the presenting feature.

Pallor and lack of activity reflect the anemia that develops from the disturbed erythropoiesis. Occult or overt hemorrhage due to thrombocytopenia may contribute significantly to the anemia. Mucous membranes and the skin are particularly affected, and retinal hemorrhages, exudates, and infiltrates may be present.

Stridor and superior vena caval obstruction, caused by a large mediastinal mass, may be the presenting symptoms of ALL of T-cell type. Pleural effusions are a common accompaniment.

Diagnosis and Treatment. Bone marrow aspiration is essential to confirm the diagnosis and to permit identification of the specific subtype.

The initial treatment is intensive and may require several weeks of hospitalization. Subsequent therapy and investigations can be offered on a largely outpatient ambulatory basis.

Severe anemia may be present at diagnosis or during therapy and is treated with blood transfusions. Severe thrombocytopenia may necessitate support with platelet concentrates. Infection may seriously complicate treatment at all stages. It is generally caused by coagulase-positive staphylococcal, gram-negative, or other bacterial infections in the presence of neutropenia. Any symptoms indicating infection in a neutropenic child should be treated immediately with broad-spectrum antibiotics such as gentamicin, floxacillin, and azlocillin. Fungal infections should receive vigorous treatment.

The basic pattern of ALL treatment is shown in Table 18–2.

The prognosis for ALL has greatly improved over the last 20 years, and some 60 percent of patients are now cured. The treatment of AML is less successful, but cure rates exceeding 40 percent are being obtained with some chemotherapy protocols.

The treatment of all leukemias is demanding and produces stresses in affected families, with marital strain and anxieties compounding those of the patient. Experienced personnel within a dedicated team of physicians, nurses, and social

Table 18–2. TYPICAL PLAN OF THERAPY IN ACUTE LYMPHOCYTIC LEUKEMIA (1991)

Induction/Remission	CNS Prophylaxis	Intensification	Continued Therapy
Induction 3–4 weeks	Given after remission achieved, usually after first intensification block	5th and 20th weeks (approx)	2 years
Steroids		Steroids	Courses of steroids Vincristine 6-Mercaptopurine Methotrexate
IV Cytotoxics Vincristine Daunorubicin L-Asparaginase	Intrathecal methotrexate Cranial irradiation *or* high dose IV methotrexate with folinic acid rescue	Cytotoxics, e.g.: Etoposide Thioguanine Vincristine Cystosine arabinoside	
IT Methotrexate Intensive support required: blood transfusion and products antibiotics nutritional care		Patients unwell for days because of pancytopenia	
		Co-trimoxazole given indefinitely as prophylaxis against *Pneumocystis*	Co-trimoxazole

workers are important factors in securing compliance with therapy and ensuring appropriate psychological adjustments.

Hematological relapse and central nervous system and testicular metastases sometimes occur despite therapy and may be confirmed by marrow aspiration, examination of the cerebrospinal fluid, and testicular biopsy.

Anesthetic Management. The anesthesiologist may become involved with leukemia patients at diagnosis, during therapy, or for related or unrelated surgical therapy. In British pediatric practice, bone marrow aspirations and some other painful medical procedures are often performed with patients under general anesthesia. Thus, the first contact of anesthesiologist and leukemic child may be at presentation, before confirmation of the diagnosis. Should the diagnosis be confirmed, repeated anesthetics may be requested frequently over the next few weeks and intermittently for a period of perhaps several years. It is therefore advantageous that an anesthesiologist be part of an identified team of clinicians involved in pediatric hematological and oncological practice and that every effort be made by him or her to secure for the child not only the safest but the most agreeable experience of anesthesia possible. The anesthetic management of the child with leukemia, even when minor intervention only is envisaged, can be critical to the child's acceptance of treatment.

Anesthesia for Investigative and Treatment Procedures. The preoperative visit assesses both the status of the child and the personality of the parents. Explanations of the role of the anesthesiologist "to stop it hurting" are given. The treatment area of the relevant children's ward can be equipped with facilities for anesthesia and resuscitation. The older child is given explanations and is invited, with parents, to view the apparatus and to try on a face mask. Assessment of the child's willingness to cooperate either on a parent's knee or on the treatment table is assessed, but on this occasion as a rule no anesthetic is administered. Premedication is prescribed if deemed essential but is rarely required.

Later, when the pediatrician and hematologist are in attendance and the child is adequately fasted, an inhalation induction is performed. Halothane and oxygen are given together with nitrous oxide if the hemoglobin level seems appropriate (more than 9 g/dl). (For children with an intravenous infusion, a central catheter (e.g., Broviac), or those experienced children expressing a preference for "a needle," induction is performed by the intravenous route). Deep sedation with propofol is very satisfactory combined with local analgesia. When light surgical anesthesia is achieved, children aged 2 years or older are turned onto the left side and positioned to facilitate bone marrow puncture from a posterior iliac crest. Tibial specimens

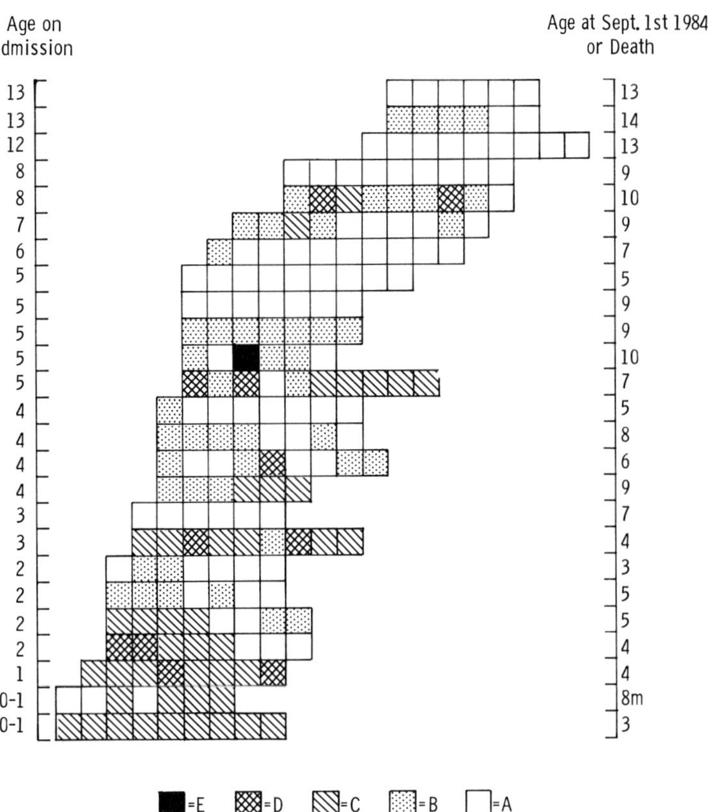

FIGURE 18–2. Mood at induction of anesthesia in 25 patients receiving 6 to 10 anesthetics, May 1980 to August 1984, at Nottingham Pediatric Oncology/Anesthesia Clinic. Serial anesthetics for each patient are represented by blocks adjacent horizontally. Patients are ranked vertically according to date of birth, with the most recently born at the lowest level. The greatest density of print, indicating the least cooperative behavior (see text), is seen in the youngest patients at the start of treatment. Maintenance or improvement of cooperation is seen most readily in older patients. (From Hain WR, Tomlinson JH, Barbor PRH: Anaesthesia for minor procedures in children with malignant disease. J R Soc Med *78*:715–720, 1985. Reproduced by permission of the Editor.)

suffice in the very young. If required and not already undertaken, an intravenous infusion is set up and blood samples are taken. Sometimes lumbar puncture is also performed on this occasion. The period of anesthesia required rarely exceeds 15 to 20 minutes, and work in progress suggests that no impairment of respiratory exchange due to the extreme posture need be anticipated (unpublished observations). The patient's condition, anesthetic, and mood at induction of anesthesia are recorded, together with the relevant anesthetic history both in the case records and on file in the treatment area. Mood is assessed on a five-point scale (A, cheerful and cooperative; B, apprehensive but cooperative; C, tearful, cooperates with difficulty; D, uncooperative; E, terrified and virtually unmanageable).

Once the diagnosis of leukemia is confirmed treatment begins, usually within 24 hours. A request for general anesthesia may be made for this and subsequent occasions. An anesthetic routine is established by the anesthesiologist in accord with the child's reactions and expressed views. When inhalation induction proves stormy, rated C or worse on the mood scale, an intravenous approach is essayed on a subsequent occasion. Any apparent or expressed preference for route of induction is adhered to. The risk of hepatitis from repeated halothane exposure is very small,[31] but it may be wise to alternate halothane with enflurane or isoflurane when repeated anesthesia is necessary.

Both radiotherapy and cytotoxic therapy promote nausea and vomiting. Antiemetics, such as prochlorperazine, may be administered prophylactically while the anesthetic is still in progress. Thrombocytopenia is common in leukemic children, and intramuscular drug administration should be avoided.

With this informal, ward-based interactive approach, it is found among older children particularly that cooperation without premedication can be achieved, maintained, and even improved, as can be seen from Figures 18–2 and 18–3.

Central Vein Access. The hematological, antibiotic, and nutritional support essential to the leukemic child under therapy may necessitate direct access to the central circulation on a long-term basis. Right atrial catheters, such as Hickman's or Broviac's, or a subcutaneous Vascuport can be used to secure such access, and general anesthesia may be required.[32]

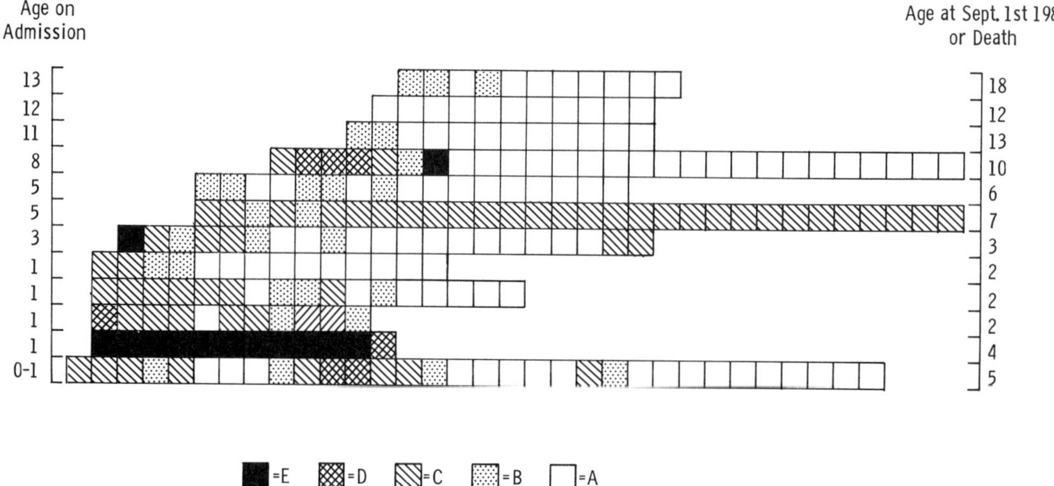

FIGURE 18–3. Mood at induction of anesthesia in 12 patients receiving more than 10 anesthetics, May 1980 to August 1984, at Nottingham Pediatric Oncology/Anesthesia Clinic. See legend of Figure 18–2 for discussion. (From Hain WR, Tomlinson JH, Barbor PRH: Anaesthesia for minor procedures in children with malignant disease. J R Soc Med *78*:715–720, 1985. Reproduced by permission of the Editor.)

In older children the cephalic vein may be used and a simple inhalation anesthetic with appropriate FIO_2 may be given as for other minor procedures described earlier. In children under 5 years of age, the diameter of the cephalic vein is insufficient, however, and the internal jugular vein is used. Endotracheal intubation is then advisable, and particular care should be taken, including transfusion of platelets, if there is thrombocytopenia.

There is a possibility of lowered plasma cholinesterase prolonging suxamethonium apnea. An anesthetic technique should be chosen to minimize the risks of air embolus when a central vein is being cannulated under direct vision. Infection is an important hazard of indwelling catheters and cannulas, particularly in immunocompressed patients. Rigorous precautions should be taken by the anesthesiologist to avoid contamination of the operative site.

Anesthesia and Leukemia Therapy. A large number of cytotoxic drugs are used in various combinations to treat leukemia and other malignancies in both adults and children. All cause bone marrow suppression, and anemia, thrombocytopenia, and neutropenia are regular complications of therapy. These agents can affect virtually all systems of the body adversely, with different classes of agent acting adversely on particular organs.[33]

Patients receiving therapy currently or in the past should be minutely screened for adverse effects. Selvin has identified seven classes of agents.[34] Some examples of each class—by no means an exhaustive list—are given in Table 18–3.

Armed with a knowledge of what class(es) of agent the patient has received, the anesthesiologist must proceed to consider each body system in turn, directing particular attention to any problems known to accompany such therapy.

Table 18–4 shows some of the known system lesions complicating therapy with particular

Table 18–3. CLASSES OF CYTOTOXIC AGENTS

Class	Examples
Alkylating Agents (AA)	*Cyclophosphamide Thiotepa *Methotrexate *Cytosine arabinoside *Thioguanine *6-Mercaptopurine Fluorouracil
Plant alkaloids (PA)	*Vincristine Vinblastine *Adriamycin *Daunorubicin Bleomycin Mithramycin Mitomycin C
Nitrosoureas (NU)	Carmustine (BCNU) Lomustine Streptozocin
Enzyme (EZ)	*L-Asparaginase
Random synthetics (RS)	Cisplatin Dacarbazine Procarbazine

*Used in treatment of leukemia.

Table 18–4. ADVERSE EFFECTS OF CYTOTOXIC THERAPY

Organ/System Effect	Specific Drug as Example	Comment/Anesthetic Implications
Bone marrow suppression	All cytotoxics	Anemia, leukopenia, and thrombocytopenia occur to a variable degree
Nonthrombocytopenic bleeding	Mithramycin	Hemorrhagic pancreatitis
Lungs. Fibrosis and/or pneumonitis	Bleomycin	O_2 toxicity particularly associated with high doses. Postoperative ARDS reported with high inspired O_2 concentrations and excessive IV fluids ?Synergistic with radiotherapy
	Mitomycin C Carmustine (BCNU) Procarbazine	
Heart. Cardiopathy, ECG and echo changes	Cyclophosphamide	
	Adriamycin	Cardiopathy months after therapy
	Daunorubicin, epirubicin	Echocardiographic changes may occur
	Cisplatin	Rarely
	Mitoxantrone	Cardiotoxic
Nervous system		
Central	Ifosfamide	Corneal effects
	Fluorouracil	Cerebellar ataxia
	Vincristine Vinblastine	Encephalopathy. Impaired sensorium, lethargy, convulsions, stroke. Inappropriate ADH secretion
	L-Asparaginase Cisplatin Procarbazine	
Peripheral neuropathy	Vincristine, vinblastine Cisplatin, procarbazine	
Autonomic	Vincristine, vinblastine	Can lead to surgical abdominal crisis
Liver. Dysfunction	6-Mercaptopurine	
	Methotrexate	Common
	Streptozocin	
	Dacarbazine	Uncommon
Kidneys. Dysfunction	All drugs	Uric acid nephropathy at start of treatment. Prophylactic allopurinol and fluid therapy necessary
	Ifosfamide	Tubular and glomerular damage
	Vincristine & vinblastine	Inappropriate ADH secretion
	Mithramycin	
	BCNU and CCNU	Glomerular damage, dose-related
	Cisplatin	Glomerular and tubular damage, dose-related Maybe low calcium and magnesium blood levels
Gastrointestinal epithelium	Methotrexate Fluorouracil Bleomycin	Stomatitis, diarrhea, cachexia, mucous membrane ulceration
Skin	Bleomycin	Eruption may parallel pulmonary toxicity
	Procarbazine	Rash
Immune status suppression	Antimetabolites	Possible increased requirement for nondepolarizing relaxants
Endocrine	Alkylating agents	Inhibition of plasma cholinesterase. Possible increased apnea from suxamethonium
	Mithramycin	Electrolyte disturbances
	Streptozocin	Hypoinsulinism
General	Procarbazine	MAO inhibitor status. Care with vasopressors, sedatives, narcotics Influenza symptoms can be present

Data from Selvin BL: Cancer chemotherapy: Implications for the anesthesiologist. Anesth Analg *60*:425, 1981; and Chung F: Cancer chemotherapy and anaesthesia. Can Anaesth Soc J *29*:364, 1982.

cytotoxic agents. Of critical concern to the anesthesiologist will be the association of bleomycin therapy with pulmonary toxicity and of daunorubicin and Adriamycin with cardiopathy. Muscle relaxants may prove unpredictable, especially since electrolyte abnormalities are common, often in combination with dehydration. The central nervous system may be depressed in some patients, and, for example, seizures may complicate vincristine therapy. Liver function and renal function will require specific investigation and attention. It is essential to consider blood transfusion, platelet concentrates, and measures to combat infection for all patients with antecedent or current cytotoxic therapy.

Anesthetic Considerations in Bone Marrow Transplantation. Patients in first remission with AML and second or later remission with ALL may be considered for bone marrow transplantation (BMT), a form of therapy also given preferentially to children with severe combined immunodeficiency disease and aplastic anemia.[35]

Ideally, syngeneic grafting from an identical twin would be performed, but this is rarely possible. Allogeneic grafting, however, is commonly feasible, usually between the patient and a nonidentical sibling or another near relative, but sometimes using a nonrelated donor with compatible lymphocytic antigens. Autologous marrow grafting, in which the recipient acts as donor, requires only that the marrow is largely free of malignant cells. Marrow is taken from the patient in remission and stored for 12 to 24 hours until intensive antitumor therapy is completed. It can also be cryopreserved for use at a later time.

Anesthesia for Donors. Filshie and colleagues[36] have described their anesthetic management of donors for BMT harvest, and a broad outline is given here.

Securing consent from a suitable donor is not usually a problem; parental consent after full discussion is required when the donor is a minor. Older children may be asked to sign a consent form.

General anesthesia is usually required, especially in children, but spinal anesthesia can be used in some adults. The donor should be fit, but stable intercurrent illness is not a contraindication to the procedure. A unit of blood is taken from most older children or adult donors prior to the procedure and stored for reinfusion during the harvest. In younger children and in those having autologous transplants, blood is cross-matched the day before the harvest and irradiated to avoid the infusion of viable lymphocytes.

Steroid cover is necessary for many of the autograft patients because of concurrent therapy. Premedication is advisable, especially in children, and the oral route is preferred. Induction of anesthesia may be by the intravenous route in adults and older children, but smaller children may prefer an inhalational technique, especially if they are used to this. The procedure may take up to 2 hours or more, and the patient is prone for some of the time, so intubation and a relaxant technique are advisable. Supplementary analgesics such as fentanyl are used and occasionally a low concentration of a gas. Good intravenous access and standard monitoring are essential. Prior to harvesting, intravenous heparin, 1500 IU/m^2, is given to prevent any clotting of the marrow, and further doses are added if necessary. Marrow aspirations are made from the posterior iliac crests with the patient prone, then from the anterior iliac crests and sternum with the patient supine. About 750 to 1000 ml of marrow and blood are harvested in an adult and proportionately less in a child. Autologous blood can be reinfused into the patient during the procedure at any time. Cross-matched blood is transfused only after harvesting is complete, and then only if indicated. Adequate fluid replacement is essential during the procedure. It has been suggested that hemodilution during bone marrow harvesting in children may reduce the need for blood transfusion.

After reversal and extubation the patient continues with oxygen, if necessary, and intravenous fluids into the postoperative period. Analgesia may be required, and antiemetics are given as necessary. Iron supplements may be given to donors for up to 2 months postoperatively.

Fat embolism is a possible complication of bone marrow harvest although heparin may be protective. Filshie and coworkers report greater cardiovascular instability in patients who did not receive heparin, and postoperative reductions in diffusing capacity of the lungs in both general and spinal anesthetic patients.[36]

Nitrous oxide is not contraindicated at present. Its capacity to affect bone marrow is time dependent and not usually apparent before 5 to 6 hours' duration, except possibly in the very ill.

THE LYMPHOMAS

The malignant lymphomas are a form of neoplasm arising in the lymph nodes or other lymphoid tissues (tonsils, thymus, Peyer's patches).

These diseases are rarer in children than the leukemias but constitute about 10 percent of all childhood cancers. The two common lymphomas usually are classified into Hodgkin's disease and non-Hodgkin's lymphoma (NHL), the latter including diseases formerly termed lymphosarcoma, and reticulum cell sarcoma.

HODGKIN'S DISEASE

This disease classically progresses from involvement of a single node or group of nodes to involve the spleen, liver, lungs, and bone marrow. Other organs also may be involved and hence the manifestations of the advanced disease are varied. The disease is rare in young children, but after 5 years of age there is a gradual increase in incidence until adolescence when there is a marked increase in the number of cases. Males are more commonly affected than females.

The disease usually presents as painless, progressive enlargement of one or more superficial lymph nodes, most commonly in the neck (60 percent). Abdominal pain may result from mesenteric and retroperitoneal node enlargement. As the disease advances, systemic symptoms include a low-grade, intermittent fever (Pel-Ebstein), anorexia, nausea, and weight loss. Early in the disease there may be no hematologic abnormalities, but later anemia develops, together with leukocytosis. In late cases leukopenia and lymphopenia occur, and Reed-Sternberg cells, which are a classic component of the disease, may be seen in a peripheral blood smear.

The child may present for anesthesia for lymph node biopsy or for "staging" laparotomy, the latter to determine the extent of the disease and appropriate therapy. Staging laparotomy involves a biopsy of the liver and spleen and mesenteric and para-aortic nodes. Anesthesia management will be discussed later.

Subsequent therapy for Hodgkin's disease is by a combination of radiotherapy and chemotherapy, including corticosteroids.

Non-Hodgkin's lymphoma (NHL) is composed of a heterogeneous group of malignant disorders of the lymphatic system. NHL is three to four times as common as Hodgkin's disease and more common in boys, with a peak incidence at 9 to 11 years of age. The histologic classification of these diseases is being continually revised, but it can be stated that the cells tend to be poorly or not differentiated and the pattern of infiltration diffuse and widespread. Early dissemination occurs, therapy is less effective, and consequently the mortality rate is high.

The presentation of NHL is much more varied than that of Hodgkin's lymphoma and depends upon the site of node involvement. The disease may present with abdominal symptoms (often as intussusception) or with cardiorespiratory symptoms due to mediastinal lymphadenopathy. The disease commonly progresses to involve the bone marrow and the central nervous system. Patients who have extensive marrow infiltration may present with a blood picture essentially similar to that of acute leukemia.

A special form of NHL is the Burkitt type. This is rare in Western countries but is common in Africa. The child classically presents with involvement of the jaw, plus abdominal swelling and central nervous system symptoms. Mediastinal node involvement is rare in Burkitt's lymphoma.

The treatment of NHL lymphoma is with combined radiotherapy and chemotherapy, and success rates for those with early disease have been improving over the past decade.

MANAGEMENT OF ANESTHESIA

The anesthesiologist usually becomes involved with patients with lymphoma who require a biopsy to confirm and further define the tissue diagnosis. In addition to all the other considerations that apply to patients with childhood malignancies, patients with lymphoma are at special risk of the cardiorespiratory complications of mediastinal node enlargement. The risks of general anesthesia are now widely recognized and include acute airway obstruction and cardiovascular compression causing circulatory failure, which may progress to death.[37] Tracheal or bronchial obstruction may occur suddenly; this typically follows induction of anesthesia, positioning the patient, or extubation. This may result in severe hypoxemia, and in some cases it may be impossible to ventilate the patient at all, even with an endotracheal tube well placed in the trachea. In other patients, profound cardiovascular collapse has occurred as a result of tamponade of the heart and great vessels by the tumor mass.

Because of these hazards, all patients with a possible diagnosis of lymphoma must be very carefully assessed prior to anesthesia, even for the simplest minor procedure (e.g., node biopsy). Whenever possible, simple procedures should be carried out under local analgesia.

A preoperative chest radiograph should be

Table 18–5. INCIDENCE OF COMMON HEMOGLOBINOPATHIES IN THE UNITED KINGDOM, UNITED STATES, AND JAMAICA

Location	Total Births	% Black Births	% of All Infants with Genotype:				
			AS	*AC*	*SS*	*SC*	*CC*
UK: London	3,165	22.0	2.8	0.9	0.15	0.09	0.090
Birmingham	43,500	10.0	1.19	0.46	0.06	0.06	—
Manchester	7,691	3.8	0.38	—	—	—	—
USA: New York	106,223	35.0	3.26	0.83	0.18	0.12	0.002
Jamaica	8,000	95.0	8.60	2.89	0.30	0.20	0.003

From Henthorn J, Anionwu E, Brozovic M: Screening cord blood for sickle haemoglobinopathies in Brent. Br Med J *289*:479, 1984.

obtained in every case. If there is evidence of an anterior mediastinal mass, further detailed investigation is required. A history of dyspnea or postural dyspnea should be sought. In asymptomatic patients, a CAT scan or MRI imaging is advised to determine the presence of airway or cardiac compression. Flow volume loops and an echocardiogram should be obtained in the upright and supine positions. If any of these investigations are abnormal, general anesthesia should be avoided; biopsy should be performed under local analgesia or the patient re-evaluated after a course of radiotherapy or chemotherapy. If it is deemed essential to provide general anesthesia to a patient with an untreated anterior mediastinal mass, the following precautions are suggested: The patient should be anesthetized in a semi-Fowler's position, spontaneous ventilation should be maintained if possible, and muscle relaxants should be avoided. Provision should be made to change the position of the patient rapidly to a lateral or prone position if acute obstruction develops. A standby rigid bronchoscope should be available at the time of induction.

It has also been recommended that femoral vein-to-artery cardiopulmonary bypass be available on standby for the induction period in high-risk patients.[37]

HEMOLYTIC ANEMIAS

HEMOGLOBINOPATHIES

Hemoglobinopathies are inherited as autosomal codominant traits. Over 100 such disorders have been detected and described. Disordered function usually follows from the abnormal structure of the hemoglobin. A familiar example is sickle cell hemoglobin (Hb S), which is less soluble than normal hemoglobin (Hb A) when deoxygenation occurs. Crystals then form, leading to deformation and increased rigidity of the cells: this process is known as "sickling."

SICKLE CELL DISEASE

Hb S is produced under the influence of a single gene that, when present, affects the constitution of the beta-chain of hemoglobin, substituting valine for glutamic acid at position 6. The gene is allelomorphic with that for Hb A and with those for many other hemoglobin variants. The proportion of Hb S within a red cell is greater in the Hb S homozygote than in the heterozygote.

The severity of the disease is directly related to the proportion of Hb S within the cell but is also influenced by other factors, notably the proportions of Hb A and fetal hemoglobin (Hb F) and interaction with beta-thalassemia.[38]

Other alleles may complicate the picture. The genes for Hb C, Hb D, Hb Punjab, and Hb E may be inherited. Allelomorphic pairs may thus include:

Hb A/Hb A—normal
Hb A/Hb S—sickle cell trait (SCT)
Hb S/Hb S—sickle cell anemia (SCA) (SCD)*
Hb C/Hb S—sickle cell Hb C disease
Hb C/Hb C—Hb C disease

Many other combinations occur; some, such as Hb E/Hb E, also have clinical manifestations.[40]

The Hb S gene is present in about 10 percent of the black population of Britain and North America (Table 18–5) and in 20 to 40 percent of the black African populations. It is also found in the Middle East, the Mediterranean basin, the hill tribes of the Indian subcontinent, and in South America.[38, 40] Infants with Hb S appear to have relative immunity from falciparum ma-

*In this text, SCD denotes conditions in which sickling may arise.[38, 39] SCA denotes the clinical expression of the homozygous state for Hb S and SCT that of the heterozygous, Hb S/Hb A genotype.

laria, probably accounting for the prevalence of SCD within Africa.

In West Africa, 1 to 2 percent of the population is homozygous for Hb S, and of those 80 percent die before the age of 2 years.[3] Improved better health care is presumed to account for a better prognosis in the United States.

Low cost programs for cord blood electrophoretic screening for families at risk have been established in many centers.[41] Anesthesiologists should have an interest in encouraging the growth of such programs.

Sickle Cell Anemia (SCA). In the homozygous genotype, the high proportion of Hb S within the red cells leads to sickling. This process, which occurs when the hemoglobin is deoxygenated, is initially reversible with restoration of oxygenation but becomes irreversible as membrane changes occur.

Sickling has two important clinical effects: an abnormally high rate of hemolysis and the formation of sickle cell aggregates, with microembolic vaso-occlusion leading to organ infarctions.

A severe hemolytic anemia (Hb 5 to 7 g/dl) is the consequence of the rapid clearance of sickled cells from the circulation by the reticuloendothelial system. Splenic enlargement, jaundice, bone marrow cavity enlargement, and reticulosis are common sequelae. Pigment gallstones can also occur.

The manifestations of vaso-occlusion are widely varied. The kidneys and spleen are especially liable to repeated infarction, with transient pain and fever but permanent loss of function. Lungs, bone, brain, and liver are also prone to this complication.

Clinical Manifestations. While hemolysis and infarctions represent the basic features of SCA at any age, there are differences in presentation characteristics of different age groups.[38] True hemolytic crises are rare and occur predominantly in those patients who also have glucose-6-phosphate dehydrogenase deficiency.

Infancy. Seventy percent of the hemoglobin in a neonate is Hb F, and although this proportion falls in the first few months of life, it exerts a protective effect on the patient with SCA, so that clinical problems are rare in small babies.

Dactylitis from vaso-occlusion is a common presentation, and the hand-foot syndrome, which involves the dorsum of hands or feet or both, may develop. Growth of the metacarpals and metatarsals may be impaired.

Splenomegaly occurs in most babies with SCD. In SCA, episodic infarction of the spleen, accompanied by pain and audible splenic rubs on auscultation, can lead eventually to autosplenectomy by 4 to 5 years of age.[38] Prior to autosplenectomy, death from peripheral circulatory failure may ensue from acute splenic sequestration. This condition has a peak incidence between 6 and 18 months of age and is heralded by such nonspecific symptoms as cough, fever, diarrhea, vomiting, pallor, and drowsiness. There is acute splenic enlargement and a fall in hemoglobin concentration exceeding 2 g/dl from erythrocyte trapping within the spleen.

Childhood. Acute episodes of vaso-occlusion (sickling crises) develop, and pain, usually of the limbs, may demand hospitalization. Anorexia and constitutional upset with pyrexia and tachycardia compound mild dehydration, which aggravates vascular sludging.

Episodes of bone marrow hypoplasia (aplastic crises) can also occur, with falls in the hemoglobin level of 2 mg/dl without reticulocyte response. Various infections and folic acid deficiency have been incriminated. Indeed, infections, particularly osteomyelitis and meningitis, are recurring problems usually involving *Streptococcus pneumoniae*.

Progressive loss of the concentrating power of the kidney develops rapidly in the early years. Polyuria with enuresis occurs. Transfusion may restore kidney function temporarily in the young, but by age 15 years the condition is irreversible. Mild hematuria is seen and commonly is due to bleeding from one kidney, occurring four times more frequently on the left than on the right. Renal blood flow, glomerular filtration rate, and the ability to produce dilute urine are all unaffected. Progression to serious renal disease is rare during childhood.[42]

CNS disturbances can arise, with seizures, stroke or temporary or permanent intellectual impairment.

Adolescence. Sickling crises and susceptibility to infection continue into adolescence and beyond. Growth problems are seen, with reduced height and weight due to delayed puberty. A characteristic "sickle habitus" includes overgrowth of the maxillae and skull. Chest pain and cough may indicate "sickle chest syndrome" in which signs and x-ray changes of lung consolidation, unilateral or bilateral, may be found to develop over several days. Spreading leg ulcers and also priapism, often leading to impotence, may develop in this age group.

Treatment. The mainstay of therapy for patients with SCA is early treatment of infections and the avoidance of hypoxia, dehydration, and chilling.[43] Tranfusion may be required in aplastic crises and during severe infections, such as the sickle chest syndrome and septicemia, and may be given repeatedly in patients who have had strokes to prevent further damage. Repeated transfusions increase the risk of alloimmunization[44] and infection, and ultimately lead to hemosiderosis.

Prophylactic penicillin therapy in patients up to the age of 3 years has been shown to decrease the incidence of *Streptococcus pneumoniae*, and such therapy beyond this age group is recommended.[45] Immunization against pneumococcus should be considered. Splenectomy has been advocated for infants who have had at least one episode of acute splenic sequestration.[46]

Patients with painful sickling crises may require bed rest in hospital, analgesics, intravenous fluids, and antibiotics if infection is present. The sickle chest syndrome, in which the $Pa{O_2}$ is less than 8 kPa with the patient breathing air, demands vigorous treatment with antibiotics, physiotherapy, oxygen, and transfusion. Caution is needed with narcotic analgesia in this condition as respiratory depression can be lethal. Monitoring of $TcP{O_2}$ is useful. Hydroxyurea has been used to ameliorate the painful crisis[47] by increasing the percentage of Hb F.

Anesthetic Management. Patients with SCA present relatively frequently for surgical therapy. Operation may be required to remove pigment gallstones. Although priapism may respond to hospitalization, analgesics, and exchange transfusion, some sufferers require surgical drainage or shunt procedures. Other surgical procedures directly related to SCA include grafting for leg ulcers and cautery procedures for epistaxis. Orthodontic treatment may be required for excessive growth of maxillary teeth in adolescents.

Patients with SCA additionally may be considered for surgical therapy, however, when vaso-occlusive incidents give pain mimicking osteomyelitis particularly frequently and acute abdominal emergencies. Increasing surgical awareness of these presentations in SCA can reduce the incidence of unnecessary operation.[48] However, many unrelated surgical conditions can also arise in patients with SCA. Umbilical hernia is particularly prevalent in black populations.

General Considerations. The hazards of general anesthesia for patients with SCD appear to have diminished with increased preoperative recognition and assessments of the factors that precipitate sickling crises.

Hypoxia and vascular stasis are the principal dangers. It is relatively easy to avoid hypoxia from respiratory causes in patients intraoperatively while an anesthesiologist is present. However, general anesthesia predisposes to hypoxia, and local techniques can seldom be used alone in children. Complications arise more frequently in the postoperative period than intraoperatively.[49]

Vascular stasis is favored by the increased viscosity of blood carrying sickle cells, particularly if that blood cools, and by other factors reducing tissue blood flow—dehydration, reduced cardiac output, and hypovolemia.

In SCA hemoglobin levels vary, 7 to 9 g/dl being normal. In minor operations, transfusion preoperatively is not necessary if the patient has been free of crises and infection. For major operations in which blood loss may be significant, preoperative transfusion is indicated to reduce the Hb S level to below 30 percent and to increase the hemoglobin to 10 g/dl or more.[48, 50] Serial transfusions can be given, the last one 2 to 3 days prior to operation so that 2,3-DPG levels are normal.[3] In an emergency, exchange transfusion may be considered.

The use of dextrans in sickle cell crises is controversial,[3, 39, 48] but they can be used to expand the circulation provided tissue hydration is adequate.

Spinal anesthesia has been discouraged by some workers[40, 48] because of the danger of hypotension and consequent decreased tissue perfusion. However, hypotension is less likely to occur in infants and young children with spinal anesthesia. Certainly local infiltration techniques and regional blocks can be considered.

Vascular stasis increases arteriovenous oxygen tension differences and therefore favors sickling, leading to a vicious cycle of sickling-stasis-tissue hypoxia-sickling. Some workers recommend avoidance of tourniquets,[48, 51] whereas others believe that proper application and careful exsanguination can permit safe use of tourniquets.[40, 52] Danger from the use of tourniquets in SCA has not been proved.

Specific Recommendations. All black children should be screened for SCD. Antenatal diagnosis is possible at certain centers in Europe, America, Israel, and Australia but is rarely requested.[53] More usually, the presence of Hb S is identified in a small sample of blood. Under a microscope such a sample may be seen to demonstrate sickling when a reducing agent is added. The Sickledex test is a very reliable method but is qualititative only and does not distinguish SCA from SCT. If the test is positive, genotyping by hemoglobin electrophoresis should be undertaken. In an emergency, SCA should be assumed when anemia, a positive sickle cell test, the history, and clinical findings are all compatible with that diagnosis.

An immediate preoperative hemoglobin estimation is advisable whether or not transfusion has been used in the preparation for operation. Changes in hemoglobin levels can occur rapidly, particularly when sequestration occurs.[48] Surgical procedures undertaken during a sickling crisis are nearly always fatal.[54]

All patients should have a thorough physical examination before operation. Any infection should be rigorously treated and prophylactic antibiotic therapy instituted.[48]

Premedication regimens have varied widely or been omitted without observed problems.[50, 55] However, promethazine appears to offer specific advantages for these patients: it does not depress respiration, it produces some drying of the mouth, and it has a fairly prolonged length of action in children. Moreover, promethazine has an antihistamine effect, which may help prevent a transfusion reaction, and it may inhibit the reduction of Hb S.[3] A suitable dose is 1 mg/kg 1 to 2 hours preoperatively by mouth.

Prolonged preoperative starvation should be avoided when feasible, to reduce the possibility of dehydration. Clear fluids can be given up to 4 hours preoperatively in elective cases.

Operative management is summarized in Table 18–6.

The choice of agents seems not to be critical. A supposition that suxamethonium fasciculations may be associated with local hypoxia and hence precipitate a sickling crisis appears to be theoretical, and this effect is evidently not seen in practice.[49] The newer short-acting nondepolarizing relaxants may be the drugs of choice when relaxation is required, as they wear off quickly and muscle power is rapidly regained at the end of operation.

Postoperative Management. Observation in an intensive care unit is desirable except for patients undergoing minor operations. Hypoxia must be avoided. Hypoventilation due to residual muscle paralysis or anesthetic agents requires prompt attention. Pain relief is essential, but caution should be exercised when using opiates, and frequent observations must be made. A pulse oximeter is valuable, and after a major operation arterial blood gas estimations may be required.

Oxygen should be administered for up to 24 hours, although this may prove impossible in the young child undergoing a minor operation. Prolonged oxygen therapy is unnecessary in most patients and may depress erythropoiesis.[3] Older children will usually tolerate a face mask, especially when the necessity has been explained beforehand, but younger children may prefer nasal prongs or a single nasal cannula. The inspired oxygen should be adjusted to give 30 to 50 percent.

Infection is a major perioperative hazard, and careful aseptic techniques should be practiced for intravenous cannulation.[48] Oral intake may be reduced by preoperative starvation and postoperative nausea, so intravenous fluids are mandatory until the patient can tolerate adequate amounts by mouth. Patients with reduced renal function may have high obligatory urine volumes.[42]

Table 18–6. OPERATIVE MANAGEMENT IN SICKLE CELL ANEMIA

Problem	Management
Hypothermia	Warm OR, blankets, humidification
Dehydration	Perioperative intravenous infusions
Blood loss	
Minor	Dextrans and/or crystalloid solutions IV
Major	Prompt replacement, fresh blood
Hypoxia	
Induction	Preoxygenate—difficult in small children, but 2 minutes will suffice if mask fit is airtight Hyperventilate with oxygen/halothane prior to intubation, smooth induction, minimum doses/concentrations
Intraoperative	F_IO_2 30–50% $F_IO_2 \propto \frac{1}{F_IN_2O}$; hence more supplements needed with high F_IO_2
At extubation	Ventilate with 100% oxygen
Acidosis	Mild hyperventilation, counter hypocapnic vasoconstriction with judicious volatile agent administration
Vascular stasis	Maintain or increase circulating blood volume, maintain cardiac output, avoid peripheral vasodilatation

Sickle Cell Trait (SCT)

Patients heterozygous for Hb A and Hb S rarely present serious clinical problems. Hb S levels within the red cells are less than 50 percent. Although sickling is very rare, extreme conditions such as flying at a high altitude in unpressurized aircraft have been reported to induce sickling crises in some individuals.

Recognition of SCT patients will usually depend upon routine testing. If SCT patients are seriously anemic, the cause is unlikely to be related, and an additional cause should be sought and treated appropriately. There is, however, an age-dependent, progressive fall in the concentrating power of the kidney,[42] although during childhood the clinical significance of this must be slight.

Increased risk from anesthesia for SCT patients has not been demonstrated except in extreme situations and in major interventions such as thoracotomy.[3, 40, 51, 55, 56] In such cases, and when such doubts exist concerning the heterozygous status of the patient, or if thalassemia coexists (see later), the recommendations for SCA patients should be followed. Otherwise, no specific plan for anesthesia need be envisaged. The patient's general condition should be optimal before elective operation, and if anemia is present it should be corrected. Appropriate premedication, smooth induction, eucapnic and nonhypoxic maintenance, with special attention to maintenance of cardiovascular performance and adequate hydration, and a well-supervised recovery form the basis of safe management.

Oxygen therapy in the postoperative period is largely unnecessary except after major operations. SCT children who are fit and whose Hb levels are normal can be considered for minor outpatient procedures.

THALASSEMIA

Unlike SCD and many other hemoglobinopathies, thalassemia does not result from amino acid substitution but from a retarded synthesis of either the alpha-chain or the beta-chain, leading to imbalance (alpha- and beta-thalassemia, respectively). The synthesis is governed by a pair of allelomorphic autosomal codominant genes, so that both homozygous (major) and heterozygous (minor) forms occur, presenting clinical features of differing severity. The disease has spread well beyond the geographical confines of countries bordering the Mediterranean Sea.

Alpha-thalassemia occurring in heterozygotes is relatively common and presents as mild anemia in American and African blacks. Jaundice and slight splenomegaly may be present, and occasionally episodes of severe anemia may require blood transfusion. Severe homozygous disorders of the alpha-chain cause intrauterine death, since they affect Hb F production. Therefore, the major thalassemias that present clinical problems in childhood are disorders of the beta-chain.[53]

Clinical Manifestations of Beta-Thalassemia. The homozygous form of beta-thalassemia (Cooley's or Mediterranean anemia) presents with very severe anemia (hemoglobin less than 7 g/dl) in children over 6 months of age. Chronic hemolysis and defective erythropoiesis lead to gross marrow hyperplasia. Extramedullary erythropoiesis can lead to characteristic deformities, especially of the skull and face. Growth is impaired and, in survivors, puberty is delayed.

Untreated children die after 1 to 6 years of chronic illness. Although transfusion therapy maintains good health in the short term, the consequent iron overload can lead to death from intractable heart failure in childhood or adolescence. Nightly subcutaneous infusions of desferrioxamine can control the overload, but there is difficulty in securing compliance with this treatment. Hemosiderosis, with brown pigmentation of the skin and cirrhosis of the liver, may develop in patients receiving frequent transfusions. Anemic crises from aplasia or folic acid deficiency can occur.

Hypersplenism (the combination of gross splenomegaly, excessive erythrocyte destruction, and thrombocytopenia) may require splenectomy to reduce transfusion requirements. The subsequent increased risk of infection necessitates prolonged prophylactic antibiotic therapy.

The heterozygous form, thalassemia minor, presents little clinical problem, and Hb C thalassemia is relatively mild. However, association with a sickling genotype may result in severe problems. Hb E thalassemia is associated with very severe anemia.

Anesthetic Management. Particular attention must be paid to the severity of the anemia in patients with thalassemia major. Iron therapy is absolutely contraindicated. Preoperative transfusion to adequate levels should be performed. Liver function and cardiac status must be carefully assessed preoperatively, and any deficiency must be borne in mind in designing the anesthetic technique. If present, cardiac failure must be treated. Hypoxia, cardiovascular depression, and hemoglobinuria should be avoided.

Preoperative blood transfusions may be augmented intraoperatively during splenectomy by autotransfusion of some of the blood sequestrated within the spleen. The splenic artery is clamped first, and epinephrine is injected provided halothane has not been used.[14]

Uncomplicated thalassemia minor may require no specific precautions from the anesthe-

Table 18–7. AGENTS THAT MAY CAUSE HEMOLYSIS IN G-6-PD–DEFICIENT SUBJECTS

Aminoquilones	Sulfones
Primaquine	Dapsone
Pamaquine	Sulfoxone
Chloroquine	Thiazosulfone
Pentaquine	Diaminodiphenylsulfone
Quinocide	
Quinacrine	Miscellaneous
Plasmoquine	Vitamin K (water-soluble analogues)
Analgesics and Antipyretics	Naphthalene
Acetylsalicylic acid	Probenecid
Acetanilid	Nalidixic acid
Aminopyrine*	Dimercaprol
Phenacetin	Methylene blue
	Trinitrotoluene*
Nitrofurans	Acetylphenylhydrazine
Nitrofurantoin	Phenylhydrazine
Furazolidone	Isoniazid
Nitrofurazone*	Para-aminosalicylic acid
Furaltadone	Tolbutamide
Sulfonamides	Neoarsphenamine
Sulfanilamide	Diabetic acidosis
Sulfacetamide	Fava beans*
Sulfasoxazole	Infections (respiratory viruses, infectious hepatitis, infectious mononucleosis, bacterial pneumonias)
Sulfamethoxypyridazine	
N^2-Acetylsulfanilamide	
Sulfisoxazole	
Sulfapyridine	
Sulfasalazine	Quinine*
	Quinidine*
	Chloramphenicol*

*Not believed hemolytic in blacks.

siologist beyond the general duty to assess thoroughly, to take care, to monitor, and to treat incidents meticulously and promptly. Any association of Hb S with thalassemia mandates the full precautionary approach detailed for SCA in the preceding section.

SPHEROCYTOSIS (ACHOLURIC JAUNDICE)

This dominantly inherited hemolytic anemia is believed to be due to an abnormality of the red cell membrane affecting sodium ion entry into the cell. Energy- and glucose-consuming processes may fail during splenic stagnation, and the cell loses viability.

Clinical Features. Many cases are manifested in the neonatal period, mimicking hemolytic disease of the newborn, but most commonly spherocytosis is first diagnosed in school children. Jaundice (1 to 4 ml/dl unconjugated bilirubin) is often slight and intermittent in older children. Kernicterus is reported in the neonate.

Anemia is also moderate and episodic. There may be aplastic or hemolytic "crises" with marked anemia, dyspnea, vomiting, abdominal pain, extreme lassitude, and fever. Such crises may be precipitated by infection or folic acid deficiency. Chronic anemia may be accompanied by impaired growth and mental retardation.

Splenomegaly is usual. After infarction or hemolytic crises, the spleen may be tender.

Treatment. Most frequently this consists of splenectomy, usually deferred until the child is 3 to 4 years old. Folic acid and blood transfusions may be needed to treat crises. Steroids have no place in treatment.

Anesthetic Management. Preoperative transfusion should seldom be required, since anemia is usually moderate and accompanied by increases in 2,3-DPG, facilitating oxygen delivery to the tissues. Careful conduct using standard modern anesthetic techniques is recommended.

GLUCOSE-6-PHOSPHATE DEHYDROGENASE (G-6-PD) DEFICIENCY

Black, Mediterranean, and North European races demonstrate different clinical pictures in response to glucose-6-phosphate dehydrogenase (G-6-PD) deficiency, which is a congenital defect of the pentose shunt pathway. All forms are inherited as sex-linked characteristics with intermediate dominance.

The racial incidence varies greatly, from 10 percent in African Americans to 1 to 35 percent in the different Mediterranean races. It is believed that at least 100 million persons in the world are G-6-PD deficient.[57]

Clinical Features. Hemolytic anemia may follow ingestion of drugs and chemicals, including antimalarials, sulfonamides, nitrofurans, analgesics (notably aspirin), and para-aminosalicylic acid (PAS) (Table 18–7). There is a variable mild, chronic hemolytic anemia in affected patients.

Anesthetic Management. Great care must be taken to avoid administration of any of the drugs that have been implicated as causing hemolysis in G-6-PD–deficient patients[4, 57–60] (Table 18–7). Prilocaine is contraindicated,[19] but with careful conduct of anesthesia, on present evidence no specific problem need be anticipated. Folic acid supplementations may be desirable perioperatively.

Table 18–8. THERAPEUTIC MATERIALS FOR HEMOPHILIA MANAGEMENT

Dried factor VIII fraction BP	BPL8Y Hemofil Monoclate Kryobulin Profilate Humate-P	Easily soluble in isotonic saline Low reaction rate
Porcine factor VIII	Hyate:C	For cases with antibodies to human factor VIII Occasional severe reactions
Dried factor IX fraction BP	Mononine Prothromplex Proplex	For hemophilia B
Desmopressin (DDAVP)		Increases factor VIII and von Willebrand's factor level Tachyphylaxis occurs For mild cases only
Tranexamic acid	Cyclokapron	Inhibits plasminogen activation, interferes with fibrinolysis

Adapted from Rizza CR: Haemophilia A and B. Prescribers' J *24*:71, 1984. With permission of the Controller of Her Britannic Majesty's Stationery Office.

COAGULOPATHIES

HEMOPHILIA

Hemophilia exists throughout the world, with an estimated incidence in developed countries approximating 1 in 10,000.[54] Hemophilia A (factor VIII deficiency) is clinically indistinguishable from the much rarer hemophilia B (factor IX deficiency). Both disorders occur as X-linked recessive traits. The disease thus affects only males but is carried by heterozygous females.

A level of factor VIII activity below 3 percent of normal is associated with severe hemophilia, but in 5 to 10 percent of cases the deficiency is less marked, and a milder form is seen.

Factor VIII deficiency also occurs in Von Willebrand's disease, together with abnormal capillary fragility. The rare homozygous form is manifested as a grave bleeding disorder.

Clinical Manifestations. Patients with severe forms of hemophilia usually manifest a bleeding tendency within the first year of life, sometimes at circumcision. Hemarthroses may develop in the first 3 years. Spontaneous hemorrhages characterize childhood and, in contrast to those hemorrhages developing in platelet and capillary disorders, the deeper tissues are more usually involved: intramuscular hematomas in the psoas, retroperitoneal bleeding, hemarthroses, and hematuria.

Early manifestations and joint involvement may not be seen in the milder form, with hematomas developing only after more severe trauma. Excessive bleeding follows dental extraction or other operation.

Treatment. The diagnosis may be made antenatally[53] or may be suspected at birth from a family history of affected males. However, 30 percent of males show no family history.[61] Screening coagulation tests on capillary samples are used in small children. The clotting time is prolonged, with a normal bleeding time. Full hematological investigation and factor VIII assay must follow any positive or borderline result.

Replacement Therapy. Prior to any surgical procedure, factor VIII levels should be augmented. This implies the administration as needed of factor VIII. One unit of factor VIII (antihemophilic globulin, AHG) is the activity present in 1 ml of fresh pooled normal plasma. One guide to dosage is that the number of units of factors required equals

$$\text{Body weight (kg)} \times \text{desired percentage increase in activity} \div 1.5.$$

Therapeutic materials used in hemophilia management[62, 63] are listed in Table 18–8.

Fifty percent of severely affected hemophiliacs in the United Kingdom are now on home therapy.[62] For minor spontaneous hemorrhages nonspecific measures, such as bed rest, immobilization, sedation, and analgesics (but not aspirin) are used, but replacement therapy is given at home or in the hospital if these measures are ineffective.

Even minor cuts will warrant hospital management. Topical thrombin application by light pressure dressings is advised. If sutures are required, if mild hemorrhage is continuing, or if recurrence would endanger a structure or function (for example, of the orbit), replacement therapy, 15 units/kg, is given every 12 hours, usually for several days. The aim is to maintain factor VIII activity at greater than 20 percent of normal.

More severe hemorrhages command more generous therapy, comparable with that recommended to cover major operations (see following).

Anesthetic Management. Patients with hemophilia may present for related operations (for example, for hemarthrosis), for dental extraction, or for unrelated surgical conditions.

In the following discussion, hemophilia A is considered. The principles apply also to hemophilia B. Full consultation with a hematologist is mandatory in the management of surgical therapy in hemophiliacs. At no time should intramuscular injections be given. Care should always be taken to preserve veins for further use when required. Large vessels such as the femoral, internal jugular, and axillary veins should be avoided for venipuncture because of the difficulties of securing hemostasis afterward.

All patients should be tested for the presence of antibody to factor VIII. In patients whose test results are positive, only life-threatening conditions should be treated surgically, although porcine factor VIII sometimes can be used to provide cover. If this is used, full facilities for treating an anaphylactic reaction must be instantly available.[62]

Patients should be tested for the presence of hepatitis B surface antigen, as 50 percent or more of patients are carriers. Most units now pursue a policy of vaccinating all newly diagnosed hemophiliacs against hepatitis B, and anesthesiologists who have regular contact with hemophiliacs are advised to seek vaccination themselves.[64, 65] Most hemophiliacs are also screened for hepatitis C.

Many hemophiliacs who have received multiple transfusions or contaminated factor VIII are HIV positive and may develop the acquired immunodeficiency syndrome (AIDS). Antibody testing for HIV is now routine in many centers. Strict precautions should be taken with these high-risk patients, and it is recommended that anesthesiologists wear gowns, gloves, and goggles.[66] All equipment should be disposable or autoclavable, and unnecessary personnel, furniture, and equipment should be kept out of the operating room.

Prior to operation the hemostatic defect should be corrected by infusion of the appropriate factor. Pre- and postinfusion factor levels are usually estimated. In an emergency, recently thawed fresh-frozen plasma (20 ml/kg) can be given if no suitable concentrate is available.

Hemarthrosis. Prompt home or hospital therapy has reduced the incidence of severe arthroses. Occasionally in young children joint aspiration, prior to pressure bandaging, may indicate general anesthesia. Pain and distress require attention. Oral, rectal, or intravenous routes may be used to administer selected analgesics and sedatives, as needed. Replacement therapy is given prior to aspiration. No special technique of anesthesia is required, but particular care in handling the patient and avoidance of any airway trauma are desirable. If their use is essential, artificial airways should be well lubricated and inserted and removed gently.

Dental Surgery. Extractions and conservations are usually performed under general anesthesia, as local anesthetic injections can be hazardous. Meticulous replacement therapy is required even for the shortest procedure. Tranexamic acid, 10 mg/kg, may be given preoperatively by intravenous infusion, and continued postoperatively by the oral route. Prophylactic antibiotics are often prescribed.

Anesthetic technique depends on the extent of the dental operation. The extraction of a small number of deciduous teeth can be performed without intubation. Nasotracheal intubation is contraindicated because of the risks of hemorrhage from the nose and adenoids, so the oral route should always be used.

When undergoing a minor operation, patients with mild hemophilia and some with von Willebrand's disease may be treated with desmopressin, a vasopressin analogue. This obviates the use of factor VIII concentrates. A three- to sixfold rise in factor VIII activity follows administration of 0.4 to 0.5 μg/kg intravenously. Desmopressin is of no value in the management of severe hemophilia.[62]

Major Operation. For more extensive dental or other operation, more intensive and prolonged therapy is required. Anesthesia should not begin until the level of factor VIII activity is 50 percent of normal, and factor VIII activity must be maintained at or above the 30 percent level for several days, by infusions of factor VIII concentrates every 12 hours.

Assays of factor VIII activity as well as the clinical course of the patient will dictate management, since the activity of the therapeutic materials is not wholly dependable. Sequestration and consumption of infused factor VIII are also unpredictable variables. Daily infusions may be needed from the seventh to the twentieth day postoperatively.

Despite the provision of adequate factor VIII levels possible today, the anesthesiologist will wish to avoid inflicting damage that could later lead to hemorrhage. Instrumentation of the upper airway should be avoided whenever possible. Artificial airways, endotracheal tubes, and monitoring probes should be generously lubricated and extreme care used in their placement and removal.

VON WILLEBRAND'S DISEASE

This disease is inherited with an autosomal dominant pattern as opposed to the sex-linked recessive inheritance of hemophilia.[67] The disease process varies from a very mild form that may occur in as many as 2 to 3 percent of the population to a severe form that affects 1 in 10,000 (i.e., the severe form has an incidence similar to that of hemophilia). The basic defect in Von Willebrand's disease is the lack of a plasma cofactor necessary for normal platelet function. Von Willebrand's factor is present in the plasma in a complex with factor VIII, and in more severe forms of the disease there is also a reduced level of factor VIIIC.

The disease is usually classified into three types, which determine the severity and also indicate appropriate therapy. Type I is the commonest and mildest form; the prothrombin time and partial thromboplastin time are usually normal. Type II is divided into two subtypes, a and b. In type IIb there is an associated thrombocytopenia due to decreased platelet survival time. Type III disease is the most severe form, in which both Von Willebrand's factor and factor VIIIC levels are undetectable.

The usual clinical manifestations of the disease are cutaneous and mucous membrane bleeding, but patients with severe forms also experience muscle and joint bleeding. A history of superficial bleeding, easy bruising, or bleeding after dental extraction should prompt baseline laboratory tests of platelet count, prothrombin time, partial thromboplastin time, and bleeding time. If any of these are abnormal, referral to a hematologist for more detailed testing is indicated. Special tests for Von Willebrand's disease include the glass bead adhesion test and the ristocetin cofactor test.

Treatment traditionally has been achieved by replacement of the Von Willebrand's factor using cryoprecipitate or fresh frozen plasma. Platelet infusions will not correct the defect but may be required if there is an associated thrombocytopenia. Recently the use of DDAVP (1-deamino-8-D-arginine vasopressin) has proved effective in some patients with Von Willebrand's disease, most notably those with type I disease. DDAVP is much less effective in patients with type III disease and produces a variable response in type II disease. It should not be given to patients with type IIb disease; these patients have a thrombocytopenia that will be exacerbated by DDAVP. In practice, if the type of Von Willebrand's disease is unclear preoperatively, it is suggested[67] that the response of the patient's coagulation indices to a test dose of the drug should be assessed. DDAVP in a dose of 0.3 μg/kg should be administered intravenously over 20 minutes and the coagulation studies reassessed after 1 hour. If they are improved, DDAVP should be administered at the time of operation. DDAVP is a synthetic analogue of antidiuretic hormone, hence fluid balance should be carefully monitored when the drug is administered, especially if repeat doses are given. It is recommended that no more than three doses should be given in a 48-hour period.

If DDAVP is ineffectual, treatment with cryoprecipitate or fresh-frozen plasma will be required.

THROMBOCYTOPENIA (PLATELET DEFICIENCY)

The normal level of circulating platelets is 150,000 to 500,000/μl. Hemostasis becomes defective when the level falls below 100,000, but spontaneous widespread purpura is unusual with levels above 25,000/μl.

In contrast to hemophilia, the ability of plasma to coagulate at sites of vascular damage is unimpaired in thrombocytopenia. Once active bleeding is arrested (for example, by pressure), coagulation can proceed, and recurrence of bleeding is unlikely.

Causes. Reduced platelet production occurs in many blood disorders, including aplastic anemia, megaloblastic anemia, and marrow infiltrations. These conditions are discussed earlier in this chapter.

Increased peripheral destruction of platelets is seen in childhood in idiopathic thrombocytopenic purpura (ITP), in hypersplenism (see page 667), and in consumption coagulopathies. Dilutional thrombocytopenia can result from massive blood transfusion or cardiopulmonary bypass.

Idiopathic Thrombocytopenic Purpura

Idiopathic thrombocytopenic purpura (ITP) is an autoimmune disorder, presenting acutely in children and usually following infection. The prognosis is good, and 80 percent of patients will have a spontaneous and permanent remission within 12 months.[68] The other 20 percent require treatment.

Clinical Features. Bleeding is usually cutaneous, with petechiae, purpura, and mucosal hemorrhage from the nose and mouth. Hematuria and gastrointestinal bleeding may occur, and there is a risk of intracranial hemorrhage, especially when the platelet count is less than 20,000/μl.[68] Diagnosis is made from the history, full blood count, and marrow aspiration.

Treatment. For many years steroid therapy has been the initial treatment of choice in the 20 percent of children with severe and persistent ITP. This is usually given as prednisolone, 40 mg/m^2 in divided doses for 10 days. Therapy failures may be treated with cytotoxic agents and occasionally by splenectomy. Both these latter treatments have inherent risks. More recently, successful remissions have been achieved using intravenous immunoglobulin (IgG) alone,[69] and in many instances this is the initial treatment of choice, especially if bleeding is a major problem.

Anesthetic Management. Until bone marrow aspirates are examined, the diagnosis usually remains uncertain, and acute leukemia may be suspected. Anesthetic management for such patients requiring diagnostic bone marrow puncture is fully described in the section on Marrow Infiltrations earlier in this chapter.

Patients may present for unrelated operations, and those refractory to all treatment, for splenectomy. Steroid augmentation may be necessary, and IgG is often given preoperatively. Platelets must be available for infusion.

As in hemophilia, all intramuscular injections are contraindicated. The anesthetic technique chosen and the application of monitoring devices should avoid risk from trauma to the upper airway. Endotracheal tubes or other tubes should be well lubricated, and both placement and removal should be secured as atraumatically as possible. Bleeding from attempted venipuncture sites responds to light pressure maintained for 4 minutes.

Platelet concentrates can be given in a dose of 1 unit/5 kg, when indicated, to correct thrombocytopenia.[64] Cross-matching for ABO compatibility is necessary. Microfilters remove platelets and therefore should not be used for platelet infusions. When splenectomy is to be performed, platelet infusion is reserved until after the splenic pedicle is clamped.

Postoperatively, intramuscular injections should be avoided. Further platelet infusions are given only if specifically indicated.

Overwhelming infection is a recognized hazard following splenectomy in childhood. Severe meningitis and septicemia may develop insidiously following splenectomy.[70] Prophylactic antibiotic therapy (for example, oral penicillin) is often prescribed, sometimes for life, but there may be considerable noncompliance in taking it. The importance of infection and its early recognition and treatment should be stressed to parents and patient. More recently, vaccination of splenectomized patients against pneumococcus has been advocated.[71]

Patients who have had splenectomy in the past may present for unrelated operation. Antibiotic cover should be given and care taken with invasive anesthetic procedures.

POLYCYTHEMIA

The diagnosis of polycythemia implies a hemoglobin concentration persistently greater than 17 g/dl in childhood or 22 g/dl in the neonate.

Both primary and secondary forms occur, but polycythemia rubra vera, which has surgical implications,[72] is a disease limited to middle age. Polycythemias are indeed extremely rare in childhood, save those secondary to prolonged arterial oxygen desaturation. Cyanotic congenital heart disease (CHD) is the usual cause, but chronic pulmonary disease as well as residence at high altitude also can lead to enhanced erythropoietin production and consequent polycythemia.

Cyanotic Congenital Heart Disease

The anesthetic management of patients with cyanotic CHD is discussed in Chapter 6.

In severe cases the polycythemia is characterized by absence of the usual postnatal fall in hemoglobin concentration. Anemia develops a few months later, but if it is treated with iron therapy, the hematocrit may rise to 75 percent or more, with accentuation of symptoms.

Red cell mass increases disproportionately as the hematocrit rises, and an increased blood volume ensues. The increase in oxygen-carrying capacity and cardiac output are potential advantages. However, above a critical hematocrit of

Table 18–9. ORAL ANALGESICS (IN ORDER OF POTENCY)

Drug	Starting Dose	Frequency
Paracetamol	15 mg/kg	q 4 hours
Dihydrocodeine or codeine linctus*	0.5–1 mg/kg	q 4 hours
NSAID*—Naproxen	5–10 mg/kg	q 12 hours
Ibuprofen	10 mg/kg	q 12 hours
Morphine sulfate	0.15–0.2 mg/kg	q 3–4 hours
MST (morphine sustained-release)*	10–30 mg	q 12 hours
Diacetylmorphine	0.1 mg/kg	q 3–4 hours

*Not suitable for children under 2 years of age.

Modified from the Guidelines for Terminal Care, Department of Oncology, Children's Hospital, Birmingham, U.K. Courtesy of Dr. M. Stevens.

70 percent, these are offset by a marked increase in blood viscosity, which hinders blood flow and predisposes to stroke.

Pulmonary Disease

In the absence of heart disease, children found to be polycythemic should undergo pulmonary function investigation. The anesthetic management of children with disease of the respiratory system is discussed in Chapter 5.

Neonatal Polycythemia

Polycythemia in neonates may result from twin-to-twin or other intrauterine transfusion, or from fetal hypoxia. Severe cases may present convulsions, heart failure, and respiratory distress. Thrombosis of peripheral blood vessels or of the renal vein, brain damage, and necrotizing enterocolitis are serious complications.

The condition is more commonly seen in babies small for gestational age, in Down's syndrome, and in babies with gastroschisis.

Whether symptoms are present or not, if the hematocrit (hem.) exceeds 60 percent hypovolemia should be corrected by infusions free of red cells, while both normovolemia and the more characteristic hypervolemia should be treated with partial exchange transfusion using fresh frozen plasma or 5 percent albumin solution.[73]

$$\text{Volume of exchange} = \frac{\text{Blood vol. (Dl/kg)} \times \text{(Observed hem.} - \text{Desired hem.)}}{\text{Observed hem.}}$$

TERMINAL CARE OF CHILDREN WITH CANCER

Despite ever-improving results of therapy, it is inevitable that some children will fail to respond to treatment or will relapse. Active treatment is then withdrawn and terminal care instituted. The aims of care are twofold: to make the patient as comfortable as possible, and to support the parents and family of the dying child.

Anesthesiologists may have some involvement in pain relief, although most oncology departments are self-contained and manage the entire course. Many children will be nursed at home by their parents with the active support of nurses and medical staff. It is important that any involvement by clinicians is extended to the home situation and that continuous practical help and advice is always available.

The symptoms of terminal cancer vary from child to child and depend to a large extent on the initial pathology. Pain is obviously one of the most distressing to child and parents. When possible, oral analgesics should be prescribed unless the child is vomiting (Table 18–9).

Bone Pain. This is a common symptom of terminal leukemia and other malignancies. The nonsteroidal anti-inflammatory drugs are particularly useful, as is dexamethasone 1 to 4 mg daily, and radiotherapy. Diclofenac can also be given as a suppository.

Nerve Root Pain. This usually presents as a constant burning pain and can often be relieved by the use of corticosteroids—dexamethasone and prednisolone—which reduce perineural edema.

Nerve blocks may be useful in a cooperative child.

Raised Intracranial Pressure. Persistent headache and vomiting may be alleviated by corticosteroids. High doses of dexamethasone or betamethasone should be used in the first instance to obtain relief and then the dose reduced to the lowest tolerated. This is to avoid the excessive weight gain that accompanies high-dose steroids and makes nursing difficult.

Intrathecal methotrexate is also helpful in

relieving symptoms caused by leukemic deposits in the meninges.

Parenteral Administration. This may be necessary because of unrelieved pain, nausea, vomiting, or an unwillingness to take oral medication. Intramuscular injections are distressing to the child, parents, and nursing staff, and so continuous infusions of analgesics should be considered, even at home. The subcutaneous route is generally preferred; a winged needle or fine plastic cannula attached by a length of tubing to a battery-operated syringe driver is the most practical way of delivering the infusion.

Morphine sulfate or diacetylmorphine is the most suitable narcotic and should be made up in solution to last for 24 hours. The infusion site requires changing only if the area becomes inflamed or painful. Some syringe drivers have a boost button to deliver an additional fixed amount of the drug, which can be useful if nursing procedures cause pain. Patient-controlled analgesia (PCA) devices are more sophisticated and bulky but may be helpful in the older, alert child. Parents can be taught to refill the syringes and manage the infusion if they have recourse to immediate help.

When changing from oral narcotics to a continuous infusion it may be prudent to reduce the total 24-hour dose at first. However, tolerance does soon develop, and increasing doses may be required. This should never present a problem, as the aim of treatment is the relief of pain.

Other soluble drugs can be added to the infusion to alleviate additional symptoms.

Hydrocortisone, 50 mg into each syringe, will reduce local skin reactions.

Cyclizine or other antiemetics can be added in appropriate dose.

Hyoscine 120μ/kg will reduce airway and salivary secretions in the semiconscious child.

Phenothiazines, which also have an antiemetic effect, can be added for sedation.

Other Symptoms. *Itching* may be the result of obstructive jaundice or morphine administration, especially if morphine is given by continuous infusion.

Antihistamines or local antipruritic lotion often may give relief.

Constipation invariably accompanies the use of dihydrocodeine or morphine, and laxatives should be prescribed early.

Depression is quite common, and can be improved by giving amtitriptyline at night. Steroids may cause euphoria and increase appetite.

Fits from cerebral infiltration usually can be controlled by phenytoin in standard doses.

With the range of drugs available and individual attention, the objective is to alleviate as much as possible the child's symptoms and the parents' distress.

REFERENCES

1. Harrison MJ, Healy TEJ, Thornton JA: Aids to Anaesthesia. Vol 2: Clinical Practice. Edinburgh, Churchill-Livingstone, 1984.
2. Brain MC: The anemias. *In* Beeson JB, McDermott W, Wyngaarden JB (eds): Cecil Textbook of Medicine. 15th ed. Philadelphia, WB Saunders, 1979.
3. Kaufman L, Sumner E: Medical Problems and the Anesthetist. London, Edward Arnold, 1979, pp 139–151.
4. Willoughby MLN: Paediatric Haematology. Edinburgh, Churchill-Livingstone, 1977.
5. Webb DKH: Aplastic anaemia: Continued cause for concern (editorial). Arch Dis Child *65*:1105, 1990.
6. Marsh JCW, Hows JM, Bryett KA, Gordon-Smith EC: Young age and outcome of treatment with anti-lymphocytic globulin for aplastic anaemia. Bone Marrow Transplant *3*(Suppl I):238, 1988.
7. Hows JM: Severe aplastic anaemia: The patient without a HLA-identical sibling (clinical annotation). Br J Haematol *77*:1, 1991.
8. Birkhill FR, Maloney MA, Levenson SM: Effect of transfusion polycythaemia upon bone marrow activity and erythrocyte survival in man. Blood *6*:1021, 1951.
9. Emlinger PJ, Huff RL, Oda JM: Depression of red cell iron turnover by transfusion. Proc Soc Exp Biol Med *79*:16, 1952.
10. Roche Products Ltd: *In* Bailey AJM, Taylor W (Compilers): A.B.P.I. Data Sheet Compendium 1984–85. London, Datapharm Publications Ltd.
11. Jarvik EM: Drugs used in the treatment of psychiatric disorders. *In* Goodman LS, Gilman A: The Pharmacological Basis of Therapeutics. 4th ed. New York, Macmillan, 1970.
12. Amos RJ, Amess SAL, Hinds CJ, et al: Incidence and pathogenesis of acute megaloblastic bone marrow change in patients receiving intensive care. Lancet *2*:835, 1982.
13. Donald JR: Induced hypotension and blood loss during surgery. J R Soc Med *75*:149, 1982.
14. Brown TCK, Fisk GC: Anaesthesia for Children. Oxford, Blackwell Scientific, 1979.
15. Eschbach JW, Egrie JC, Downing MR, et al: Correction of the anemia of end-stage renal disease with recombinant human erythropoietin. Results of a combined phase I and II clinical trial. N Engl J Med *316*:73, 1987.
16. Wharton B: Nutrition and nutritional disorders. *In* Forfar JO, Arneil GC (eds): Textbook of Paediatrics. 2nd ed. Edinburgh, Churchill-Livingstone, 1978.
17. Rennie JS, MacDonald DG, Dagg JH: Iron and the oral epithelium: A review. J R Soc Med *77*:602, 1984.
18. Howells TH, Pettit JE: Haematological disorders. *In* Vickers MD (ed): Medicine for Anaesthetists. 2nd ed. London, Churchill-Livingstone, 1982, pp 335–385.
19. Howells TH: Anaesthesia and blood diseases. *In* Hewer CL, Atkinson RS (eds): Recent Advances in Anaesthesia and Analgesia. Vol 12. London, Churchill-Livingstone, 1975, pp 120–130.
20. Severinghaus JW, Koh SD: Effect of anemia on pulse

oximeter accuracy at low saturation. J Clin Monit *6*:85, 1990.
21. Barltrop D: Nutrition and nutritional disorders. *In* Forfar JC, Arneil GC (eds): Textbook of Paediatrics. 2nd ed. Edinburgh, Churchill-Livingstone, 1978.
22. Co-trimoxazole and blood (editorial). Lancet *21*:950, 1973.
23. Herbert V: Megaloblastic anemias. *In* Beeson PB, McDermott W, Wyngaarden JB (eds): Cecil Textbook of Medicine. 15th ed. Philadelphia, WB Saunders, 1979, pp 1719–1729.
24. Lawson DH, Murray RM, Parker JLW: Early mortality in the megaloblastic anaemias. Q J Med *41*:1, 1972.
25. Megaloblastic anaemia and sudden death (editorial). Br Med J *1*:525, 1972.
26. Amess JAL, Burman JF, Rees JM, et al: Megaloblastic haemopoiesis in patients receiving nitrous oxide. Lancet *2*:339, 1978.
27. Amos RJ, Amess JAL, Nancekievill DG, et al: Prevention of nitrous oxide–induced megaloblastic changes in bone marrow using folic acid. Br J Anaesth *56*:103, 1984.
28. Parkin DM, Stiller CA, Draper GJ, et al (eds): International Incidence of Childhood Cancer. Lyon, International Agency for Research on Cancer, 1988. (IARC Scientific Publications No. 87)
29. Linet MS, Deresa SS: Descriptive epidemiology of childhoood leukaemia. Br J Cancer *63*:424, 1991.
30. Roman E, Beral V: Possible aetiological factors in childhood leukaemia. Arch Dis Child *66*:179, 1991.
31. Wark HJ: Postoperative jaundice in children: the influence of halothane. Anaesthesia *38*:237, 1983.
32. Thomas M: The use of the Hickman catheter in the management of patients with leukaemia and other malignancies. Br J Surg *66*:673, 1979.
33. Chung F: Cancer chemotherapy and anaesthesia. Can Anaesth Soc J *29*:364, 1982.
34. Selvin BL: Cancer chemotherapy: Implications for the anesthesiologist. Anesth Analg *60*:425, 1981.
35. Serota FT, August CS, Koch PA, et al: Pulmonary function in patients undergoing bone marrow transplantation. Med Pediatr Oncol *12*:137, 1984.
36. Filshie J, Pollock AN, Hughes RG, et al: The anaesthetic management of bone marrow harvest for transplantation. Anaesthesia *39*:480, 1984.
37. Neuman GG, Weingarten AE, Abromowitz RM, et al: The anesthetic management of the patient with an anterior mediastinal mass. Anesthesiology *60*:144, 1984.
38. Davies SC, Hewitt PE: Sickle cell disease. Br J Hosp Med *31*:440, 1984.
39. Salem MR: Anesthesia for orthopedic surgery. *In* Gregory GA (ed): Pediatric Anesthesia. Vol 2. New York, Churchill-Livingstone, 1983, pp 851–898.
40. Howells TA, Huntsman RG, Boys JE, et al: Anaesthesia and sickle cell haemoglobin. Br J Anaesth *44*:975, 1972.
41. Henthorn J, Anionwu E, Brozovic M: Screening cord blood for sickle haemoglobinopathies in Brent. Br Med J *289*:479, 1984.
42. Berry FA: Anesthesia for genitourinary surgery. *In* Gregory GA (ed): Pediatric Anesthesia. Vol 2. New York, Churchill-Livingstone, 1983, pp 727–771.
43. Davies SC: The vaso-occlusive crisis of sickle cell disease (editorial). Br Med J *302*:1551, 1991.
44. Davies SC, McWilliam AC, Hewitt PE, et al: Red cell alloimmunization in sickle cell disease. Br J Haematol *63*:241, 1986.
45. John AB, Ramlal A, Jackson H, et al: Prevention of pneumococcal infection in children with homozygous sickle cell disease. Br Med J *288*:1567, 1984.
46. Topley JM, Rogers DW, Stevens MCG, et al.: Acute splenic sequestration and hypersplenism in the first five years in homozygous sickle cell disease. Arch Dis Child *56*:765, 1981.
47. Goldberg MA, Brugnata C, Dover GJ, et al: Treatment of sickle cell anaemia with hydroxyuria and erythropoietin. N Engl J Med *323*:366, 1990.
48. Bentley PC, Howard ER: Surgery in children with homozygous sickle cell anemia. Ann R Coll Surg Engl *61*:55, 1979.
49. Homi J, Reynolds J, Skinner A, et al: General anaesthesia in sickle cell disease. Br Med J *1*:1599, 1979.
50. Furman EB: Blood and fluid replacement for paediatric patients. *In* Steward DJ (ed): Some Aspects of Paediatric Anaesthesia. Amsterdam, Excerpta Medica, 1982.
51. Janik J, Seeler RA: Perioperative management of children with sickle hemoglobinopathy. J Pediatr Surg *15*:117, 1980.
52. Browne RA: Anaesthesia in patients with sickle cell anaemia. Br J Anaesth *37*:181, 1965.
53. Modell B, Mibashan RS: Antenatal diagnosis of haemoglobinopathies. *In* Willoughby M, Siegel SE (eds): Hematology and Oncology. London, Butterworth, 1982, pp 162–195.
54. Letsky EA: Inherited red cell defects which may complicate surgical treatment. *In* Wilkinson AW (ed): Recent Advances in Paediatric Surgery. Vol 3. London, Churchill-Livingstone, 1975, pp 11–20.
55. Oduro KA, Searle JF: Anaesthesia in sickle cell states—a plea for simplicity. Br Med J *4*:596, 1972.
56. Searle JF: Anaesthesia in sickle cell states. Anaesthesia *28*:48, 1973.
57. Jacob HS: Hemolysis due to intracorpuscular abnormalities. *In* Beeson PB, McDermott W, Wyngaarden JS (eds): Cecil Textbook of Medicine. 15th ed. Philadelphia, WB Saunders, 1979, pp 865–869.
58. Keller DF: G-6-PD Deficiency. London, Butterworth, 1971.
59. Wintrobe MM (ed): Clinical Hematology. 7th ed. Philadelphia, Lea and Febiger, 1974, p 785.
60. Weatherall DJ: Haemolytic anaemias. *In* Weatherall DJ, Ledingham JG, Warrell DA (eds): Oxford Textbook of Medicine. Oxford, Oxford University Press, 1983.
61. Atkinson RS, Rushman GB, Lee JA: A Synopsis of Anaesthesia. 8th ed. Bristol, John Wright, 1977.
62. Rizza CR: Haemophilia A and B. Prescribers' J *24*:71, 1984.
63. Chessells JM: Management of haemophilia and allied disorders. *In* Wilkinson AW (ed): Recent Advances in Paediatric Surgery. Vol 3. London, Churchill-Livingstone, 1975, pp 22–30.
64. Horsey PJ: Blood transfusion. *In* Atkinson RS, Langton Hewer C: Recent Advances in Anaesthesia. Vol 15. London, Churchill-Livingstone, 1982.
65. Trimmer EJ: Hepatitis B immunisation. Br J Parenter Ther *5*:135, 1984.
66. Department of Health and Social Security (U.K.): Guidance for surgeons, anaesthetists, dentists and their teams dealing with patients infected with HTLV III. Chief Medical Officer *86*:7, 1986.
67. Cameron CB, Kobrinsky N: Perioperative management of patients with Von Willebrand's disease. Can J Anaesth *37*:341, 1990.
68. Newland AC: Idiopathic thrombocytopenic purpura and IgG: A review. J Infect *15* (Suppl I):41, 1987.
69. Imbach P, D'Apuzzo B, Hirt A, et al: High dose intravenous gammaglobulin for idiopathic thrombocytopenic purpura in childhood. Lancet *1*:1228, 1981.

70. Eraklis AJ: Spleen and portal circulation. *In* Welch B (ed): Complications of Pediatric Surgery. Philadelphia, WB Saunders, 1982, pp 264–273.
71. Austrian R: Prevention of fatal bacterial infection in patients with anatomic or functional asplenia (editorial). Ann Intern Med *96*:117, 1982.
72. Fitts WTJ, Erde A, Peskin GW, et al: Surgical implications of polycythemia vera. Ann Surg *152*:548, 1960.
73. Rowe MI: Shock and resuscitation. *In* Welch B (ed): Complications of Pediatric Surgery. Philadelphia, WB Saunders, 1982, p 20.

CHAPTER

19 Neuromuscular Diseases

PETER G. DUNCAN, M.D.

Neuromuscular diseases in infants and children are relatively rare, yet their presentation to the pediatric anesthesiologist is not unusual, since the need for diagnostic procedures or palliative orthopedic operation occurs with many of these entities. While some of the diseases have profound and well-described anesthetic implications, others, because of their rarity, do not. Consequently, discussion of anesthetic management must be based on the medical description of the pathogenesis and extrapolation of anesthetic implications of related diseases.

Numerous classifications of neuromuscular diseases exist, depending on the interest of the writer.[1,2] From the anesthesiologist's viewpoint, diseases are best classified according to the site of the anatomical lesion and hence the likely nature of any adverse occurrence during an operative procedure.[3]

DISEASES OF THE SPINAL CORD AND ANTERIOR HORN CELLS

Primary diseases of the anterior horn cells or the motor nuclei of the cranial nerves present a uniform clinical syndrome of profound weakness, neurogenic muscle atrophy, absent deep tendon reflexes, and fasciculations in the region of the denervated muscle groups. They are differentiated from peripheral nerve damage by the normality of sensation. In infants, the fasciculations and muscle atrophy may be difficult to recognize because of generous subcutaneous fat, and marked hypotonia may be the predominant sign. Segmental involvement of the spinal cord with disease may present with regional signs of the lower motor neuron disease at the level of involvement combined with upper motor signs below the level of the lesion. In the latter situation, the clinical implications to the anesthesiologist will depend upon the extent of cord involvement.

In any lesion involving the motor nuclei of the spinal cord, the anesthesiologist must be concerned about compromised respiratory reserve secondary to muscle weakness, positioning difficulty due to muscle atrophy and contractures, aspiration due to pharyngeal muscle involvement, and altered effects of neuromuscular blocking drugs. Experience with relaxants in all clinical entities has not been reported,[4] yet there have been numerous case reports of life-threatening hyperkalemia following succinylcholine administration to paraplegics[5] or patients with lower motor neuron disease.[6] Experimentally, the susceptibility begins 14 days after cord or peripheral nerve transection and is present up to 1 year after injury.[7] Beyond a year in patients with stable neurological lesions the induced hyperkalemia is less marked, probably owing to reduction of the muscle bulk;[8] children with cerebral palsy do not seem to be at risk for hyperkalemia after succinylcholine.[9] Prior administration of nondepolarizing relaxants does not consistently protect against the phenomenon.[10] Since other rapid-onset, short-duration, nondepolarizing muscle relaxants are available, the use of succinylcholine should be limited, except in emergency situations.

Primary anterior horn cell disease of longstanding duration may also be associated with altered responses to nondepolarizing muscular relaxants. It has been shown in animals[11] and in humans[12] with lower motor neuron and upper motoneuron diseases, respectively, that denervation results in a resistance of affected muscle to such relaxants. It has been suggested that denervation results in an increased number of acetylcholine receptors along the muscle beyond the neuromuscular membrane, resulting in extrajunctional chemosensitivity to acetylcholine. In addition to this quantitative change in receptor number, there is a qualitative change in the receptors from a modification of subunit composition.[13] These denervation-induced acetylcholine receptors have embryonic-like channel properties[14] such that, when stimulated, their channels stay open longer and conduct less current than adult endplate receptors. The overall result is a sensitivity to acetylcholine (and other agonists such as succinylcholine) and reduced binding and blocking effectiveness of D-tubocurarine at any given concentration.[15]

In the developmental regulation of embryonic acetylcholine receptors, the stimulation of denervated muscle prevents or reverses this extrajunctional chemosensitivity, resulting in receptors of more normal, longer half-life.[16] Although newborn muscle contains virtually 100 percent immature, slow ion-channel receptors at birth, the percentage falls to below 20 percent 3 weeks later.[13] If muscles are denervated from birth, the normal fast channels do not develop; if denervated after birth, the endplate regions regress in 2 to 14 days to become primary slow (embryonic) channels. In time, totally denervated muscles become too atrophied and covered with connective tissue to be functional. However, the time of receptor modification corresponds well to the period of clinical susceptibility to altered muscle relaxant effects.

In a given patient it is unknown how much extrajunctional chemosensitivity will antagonize nondepolarizing relaxants, or how much atrophy will potentiate their clinical efforts.[17] Although nondepolarizing relaxants are preferable to the depolarizing group (with their attendant hyperkalemia), judicious tempering of the dose and appropriate monitoring are essential for safety.

SYRINGOMYELIA

This slowly progressive, degenerative disease involves the spinal cord, the medulla (syringobulbia), or both. A progressive cavitation occurs, usually in the cervical and lumbar segments of the cord, and primarily in the anterior white commissure. Initially there is loss of pain and temperature sensation as the crossed fibers of the lateral spinothalamic tract are disrupted. As the cavitation extends it may involve the long motor tracts, including the corticospinal tract. The lower motor neurons of the medulla and cord are similarly secondarily affected. Progressive dilatation in the cervical region may lead to impaired cerebrospinal fluid (CSF) drainage, elevation of intracranial pressure, and hydrocephalus.

The pathophysiology of the lesion is unknown. It could be due to incomplete closing of the neural tube in the fourth week of gestation. Alternatively, fluid accumulation in the fourth ventricle may result from failure of the foramen of Magendie to open in prenatal life. Most likely, there is a defect in the intermedullary vascular supply, leading to infarction or hemorrhage. The inadequate circulation results in cavitation. Occasionally the syndrome occurs in the small muscles of the hands, and fasciculations are common. Papilledema may accompany the elevated intracranial pressure. Associated physical findings include cervical ribs, kyphoscoliosis, and the Klippel-Feil syndrome.

The primary management has been surgical, either laminectomy or suboccipital craniotomy, but the results have been variable and have included a death rate of up to 15 percent. Orthopedic surgery also may be used to control the scoliosis. Anesthetic concerns in such procedures include a possibility of raised intracranial pressure, inadequacy of bulbar reflexes protecting the airway, the degree of impairment of ventilatory function due to the kyphoscoliosis, and the extent of preexisting debility of a chronically ill patient. Defective sweating mechanisms may result from autonomic nervous system compromise, and perioperative thermal regulation may be difficult.

DIASTEMATOMYELIA

In this entity a mesodermal septum divides the cord laterally into equal portions. The septum, composed of cartilage, fibrous tissue, and bone, is attached to the posterior aspect of the vertebral bodies and passes through the neural canal to the posterior arch. The lesion may occur in the thoracic or lumbar area and may be associated with skeletal changes such as spina bifida or kyphoscoliosis. Skin lesions, including lipomas, sacrococcygeal sinus, meningomyelocele, nevi, and hemangiomas may occur over the spine.

Clinically the patient presents with signs and symptoms in the lower legs and feet, together with bladder atony. Disruption of the anterior horn cells results in weakness and atrophy, while interference with crossing fibers may impair pain and temperature sensations.

The treatment of the lesion is surgical to prevent or retard progression of symptoms. Specific anesthetic implications have not been reported.

SPINAL CORD LESIONS

Spinal cord injury in children can result from several causes. It can occur from birth injury or at any age from falls, car accidents, or direct blows to the spine. Vascular injury may result in decreased flow in the anterior spinal artery, which may also occur during repair of coarctation of the aorta. Inflammatory lesions may result in transverse myelitis secondary to viral infections or hyperimmune response to immunization. Whatever the etiology, the patient is left in the initial phase of spinal shock with distal flaccidity and loss of bladder and bowel function, followed in a later phase by spasticity and secondary contracture. Sensation is impaired below the lesion, and autonomic regulation of temperature and circulatory dynamics is compromised.

The anesthetic implications depend on the duration of the lesion.[18] During the acute phase (less than 3 weeks), there may be considerable cardiovascular instability due to impaired sympathetic reflexes and fluctuating vascular volumes. In the intermediate phase (3 days to 3 months), excessively high serum potassium levels occur with the use of depolarizing muscle relaxants (denervation hypersensitivity). With the availability of short-acting, nondepolarizing muscle relaxants, the need for succinylcholine is limited.[5, 19] In the chronic state, the patients are prone to secondary musculoskeletal abnormalities, which may compromise positioning for surgery, restrict pulmonary function, and contribute to the development of decubitus ulcers through impairment of sensation over bony prominences. Renal complications, including infection and calculi, are common in patients with long-standing cord lesions.

The level of the lesion is the critical factor determining anesthetic problems. Patients with lesions affecting sympathetic outflow may have significant cardiovascular, thermal, and respiratory difficulties. Autonomic hyperreflexia may occur in response to stimulation such as pain or a distended bladder. Control of this potentially fatal complication can be attempted by ensuring adequate depths of anesthesia and the use of vasodilating drugs such as sodium nitroprusside to treat hypertension.[20, 21] Hypotensive responses can be controlled by correcting hypovolemia and by the use of vagal blocking drugs to abolish unopposed vagal tone causing bradycardia or heart block. Lack of sympathetic control of sweating and cutaneous blood flow compromises body temperature control, demanding prudent monitoring and maintenance of temperature perioperatively. Finally, lesions in the thoracic cord or above may decrease the function of accessory respiratory muscles, lowering vital capacity and expiratory reserve volumes and predisposing to postoperative pulmonary complications.

PROGRESSIVE INFANTILE SPINAL MUSCLE ATROPHY

This disease, also known as *Werdnig-Hoffmann disease,* is an autosomal recessive degenerative disease of the anterior horn cells and cranial nerve motor nuclei. Clinically the course of the illness varies according to the age of onset. Neonates or patients in the first 6 months of life experience a rapidly progressive course, with death from respiratory complications by the age of 2 years. Those who become symptomatic after 1 year experience a less fulminating course and may survive into the second decade. No medical treatment is available, although orthopedic surgery may be attempted to stabilize the unsupported spine and thus slow the progression to respiratory failure.

The clinical picture is uniform in these patients. They demonstrate generalized muscle weakness and hypotonia, although sparing of the facial and extraocular muscles allows an alert facial expression to be maintained. Secondary skeletal changes of pectus excavatum and kyphoscoliosis invariably occur. Sensation remains intact despite a marked atrophy of the skeletal muscles. Later bulbar involvement develops and leads to problems with secretion control and recurrent aspiration pneumonia.

Numerous syndromes have been described with similar hereditary degeneration of anterior horn cells. Juvenile proximal hereditary muscular atrophy (*Kugelberg-Welander disease*) has its onset in the first or second decade and progresses slowly over the next 20 to 40 years to total debility. Cardiac arrhythmias and congestive heart failure may occur.[22] *Facioscapulohumeral neurogenic atrophy, scapuloperoneal atrophy,* and *chronic spinal muscular atrophy* are inherited syndromes with predominantly regional involvement beginning at the first decade of life. Progressive bulbar paralysis of childhood (*Fazio-Londe disease*) is a progressive degeneration of the anterior horn cells in the bulbar nuclei and cervical and upper thoracic cord. *Möbius' syndrome,* on the other hand, is a nonprogressive deterioration of the motor nuclei of cranial nerves VI and VII.[23]

Amyotrophic lateral sclerosis is a progressive degenerative disease affecting the cortical spinal tracts, motor nuclei of the lower medulla, and anterior horn cells of the spinal cord. While mainly a disease of adults, it may begin in the first two decades of life and then rapidly progress. Death usually occurs within several years after diagnosis as a result of bulbar involvement.

The anesthesia literature in regard to these degenerative entities is sparse. There are numerous documented reports of succinylcholine-induced hyperkalemia[6, 10] with subsequent cardiovascular collapse, and this drug is therefore contraindicated. Motor nerve degeneration and subsequent recruitment by neighboring fibers may cause a change in the neuromuscular junction, resulting in altered sensitivity to all nondepolarizing relaxants.[4] Hence all relaxants of this type should be used in titrated doses with appropriate monitoring. While there is no evidence that respiratory drive is impaired in these diseases, respiratory reserve is definitely reduced from muscle weakness and skeletal changes. Aspiration is a clear danger in the presence of pharyngeal involvement, particularly in the anesthetic and postoperative periods when muscular deficits may be exaggerated.[23] If there is any doubt of the ability of the patient to protect the airway or sustain an adequate minute ventilation, mechanical support should be continued well into the postoperative period. Whenever possible, relaxants are best avoided, and any muscle relaxation that is needed should be achieved by use of volatile anesthetics that have significant relaxant properties.

ARTHROGRYPOSIS MULTIPLEX CONGENITA

Arthrogryposis is a syndrome present from birth that is characterized by multiple contractures of the arms and legs. The mechanism of inheritance is unknown. In some cases the contractures may be secondary to degeneration of nerve roots or myopathies, but the most common form stems from profound reductions in the number of anterior horn cells in the cervical and lumbar enlargements of the cord.[1] The weak, hypotonic musculature results in multiple deformities of the limbs and permanent contractures. Associated abnormalities include cardiac malformations, inguinal hernias, cleft palate, scoliosis, and rigidity of the temporomandibular joints.

Patients with this rare syndrome need anesthesia for release of contractures or correction of associated defects. Preoperatively, the ability to open the mouth and control the airway must be assured. Clinical and radiographic examination of the mandible and upper airway may be indicated, and ancillary devices for intubation may be needed. Slow induction by mask with oxygen and volatile agents rather than precipitous intravenous induction is preferred. Although adverse reactions to relaxants has not been reported, apprehension exists about the safety of depolarizing drugs with all anterior horn cell diseases.

Positioning for operation may pose a considerable problem because of the extensive flexion contractures. Care must be taken to protect skin over bony points and to prevent pathological fractures.

POLIOMYELITIS

Fortunately less common since the introduction of immunization, the infective destruction of anterior horn cells by the polio virus leaves a clinical picture similar to that of the degenerative diseases of the anterior horn cells. Anesthetic concerns are similar, with sensitivity to depolarizing drugs to be expected. If nondepolarizing relaxants are used, one must be careful to monitor respiratory musculature carefully and to avoid erroneous conclusions drawn from assessment of noninvolved muscle groups.[4]

DISORDERS OF PERIPHERAL NERVES AND SPINAL NERVE ROOTS

GUILLAIN-BARRÉ SYNDROME

Usually following a nonspecific illness or infection, this syndrome consists of a gradual onset of symmetrical paralysis ascending from the feet. In half the cases the disease involves the cranial nerves, with resultant compromise of respiratory and bulbar function. Patchy sensory loss occurs as well, although it is less prominent than the motor deficit. Autonomic dysfunction is common, with variable heart rates, labile blood pressures, and electrocardiographic changes.[24] Pathologically, there is demyelination of the axons with lymphocyte infiltration. IgM antibodies in the myelin sheaths suggest an immunological mechanism.

The clinical course is variable, with slow progression over days or weeks or rapid progression to flaccid quadriplegia. Recovery occurs in 2 to 8 weeks, being complete in 65 percent of those afflicted and leaving residual weakness in the remainder. Mortality is quoted at 3 to 4 percent of cases, mainly from complications of respiratory muscle paralysis. Treatment is supportive only; steroid therapy is of equivocal value.

Anesthetic considerations in Guillain-Barré syndrome revolve around the instability of the cardiovascular system and impaired respiratory reserve. Techniques should be employed that cause minimal disruption of compensatory cardiovascular reflexes, intravascular volumes must be carefully maintained, and drugs potentiating catecholamine-induced arrhythmias must be avoided.[25] During positive-pressure ventilation, the cardiovascular system must be carefully monitored to detect alterations in cardiac output.

TOXIC POLYNEUROPATHIES

Postimmunization neuropathies have been reported after use of virtually all preparations and can affect any of the peripheral nerves. Following rubella immunization, the syndrome develops after a latency of 7 to 99 days, usually as a painful sensation in the arm or leg. Recovery is usually complete.

Heavy metal intoxication similarly can result in peripheral neuropathies. Lead intoxication usually produces an encephalopathy but may be associated with a motor neuropathy with minimal sensory changes. Arsenic, as found in insecticides, produces acute gastrointestinal distress but chronic paresthesias, weakness, and tropic skin changes. Treatment is with chelating drugs.

The bacterial infections of *diphtheria* and *botulism* may each be responsible for a neuropathy in susceptible children. In unimmunized subjects *Corynebacterium diphtheriae* produces weakness, classically beginning with swallowing difficulty (paralysis of the palate), blurred vision (paralysis of the ciliary muscles), and diplopia (paralysis of the extraocular muscles). Subsequently weakness and paresthesias develop in the trunk and extremities. Diphtheritic myocarditis will cause ECG changes varying from slow conduction to AV block. Therapy includes use of antibiotics and antitoxin and supportive management. Botulism is caused by acute food poisoning with the toxin of *Clostridium botulinum;* in infants this classically results from ingestion of home-preserved honey. Progressive weakness beginning in the cranial nerves results in swallowing and respiratory problems requiring medical support. Autonomic nervous system involvement results in ileus and delayed gastric emptying. Recovery is usually complete but may take months.

METABOLIC NEUROPATHIES

Diabetes is associated with several peripheral neuropathic syndromes, ranging from a slowly progressive symmetrical distal sensory neuropathy to single or multiple polyneuropathies. Autonomic neuropathy may lead to impaired compensatory cardiovascular reflexes. Such syndromes usually occur in adults but have been noted in up to 10 percent of diabetic children, particularly when disease control is poor.

Acute intermittent porphyria is an autosomal dominant inherited disorder of porphyrin metabolism.[26] Increased levels of delta-aminolevulinic acid synthetase result in increased delta-aminolevulinic acid and porphobilinogen excretion. The former causes patchy demyelination of peripheral nerves, and axonal degeneration results in flaccid paralysis or weakness of skeletal muscle. The disease usually has an onset about the time of puberty and may present either as a "surgical emergency" with severe, colicky abdominal pain or with psychiatric disturbances. Many drugs, including barbiturates, have been associated with enzyme induction that worsens the syndrome; these drugs must be avoided. While some workers have noted that thiopental has been used inadvertently without problems in the latent periods,[27] others have noted a deterioration in symptoms if it is used during an acute episode. In a review of anesthetic exposures to patients with inducible porphyrias, Mustajoki and Heinonen report that it is rare indeed for any anesthetic drug, including thiopental, to induce symptoms in latent porphyria.[28] During acute attacks it is probable that drugs may be harmful only in association with other factors precipitating the development of symptoms—surgical therapy may worsen an acute attack even without the administration of precipitating drugs. In experimental animals, numerous anesthetics have been shown to induce porphyria synthesis, including barbiturates (thiopental and methohexital), steroids, alfaxalone (Althesin), etomidate, chlordiazepoxide, pentazocine, enflurane, and methoxyflurane. Ketamine is without effect in the rat but induces delta-aminolevulinic acid synthetase in the chick embryo liver. It has been used without adverse sequelae in humans. It is probably advisable on a theoretical basis to avoid these drugs if alternative agents are available. No harmful effect is expected with opiates, local anesthetics, or inhalational anesthetics (nitrous oxide, halothane, isoflurane). Propofol is reported[28a] to be safe for use as an anesthetic induction agent in patients with porphyria. Regional anesthetic techniques may be appropriate during an acute attack, although the etiology of residual neurological deficits may be obscured by major conduction techniques.

Disorders of fat metabolism are associated with various syndromes of peripheral nerve impairment. Abetalipoproteinemia, or *Bassen-Kornzweig's syndrome,* is a deficiency of low-density lipoprotein and chylomicrons. Peripheral sensory neuropathy is associated with cardiac failure, arrhythmia, or diarrhea. Familial alpha-lipoprotein deficiency, or *Tangier disease,* is a deficiency of high-density lipoproteins with excessive accumulation of cholesterol ester and triglycerides. The syndrome of *metachromatic leukodystrophy* is characterized by demyelination and intracellular storage of sulfatide in the brain, nerves, liver, and kidney. *Refsum's disease* represents a disorder of fatty acid metabolism resulting in excessive storage of phytanic acid in brain, nerves, liver, kidney, and heart. Globoid cell leukodystrophy, or *Krabbe's disease,* is a primary deficiency of the enzyme galactocerebrosidase resulting in demyelination and the presence of inclusion bodies in Schwann's cells. This disease results in a progressive development of spasticity from infancy, then ultimately a flaccid paralysis and death.

There is no information regarding the effect of anesthesia on these metabolic conditions or on the safety of anesthetic drugs in their presence. It is speculated that positioning and protection of the patient's skin may be difficult during prolonged procedures. Cardiovascular tolerance may be reduced owing to infiltrative involvement of the myocardium and abolition of compensatory sympathetic reflexes. Potent cardiac depressants are best avoided, and hydration must be watched carefully. Respiratory muscle innervation may be affected, and compensation for respiratory embarrassment reduced; if doubt exists, ventilation should be controlled until adequate. Gastroparesis, with delayed emptying after normal fasting periods, may accompany autonomic involvement. Involvement of liver or kidney by fat accumulation may predispose the patient to fasting hypoglycemia, as well as altered fixed drug metabolism and excretion. Careful monitoring for the residual effects of narcotics and relaxants is essential. Although the neuromuscular junction is not primarily affected, denervation hypersensitivity will exist to depolarizing drugs, whereas reduced reserves exist for nondepolarizing substances.[4]

HEREDITARY NEUROPATHIES

Hereditary neuropathies are often found associated with other degenerative disorders. The lesions are primarily in the peripheral nerves, resulting in a mixed picture of lower motor neuron disease and sensory deprivation. Secondary neurogenic muscle atrophy occurs, while denervation hypersensitivity can be expected to cause a hyperkalemic response to succinylcholine.

Charcot-Marie-Tooth disease (peroneal muscle atrophy) is an autosomal dominant disorder with onset in the second decade. Weakness is confined to the limbs, particularly the legs and feet. Involvement of the sympathetic postganglionic fibers impairs autonomic function, particularly the control of temperature by sweating. Although the primary lesion is demyelination of the peripheral axon, secondary loss of anterior horn cells and degeneration of the posterior columns occur. Life expectancy is not affected, although the degree of debility may be severe. The anesthetic implications are similar to those of other denervating syndromes.[29]

Hypertrophic interstitial neuritis (*Déjérine-Sottas disease*) has its onset in infancy, with delayed motor development and an undulating but progressive course. Weakness and atrophy involve the entire motor system, including bulbar muscles; sensory changes are more profound. Autonomic changes with thermal lability and mottled cyanosis of the extremities are common. A similar entity, but associated with more severe demyelination, is congenital hypomyelination neuropathy.

Friedreich's ataxia is an autosomal recessive disease often with onset in childhood, resulting in progressive degeneration throughout the central nervous system. Clinically there is mental deterioration, ataxia from degeneration of the spinocerebellar tract, and loss of the large myelinated fibers and cells from the dorsal root ganglia. Skeletal abnormalities such as scoliosis and hammer toe are common. The myocardium is involved in 30 percent of cases, with necrosis and degeneration of muscle causing arrhythmias and murmurs.[30] The safe use of spinal anesthesia for cesarean section has been described.[31]

Numerous syndromes, the hereditary sensory neuropathies, have been described in which the sensory modality is affected without significant muscle weakness. Patients with these disorders are prone to skeletal and cutaneous injury and also to thermal lability. The lesion usually lies in the dorsal root ganglion or in the myelination of sensory nerves.

One clinical entity with a significant sensory neuropathy is familial dysautonomia (*Riley-Day syndrome*). Occurring predominantly in Ashkenazi Jews, it presents a clinical complex of deficient tear production, absent corneal and deep tendon reflexes, hypotonia, lability of the cardiovascular system, insensitivity to pain, and emotional lability. Absence of fungiform papillae on the tongue may suggest the diagnosis. Pathologically, there is focal demyelination of the posterior columns of the spinal cord and degeneration of dorsal root ganglia. The defect in the autonomic nervous system is unknown, although it may represent an imbalance between sympathetic and parasympathetic tone or insufficiency of acetylcholine and catecholamine release. A defect in the formation of norepinephrine from levodopa has also been postulated.

The anesthetic management of Riley-Day syndrome has been described by several investigators.[32–36] The fundamental difficulty is the lack of compensatory cardiovascular reflexes, especially in the presence of potent cardiovascular depressant anesthetic drugs. Hypovolemia is also not compensated, and blood volumes must be carefully monitored. Insensitivity to pain may reduce the anesthetic requirement, although lack of cardiovascular signs of blood pressure and pulse rate changes make assessment of anesthetic depth difficult. Careful monitoring and control of body temperature are imperative.

Emotional lability with severe perioperative anxiety is common, and appropriate sedation preoperatively is recommended. Phenothiazines have been recommended because of their alpha-adrenergic blocking effect, thereby minimizing the hypertensive response to circulating catecholamines. Preoperative use of propranolol has been similarly advocated. Difficulty in assessing anesthetic depth, in addition to possible disturbed control of ventilation,[37] leads one to advocate controlled ventilation during general anesthesia. No abnormality has been reported with the use of muscle relaxants. Vomiting and aspiration is a significant hazard postoperatively.

A disease of significance to anesthetic practice is neurofibromatosis (*von Recklinghausen's disease*).[38, 39] Its incidence is 1 in 3000 live births, although the mode of inheritance is uncertain. The syndrome consists of café-au-lait spots, moles, and benign neurocutaneous tumors. Such neurofibromas can achieve a considerable size, causing secondary compromise of nerve or organ function. Lesions in the larynx have been associated with anesthetic disasters. Lesions impinging on bones cause erosion. Fifty percent of patients have kyphoscoliosis. Associated findings may include honeycomb cystic lung changes[40] and renal artery dysplasia with hypertension.[41] Because of common embryonic origins, there is an association of this disease with medullary thyroid tumors and pheochromocytoma; such tumors occur in up to 25 percent of cases and may be undetected preoperatively. Anesthetic management of patients with von Recklinghausen's disease must include preoperative calcium and blood pressure determinations, as well as a chest radiograph to rule out related abnormalities. The conduct of the anesthetic should be similar to that for a patient with a pheochromocytoma, avoiding physiological trespass and monitoring closely for unexpected blood pressure changes. Prolonged paralysis with depolarizing relaxants has been reported, although the reasons have not been investigated.[42, 43]

NEUROPATHIES ASSOCIATED WITH OTHER CONDITIONS

Connective tissue or collagen vascular diseases have frequently been associated with central nervous system findings, probably owing to interference with nervous blood supply. In *polyarteritis nodosa* there are signs of peripheral neuropathy in up to 50 percent of patients. *Systemic lupus erythematosus* is commonly associated with central nervous system signs in adults, although these are rare in children.

Tumors and neoplasms may cause neuropathies in any age group. *Leukemia,* the most common malignant disease in children, may infiltrate the cranial and peripheral nerves. *Neuroblastoma,* the most common solid tumor, may be associated with a diffuse nervous syndrome consisting of bewildering athetoid movements. Any other tumor may infiltrate peripheral nerves or nerve roots locally, leading to sensory or motor neuropathies.

DISORDERS OF THE NEUROMUSCULAR JUNCTION

MYASTHENIA GRAVIS

Myasthenia gravis is a neuromuscular disorder manifested by weakness and fatigability of voluntary muscles. The ocular muscles are most commonly involved, causing ptosis and diplopia. Cranial nerve problems are usual, resulting in dysarthria and dysphagia. Respiratory muscle weakness is less common but may be profound during a crisis. The symptoms fluctuate and are worsened by exercise and improved by rest. Similarly, electrical stimulation of involved musculature shows fatigue of contraction on repeated stimulation and exhaustion after a tetanic burst.[44]

The basic mechanism of the disease appears to be autoimmune, with a reduction in the number of available acetylcholine receptors at the neuromuscular junction. Antibodies to the receptors have been demonstrated.[45] There is an association with other immunological diseases, particularly thyroid disease. However, a poor relationship of the antibody titers to the clinical state has been documented. The muscles are small, probably owing to neurogenic atrophy, but are structurally normal. Aggregations of lymphocytes about the neuromuscular junctions are again perceived as support for the hypothesis of an autoimmune etiology.

The incidence of the disease is 3 per 100,000, and about 10 percent of patients are under 16 years of age. Pediatric cases are described as one of three types:

1. *Neonatal transient myasthenia,* affecting the infant of a mother with the disease. Symptoms persist for 1 to 8 weeks and consist of weakness and difficulty in feeding. The severity of the disease in the infant does not correlate with the mother's symptoms, and only 10 to 15 percent of newborn infants of affected mothers will be affected; however, medical therapy with an anticholinesterase drug may be needed.
2. *Congenital myasthenia gravis,* affecting an infant in the first few months of life. The mother does not have the disease, and the child will persist with symptoms, which are usually mild, for life.
3. *Juvenile myasthenia gravis,* affecting those over the age of 10 years, usually girls, with a presentation similar to that in adults. Cases in juvenile and adult patients have been classified by involvement as "ocular," affecting the eye only, or "generalized," affecting all voluntary muscles.

The treatment of myasthenia gravis consists of elevating the level of acetylcholine at the neuromuscular junction by the inhibition of cholinesterase.[46] The most commonly used preparations are oral pyridostigmine and neostigmine. These drugs improve the symptoms but also increase airway secretions and potentiate the effects of narcotics.[47] They also will inhibit the degradation of succinylcholine and the ester type of local anesthetics. Steroid hormones are used to suppress the immune response, and although the patients may feel better subjectively, the sensitivity to nondepolarizing muscle relaxants may persist.[48] The use of other forms of immunosuppression with cytotoxic drugs such as cyclosporin has also been considered,[49] but the failure to induce permanent remission and the high incidence of side effects have limited its use. The third therapeutic option, plasma exchange, is useful for inducing short-term improvement, whereas thymectomy has been gaining wider acceptance.[50]

Much debate can be found in the anesthetic literature concerning the optimal medical regimen in the perioperative period. It is suggested that, in ocular disease, if the patient does not absolutely require the anticholinesterase medication, one should omit treatment on the day of operation to avoid interaction with anesthetic drugs, potentiated vagal tone, and copious bronchial secretions. If patients are dependent on anticholinesterase therapy and have symptoms other than ocular symptoms, it is appropriate to continue their usual therapy preoperatively. When the therapeutic requirement is expected to change following thymectomy, it is suggested that withdrawal of anticholinesterase drugs with bed rest for at least 24 hours preoperatively is the preferred regimen.[51] Postoperative anticholinesterase therapy is then based on the results of repeated edrophonium tests (0.2 mg/kg) as the requirements change in the postoperative period.

The best results of thymectomy for myasthenia are seen in young females with a short history of the disease and no evidence of thymoma. Complications of the procedure are diminished if anticholinesterase therapy is discontinued preoperatively.[46] Improvement can be expected in most cases, with up to 25 percent of patients requiring no further drug therapy. Leventhal and associates predicted that the need for postoperative mechanical ventilation after this procedure would depend upon the duration of the disease, the presence of pulmonary complications, pyridostigmine dosage, and vital capacity.[52] However, others have suggested that these predictors are valid only after thymectomy and are unreliable after other surgery.[53] Given the sensitivity of these patients to postoperative narcotics and their fluctuating postoperative anticholinesterase requirements, it is usually more appropriate to allow them to demonstrate adequate neuromuscular strength (head lift), vital capacity (greater than 15 ml/kg) and inspiratory force (greater than 30 cm H_2O) before assuming that ventilation will be sufficient. The need for continued use of an artificial airway postoperatively will be predicted by the patient's ability to handle secretions, especially with the involvement of bulbar muscles.

It is preferable to omit preoperative sedation because of the risk of potentiated effects. Induction can be performed with thiopentone, although preservation of spontaneous respiration during mask induction will avoid the need for relaxants for intubation. Halothane, as opposed to drugs with more potent muscle relaxant effects (enflurane, isoflurane), is preferred until the airway is secured. If really necessary, muscle relaxants can be used with recognition of their altered action in these patients: Patients may be "resistant" to succinylcholine to induce muscle paralysis[54] and require a dose 2.6 times normal for 95 percent blockade.[55] In turn, they may be more susceptible to dual block from anticholinesterase therapy. Nondepolarizing drugs should be given in doses that are one twentieth of normal, with careful monitoring;[51] even when short-acting preparations were used, effective doses are 10 to 20 percent of normal.[56] However it is preferable to avoid their use altogether by using one of the volatile agents to secure any relaxation needed for operation.[57] Narcotics are to be used with caution owing to the described respiratory sensitivity[47] and are better titrated to requirement in the postoperative period. Although reversal of the anesthetic drugs and relaxants may be attempted postoperatively, it must be remembered that the patients may require ventilation even after peripheral operation (and even without relaxants) owing to changing anticholinesterase requirements. Note that hypothermia, by increasing ventilatory requirements, and hypokalemia, by affecting resting membrane potentials, will further impair marginal respiratory function.

General anesthesia can be safely used, but regional or local anesthesia should be considered whenever possible, although it may be difficult to secure cooperation in many pediatric patients. Under such circumstances, management will depend on the severity of the disease, with postoperative care following the foregoing principles.

MYASTHENIC SYNDROME

Myasthenic syndrome, also called Eaton-Lambert syndrome, is characterized by a reduction of acetylcholine release at the motor nerve endplate, presumably due to impaired acetylcholine esterase activity. Associated diseases are common, including hyper- or hypothyroidism. In adults there is an association with small cell carcinoma of the lung, whereas in children myasthenic syndrome may occur with leukemia, neuroblastoma, systemic lupus erythematosus, or rheumatoid arthritis.

Clinically, myasthenic syndrome differs from myasthenia gravis in that in the former, proximal limb muscles and rarely the bulbar or ocular muscles are involved, and the muscles become stronger with activity. The patients are extremely sensitive to both nondepolarizing and depolarizing relaxants; these are best avoided by the use of volatile anesthetics to produce any relaxation required.

The anesthetic considerations are similar to those for myasthenia gravis.

ORGANOPHOSPHATE POISONING

The insecticides parathion and malathion are potent inhibitors of cholinesterase throughout the body. They can be rapidly absorbed by the skin or respiratory tract and essentially produce a cholinergic crisis throughout the body. Respiratory support may be necessary owing to profound weakness. Treatment consists of large doses of atropine to inhibit muscarinic effects and 2-pyridine aldoxime methylchloride (2-PAM chloride), which reactivates the inhibited cholinesterase and binds and inactivates the poison.

PROGRESSIVE MUSCULAR DYSTROPHIES

Myopathies are primary diseases of striated muscles in which biochemical, morphological, or neurophysiological changes occur singly or in combination. Dystrophies are hereditary myopathies characterized by progressive muscle degeneration and weakness. Little is known of the primary defects in these disorders, and classification is based on historic descriptions or clinical similarities. Many eponyms have been given to the entities; the most common are listed in Table 19–1.

DUCHENNE'S MUSCULAR DYSTROPHY

The most common form, Duchenne's muscular dystrophy, or pseudohypertrophic muscular dystrophy, is inherited as an X-linked recessive characteristic. The incidence is reported as 3 per 10,000 births. Although defects can be found as early as the second trimester in the fetus, the usual presentation is at age 3 to 5 years. The child develops a waddling gait, lumbar lordosis, and difficulty climbing stairs. Gowers' sign, the use of the arm to assist in standing up, reflects the pronounced weakness of the hip girdle. The proximal muscles are affected first, while the distal muscles may appear hypertrophied, particularly in the calves. Contractures develop in the limbs, and progressive kyphoscoliosis restricts pulmonary function. The patient is usually wheelchair-bound by the early teens, with death occurring before 20 years of age. Respiratory weakness, often combined with difficulty swallowing secretions from pharyngeal involvement, often leads to pneumonia as a terminal event. However, diaphragmatic involvement is late, and central control of ventilation is maintained.[58] Cardiac involvement occurs in up to 70 percent of cases, although it is clinically significant in only 10 percent—usually during the terminal stages. Arrhythmias and impaired contractility due to involvement of the muscle of the left ventricle may lead to heart failure and sudden death,[59] whereas nocturnal oxygen desaturation and sleep apnea may predispose patients to pulmonary hypertension.[60]

Pathological findings are similar in the muscular dystrophies. Muscle bulk is reduced, to be replaced by fat and connective tissue. The basic defect is unknown, although altered muscle membrane permeability leads to large elevations of serum enzymes (particularly creatine phosphokinase [CPK]) and myoglobin. The enzyme concentration is highest early in the disease, then falls as muscle atrophy occurs. The cardiac muscle component is also increased, although the level correlates poorly with cardiac involvement. The female carriers of the condition also show elevated serum enzymes, although they are asymptomatic.

There is no specific treatment for the disease. Physiotherapy and such activity as is possible are suggested to prevent contractures; the patient deteriorates with bed rest. Surgical treatment may be recommended for contractures, and stabilization of the spine may slow the compromise of pulmonary function secondary to kyphoscoliosis.[58] It appears that the rate of deterioration of pulmonary function, as assessed by vital capacity measurements, can be reduced from 20 percent to 5 percent per year by spinal fusion. The risk of operation varies with vital capacity. If vital capacity is greater than 45 percent of predicted, mechanical ventilation is

Table 19–1. SYNONYMS FOR PROGRESSIVE MUSCULAR DYSTROPHIES

Duchenne's muscular dystrophy
Aran-Duchenne dystrophy
Progressive muscular dystrophy
Pseudohypertrophic muscular dystrophy
Late-onset, X-linked muscular dystrophy
Becker's dystrophy
Facioscapulohumeral dystrophy
Landouzy-Déjérine dystrophy
Limb-girdle muscular dystrophy
Erb's dystrophy
Erb's limb-girdle dystrophy
Juvenile dystrophy of Erb
Leyden-Möbius dystrophy
Myotonic dystrophy
Steinert's disease
Steinert's dystrophy
Hoffmann's disease
Batten-Curschmann disease

not needed postoperatively; if it is less than 30 percent of predicted, serious postoperative complications ensue even with mechanical support. Similar predictive figures have been produced by others.[61] The presence of obesity or cardiovascular involvement implies greater risk.

Anesthetic experiences have been reported in Duchenne's muscular dystrophy with a wide variety of anesthetic agents and techniques.[62, 63] Anesthetic difficulties seem to parallel the severity of illness, particularly the degree of restrictive lung disease. The earlier medical literature also warned of the appearance of acute gastric dilatation with cardiovascular compromise, now known to be a function of gastric hypomobility,[63, 64] suggesting the routine insertion of a nasogastric tube.[65]

More recently numerous reports have questioned the safety of succinylcholine in Duchenne's muscular dystrophy: acute rhabdomyolysis, myoglobinuria, hyperkalemia, and cardiac arrest have been reported after its administration.[66, 67] Similar events have occurred even in the absence of a clinical myopathy[68] and in the distant relative of an affected patient.[69] These events were not associated with a temperature elevation. In addition, susceptibility to malignant hyperthermia has been suggested by biopsy in Duchenne-type muscular dystrophy, although early therapy prevented significant temperature elevations in the reported cases.[70–72] Undoubtedly the muscle membrane in these patients is damaged by depolarizing relaxants, and their use therefore is contraindicated. Halothane alone can elicit a similar response,[73] although the similarity to the syndrome of malignant hyperthermia and the high complication rate after halothane and succinylcholine use[74–76] suggest that the volatile agents should not be used. The occurrence of hyperkalemia with cardiac arrest in the recovery room after an uneventful operation suggests that continued vigilance is necessary for some hours postoperatively.[65] Routine prophylaxis with dantrolene sodium is not indicated for all patients with muscular dystrophy and indeed might cause serious weakness. The drug in parenteral form should be available to treat malignant hyperpyrexia if it should be present. Preoperative sedation, if used, should include only very small doses of opiates or barbiturates. Atropine and scopolamine are to be avoided if possible. Induction and maintenance of anesthesia with barbiturates, opiates, nitrous oxide, and nondepolarizing relaxants (if necessary) is the preferred technique. Postoperative ventilation may be required.

LATE-ONSET X-LINKED MUSCULAR DYSTROPHY

This syndrome resembles Duchenne's muscular dystrophy but has a later onset, usually in the second decade, and a slower progression of debility. Whereas most patients can still walk by the late teens, only 50 percent survive to age 40 years. Anesthetic experiences have not been outlined, but the considerations should resemble those in Duchenne's muscular dystrophy.

LIMB-GIRDLE MUSCULAR DYSTROPHY

This group of clinical syndromes is inherited as an autosomal recessive trait that affects primarily the hips and shoulders. The onset is in the second decade, presenting as weakness in the neck, pectoral, and arm muscles with loss of muscle mass. Later the legs are affected, resulting in wheelchair dependence by age 30 years. Involvement of the myocardium is variable.

FACIOSCAPULOHUMERAL DYSTROPHY

An autosomal dominant disease, facioscapulohumeral dystrophy has an onset in the second decade with inability to raise the arms, drooping shoulders, winging of the scapulas, and weakness of the facial musculature. Later involvement of the hips and back may cause kyphoscoliosis. The course is long and insidious, with a normal life span in many cases. Cardiac involvement is less common than in Duchenne's muscular dystrophy, but atrial paralysis (absent atrial electrical activity that cannot be paced) with severe bradycardia has been reported. Ventricular pacing may be required. Involvement of the accessory muscles of respiration may cause reduced vital capacity and recurrent respiratory infections, predisposing to perioperative complications. However, the response to nondepolarizing relaxants appears normal.[77]

OCULAR MUSCULAR DYSTROPHY

This form of muscular dystrophy is seen before the age of 30 years, with weakness of the extraocular muscles and ptosis but rarely diplopia. The muscle pathology resembles that of other dystrophies, but progression is slow and involvement of other muscles is limited. In addition, patients with ocular muscular dystrophy have a similarity to myasthenics in their exquisite sensitivity to curare—doses of 10 percent of the usual may result in complete paralysis.[78]

MYOTONIC DYSTROPHY

Myotonia implies an abnormal persistence of induced or voluntary muscle contractions and may appear as part of several syndromes, such as periodic paralysis, hypothyroidism, or polymyositis. The syndrome of myotonic dystrophy is inherited as an autosomal dominant trait, with a frequency of 5 per 100,000 births. The myotonia affects predominantly the limb muscles, but extraocular and facial muscles are also involved. The myotonia is thought to be due to a generalized membrane defect in which biological membranes have normal resting potentials but increased resistance to electrical conduction. The myotonia persists even after denervation or paralysis.

The clinical picture varies with the age of the subject. The neonate may show poor sucking or swallowing, facial weakness, ptosis, and arthrogryposis. The older chid may have muscle atrophy, poor gait, and atrophy of the distal limb muscles. In older subjects cataracts, baldness, gonadal atrophy, and mental retardation form the symptom complex. Swallowing difficulties may lead to aspiration; at all stages CPK is elevated in the serum, while thc clcctromyogram shows high-frequency repetitive discharges. The myotonia is made worse by exercise or cold.

Many of the patients have abnormal electrocardiograms, with bradycardias and delayed intraventricular conduction. Death from arrhythmias is common, and the degree of cardiac abnormality does not correlate with the severity of skeletal muscle involvement. Carbon dioxide retention due to a depressed CO_2 response curve, together with pulmonary hypertension, may complicate anesthetic management.[79] Relative resistance to insulin may result in hyperglycemia. Treatment depends upon stabilization of muscle membranes; phenytoin, procainamide, and quinine are the drugs of choice.

A related progressive myotonic dystrophy called *Schwartz-Jampel syndrome* (myotonic chondrodystrophy) is an autosomal recessive trait characterized by dwarfism, skeletal abnormalities, and muscle stiffness. Thermal regulatory dysfunction with a picture resembling malignant hyperpyrexia has been reported following administration of curare.[80] No evidence exists for a similar predisposition to malignant hyperthermia in other myotonic diseases.[90]

Two other myotonic syndromes that are not progressive are myotonia congenita (*Thomsen's disease*) and paramyotonia. In *myotonia congenita* there are myotonia and hypertrophy of some voluntary muscles. The myotonia is most severe following rest and decreases with exercise. There is no dystrophic change, and no involvement of cardiac muscle. The disease begins in childhood, with little progression through life. Inheritance is autosomal dominant.

Paramyotonia is the rarest of the myotonic syndromes, with signs similar to myotonia congenita but with myotonia appearing only on exposure to cold. Both forms of nonprogressive myotonia respond to quinidine therapy.

Dystonia musculorum deformans is a progressive disease beginning as abnormal movements resulting in sustained postures of the extremities and trunk, including the neck and jaw. Over time, tendon shortening and muscle fibrosis result in fixed deformities. It may occur secondarily to neurological disease affecting the extrapyramidal tracts, or as an autosomal recessive primary disease with a usual onset between 5 and 15 years of age. Anesthetic concerns relate to the anatomical deformity and associated airway hazard; as a primary neurological disease the response to muscle relaxants appears normal.[81]

The *Freeman-Sheldon syndrome* is another rare congenital myopathy with increased muscle tone leading to fibrotic contractures and skeletal deformity. Difficulties with intubation (microstomia and micrognathia causing a "whistling face"), intravenous access (limb deformities and thickened subcutaneous tissue), and truncal involvement (kyphoscoliosis and intercostal myopathy) may complicate anesthesia.[82]

Anesthetic experience with myotonic syndromes has been reported only with myotonic dystrophy.[83–85] The initial hazard is inability to secure the airway due to spasm of the muscles of the jaw, or inability to ventilate due to respiratory muscle myotonic spasm. The patient may be markedly sensitive to the effects of respiratory depressants, including narcotics, thiopentone, halothane, and diazepam, and apnea from low doses and delayed recovery are common.[83, 85] Succinylcholine should be avoided, as it may induce a myotonic response. General anesthesia, spinal anesthesia, and depolarizing relaxant drugs cannot break a myotonic contracture, but the effect of using a nondepolarizing relaxant for operation appears to be normal.[85, 86] Although theoretically the reversal of relaxation with neostigmine and atropine might cause a myotonic spasm, the response is usually normal.[85] The added risk of uterine hemorrhage exists in the parturient patient with myotonic syndromes.[87]

No preoperative sedatives or analgesics should be given to patients with myotonic dystrophy without close, continuous observation. If necessary, the airway should be secured with the patient in the awake state under topical anesthesia. Otherwise, induction can be achieved with thiopental, anesthesia continued with halothane, and the airway secured without relaxants. Although halothane can be safely used, apnea will occur at low concentrations, and ventilation must be supported. Cardiac monitoring[88] and avoidance of cold stress are essential. Postoperatively, the ventilation and airway must be supported until the patient demonstrates adequate recovery. Provision must be made for prolonged recovery from fixed drugs. Myotonia may compromise the ability to cough effectively and thus create a predisposition to pulmonary complications.

CONGENITAL DEFECTS OF MUSCLES

Congenital myopathies are a group of diseases defined by a pathological defect or a clinical picture of profound weakness and hypotonia from birth. In many cases the pathogenesis is incompletely understood. Weakness is usually of the proximal muscle groups, particularly the hips and shoulder girdle. In most cases the disease is not progressive, but muscle wasting and weakness are associated with secondary skeletal changes or dysmorphic features. Limited experience with each entity precludes definitive statements, yet most would consider depolarizing relaxants contraindicated in primary muscle disease. However, if data from adult patients with polymyositis can be extrapolated, the response to nondepolarizing drugs is anticipated to be normal.[89]

CENTRAL CORE DISEASE

Central core disease is a nonprogressive congenital myopathy inherited as an autosomal dominant trait. The intellect is normal. Weakness of the proximal muscles leads to difficulty climbing stairs or rising from chairs. Muscles supplied by the cranial nerves are not involved. Secondary skeletal changes include hip dislocation, kyphoscoliosis, funnel chest, mandibular hypoplasia, and a short neck. Serum enzymes are usually normal.

Pathologically there is aberration of type I fibers, with a central core of abnormal fibrillary material. Biochemically there is reduced phosphorylase activity, as well as reduced actomyosin and magnesium-activated ATPase activity of the sarcoplasmic reticulum. The net effect is a reduction in the rate of calcium uptake by the sarcoplasmic reticulum, leading to an elevated calcium concentration in the muscle fiber.

The importance of recognizing this entity in anesthesia results from its known association with malignant hyperthermia.[90, 91] The association of many myopathic disorders with the syndrome remains to be established, but patients with central core disease are most certainly at risk. The increased calcium level within the muscle fiber probably leads to a plasmalemmal susceptibility to triggering drugs. All precautions to avoid malignant hyperthermia must be taken when anesthetizing individuals with this diagnosis.

NEMALINE MYOPATHY

Named for the unique rodlike or threadlike structures that run in biopsied muscles, this disease is inherited as an autosomal dominant. The infants are born weak and hypotonic at birth and may develop respiratory difficulty. The weakness persists into adult life and is associated with dysmorphic skeletal features, scoliosis, and the potential for perioperative respiratory complications.[92] The weakness may be severe enough to cause recurrent pneumonias or seriously limit respiratory reserves. No cardiac or smooth muscle involvement has been described. In one reported anesthetic experience there was a slight resistance to succinylcholine, with no abnormal hyperkalemia and a normal response to pancuronium,[93] although others consider depolarizing drugs contraindicated.[92]

Numerous other myopathies due to defects in the sarcolemmal structure have been described.[1] However, their occurrence is rare indeed and anesthetic experience is not available.

LIPID MYOPATHIES

Several disease states have been described in which biochemical abnormalities in lipid metabolism result in excessive storage of material in skeletal muscles. *Carnitine* is required as a cofactor in the transport of long-chain fatty acids into mitochondria for oxidation. A deficiency state has been described that results in reduced fatty acid oxidation and excessive formation of triglycerides. Progressive weakness begins in the first or second decade and may be associated with a cardiomyopathy. A potentially fatal systemic form with hepatomegaly and episodic acidosis has also been described. Treatment is by dietary supplement and steroids. Anesthetic management dictates adequate rehydration, avoidance of hypoglycemia, and continued carnitine therapy.[94, 95]

Episodic muscle cramps and myoglobinemia characterize *carnitine palmitoyl transferase deficiency,* particularly after exercise. Weakness is not remarkable. The biochemical lesion results in elevated cholesterol, triglyceride, and free fatty acid concentrations in the serum and muscles. Avoidance of succinylcholine as well as glucose infusions is advised to prevent rhabdomyolysis associated with surgical therapy, at times of sufficient severity to precipitate acute renal failure.[96]

Pyruvate decarboxylase deficiency causes a syndrome of intermittent ataxia associated with choreoathetosis, particularly with stress or febrile illness. It and a related syndrome, pyruvate dehydrogenase deficiency, may result in lactic acidosis, particularly in the presence of hypocapnia. On a theoretical basis, glucose loading and halothane, by inhibiting gluconeogenesis, may be contraindicated.[97]

Avoidance of prolonged fasting (and hence dependence on lipids for metabolism) and excessive muscle activity such as fasciculations and shivering appear prudent.

MITOCHONDRIAL MYOPATHIES

Several myopathies have been described that involve abnormalities of the mitochondria. Indeed, 12 percent of all patients with clinical myopathies have mitochondrial abnormalities, but their significance in the pathogenesis is unknown. The syndromes usually present as a long-term myopathy, usually beginning at birth or in childhood, but more precipitous variants are described.[98]

In *Luft's disease* there are an increased number of mitochondria, with an increased amount of cristae, resulting in increased muscle enzyme activity. The increased mitochondrial respiration with loosely coupled oxidative phosphorylation results in the clinical signs of hypermetabolism. Excessive sweating, polydipsia, polyphagia, and heat intolerance present a clinical picture resembling that of hyperthyroidism. Treatment is with chloramphenicol, which reduces mitochondrial synthesis.

Anaesthetic experiences have not been documented, but the high metabolic rate with high oxygen consumption suggests the importance of maintaining maximal oxygenation, preserving cardiac output and minute ventilation, and carefully monitoring temperature to recognize hyperthermia with its metabolic consequences.

Other mitochondrial myopathies have been described with structural mitochondrial abnormalities, but the metabolic consumption of oxygen is normal. Anesthetic experiences are limited, but minimal muscular reserve with stress would be expected in view of the muscle fatigue with exercise. Severe encephalomyopathies can be associated with skeletal and cardiac muscle abnormalities and also metabolic acidosis.[99] The response to nondepolarizing relaxants appears normal.[100]

GLYCOGEN STORAGE DISEASES

Glycogen storage diseases are a group of diseases characterized by the accumulation of glycogen of normal or abnormal configuration in various tissues. Each type of disease is caused by the inherited deficiency or absence of a specific enzyme in the metabolic pathway of glycogen. The signs and symptoms result from the excessive glycogen storage, plus the secondary free glucose deficiency with ensuing hypoglycemia. Many of the diseases do not primarily involve muscle; nevertheless, they may be associated with an unexplained weakness and hypotonia. Only those types primarily involved with muscle will be considered here.

1. *Acid maltase deficiency (Pompe's disease, or Cori's type II disease)* is characterized by hypotonia and cardiac involvement in the neonate. Difficulty in swallowing secretions, respiratory distress from the large tongue and weak muscles, and congestive cardiac failure lead to death by 1 year of age. Late infantile and adult forms have also been described in which the enzyme deficiency is incomplete, the myopathy is slower to develop, and involvement of the heart and tongue is absent. There is no effective treatment.
2. *Amylo-1,6-glucosidase deficiency (Forbes'*

disease, or Cori's type III disease) results in neonatal symptoms of hypotonia, failure to thrive, hepatomegaly, and hypoglycemia. An adult type with chronic progressive myopathy has also been described. Fasting creates severe hypoglycemia due to limitation of glycogen breakdown, and glucose supplies are then dependent on gluconeogenesis. Ketonuria and hyperlipidemia are frequently present.

3. *Amylo-1,4-1,6-transglucosidase deficiency (Andersen's disease, or Cori's type IV disease)* causes rapid exhaustion with exercise of otherwise normal muscles. Myoglobinuria may follow moderate or strenuous exercise, while lactic acid cannot be produced with exertion. Cardiac muscle may be involved, with bradycardia, increased amplitude of QRS complex, and T wave inversion. CPK elevation occurs with exercise.
4. *Muscle phosphofructokinase deficiency (Tarui's disease), phosphoglucomutase deficiency (Thomsen's disease),* and *phosphohexoisomerase deficiency (Satoyoshi's disease)* all produce exercise intolerance from pain and fatigue without further abnormalities of muscle. Lactic acid cannot be produced. The clinical significance of these abnormalities is equivocal.

Little is known of the effect of anesthesia on these entities.[101, 102] The major consideration involves the biochemical abnormalities, particularly hypoglycemia with fasting. Reduced tolerance to exercise implies a reduced respiratory reserve, which dictates careful monitoring and support of ventilatory function perioperatively. No data are available on the effects of muscle relaxants in these diseases. Cardiac and hepatic involvement, when present, will influence the choice of pharmacological agents for anesthesia. The inability to withstand exercise implies that ischemia is poorly tolerated, and operative tourniquets should not be used. Myoglobinuria must be treated when it occurs, and succinylcholine must be avoided to prevent simulating severe exercise. For similar reasons shivering triggered by inadvertent hypothermia or halothane administration should be prevented if possible.

FAMILIAL PERIODIC PARALYSIS

Episodic weakness can occur with several clinical diseases. Often it is associated with a reduced plasma potassium concentration, as is seen in thyrotoxicosis, renal disease, diabetic acidosis, or diuretic ingestion. Hyperaldosterone excess, as occurs with primary hyperaldosteronism (*Conn's syndrome*), or pseudoaldosteronism from licorice ingestion also may cause episodic weakness. Periodic weakness is also common in McArdle's disease, paramyotonia congenita, and certain mitochondrial myopathies, although no potassium deficit is documented.

Familial periodic paralysis is inherited as an autosomal dominant trait. Two forms have been described, depending upon serum potassium levels. In the *hypokalemic* form, weakness begins in the second decade and tends to be made worse by high-carbohydrate meals or salt loading or after a period of rest following strenuous exercise. The flaccid paralysis may be severe and may last up to 36 hours, but it spares the cranial and respiratory musculature. Hypokalemia is usually present, with serum levels of 2 to 3 mEq/L, and electrocardiographic manifestations occur, including sinus arrhythmia and QRS and T wave changes. The severity of the weakness correlates poorly, however, with the level of potassium in the serum. Acute attacks can be treated by potassium infusions; prevention depends on avoiding large meals and salt. Drug therapy with spironolactone or acetazolamide is helpful in maintaining serum potassium levels.

Anesthetic management depends upon the recognition that, no matter how minor the operative procedure, anesthesia and surgical therapy do something (as yet undefined) to initiate an episode of weakness. To minimize occurrence of the event, preoperative electrolytes must be carefully checked. The patient must be instructed not to overeat, and infusions of glucose and sodium are kept to a minimum. Hypothermia can precipitate an attack, so temperature monitoring is critical. The relationship between muscle relaxants and this disease suggests that nondepolarizers can be used normally.[103, 104] Prolonged postoperative monitoring is essential even with a benign intraoperative course and normal serum potassium levels.[105–107]

Hyperkalemic periodic paralysis is also an autosomal dominant trait with onset usually under the age of 10 years. Attacks are similar to those in the hypokalemic form but tend to be shorter-lasting (1 to 2 hours), and patients may have difficulty swallowing or coughing, though respiratory muscles are usually spared. Myotonia may be present. Biochemically, the elevation of serum potassium may be transient and mild and probably represents a hypersensitivity of the muscle membrane to acetylcholine or mechanical stimulations. The treatment of the acute attack is infusion of calcium and insulin/glucose therapy, whereas paradoxically acetazolamide is effective in prophylaxis.

Anesthetic exposures have been reported in patients with the hyperkalemic form, with paralysis lasting several hours postoperatively.[108, 109] It is more essential to prevent carbohydrate depletion by starting a dextrose infusion the night before. All intravenous solutions should be dextrose-rich and potassium-free. ECG monitoring is essential. Muscle relaxants should be avoided, since succinylcholine may induce a hyperkalemic response, and neostigmine administered to reverse nondepolarizing drugs may induce myotonia from excessive acetylcholine elevation. Thermal control is essential.

A third, *normokalemic* form of periodic paralysis has been described in early childhood, with severe weakness and loss of cough reflex. The attack may last many days and is associated with cardiac tachyarrhythmias. The same anesthetic concerns pertain as are suggested for the hypokalemic form.

MYOSITIS OSSIFICANS

This familial disease starts in childhood, with cystlike nodules developing under the skin after minor trauma. Later, bone develops in the area, hardening the muscle. The disease becomes widespread, with death occurring in the second to fourth decade. At the end, the patients develop severe limitation in the motion of the chest, with secondary respiratory and cardiac failure. Associated skeletal abnormalities are common.

Anesthetic problems relate to the difficulty in opening the mouth or bending the neck; mouth and neck are fixed by ossification of muscle. Tracheostomy or blind nasotracheal intubation may be necessary. Limitation of thoracic wall compliance can become a problem in later stages of the disease.

INFLAMMATORY MYOPATHIES

Myositis defines a group of conditions characterized by inflammation of muscles. While it may be related to specific diseases such as scleroderma, lupus erythematosus, polyarteritis, or rheumatoid arthritis, myositis also may occur as the primary presentation.

Dermatomyositis is a relatively rare condition affecting the skin and muscles. It occurs in both children and adults; the childhood form is generally more severe. Commonly, pain and weakness begin in the hips with fever, and the weakness may progress to involve the pharyngeal muscles. Swallowing difficulties may prove fatal, and perforation of the gastrointestinal tract is a common cause of death. Myocardial insufficiency with arrhythmias may occur. Recovery may leave residual atrophy with calcification of involved muscles.

Pathologically, there is a diffuse angiopathic process involving the skin, muscle, gastrointestinal tract, and small nerves. Obstruction of the intima of arteries leads to cellular necrosis with elevation of muscle enzymes. The disease is probably immunological in etiology, perhaps triggered by a virus of the myxovirus or picornavirus group. Treatment is with steroid hormones and immunosuppression. The association with malignancy seen in adults is uncommon in children.

No information is available about the implications for anesthesia. However, the inflammatory process of the musculature suggests caution with depolarizing relaxants for they may be expected to increase membrane leakage, leading to hyperkalemia and myoglobinuria. Nondepolarizing relaxants appear to be safe.[89]

RHABDOMYOLYSIS AND MUSCLE DISEASE

Rhabdomyolysis with myoglobinuria is a condition of diverse etiology characterized by the sudden onset of muscle pain and weakness followed by passage of dark urine. There is extreme necrosis of muscle cells, without an interstitial inflammatory reaction, and alteration of muscle membrane permeability to intracellular enzymes and proteins. The muscles become swollen and tender, and systemic signs of fever, chills, and general malaise ensue. Therapy is based upon prevention of complications such as renal failure, sudden death from arrhythmias secondary to electrolyte disturbances or myocardial involvement, and respiratory failure from respiratory muscle involvement. The clinical entities associated with rhabdomyolysis-myoglobinuria are listed in Table 19–2.[110] While up to 40 percent of normal children will demonstrate myoglobinemia after a single dose of succinylcholine,[111–113] an occasional case occurs of severe rhabdomyolysis induced by such a dose in the absence of temperature change.[114, 115] Whether this situation represents a variant of

Table 19–2. CLASSIFICATION OF RHABDOMYOLYSIS

Defined enzymatic defects
Muscle phosphorylase deficiency
Phosphofructokinase deficiency
Carnitine palmitoyl transferase deficiency
Presumed metabolic defects
Fasting/exercise precipitant
Malignant hyperthermia
Familial periodic paralysis (hypokalemic)
Cellular metabolic toxins
Alcohol
Heroin
Amphotericin B
Unavailability of adequate substrate or oxygen
Ischemic compression–crush syndrome
Intense muscular activity
Heat stress
Succinylcholine
Intrinsic muscle disease
Dermatomyositis
Progressive muscular dystrophies
Infections (influenza and coxsackievirus)

malignant hyperpyrexia or the unmasking of an occult myopathy remains to be determined.[116]

MALIGNANT HYPERTHERMIA

The syndrome of malignant hyperthermia is a rare but lethal complication of anesthetic drug administration.[117] After administration of inciting drugs, the patient develops a rapid rise in temperature, a hypermetabolic state outstripping oxygen delivery, and diffuse rhabdomyolysis usually with muscle rigidity. The syndrome has been associated with other myopathic entities, including muscular dystrophy[118] and central core myopathy, but the majority of patients probably have a mild subclinical myopathy that is yet to be clearly defined. Inheritance is probably autosomal dominant, although penetrance is often incomplete.[119]

The incidence of malignant hyperthermia is reported as 1 in 4200 instances of anesthesia induced in the presence of triggering drugs[120] in children—about five times that in adults. These statistics do not reflect the true incidence of susceptibility, since 50 percent of patients who have had the syndrome have had prior anesthesia without the syndrome developing.[121] The disease may present in children as young as 3 months of age,[122] after over 24 hours' exposure to a prolonged anesthetic,[123] or many hours after the termination of an exposure.[124] It has been suggested that other catastrophic events, such as sudden infant death syndrome, may represent malignant hyperthermic episodes occurring independent of exposure to anesthesia.[125]

The underlying defect seems to be an idiopathic increase in the sarcoplasmic concentration of calcium ion.[126] As a consequence, during anesthesia with inciting drugs, total body oxygen consumption in susceptible patients is two to three times that of normal patients, and body temperature rises to as high as 43°C at a rate up to 1°C every 5 minutes. It is most frequently associated with the administration of halogenated inhalational anesthetic drugs and the muscle relaxant succinylcholine. Physical or emotional stress can trigger the syndrome in awake subjects, as can psychotropic drugs.[127] Both recrudescence and an initial attack can occur during recovery from general anesthesia.[128–131]

Development of the syndrome can vary from insidious to fulminant. Features of the slowly developing entity include tachycardia and other arrhythmias. Arterial blood gas analysis will demonstrate metabolic acidosis and an inappropriately low oxygen tension. Hyperpnea occurs owing to rising carbon dioxide production; core temperature begins to rise, while muscle rigidity occurs late in the crisis.

The more fulminant form of the disease is usually associated with administration of succinylcholine, followed by a halothane anesthetic. The onset of muscle rigidity occurs immediately after the relaxant, and may be global or limited to the masseter muscles. Tracheal intubation may be difficult or impossible but sometimes is readily accomplished. Cardiac arrhythmias and a malignant hypermetabolic state with vasoconstriction and cyanosis rapidly ensue—probably secondary to the metabolic state rather than from primary cardiac involvement[132]—unless prompt therapy is rendered.

Masseter spasm may be the initial indication of an imminent crisis, although increased masseter muscle tone after succinylcholine has been found to be the normal response in halothane-anesthetized children,[133, 134] including those undergoing strabismus operation.[135, 136] In contrast, masseter muscle rigidity is relatively rare following succinylcholine in infants and children after a thiopental induction without halothane.[137] The early recommendations[138–140] suggested, from the observation that a high proportion (up to 70 percent) of subjects with masseter spasm will be subsequently biopsy positive for malignant hyperthermia,[141–144] that such spasm should dictate immediate abortion of the procedure.[145] However, such suggestions may stem from lack of standardization of the contracture test,[146] the definition of masseter spasm,[147, 148] or reflect the referral population to the test center, and no longer may be justified. Indeed, continuing the anesthetic after isolated masseter spasm, albeit with careful monitoring, was reported to be not associated with appearance of the full malignant hyperthermia syndrome.[149]

Rhabdomyolysis occurs later in the course of the syndrome, producing gross elevations in serum creatine kinase and myoglobin.[150, 151] Electrolyte disturbances are severe, with acute hyperkalemia and hypocalcemia developing from altered muscle cellular permeability to these ions. During the postcrisis diuresis the reverse occurs, with hypokalemia and hypercalcemia ensuing. Renal failure is common, as is disseminated intravascular coagulation. The mortality is approximately 7 percent even with optimal therapy.

Management of the crisis must be prompt. The volatile anesthetic agents must be discontinued immediately and exposed circuitry replaced. Hyperventilation with oxygen must match metabolic requirements, with a minute ventilation of at least three times normal. Sodium bicarbonate is indicated for the metabolic acidosis while active cooling by surface and body cavity is begun. Chilled saline is the recommended intravenous fluid. Cardiovascular monitoring is imperative, and arrhythmias should be treated with procainamide if they are not abolished by metabolic correction. Volume loading and osmotic diuretics are given to induce a brisk diuresis to avoid myoglobin deposition and renal failure. Intravascular monitoring of cardiac filling and arterial pressures is desirable, and vascular access is necessary for frequent blood gas and biochemical monitoring. Glucose should be given as an energy substrate. Surgical procedures must be terminated as soon as possible, but the patient should not be moved until the crisis is over.

Dantrolene sodium is currently the drug of choice.[152, 153] This acts directly on skeletal muscle and probably blocks transfer of the excitation from the sarcolemmal membrane to release calcium from storage sites in the sarcoplasmic reticulum. There is no effect on cardiac muscle. Responses to treatment have occurred at doses of between 1 and 10 mg/kg intravenously. For practical purposes an initial dose of 2.4 mg/kg should be given;[154] if this is unsuccessful, the patient should then be given 10 mg/kg. A repeat dose of 1.2 mg/kg is necessary 6 hours later to sustain a plasma level in children.[155] Serious cardiopulmonary depression does not usually occur at that dosage, unless there is potentiation by other drugs. Verapamil, a potent calcium channel blocker, is particularly dangerous in this situation.[156]

Preoperative preparation with dantrolene is recommended for patients known to have malignant hyperthermia. For elective surgical therapy the drug can be given orally in a total dose of 5 mg/kg, divided into four doses every 6 hours, with the last dose given 4 hours before anesthesia. For emergency operation the administration of 2.5 mg/kg intravenously is recommended. The elimination half-life is 12 hours.[157] It has been reported that such prophylaxis is not absolute protection from the syndrome,[158, 159] so all other precautions are indicated.

Patients known to be susceptible to malignant hyperthermia, and their relatives, need not be denied anesthesia. Drugs not associated with the syndrome include barbiturates, narcotics, diazepam, droperidol, nitrous oxide, and ester-type local anesthetics. The use of amide-type local anesthetics and ketamine has also been shown to be safe.[160–162] Skeletal muscle paralysis can be accomplished with nondepolarizing drugs. Reversal of paralysis with atropine and neostigmine has not been reported to be associated with difficulties. Since calcium flux across the sarcoplasmic membrane may be regulated by the cyclic-AMP system, the use of sympathomimetics theoretically is not recommended.[153]

The muscles from patients with susceptibility to malignant hyperthermia may be structurally and biochemically normal upon biopsy. Although the frequency of musculoskeletal abnormalities such as scoliosis, strabismus, and hernia is reported as greater in patients with malignant hyperthermia, there is nothing diagnostic in their presence. A high index of suspicion must exist whenever there is a family or personal history of anesthetic or surgical disaster. Muscle enzyme elevations in the serum, while increased in 70 percent of subjects, may be normal in 30 percent of those with documented susceptibility.[163, 164] The level of CPK also may be elevated by exercise in other myopathic conditions, and hence its value is limited. HLA typing of family members susceptible to the condition has not proved useful.[165] Since this disease may represent a generalized defect of membrane function, evaluation of more accessible membranes such as those of blood platelets has been attempted in vitro.[166] However, the results have not been sufficiently reliable to prove diagnostic.[167–172] The future, however, may offer noninvasive diagnostic tests using either nuclear magnetic resonance spectroscopy[173, 174] or molecular genetic diagnosis.[175]

It has been shown that caffeine is capable of producing contracture of skeletal muscle in vitro, by causing the release or efflux of calcium from the sarcoplasmic reticulum. It was demonstrated that muscle from patients with malignant hyperthermia undergoes a hypercontracture to caffeine, and that this can be potentiated by halothane and blocked by dantrolene. This forms the basis for the only currently reliable test for susceptibility.[176, 177] Skeletal muscle is obtained by open biopsy and suspended between force transducers in a physiological bath. Susceptible muscle demonstrates a contracture of 1 gram at a much lower caffeine concentration (1 to 2 mM of caffeine) than does normal muscle (less than 4 mM). Halothane 3 percent, bubbled through the specimen bath of susceptible individuals, also may elicit a large contracture. Patients demonstrating either of these phenomena are susceptible to malignant hyperthermia and are described as having H-type phenotypes. The combined use of caffeine and halothane to elicit a response defines the K-type phenotype and a more equivocal susceptibility to the disease.[178, 179] Although the diagnostic testing is perhaps imperfect and depends considerably on laboratory interpretation and biopsy characteristics,[180, 181] few false negative results have been reported from any laboratory, and the sensitivity is sufficient that patients testing negative probably can be given triggering drugs safely.[182] Those who have been H-typed are conclusively susceptible; K-type responders should be assumed to have a variant of the disease but to be nevertheless susceptible in the presence of inciting drugs.

REFERENCES

1. Swainman KF, Wright FS: Pediatric Neuromuscular Diseases. St. Louis, CV Mosby, 1979.
2. Dubowitz V: Muscle Disorders in Childhood. Philadelphia, WB Saunders, 1978.
3. Ellis RF: Neuromuscular disease and anaesthesia. Br J Anaesth *46*:603, 1974.
4. Azar I: The response of patients with neuromuscular disorders to muscle relaxants: A review. Anesthesiology *61*:173, 1984.
5. Tobey RE: Paraplegia, succinylcholine, and cardiac arrest. Anesthesiology *32*:359, 1970.
6. Beach TP, Stone WA, Hamelberg W: Circulatory collapse following succinylcholine: Report of a patient with diffuse motor neuron disease. Anesth Analg *50*:431, 1971.
7. Stone WA, Beach TP, Hamelberg W: Succinylcholine-induced hyperkalemia in dogs with transected sciatic nerves or spinal cords. Anesthesiology *32*:515, 1970.
8. Cooperman LH: Succinylcholine-induced hyperkalemia in neuromuscular disease. JAMA *213*:1867, 1970.
9. Dierdorf SF, McNiece WL, Rao CC, et al: Effect of succinylcholine on plasma potassium in children with cerebral palsy. Anesthesiology *62*:88, 1985.
10. Smith RB: Hyperkalemia following succinylcholine administration in neurologic disorders: A review. Can Anaesth Soc J *18*:199, 1971.
11. Hogue CW, Itani MS, Martyn JA: Resistance to D-tubocurarine in lower motor neuron injury is related to increased acetylcholine receptors at the neuromuscular junction. Anesthesiology *73*:703, 1990.
12. Shayevitz JR, Matteo RS: Decreased sensitivity to metocurine in patients with upper motoneuron disease. Anesth Analg *64*:767, 1985.
13. Schuetze SM, Role LW: Developmental regulation of nicotinic acetylcholine receptors. Annu Rev Neurosci *10*:403, 1987.
14. Goudsouzian NG, Standaert FG: The infant and the myoneural junction. Anesth Analg *65*:1208, 1986.
15. Lorkovic H: Sensitivity of rodent skeletal muscles to dicholines: Dependence of innervation and age. Neuropharmacology *28*:373, 1989.
16. Shyng SL, Salpeter MM. Effect of reinnervation on the denervation rate of junctional acetylcholine receptors synthesized in denervated skeletal muscles. J Neurosci *10*:3905, 1990.
17. Rosenbaum KJ, Neigh JL, Strobel GE: Sensitivity to nondepolarizing muscle relaxants in amyotrophic lateral sclerosis: Report of two cases. Anesthesiology *35*:638, 1971.
18. Desmond J: Paraplegia: Problems confronting the anesthesiologist. Can Anaesth Soc J *17*:435, 1970.
19. Gode GR: Paraplegia and cardiac arrest: Case reports. Can Anaesth Soc J *17*:452, 1970.
20. Ciliberti BJ, Goldfine J, Rovenstine EA: Hypertension during anesthesia in patients with spinal cord injuries. Anesthesiology *15*:273, 1954.
21. Drinker AS, Helrich M: Halothane anesthesia in the paraplegic patient. Anesthesiology *24*:399, 1963.
22. Tanaka H, Uemura N, Toyama Y: Cardiac involvement in the Kugelberg-Welander syndrome. Am J Cardiol *38*:528, 1976.
23. Edwards AE, Bras JF: The enhancement of neurologic signs under anaesthesia. Br J Anaesth *42*:337, 1970.
24. Lichtenfeld P: Autonomic dysfunction in Guillain-Barré syndrome. Am J Med *50*:72, 1971.
25. Perel A, Reche A, Davidson JT: Anaesthesia in the Guillain-Barré syndrome. Anaesthesia *32*:257, 1977.
26. Summer E: Porphyria in relation to surgery and anaesthesia. Ann R Coll Surg Engl *56*:81, 1975.
27. Ward RJ: Porphyria and its relation to anesthesia. Anesthesiology *26*:212, 1965.
28. Mustajoki P, Heinonen J: General anesthesia in "inducible" porphyrias. Anesthesiology *53*:15, 1980.
28a. Harrison F: Propofol anaesthesia in pharmacogenetic states. In Prys-Roberts C (ed.): Focus on Infusion. London, Current Medical Literature, 1991, pp 186–190.
29. Greenberg RS, Parker SD: Anesthetic management for the child with Charcot-Marie-Tooth disease. Anesth Analg *74*:305, 1992.
30. Huxtable R: Cardiac pharmacology and cardiomyopathy in Friedreich's ataxia. J Can Sci Neurol *5*:83, 1978.
31. Kubal K, Pasricha SK, Bhargava M: Spinal anesthesia in a patient with Friedreich's ataxia. Anesth Analg *72*:257, 1991.
32. McCaughey TJ: Familial dysautonomia as an anaesthetic hazard. Can Anaesth Soc J *12*:558, 1965.
33. Meridy HW, Creighton RE: General anaesthesia in eight patients with familial dysautonomia. Can Anaesth Soc J *18*:563, 1971.

34. Bortels JM: Familial dysautonomia. JAMA *212*:318, 1970.
35. Kritcheman MM, Swartz J, Papper E: Experience with general anesthesia in patients with familial dysautonomia. JAMA *170*:529, 1959.
36. Inkster JS: Anaesthesia for a patient suffering from familial dysautonomia. Br J Anaesth *43*:509, 1971.
37. Filler J, Smith AA, Stone S, et al: Respiratory control in familial dysautonomia. J Pediatr *66*:509, 1965.
38. Humble RM: Pheochromocytoma, neurofibromatosis, and pregnancy. Anaesthesia *22*:296, 1967.
39. Fisher MD: Anaesthetic difficulties in neurofibromatosis. Anaesthesia *30*:648, 1975.
40. Massaro D, Katz S, Matthews MJ, et al: Von Recklinghausen's neurofibromatosis associated with cystic lung disease. Am J Med *38*:233, 1965.
41. Bourke E, Fatenby PBB: Renal artery dysplasia with hypertension in neurofibromatosis. Br J Med *3*:681, 1971.
42. Magbagbeola JA: Abnormal responses to muscle relaxants in a patient with von Recklinghausen's disease. Br J Anaesth *42*:710, 1970.
43. Manser J: Abnormal responses in von Recklinghausen's disease. Br J Anaesth *42*:183, 1970.
44. Drachman DB: Myasthenia gravis. N Engl J Med *298*:136, 1978.
45. Appel SH, Almon RR, Levy N: Acetylcholine receptor antibodies in myasthenia gravis. N Engl J Med *293*:760, 1975.
46. Flacke W: Treatment of myasthenia gravis. N Engl J Med *288*:27, 1973.
47. Head JM: Respiratory failure after thymectomy for myasthenia gravis. Ann Surg *160*:123, 1964.
48. Lake CL: Curare sensitivity in steroid-treated myasthenia gravis. Anesth Analg *56*:132, 1978.
49. Tindall RSA, Rollins JA, Phillips JT, et al: Preliminary results of a double-blind, randomized, placebo-controlled trial of cyclosporine in myasthenia gravis. N Engl J Med *316*:719, 1987.
50. Drachman DB: Present and future treatment of myasthenia gravis. N Engl J Med *316*:743, 1987.
51. Davies DW, Steward DJ: Myasthenia gravis in children and anaesthetic management for thymectomy. Can Anaesth Soc J *20*:253, 1973.
52. Leventhal SR, Orkin F, Hirsh R: Prediction of the need for postoperative mechanical ventilation in myasthenia gravis. Anesthesiology *53*:26, 1980.
53. Grant RP, Jenkins LC: Prediction of the need for postoperative mechanical ventilation in myasthenia gravis: Thymectomy compared to other surgical procedures. Can Anaesth Soc J *29*:112, 1982.
54. Dalal FY, Bennett EJ, Gregg WS: Congenital myasthenia gravis and minor surgical procedures. Anaesthesia *27*:61, 1972.
55. Eisenkraft JB, Book WJ, Mann SM, et al: Resistance to succinylcholine in myasthenia gravis: A dose-response study. Anesthesiology *69*:760, 1988.
56. Baraka A, Tabboush Z: Neuromuscular response to succinylcholine-vecuronium sequence in three myasthenic patients undergoing thymectomy. Anesth Analg *72*:827, 1991.
57. Wahlin A, Havermark KG: Enflurane anesthesia in patients with myasthenia gravis. Acta Anaesth Belg *2*:215, 1974.
58. Jenkins JG, Bohn D, Edmonds JF, et al: Evaluation of pulmonary function in muscular dystrophy patients requiring spinal surgery. Crit Care Med *10*:645, 1982.
59. Sanyal SK, Tierney RC, Rao PS, et al: Systolic time interval characteristics in children with Duchenne's progressive muscle dystrophy. Pediatrics *70*:958, 1982.
60. Smith PEM, Calverly PMA, Edwards RHT, et al: Practical problems in the respiratory care of patients with muscular dystrophy. N Engl J Med *316*:1197, 1987.
61. Milne B, Rosales JK: Anaesthetic considerations in patients with muscular dystrophy undergoing spinal fusion and Harrington rod insertion. Can Anaesth Soc J *29*:250, 1982.
62. Cobham JG, Davis HS: Anesthesia for muscular dystrophy patients. Anesth Analg *43*:22, 1964.
63. Richards WC: Anaesthesia and serum creatine phosphokinase levels in Duchenne's pseudohypertrophic muscular dystrophy. Anaesth Intens Care *1*:150, 1972.
64. Barohn RJ, Levine EJ, Olson JO, Mendell JR: Gastric hypomobility in Duchenne's muscular dystrophy. N Engl J Med *319*:15, 1988.
65. Wislicki L: Anaesthesia and post-operative complications in progressive muscular dystrophy. Anaesthesia *17*:482, 1962.
66. Kelfer HM, Singer WD, Reynolds RN: Malignant hyperthermia in a child with Duchenne muscular dystrophy. Pediatrics *71*:118, 1983.
67. Seay AR, Ziter FA, Thompson JA: Cardiac arrest during induction of anesthesia in Duchenne muscular dystrophy. J Pediatr *93*:88, 1978.
68. Henderson WAV: Succinylcholine-induced cardiac arrest in unsuspected Duchenne muscular dystrophy. Can Anaesth Soc J *31*:444, 1984.
69. Lewandowski KB: Strabismus as a presenting sign of subclinical muscular dystrophy predisposing to rhabdomyolysis and myoglobinuria. Can Anaesth Soc J *29*:372, 1982.
70. Oka S, Igarashi Y, Takagi A, et al: Malignant hyperpyrexia and Duchenne muscular dystrophy: A case report. Can Anaesth Soc J *29*:627, 1982.
71. Brownell AKW, Paasuke RT, Elash A: Malignant hyperthermia in Duchenne muscular dystrophy. Anesthesiology *58*:180, 1983.
72. Wang JM, Stanly TH: Duchenne muscular dystrophy and malignant hyperthermia—two case reports. Can Anaesth Soc J *33*:492, 1986.
73. Sethna NF, Rockoff MA: Cardiac arrest following inhalation induction of anaesthesia in a child with Duchenne's muscular dystrophy. Can Anaesth Soc J *33*:799, 1986.
74. Sethna NF, Rockoff MA, Worthen MM, Rosnow JM: Anesthesia-related complications in children with Duchenne muscular dystrophy. Anesthesiology *68*:462, 1988.
75. Larsen UT, Juhl B, Hein-Sorensen O, de Fine Olivarius B: Complications during anesthesia in patients with Duchenne's muscular dystrophy (a retrospective study). Can J Anaesth *36*:418, 1989.
76. Worthen HM, Kuban KCK, Sullivan KF, Bresnan MJ: A national survey of anesthetic complications in children with Duchenne's muscular dystrophy. Anesth Analg *66*:S190, 1987.
77. Dresner DL, Ali HJH. Anaesthetic management of a patient with facioscapulohumeral muscular dystrophy. Br J Anaesth *62*:331, 1989.
78. Jacob JG, Varkey GP: Curare sensitivity in ocular myopathy. Can Anaesth Soc J *13*:449, 1966.
79. Gillam PMS, Heaf PJD, Kaufman L, Lucas BGB: Respiration in dystrophia myotonia. Thorax *19*:112, 1964.
80. Seay AR, Ziter FA: Malignant hyperthermia in a patient with Schwartz-Jampel syndrome. J Pediatr *93*:83, 1978.
81. Walajahi FH, Karasic LH. Anesthetic management of a patient with dystonia musculorum deformans. Anesth Analg *63*:616, 1984.

82. Laishley RS, Roy WL: Freeman-Sheldon syndrome; Report of three cases and the anaesthetic implications. Can Anaesth Soc J *33*:388, 1986.
83. Dundee JW: Thiopentone in dystrophia myotonica. Anesth Analg *31*:257, 1952.
84. Ravin M, Newmark Z, Saviello G: Myotonia dystrophica—an anesthetic hazard. Anesth Analg *54*:216, 1975.
85. Mitchell MM, Ali HH, Savarese JJ: Myotonia and neuromuscular blocking agents. Anesthesiology *49*:44, 1978.
86. Stert JA, Stone DJ, Weinberg G, et al: Atracurium in a child with myotonic dystrophy. Anesth Analg *64*:369, 1985.
87. Paterson RA, Tousignant M, Skene DS. Caesarean section for twins in a patient with myotonic dystrophy. Can Anaesth Soc J *32*:418, 1985.
88. Myers MB, Barash PG: Cardiac decompensation during enflurane anesthesia. A patient with myotonia dystrophica. Anesth Analg *55*:433, 1976.
89. Saarnivaara LHM: Anesthesia for a patient with polymyositis undergoing myectomy of the cricopharyngeal muscle. Anesth Analg *67*:701, 1988.
90. Eng GD, Epstein BS, Engel WK, et al: Malignant hyperthermia and central core disease in a child with congenital dislocating hips. Arch Neurol *35*:189, 1978.
91. Denborough MA, Dennett X, Anderson R: Central core disease and malignant hyperpyrexia. Br Med J *1*:272, 1973.
92. Cunliffe M, Burrows FA: Anaesthetic implications of nemaline rod myopathy. Can Anaesth Soc J *32*:543, 1985.
93. Heard SO, Kaplan RF: Neuromuscular blockade in a patient with nemaline myopathy. Anesthesiology *59*:588, 1983.
94. Rowe RW, Helander E: Anesthetic management of a patient with systemic carnitine deficiency. Anesth Analg *71*:295, 1990.
95. Beilin B, Shulman D, Schiffman Y: Anaesthesia in myopathy of carnitine deficiency. Anaesthesia *41*:92, 1986.
96. Katsuya H, Misumi M, Ohtani Y, Muki T: Postanesthetic acute renal failure due to carnitine palmityl transferase deficiency. Anesthesiology *68*:945, 1988.
97. Dierdorff SF, McNiece WL. Anaesthesia and pyruvate dehydrogenase deficiency. Can Anaesth Soc J *30*:413, 1983.
98. Schapira AHV: Mitochondrial myopathies. Br Med J *298*:1127, 1989.
99. Burns AM, Shelly MP: Anaesthesia for patients with mitochondrial myopathy. Anaesthesia *44*:975, 1989.
100. Wiesel S, Bevan JC, Samuel J, Donati F: Vecuronium neuromuscular blockade in a child with mitochondrial myopathy. Anesth Analg *72*:696, 1991.
101. Cox JM: Anesthesia and glycogen storage disease. Anesthesiology *29*:1221, 1968.
102. Kaplan R: Pompe's disease presenting for anesthesia. Anesth Rev 7:21, 1980.
103. Rooney RT, Shanahan EC, Sun T, Nally B: Atracurium and hypokalemic familial periodic paralysis. Anesth Analg *67*:782, 1988.
104. Lema G, Urzua J, Moran S, Canessa R: Successful anesthetic management of a patient with hypokalemic familial periodic paralysis undergoing cardiac surgery. Anesthesiology *74*:373, 1991.
105. Melnick B, Chang JL, Larson CE, et al: Hypokalemic familial periodic paralysis. Anesthesiology *58*:263, 1983.
106. Siler JN, Discavage WJ: Anesthetic management of hypokalemic periodic paralysis. Anesthesiology *43*:489, 1975.
107. Horton B: Anesthetic experiences in a family with hypokalemic periodic paralysis. Anesthesiology *47*:308, 1977.
108. Egan TJ, Klein R: Hyperkalemic familial periodic paralysis. Pediatrics *24*:761, 1959.
109. Aarons JJ, Moon RE, Camporesi EM: General anesthesia and hyperkalemic periodic paralysis. Anesthesiology *71*:303, 1989.
110. Robotham JL, Haddow JE: Rhabdomyolysis and myoglobinuria in childhood. Pediatr Clin North Am *23*:279, 1976.
111. Ryan JF, Hagen LJ, Heyman AI: Myoglobinemia after a single dose of succinylcholine. N Engl J Med *285*:824, 1971.
112. Asari H, Inoue K, Maruta H, Hirose Y: The inhibitory effect of intravenous D-tubocurarine and oral dantrolene on halothane-succinylcholine induced myoglobinemia in children. Anesthesiology *61*:332, 1984.
113. Blanc VF, Vaillancourt G, Brisson G: Succinylcholine, fasciculations, and myoglobinemia. Can Anaesth Soc J *33*:178, 1986.
114. Schaer H, Steinman B, Jerusalem S, et al: Rhabdomyolysis induced by anaesthesia with intraoperative cardiac arrest. Br J Anaesth *49*:495, 1977.
115. Younker D, De Vore M, Hartlage P: Malignant hyperthermia and glucose-6-phosphate dehydrogenase deficiency. Anesthesiology *60*:601, 1984.
116. Rubrano R, Chang JL, Carroll J, Sonbolian N, Larson CE: Acute rhabdomyolysis following halothane anesthesia without succinylcholine. Anesthesiology *67*:856, 1987.
117. Merz B: Malignant hyperthermia: Nightmare for anesthesiologists—and patients. JAMA *255*:709, 1986.
118. McKishnie JD, Muir JM, Girvan DP: Anaesthetic-induced rhabdomyolysis. Can Anaesth Soc J *30*:295, 1983.
119. King JO, Denborough MA, Zapp PW: Inheritance of malignant hyperpyrexia. Lancet *1*:365, 1972.
120. Ording H. Incidence of malignant hyperthermia in Denmark. Anesth Analg *64*:700, 1985.
121. Britt BA, Kalow W: Malignant hyperthermia: a statistical review. Can Anaesth Soc J *17*:293, 1970.
122. Bailey AG, Block EC: Malignant hyperthermia in a three-month-old American Indian infant. Anesth Analg *66*:1043, 1987.
123. Murphy AL, Conlay L, Ryan JF, Roberts JT: Malignant hyperthermia during a prolonged anesthetic for reattachment of a limb. Anesthesiology *60*:149, 1984.
124. Lee DS, Adams JP, Zimmerman JE: Malignant hyperthermia—a possible new variant. Can Anaesth Soc J *32*:268, 1985.
125. Peterson DR, Davis N: Malignant hyperthermia diathesis and the sudden infant death syndrome. Anesth Analg *65*:209, 1986.
126. Blanck TJ, Gruener R, Suffecool S, et al: Calcium uptake by isolated sarcoplasmic reticulum: Examination of halothane inhibition, pH dependence, and calcium dependence of normal and malignant hyperthermic human muscle. Anesth Analg *60*:492, 1981.
127. Gronert FA, Thompson GL, Onofrio BM: Human malignant hyperthermia: Awake episodes and correction by dantrolene. Anesth Analg (Paris) *59*:377, 1980.
128. Mathieu A, Bogosian AJ, Ryan JF, et al: Recrudescence after survival of an acute episode of malignant hyperthermia. Anesthesiology *51*:454, 1979.
129. Schulte-Sasse U, Hess W, Eberlien HJ: Postoperative malignant hyperthermia and dantrolene therapy. Can Anaesth Soc J *30*:635, 1983.
130. Grinberg R, Edelist G, Gordon R: Postoperative malignant hyperthermia episodes in patients who received safe anaesthetics. Can Anaesth Soc J *30*:273, 1983.

131. Kripke BJ, Blanck TJ, Sizemore DA, et al: Association of post-anaesthetic hyperthermia with abnormal muscle characteristics. Can Anaesth Soc J *30*:290, 1983.
132. Kowamoto M, Yugi O, Kikuchi H, et al: No myocardial involvement in non-rigid malignant hyperthermia. Anesthesiology *64*:93, 1986.
133. Van der Spek AFL, Fang WB, Ashton-Miller JA, et al: The effects of succinylcholine on mouth opening. Anesthesiology *67*:459, 1987.
134. Plumley MH, Bevan JC, Sadder JM, et al: Dose-related effects of succinylcholine on the adductor pollicis and masseter muscles in children. Can J Anaesth *37*:15, 1990.
135. Saddler JM, Bevan JC, Plumley MH, et al: Jaw muscle tension after succinylcholine in children undergoing strabismus surgery. Can J Anaesth *37*:21, 1990.
136. Carroll JB: Increased incidence of masseter spasm in children with strabismus anesthetized with halothane and succinylcholine. Anesthesiology *67*:559, 1987.
137. Lazzell VA, Lerman J, Burrows FA, Creighton RE: The effect of thiopental on the incidence of masseter muscle rigidity following succinylcholine in infants and children. Can J Anaesth *36*:S98, 1989.
138. Flewellen EH, Nelson TE: Masseter spasm induced by succinylcholine in children: Contracture testing for malignant hyperthermia. Can Anaesth Soc J *29*:42, 1982.
139. Flewellen EH, Nelson TE: Halothane-succinylcholine induced masseter spasm: Indicative of malignant hyperthermia susceptibility? Anesth Analg *63*:693, 1984.
140. Badgwell JM, Heavner JE: Masseter spasm heralds malignant hyperthermia—current dilemma or merely academia gone mad? Anesthesiology *61*:230, 1984.
141. Schwartz L, Rockoff MA, Koka BV: Masseter spasm with anesthesia: Incidence and implications. Anesthesiology *61*:772, 1984.
142. Rosenberg H, Fletcher JE: Masseter muscle rigidity and malignant hyperthermia susceptibility. Anesth Analg *65*:161, 1986.
143. Allen GC, Rosenberg H: Malignant hyperthermia susceptibility in adult patients with masseter muscle rigidity. Can J Anaesth *37*:31, 1990.
144. Rosenberg H: Trismus is not trivial. Anesthesiology *67*:453, 1987.
145. Fletcher J, Rosenberg H: In vitro interaction between halothane and succinylcholine in human skeletal muscle: Implications for malignant hyperthermia and masseter muscle rigidity. Anesthesiology *63*:190, 1985.
146. Ellis FR, Halsall PJ: Improper diagnostic test may account for high incidence of malignant hyperthermia associated with masseter spasm. Anesthesiology *64*:291, 1986.
147. Van der Spek AFL, Spargo PM, Nahrwold ML: Masseter spasm and malignant hyperthermia are not the same thing. Anesthesiology *64*:291, 1986.
148. Gronert GA: Management of patients in whom trismus follows succinylcholine. Anesthesiology *68*:653, 1988.
149. Littleford JA, Patel LR, Bose D, et al: Masseter muscle spasm in children—implications of continuing the triggering anesthetic. Anesth Analg *72*:151, 1991.
150. Larach MG, Rosenberg H, Larach DR, Broennle AM: Prediction of malignant hyperthermia susceptibility by clinical signs. Anesthesiology *66*:547, 1987.
151. Birmingham PK, Stevenson SW, Uejima T, Hall SC: Isolated postoperative myoglobinuria in a pediatric outpatient: A case report of malignant hyperthermia. Anesth Analg *69*:846, 1989.
152. Kolb ME, Horne ML, Martz R: Dantrolene in human malignant hyperthermia: A multicenter study. Anesthesiology *56*:254, 1982.
153. Gronert GA: Malignant hyperthermia. Anesthesiology *53*:395, 1980.
154. Flewellen EH, Nelson TE, Jones WP, et al: Dantrolene dose response in awake man: Implications for management of malignant hyperthermia. Anesthesiology *59*:275, 1983.
155. Lerman J, McLeod ME, Strong HA: Pharmacokinetics of intravenous dantrolene in children. Anesthesiology *70*:625, 1989.
156. Saltzman LS, Kates RA, Corke BC, et al: Hyperkalemia and cardiovascular collapse after verapamil and dantrolene administration in swine. Anesth Analg *63*:473, 1984.
157. Allen GC, Cattrac CB, Peterson RG, et al: Plasma levels of dantrolene following oral administration in malignant hyperthermia–susceptible patients. Anesthesiology *69*:900, 1988.
158. Fitzgibbons DC: Malignant hyperthermia following preoperative oral administration of dantrolene. Anesthesiology *54*:73, 1981.
159. Ruhland G, Hinkle AJ: Malignant hyperthermia after oral and intravenous pretreatment with dantrolene in a patient susceptible to malignant hyperthermia. Anesthesiology *60*:159, 1984.
160. Berkowitz A, Rosenberg H: Femoral block with mepivacaine for muscle biopsy in malignant hyperthermia patients. Anesthesiology *62*:651, 1985.
161. Paasuke RT, Brownell AKW: Amide local anesthetics and malignant hyperthermia. Can Anaesth Soc J *33*:126,1986.
162. Dershwitz M, Sreter FA, Ryan JF: Ketamine does not trigger malignant hyperthermia in susceptible swine. Anesth Analg *69*:501, 1989.
163. Ellis FR, Clarke IMC, Modgill M, et al: Evaluation of creatine phosphokinase in screening patients for malignant hyperpyrexia. Br Med J *3*:511, 1975.
164. Lingaraju N, Rosenberg H: Unexplained increases in serum creatine kinase levels: its relation to malignant hyperthermia susceptibility. Anesth Analg *72*:702, 1991.
165. Lutsky I, Witkowski H, Henschel E: HLA typing in a family prone to malignant hyperthermia. Anesthesiology *56*:224, 1982.
166. Solomons C, McDermott N, Mahowald M: Screening for malignant hyperthermia with a platelet bioassay. N Engl J Med *303*:642, 1980.
167. Rosenberg H, Fisher CA, Reed S, et al: Platelet aggregation in patients susceptible to malignant hyperthermia. Anesthesiology *55*:621, 1981.
168. Giger U, Kaplan R: Halothane-induced ATP depletion from patients susceptible to malignant hyperthermia and from controls. Anesthesiology *58*:347, 1983.
169. Britt BA, Scott EA: Failure of the platelet-halothane nucleotide deletion test as a diagnostic or screening test for malignant hyperthermia. Anesth Analg *65*:171, 1986.
170. Kistler P, Fletcher JE, Rosenberg H: Erythrocyte fragility screening is not a tool for diagnosis of human malignant hyperthermia. Anesth Analg *66*:1004, 1987.
171. Walsh MP, Brownell AKW, Littman V, et al: Electrophoresis of muscle proteins is not a method for diagnosis of malignant hyperthermia susceptibility. Anesthesiology *64*:473, 1986.
172. Britt BA, Scott EA, Kleiman A, et al: Failure of the tourniquet-twitch test as a diagnostic or screening test for malignant hyperthermia. Anesth Analg *65*:1047, 1986.
173. Olgin J, Argov Z, Rosenberg H, et al: Noninvasive evaluation of malignant hyperthermia susceptibility with phosphorus nuclear magnetic resonance spectroscopy. Anesthesiology *68*:507, 1988.

174. Olgin J, Rosenberg H, Allen G, et al: A blinded comparison of noninvasive, in vivo phosphorus nuclear magnetic resonance spectroscopy and the in vitro halothane/caffeine contracture test in the evaluation of malignant hyperthermia susceptibility. Anesth Analg *72*:36, 1991.
175. MacKenzie AE, Allen G, Lahey D, et al: A comparison of the caffeine-halothane muscle contracture test with the molecular genetic diagnosis of malignant hyperthermia. Anesthesiology *75*:4, 1991.
176. Britt BA, Frodis W, Scott E, et al: Comparison of the caffeine skinned fibre tension (CST) test with the caffeine-halothane contracture test in the diagnosis of malignant hyperthermia. Can Anaesth Soc J *29*:550, 1982.
177. Hackl W, Mauritz W, Schemper M, et al: Prediction of malignant hyperthermia susceptibility: Statistical evaluation of clinical signs. Br J Anaesth *64*:425, 1990.
178. Rosenberg H, Reed S: In vitro contracture tests for susceptibility to malignant hyperthermia. Anesth Analg *62*:415, 1983.
179. Nelson TE, Flewellen EH, Gloyna DF: Spectrum of susceptibility to malignant hyperthermia—diagnostic dilemma. Anesth Analg *62*:545, 1983.
180. Brownell AKW, Szabo M: The in vitro caffeine contracture test: Influence of the muscle histochemical profile on test results. Can Anaesth Soc J *29*:218, 1982.
181. Melton AJ, Martucci RW, Kien ND, et al: Malignant hyperthermia in humans—standardization of contracture testing protocol. Anesth Analg *69*:437, 1989.
182. Allen GC, Rosenberg H, Fletcher JE: Safety of general anesthesia in patients previously tested negative for malignant hyperthermia susceptibility. Anesthesiology *72*:619, 1990.

INDEX

Note: Page numbers in *italics* refer to illustrations; page numbers followed by (t) refer to tables.